LABORATORY
TESTS AND
DIAGNOSTIC
PROCEDURES
SECOND EDITION

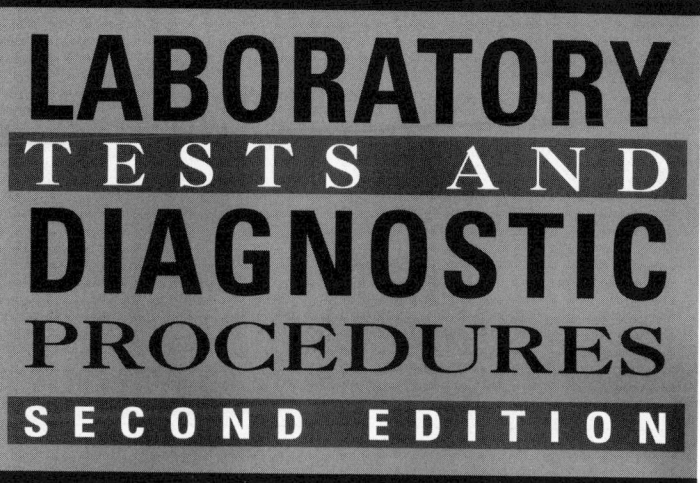

LABORATORY TESTS AND DIAGNOSTIC PROCEDURES

SECOND EDITION

Edited by

Cynthia C. Chernecky, PhD, RN, CNS
Clinical Nurse Specialist
Associate Professor of Nursing
Medical College of Georgia
Augusta, Georgia

Barbara J. Berger, MSN, RN, CCRN
Clinical Nurse Specialist
University Hospitals Health Systems
Bedford Medical Center
Bedford, Ohio

W.B. Saunders Company
A Division of Harcourt Brace & Company
Philadelphia • London • Toronto •
Montreal • Sydney • Tokyo

W.B. SAUNDERS COMPANY

A Division of Harcourt Brace & Company

The Curtis Center
Independence Square West
Philadelphia, Pennsylvania 19106

Library of Congress Cataloging-in-Publication Data

Laboratory tests and diagnostic procedures / [edited by] Cynthia C. Chernecky,
Barbara J. Berger. — 2nd ed.
  p.   cm.
  Includes bibliographical references and index.
  ISBN 0–7216–6793–7
    1. Diagnosis, Laboratory—Handbooks, manuals, etc.   2. Diagnosis,
Laboratory—Encyclopedias.   I. Chernecky, Cynthia C.   II. Berger,
Barbara J.
    [DNLM: 1. Diagnosis. Laboratory—methods—handbooks.   QY 39 L1229
1997]
  RB38.2.L33   1997
DNLM/DLC
                                                        96–43069

Laboratory Tests and Diagnostic Procedures   ISBN 0–7216–6793–7

Printed in United States of America

Last digit is the print number: 9   8   7   6   5   4   3   2

Contributors

Barbara J. Berger, MSN, RN, CCRN
Clinical Nurse Specialist
University Hospitals Health Systems
Bedford Medical Center
Bedford, Ohio

Cynthia C. Chernecky, PhD, RN, CNS
Associate Professor of Nursing
Medical College of Georgia
Augusta, Georgia

Maureen R. Denk, MSN, RN, LHRM
Professional Nursing Development Coordinator
Shands Teaching Hospital at the University of Florida
Gainesville, Florida

Anthony L. D'Eramo, MSN, RN
Adjunct Faculty, School of Nursing
Kent State University
Kent, Ohio
and
Staff Development Specialist
Department of Veterans Affairs Medical Center
Cleveland, Ohio

Irene Glanville, RN, PhD, CFNP
Adjunct Assistant Professor of Nursing
University of Akron
Akron, Ohio
and
Staff Development Specialist
Certified Family Nurse Practitioner
Department of Veterans Affairs Medical Center
Cleveland, Ohio

Susan M. Groh, RN, AA Nursing
Project Nurse, Department of Surgery
St. Joseph Hospital
Orange, California

Janice L. Hickman, RN, MSN, CS
Clinical Nurse Specialist
Neuroscience Intensive Care Unit
University Hospitals of Cleveland
Cleveland, Ohio

Catherine A. Kefer, RN, MJ, OCN
Manager, Protocol Office
Rush–Presbyterian–St. Luke's Medical Center
Rush Cancer Institute
Chicago, Illinois

Catherine A. Kernich, MSN, RN
Clinical Nurse Specialist, Department of Neurology
University Hospitals of Cleveland
Cleveland, Ohio
and
Clinical Faculty
Frances Payne Bolton School of Nursing
Case Western Reserve University
Cleveland, Ohio

Mary Ann Lamont Krall, BS, MS, MSN, RN
Quality Management Nurse, Medicine and Intensive Care
Department of Veterans Affairs Medical Center
Cleveland, Ohio
and
Clinical Faculty
Frances Payne Bolton School of Nursing
Case Western Reserve University
Cleveland, Ohio

Deborah Marantides, MSN, RN
Clinical Instructor
Frances Payne Bolton School of Nursing
Case Western Reserve University
Cleveland, Ohio

Jeffrey Edward Molter, RN, BSN, CCRN
Clinical Nurse, Cardiac Intensive Care Unit
University Hospitals of Cleveland
Cleveland, Ohio
and
Clinical Instructor/Preceptor
Frances Payne Bolton School of Nursing
Case Western Reserve University
Cleveland Ohio

Karen A. Pfeifer, MSN, RN, CNA, OCN
Doctoral Student and Graduate Research Assistant
College of Nursing
Texas Woman's University
Denton, Texas

Kelly E. Randolph, RN, ADN
Cardiac Catheterization Laboratory
St. Anthony Hospital
Michigan City, Indiana

Jeanene (Gigi) Robison, MSN, RN, OCN
Oncology Clinical Nurse Specialist
The Christ Hospital
Cincinnati, Ohio

Andrea M. Russo, BSN, RN
Quality Improvement Project Coordinator
University Hospitals of Cleveland
Cleveland, Ohio

Sandra Read Schurdell, BSN, RN
Nurse Case Manager, Medicine
Department of Veterans Affairs Medical Center
Cleveland, Ohio

Jane E. Trayte, BS, ND
Critical Care Instructor, Medical–Surgical Nursing
University Hospitals of Cleveland
Cleveland, Ohio
and
Assistant Clinical Professor of Nursing
Frances Payne Bolton School of Nursing
Case Western Reserve University
Cleveland, Ohio

Susanne Vendlinski, RN, BSN, MSN
Instructor in Nursing, Undergraduate Program
The University of Akron
Akron, Ohio
and
Staff Nurse
Akron General Medical Center
Akron, Ohio
and
Staff Nurse
Hospice Care Center of Visiting Nurse Service
Copley, Ohio

Clinical Expert Consultants

The editors acknowledge the expertise shared for selected tests by the following clinical experts from University Hospitals of Cleveland:

Peter Faulhaber, MD
Department of Radiology/Nuclear Medicine
Bette K. Idemoto, MSN, RN, CS, CCRN
Clinical Nurse Specialist/Case Manager, Vascular Service
Claudia Kraly, CRMT
Manager, Nuclear Medicine/Positive Emission Tomography
Marilyn Kabb, RN, MSN, JD
Clinical Nurse Specialist, Medical–Surgical Nursing
Michael Lewis, RN, ACN
Angio-interventional Radiology
Hugo Montenegro, MD
Medical Director, Medical Intensive Care Unit
Mary Jo Nelisse, RN, BSN
Advanced Practice Nurse, Noninvasive Cardiology
Peter Sachs, MD
Angio-interventional Radiology

Contributors to the First Edition

The editors acknowledge the contributors to the first edition because their work provided a foundation for the publication of this text:

Barbara J. Berger, MSN, RN, CCRN
Cynthia C. Chernecky, PhD, RN
Olga Chernecky, LPN (Retired)
Kimberly L. Cunningham, BSN, RN
Mary C. Dellorso, BSN, RN, C
Margaret Harrison, BA, RN
Gail A. Kiser, PhD, RN
Mary Ann Lamont Krall, MSN, RN
Ruth L. Krech Fritskey, MSN, RN
Lynnette Paver, MSN, RN
Sandra A. Read Schurdell, BSN, RN
Kathleen A. Singleton, MSN, RN

NOTICE

Medical-surgical nursing is an ever-changing field. Standard safety precautions must be followed, but as new research and clinical experience broaden our knowledge, changes in treatment and drug therapy become necessary or appropriate. The editors of this work have carefully checked the generic and trade drug names and verified drug dosages to ensure that the dosage information in this work is accurate and in accord with the standards accepted at the time of publication. Readers are advised, however, to check the product information currently provided by the manufacturer of each drug to be administered to be certain that changes have not been made in the recommended dose or in the contraindications for administration. This is of particular importance in regard to new or infrequently used drugs. It is the responsibility of the treating physician, relying on experience and knowledge of the patient, to determine dosages and the best treatment for the patient. The editors cannot be responsible for misuse or misapplication of the material in this work.

THE PUBLISHER

Acknowledgments

As the saying goes, "No one does it alone." Nothing is more truthful than this when it comes to this book. I have so many to thank for their love, encouragement, support, and spirit of wisdom and for exemplifying the true meaning of family: my mother Olga (Budnik) Chernecky, late father Edward Chernecky, brother Richard Chernecky, godmother Helen (Budnik) Prohorik, godson Johnathon Tarutis, nieces Ellie and Annie Chernecky, nephew Michael Chernecky, cousins Paula Smart and Karyn Tarutis, Aunt Julie Dewey, and late Uncle Charles "Chuck" Dewey. I want you to know that you all bring a smile to my heart and love to my soul. My co-editor and co-author, Barb, who was a true colleague understands unconditional trust, hard work, computer technology, the nature of good wine, the need for humor, and a heart full of respect. My colleagues at the universities that I have been affiliated with: the University of Connecticut, the University of Pittsburgh, Clemson University, Case Western Reserve University, the University of Wisconsin Oshkosh, and the Medical College of Georgia. To Ruth Krech-Fritskey, co-author of the first edition, and to all the past and current contributors to this book, who worked endlessly in pursuit of an outcome of knowledge that adds true meaning to life, you have my respect, admiration, and humble thanks.

To Barbara Nelson Cullen, Senior Editor, and Marie Pelcin, Editorial Assistant, at W.B. Saunders, who were there for all our questions and time frames; you made the project a joy. To nurses, physicians, and other health care professionals who give meaning to this entire project, we welcome and respect your feedback. You have been truly amazing! Then there are the words of wisdom that I feel I must share with those of you who contemplate a project such as this: You will require at least one dog to put things into perspective (thanks, Sasha, Josh, and Cleo); a computer with 32 MB of RAM; a clock that is broken and always reads 9 o'clock, no matter how long you have been working; a taste for wine; an endless sense of humor; a case of diskettes; e-mail; a phone with lots of memory dials; endless organizational skills that include baskets labeled with phrases like "to be edited," "first edit," "second edit," "final revisions," and—can you believe it—"ready to print"; and a time frame that includes such things as taking the computer apart and adding more memory and allowing an entire day for nonstop printing. Such is life!

There are several people who have touched my life and whose kindness has come from the heart, and I wish to thank them publicly: His Eminence Archbishop DMITRI of Texas, Archpriest John and Matushka Barbara Townsend and Priest Peter (Catalin) and Preotassa Felicia Mot of St. Mary of Egypt Orthodox Church in Georgia; Priest Gregory and Presbytera Raisa Koo of St. John the Theologian Orthodox Mission Church in Georgia; Priest Jason and Matushka Kappanadze of St. Theodosius Orthodox Cathedral in Ohio; Priest Alexis and Matushka Venogradov of St. Gregory the Theologian Orthodox Church in New York; Priest Michael and Matushka Herrick of St. Matthew's Orthodox Church in Wisconsin; Choir Director Dr. Jeff Zdrale; Bonita Zdrale; Abigail Zdrale; Elaine Calugar; Judy Zynko; Choir Director Phyllis Skiba; Monk Sergius; Jack, Rebecca, and Mary Beth Chaoussoglou; Mike, Lydia, and Nina Mytrohovich; Tom and LaVerne Jacobson; Dr. Leon and Barbara Sheehan; Claire and Phyllis Gindlesperger; Flossie Seargent; Sue McIssic; Carol Matthews; Dr. Rosemary Smith; Dr. Claire Meisenheimer; Dr. Vickie Lambert (Dean); Dr. Patricia Lillis; Dr. Lore Wright; Dr. Katherine Nugent; Dr. Virginia Kemp; David and Janice Douglass; Ursula Grimmett; Kathleen Haverlack of St. Vladimir's Orthodox Theological Seminary; and cousins George and Valentina Yelenovsky. To those who have supported me on my quest for truth on the road to eternal life; to Orthodoxy worldwide; to His Holy, Catholic, and Apostolic Church; to the Episcopate of the Orthodox Church whose preservation and continuation of the word of truth are truly inspiring; and to Orthodox Christians everywhere who have found the true faith: May God Grant You Many Years!

Cynthia (Cinda) Cecilia Chernecky

It is with extreme gratitude that I thank the many people and organizations that helped this second edition of *Laboratory Tests and Diagnostic Procedures* go to press. My contributing colleagues in town and across the country helped expand the content where needed, condense the content where wordiness impeded clarity, and add the special features that set this book apart from others on the market. Each contributor tapped experts in his or her region of the country so that we could include the most timely information on the current and new tests and procedures. This edition shines as a result of all of the contributors' efforts. Special thanks to our consultants at University Hospitals of Cleveland (listed within), who were heavily queried for information. I also thank the employees of organizations such as the Allen Memorial Library at Case Western Reserve University, the National Library of Medicine, the National Cancer Institute, and the Poison Control Center of Greater Cleveland. They readily shared their time and expertise to help us locate the specific literature and research information that we needed for clarification and synthesis of content. Barbara Nelson Cullen, our editor at W.B. Saunders, and her assistant, Marie Pelcin, are to be thanked for helping us keep the numerous details of the coordination of this edition on the straight-and-narrow time line. Likewise, Fran Bartlett and her staff provided meticulous copyediting that greatly improved the continuity of this edition. We are also indebted to Jeanne Borczuk for the attractive page layouts. Thanks to Pentium technology, this edition brought only one computer to a standstill, easily remedied by additional RAM, so thank you Intel and Acer America! Thank you to my husband, Stephan Berger, who once again provided so many small comforts that added up to a LOT of support for this project. My parents,

Alice and Arlington Adams, also provided moral support and encouragement as I waded through my share of details and editing. Finally, thanks to Cinda Chernecky, my co-editor and friend, without whom I surely would have forgotten that teamwork comes in handy when you're bleary-eyed, that some people don't need much (any?) sleep, and that humor can be found in everything to help provide balance in one's life.

Barbara J. Berger

References

The editors acknowledge the authors, editors, and publishers of the following texts, which were frequently consulted in the preparation of the manuscript.

American Hospital Formulary Service. Baltimore, MD, American Society of Health-System Pharmacists, 1993.

Bakerman P. Bakermans ABC's of Interpretive Laboratory Data, 3rd ed. Myrtle Beach, SC, Interpretive Laboratory Data, Inc., 1994.

Baron EJ, Peterson LR, Finegold SM (eds): Diagnostic Microbiology, 9th ed. St. Louis, MO, CV Mosby, 1994.

Barondess JA, Carpenter CC: Differential Diagnosis. Philadelphia, A. Waverly, 1994.

Black JM, Matassarin-Jacobs E: Luckmann and Sorensen's Medical-Surgical Nursing: A Psychophysiological Approach, 4th ed. Philadelphia, WB Saunders, 1993.

Boyd R, Hooene BS: Basic Medical Microbiology, 4th ed. Boston, MA, Little, Brown, 1991.

Breger B, Bruguera C, Gharbi H, Goldberg B, Tan F, Wachira W, Weil F (Palmer P, ed): Manual of Diagnostic Ultrasound. USA, World Health Organization, 1995.

Bunzel NA: Fundamentals of Urine and Body Fluid Analysis. Philadelphia, WB Saunders, 1994.

Calbreath DF: Clinical Chemistry: A Fundamental Textbook. Philadelphia, WB Saunders, 1992.

Conn RB: Current Diagnosis. Philadelphia, WB Saunders, 1992.

Cooper GM: Oncogenes. Boston, MA, Jones and Bartlett, 1990.

Cooper NG: The Human Genome Project: Deciphering the Blueprint of Heredity. Mill Valley, CA, University Science Books, 1994.

Copstead LE: Perspectives on Pathophysiology. Philadelphia, WB Saunders, 1995.

Corbett JV: Laboratory Tests and Diagnostic Procedures with Nursing Diagnoses. Norwalk, CT, Appleton and Lange, 1987.

Corbett JV: Laboratory Tests and Diagnostic Procedures with Nursing Diagnoses. Norwalk, CT, Appleton and Lange, 1992.

Crawford MV, Spence MI: Commonsense Approach to Coronary Care, 6th ed. St. Louis, MO, CV Mosby, 1995.

Darovic GO: Hemodynamic Monitoring: Invasive and Noninvasive Clinical Application. Philadelphia, WB Saunders, 1995.

Edmunds MA (ed): Nursing Drug Reference: A Practitioners's Guide. Bowie, MD, Brady Communications Company, 1985.

Fandek N, Moreau D, Newell K, Ofner A (eds): Clinical Laboratory Tests: Values and Implications, 2nd ed. Springhouse, PA, Springhouse Corporation, 1995.

Fischbach FT: A Manual of Laboratory and Diagnostic Tests. Philadelphia, JB Lippincott, 1992.

Flomenbaum N, Goldfrank L, Jacobson S: Emergency Diagnostic Testing, 2nd ed. St. Louis, MO, CV Mosby, 1995.

Friedman HH (ed): Problem Oriented Medical Diagnosis. Boston, MA, Little, Brown, 1991.

Golish J (ed): Diagnostic Procedure Handbook: With Key Word Index. Baltimore, MD, Williams and Wilkins, 1994.

Gulrani ER, Faster V, Gersch BJ, McGoon MD, McGoon DC: Cardiology Fundamentals and Practice, Vols. I and II. St. Louis, MO, Mosby Year Book, 1991.

Hathaway WE, Groothuis JR, Hay WW, Paisley JW: Current Pediatric Diagnosis and Treatment, 10th ed. Norwalk, CT, Appleton and Lange, 1991.

Hayward CPM, Lawson GM, Santrach PJ: Clinical Laboratory Tests: Values and Implications, 2nd ed. Springhouse, PA,: Springhouse Corporation, 1995.

Henrich WL: Principles and Practice of Dialysis. Baltimore, MD, Williams and Wilkins, 1995.

Hickey JV: Clinical Practice of Neurological and Neurosurgical Nursing, 3rd ed. Philadelphia, JB Lippincott, 1992.

Hodgson BB, Kizior RJ, Kingdon RT: Nurse's Drug Handbook. Philadelphia, WB Saunders, 1995.

Hodgson BB, Kizior RJ, Kingdon RT (eds): Nurse's Drug Handbook. Philadelphia, WB Saunders, 1996.

Howanitz J, Howanitz P: Laboratory Medicine: Test Selection and Interpretation. New York, Churchill Livingstone, 1991.

Isenberg HD (ed-in-chief): Clinical Microbiology Procedures Handbook, Vols. I and II. Washington, DC, American Society for Microbiology, 1992.

Jacobs D, Demott W, Finley P, Horvat R, Kasten JRB, Tilzer L: Laboratory Test Handbook, 3rd ed. Hudson, OH, Lexi-Comp, 1994.

Krenhau FW: Diagnostic Ultrasound Principles and Instruments. Philadelphia, WB Saunders, 1993.

Lefever Kee, JL: Handbook of Laboratory and Diagnostic Tests with Nursing Implications, 2nd ed. Norwalk, CT, Appleton and Lang, 1994.

Lefever Kee, JL: Laboratory and Diagnostic Tests with Nursing Implications, 4th ed. Norwalk, CT, Appleton and Lange, 1995.

Linne JJ, Ringsrud KM: Basic Techniques in Clinical Laboratory Science. St. Louis, MO, Mosby Year Book, 1993.

Loeb S (ed): Illustrated Guide to Diagnostic Tests. Springhouse, PA, Springhouse Corporation, 1994.

Luckmann and Sorensen's Medical-Surgical Nursing: A Psychophysiological Approach, 4th ed. Philadelphia, WB Saunders, 1995.

Malarkey LM, McMorrow ME: Nurse's Manual of Laboratory Tests and Diagnostic Procedures. Philadelphia, WB Saunders, 1996.

May KA, Madlemeister LR: Maternal and Neonatal Nursing, 3rd ed. Philadelphia, JB Lippincott, 1994.

McClatchey KD: Clinical Laboratory Medicine. Baltimore, MD, Williams and Wilkins, 1994.

McEvoy G (ed): Drug Information. Bethseda, MD, American Hospital Formulary Service, 1996.

Meietes S (ed-in-chief): Pediatrics Clinical Chemistry. Washington, DC, American Association of Clinical Chemistry Press, 1989.

Monahan FD, Drake T, Neighbors M: Nursing Care of Adults. Philadelphia, WB Saunders, 1994.

Nichols DH, Sweeney PJ: Ambulatory Gynecology, 2nd ed. Philadelphia, JB Lippincott, 1995.

Noe DA, Rock RC (eds): The Selection and Interpretation of Clinical Laboratory Studies. Baltimore, MD, Williams and Wilkins, 1994.

Pagana KD, Pagana TJ: Diagnostic Tests and Nursing Implications: A Case Study Approach, 3rd ed. St. Louis, MO, CV Mosby, 1990.

Pagana KD, Pagana TJ: Diagnostic Testing and Nursing Implications: A Case Study Approach, 4th ed. St. Louis, MO, Mosby Year Book, 1994.

Randol L, Barker E, Burton JR, Zieve PD: Principles of Ambulatory Medicine. Baltimore, MD, Williams and Wilkins, 1991.

Ravel R: Clinical Application of Laboratory Data, 5th ed. Chicago, Year Book Medical Publishers, 1989.

Ravel R: Clinical Laboratory Medicine: Clinical Application of Laboratory Data, 6th ed. St. Louis, MO, Mosby Year Book, 1995.

Ryan K (ed): Sherries Medical Microbiology: An Introduction to Infectious Diseases. Norwalk, CT, Appleton and Lange, 1994.

Simmons WD, Johnson CA: Dialysis of Drugs. New York, The McMahon Group, 1994.

SmithKline Beecham Clinical Laboratories, Directory of Services. Philadelphia, 1993.

SmithKline Beecham Clinical Laboratories, Directory of Services. Philadelphia, 1995.

Society of Gastroenterology Nurses and Associates: Gastroenterology Nursing: A Core Curriculum (Nancy G. Evans, et al., eds). St. Louis, MO, Mosby Year Book, 1993.

Soldin SJ, Hicks JM (eds): Pediatric Reference Ranges. Washington, DC, American Association of Clinical Chemistry Press, 1995.

Springhouse Corporation: Illustrated Guide to Diagnostic Tests. Springhouse, PA, Springhouse Corporation, 1994.

Stillwell SB: Mosby's Critical Care Nursing Reference. St. Louis, MO, Mosby Year Book, 1992.

Stillwell SB: Mosby's Critical Care Nursing Reference, 2nd ed. St. Louis, MO, Mosby Year Book, 1996.

Thelan L, David JK, Urdern LD, Lough ME: Critical Care Nursing Diagnosis and Management. St. Louis, MO, Mosby Year Book, 1994.

Thomas CL (ed): Taber's Cyclopedic Medical Dictionary. Philadelphia, FA Davis, 1993.

Tierney LM, McPhee SJ, Papadakis MA: Current Medical Diagnosis and Treatment, 3rd ed. Norwalk, CT, Appleton and Lange, 1994.

Tietz NW (Burtis CA, Ashwood ER [eds]): Tietz Textbook of Clinical Chemistry, 2nd ed. Philadelphia, WB Saunders, 1994.

Tietz NW (ed): Clinical Guide to Laboratory Tests, 3rd ed. Philadelphia, WB Saunders, 1995.

Treseler KM: Clinical Laboratory and Diagnostic Tests, Significance and Nursing Implications, 3rd ed. Norwalk, CT, Appleton and Lange, 1995.

Turgeon ML: Clinical Hematology Theory and Procedures. Boston, MA, Little, Brown, 1993.

Pathology Laboratory Manual. Cleveland, OH, University Hospitals of Cleveland, 1993.

Wallach J: Interpretation of Diagnostic Tests, 5th ed. Boston, MA, Little, Brown, 1992.

Watson J, Jaffe MS: Nurse's Manual of Laboratory and Diagnostic Tests, 2nd ed. Philadelphia, FA Davis, 1995.

Wilson JD, et al.: Harrison's Principles of Internal Medicine. New York, McGraw-Hill, 1991, pp 291–293, 953–954.

Woodley M, Whelan A: The Washington Manual of Medical Therapeutics. Boston, Little, Brown, 1992.

Woods GJ, Gutierrez Y (eds): Diagnostic Pathology of Infectious Diseases. Philadelphia, Lea and Febiger, 1993.

Woods SL, Froelicher ESS, Halpenny CJ, Motzer SU: Cardiac Nursing, 3rd ed. Philadelphia, JB Lippincott, 1995.

Wyngaarden JB, Smith LH, Bennett JC: Cecil Textbook of Medicine. Philadelphia, WB Saunders, 1992.

Yamada T: Textbook of Gastroenterology, 2nd ed. Philadelphia, JB Lippincott, 1995.

Preface

We are pleased to announce the arrival of the second edition of *Laboratory Tests and Diagnostic Procedures*. The text is completely alphabetical, fully cross-referenced, and indexed. There is no need to know which body system is tested or whether the test uses blood or urine, or is diagnostic in order to locate the test. The best advantage, we believe, is that all of the information is complete and contained within one cover. There is no need to waste valuable time referring to multiple texts or flipping between sections to obtain test-specific information. Several of the special features are inclusion of medicolegal implications; panic levels and symptoms and emergency treatment for panic levels; client and family teaching; risks of and contraindications for procedures; and whether written consent is needed. The content is basic enough for novices and complete enough for seasoned practitioners. It has significant value for both students and practitioners of medical technology, medicine, and nursing and is the kind of reference to use throughout one's career. It is appropriate for the many specialties within the professions, and it includes information from across the lifespan.

The text is organized into two parts. Part One is designed to help the practitioner confirm a suspected diagnosis or condition, as well as to provide additional conditions that may demonstrate similar symptoms. Part Two lists the tests and diagnostic procedures in alphabetical order with normal values; panic level symptoms and treatment, including whether the substance is dialyzable; usage and/or conditions in which the values may be abnormal; and a concise description of the test and its significance. This edition also includes expanded information on consent requirements, risks and contraindications, client and family teaching, and the details of the test and client care, as well as integration of the most current scientific literature. Other new features include the addition of shading in Part Two for ease of use, reduction of blood sample volumes to the minimum amount required (to help avoid iatrogenic anemia), information on whether blood samples can be drawn during hemodialysis, expansion of age-specific norms, and improved quality-assurance information on factors that interfere with results. Finally, a comprehensive, international, up-to-date bibliography of specific resources is included to direct practitioners to additional information about each test or procedure.

Other features of this edition include the newest tests in cardiology, human immunodeficiency virus diagnosis and monitoring, ultrafast computed tomography, *Helicobacter pylori* diagnosis, genetic tests, oncology, obstetrics, and nuclear medicine. Cross-referencing of the test and procedure names has been expanded to include all associated acronyms to expedite the location of each. The index now includes a synthesis of diseases, tests, and procedures for the entire book in one place. The format of this text is the product of years of clinical practice and expertise. It has been written *by* practitioners *for* practitioners. The invaluable contributions of a large number of clinical experts and their contacts who freely shared the most up-to-date information about the tests, procedures, and medical conditions are a most valued feature of this edition.

The purpose of this text is to provide complete information to guide practitioners or students in the clinical care of clients. Applicability of information in a text of this type is relative. Although we have used reliable and current sources in the compilation of the book, variations in laboratory techniques and client conditions must be considered for interpretation. The normal and panic levels listed are not meant to be used as rigid separations of normal and abnormal, but rather as guidelines for consideration within the context of individual client conditions and laboratory specifications.

We have provided information regarding procedures that may require separate consent forms, or those beyond the general institutional consent form. Certainly, there is much variation among institutions regarding whether a consent form is necessary. At the minimum, verbal consent is generally documented. We have provided what is general practice according to the literature and the experience of our expert contributors across the country. However, we caution that institutional protocols vary and should, of course, be consulted and followed. Regardless of whether formal consent is obtained, it is the responsibility of all health care professionals to educate clients undergoing *any* test or procedure. Teaching about the test or procedure must be tailored to the client's and the client's family's condition, language, comprehension, anxiety level, clinical goals, and other specific needs.

Most drugs in this text are listed by their generic names. This includes specific tests to determine drug levels in either blood or urine, and includes within these tests names of drugs that may interfere with the test results. Generic names have been used to save valuable printed space and to avoid confusion due to multiple trade names. We must stress that in judging possible drug interferences, the clinical evaluation of the client should remain primary in the process of interpreting test values. Clearly, it is impractical to discontinue all medications in order to get a "pure value." If, however, a drug is known to cause severe interferences with the test results, it is clearly stated, and the drug should be discontinued when possible.

With concern about the transmission of blood-borne pathogens, and in view of the content of this text, it is imperative to address the safe handling of specimens. In 1994, the Centers for Disease Control (CDC) published "Standard Precautions," which include guidelines for isolation precautions in hospitals, designed to prevent the transmission of the hepatitis B virus and the human immunodeficiency virus (HIV). A condensed version of these recommendations is provided. Most institutions currently follow these guidelines in some version, and we recommend referral to individual institutional protocol.

Years of research and writing went into the completion of this text. It could not have been done without our many dedicated professional contributors, without the assistance and support of Barbara Nelson-Cullen and Marie Pelcin at WB Saunders, and without the support of our families, friends, and professional colleagues. We know that we have acquired much knowledge through the process of writing and editing this book. We believe the book is a valuable tool for all health care professionals.

Cynthia C. Chernecky
Barbara J. Berger

How to Use This Book

This section of the book is designed to assist in full mastery of the format. Although its strictly alphabetical format makes the book easy to use, the following examples may clarify any confusion.

PART ONE:

The purpose of this section is to assist practitioners in diagnosing and monitoring the progress of illness or wellness.

Part One is a selected alphabetical listing of diseases, conditions, and symptoms. Beneath each topic in the left column is a list of laboratory and diagnostic tests, also in alphabetical order. It is not expected that all of the tests listed would necessarily be required or be abnormal for any one disease, condition, or symptom. Rather, any of the listed tests or a combination of tests would likely be performed to aid, confirm, monitor, or rule out that diagnosis or condition.

EXAMPLES:

HYPERNATREMIA
- Cholesterol, Blood
- Electrolyte, Blood or Urine
- Glucose, Fasting (FBS), Blood
- Glucose, Quantitative, 24-Hour, Urine
- Glucose, Random, Serum
- Osmolality, Serum
- Sodium, Plasma or Serum
- Sodium, Urine
- Triglycerides, Blood

ADDITIONAL CONDITIONS
- Dehydration
- Diabetes Insipidus
- Diabetic Ketoacidosis
- HHNK
- Hypotension
- Tachycardia

The "Additional Conditions" column includes other related diseases or conditions that should be considered when postulating the diagnosis in the left column. Many of these additional conditions are, in fact, listed in the left column elsewhere in the section with their own battery of tests (see below).

DIABETES INSIPIDUS
- Antidiuretic Hormone, Serum
- Chloride, Sweat, Specimen
- Concentration Test, Urine
- Cyclic Adenosine Monophosphate (cAMP), Urine
- Electrolyte, Blood or Urine
- Osmolality, Serum
- Osmolality, Urine
- Sodium, Plasma or Serum
- Sodium, Urine
- Specific Gravity, Urine

ADDITIONAL CONDITIONS
- Amyloidosis, Renal
- Breast Cancer
- Encephalitis
- Hand-Schuller-Christian Disease
- Lung Cancer
- Pyelonephritis
- Sickle Cell Anemia
- Sjögren's Syndrome
- Syphilis
- Tuberculosis

PART TWO:

The purpose of this section is to provide a comprehensive, concise, ready reference of practitioner "need-to-know" information about laboratory tests and diagnostic procedures. Features of this section include:

ALPHABETICAL LIST
of laboratory tests and diagnostic procedures.

ABDOMINAL AORTA SONOGRAM, DIAGNOSTIC
ABO GROUP AND Rh TYPE, BLOOD

NORMS:
Norms specific to all known units and all age groups.

UREA NITROGEN, PLASMA OR SERUM

Norm:

		SI Units
Young adult (<40)	5–18 mg/dl	1.8–6.5 mmol/L
Adult	5–20 mg/dl	1.8–7.1 mmol/L
Elderly >60	8–21 mg/dl	2.9–7.5 mmol/L
Mild azotemia	20–50 mg/dl	7.1–17.7 mmol/L
Children		
Cord blood	21–40 mg/dl	7.5–14.3 mmol/L
Premature infant, first 7 days	3–25 mg/dl	1.1–8.9 mmol/L
Full-term newborn	4–18 mg/dl	1.4–6.4 mmol/L
Infant	5–18 mg/dl	1.8–6.4 mmol/L
Child	5–18 mg/dl	1.8–6.4 mmol/L
Panic level	>100 mg/dl	>35.7 mmol/L

PANIC LEVELS SYMPTOMS AND TREATMENT:
Toxic levels and panic levels with associated signs, symptoms, and emergency treatment.

THEOPHYLLINE (AMINOPHYLLINE), BLOOD

Norm:

		SI Units
Therapeutic	10–20 mg/ml	44–111 mmol/L
Toxic level	>20 mg/ml	>111 mmol/L
Panic level	>30 mg/ml	>160 mmol/L

Panic Level Symptoms and Treatment:

Symptoms: Dysrhythmias, gastrointestinal bleeding, headache, hypotension, nausea, restlessness, seizures, syncope, tachycardia, and vomiting.

Treatment:
Maintain a patent airway.
Withhold the drug.
Perform gastric lavage.
Give activated charcoal.
Hydrate.

Give diazepam for convulsions.
40% of theophylline may be removed by hemodialysis.
Peritoneal dialysis will NOT remove theophylline.

USAGE:
Typical conditions or monitoring for which the test or procedure is commonly used.

CARDIAC CATHETERIZATION, DIAGNOSTIC

Usage: Identification, documentation, and quantitation of congenital disorders of the heart and diseases and disorders of the greater vessels of the heart; evaluation of cardiac muscle function; evaluation of coronary artery patency; identification of ventricular aneurysms; and identification and quantitation of the severity of acquired or congenital cardiac valve disease.

INCREASED, DECREASED or POSITIVE, NEGATIVE:
Conditions that cause abnormal results.

COOMBS', DIRECT (DIRECT ANTIGLOBULIN TEST), SERUM

Norm: Negative.

Positive: Arthritis (rheumatoid), elderly clients, erythroblastosis fetalis, hemolytic anemia (autoimmune, drug-induced), infection, neoplasm, renal disorders, systemic lupus erythematosus, and transfusion reaction. Drugs include (possibly due to IgG erythrocyte sensitization by the drugs) aminopyrine, cephalosporins, chlorpromazine, dipyrone, ethosuximide, hydralazine hydrochloride, insulin, isoniazid, levodopa, mefenamic acid, melphalan, methyldopa, methyldopate hydrochloride, oxyphenisatin, *para*-aminosalicylic acid, penicillins, phenacetin, phenytoin, phenytoin sodium, procainamide hydrochloride, quinidine gluconate, quinidine polygalacturonate, quinidine sulfate, rifampin, streptomycin sulfate, sulfonamides, and tetracyclines.

Negative: Hemolytic anemia (nonautoimmune, non–drug-induced). Normal finding.

DESCRIPTION:
Concise description of the test or procedure, including interpretation of results and significance for various conditions.

UREA BREATH TEST (UBT), DIAGNOSTIC

Description: This simple, noninvasive test involves the measurement of gas released in the breath after ingestion of a radiolabeled urea isotope. The urease of *Helicobacter pylori* bacteria in the stomach generates labeled carbon dioxide (CO_2), known as 13C, within 10–30 minutes. This 13C is measured in the client's breath with a sensitivity of 95–98% and a specificity of 97% for the diagnosis of gastric *H. pylori* colonization. This test is useful in pediatrics and is a sensitive indicator of *H. pylori* eradication six weeks after treatment with antibiotics.

PROFESSIONAL CONSIDERATIONS:
Includes seven types of information.

---

❶ *Consent, risks, and contraindications:* Whether or not a separate special consent form IS or is NOT required. Where tests or procedures carry significant risks, the risks that should be explained to the client are included in a highlighted alert box. Contraindications are a list of generally accepted conditions (in a highlighted alert box) in which the test or procedure should not be performed or relative contraindications in which the test or procedure should be modified, where applicable.

TRANSESOPHAGEAL SONOGRAM (TRANSESOPHAGEAL ECHOCARDIOGRAM), DIAGNOSTIC

1. Consent form IS required.

Risks:
Vasovagal bradycardia (common), drug-induced tachycardia (common), transient hypoxemia (common), esophageal perforation and pulmonary aspiration are possible.

TRANSESOPHAGEAL ECHOCARDIOGRAM, DIAGNOSTIC

Contraindications:
Esophageal obstructions, stenosis, or fistula; history of radiation therapy to the esophagus or surrounding area; acute penetrating chest injuries. Neonates and young children are not candidates due to the unavailability of pediatric-sized TEE scopes.

---

❷ *Preparation:* Includes supplies needed, assessment for allergies, unusual scheduling requirements, procedural preparation requirements, such as establishing intravenous access, and medico-legal handling.

HEPATOBILIARY SCAN, DIAGNOSTIC

A. Assess for allergy to radionuclide dye, iodine, or shellfish.
B. Establish intravenous access.
C. Have emergency equipment readily available for use in the event of an anaphylactic reaction to the radionuclide

❸ *Procedure:* Step-by-step description of specimen collection or procedural steps, including client positioning and participation, and monitoring required during the procedure. *Note:* For blood samples, minivolumes (1–3 ml) are listed for tests in which special manual tests may be run in smaller volumes for clients in whom blood preservation is essential. For clients not at risk for iatrogenic anemia due to frequent blood sampling, the quickest turnaround times are achieved with higher volumes, which enable automated testing.

I-125-LABELED FIBRINOGEN (FIBRINOGEN UPTAKE), LEG SCAN, DIAGNOSTIC

A. The client's legs are elevated during the scanning to prevent pooling of blood in the veins of the legs.

B. Iodine-125-labeled fibrinogen is injected intravenously, and serial scans are performed on each leg 1, 4, 24, and 48 hours afterward. Surface radioactivity may be measured daily for as long as 2 days.

C. Assess for allergic reaction after dye injection.

D. The extremity is marked in segments along the course of the vein tract.

E. Areas of fibrinogen incorporation into a thrombus are detected with the counter as areas exhibiting increased radioactivity, indicating increased concentration of radioactive tracer.

❹ *Postprocedure care:* Aftercare instructions regarding specimen handling, site dressing, activity restriction, vital signs, and postsedation monitoring.

BRONCHOSCOPY, DIAGNOSTIC

4. Postprocedure care:

A. No food or fluids until the gag reflex has returned, about 2 hours after the procedure.

B. The client should not attempt to swallow saliva until the gag reflex has returned. Saliva should be expectorated into an emesis basin. Observe the client's sputum for blood if a biopsy was performed. If a tumor is suspected, collect postbronchoscopy sputum specimens for cytology.

C. Observe postanesthesia precautions if a sedative was given. If deep sedation was used, follow institutional protocol for postsedation monitoring. Typical monitoring includes continuous ECG monitoring and pulse oximetry, with continual assessments (q 5–15 minutes) of airway, vital signs, and neurologic status until the client is lying quietly awake and responds to commands spoken in a normal voice.

D. Observe closely for postprocedure complications listed above under *Risks*.

❺ *Client and family teaching:* Instructions the client and/or family should have associated with precare, procedural care, and aftercare and monitoring, as well as disease-specific information, time frame for test results, and follow-up recommendations.

VENEREAL DISEASE RESEARCH LABORATORY TEST (VDRL), SERUM

5. Client and family teaching:

A. Syphilis is a sexually transmitted disease where information regarding sexual partners is necessary for control of the disease.

  B. If testing positive for syphilis and diagnosis is confirmed:
    i. Notify all sexual contacts from the last 90 days (if early stage) to be tested for syphilis.
    ii. Syphilis can be cured with antibiotics. These may worsen the symptoms for the first 24 hours.
    iii. Do not have sexual relations for 2 months and until after repeat testing has confirmed that the syphilis is cured. Use condoms after that for 2 years. Return for repeat testing every 3–4 months for the next 2 years to make sure the disease is cured.
    iv. Do not become pregnant for 2 years, because syphilis can be transmitted to the fetus.
    v. If left untreated, syphilis can damage many body organs, including the brain, over several years time.

---

❻ *Factors that affect results:* Quality assurance information about items that will interfere with the accuracy of results, such as improper collection techniques, improper specimen handling, drugs that cause false-positive or false-negative results, and cross-reactivity of other diseases or conditions.

UROBILINOGEN, URINE

6. Factors that affect results:
  A. Drugs that may cause falsely increased results include acetazolamide, aminosalicylic acid, antipyrine, aspirin, Bromsulphalein, cascara, chlorpromazine, 5-hydroxyindoleacetic acid, phenazopyridine, phenothiazines, and sulfonamides.
  B. Urine alkalinization increases the excretion rate of urine urobilinogen. Urine acidification decreases the excretion rate of urine urobilinogen.
  C. Dipstick methods can detect only abnormally high levels, not abnormally low levels.
  D. The level may be normal in clients with incomplete common bile duct obstruction.
  E. False-positive or falsely increased results may occur in porphyria.

---

❼ *Other data:* Selected information from current research that may not yet be generalizable, but could be helpful in decision-making for individuals or groups of clients; recommendations for confirmatory testing if the results are positive; direction to other tests related to the same diagnosis or condition and known association between tests; and national guideline information and recommendations, when available.

COOMBS', DIRECT (DIRECT ANTIGLOBULIN TEST), SERUM

  A. This test does not delineate the nature of the antibodies identified.
  B. The test must be completed within 24 hours of specimen collection.
  C. DeAngelis et al. found a high incidence of positive results in clients with antibodies to HIV and suggests that this test may be helpful as a prognostic indicator for the disease course.
  D. *See also Antibody Identification, Red Cell, Serum.*

BIBLIOGRAPHY:
Includes listings of current and updated research and literature from both national and international perspectives.

RETROSYNCYNTIAL VIRUS (RSV), CULTURE

Bibliography:

Becker S, Soukup J, Yankaskas JR: Respiratory syncytial virus infection of human primary nasal and bronchial epithelial cell cultures and bronchoalveolar macrophages. Am J Respir Cell Mol Biol 6(4):369–374, 1992.

Isselbacher KJ, et al.: Harrison's Principles of Internal Medicine, 13th ed. New York: McGraw-Hill, 1994, pp 805–806.

Mendoza J, Rojas A, Navarro JM, de la Rosa M: Evaluation of three rapid enzyme immunoassays and cell culture for detection of respiratory syncytial virus. Eur J Clin Microbiol Infect Dis 11(5):452–454, 1992.

The Merck Manual, 16th ed. Rahway, NJ, Merck & Co., 1992, pp 2177–2178.

Wyngaarden JB, Smith LH, Bennett JC: Cecil Textbook of Medicine, 19th ed. Philadelphia, WB Saunders, 1992, pp 1845–1851.

The information presented in the above examples was excerpted from the text to illustrate the format. Please refer to the Preface for additional information regarding inclusions and exclusions. We hope you find this book as useful in your practice as it has been in ours.

Standard Precautions

Based on new information that is epidemiologically sound, a need for a user-friendly system, and a design to reduce the risk of transmission of micro-organisms from recognized and unrecognized sources, the Centers for Disease Control (CDC) has introduced its "Standard Precautions." These guidelines synthesize the major features of universal precautions and body substance isolation. The precautions apply to *all blood and body fluids and secretions, nonintact skin, and mucous membranes.* The following instructions should be followed according to "Standard Precautions":

1. Gloves should be worn during phlebotomy and any time there is a risk of exposure to blood and/or body fluids.
2. Needles and sharps shall be properly disposed of in puncture-resistant containers. Needles shall not be recapped or otherwise manipulated by hand after use.
3. Hands shall be washed immediately and thoroughly with antiseptic cleanser after any contamination with blood or body fluids and after glove removal.
4. Protective clothing and eyewear should be worn if there is a potential for splashing of fluids.
5. Spills should be cleaned while wearing gloves with an EPA-approved germicide or a 1:100 solution of household bleach.
6. Soiled linen should be handled as little as possible and bagged at the location where it was used.
7. Infective waste should be disposed of according to institutional and local protocol.
8. When possible, persons with highly transmittable or epidemiologically important organisms are placed in a private room with separate toilet and handwashing facilities.
9. Transportation of infected persons requires the use of appropriate barriers such as masks and impervious dressings.

Reference:

Condensed from The Centers for Disease Control. Draft Guidelines for Isolation Precautions in Hospitals: Part I and Part II. Federal Register *59*(214):55552–55570, 1994.

Contents

PART ONE

Diseases, Conditions, and Symptoms

ABDOMINAL AORTIC ANEURYSM
(see Aneurysm, Abdominal Aortic; Aneurysm, Cerebral; or Aneurysm, Thoracic Aortic)

ABORTION
Alpha-Fetoprotein, Blood
Amniotic Fluid, Alpha$_1$-Fetoprotein, Specimen
Amniotic Fluid, Chromosome Analysis, Specimen
Amniotic Fluid, Erythroblastosis Fetalis, Specimen
Chorionic Villi Sampling, Diagnostic
Endometrium, Anaerobic, Culture
Estriol, Serum or 24-Hour Urine
Glucose Tolerance Test, Blood
Histopathology, Specimen
Human Chorionic Gonadotropin, Beta-Subunit, Serum
Pregnancy Test, Routine, Serum
Progesterone, Serum
Type and Crossmatch, Blood

ADDITIONAL CONDITIONS
Ectopic Pregnancy
Pelvic Inflammatory Disease

ABSCESS
Abscess, Anaerobic Culture
Actinomyces, Culture
Biopsy, Anaerobic, Culture
Biopsy, Fungus, Culture
Body Fluid, Anaerobic, Culture
Bronchial Aspirate, Routine, Culture
Histopathology, Specimen
Magnetic Resonance Imaging, Diagnostic
Skin, *Mycobacteria,* Culture
Sputum, Routine, Culture
Wound, Culture
Wound, Fungus, Culture
Wound, *Mycobacteria,* Culture

ADDITIONAL CONDITIONS
Bronchiectasis
Dental Problems
Empyema
Fever
Foreign Body
Otitis Media
Pelvic Inflammatory Disease
Postoperative
Rheumatic Heart Disease
Scarlet Fever
Sinusitis
Urinary Tract Infection

ACHLORHYDRIA
Acid Perfusion Test, Diagnostic
Gastric Analysis, Specimen
Gastrin, Serum
Histopathology, Specimen
Intrinsic Factor Antibody, Blood
Parietal Cell Antibody, Blood
Pepsinogen-1 Antibody, Blood
pH, Urine
Schilling Test, Diagnostic
Urinalysis, Urine
Vitamin B$_{12}$, Serum

ADDITIONAL CONDITIONS
Gastric Cancer
Gastric Ulcer
Peptic Ulcer

ACIDOSIS
(see Metabolic Acidosis or Respiratory Acidosis)

ACNE VULGARIS
Biopsy, Anaerobic, Culture
Histopathology, Specimen

ADDITIONAL CONDITIONS
Hormonal Changes
Puberty
Stress

ACQUIRED IMMUNE DEFICIENCY SYNDROME (AIDS)
Acquired Immune Deficiency Syndrome Evaluation Battery, Diagnostic
Beta₂-Microglobulin, Blood and 24-Hour Urine
Biopsy, Site-Specific, Specimen
Bronchial Culture
Bronchoscopy, Diagnostic
Cerebrospinal Fluid, Routine, Culture and Cytology
Chest X-Ray, Diagnostic
Cryptococcal Antigen Titer, Cerebrospinal Fluid, Specimen
Cryptococcal Antigen Titer, Serum
Cryptococcal Antibody Titer, Serum
Cryptosporidium Diagnostic Procedures, Stool
Cytomegalovirus Antibody, Serum
Hepatitis B Surface Antigen, Blood
Lymphocyte Subset Enumeration, Blood
Magnetic Resonance Spectography, Diagnostic
Mantoux Skin Test, Diagnostic
Pneumocystis IFA, Serum
Skin *Mycobacteria,* Culture
T- and B-Lymphocyte Subset Assay, Blood
Throat Culture for *Candida albicans,* Culture
Toxoplasmosis Serology, Serum

ADDITIONAL CONDITIONS
Anemia
Blood Transfusion that is Allogenic
Candidiasis
Cervical Cancer
Coccidioidomycosis
Cryptococcosis
Cryptosporidium
Cytomegalovirus
Diarrhea
Drug Abuse
Encephalopathy
Esophagitis
Hemophilia
Herpes Simplex
Histoplasmosis
Hypocalcemia
Isosporiasis
Kaposi's Sarcoma
Leukoencephalopathy, Multifocal
Lymphoma
Mycobacterium TB
Pneumonia
Septicemia
Sexual Promiscuity
Stomatitis
Thrombocytopenia
Toxoplasmosis of the Brain
Washing Syndrome Due to HIV

ACROMEGALY
(see also Hyperpituitarism)
Alkaline Phosphatase, Serum
Alkaline Phosphatase Isoenzymes, Serum
Calcium, Total, Serum
Calcium, Urine
Glucose, Blood
Growth Hormone, Blood
Hydroxyproline, Total, 24-Hour, Urine
Insulin-Like Growth Factor-I, Blood
Phosphorus, Serum

ADDITIONAL CONDITIONS
Adenomas
Bronchial Carcinoids
Gangliocytomas
Intestinal Carcinoids
Lung Carcinoma

ACTINOMYCOSIS
Abscess, Anaerobic Culture
Acid-Fast Stain, *Nocardia* Species, Culture
Actinomyces, Culture

ADDITIONAL CONDITIONS
Abscess of Lung
Pelvic Inflammatory Disease
Sinus Infection
Tooth Extraction

Biopsy, Anaerobic, Culture
Biopsy, Routine, Culture
Biopsy, Fungus, Culture
Bronchial Aspirate, Routine, Culture
Bronchial Washing, Specimen,
    Diagnostic
Brushing Cytology, Specimen,
    Diagnostic
Cervical/Vaginal Cytology, Specimen
Endometrium, Anaerobic, Culture
Foreign Body, Routine, Culture
Histopathology, Specimen
Sputum Fungus, Specimen
Wound Culture

ACUTE MYOCARDIAL INFARCTION
(see Myocardial Infarction)

ACUTE RESPIRATORY DISTRESS SYNDROME (ARDS)
Blood Gases, Arterial, Blood
Chest X-Ray, Diagnostic
C-Reactive Protein, Serum
Complete Blood Count, Blood
Oximetry, Diagnostic
Prothrombin Time and International
    Normalized Ratio, Serum
Pulmonary Artery Catheterization,
    Diagnostic
Pulmonary Function Test, Diagnostic
Sputum Culture and Sensitivity,
    Specimen

ADDITIONAL CONDITIONS
Aspiration of Gastric Contents
COPD
Hypoxemia
Multiple Blood Transfusions
Near Drowning
Pancreatitis
Pneumonia
Pulmonary Infiltrate
Sepsis
Trauma

ACUTE TUBULAR NECROSIS
(see Renal Failure)

ADDISON'S DISEASE
Alkaline Phosphatase, Serum
Alkaline Phosphatase Isoenzymes,
    Serum
Calcium, Total, Serum
Calcium, Urine
Glucose, Blood
Growth Hormone, Blood
Hydroxyproline, Total, 24-Hour,
    Urine
Insulin-Like Growth Factor-I, Blood
Magnesium, Serum
Metyrapone Test, Serum
Metyrapone, 24-Hour, Urine
Parietal Cell Antibody, Blood
Phosphorus, Serum

ADDITIONAL CONDITIONS
ACTH Deficiency
Adrenoleukodystrophy
Amyloidosis
Adrenal Hyperplasia
Anticoagulant Therapy
Candidiasis (Thrush)
Cushing's Syndrome
Diabetes Mellitus
Hypogonadism
Hypoparathyroidism
Lymphoid Hyperplasia
Metastasis, Breast or Lung Cancer
Pernicious Anemia
Schmidt Syndrome
Thyroiditis

ADENOVIRUS INFECTION
Adenovirus Antibody Titer, Serum
Adenovirus Immunofluorescence,
  Diagnostic
Ocular Cytology, Specimen
Viral Culture, Specimen

ADDITIONAL CONDITIONS
Acute Hemorrhagic Cystitis
Common Cold
Nonstreptococcal Pharyngitis

ADRENAL HYPERPLASIA OR TUMOR
Luteinizing Hormone, Blood
Magnetic Resonance Imaging, Brain,
  Diagnostic

ADDITIONAL CONDITIONS
Addison's Disease
Alcoholism
Congenital Adrenal Hyperplasia
Cushing's Syndrome
Hirsutism
Infertility
Menstrual Irregularities
Renal Failure

ADRENALECTOMY
Magnesium, Serum

ADDITIONAL CONDITIONS
Adrenal Adenoma
Adrenal Carcinoma
Waterhouse-Friderichsen Syndrome

ADULT RESPIRATORY DISTRESS SYNDROME
(see Acute Respiratory Distress Syndrome [ARDS])

AGRANULOCYTOSIS
Blood Culture, Blood
Bone Marrow Aspiration Analysis,
  Specimen
Culture, Skin, Specimen
Culture, Urine
Differential Leukocyte Count,
  Peripheral Blood

ADDITIONAL CONDITIONS
Anemia
Leukemia

AHAPTOGLOBINEMIA
Haptoglobin, Serum

ADDITIONAL CONDITIONS
Hemolytic Transfusion Reaction

AIDS
(see Acquired Immune Deficiency Syndrome)

ALBRIGHT'S SYNDROME
Alkaline Phosphatase, Serum
Bone X-Ray, Diagnostic
Hydroxyproline, Total, 24-Hour,
  Urine

ADDITIONAL CONDITIONS
Acromegaly
Cushing's Syndrome
Hyperthyroidism
Osteomalacia
Ovarian Cysts

ALCOHOLISM
Alanine Aminotransferase, Serum
Albumin, Serum, Urine, and 24-Hour
  Urine
Alcohol, Blood

ADDITIONAL CONDITIONS
Anemia
Brain Encephalopathy
Bronchitis
Cirrhosis

Alkaline Phosphatase, Serum
Alkaline Phosphatase Isoenzymes,
    Serum
Ammonia, Blood
Amylase, Serum and Urine
Anion Gap, Blood
Aspartate Aminotransferase, Serum
Bilirubin, Direct, Serum
Bilirubin, Total, Serum
Blood Indices (MCV), Blood
Chemistry Profile, Blood
Complete Blood Count, Blood
Differential Leukocyte Count,
    Peripheral Blood
Electrolyte, Blood
Folic Acid, Serum
Gamma-Glutamyl Transpeptidase,
    Blood
Glucose, Blood
Heavy Metals, Blood and 24-Hour Urine
Histopathology, Specimen
Ketone Bodies, Blood
Ketones, Semiquantitative, Urine
Lactic Acid, Blood
Lactate Dehydrogenase, Blood
Lactate Dehydrogenase, Isoenzymes,
    Blood
Lipid Profile, Blood
Liver Battery, Serum
Magnesium, Serum
5'Nucleotidase, Serum
Occult Blood, Stool, Diagnostic
Osmolality, Serum
pH, Blood
Phosphorus, Serum
Platelet Count, Blood
Prothrombin Time and International
    Normalized Ratio, Serum
4-Pyridoxic Acid, Urine
Red Blood Cell Morphology, Blood
Schilling Test, Diagnostic
Sedimentation Rate, Erythrocyte,
    Blood
Toxicology, Volatiles Group by GLC,
    Blood or Urine
Triglycerides, Blood
Uric Acid, Serum
Vitamin B_{12}, Serum
Zinc, Blood

COPD
Depression
Dermatitis
Dysfunctional Family
Gastritis
Hepatomegaly
Hypertension
Hypertriglyceridemia
Hypocalcemia
Hypomagnesemia
Hypophosphatemia
Malabsorption
Malnutrition
Organic Brain Syndrome
Pancreatitis
Seizures
Thrombocytopenia

ALKALOSIS
*(see Metabolic Alkalosis or
Respiratory Alkalosis)*

ALZHEIMER'S DISEASE
Bromides, Serum
Cerebrospinal Fluid Immunoglobulin
    G, Immunoglobulin G Ratios and
    Immunoglobulin G Index,

ADDITIONAL CONDITIONS
AIDS
Dementia
Malnutrition
Organic Brain Syndrome

Immunoglobulin G Synthesis
Rate, Specimen
Cerebrospinal Fluid, Oligoclonal
Bands, Specimen
Cerebrospinal Fluid, Protein,
Specimen
Cerebrospinal Fluid, Routine
Analysis, Specimen
Ceruloplasmin, Serum
Computed Tomography of the Brain,
Diagnostic
Copper, Serum
Copper, Urine
Heavy Metals, Blood and 24-Hour
Urine
Neurological Examination,
Diagnostic
Positron Emission Tomography,
Diagnostic
Protein Electrophoresis,
Cerebrospinal Fluid, Specimen
Single Photon Emission Computed
Tomography, Brain, Diagnostic

AMAUROSIS FUGAX

Viscosity, Serum

ADDITIONAL CONDITIONS

Arteriosclerotic Heart Disease
Arteritis, Temporal
Cerebrovascular Accident
Rheumatic Heart Disease
Sepsis
Transient Ischemic Attacks

AMENORRHEA

Adrenocorticotropic Hormone,
Serum
Chromosome Analysis, Blood
Cortisol, Plasma or Serum
Cortisol, Urine
Estradiol, Serum
Estrogens, Serum and 24-Hour Urine
Follicle-Stimulating Hormone,
Serum
Histopathology, Specimen
Hormonal Evaluation, Cytologic,
Specimen
17-Hydroxycorticosteroids, 24-Hour,
Urine
17-Ketogenic Steroids, Total, 24-
Hour, Urine
17-Ketosteroid Fractionation, 24-
Hour, Urine
Luteinizing Hormone, Blood
PAP Smear, Diagnostic
Pregnancy Test, Routine, Serum
Prolactin, Serum
Testosterone, Total, Blood
Thyroid-Stimulating Hormone, Blood
Thyroid Test: Free Thyroxine Index,
Serum

ADDITIONAL CONDITIONS

Acromegaly
Anorexia Nervosa
Azotemia
Cushing's Syndrome
Excessive Exercise
Galactorrhea
Herpes Zoster
Hypothyroidism
Menopause
Menstrual Irregularity
Perimenopause
Pituitary Tumor
Pregnancy
Renal Failure
Stress

AMIKACIN
(see Aminoglycoside Toxicity)

AMINOGLYCOSIDE TOXICITY
(Amikacin, Gentamicin, Kanamycin, Neomycin, Spectinomycin, Streptomycin, Tobramycin)
Amikacin Sulfate, Blood
Beta$_2$-Microglobulin, Blood and 24-Hour Urine
Bicarbonate, Serum
Blood Gases, Arterial, Blood
Blood Volume, Blood
Blood Urea Nitrogen/Creatinine Ratio, Blood
Creatinine Clearance, Serum, Urine
Creatinine, Serum
Gentamicin, Blood
Osmolality, Serum
Osmolality, Urine
pCO$_2$, Blood
Sodium, Plasma, Serum, or Urine
Specific Gravity, Urine
Tobramycin, Serum
Urinalysis, Urine

ADDITIONAL CONDITIONS
Deafness
Renal Dysfunction

AMNIOCENTESIS
Chronic Villi Sampling, Diagnostic

ADDITIONAL CONDITIONS
Genetic Testing of Fetus
Pregnancy

AMPUTATION
(see Surgery, Preoperative and Surgery, Postoperative)

AMYLOIDOSIS
Bone Marrow Aspiration Analysis, Specimen
Chemistry Profile, Blood
Concentration Test, Urine
Creatinine Clearance, Serum, Urine
Creatinine, Serum
Cytologic Study of Gastrointestinal Tract, Diagnostic
d-Xylose Absorption Test, Diagnostic, Serum or Urine
Globulin, Serum
Histopathology, Specimen
Immunoelectrophoresis, Serum and Urine
Leukocyte Cytochemistry, Specimen
Liver Biopsy, Diagnostic
Liver I-131 Scan, Diagnostic
Protein, Electrophoresis, Serum
Protein, Electrophoresis, Urine
Protein, Quantitative, Urine
Protein, Semiquantitative, Urine
Skin *Mycobacteria*, Culture

ADDITIONAL CONDITIONS
Cardiomegaly
Cardiomyopathy
Carpal Tunnel Syndrome
Chronic Renal Failure
Endocrine Gland Abnormality
Intestinal Obstruction
Macroglossia
Nephrotic Syndrome
Peripheral Neuropathy
Respiratory Failure

Urea Nitrogen, Plasma or Serum
Urinalysis, Urine

AMYOTROPHIC LATERAL SCLEROSIS (ALS)

Biopsy, Site-Specific (Muscle), Specimen
Creatine Kinase, Serum
Creatinine Clearance, Serum, Urine
Electromyogram and Nerve Conduction (Electromyelogram) Studies, Diagnostic

ADDITIONAL CONDITIONS

Dementia
Neurological Diseases
Parkinsonism

ANAPHYLAXIS

(see Shock)

ANEMIAS

(see Aplastic, Dyserythropoietic, Folic Acid, G-6-PD Deficiency, Galactokinase Deficiency, Heinz Body, Hemolytic, Iron [hypochromic] Deficiency, Megaloblastic, Pernicious, or Sickle Cell Anemias)

ANESTHESIA

(see also Surgery, Preoperative and Surgery, Postoperative)
Blood Gases, Arterial, Blood
Chest X-Ray, Diagnostic
Complete Blood Count, Blood
Electrocardiogram, Diagnostic
Electrolyte, Blood

ADDITIONAL CONDITIONS

Pregnancy, Cesarean
Surgery
Trauma

ANEURYSM

(see Aneurysm, Abdominal Aortic; Aneurysm, Cerebral; or Aneurysm, Thoracic Aortic)

ANEURYSM, ABDOMINAL AORTIC

Cardiac Catheterization, Diagnostic
Chest X-Ray, Diagnostic
Computed Tomography of the Body, Diagnostic
Fluorescent Treponemal Antibody-Absorbed Double-Stain Test, Serum
Lipid Profile, Blood
Magnetic Resonance Angiography, Diagnostic
Magnetic Resonance Imaging, Diagnostic
Rapid Plasma Reagin Test, Blood
Venereal Disease Research Laboratory Test, Serum

ADDITIONAL CONDITIONS

Aortitis
Arteriosclerosis
Congenital Defects
Congestive Heart Failure
Hypertension
Local Infection
Marfan's Syndrome
Pregnancy
Syphilis
Trauma

ANEURYSM, CEREBRAL

Cerebral Angiogram, Diagnostic
Cerebral Computed Tomography,
  Diagnostic
Cerebrospinal Fluid, Protein,
  Specimen
Doppler Ultrasound Flow Studies,
  Diagnostic
Magnetic Resonance Angiography,
  Diagnostic
Magnetic Resonance Imaging of the
  Brain, Diagnostic
Partial Thromboplastin Time, Plasma
Prothrombin Time and International
  Normalized Ratio, Serum

ADDITIONAL CONDITIONS

Arteriosclerosis
Congestive Heart Failure
Hypertension
Local Infection
Syphilis
Trauma

ANEURYSM, THORACIC AORTIC

Fluorescent Treponemal Antibody-
  Absorbed Double-Stain Test, Serum
Lipid Profile, Blood
Magnetic Resonance Angiography,
  Diagnostic
Pulmonary Angiogram, Diagnostic
Rapid Plasma Reagin Test, Blood
Venereal Disease Research Laboratory
  Test, Serum

ADDITIONAL CONDITIONS

Arteriosclerosis
Congestive Heart Failure
Hypertension
Local Infection
Syphilis
Trauma

ANGINA PECTORIS

Anticardiolipin Antibody, Serum
Antimyocardial Antibody, Serum
Aspartate Aminotransferase, Serum
Cardiac Catheterization, Diagnostic
Coronary Intravascular Ultrasound,
  Diagnostic
Creatine Kinase, Serum
Creatine Kinase Isoenzymes, Serum
D-Dimer Test, Blood
Electrocardiogram, Diagnostic
Ergonovine Provocation Test,
  Diagnostic
Heart Scan, Diagnostic
Holter Monitor, Diagnostic
Lactate Dehydrogenase Isoenzymes,
  Blood
Lipid Profile, Blood
Positive Emission Tomography,
  Diagnostic
Stress/Exercise Test, Diagnostic
Stress Test, Pharmacologic, Diagnostic
Troponin I, Serum
Troponin T, Serum

ADDITIONAL CONDITIONS

Aortic Stenosis
Cervical Spine/Disc Disease
Diabetes Mellitus
Gallbladder Disease
Herpes Zoster
Hypertension
Mitral Valve Prolapse
Myocarditis
Myocardial Infarction
Pericarditis
Peripheral Vascular Disease
Reflux Esophagitis
Rheumatic Fever
Thyrotoxicosis
Xanthelasma
Xanthomas

ANKYLOSING SPONDYLITIS

Human Leukocyte Antigen B-27,
  Blood
Protein, Electrophoresis, Serum
Rheumatoid Factor, Blood

ADDITIONAL CONDITIONS

Aortic Insufficiency
A-V Conduction Defects
Pulmonary Fibrosis
Rheumatoid Arthritis

Sedimentation Rate, Erythrocyte,
  Blood
Tissue Typing, Blood
X-Ray, Diagnostic

ANOREXIA NERVOSA

Estradiol, Serum
17-Hydroxycorticosteroids, 24-Hour,
  Urine
Low-Density Lipoprotein, Blood
Luteinizing Hormone, Blood
Phenolphthalein Test, Diagnostic
Potassium, Serum
Protein-Bound Iodine, Blood
Thyroid Test: Free Thyroxine Index,
  Serum
Thyroid Test: Triiodothyronine, Blood
Thyroid Test: Thyroxine, Blood

ADDITIONAL CONDITIONS

Amenorrhea
Anovulation
Anxiety
Depression
Endocrine Disorders
Hypotension
Malnutrition

ANOXIA

Blood Gases, Arterial, Blood
Bicarbonate, Serum
Blood Gases, Capillary, Blood
Blood Gases, Venous, Blood
Bronchography, Diagnostic
Carbon Dioxide, Partial Pressure,
  Blood
Carbon Dioxide, Total Content, Blood
Chest X-Ray, Diagnostic
Single Photon Emission Computed
  Tomography, Brain, Diagnostic

ADDITIONAL CONDITIONS

Anemia
Asthma
Carbon Monoxide Poisoning
Congestive Heart Failure
Diabetes Mellitus
Emphysema
Empyema
Head Trauma
Hypertension
Seizures

ANTHRAX

Blood Culture, Blood
Chest X-Ray, Diagnostic
Culture, Skin, Specimen
Differential Leukocyte Count,
  Peripheral Blood

ADDITIONAL CONDITIONS

Cyanosis
Fever
Headache
Hemorrhagic Meningitis
Nausea
Pneumonia
Sepsis
Shock
Vomiting

ANTIGENS
(see Immunoglobulins)

ANXIETY

Blood Gases, Arterial, Blood
Electrocardiogram, Diagnostic
Epinephrine, Blood
Norepinephrine, Serum
Toxicology Screen, Urine

ADDITIONAL CONDITIONS

Alcoholism
Depression
Drug Abuse
Hyperventilation
Mitral Valve Prolapse
Phobias
Sleep Disturbances
Stress
Tachycardia

AORTIC ANEURYSM
(see Aneurysm, Abdominal Aortic)

AORTIC VALVULAR STENOSIS

Blood Gases, Arterial, Blood
Cardiac Catheterization, Diagnostic
Chest X-Ray, Diagnostic
Digital Subtraction Angiography and
Transvenous-Digital Subtraction,
Diagnostic
Electrocardiogram, Diagnostic
Magnetic Resonance Angiography,
Diagnostic
Transesophageal Sonogram,
Diagnostic

ADDITIONAL CONDITIONS

Angina
Deep Vein Thrombosis
Dysrhythmias
Cerebrovascular Accident
Congenital Aortic Narrowing
Myocardial Infarction
Rheumatic Fever
Syncope

AORTITIS

Abdominal Aortic Sonogram,
Diagnostic
Complete Blood Count, Blood
Lipid Profile, Blood
Rapid Plasma Reagin Test, Blood
Venereal Disease Research Laboratory
Test, Serum

ADDITIONAL CONDITIONS

Endocarditis
Rheumatic Heart Disease
Scarlet Fever
Sepsis

APLASTIC ANEMIA

Bone Marrow Biopsy, Diagnostic
Mixed Leukocyte Culture, Specimen
Red Blood Cell Morphology, Blood
Red Cell Count, Serum

ADDITIONAL CONDITIONS

Hypoplastic Bone Marrow
Leukemia
Pancytopenia
Systemic Lupus Erythematosus
(SLE)

APPENDICITIS

Abscess, Anaerobic Culture
Complete Blood Count, Blood
Differential Leukocyte Count,
Peripheral Blood
Histopathology (Postoperatively),
Specimen
Infectious Mononucleosis Screening
Test, Blood
Occult Blood, Stool
Urinalysis, Urine

ADDITIONAL CONDITIONS

Abscess
Acute Pain, RLQ Abdomen
Amebiasis
Crohn's Disease
Enteritis
Leukocytosis
Peritonitis

ARDS
(see Acute Respiratory Distress Syndrome)

ARRHYTHMIAS
(see Dysrhythmias)

ARTERIAL ISCHEMIC LEG ULCER
(see Peripheral Vascular Disease)

ARTERIAL OCCLUSION
(see Occlusion, Acute Arterial)

ARTERIAL THROMBOSIS
(see Thrombosis or Embolism)

ARTERIOSCLEROSIS
Anticardiolipin Antibody, Serum
Cholesterol, Blood
Coronary Intravascular Ultrasound,
    Diagnostic
Doppler Ultrasound Flow Studies,
    Diagnostic
High-Density Lipoprotein
    Cholesterol, Blood
Lipid Profile, Blood
Lipoprotein Electrophoresis, Serum
Low-Density Lipoprotein Cholesterol,
    Blood
Mean Platelet Volume, Blood
Stress Test, Pharmacologic,
    Diagnostic
Stress/Exercise Test, Diagnostic
Triglycerides, Blood
Ultrafast Computed Tomography,
    Diagnostic

ADDITIONAL CONDITIONS
Arteriosclerotic Heart Disease
Arteriosclerosis Obliterans
Coronary Heart Disease
Hypertension
Organic Brain Syndrome
Transient Ischemic Attacks

ARTERIOSCLEROTIC HEART DISEASE
(see Arteriosclerosis)

ARTERITIS
Biopsy, Site-Specific (Temporal
    Artery), Specimen
Complete Blood Count, Blood
Sedimentation Rate, Erythrocyte,
    Blood

ADDITIONAL CONDITIONS
Anorexia
Atherosclerosis
Brain Tumor
Headache
Multiple Sclerosis
Transient Ischemic Attack
Vision Loss

ARTHRITIS, OSTEO
Body Fluid Cytology, Specimen
Bone Scan, Diagnostic
Histopathology, Specimen
Mucin Clot Test (Synovial Fluid),
    Specimen
Synovial Fluid Analysis, Diagnostic
X-Ray of Long Bones, Diagnostic

ADDITIONAL CONDITIONS
Metastasis from Cancer
Multiple Myeloma
Osteoporosis
Rheumatoid Arthritis

ARTHRITIS, RHEUMATOID
Anti-DNA, Serum
Antinuclear Antibody, Serum
Antistreptolysin-O Titer, Blood
Body Fluid, Routine, Culture
C4 Complement, Serum
Chemistry Profile, Blood
Complement Components, Serum
Complement, Total, Serum
C-Reactive Protein, Serum
Extractable Nuclear Antigen, Serum

ADDITIONAL CONDITIONS
Amyloidosis
Lymphadenopathy
Pericarditis
Pleural Effusion
Raynaud's Phenomenon
Splenomegaly
Vasculitis

Genital, *Candida albicans,* Culture
Genital, *Neisseria gonorrhoeae,*
    Culture
Genital, Routine, Culture
Human Leukocyte Antigen B-27,
    Blood
Immune Complex Assay, Blood
Lupus Test, Blood
Mean Platelet Volume, Blood
Mucin Clot Test (Synovial Fluid),
    Specimen
Protein, Electrophoresis, Serum
Rheumatoid Factor, Blood
Sedimentation Rate, Erythrocyte,
    Blood
Sjögren's Antibodies, Blood
Synovial Fluid Analysis, Diagnostic
Tissue Typing, Blood
Uric Acid, Serum
Uric Acid, Urine

ASBESTOSIS
(see Industrial-Related Diseases)

ASCITES
Albumin, Serum, Urine, and 24-Hour
    Urine
Body Fluid Analysis, Cell Count,
    Specimen
Body Fluid Cytology, Specimen
KUB, Diagnostic
Liver Battery, Serum
Paracentesis, Diagnostic
Synovial Fluid Analysis, Diagnostic

ADDITIONAL CONDITIONS
Alcoholism
Burns
Congestive Heart Failure
Cirrhosis
Myxedema
Ovarian Cancer
Pancreatitis
Peritonitis
Pleural Effusion
Wilson's Disease

ASHD/ARTERIOSCLEROTIC HEART DISEASE
(see Arteriosclerosis)

ASPIRATION PNEUMONIA
(see Pneumonia)

ASPIRIN POISONING
(see Poisoning, Salicylate)

ASTERIXIS
(see Liver Failure)

ASTHMA
Acid Perfusion Test (Nocturnal
    Asthma), Diagnostic
Allergen-Specific IgE Antibody, Serum
Bicarbonate, Serum
Blood Gases, Arterial, Blood
Carbon Dioxide, Partial Pressure,
    Blood

ADDITIONAL CONDITIONS
Allergies
Beta Blockade
Bronchitis
COPD
Pneumonia
Pneumonitis
Pulmonary Infection

Carbon Dioxide, Total Content, Blood
Chest X-Ray, Diagnostic
Complete Blood Count, Blood
Differential Leukocyte Count,
    Peripheral Blood
Eosinophil Count, Blood
Eosinophil Smear
    (Fecal/Nasal/Sputum), Specimen
Hypersensitivity Pneumonitis
    Serology, Blood
Immunoglobulin E, Serum
Low-Density Lipoprotein, Blood
Ova and Parasites, Stool
Pulmonary Function Test,
    Diagnostic
4-Pyridoxic Acid, Urine
Spirometry, Diagnostic
Sputum Cytology, Specimen
Theophylline, Blood

Stress
Tachycardia

ATAXIA
Alcohol, Blood
Antistreptolysin-O Titer, Serum
Benzodiazepines, Plasma and Urine
    (Urine)
Heavy Metals, Blood and 24-Hour
    Urine
Lead, Blood and Urine
Magnesium, Serum
Neurological Examination,
    Diagnostic
Phenothiazines (Chlorpromazine,
    Compazine, Fluphenazine,
    Mellaril, Mesoridazine,
    Prochlorperazine, Prolixin,
    Serentil, Stelazine, Thioridazine,
    Thorazine, Trifluoperazine),
    Blood
Phenytoin, Serum
Streptozyme, Blood
Venereal Disease Research
    Laboratory Test, Cerebrospinal
    Fluid, Specimen

ADDITIONAL CONDITIONS
Aminoglycoside Reaction
Aspirin Toxicity
Brain Tumor
Cerebrovascular Accident
Labyrinthitis
Meniere's Disease
Multiple Sclerosis
Transient Ischemic Attack

ATELECTASIS
Blood Gases, Arterial, Blood
Chest X-Ray, Diagnostic
Complete Blood Count, Blood

ADDITIONAL CONDITIONS
Chest Trauma
COPD
Empyema
Postoperative
Pulmonary Embolism

ATHEROSCLEROSIS
(see Arteriosclerosis)

ATHLETE'S FOOT
Culture, Skin, Specimen

ADDITIONAL CONDITIONS
Lymphadenitis
Lymphangitis

ATRIAL SEPTAL DEFECT (ASD)
Blood Gases, Arterial, Blood
Cardiac Catheterization, Diagnostic
Chest X-Ray, Diagnostic
Complete Blood Count, Blood
Echocardiogram, Diagnostic
Electrocardiogram, Diagnostic
Heart Scan, Diagnostic
Pulmonary Artery Catheterization,
    Diagnostic

AUSTRALIAN ANTIGEN
(see Hepatitis)

AUTOIMMUNE DISEASES
*(see Amyloidosis, Ankylosing
Spondylitis, Goodpasture's
Syndrome, Myasthenia Gravis,
Raynaud's Disease, Rheumatic Fever,
Rheumatoid Arthritis, Scleroderma,
Sjögren's Syndrome, Systemic Lupus
Erythematosus {SLE}, or Vasculitis)*

AZOTEMIA
Blood Urea Nitrogen/Creatinine
    Ratio, Blood
Calcium, Total, Serum
Chemistry Profile, Blood
Creatinine Clearance, Serum, Urine
Creatinine, Serum
Electrolytes, Blood or Urine
Occult Blood, Stool
Osmolality, Serum
Osmolality, Urine
Phosphorus, Serum
Phosphorus, Urine
Protein, Semiquantitative, Urine
Urea Nitrogen, Plasma or Serum
Uric Acid, Serum
Urinalysis, Urine

BACTEREMIA
(see Sepsis)

BACTERIAL ENDOCARDITIS
(see Endocarditis)

BELL'S PALSY
Electromyogram and Nerve
    Conduction Studies, Diagnostic

BENIGN PROSTATIC HYPERTROPHY (BPH)
Acid Phosphatase, Serum
Alkaline Phosphatase, Serum

ADDITIONAL CONDITIONS
Bundle Branch Block
Cleft Mitral Valve Leaflet

ADDITIONAL CONDITIONS
Amenorrhea
Anemia
Congestive Heart Failure
Hyperglycemia
Hyperparathyroidism
Hypertension
Hypothyroidism
Impotence
Infertility
Metabolic Acidosis
Osteomalacia
Pericarditis
Pulmonary Edema
Renal Failure
Uremia

ADDITIONAL CONDITION
Herpes Simplex Virus

ADDITIONAL CONDITIONS
Uremia
Urinary Retention

Bicarbonate, Serum
Chemistry Profile, Blood
Complete Blood Count, Blood
Electrolyte, Blood
Occult Blood, Urine
Urinalysis, Urine

BERGER'S DISEASE
Biopsy, Site-Specific (Renal),
    Specimen
Creatinine Clearance, 12- or 24-Hour,
    Urine
Immunoglobulin A, Serum
Intravenous Pyelography, Diagnostic
Urinalysis, Urine

ADDITIONAL CONDITIONS
Hematuria
Hypertension
Immune Complex Glomerulopathies
Proteinuria
Upper Respiratory Tract Disease

BERIBERI
Chest X-Ray, Diagnostic
Electrocardiogram, Diagnostic
Electromyogram and Nerve
    Conduction Studies, Diagnostic
Vitamin B_1, Serum or Urine

ADDITIONAL CONDITIONS
Cardiomegaly
Congestive Heart Failure
Pulmonary Edema
Tachycardia

BERNARD-SOULIER SYNDROME
Platelet Adhesion Test, Diagnostic
Platelet Aggregation, Blood, Platelet
    Aggregation, Hypercoagulable
    State, Blood
Platelet Count, Blood
von Willebrand Factor Assay, Blood

ADDITIONAL CONDITION
Postoperative Bleeding

BETA-GLUCURONIDASE SYNDROME
Mucopolysaccharides, Qualitative,
    Urine

ADDITIONAL CONDITIONS
Amyloidosis
Leukemia

BILIARY CALCULI
Bile, Urine
Urobilinogen, Urine

ADDITIONAL CONDITIONS
Cholecystitis
Jaundice

BILIRUBINURIA
Bile, Urine
Gallbladder and Biliary System
    Sonogram, Diagnostic

ADDITIONAL CONDITIONS
Jaundice
Renal Failure

BLACK LUNG DISEASE
(see Silicosis)

BLEPHARITIS
Culture (Eye Margin), Routine,
    Specimen

ADDITIONAL CONDITIONS
Herpes Zoster
Seborrhea

BOTULISM
Abscess, Anaerobic Culture
Botulism, Diagnostic Procedures, Stool
Clostridium difficile Toxin Assay,
    Stool
Complete Blood Count, Blood
Culture, Stool, Specimen
Electromyogram and Nerve
    Conduction Studies, Diagnostic

ADDITIONAL CONDITIONS
Fever
Gastritis
Paralytic Ileus

BOWEL OBSTRUCTION
(see Obstruction)

BRADYCARDIA
Digitoxin, Serum
Digoxin, Serum
Disopyramide Phosphate, Serum
Echocardiogram, Diagnostic
Electrocardiogram, Diagnostic
Electrolyte, Blood
Propranolol, Blood
Quinidine, Serum
Thyroid Profile, Blood

ADDITIONAL CONDITIONS
A-V Heart Block
Coronary Artery Disease
Dilantin, Rapid Intravenous Usage
Infections, Severe
Jaundice
Myocardial Infarction
Sinus Arrest

BRAIN ABSCESS
(see Abscess)

BRAIN CANCER
Brain Biopsy, Diagnostic
Computed Tomography of the Brain,
    Diagnostic
Electroencephalogram, Diagnostic
Magnetic Resonance Imaging,
    Diagnostic
Magnetic Resonance Spectography,
    Diagnostic
Positron Emission Tomography,
    Diagnostic

ADDITIONAL CONDITIONS
Nausea
Personality Changes
Seizures

BRAIN DEATH
Autopsy, Diagnostic
Electroencephalogram, Diagnostic
Neurologic Examination, Diagnostic
pCO_2, Blood

ADDITIONAL CONDITIONS
Cerebral Hemorrhage
Multiple System Organ Failure
Trauma

BRAIN TUMORS
Brain Biopsy, Diagnostic
Carcinoembryonic Antigen, Serum
Cerebral Angiogram, Diagnostic
Cerebrospinal Fluid, Protein, Specimen
Cerebrospinal Fluid, Routine
    Analysis, Specimen
Computed Tomography of the Brain,
    Diagnostic
Doppler Ultrasound Flow Studies,
    Diagnostic

ADDITIONAL CONDITIONS
Epilepsy
Hallucinations
Nausea
Personality Changes
Seizures

Histopathology, Specimen
Homovanillic Acid, 24-Hour, Urine
Ki-67, Antigen, Blood
Magnetic Resonance Imaging,
    Diagnostic
Metanephrines, Total, 24-Hour, Urine
Neurologic Examination, Diagnostic
Vanillylmandelic Acid, Urine

BREAST CANCER
Alanine Aminotransferase, Serum
Alkaline Phosphatase, Serum
Alpha-Fetoprotein, Blood
Breast Cysts and Abscesses, Specimen
CA 15–3, Serum
CA 50, Blood
Calcitonin, Plasma or Serum
Calcium, Total, Serum
Carcinoembryonic Antigen, Serum
Cathepsin D, Serum
DNA Ploidy, Specimen
Estradiol Receptor and Progesterone
    Receptor in Breast Cancer,
    Diagnostic
Follicle-Stimulating Hormone,
    Serum
HER-2-Neu Oncogene, Specimen
Ki-67 Proliferation Marker, Specimen
Liver Battery, Serum
Mammography, Diagnostic
Methotrexate, Serum
Mucin-Like Carcinoma-Associated
    Antigen, Blood
Progesterone Receptor Assay, Blood
Prolactin, Serum
Proliferation Marker MIB 1–3,
    Specimen
Stereotactic Breast Biopsy, Specimen

ADDITIONAL CONDITIONS
Chronic Mastitis
Fibrocystic Breast Disease
Gynecologic Cancer
Metastasis
Paget's Disease, Breast

BRONCHITIS, ACUTE OR CHRONIC
Bicarbonate, Serum
Blood Gases, Arterial, Blood
Blood Gases, Venous, Blood
Bronchial Aspirate, Fungus, Culture
Bronchial Aspirate, Routine
    (Anaerobic), Culture
Bronchoscopy, Diagnostic
Carbon Dioxide, Partial Pressure,
    Blood
Carbon Dioxide, Total Content, Blood
Chest X-Ray, Diagnostic
Chloride, Sweat, Specimen
Complete Blood Count, Blood
Low-Density Lipoprotein, Blood
Pulmonary Function Test, Diagnostic
Sputum, Routine, Culture
Theophylline, Blood

ADDITIONAL CONDITIONS
Allergies
Chemical Irritation
COPD
Upper Respiratory Infections

BRUCELLOSIS

Bone Marrow Aspiration Analysis,
  Specimen
Brucellosis Agglutinins, Blood
Brucellosis Skin Test, Diagnostic
Differential Leukocyte Count,
  Peripheral Blood
Liver Battery, Serum

ADDITIONAL CONDITIONS

Anemia
Fever
Lymphadenopathy
Pain in Joints
Splenomegaly

BUERGER'S DISEASE
(see Thromboangiitis Obliterans)

BUFFER SYSTEM
*(see Carbonic Acid Bicarbonate
System, Protein Buffer System,
Phosphate Buffer System, and
Respiratory Control of H⁺ Balance)*

BULIMAREXIA
(see Anorexia and Bulimia)

BULIMIA

Electrolyte, Blood
Glucose, Blood
Phenolphthalein Test, Diagnostic
Protein, Total, Serum

ADDITIONAL CONDITIONS

Alcoholism
Anxiety
Constipation
Dental Caries
Depression
Electrolyte Imbalance
Esophagitis
Malnutrition
Post-Traumatic Stress Disorder
Stress
Upper GI Bleeding

BURNS

Albumin, Serum
Albumin/Globulin Ratio, Serum
Blood Culture, Blood
Blood Gas, Arterial, Blood
Blood Urea Nitrogen/Creatinine
  Ratio, Blood
Complete Blood Count, Blood
Electrolyte, Blood or Urine
Hemoglobin, Plasma and Qualitative,
  Urine (Urine)
Occult Blood, Urine
Osmolality, Serum
Protein, Total, Serum
Wound Culture

ADDITIONAL CONDITIONS

Alcoholism
Chemical Irritant Exposure
Diabetes Mellitus
Dysrhythmias
Electrolyte Imbalance
High-Voltage Injury
Lightning Injury
Psychiatric Illness
Renal Failure
Respiratory Failure
Smoke Inhalation

BURSITIS

Body Fluid Analysis, Cell Count,
  Specimen
X-Ray, Diagnostic

ADDITIONAL CONDITIONS

Gout
Rheumatoid Arthritis

CABG
(see Coronary Artery Bypass Graft)

CACHEXIA
(see Kwashiorkor and Marasmus)

CALCULI
(see Renal Calculi or Biliary Calculi)

CANCER
*(see specific type of Cancer and
Ganglioneuroblastoma, Hodgkin's
Disease, Leukemia, Lymphoma,
Metastasis, Neuroblastoma, or
Wilm's Tumor)*

CANDIDIASIS
(see Thrush)

CANNABIS DRUG ABUSE
(see Drug Abuse)

CARBON MONOXIDE POISONING
Blood Gases, Arterial, Blood
Carbon Monoxide, Blood
Carboxyhemoglobin, Blood
Electrocardiogram, Diagnostic
Oximetry, Diagnostic

ADDITIONAL CONDITIONS
Coma
Hypoxia
Psychiatric Illness

CARBONIC ACID-BICARBONATE SYSTEM
Bicarbonate, Serum
Blood Gases, Arterial, Blood

ADDITIONAL CONDITIONS
Cardiac Failure
Diabetes Mellitus
Drug Overdose
Renal Failure
Shock

CARCINOMA
(see Cancer)

CARDIOGENIC SHOCK
(see Shock)

CARDIOMYOPATHY
Alanine Aminotransferase, Serum
Aspartate Aminotransferase, Serum
Cardiac Enzymes/Isoenzymes, Blood
Cardiac Output, Diagnostic
Cardiac Radiography, Diagnostic
Chest X-Ray, Diagnostic
Coronary Intravascular Ultrasound,
   Diagnostic
Creatine Kinase, Serum
Echocardiogram, Diagnostic
Electrocardiogram, Diagnostic

ADDITIONAL CONDITIONS
Congestive Heart Failure
Endocarditis
Familial Trait
Hypertension, Chronic
Inflammatory Processes
Neuromuscular Disease
Post Heart Transplant
Radiation
Valvular Regurgitation
Valvular Stenosis
Viral Infection

Electron Microscopy, Diagnostic
(for Cardiomyopathy)
Histopathology, Specimen
Hydroxybutyrate Dehydrogenase,
Blood
Lactate Dehydrogenase, Blood
Lactate Dehydrogenase Isoenzymes,
Blood
Transesophageal Sonogram,
Diagnostic
Viral Culture, Specimen

CARPAL TUNNEL SYNDROME

Electromyogram and Nerve
Conduction Studies, Diagnostic
4-Pyridoxic Acid, Urine
Nerve Conduction Studies,
Diagnostic

ADDITIONAL CONDITIONS

Alcoholism
Amyloidosis
Diabetes Mellitus
Hyperparathyroidism
Leukemia
Myxedema
Rheumatoid Arthritis
Sarcoidosis
Synovitis

CAT SCRATCH DISEASE

Biopsy, Site-Specific (Lymph Node),
Specimen
Differential Leukocyte Count,
Peripheral Blood
Rochalimaea henselae, Antibody,
Serum
Sedimentation Rate, Erythrocyte,
Blood
Skin Test for Hypersensitivity,
Diagnostic

ADDITIONAL CONDITIONS

Encephalitis
Lymphadenopathy

CATARACTS

Galactokinase, Blood

ADDITIONAL CONDITIONS

Congenital Abnormality
Diabetes Mellitus
Trauma

CELIAC SPRUE

Barium Enema, Diagnostic
Complete Blood Count, Blood
Fecal Fat, Quantitative, 72-Hour,
Stool
Sigmoidoscopy, Diagnostic

ADDITIONAL CONDITIONS

Enteritis
Gastric Fistula
Lymphoma
Whipple's Disease

CEREBRAL ANEURYSM

(see Aneurysm, Cerebral)

CEREBRAL ARTERIOVENOUS MALFORMATIONS

Magnetic Resonance Angiography,
Diagnostic

ADDITIONAL CONDITIONS

Congenital Disease
Lung Cancer
Polycythemia, Secondary

CEREBRAL INFARCTION
(see Cerebrovascular Accident)

CEREBRAL INFECTIONS
(see Encephalitis or Meningitis)

CEREBRAL PALSY
Chloride, Serum
Computed Tomography of the Brain,
    Diagnostic
Electroencephalogram, Diagnostic
Magnetic Resonance Imaging,
    Diagnostic
Neurologic Examination, Diagnostic
Potassium, Serum
Sodium, Plasma, Serum, or Urine

ADDITIONAL CONDITIONS
Anemia
Cerebrovascular Accident
Drug Abuse
Hyperbilirubinemia
Meningitis
Rubella
Toxemia
Toxoplasmosis

CEREBROVASCULAR ACCIDENT (CVA)
Brain Scan, Cerebral Flow and
    Pathology, Diagnostic
Carotid Doppler Ultrasound,
    Diagnostic
Cerebral Computed Tomography,
    Diagnostic
Cerebrospinal Fluid, Lactic Acid,
    Specimen
Cerebrospinal Fluid, Routine
    Analysis, Specimen
Doppler Ultrasound Flow Studies,
    Diagnostic
Magnetic Resonance Angiography,
    Diagnostic
Magnetic Resonance Imaging (of
    Brain), Diagnostic
Magnetic Resonance Spectography,
    Diagnostic
Partial Thromboplastin Time, Plasma
Platelet Count, Blood
Prothrombin Time and International
    Normalized Ratio, Serum

ADDITIONAL CONDITIONS
Arteriosclerotic Heart Disease
Brain Tumor
Cerebral Aneurysm
Emboli
Hypertension
Subdural Hemorrhage

CERVICAL CANCER
Cervical/Vaginal Cytology, Specimen
Colposcopy, Diagnostic
Conization of Cervix, Diagnostic
Ki-67 Proliferation Marker, Specimen
Pap Smear, Diagnostic
Urinary Gonadotropin Peptide, Urine

ADDITIONAL CONDITIONS
Dysmenorrhea
Herpes Virus

CERVICAL SPONDYLOSIS
Computed Tomography of Body
    (Spine), Diagnostic
Magnetic Resonance Imaging,
    Diagnostic
X-Ray (Cervical Discs of Spine),
    Diagnostic

ADDITIONAL CONDITIONS
Myelopathy
Trauma to Spine

CERVICITIS
Cervical/Vaginal Cytology, Specimen
Chlamydia Culture
Genital, *Neisseria gonorrhoeae,*
    Culture
Genital, Routine, Culture
Herpes Virus Antigen, Direct
    Fluorescent Antibody, Specimen
Histopathology, Specimen
Rapid Plasma Reagin Test, Blood
Trichomonas Preparation, Specimen
Urinary Gonadotropin Peptide,
    Urine
Venereal Disease Research Laboratory
    Test, Serum

ADDITIONAL CONDITIONS
Abortion
Gonorrhea
Herpes Virus

CHANCROID
Genital, Bacillus *Haemophilus
    ducreyi,* Culture

ADDITIONAL CONDITION
Adenitis

CHEST PAIN
*(see Angina, Myocardial Infarction,
Pleurisy, or Pneumonia)*

CHICKENPOX
Differential Leukocyte Count,
    Peripheral Blood
Varicella-Zoster Virus Serology,
    Serum

ADDITIONAL CONDITIONS
Herpes Zoster
Leukopenia

CHLAMYDIA
Cervical/Vaginal Cytology,
    Specimen
Chlamydia Culture
Chlamydia Group Titer (Tachoma
    Titer), Serum
Lymphogranuloma Venereum Titer,
    Blood
Ocular Cytology, Specimen
Psittacosis Titer, Blood

ADDITIONAL CONDITIONS
Keratoconjunctivitis
Lymphogranuloma venereum
Pneumonia
Proctitis
Vaginitis

CHOLECYSTITIS
Amylase, Serum and Urine
Bile, Urine
Bilirubin, Urine
Endoscopic Retrograde
    Cholangiopancreatography,
    Diagnostic
Gallbladder and Biliary System
    Sonogram, Diagnostic
Gamma-Glutamyl-Transpeptidase,
    Blood
Glucose, Blood
Histopathology, Specimen
Ornithine Carbamoyltransferase,
    Blood

ADDITIONAL CONDITIONS
Gallstones
Pancreatitis

CHOLELITHIASIS

Bile Fluid Examination, Diagnostic
Bile, Urine
Chemistry Profile, Blood
Chorionic Villi Sampling, Diagnostic
Endoscopic Retrograde
    Cholangiopancreatography,
    Diagnostic
Gallbladder and Biliary System
    Sonogram, Diagnostic
Histopathology, Specimen
Leucine Aminopeptidase, Blood
T-tube Cholangiography
    (Postoperative), Diagnostic

CHRONIC OBSTRUCTIVE PULMONARY DISEASES

(see Asthma, Bronchitis, or Emphysema)

CIRRHOSIS

Alanine Aminotransferase, Serum
Albumin, Serum, Urine, and 24-Hour
    Urine
Albumin/Globulin Ratio, Serum
Aldosterone, Serum and Urine
Alkaline Phosphatase, Heat Stable,
    Serum
Alkaline Phosphatase Isoenzymes,
    Serum
Alkaline Phosphatase, Serum
Alpha$_1$-Antitrypsin, Serum
Ammonia, Blood
Antimitochondrial Antibody, Blood
Antinuclear Antibody, Serum
Anti-Smooth Muscle Antibody,
    Serum
Antithrombin III Test, Diagnostic
Aspartate Aminotransferase, Serum
Bilirubin, Direct, Serum
Ceruloplasmin, Serum
Chemistry Profile, Blood
Cold Agglutinin Titer, Serum
Copper, Serum
Copper, Urine
Cryoglobulin, Qualitative, Serum
Endoscopic Retrograde
    Cholangiopancreatography,
    Diagnostic
Gamma-Glutamyl Transpeptidase,
    Blood
Hepatitis B Surface Antibody, Blood
Hepatitis B Surface Antigen, Blood
Histopathology, Specimen
Immunoglobulin M, Serum
Iron, Serum
Lactate Dehydrogenase, Blood
Lactate Dehydrogenase Isoenzymes,
    Blood

ADDITIONAL CONDITIONS

Enteritis
Pregnancy

ADDITIONAL CONDITIONS

Alcoholism
Anasarca
Hepatitis
Jaundice
Osteomalacia
Pleural Effusion

Leucine Aminopeptidase, Blood
Liver Battery, Serum
Mixing Study (Circulating
 Anticoagulants), Plasma
Mucin-Like Carcinoma-Associated
 Antigen, Blood
5'-Nucleotidase, Blood
Ornithine Carbamoyltransferase,
 Blood
Prothrombin Time and International
 Normalized Ratio, Serum
Red Blood Cell Morphology, Blood
Sodium, Plasma, Serum, or Urine
Total Iron Binding Capacity, Serum
Transferrin, Serum
Urobilinogen, Urine
Zinc, Blood

CLAUDICATION
(see Venous Insufficiency)

COARCTATION OF THE AORTA
Blood Gases, Arterial, Blood
Cardiac Catheterization,
 Diagnostic
Chest X-Ray, Diagnostic
Echocardiogram, Diagnostic
Electrocardiogram, Diagnostic

ADDITIONAL CONDITIONS
Dizziness
Endocarditis
Epistaxis
Hypertension

COCCIDIOIDOMYCOSIS
Abscess, Anaerobic Culture
Biopsy, Site-Specific (Lymph Node),
 Specimen
Blood Culture, Blood
Bone Scan, Diagnostic
Chest X-Ray, Diagnostic
Eosinophil Count, Blood
Sedimentation Rate, Erythrocyte,
 Blood

ADDITIONAL CONDITIONS
Cervical Adenopathy
Fever
Friction Rub
Pleural Effusion

COCCIDIOSIS
Acquired Immune Deficiency
 Syndrome Evaluation Battery,
 Diagnostic
Biopsy, Site-Specific (Duodenum),
 Specimen
Stool Culture, Routine, Stool

ADDITIONAL CONDITION
AIDS

COLD, COMMON
(see also Rhinitis)
Complete Blood Count, Blood
Viral Culture, Specimen

ADDITIONAL CONDITIONS
Allergic Response
Diarrhea
Enteritis
Fever
Sinusitis

COLITIS
(see Ulcerative Colitis)

COLLAGEN DISEASES
(see Arthritis, Autoimmune Diseases, Rheumatoid Arthritis, Scleroderma, Sjögren's Syndrome, and Systemic Lupus Erythematosus)

COLON CANCER
Brushing Cytology, Specimen, Diagnostic
CA 50, Blood
Carcinoembryonic Antigen, Serum
Colorectal Cancer Allelotyping for Chromosome 17p and 18q, Specimen and Blood
Histopathology, Specimen
Ki-67 Proliferation Marker, Specimen
Occult Blood, Stool
Sedimentation Rate, Erythrocyte, Blood

ADDITIONAL CONDITIONS
Anemia
Ascites
Hypoalbuminemia
Hypokalemia
Low-Fiber Diet
Rectal Bleeding

COLOSTOMY
(see Ostomies)

CONDYLOMA LATUM
Condyloma Latum, Vulvar or Anal Culture for Cytology, Specimen

ADDITIONAL CONDITION
Syphilis

CONGENITAL HEART DISEASE
Magnetic Resonance Angiography, Diagnostic
Magnetic Resonance Imaging, Diagnostic
Mean Platelet Volume, Blood

ADDITIONAL CONDITIONS
Bacterial Endocarditis
Carcinoid Syndrome
Marfan's Syndrome
Rheumatic Valvular Disease
Syphilis

CONGESTIVE HEART FAILURE
Alanine Aminotransferase, Serum
Albumin, Serum, Urine, and 24-Hour Urine
Aspartate Aminotransferase, Serum
Atrial Natriuretic Hormone, Blood
Body Fluid Analysis, Cell Count, Specimen
Cardiac Enzymes/Isoenzymes, Blood
Chemistry Profile, Blood
Chest X-Ray, Diagnostic
Complete Blood Count, Blood
Creatine Kinase, Serum
Creatine Kinase, Isoenzymes, Serum
Digitoxin, Serum
Digoxin, Serum
Disopyramide Phosphate, Serum
Echocardiography, Diagnostic
Electrocardiogram, Diagnostic
Electrolyte, Blood or Urine
Gamma-Glutamyl Transpeptidase, Blood

ADDITIONAL CONDITIONS
Aortic Dissection
Ascites
Cardiac Disease
Dysrhythmias
Edema
Electrolyte Imbalance
Hepatomegaly
Hypercholesterolemia
Hyperglycemia
Hypocholesterolemia
Hypomagnesemia
Jaundice
Myocardial Infarction
Myocarditis
Pleural Effusion
Pulmonary Hypertension
Renal Disease
Rheumatic Heart Disease
Systemic Hypertension
Valvular Dysfunction

Heart Scan, Diagnostic
Lactate Dehydrogenase Isoenzymes,
    Blood
Lidocaine, Serum
Osmolality, Serum
Osmolality, Urine
Positron Emission Tomography,
    Diagnostic
Procainamide, Serum
Propranolol, Blood
Protein, Quantitative, Urine
Sedimentation Rate, Erythrocyte,
    Blood
Sodium, Plasma or Serum
Thyroid Profile, Blood
Transesophageal Sonogram, Diagnostic
Urea Nitrogen, Plasma or Serum

CONJUNCTIVITIS
Adenovirus Immunofluorescence,
    Diagnostic
Chlamydia Culture
Conjunctival, Fungus, Culture
Conjunctival, Routine, Culture
Ocular Cytology, Specimen
Periodic Acid Schiff, Specimen
Sjögren's Antibodies, Blood

ADDITIONAL CONDITIONS
Allergies
Rheumatoid Arthritis
Sjögren's Syndrome

CONSTRICTIVE PERICARDITIS
(see Pericarditis)

CONVULSIONS
(see Seizures)

COPD
(see Asthma, Bronchitis, or Emphysema)

CORONARY ARTERY BYPASS GRAFT (CABG)
Activated Coagulation Time,
    Automated, Blood
Blood Gases, Arterial, Blood
Cardiac Catheterization, Diagnostic
Cardiac Output, Diagnostic
Coronary Intravascular Ultrasound,
    Diagnostic

ADDITIONAL CONDITIONS
Angina
Coronary Artery Disease

CORONARY ARTERY DISEASE
(see Arteriosclerosis)

COUGH
Chest X-Ray, Diagnostic
Sputum Acid-Fast Bacteria, Culture

ADDITIONAL CONDITIONS
ACE-Inhibitor Therapy
Allergies

Sputum Culture and Sensitivity,
   Specimen
Sputum, Gram Stain, Diagnostic

Anticholinergic Therapy
ARDS
COPD
Industrial-Related Diseases
Lung Cancer
Pneumonia

CRETINISM
(see Hypothyroidism)

CROHN'S DISEASE
Albumin, Serum, Urine, and 24-Hour
   Urine
Chemistry Profile, Blood
Complete Blood Count, Blood
C-Reactive Protein, Serum
Cytologic Study of the
   Gastrointestinal Tract, Diagnostic
Fecal Fat, Quantitative, 72-Hour,
   Stool
Histopathology, Specimen
KUB, Diagnostic
Methylene Blue Stain, Stool
Muramidase, Serum and 24-Hour,
   Urine
Occult Blood, Stool
Oxalate, 24-Hour, Urine
Sedimentation Rate, Erythrocyte,
   Blood
Small Bowel Series, Diagnostic
Yersinia enterocolitica Antibody,
   Blood

ADDITIONAL CONDITIONS
Appendicitis
Anal/Rectal Fistula or Abscess
Ankylosing Spondylitis
Granuloma
Malnutrition
Polyarthritis
Seizures
Stress

CUSHING'S SYNDROME
Adrenocorticotropic Hormone, Serum
Aldosterone, Serum and Urine
Androstenedione, Serum
Calcitonin, Plasma or Serum
Calcium, Urine
Chemistry Profile, Blood
Chloride, Urine
Complete Blood Count, Blood
Computed Tomography of the Body
   (Kidney), Diagnostic
Cortisol, Plasma or Serum
Cortisol, Urine
Differential Leukocyte Count,
   Peripheral Blood
Electrolyte, Blood or Urine
Glucose, Blood
Glucose Tolerance Test, Blood
Histopathology, Specimen
17-Hydroxycorticosteroids, 24-Hour,
   Urine
17-Ketogenic Steroids, 24-Hour,
   Urine
17-Ketosteroid Fractionation, 24-
   Hour, Urine

ADDITIONAL CONDITIONS
ACTH-Secreting Adenoma
Adrenal Hyperplasia
Adrenal Tumor
Amenorrhea
Hyperglycemia
Hypertension
Hypothalamus Lesion
Impotence
Nephrolithiasis
Osteoporosis
Ovarian Cancer
Virilization

17-Ketosteroids, Total, 24-Hour, Urine
Low-Density Lipoprotein, Blood
Metyrapone Test, Serum
Metyrapone, 24-Hour, Urine
Magnetic Resonance Imaging,
    Diagnostic
Renin, Plasma
Sodium, Serum or Plasma
Testosterone, Total, Blood

CVA
(see Cerebrovascular Accident)

CYANOSIS
Bicarbonate, Serum
Blood Gases, Capillary, Blood
Blood Gases, Venous, Blood
Carbon Dioxide, Partial Pressure,
    Blood
Carbon Dioxide, Total Content, Blood
Carboxyhemoglobin, Blood
Glucose, Blood
Heavy Metals, Blood and 24-Hour,
    Urine (Urine)
5-Hydroxyindoleacetic Acid,
    Quantitative, 24-Hour, Urine
Methemoglobin, Blood
Serotonin, Plasma

ADDITIONAL CONDITIONS
Anemia
Cardiac Diseases
Peripheral Vascular Disease
Polycythemia
Pulmonary Diseases

CYSTECTOMY
Chemistry Profile, Blood
Complete Blood Count, Blood
Type and Crossmatch, Blood
Urinalysis, Urine

ADDITIONAL CONDITIONS
Cholecystitis
Urinary Carcinoma

CYSTIC FIBROSIS
Albumin, Serum, Urine, and 24-Hour
    Urine
Chloride, Sweat, Specimen
Chest X-Ray, Diagnostic
d-Xylose Absorption Test, Diagnostic,
    Serum or Urine
Electrolyte, Blood
Fat, Semiquantitative, Stool
Liver Battery, Serum
Pulmonary Function Test, Diagnostic
Semen Analysis, Specimen
Sputum for *Haemophilus* Species,
    Culture
Sputum, Routine, Culture
Trypsin, Plasma or Serum
Trypsin, Stool
Vitamin E_1, Serum

ADDITIONAL CONDITIONS
Atelectasis
Azoospermia
Biliary Cirrhosis
Cholelithiasis
COPD
Cor pulmonale
Hemoptysis
Intussusception
Pancreatitis
Pneumonia
Pneumothorax
Steatorrhea

CYSTITIS
Gram Stain, Diagnostic (Urine)
Histopathology, Specimen

ADDITIONAL CONDITIONS
Cervicitis
Cyclophosphamide Medication

Nitrite, Bacteria Screen, Urine
Occult Blood, Urine
Urinalysis, Urine
Urinalysis, Fractional, Urine
Urine Anaerobic Culture, Suprapubic
    Puncture, Culture
Urine Culture, Routine, Catheterized,
    Urine
Urine Culture, Routine, Clean-Catch,
    Urine
Urine Culture, Routine, Suprapubic
    Puncture, Urine
Urine Cytology, Urine
Urine, Fungus, Culture

Pregnancy
Pyelonephritis
Urinary Tract Infection
Vaginitis

CYTOMEGALIC INCLUSION DISEASE
(see Cytomegalovirus)

CYTOMEGALOVIRUS

Acquired Immune Deficiency Syndrome
    Evaluation Battery, Diagnostic
Blood Indices, Blood
Brushing Cytology, Specimen,
    Diagnostic
Chemistry Profile, Blood
Complete Blood Count, Blood
Cytomegalic Inclusion Disease,
    Cytology, Urine
Cytomegalovirus Antibody, Serum
Differential Leukocyte Count,
    Peripheral Blood
Heterophile Agglutinins, Blood
Histopathology, Specimen
Infectious Mononucleosis Screening
    Test, Blood
Red Cell Count, Serum
Sputum Cytology, Specimen
Toxoplasmosis, Rubella,
    Cytomegalovirus, Herpes Virus
    Serology (TORCH), Blood
Urine Culture, Routine or Clean-
    Catch, Urine
Urine Cytology, Urine

ADDITIONAL CONDITIONS

AIDS
Immunocompromised Persons
Liver Dysfunction
Massive Blood Transfusions
Pneumonia

DEAFNESS
(see Hearing Disorders)

DECUBITI

Biopsy, Anaerobic, Culture
Biopsy, Routine, Culture
Wound Culture

ADDITIONAL CONDITIONS

Chronic Bedrest
Malnutrition
Paralysis

DEEP VEIN THROMBOSIS (DVT)

Antithrombin III Test, Diagnostic
Arteriogram, Diagnostic

ADDITIONAL CONDITIONS

Atherosclerosis
Chronic Bedrest
Postoperative

D-Dimer Test, Plasma
Doppler, Duplex, Doppler, Ultrasound,
   Diagnostic
Doppler Ultrasound Flow Studies,
   Diagnostic
I-125-Labeled Fibrinogen Leg Scan,
   Diagnostic
Partial Thromboplastin Time, Plasma
Plasminogen Assay, Blood
Prothrombin Time and International
   Normalized Ratio, Serum
Venography (Phlebography),
   Diagnostic

DEGENERATIVE ARTHRITIS
(see Cervical Spondylosis)

DEGENERATIVE DISORDERS OF NERVOUS SYSTEM
(see Alzheimer's Disease)

DEGENERATIVE JOINT DISEASE
(see Arthritis, Osteo)

DEHYDRATION
(see Hypovolemia)

DELIRIUM TREMENS
Alcohol, Blood
Magnesium, Serum
Potassium, Serum

ADDITIONAL CONDITIONS
Alcoholism
Convulsions
Drug Abuse

DEMENTIA
Brain Scan, Cerebral Flow and
   Pathology, Diagnostic
Chest X-Ray, Diagnostic
Computed Tomography of the Brain,
   Diagnostic
Electroencephalogram, Diagnostic
Magnetic Resonance Imaging,
   Diagnostic
Thyroid Profile, Blood
Vitamin B_1, Serum or Urine
Vitamin B_{12}, Serum

ADDITIONAL CONDITIONS
AIDS
Alzheimer's Disease
Cerebrovascular Accident
Hypothyroidism
Organic Brain Syndrome

DEMYELINIZATION
(see Multiple Sclerosis)

DENGUE FEVER
Differential Leukocyte Count,
   Peripheral Blood
Immune Complex Assay, Blood

ADDITIONAL CONDITIONS
Fever
Headache
Leukopenia
Rash

DEPRESSANT DRUG ABUSE
*(see Drug Abuse: Barbiturates,
Chloral Hydrate, Meprobamate,
Methaqualone)*

DEPRESSION
Chromosome Analysis, Blood
Cortisol, Plasma or Serum
Dexamethasone Suppression Test,
   Diagnostic
Electroencephalogram, Diagnostic

ADDITIONAL CONDITIONS
Alzheimer's Disease
Anxiety
Chronic Illness
Dementia
Insomnia
Schizophrenia

DERMATITIS
Allergen-Specific IgE, Serum
Antinuclear Antibody, Serum
Chromium, Serum
Complete Blood Count, Blood
Differential Leukocyte Count,
   Peripheral Blood
Eosinophil Count, Blood
Heavy Metals, Blood and 24-Hour,
   Urine (Urine)
Histopathology, Specimen
Immunoglobulin E, Serum
Potassium Hydroxide Preparation,
   Serum
Porphyrins, Quantitative, Blood
Skin Fungus Culture

ADDITIONAL CONDITIONS
Allergic Reactions
Arthropod Bite
Athlete's Foot
Eczema
Herpes Simplex or Zoster
Impetigo
Kaposi's Sarcoma
Malignant Melanoma
Pemphigus
Pruritus
Psoriasis
Rash
Seborrhea
Skin Cancer
Systemic Lupus Erythematosus
   (SLE)
Tinea Capitis
Tinea Cruris

DIABETES GESTATIONAL
Glucose Tolerance Test, Blood

ADDITIONAL CONDITIONS
Pregnancy

DIABETES INSIPIDUS
Antidiuretic Hormone, Serum
Chloride, Sweat, Specimen
Concentration Test, Urine
Cyclic Adenosine Monophosphate,
   Serum and Urine
Electrolyte, Blood or Urine
Osmolality, Serum
Osmolality, Urine
Sodium, Plasma, Serum, or
   Urine
Specific Gravity, Urine

ADDITIONAL CONDITIONS
Amyloidosis, Renal
Breast Cancer
Encephalitis
Hand-Schuller-Christian Disease
Lung Cancer
Pyelonephritis
Sickle Cell Anemia
Sjögren's Syndrome
Syphilis
Tuberculosis

DIABETES MELLITUS
Anion Gap, Blood
Chemistry Profile, Blood
Complete Blood Count, Blood
C-Peptide, Serum
Creatinine Clearance, Serum, Urine
Differential Leukocyte Count,
   Peripheral Blood

ADDITIONAL CONDITIONS
Addison's Disease
Atherosclerosis
Cancer
Cushing's Syndrome
Fanconi's Syndrome
Gangrene
Glucagonoma

Electrolyte, Blood or Urine
Fructosamine, Serum
Glucagon, Plasma
Glucose, Blood
Glucose Monitoring Machines,
    Diagnostic
Glucose, Qualitative,
    Semiquantitative, Urine
Glucose, Quantitative, 24-Hour, Urine
Glucose Tolerance Test, Blood
Glucose, 2-Hour Postprandial, Serum
Glycosylated Hemoglobin, Blood
Insulin Assay (RIA), Blood
Ketone Bodies, Blood
Ketone, Semiquantitative, Urine
Lactic Acid, Blood
Lipid Profile, Blood
Magnesium, Serum
Magnetic Resonance Spectography,
    Diagnostic
Mean Platelet Volume, Blood
Osmolality, Urine
pH, Blood
Phosphorus, Serum
Potassium, Serum
Protein Electrophoresis, Serum
4-Pyridoxic Acid, Urine
Red Cell Count, Serum
Tissue Typing (HLA-B8), Blood
Triglycerides, Blood
Urinalysis, Urine
Urine Culture, Routine, Catheterized,
    Urine
Urine Culture, Routine, Clean-Catch,
    Urine
Urine, Fungus, Culture

Hemochromatosis
Human Leukocyte Antigen DR_3 or
    DR_4
Liver Disease
Obesity
Phenytoin Medication
Pheochromocytoma
Pregnancy
Stress
Thiazide Diuretic Medications
Thyrotoxicosis

DIABETIC GLOMERULOSCLEROSIS

Creatinine Clearance, Serum, Urine
Creatinine, Serum
Kidney Biopsy, Specimen
Protein, Quantitative, Urine
Urea Nitrogen, Plasma or Serum

ADDITIONAL CONDITIONS

Atherosclerosis
Diabetes Insipidus
Diabetes Mellitus
Scleroderma

DIABETIC KETOACIDOSIS (DKA)

Blood Gases (pH), Arterial, Blood
Glucose, Serum
Osmolality, Serum
Phosphate, Serum
Potassium, Serum
Urea Nitrogen, Blood

ADDITIONAL CONDITIONS

Acute Illness
Infection
Steroid Usage
Stress
Type I Diabetes
Trauma

DIALYSIS, HEMO

Activated Coagulation Time,
    Automated, Blood
Complete Blood Count, Blood

ADDITIONAL CONDITIONS

Diabetes Mellitus
Heart Failure
Hypercalcemia

Creatinine, Serum
Electrolyte, Blood
Lee-White Clotting Time, Blood
Parathyroid Hormone, Blood
Partial Thromboplastin Time, Serum
Urea Nitrogen, Plasma or Serum

Multiple Myeloma
Nephrosis
Poisoning
Renal Failure
Systemic Lupus Erythematosus (SLE)
Uremia

DIALYSIS, PERITONEAL

Complete Blood Count, Blood
Creatinine, Serum
Electrolyte, Blood
4-Pyridoxic Acid, Urine
Urea Nitrogen, Plasma or Serum

ADDITIONAL CONDITIONS

Diabetes Mellitus
Heart Failure
Hypercalcemia
Multiple Myeloma
Nephrosis
Poisoning
Renal Failure
Systemic Lupus Erythematosus (SLE)
Uremia

DIARRHEA

Albumin, Serum, Urine, and 24-Hour
    Urine
Carotene, Serum
Chemistry Profile, Blood
Clostridial Toxin, Serum
Clostridium difficile Toxin Assay, Stool
Cortisol, Plasma or Serum
Cryptosporidium Diagnostic
    Procedures, Stool
d-Xylose Absorption Test, Diagnostic,
    Serum or Urine
Electrolyte (CO_2, Cl, K, Na), Blood
Entamoeba histolytica Serological
    Test, Blood
Fat, Semiquantitative, Stool
Fecal Fat, Quantitative, 72-Hour, Stool
Fecal Leukocytes, Stool, Diagnostic
Gastrin, Serum
Glucagon, Plasma
Glucose, 2-Hour Postprandial, Serum
Histopathology, Specimen
Homovanillic Acid, 24-Hour, Urine
5-Hydroxyindoleacetic Acid,
    Quantitative, 24-Hour, Urine
Magnesium, Serum
Methylene Blue Stain, Stool
Milk Precipitins, Blood
Mycoplasma Titer, Blood
Occult Blood, Stool
Osmolality, Serum
Osmolality, Urine
Ova and Parasites, Stool
Phenolphthalein Test, Diagnostic
pH, Stool
Reducing Substances, Stool
Rotavirus Antigen, Stool
Schilling Test, Diagnostic
Serotonin (5-Hydroxytryptamine), Plasma
Specific Gravity, Urine
Stool Culture, Routine, Stool

ADDITIONAL CONDITIONS

AIDS
Anorexia Nervosa
Botulism
Bulimia
Chlamydia
Cholera
Colitis
Colon Cancer
Crohn's Disease
Cytomegalovirus
Diabetes Mellitus
Diverticulitis
Diverticulosis
Gastroenteritis
Giardiasis
Hepatitis
Hyperthyroidism
IgA Deficiency
Kwashiorkor
Malabsorption
Marasmus
Metabolic Acidosis
Neisseria gonorrhoeae
Toxic Shock Syndrome
Transplant Rejection
Traveler's Diarrhea
Tube Feeding

Thyroid Profile, Blood
Vasoactive Intestinal Polypeptide,
  Blood
Yersinia enterocolitica Antibody, Blood

DIC
*(see Disseminated Intravascular
Coagulation)*

DIPHTHERIA
Throat Culture for *Corynebacterium
  diphtheriae,* Culture

ADDITIONAL CONDITIONS
Myocarditis
Neuritis
Proteinuria

DISACCHARIDE
DEFICIENCIES
d-Xylose Absorption Test,
  Diagnostic,Serum or Urine
pH, Stool
Reducing Substances, Stool
Rotavirus Antigen, Stool

ADDITIONAL CONDITIONS
Celiac Disease
Colitis
Cystic Fibrosis
Diarrhea
Giardiasis

DISCOID LUPUS
ERYTHEMATOSUS
*(see Systemic Lupus Erythematosus:
[SLE])*

DISSEMINATED
INTRAVASCULAR
COAGULATION (DIC)
Activated Coagulation Time,
  Automated, Blood
Antithrombin III Test, Diagnostic
C3 Proactivator, Serum
Clot Retraction, Serum
D-Dimer Test, Blood
Diluted Whole Blood Clot Lysis, Blood
Euglobulin Clot Lysis, Blood
Fibrin Breakdown Products, Blood
Fibrin Split Products, Protamine
  Sulfate Test, Blood
Fibrinogen, Plasma
Intravascular Coagulation Screen, Blood
Mixing Study (Circulating
  Anticoagulants), Plasma
Partial Thromboplastin Time, Plasma
Plasminogen Assay, Blood
Platelet Count, Blood
Prothrombin Time and International
  Normalized Ratio, Serum
Red Blood Cell Morphology, Blood
Thrombin Time, Serum

ADDITIONAL CONDITIONS
Abortion, Septic
Amniotic Fluid Embolus
Anaphylaxis
Antibiotic Therapy
Anticoagulant Therapy
Blood Transfusion Reaction
Burns
Cancer
Head Injury (penetrating)
Hemophilia
Hypothermia
Liver Failure
Malnutrition
Obstetrical Complications
Renal Failure
Sepsis
Shock
Snake Venom
Thrombocytopenia
Thrombolytic Therapy
Trauma
Von Willebrand's Disease

DIVERTICULITIS
Barium Enema, Diagnostic
Blood Indices (Red Blood Cells), Blood
Complete Blood Count, Blood

ADDITIONAL CONDITIONS
Abscess
Bowel Obstruction
Constipation

Differential Leukocyte Count,
  Peripheral Blood
Histopathology, Specimen
Occult Blood, Stool
Red Cell Count, Serum
Sigmoidoscopy, Diagnostic

Diarrhea
Sepsis

DIVERTICULOSIS

Barium Enema, Diagnostic
Blood Indices (Red Blood Cells), Blood
Complete Blood Count, Blood
Differential Leukocyte Count,
  Peripheral Blood
Histopathology, Specimen
Occult Blood, Stool
Red Cell Count, Serum
Sigmoidoscopy, Diagnostic

ADDITIONAL CONDITIONS

Constipation
Fever
Fistula, Bladder

DOWN SYNDROME

Amniotic Fluid, Chromosome
  Analysis, Specimen
Chorionic Villi Sampling, Specimen
Chromosome Analysis (#21
  Chromosome), Blood
Pelvic X-Ray for Flat Ileum, Diagnostic
Urinary Gonadotropin Peptide, Urine

ADDITIONAL CONDITIONS

Mental Retardation

DRACUNCULIASIS

Culture, Skin, Specimen
Eosinophil Count, Blood
X-Ray, Diagnostic

ADDITIONAL CONDITIONS

Abscess
Pruritus
Tetanus

DROWNING, NEAR

Blood Gases, Arterial, Blood
Chest X-Ray, Diagnostic
Complete Blood Count, Blood
Computed Tomography of the Brain,
  Diagnostic
Drug Screen, Blood
Electroencephalogram, Diagnostic
Electrolyte, Blood
Toxicology, Drug Screen, Urine

ADDITIONAL CONDITIONS

Alcoholism
Anaphylaxis
Brain Death
Cyanosis
Drug Abuse
Myocardial Infarction
Pulmonary Edema
Spinal Cord Injury

DRUG ABUSE

(includes Cannabis, Depressants,
  Ethanol, Hallucinogenics,
  Narcotics, Stimulants)
Acetaminophen, Serum
Alcohol, Blood
Barbiturates, Quantitative, Blood
Blood Fungus, Culture
Cannabinoids (Marijuana, THC),
  Qualitative, Blood or Urine
Carbamazepine, Blood
Chlordiazepoxide, Blood
Clonazepam, Blood

ADDITIONAL CONDITIONS

AIDS
Alcoholism
Anxiety
Depression
Endocarditis
Insomnia
Malnutrition
Mitral Valve Prolapse
Rhabdomyolysis

Cocaine, Blood
Cytologic Study of the
    Gastrointestinal Tract, Diagnostic
Diazepam, Serum
Ethchlorvynol, Blood
Ethosuximide, Blood
Flurazepam, Serum
Fluorescent Treponemal Antibody-
    Absorbed Double-Stain Test, Serum
Glutethimide, Blood
Hepatitis B Surface Antigen, Blood
Lidocaine, Serum
Lithium, Serum
Liver Battery, Serum
Meprobamate, Blood
Methaqualone, Blood
Methotrexate, Serum
Methyprylon, Serum
Morphine, Urine
Phencyclidine, Qualitative, Urine
Phenobarbital, Plasma or Serum
Phenothiazines (Chlorpromazine,
    Compazine, Fluphenazine,
    Mellaril, Mesoridazine,
    Prochlorperazine, Prolixin,
    Serentil, Stelazine, Thorazine,
    Trifluoperazine), Blood
Phenytoin, Serum
Primidone, Serum
Propoxyphene, Blood
Rapid Plasma Reagin Test, Blood
Salicylate, Blood
Toxicology, Drug Screen, Blood and
    Urine
Toxicology, Volatiles Group by GLC,
    Blood or Urine
Tricyclic Antidepressants, Plasma or
    Serum

DRUG WITHDRAWAL
(see Drug Abuse)

DUCHENNE'S MUSCULAR DYSTROPHY
Aldolase, Serum
Aspartate Aminotransferase, Serum
Creatine Kinase, Serum
Creatine Kinase, Isoenzymes, Serum
Muscle Biopsy, Specimen

DUODENAL ULCER
(see also Helicobacter pylori)
ABO Group and Rh Type, Blood
Barium Swallow, Diagnostic
Complete Blood Count, Blood
Helicobacter pylori, Quick Office
    Serology, Serum and Titer,
    Blood

ADDITIONAL CONDITIONS
Dysrhythmias
Intellectual Retardation
Skeletal Deformity

ADDITIONAL CONDITIONS
Bowel Obstruction
Gastric Ulcer
Gastritis
Hemorrhage
Peptic Ulcer

Histopathology, Specimen
Upper Gastrointestinal Series,
    Diagnostic

DWARFISM
(see Hypopituitarism)

DYSENTERY

Entamoeba Histolytica, Serological
    Test, Blood
Methylene Blue Stain, Stool
Ova and Parasites, Stool
Parasite Screen, Stool
Stool Culture, Routine, Stool

ADDITIONAL CONDITIONS

Arthritis
Dehydration
Diarrhea
Fever

DYSERYTHROPOIETIC ANEMIA

Blood Indices (Red Blood Cells),
    Blood
Bone Marrow Biopsy, Diagnostic
Complete Blood Count, Blood
Differential Leukocyte Count,
    Peripheral Blood
Ham Test, Diagnostic
Red Blood Cell Morphology, Blood
Red Cell Count, Serum
Sucrose Hemolysis Test, Diagnostic

ADDITIONAL CONDITIONS

Hemoglobinuria
Leukopenia
Sepsis
Thrombocytopenia

DYSFIBRINOGENEMIA

Fibrin Split Products, Protamine
    Sulfate Test, Blood
Fibrinogen, Plasma
Partial Thromboplastin Time, Plasma
Prothrombin Time and International
    Normalized Ratio, Serum
Thrombin Time, Serum

ADDITIONAL CONDITIONS

Burns
Hypofibrinogenemia
Leukemia
Polycythemia Vera
Syphilis
Thrombocytopenia

DYSMENORRHEA

Complete Blood Count, Blood
Dilation and Curettage, Diagnostic
Estrogens, Serum and 24-Hour Urine
Iron, Serum
Laparoscopy, Diagnostic
Total Iron Binding Capacity, Serum
Urinalysis, Urine

ADDITIONAL CONDITIONS

Endometriosis
Ovarian Fibromas or Cysts
Pelvic Inflammatory Disease
Submucous Myoma

DYSPEPSIA

Gastric Analysis, Specimen
Gastric pH, Specimen

ADDITIONAL CONDITIONS

Gastritis
Hiatal Hernia
Myocardial Infarction
Ulcer

DYSPHAGIA

Acid Perfusion Test, Diagnostic
Esophageal Manometry, Diagnostic

ADDITIONAL CONDITIONS

Foreign Object Ingestion
Head and Neck Cancer

Laryngitis
Mucositis
Oral STD
Stomatitis

DYSPNEA

Bicarbonate, Serum
Blood Gases, Arterial, Blood
Carbon Monoxide, Blood
Carboxyhemoglobin, Blood
Chest X-Ray, Diagnostic
Complete Blood Count, Blood
Heavy Metals, Blood and 24-Hour
    Urine
Methemoglobin, Blood
pCO_2, Blood

ADDITIONAL CONDITIONS

Anxiety
Cardiac Disease
COPD
Obesity
Pulmonary Edema

DYSPROTEINEMIA

Blood Indices (Red Blood Cells),
    Blood
Bone Marrow Biopsy, Diagnostic
Chemistry Profile, Blood
Complete Blood Count, Blood
Differential Leukocyte Count,
    Peripheral Blood
Globulin, Serum
Immunoelectrophoresis, Serum and
    Urine
Immunoglobulin A, Serum
Immunoglobulin D, Serum
Immunoglobulin E, Serum
Immunoglobulin M, Serum
Platelet Aggregation, Blood; Platelet
    Aggregation, Hypercoagulable
    State, Blood
Platelet Count, Blood
Protein, Electrophoresis, Serum
Protein, Electrophoresis, Urine
Red Cell Count, Serum
Urinalysis, Urine
Viscosity, Serum

ADDITIONAL CONDITIONS

Epistaxis
GI Hemorrhage
Multiple Myeloma
Purpura
Waldenstrom's Macroglobulinemia

DYSRHYTHMIAS

Amiodarone, Plasma or Serum
Bicarbonate, Serum
Blood Gases, Arterial, Blood
Calcium, Total, Serum
Digitoxin, Serum
Digoxin, Serum
Disopyramide Phosphate, Serum
Echocardiogram, Diagnostic
Electrocardiogram, Diagnostic
Electrolyte, Blood
Electrophysiologic Study, Diagnostic
Flecainide, Plasma or Serum
Holter Monitor, Diagnostic
Lidocaine, Serum
Magnesium, Serum

ADDITIONAL CONDITIONS

Acid/Base Imbalance
Anemia
Anoxia
Anxiety
Cardiomyopathy
Cerebrovascular Accident
Chest Trauma
Congestive Heart Failure
COPD
Digitalis Toxicity
Drug Side Effects
Electrolyte Imbalances
Emboli
Hepatomegaly
Hypertension

pCO$_2$, Blood
Potassium, Serum
Procainamide, Serum
Propranolol, Blood
Quinidine, Serum
Signal-Averaged Electrocardiogram,
    Diagnostic

Hypoxia
Pacemaker Failure
Pericarditis
Pheochromocytoma
Quinidine Toxicity
Sepsis
Stress
Theophylline Toxicity
Thyroid Dysfunction
Trauma
Valvular Disease
Vertigo

DYSURIA

Chlamydia Culture
Cystoscopy, Diagnostic
Nitrite, Bacteria Screen, Urine
Occult Blood, Urine
Trichomonas Preparation, Specimen
Urinalysis, Urine
Urine Culture, Routine, Catheterized,
    Urine
Urine Culture, Routine, Clean-Catch,
    Urine

ADDITIONAL CONDITIONS

Bladder Infection
Prostate Infection
Urinary Tract Infection

ECCHYMOSIS (SPONTANEOUS)

Bleeding Time, Duke, Blood
Bleeding Time, Ivy, Blood
Capillary Fragility Test (In Vivo),
    Diagnostic
Factor VIII, Blood
Factor VIII R:Ag, Blood
Fibrin Breakdown Products, Blood
Fibrinogen, Plasma
Partial Thromboplastin Time,
    Plasma
Platelet Aggregation, Blood; Platelet
    Aggregation, Hypercoagulable
    State, Blood
Platelet Count, Blood
Prothrombin Time and International
    Normalized Ratio, Serum
Salicylate, Blood

ADDITIONAL CONDITIONS

Cancer
Chemotherapy Drug Usage
Disseminated Intravascular
    Coagulation (DIC)
Idiopathic Thrombocytopenic
    Purpura (ITP)
Leukemia

ECHINOCOCCOSIS

Bile Fluid Examination, Diagnostic
Cerebrospinal Fluid, Cytology
    Specimen
Echinococcosis Serological Test,
    Blood
Histopathology, Specimen

ADDITIONAL CONDITIONS

Cyst on the Liver
Jaundice
Shock

ECLAMPSIA (TOXEMIA)

Albumin, Serum, Urine, and 24-Hour
    Urine (24-Hour Urine)
D-Dimer Test, Blood

ADDITIONAL CONDITIONS

Collagen Disorder
Diabetes Mellitus
Hydatidiform Mole

Glucose, Qualitative and
    Semiquantitative, Urine
Hematocrit, Blood
Low-Density Lipoprotein, Blood
Protein, Quantitative, Urine
Sodium, Plasma, Serum, or Urine
Uric Acid, Serum

Hypertension
Multiple Pregnancy
Renal Failure

ECTOPIC HYPERPARATHYROIDISM

Calcium, Ionized, Blood
Calcium, Total, Serum
Calcium, Urine
Chemistry Profile, Blood
Parathyoid Hormone, Blood
Phosphorus, Serum
Phosphorus, Urine
Sputum Cytology, Specimen

ADDITIONAL CONDITIONS

Hypercalcemia
Hypophosphatemia
Nephrolithiasis
Renal Failure

ECTOPIC PREGNANCY

Histopathology, Specimen
Human Chorionic Gonadotropin,
    Beta Subunit, Serum
Pregnancy Test, Routine, Serum

ADDITIONAL CONDITIONS

Abortion
Amenorrhea
Appendicitis
Pain, Abdominal
Salpingitis
Shock
Urinary Tract Infection

ECZEMA

Allergen-Specific IgE Antibody, Serum
Eosinophil Count, Blood
Histopathology, Specimen
Immunoglobulin E, Serum

ADDITIONAL CONDITIONS

Allergic Rhinitis
Asthma
Cataracts
Pruritus

EDEMA

Albumin/Globulin Ratio, Serum
Chemistry Profile, Blood
Electrolyte, Blood
Magnetic Resonance Imaging,
    Diagnostic
Osmolality, Serum
Osmolality, Urine
Protein, Total, Serum

ADDITIONAL CONDITIONS

Cardiac Diseases
Cellulitis
Deep Vein Thrombosis
High-Altitude Living
Kwashiorkor
Pulmonary Disease

EFFUSIONS, ABDOMINAL

Body Fluid, Amylase, Specimen
Body Fluid, Anaerobic, Culture
Body Fluid, Glucose, Specimen
Body Fluid Analysis, Cell Count,
    Specimen
Body Fluid Cytology, Specimen
Gram Stain (Effusion Specimen),
    Diagnostic
KUB, Diagnostic
Paracentesis, Diagnostic
Sputum, Routine, Culture
Synovial Fluid Analysis, Diagnostic

ADDITIONAL CONDITIONS

Ascites
Empyema
Metastasis

EFFUSIONS, PERICARDIAL

Body Fluid Cytology, Specimen
Chest X-Ray, Diagnostic
Echocardiogram, Diagnostic
Electrocardiogram, Diagnostic
Pericardiocentesis, Diagnostic

ADDITIONAL CONDITIONS

AIDS
Cancer
Congestive Heart Failure
COPD
Tachycardia
Trauma

EFFUSIONS, PLEURAL

Blood Gases, Arterial, Blood
Body Fluid, Anaerobic, Culture
Body Fluid, Glucose, Specimen
Body Fluid Analysis, Cell Count,
    Specimen
Body Fluid Cytology, Specimen
Chest X-Ray, Diagnostic
Fluoroscopy, Diagnostic
Gram Stain (Effusion Specimen),
    Diagnostic
Sputum, Routine, Culture
Synovial Fluid Analysis, Diagnostic
Thoracentesis, Diagnostic

ADDITIONAL CONDITIONS

Ascites
Congestive Heart Failure
Empyema
Esophageal Perforation
Lung Cancer
Pulmonary Emboli
Tuberculosis

EMBOLECTOMY

*(see Fat Embolism or Pulmonary
Embolism)*

EMPHYSEMA

Alpha1-Antitrypsin, Serum
Bicarbonate, Serum
Blood Gases, Arterial, Blood
Carbon Dioxide Partial Pressure,
    Blood
Carbon Dioxide, Total Content, Blood
Chest X-Ray, Diagnostic
Digoxin, Serum
Electrolyte, Blood
Histopathology, Specimen
Low-Density Lipoprotein, Blood
Pulmonary Function Test, Diagnostic
Red Cell Mass, Blood
Sputum Cytology, Specimen
Theophylline, Blood

ADDITIONAL CONDITIONS

Asthma
Bronchitis
Cor pulmonale
Dyspnea
Pneumonia

EMPYEMA

Abscess, Anaerobic Culture
Blood Gases, Arterial, Blood
Body Fluid, Anaerobic, Culture
Body Fluid Cytology, Specimen
Body Fluid, Fungus, Culture
Body Fluid, *Mycobacteria,* Culture
Body Fluid, Routine, Culture
C-Reactive Protein, Serum
Chest X-Ray, Diagnostic
Gram Stain (Empyema Specimen),
    Diagnostic
Thoracentesis, Diagnostic

ADDITIONAL CONDITIONS

Acute Respiratory Distress Syndrome
COPD
Lung Abscess
Pleural Effusion
Pneumonia

ENCEPHALITIS

California Encephalitis Virus Titer, Serum
Cerebrospinal Fluid, Immunoglobulin G, Immunoglobulin G Ratios and Immunoglobulin G Index, Immunoglobulin G Synthesis Rate, Specimen
Cerebrospinal Fluid, Protein, Specimen
Cerebrospinal Fluid, Routine Analysis, Specimen
Eastern Equine Encephalitis Virus Titer, Specimen
Herpes Virus Antigen, Direct Fluorescent Antibody, Specimen
Rubeola Serology, Serum
St. Louis Encephalitis Virus Serology, Serum
Toxoplasmosis, Rubella, Cytomegalovirus, Herpes Virus Serology (TORCH), Blood
Toxoplasmosis Serology, Serum
Venezuelan Equine Encephalitis Virus Serology, Serum
Viral Culture, Specimen
Western Equine Encephalitis Virus Serology, Serum

ADDITIONAL CONDITIONS

Fever
Herpes Simplex Virus
Infectious Mononucleosis
Measles
Mumps
Poisoning
Polio
Rabies
Reye's Syndrome
Rubella
Sepsis
Vaccination-Induced

ENCEPHALOPATHY

Cerebral Angiography, Diagnostic
Computed Tomography of Brain, Diagnostic
Doppler Ultrasound, Diagnostic
Electroencephalogram, Diagnostic
Magnetic Resonance Imaging, Diagnostic

ADDITIONAL CONDITIONS

AIDS
Epilepsy
Hypertension
Liver Disease

ENDARTERECTOMY

(see Anesthesia, Preoperative)

ENDOCARDITIS

(see also Subacute Bacterial Endocarditis, SBE)
Anti-DNA, Serum
Antinuclear Antibody, Serum
Blood Culture, Blood
Blood Culture with Antimicrobial Removal Device, Culture
Blood Fungus, Culture
Blood Indices, Blood
C1q Immune Complex Detection, Serum
C3 Complement, Serum
C4 Complement, Serum
Cell Wall Defective Bacteria, Culture
Chemistry Profile, Blood

ADDITIONAL CONDITIONS

Abortion, Suction
Bacteremia
Coarctation of the Aorta
Drug Abuse, Intravenous
Myocarditis
Patent Ductus Arteriosus
Post Cardiac Surgery
Pulmonary Emboli
Rheumatic Fever
Tetralogy of Fallot
Valvular Heart Disease
Ventricular Septal Defect

Chest X-Ray, Diagnostic
Complement Total, Serum
Complete Blood Count, Blood
C-Reactive Protein, Serum
Differential Leukocyte Count,
    Peripheral Blood
Echocardiogram, Diagnostic
Electrocardiogram, Diagnostic
5-Hydroxyindoleacetic Acid,
    Quantitative, 24-Hour, Urine
Immune Complex Assay, Blood
Minimum Bactericidal
    Concentration, Culture
Red Cell Count, Serum
Rheumatoid Factor, Blood
Schlichter Test (Body Fluid),
    Specimen
Sedimentation Rate, Erythrocyte,
    Blood
Serotonin, Plasma
Teichoic Acid Antibody, Blood
Transesophogeal Sonogram,
    Diagnostic
Urinalysis, Urine

ENDOCRINE TUMORS
*(see also Addison's Disease, Cushing's
Syndrome, Hashimoto's Thyroiditis,
Hypothyroidism,
Hyperparathyroidism,
Hyperpituitarism, and
Hyperthyroidism)*
Immunoperoxidase Procedures,
    Diagnostic

ADDITIONAL CONDITIONS
Diabetes Mellitus
Ulcerative Colitis

ENDOMETRITIS (ENDOMETRIOSIS)
Abscess, Anaerobic Culture
CA-125, Blood
Chlamydia Culture
Endometrium, Anaerobic, Culture
Foreign Body, Routine, Culture
Genital, *Candida albicans,* Culture
Genital, *Neisseria gonorrhoeae,*
    Culture
Genital, Routine, Culture
Histopathology, Specimen
Laparoscopy, Diagnostic

ADDITIONAL CONDITIONS
Dysmenorrhea
Infertility
Ovarian Cancer
Pain, Acute
Salpingitis
Uterine Myomas

ENTERIC FEVER
Blood Culture, Blood
Methylene Blue Stain, Stool
Stool Culture, Routine, Stool

ADDITIONAL CONDITIONS
Diarrhea
Sepsis

EPIDIDYMITIS
Histopathology, Specimen

ADDITIONAL CONDITIONS
Pain, Acute
Urinary Tract Infection

EPIGLOTTITIS

Blood Culture, Blood
Nose, Routine, Culture
Penicillinase Test, Diagnostic
Sputum for *Haemophilus* Species,
  Culture
Throat Culture, Routine, Culture

ADDITIONAL CONDITIONS

Fever
Influenza B

EPILEPSY

Brain Scan, Cerebral Flow and
  Pathology, Diagnostic
Carbamazepine, Blood
Clonazepam, Blood
Computed Tomography of the Brain,
  Diagnostic
Diazepam, Serum
Electroencephalogram, Diagnostic
Ethosuximide, Blood
Magnetic Resonance Imaging,
  Diagnostic
Mephenytoin, Blood
Methsuximide, Serum
Phenobarbital, Plasma or Serum
Phenytoin, Serum
Primidone, Serum
Valproic Acid, Blood

ADDITIONAL CONDITIONS

Abscess, Brain
Alcoholism
Brain Tumor
Drug Abuse
Encephalitis, Herpes
Ganglioneuroblastoma
Meningitis
Neuroblastoma
Peripheral Vascular Disease
Phenylketonuria
Syphilis
Trauma

EPISTAXIS

Autoerythrocyte Sensitivity Test,
  Diagnostic
Bleeding Time, Duke, Blood
Bleeding Time, Ivy, Blood
Complete Blood Count, Blood
Hematocrit, Blood
Hemoglobin, Blood
Partial Thromboplastin Time,
  Plasma
Platelet Count, Blood
Red Blood Cell Morphology,
  Blood
Thrombin Time, Serum

ADDITIONAL CONDITIONS

Deviated Nasal Septum
Disseminated Intravascular
  Coagulation (DIC)
Leukemia
Rhinitis
Thrombocytopenia
Trauma

EPSTEIN-BARR VIRUS

Differential Leukocyte Count,
  Peripheral Blood
Epstein-Barr Virus, Serology,
  Blood
Heterophile Agglutinins, Blood
Infectious Mononucleosis Screening
  Test, Blood

ADDITIONAL CONDITIONS

Burkitt's Lymphoma
Encephalitis
Hepatitis
Infectious Mononucleosis
Myocarditis
Neuritis
Splenomegaly

ERYTHROBLASTOSIS FETALIS

ABO Group and Rh Type, Blood
Amniotic Fluid, Erythroblastosis
  Fetalis, Specimen

ADDITIONAL CONDITION

Pregnancy

ESOPHAGEAL ATRESIA WITH TRACHEOSEPTAL FISTULA

Blood Gases, Arterial, Blood
Flat Plate X-Ray of Abdomen,
   Diagnostic

ADDITIONAL CONDITIONS

Congenital Heart Disease
Cyanosis
Pneumonitis

ESOPHAGEAL VARICES

(see Varices)

ESOPHAGITIS

Biopsy, Fungus, Culture
Brushing Cytology, Specimen,
   Diagnostic
Esophageal Radiography, Diagnostic
Herpes Virus Antigen, Direct
   Fluorescent Antibody, Specimen
Histopathology, Specimen

ADDITIONAL CONDITIONS

AIDS
Candida albicans
Cytomegalovirus
Herpes Simplex
Hiatal Hernia
Nasogastric Tube Irritation
Obesity
Pregnancy
Raynaud's Phenomenon

ESOPHAGOSCOPY

Brushing Cytology, Specimen,
   Diagnostic
Histopathology, Specimen
Washing Cytology, Specimen

ADDITIONAL CONDITIONS

Esophageal Cancer
Esophagitis
Mallory-Weiss Syndrome
Throat Infection
Varices, Esophageal

ETHYLENE GLYCOL POISONING

Ethylene Glycol, Serum and Urine
Heavy Metals, Blood and 24-Hour
   Urine
Toxicology, Volatiles Group by GLC,
   Blood or Urine

ADDITIONAL CONDITIONS

Alcoholism
Depression

ETOH

(see Alcoholism and Drug Abuse)

FACTOR DEFICIENCY

Activated Partial Thromboplastin
   Substitution Test, Diagnostic
Coagulation Factor Assay, Blood
Factor II, Blood
Factor V, Blood
Factor VII, Blood
Factor VIII, Blood
Factor VIII R:Ag, Blood
Factor IX, Blood
Factor X, Blood
Factor XI, Blood
Factor XII, Blood
Factor XIII Blood
Factor, Fitzgerald, Plasma
Factor, Fletcher, Plasma
Fibrinogen, Plasma

ADDITIONAL CONDITIONS

Afibrinogenemia
Cancer
Disseminated Intravascular
   Coagulation (DIC)
Hemophilia
Vitamin K Deficiency

Mixing Study (Circulating
Anticoagulants), Plasma
Thrombin Time, Serum
von Willebrand Factor Assay, Blood

FACTOR IX DEFICIENCY (CHRISTMAS DISEASE)
Circulating Anticoagulant (CAC,
Lupus Anticoagulant), Blood
Coagulation Factor Assay, Blood
Factor XII, Blood
Mixing Study (Circulating
Anticoagulants), Plasma
Partial Thromboplastin Time, Plasma
Plasma Recalcification Time, Plasma

ADDITIONAL CONDITIONS
Hemorrhage
Thrombosis

FACTOR V DEFICIENCY
Mixing Study (Circulating
Anticoagulants), Plasma
Coagulation Factor Assay, Blood
Factor V, Blood

ADDITIONAL CONDITIONS
Hemorrhage
Thrombocytopenia

FACTOR XIII DEFICIENCY
Coagulation Factor Assay, Blood
Factor VIII, Blood
Factor VIII R:Ag, Blood
Mixing Study (Circulating
Anticoagulants), Plasma
Plasma Recalcification Time,
Plasma
von Willebrand Factor Assay, Blood

ADDITIONAL CONDITIONS
Cirrhosis
Hemorrhage

FAILURE TO THRIVE
Blood Gases, Arterial, Blood
Complete Blood Count, Blood
Creatinine, Serum
Fat, Semiquantitative, Stool
Growth Hormone, Blood
Ova and Parasites, Stool
Urea Nitrogen, Plasma or Serum
Urine, Culture and Sensitivity,
Urine

ADDITIONAL CONDITIONS
Alcohol Abuse During Pregnancy
Down Syndrome
Drug Abuse During Pregnancy
Galactosemia
Hypoxia

FANCONI SYNDROME
Alkaline Phosphatase, Serum
Blood Gases, Venous, Blood
Calcium, Urine
Chemistry Profile, Blood
Complete Blood Count, Blood
Electrolyte, Blood
Glucose, Semiquantitative, Urine
Ketone, Semiquantitative, Urine
pH, Urine
Phosphorus, Serum
Phosphorus, Urine
Protein, Quantitative, Urine
Uric Acid, Serum

ADDITIONAL CONDITIONS
Heavy Metal Poisoning
Osteomalacia
Renal Tubular Acidosis

FARMER'S LUNG
Chest X-Ray, Diagnostic
Hypersensitivity Pneumonitis
  Serology, Blood

ADDITIONAL CONDITIONS
Asthma
Bronchitis

FASCIOLIASIS
Differential Leukocyte Count,
  Peripheral Blood
Eosinophil Count, Blood
Liver Scan, Diagnostic

ADDITIONAL CONDITIONS
Fever
Hepatomegaly
Urticaria

FAT EMBOLISM
Bicarbonate, Serum
Blood Gases, Arterial, Blood
Carbon Dioxide, Partial Pressure,
  Blood
Carbon Dioxide, Total Content, Blood
Complete Blood Count, Blood
Fat, Urine
Lipase, Serum
Venography, Diagnostic

ADDITIONAL CONDITIONS
Anemia
Fractures, Long Bones
Thrombocytopenia

FATIGUE
*(see also Cancer, Infectious
Mononucleosis, Myasthenia Gravis,
and Systemic Lupus Erythematosus)*
Alcohol, Blood
Complete Blood Count, Blood
Liver Battery, Serum
Thyroid Profile, Blood

ADDITIONAL CONDITIONS
Anemia
Cancer
COPD
Fever of Undetermined Origin (FUO)
Hypothyroidism

FATTY LIVER
(see Liver Dysfunction)

FEBRILE DISEASES
(see Fever of Undetermined Origin)

FEMOROPOPLITEAL BYPASS GRAFT
(see Anesthesia)

FEVER OF UNDETERMINED ORIGIN (FUO)
Acid-Fast Stain, *Nocardia* Species,
  Culture
Anti-DNA, Serum
Antinuclear Antibody, Serum
Biopsy, *Mycobacteria,* Culture
Blood Culture, Blood
Blood Culture with Antimicrobial
  Removal Device, Culture
Bone Marrow Aspiration Analysis,
  Specimen
Cell Wall Defective Bacteria (Body
  Fluid), Culture

ADDITIONAL CONDITIONS
Cancer
Cat Scratch Disease
Chickenpox
Lyme Disease
Measles
Sepsis
Sinusitis
Tic Bite
Typhus
Urinary Tract Infection

C-Reactive Protein, Serum
Chest X-Ray, Diagnostic
Differential Leukocyte Count,
    Peripheral Blood
Histopathology, Specimen
Malaria Smear, Blood
Salmonella Titer, Blood
Sedimentation Rate, Erythrocyte,
    Blood
Urine Culture, Routine, Clean-Catch,
    Urine

FIBRINOLYSIS
D-Dimer Test, Blood
Euglobulin Clot Lysis, Blood
Fibrin Breakdown Products,
    Blood
Fibrinogen, Plasma
Intravascular Coagulation Screen,
    Blood
Plasminogen Assay, Blood

ADDITIONAL CONDITIONS
Cirrhosis
Disseminated Intravascular
    Coagulation (DIC)

FIBRINOPENIA
Cryofibrinogen, Serum
Fibrinogen, Plasma
Intravascular Coagulation Screen,
    Blood
Reptilase Time, Serum
Thrombin Time, Serum

ADDITIONAL CONDITIONS
Cirrhosis
Hemorrhage

FIBROCYSTIC BREAST
Estrogens, Serum and 24-Hour
    Urine
Histopathology, Specimen
Mammography, Diagnostic
Nipple Discharge Cytology,
    Specimen
Thermography, Diagnostic

ADDITIONAL CONDITIONS
Breast Cancer
Obesity
Pain, Acute

FOLIC ACID ANEMIA (FOLATE DEFICIENCY ANEMIA)
Blood Indices (Red Blood Cells),
    Blood
Bone Marrow Biopsy, Diagnostic
Differential Leukocyte Count,
    Peripheral Blood
Folic Acid, Red Blood Cell, Blood
Folic Acid, Serum
Lactate Dehydrogenase Isoenzymes,
    Blood
Platelet Count, Blood
Red Blood Cell Morphology
    (Megalocyte), Blood
Red Cell Count, Serum
Schilling Test, Diagnostic
Vitamin B_{12}, Serum

ADDITIONAL CONDITIONS
Alcoholism
Cachexia
Chronic Hemolytic Anemia
Dialysis
Exfoliative Skin Disease
Low-Fiber Diet
Pregnancy
Tropical Sprue

FORBES-ALBRIGHT SYNDROME
Prolactin, Serum

ADDITIONAL CONDITIONS
Amenorrhea
Galactorrhea
Hypogonadism
Impotence
Oligomenorrhea
Pituitary Tumor

FRACTURES
Bone X-Ray, Diagnostic
Complete Blood Count, Blood
Fat, Urine
Tomography, Diagnostic

ADDITIONAL CONDITIONS
Alcoholism
Drug Abuse
Metastasis

FUNGAL INFECTIONS
Amphotericin B, Blood
Biopsy, Fungus, Culture
Blood Fungus, Culture
Bronchial Aspirate, Fungus, Culture
Cerebrospinal Fluid, Fungus, Culture
Conjunctival, Fungus, Culture
Fungal Antibody Screen, Blood
Genital, *Candida albicans,* Culture
Genital, Routine, Culture
India Ink Preparation, Specimen
Periodic Acid Schiff, Specimen
Potassium Hydroxide Preparation,
    Serum
Skin Fungus, Culture
Sputum, Fungus, Culture
Stool Fungus Culture
Urine, Fungus, Culture
Wound, Fungus, Culture

ADDITIONAL CONDITIONS
AIDS
Cancer
Candidiasis (Thrush)
Conjunctivitis
Post Transplant

FUO
(see Fever of Undetermined Origin)

G-6-PD DEFICIENCY (GLUCOSE-6-PHOSPHATE DEHYDROGENASE)
Blood Indices (Red Blood Cells), Blood
Complete Blood Count, Blood
Differential Leukocyte Count,
    Peripheral Blood
Glucose-6-Phosphate Dehydrogenase,
    Quantitative, Blood
Glucose-6-Phosphate Dehydrogenase
    Screen, Blood
Haptoglobin, Serum
Red Cell Count, Serum
Reticulocyte Count, Blood

ADDITIONAL CONDITIONS
Anemia
Jaundice
Splenomegaly

G-CELL HYPERPLASIA
Gastrin, Serum
Histopathology, Specimen
Immunoperoxidase Procedures,
    Diagnostic
Pepsinogen-1 Antibody, Blood

ADDITIONAL CONDITIONS
Stomach Cancer
Ulcers

GALACTOKINASE DEFICIENCY

Galactose, Screening Test for
Galactosemia, Urine

ADDITIONAL CONDITIONS

Cataracts

GALACTORRHEA

Nipple Discharge Cytology, Specimen
Prolactin, Serum

ADDITIONAL CONDITIONS

Acromegaly
Myxedema
Thyrotoxicosis

GALACTOSE-1-PHOSPHATE URIDYL TRANSFERASE

Galactose, Screening Test for
Galactosemia, Urine
Galactose-1-Phosphate Uridyl
Transferase, Erythrocyte, Blood

ADDITIONAL CONDITIONS

Cataracts
Cirrhosis
Failure to Thrive
Mental Retardation

GALACTOSEMIA

Galactokinase, Blood
Galactose, Screening Test for
Galactosemia, Urine
Galactose-1-Phosphate, Blood
Galactose-1-Phosphate Uridyl
Transferase, Erythrocyte, Blood
Galactose-1-Phosphate Uridyl
Transferase, Qualitative, Blood
Glucose, Qualitative and
Semiquantitative, Urine

ADDITIONAL CONDITIONS

Cataracts
Cirrhosis
Failure to Thrive
Mental Retardation

GANGLIONEUROBLASTOMA

Bone Marrow Aspiration Analysis,
Specimen
Bone Scan, Diagnostic
Brain Biopsy, Diagnostic
Complete Blood Count, Blood
Computed Tomography of the Brain,
Diagnostic
Histopathology, Specimen
Homovanillic Acid, 24-Hour, Urine
5-Hydroxyindoleacetic Acid,
Quantitative, 24-Hour, Urine
Metanephrines, Total, 24-Hour, Urine
Magnetic Resonance Imaging, Brain,
Diagnostic
Magnetic Resonance Spectography,
Diagnostic
Vanillylmandelic Acid, Urine

ADDITIONAL CONDITIONS

Congenital Heart Disease
Diarrhea
Pain, Abdominal
Periorbital Ecchymosis
von Recklinghausen's Disease

GANGRENE

Abscess, Anaerobic Culture
Biopsy, Anaerobic, Culture
Blood Indices (Red Blood Cells), Blood
Complete Blood Count, Blood
Differential Leukocyte Count,
Peripheral Blood
Glucose, 2-Hour Postprandial, Serum
Histopathology, Specimen
Red Cell Count, Blood

ADDITIONAL CONDITIONS

Cholecystitis
Diabetes Mellitus
Peripheral Vascular Disease
Sepsis

GASTRIC CANCER
(see also Helicobacter pylori)
Barium Enema, Diagnostic
Carcinoembryonic Antigen, Serum
Gastroscopy, Diagnostic
Helicobacter pylori, Quick Office
    Serology, Serum and Titer, Blood
Iron, Serum
Mucin-Like Carcinoma-Associated
    Antigen, Blood
Occult Blood, Stool
Pepsinogen I, Blood
Upper Gastrointestinal Series,
    Diagnostic

ADDITIONAL CONDITIONS
Anemia
Malnutrition
Metastasis

GASTRIC ULCER
(see also Helicobacter pylori)
ABO Group and Rh Type, Blood
Amylase, Serum and Urine
Brushing Cytology, Specimen,
    Diagnostic
Complete Blood Count, Blood
Gastrin, Serum
Gastroscopy, Diagnostic
Helicobacter pylori, Quick Office
    Serology, Serum and Titer, Blood
Histopathology, Specimen
Occult Blood, Stool
Washing Cytology, Specimen

ADDITIONAL CONDITIONS
Gastritis
Hemorrhage
Pain, Acute

GASTRINOMA
(see Zollinger-Ellison Syndrome)

GASTRITIS
(see also Helicobacter pylori)
Brushing Cytology, Specimen,
    Diagnostic
Campylobacter-Like-Organism Test,
    Specimen
Folic Acid, Serum
Helicobacter pylori, Quick Office
    Serology, Serum and Titer, Blood
Histopathology, Specimen
Occult Blood, Stool
Pepsinogen I, Blood
Schilling Test, Diagnostic
Vitamin B_{12}, Serum

ADDITIONAL CONDITIONS
Cytomegalovirus
Crohn's Disease
Eosinophilia
Gastric Ulcer
Sarcoidosis
Schistosomiasis
Syphilis
Tuberculosis

GASTROENTERITIS
Meat Fibers, Stool
Methylene Blue Stain, Stool
Stool Culture, Routine, Stool

ADDITIONAL CONDITIONS
Fever
Immunocompromised Persons
Malnutrition
Pain, Acute

GASTROESOPHAGEAL REFLUX
Acid Perfusion Test, Diagnostic
Esophageal Acidity Test, Diagnostic

ADDITIONAL CONDITIONS
Hiatal Hernia
Stomach Cancer

Esophageal Manometry, Diagnostic
Esophageal Radiography, Diagnostic

GASTROINTESTINAL BLEEDING

Autoerythrocyte Sensitivity Test, Diagnostic
Blood Urea Nitrogen/Creatinine Ratio, Blood
Complete Blood Count, Blood
Cr-51 (Chromium) Red Cell Survival, Blood
Gastroscopy, Diagnostic
Occult Blood, Stool

ADDITIONAL CONDITIONS

Alcoholism
Ascites
Encephalopathy
Esophageal Varices
Gastritis
Hypovolemic Shock
Mallory-Weiss Syndrome
Peptic Ulcer
Thrombocytopenia

GAUCHER'S DISEASE

Acid Phosphatase, Serum
Bone Marrow Biopsy, Diagnostic
Complete Blood Count, Blood
Magnetic Resonance Imaging, Diagnostic

ADDITIONAL CONDITIONS

Anemia
Hepatosplenomegaly
Thrombocytopenia

GENITAL HERPES

Herpes Cytology, Specimen
Herpes Simplex Antibody, Blood
Histopathology, Specimen
Rapid Plasma Reagin Test, Blood
Viral Culture, Specimen

ADDITIONAL CONDITIONS

Cervicitis
Gonorrhea
Syphilis
Urinary Tract Infection
Vaginitis
Vulvar Cancer

GENTAMYCIN

(see Aminoglycoside Toxicity)

GERMAN MEASLES

(see Rubella Measles)

GESTATIONAL DIABETES

(see Diabetes, Gestational)

GIARDIASIS

Histopathology, Specimen
Ova and Parasites, Stool
Washing Cytology, Specimen

ADDITIONAL CONDITIONS

AIDS
Diarrhea
Malabsorption Syndrome

GI BLEEDING

(see Gastrointestinal Bleeding)

GLANZMANN'S DISEASE

Bleeding Time, Ivy, Blood
Bleeding Time, Mielke, Blood
Clot Retraction, Serum
Platelet Adhesion Test (Venous Blood), Diagnostic
Platelet Aggregation, Blood; Platelet Aggregation, Hypercoagulable State, Blood

ADDITIONAL CONDITIONS

Epistaxis
Menorrhagia

GLAUCOMA

Tonometry Test for Glaucoma,
Diagnostic

ADDITIONAL CONDITIONS

Pain, Acute
Visual Blurring
Visual Field Loss

GLOMERULONEPHRITIS

Addis Count, 12-Hour, Urine
Albumin/Globulin Ratio, Serum
Antideoxyribonuclease-B Titer,
Serum
Anti-DNA, Serum
Antihyaluronidase Titer, Serum
Antistreptolysin-O Titer, Serum
C1q Immune Complex Detection,
Serum
C3 Complement, Serum
C3 Proactivator, Serum
C4 Complement, Serum
Chemistry Profile, Blood
Complement Components, Serum
Complement, Total, Serum
Creatinine Clearance, Serum, Urine
Glomerular Basement Membrane
Antibody, Serum
Hepatitis B Surface Antigen, Blood
Immune Complex Assay, Blood
Intravenous Pyelography, Diagnostic
Kidney Biopsy, Specimen
Mean Platelet Volume, Blood
Occult Blood, Urine
Protein, Electrophoresis, Serum
Protein, Urine
Specific Gravity, Urine
Streptozyme, Blood
Throat Culture for Group A Beta-
Hemolytic Streptococci, Culture
Urea Nitrogen, Plasma or Serum
Urinalysis, Urine

ADDITIONAL CONDITIONS

Amyloidosis
Colon Cancer
Chickenpox
Endocarditis
Goodpasture's Syndrome
Hepatitis
Kidney Cancer
Leprosy
Lung Cancer
Malaria
Measles
Melanoma
Pneumonia
Schistosomiasis
Scleroderma
Sickle Cell Disease
Syphilis
Systemic Lupus Erythematosus
(SLE)
Toxoplasmosis

GLUCAGONOMA

Chemistry Profile, Blood
Glucagon, Plasma
Glucose, Blood
Insulin Assay, Blood

ADDITIONAL CONDITIONS

Hypoglycemia
Pheochromocytoma

GLYCOGEN STORAGE DISEASE

Bone Marrow Aspiration Analysis,
Specimen
Glucose, Blood
Glucose Tolerance Test, Blood
Glucose, 2-Hour Postprandial,
Serum
Histopathology, Specimen
Ketone Bodies, Blood
Ketones, Semiquantitative, Urine
Lipid Profile, Blood
Uric Acid, Serum

ADDITIONAL CONDITIONS

Ataxia
Congestive Heart Failure
Gout
Hepatomegaly
Hyperlipidemia
Hyperuricemia
Hypoglycemia

GLYCOGENOSIS
(see Glycogen Storage Disease)

GLYCOSURIA
Glucose, Qualitative and
Semiquantitative, Urine
Glucose, Quantitative, 24-Hour, Urine
Glucose, 2-Hour Postprandial,
Serum
Glycosylated Hemoglobin, Blood
Osmolality, Urine

ADDITIONAL CONDITIONS
Cancer
Diabetes Mellitus
Obesity

GOITER
(see Hypothyroidism)

GONOCOCCAL INFECTION OF PHARYNX
Throat Culture for *Neisseria
gonorrhoeae,* Culture

ADDITIONAL CONDITION
Pharyngitis

GONORRHEA
Chlamydia Culture
Fluorescent Treponemal Antibody-
Absorbed Double-Stain Test,
Serum
Genital, *Neisseria gonorrhoeae,*
Culture
Genital, Routine, Culture
Gram Stain, Diagnostic (Urine)
Neisseria gonorrhoeae Smear,
Specimen
Penicillinase Test, Diagnostic
Rapid Plasma Reagin Test, Blood
Throat Culture for *Neisseria
gonorrhoeae,* Culture
Urine Culture for *Neisseria
gonorrhoeae,* Urine
Venereal Disease Research Laboratory
Test, Serum

ADDITIONAL CONDITIONS
Cervicitis
Chlamydia
Conjunctivitis
Epididymitis
Prostatitis
Salpingitis
Trichomonas
Vaginitis

GOODPASTURE'S SYNDROME
Bronchial Washing, Specimen,
Diagnostic
Brushing Cytology, Specimen,
Diagnostic
Eosinophil Count, Blood
Glomerular Basement Membrane
Antibody, Serum
Kidney Biopsy, Specimen
Occult Blood, Urine
Protein, Quantitative, Urine
Protein, Semiquantitative, Urine
Sputum Hemosiderin Preparation,
Specimen
Urinalysis, Urine
Washing Cytology, Specimen

ADDITIONAL CONDITIONS
Glomerulonephritis
Hemodialysis
Hemoptysis
Hypoxia

GOUT
Body Fluid Analysis, Cell Count, Specimen
Body Fluid, Routine, Culture
Chemistry Profile, Blood
Heavy Metals, Blood and 24-Hour, Urine (Urine)
Mucin Clot Test, Specimen
Phosphorus, Serum
Synovial Fluid Analysis, Diagnostic
Uric Acid, Serum
Uric Acid, Urine

ADDITIONAL CONDITIONS
Anemia
Arthritis
Cancer
Chronic Renal Disease
Diabetes Insipidus
Diabetic Ketoacidosis
Glycogen Storage Disease
Hyperuricemia
Lead Poisoning
Lesch-Nyhan Syndrome
Multiple Myeloma
Pruritus
Psoriasis
Sarcoma

GRANULOCYTIC LEUKEMIA
(see Leukemia)

GRANULOMAS
Liver I-131, Scan, Diagnostic

ADDITIONAL CONDITIONS
Diabetes Mellitus
Hypoxemia
Pulmonary Infiltrates
Splenomegaly

GRAVES' DISEASE
(see Hyperthyroidism)

GROWTH HORMONE DEFICIENCY
Chromosome Analysis, Blood
Growth Hormone, Blood
Insulin-Like Growth Factor-I, Blood
Zinc, Blood

ADDITIONAL CONDITIONS
Cushing's Syndrome
Dwarfism
Hashimoto's Thyroiditis
Hypopituitarism
Rickets
Turner's Syndrome

GUILLAIN-BARRE SYNDROME
Cerebrospinal Fluid, Routine Analysis, Specimen
Electromyogram and Nerve Conduction (Electromyelogram) Studies, Diagnostic
Heavy Metals, Blood and 24-Hour, Urine (Urine)
Immunoglobulin G Synthesis Rate, Cerebrospinal Fluid, Specimen

ADDITIONAL CONDITIONS
Autoimmune Diseases
Malnutrition
Viral Disorder
Vitamin E Deficiency

GYNECOMASTIA
Chemistry Profile, Blood
Estradiol, Serum
Follicle-Stimulating Hormone, Serum
Histopathology, Specimen
Human Chorionic Gonadotropin, Beta-Subunit, Serum

ADDITIONAL CONDITIONS
Addison's Disease
Cirrhosis
Hyperthyroidism
Hypogonadism
Puberty
Testicular Tumors

17-Ketosteroid Fractionation,
24-Hour, Urine
Liver Battery, Serum
Prolactin, Serum
Testosterone, Total, Blood

HAEMOPHILUS INFLUENZAE INFECTION

Sputum for *Haemophilus* Species,
Culture

ADDITIONAL CONDITIONS

Croup
Meningitis
Pneumonia

HAGEMAN FACTOR

Coagulation Factor Assay, Blood
Factor XII, Blood
Partial Thromboplastin Time, Plasma

ADDITIONAL CONDITIONS

Thrombocytopenia
Vasoconstriction

HAIRY CELL LEUKEMIA

Acid Phosphatase, Serum
Bone Marrow Biopsy, Diagnostic
Histopathology, Specimen
Leukocyte Cytochemistry (Bone
Marrow), Specimen
Tartrate-Resistant Leukocyte, Blood

ADDITIONAL CONDITIONS

Fatigue
Hepatomegaly
Pancytopenia
Splenomegaly

HALLUCINOGENS: LSD, MESCALINE, MDA, PCP, PSILOCYLIN

(see Drug Abuse)

HAND-SCHULLER-CHRISTIAN DISEASE

Bone Scan, Diagnostic
Chest X-Ray, Diagnostic

ADDITIONAL CONDITIONS

Bronchiolitis
Dyspnea
Fever
Pneumothorax

HARTNUP DISEASE

Indican, Urine

ADDITIONAL CONDITIONS

Dermatitis
Renal Failure

HASHIMOTO'S THYROIDITIS

Histopathology, Specimen
Needle Aspiration Cytology (Thyroid),
Specimen
Thyroid Antimicrosomal Antibody,
Blood
Thyroid Antithyroglobulin Antibody,
Serum
Thyroid Profile, Blood
Thyroid-Stimulating Hormone, Blood

ADDITIONAL CONDITIONS

Goiter
Myxedema

HAY FEVER

Allergin-Specific IgE, Serum
Eosinophil Count, Blood
Immunoglobulin E, Serum

ADDITIONAL CONDITIONS

Nasal Polyps
Pruritus

HEAD AND NECK CANCER

Barium Swallow, Diagnostic
Biopsy, Site-Specific, Specimen
CA 15–3, Serum
CA 50, Blood (Esophagus Squamous)
Chest X-Ray, Diagnostic
Computed Tomography of the Body
(Head and Neck), Diagnostic
Esophageal Radiography, Diagnostic
Magnetic Resonance Imaging,
Diagnostic
Transesophageal Sonogram,
Diagnostic

ADDITIONAL CONDITIONS

Alcoholism
Epstein-Barr Virus
Iron Deficiency
Malnutrition

HEAD INJURIES

Cerebrospinal Fluid, Routine
Analysis, Specimen
Cervical Spine Films, Diagnostic
Complete Blood Count, Blood
Computed Tomography of the Brain,
Diagnostic
Electroencephalogram, Diagnostic
Magnetic Resonance Imaging,
Diagnostic

ADDITIONAL CONDITIONS

Concussion
Edema
Hematoma
Hemorrhage
Shock

HEADACHE

Carbon Monoxide, Blood
Carboxyhemoglobin, Blood
Cerebrospinal Fluid, Routine
Analysis, Specimen
Cold Agglutinin Screen, Blood
Cold Agglutinin Titer, Serum
Computed Tomography of the Brain,
Diagnostic
Heavy Metals, Blood and 24-Hour,
Urine (Urine)
Methemoglobin, Blood
Mycoplasma Titer, Blood
Rocky Mountain Spotted Fever
Serology, Blood
Viscosity, Serum

ADDITIONAL CONDITIONS

Allergies
Arteritis
Brain Tumor
Concussion
Coughing
Depression
Encephalitis
Horner's Syndrome
Hypertension
Photophobia
Subarachnoid Hemorrhage
Tension/Stress

HEARING DISORDERS

Fluorescent Treponemal Antibody-
Absorbed Double-Stain Test,
Serum
Hearing Test for Loudness-
Recruitment, Diagnostic
Tuning Fork Test of Weber, Rinne,
and Schwabach Tests, Diagnostic

ADDITIONAL CONDITIONS

Aminoglycoside Toxicity
Chemotherapy Induced
Diabetes Mellitus
Hypothyroidism
Measles
Mumps
Otitis Media
Renal Failure
Syphilis
Tinnitus

HEART-LUNG MACHINE

Activated Coagulation Time,
Automated, Blood
Blood Gases, Arterial, Blood

ADDITIONAL CONDITIONS

COPD
Coronary Artery Bypass Graft Surgery

Complete Blood Count, Blood
Partial Thromboplastin Time, Plasma
Prothrombin Time and International
Normalized Ratio, Serum

HEART MURMUR

Cardiac Radiography, Diagnostic
Echocardiogram, Diagnostic
Electrocardiogram, Diagnostic
Stress Test, Pharmacologic, Diagnostic
Transesophageal Sonogram,
Diagnostic

ADDITIONAL CONDITIONS

Patent Ductus Arteriosus
Rheumatic Fever
Scarlet Fever
Tetralogy of Fallot

HEART TRANSPLANT

(see Transplants)

HEAT STROKE

Calcium, Total, Serum
Platelet Count, Blood
Potassium, Serum
Prothrombin Time and International
Normalized Ratio, Serum
Urea Nitrogen, Plasma or Serum
Urinalysis, Urine

ADDITIONAL CONDITIONS

Convulsions
Hyperventilation
Myocardial Infarction
Renal Failure

HEINZ BODY ANEMIA

Blood Indices (Red Blood Cells), Blood
Complete Blood Count, Blood
Differential Leukocyte Count,
Peripheral Blood
Glucose-6-Phosphate Dehydrogenase,
Quantitative, Blood
Glucose-6-Phosphate Dehydrogenase
Screen, Blood
Heinz Body Stain, Diagnostic
Helicobacter pylori, Quick Office
Serology, Serum and Titer, Blood
Hemoglobin Electrophoresis, Blood
Hemoglobin, Unstable, Heat Labile
Test, Blood
Hemoglobin, Unstable, Isopropanol
Precipitation Test, Blood
Methemoglobin, Blood
Red Blood Cell Morphology, Blood
Red Cell Count, Serum
Reticulocyte Count, Blood
Urea Breath Test, Diagnostic

ADDITIONAL CONDITIONS

G-6-PD Deficiency
Hemoglobinemia
Hemoglobinuria
Hyperbilirubinemia
Jaundice

HELICOBACTER PYLORI

Campylobacter-Like-Organism Test,
Specimen
Cytologic Study of Gastrointestinal
Tract, Diagnostic
Gastric Acid Analysis Test, Diagnostic
Gastric Analysis, Specimen
Gastroscopy or Gastroduodenal-
jejunoscopy, Diagnostic

ADDITIONAL CONDITIONS

Botulism
Colitis
Diarrhea
Ulcers

Helicobacter pylori, Quick Office
    Serology, Serum
Helicobacter pylori, Serum and Titer,
    Blood
Immunoglobulin G, Serum
Methylene Blue Stain, Stool
Pepsinogen I, Blood
Stool Culture, Routine, Stool
Urea Breath Test, Diagnostic

HEMATURIA

Addis Count, 12-Hour, Urine
Antideoxyribonuclease-B Titer,
    Serum
Antihyaluronidase Titer, Serum
Antistreptolysin-O Titer, Serum
Creatinine, Serum
Glomerular Basement Membrane
    Antibody, Serum
Kidney Biopsy, Specimen
Kidney Stone Analysis, Specimen
Occult Blood, Urine
Streptozyme, Blood
Urea Nitrogen, Plasma or Serum
Urinalysis, Urine
Urine Culture, Routine Catheterized,
    Urine
Urine Culture, Routine, Clean-Catch,
    Urine
Urine Cytology, Urine
Urine, Fungus, Culture
Urine, *Mycobacteria,* Culture

ADDITIONAL CONDITIONS

Bladder Cancer
Disseminated Intravascular
    Coagulation
Glomerulonephrosis
Hemoglobinuria
Hemophilia
Renal Disease
Sickle Cell Disease
Trauma
Urinary Tract Infection

HEMOCHROMATOSIS

Ferritin, Serum
Glucose, Blood
Glucose Tolerance Test, Blood
Hemosiderin Stain, Urine
Histopathology, Specimen
Iron, Serum
Iron Stain, Bone Marrow, Specimen
Liver Battery, Serum
Liver Biopsy, Diagnostic
Total Iron Binding Capacity, Serum

ADDITIONAL CONDITIONS

Congestive Heart Failure
Diabetes Mellitus
Hepatomegaly
Hyperglycemia
Renal Failure

HEMOFLAGELLATES

(see Trypanosomiasis)

HEMOGLOBIN C DISEASE

Hemoglobin Electrophoresis, Blood
Red Blood Cell Morphology, Blood

ADDITIONAL CONDITIONS

Anemia
Jaundice
Retinopathy
Splenomegaly

HEMOLYTIC ANEMIA

Bilirubin, Total, Serum
Ham Test, Blood
Red Blood Cell Morphology, Blood

ADDITIONAL CONDITIONS

Burns
Disseminated Intravascular
    Coagulation

Reticulocyte Count, Blood
Sedimentation Rate, Erythrocyte,
Blood
Transferrin, Serum
Urobilinogen, Urine

G-6-PD Deficiency
Malaria
Metastasis
Sickle Cell Disease Transfusion
Reaction, Delayed or Immediate
Vasculitis

HEMOPHILIA

Activated Coagulation Time,
Automated, Blood
Aspirin Tolerance Test, Diagnostic
Circulating Anticoagulant, Blood
Complete Blood Count, Blood
Factor VIII, Blood
Factor VIII R:Ag, Blood
Mixing Study (Circulating,
Anticoagulants), Plasma
Occult Blood, Urine
Partial Thromboplastin Time,
Plasma
Plasma Recalcification Time, Plasma
Platelet Aggregation,
Hypercoagulable State, Blood

ADDITIONAL CONDITIONS

AIDS
Hemorrhage
Thrombosis

HEMOPTYSIS

Bleeding Time, Duke, Blood
Bleeding Time, Ivy, Blood
Bronchial Washing, Specimen,
Diagnostic
Bronchoscopy, Diagnostic
Brushing Cytology, Specimen,
Diagnostic
Prothrombin Time and International
Normalized Ratio, Serum
Sputum, Routine, Culture
Sputum Cytology, Specimen
Sputum, *Mycobacteria,* Culture

ADDITIONAL CONDITIONS

Bronchitis
Esophageal Varices
Lung Cancer
Tuberculosis

HEMORRHAGE

Activated Partial Thromboplastin
Time, Serum
Betke-Kleihauer Stain, Diagnostic
Chemistry Profile, Blood
Complete Blood Count, Blood
Hematocrit, Blood
Hemoglobin, Blood
Iron, Serum
Magnetic Resonance Imaging,
Diagnostic
Occult Blood, Stool
Platelet Count, Blood
Prothrombin Time and International
Normalized Ratio, Serum
Sputum Hemosiderin Preparation,
Specimen
Total Iron Binding Capacity, Serum
Type and Crossmatch, Blood
Urinalysis, Urine

ADDITIONAL CONDITIONS

Aneurysm
Brain Tumor
Burns
Cerebral Hemorrhage
Cystitis
Disseminated Intravascular
Coagulation
Esophageal Varices
Hemophilia
Leukemia
Trauma
Ulcers

HEMORRHOIDS
Complete Blood Count, Blood
Proctoscopy, Diagnostic

ADDITIONAL CONDITIONS
Anal Fissure
Anemia
Bowel Incontinence
Colon Cancer
Portal Hypertension
Pregnancy
Rectal Cancer

HEPATIC CIRRHOSIS
Liver Biopsy, Diagnostic
Liver Sonogram, Diagnostic

ADDITIONAL CONDITIONS
Alcoholism
Cystic Fibrosis
Drug Abuse
Peptic Ulcers
Sjögren's Syndrome

HEPATIC COMA
(see also Hepatitis and Jaundice)
Albumin, Serum, Urine, and 24-Hour
    Urine
Ammonia, Blood
Amylase, Serum and Urine
Antinuclear Antibody, Serum
Bilirubin, Total, Serum
Lactic Acid, Blood
Urea Nitrogen, Plasma or Serum

ADDITIONAL CONDITIONS
Encephalitis
Hepatorenal Syndrome
Poisoning, Heavy Metal
Renal Failure

HEPATIC CYSTS OR ABSCESSES
Liver Biopsy, Diagnostic
Liver I-131 Scan, Diagnostic
Liver Sonogram, Diagnostic

ADDITIONAL CONDITIONS
Echinococcosis

HEPATIC ENCEPHALOPATHY
Ammonia, Blood
Liver Battery, Serum
Liver Biopsy, Diagnostic
Liver Scan, Diagnostic
Liver/Spleen Scan, Diagnostic
Magnetic Resonance Spectography,
    Diagnostic
Paracentesis, Diagnostic
Ultrasound, Liver, Diagnostic

ADDITIONAL CONDITIONS
Gastrointestinal Bleed
Hypokalemia
Hypovolemia, Following Paracentesis
Metabolic Acidosis
Sepsis

HEPATITIS
Acetaminophen, Serum
Alanine Aminotransferase, Serum
Albumin/Globulin Ratio, Serum
Alkaline Phosphatase Isoenzymes,
    Serum
Alkaline Phosphatase, Serum
Alpha-Antitrypsin, Serum
Alpha-Fetoprotein, Serum
Antimitochondrial Antibody, Blood
Anti-Smooth Muscle Antibody,
    Serum

ADDITIONAL CONDITIONS
Alcoholism
Amenorrhea
Anemia, Hemolytic
Cirrhosis
Drug Abuse
Following Transfusion of Blood
Hepatic Coma
Hyperuricemia
Hypocholesterolemia
Jaundice
Pruritus

Aspartate Aminotransferase, Serum
Bilirubin, Direct, Serum
Bilirubin, Indirect, Serum
C1q Immune Complex Detection,
    Serum
C3 Complement, Serum
C4 Complement, Serum
Chemistry Profile, Blood
Cytomegalovirus Antibody, Serum
Epstein-Barr Virus, Serology, Blood
Gamma-Glutamyl Transpeptidase,
    Blood
Hepatitis A Antibody, IgM and IgG,
    Blood
Hepatitis B Core Antibody, Blood
Hepatitis B E Antibody, Serum
Hepatitis B E Antigen, Blood
Hepatitis B Surface Antibody, Blood
Hepatitis B Surface Antigen, Blood
Hepatitis C Antibody, Serum
Hepatitis Delta Antibody (Total Anti-
    HDV), Serum
Histopathology, Specimen
Lactate Dehydrogenase Isoenzymes,
    Blood
Liver Battery, Serum
Liver Biopsy, Diagnostic
Liver Scan, Diagnostic
Lupus Test, Blood
Methotrexate, Serum
5'Nucleotidase, Serum
Ornithine Carbamoyltransferase,
    Blood
Protein, Electrophoresis, Serum
Prothrombin Time and International
    Normalized Ratio, Serum
Salicylate, Blood
Toxoplasmosis Serology, Serum
Ultrasound, Liver, Diagnostic
Urobilinogen, Urine

HEPATOMAS
Liver I-131 Scan, Diagnostic
Liver Sonogram, Diagnostic

ADDITIONAL CONDITIONS
Cirrhosis
Endocrine Syndrome
Immunoglobulin Changes

HEPATOMEGALY
Liver Biopsy, Diagnostic

ADDITIONAL CONDITIONS
Alcohol Abuse
Cirrhosis
Leukemia
Neoplastic Disease

HERPES SIMPLEX
(COLD/FEVER SORE)
Herpes Simplex Antibody, Blood
Herpes Virus Antigen, Direct
    Fluorescent Antibody,
    Specimen

ADDITIONAL CONDITIONS
Encephalitis
Keratitis
Opthalmitis
Stress

HERPES VIRUS INFECTION

Bronchial Washing, Specimen, Diagnostic
Brushing Cytology, Specimen, Diagnostic
Cervical/Vaginal Cytology, Specimen
Herpes Cytology, Specimen
Herpes Simplex Antibody, Blood
Oral Cavity Cytology (Scrape), Specimen
Sputum Cytology, Specimen
Toxoplasmosis, Rubella, Cytomegalovirus, Herpes Virus Serology (TORCH), Blood
Varicella-Zoster Virus Serology, Serum
Viral Culture, Specimen

ADDITIONAL CONDITIONS

Cervicitis
Glaucoma
Leukemia
Stomatitis

HERPES ZOSTER (SHINGLES)

Varicella-Zoster Virus Serology, Serum

ADDITIONAL CONDITIONS

Chickenpox
Fever
Hodgkin's Disease
Leukemia
Lymphoma

HIATAL HERNIA

Barium Swallow, Diagnostic
Esophageal Radiography, Diagnostic
Upper Gastrointestinal Series, Diagnostic

ADDITIONAL CONDITIONS

Dysphagia

HIRSCHSPRUNG'S DISEASE

Barium Enema, Diagnostic
Histopathology, Specimen
Rectal Biopsy, Diagnostic

ADDITIONAL CONDITIONS

Constipation
Pain, Abdominal
Vomiting

HIRSUTISM (HYPERTRICHOSIS)

Androstenedione, Serum
Dehydroepiandrosterone Sulfate, Serum and 24-Hour Urine (Serum)
17-Hydroxycorticosteroids, 24-Hour, Urine
17-Hydroxyprogesterone, Blood
17-Ketogenic Steroids, 24-Hour, Urine
17-Ketosteroids, Total, 24-Hour, Urine
Pregnanetriol, Urine
Prolactin, Serum
Testosterone, Total, Blood

ADDITIONAL CONDITIONS

Amenorrhea
Cushing's Syndrome
Hypertension
Hypokalemia
Obesity
Ovarian Tumor
Postmenopausal Effect

HISTOPLASMOSIS

Amphotericin B, Blood
Biopsy, Fungus, Culture
Blood Fungus, Culture
Body Fluid, Fungus, Culture

ADDITIONAL CONDITIONS

Anemia
COPD
Diarrhea
Fever

Bone Marrow Biopsy, Diagnostic
Bronchial Aspirate, Routine, Culture
Bronchial Aspirate, Fungus, Culture
Bronchial Washing, Specimen,
   Diagnostic
Brushing Cytology, Specimen,
   Diagnostic
Cerebrospinal Fluid, Fungus, Culture
Complement Fixation, Serum
Flucytosine, Serum
Fungal Antibody Screen, Blood
Histopathology, Specimen
Histoplasmosis Serology, Blood
Migration Inhibition Test, Blood
Needle Aspiration Cytology (Lung),
   Specimen
Platelet Count, Blood
Sputum Cytology, Specimen
Sputum, Fungus, Culture

Hepatosplenomegaly
Immunosuppression
Pneumonia

HODGKIN'S DISEASE

Biopsy, Site-Specific, Specimen
Body Fluid Cytology, Specimen
Bone Marrow Biopsy, Diagnostic
Chemistry Profile, Blood
Chromosome Analysis, Blood
Complete Blood Count, Blood
C-Reactive Protein, Serum
Cryoglobulin, Qualitative, Serum
Differential Leukocyte Count,
   Peripheral Blood
d-Xylose Absorption Test, Diagnostic,
   Serum or Urine
Globulin, Serum
Histopathology, Specimen
Immunoelectrophoresis, Serum and
   Urine
Immunoglobulin A, Serum
Immunoglobulin G, Serum
Immunoglobulin M, Serum
Immunoperoxidase Procedures
   (for Antigens), Diagnostic
Leukocyte Cytochemistry,
   Specimen
Lymph Node Biopsy, Specimen
Lymphocyte Subset Enumeration,
   Blood
Migration Inhibition Test, Blood
Muramidase, Serum and Urine
Needle Aspiration Cytology (Mass),
   Specimen
Platelet Count, Blood
Pneumocystis IFA, Serum
Protein, Electrophoresis, Serum
Protein, Electrophoresis, Urine
T and B Lymphocyte Subset Assay,
   Blood
Terminal Deoxynucleotidyltransferase
   (TdT), Bone Marrow, Diagnostic
Uric Acid, Serum

ADDITIONAL CONDITIONS

Cat Scratch Disease
Fever
Infectious Mononucleosis
Lymphadenopathy
Night Sweats

HORMONAL THERAPY
Estradiol Receptor and Progesterone
Receptor in Breast Cancer,
Diagnostic
Progesterone Receptor Assay, Blood

ADDITIONAL CONDITIONS
Breast Cancer
Endometrial Cancer
Postmenopause
Prostate Cancer

HUMAN PAPILLOMAVIRUS
Human Papillomavirus, Specimen

ADDITIONAL CONDITIONS
AIDS
Chancroid
Chlamydia
Gonorrhea
Granuloma Inguinale
Herpes Hominus II
Human Immunodeficiency Virus
(HIV)
Lymphogranuloma Venereum
Syphilis

HUMORAL IMMUNE DEFICIENCY
Globulin, Serum
Immunoelectrophoresis, Serum and
Urine
Immunoglobulin A, Serum
Immunoglobulin G, Serum
Immunoglobulin M, Serum
Protein, Electrophoresis, Serum
T- and B-Lymphocyte Subset Assay,
Blood

ADDITIONAL CONDITIONS
Lymphoma
Multiple Myeloma
Thymoma

HUNTER'S SYNDROME
Mucopolysaccharides, Qualitative,
Urine

ADDITIONAL CONDITIONS
Arthritis, Rheumatoid
Rheumatic Fever
Scleroderma
Sjögren's Syndrome
Systemic Lupus Erythematosus

HURLER'S SYNDROME
Differential Leukocyte Count,
Peripheral Blood
Fibroblast Skin Culture
Mucoplysaccharides, Qualitative,
Urine
S Mucopolysaccharide Turnover,
Diagnostic

ADDITIONAL CONDITIONS
Corneal Blurring
Deafness
Hepatosplenomegaly
Mental Retardation
Myocarditis

HYALINE MEMBRANE DISEASE
Alpha1-Antitrypsin, Serum
Amniotic Fluid Analysis (Pulmonary
Surfactant), Specimen
Bicarbonate, Serum
Blood Gases, Arterial, Blood
Blood Gases, Capillary, Blood
Chest X-Ray, Diagnostic
pCO_2, Blood

ADDITIONAL CONDITIONS
Diabetes Mellitus in Pregnancy
Premature Infants Weighing Between
1000 and 1500 g

HYDATIDIFORM MOLE
Histopathology, Specimen
Human Chorionic Gonadotropin,
    Beta-Subunit, Serum
Obstetric Sonogram, Diagnostic
Protein, Quantitative, Urine

HYDRATION
Chemistry Profile, Blood
Complete Blood Count, Blood
Electrolyte, Blood or Urine
Osmolality, Serum
Osmolality, Urine
Parathyroid Hormone, Blood
Sodium, Plasma, Serum, or Urine

HYDRONEPHROSIS
Complete Blood Count, Blood
Computed Tomography of the Body
    (Kidney), Diagnostic
Creatinine, Serum
Creatinine Clearance, Serum, Urine
Intravenous Pyelography,
    Diagnostic
Kidney Sonogram, Diagnostic
Magnetic Resonance Imaging,
    Diagnostic
Urea Nitrogen, Plasma or Serum
Urinalysis, Urine
Urine Culture, Routine, Clean-Catch,
    Urine
Urine Cytology, Urine

HYPERALDOSTERONISM
Aldosterone, Serum and Urine
Chemistry Profile, Blood
Electrolyte, Blood
Electrolyte, Urine
Histopathology, Specimen
Kidney Profile, Specimens
Osmolality, Serum
Osmolality, Urine
Potassium, Serum
Renin, Blood
Sodium, Plasma, Serum, or Urine

HYPERALIMENTATION
Albumin, Serum, Urine, and 24-Hour
    Urine
Albumin/Globulin Ratio, Serum
Blood Fungus, Culture
Chemistry Profile, Blood
Electrolyte, Blood
Foreign Body, Routine, Culture
Glucose, Blood
Lipid Profile, Blood

ADDITIONAL CONDITIONS
Eclampsia
Hyperthyroidism
Nausea and Vomiting
Uterine Bleeding

ADDITIONAL CONDITIONS
Chemotherapy
Postoperative
Preoperative

ADDITIONAL CONDITIONS
Pyelonephritis
Ureteral Obstruction

ADDITIONAL CONDITIONS
Cirrhosis
Congestive Heart Failure
Conn's Syndrome
Headache
Hypernatremia
Hypertension
Hypokalemia
Metabolic Alkalosis
Polydipsia
Polyuria

ADDITIONAL CONDITIONS
Anorexia Nervosa
Cachexia
Cancer
Catatonia
Coma
Malnutrition

HYPERBARIC OXYGENATION
Blood Gases, Arterial, Blood

ADDITIONAL CONDITIONS
Divers' Bends

HYPERBILIRUBINEMIA
Bilirubin, Total, Serum

ADDITIONAL CONDITIONS
Cholestasis
Crigler-Najjar Syndrome
Dubin-Johnson Syndrome
Gilbert's Syndrome
Jaundice
Rotor's Syndrome

HYPERCALCEMIA
Albumin, Serum, Urine, and 24-Hour
    Urine
Alkaline Phosphatase, Serum
Anion Gap, Blood
Blood Urea Nitrogen/Creatinine
    Ratio, Blood
Calcium, Total, Serum
Calcium, Urine
Cyclic Adenosine Monophosphate,
    Serum and Urine
Magnesium, Serum
Parathyroid Hormone, Blood
Phosphorus, Serum
Phosphorus, Urine
Vitamin D_3, Plasma or Serum

ADDITIONAL CONDITIONS
Acromegaly
Cancer
Hyperparathyroidism
Hypophosphatemia
Immobilization
Metastasis to Bone
Multiple Myeloma
Paget's Disease of Bone
Sarcoidosis

HYPERCAPNIA
Bicarbonate, Serum
Blood Gases, Arterial, Blood
Blood Gases, Capillary, Blood
Blood Gases, Venous, Blood
Carbon Dioxide (CO_2), Blood
Chest X-Ray, Diagnostic
pH, Blood
Pulmonary Function Test, Diagnostic

ADDITIONAL CONDITIONS
Anesthesia
Congestive Heart Failure
COPD
Dysrhythmias
Kyphoscoliosis
Myocardial Infarction
Respiratory Acidosis

HYPERCHOLESTEROLEMIA
Cholesterol, Blood
Glucose, Blood
High-Density Lipoprotein
    Cholesterol, Blood
Lipid Profile, Blood
Phospholipids, Serum
Thyroid Profile, Blood
Triglycerides, Blood
Uric Acid, Serum

ADDITIONAL CONDITIONS
Atherosclerosis
Hypercalcemia
Hypertension
Hyperuricemia
Hypoalbuminemia
Myocardial Infarction
Obesity

HYPERGLUCAGON
SYNDROME
Glucagon, Plasma

ADDITIONAL CONDITIONS
Addison's Disease
Cirrhosis
Hypopituitarism

HYPERGLYCEMIA
Chemistry Profile, Blood
Cortisol, Plasma or Serum

ADDITIONAL CONDITIONS
Cancer
Diabetes Mellitus

Glucagon, Plasma
Glucose, Blood
Glucose, 2-Hour Postprandial Serum
Glucose Monitoring Machines,
    Diagnostic
Glucose Tolerance Test, Blood
Glycosylated Hemoglobin, Blood
Growth Hormone, Blood
Insulin Assay, Blood
Ketone Bodies, Blood
Urinalysis, Urine

HYPERGLYCEMIC HYPEROSMOLAR NONKETOTIC COMA (HHNK)

Blood Gases (pH), Arterial, Blood
Glucose, Serum
Hematocrit, Blood
Osmolality, Serum
Osmolality, Urine
Urea Nitrogen, Blood

ADDITIONAL CONDITIONS

Acute Infection
Renal Failure
Steroid Use
Stress
Trauma
Type II Diabetes Mellitus

HYPERINSULINISM

Insulin, Serum
Insulin Assay (RIA), Blood

ADDITIONAL CONDITIONS

Hypoglycemia
Insulinoma

HYPERKALEMIA

Aldosterone, Serum and Urine
Calcium, Total, Serum
Chemistry Profile, Blood
Electrocardiogram, Diagnostic
Electrolyte, Blood
Glucose, Blood
Magnesium, Serum
Potassium, Serum
Potassium, Urine

ADDITIONAL CONDITIONS

Dehydration
Hypercapnia
Hyperlipoproteinemia
Poisoning
Renal Failure

HYPERLIPOPROTEINEMIA

Cholesterol, Blood
Lipid Profile, Blood
Triglycerides, Blood

ADDITIONAL CONDITIONS

Alcoholism
Atherosclerosis
Glycogen Storage Disease
Hepatic Disease
Hypercholesterolemia
Hypothyroidism
Myocardial Infarction
Pancreatitis

HYPERMAGNESEMIA

Anion Gap, Blood
Calcium, Total, Serum
Electrolyte, Blood
Magnesium, Serum
Magnesium, 24-Hour, Urine

ADDITIONAL CONDITIONS

Adrenal Insufficiency
Antacid Abuse (containing Mg^+)
Apnea
Burns
Cathartic Abuse
Diabetic Ketoacidosis
Hypothyroidism
Hypoxia
Rhabdomyolysis
Trauma

HYPERNATREMIA
Cholesterol, Blood
Electrolyte, Blood or Urine
Glucose, Blood
Glucose, Quantitative, 24-Hour, Urine
Osmolality, Serum
Sodium, Plasma, Serum, or Urine
Triglycerides, Blood

ADDITIONAL CONDITIONS
Dehydration
Diabetes Insipidus
Diabetic Ketoacidosis
HHNK
Hypotension
Tachycardia

HYPERPARATHYROIDISM
Alkaline Phosphatase, Serum
Amylase, Serum and Urine
Calcitonin, Plasma or Serum
Calcium, Total, Serum
Calcium, Urine
Chemistry Profile, Blood
Cyclic Adenosine Monophosphate,
    Serum and Urine
Histopathology, Specimen
Magnesium, Serum
Parathyroid Hormone, Blood
Phosphorus, Serum
Phosphorus, Urine

ADDITIONAL CONDITIONS
Adrenal Glands Cancer
Hypercalcemia
Hypertension
Pancreatic Cancer
Pituitary Cancer
Renal Failure
Thyroid Cancer
Uremia
Vitamin D Deficiency

HYPERPHOSPHATEMIA
Calcium, Total, Serum
Creatinine, Serum
Electrolytes, Plasma or Serum
Phosphorus, Serum

ADDITIONAL CONDITIONS
Burns
Cathartic Abuse
Cytoxic Drugs
Hypoparathyroidism
Renal Failure
Rhabdomyolysis

HYPERPITUITARISM (ACROMEGALY OR GIGANTISM)
Adrenocorticotropic Hormone, Serum
Alkaline Phosphatase Isoenzymes,
    Serum
Alkaline Phosphatase, Serum
Calcium, Total, Serum
Calcium, Urine
Follicle-Stimulating Hormone,
    Serum
Glucose, Blood
Growth Hormone, Blood
Hydroxyproline, Total, 24-Hour, Urine
Insulin-Like Growth Factor-I, Blood
Luteinizing Hormone, Blood
Phosphorus, Serum
Prolactin, Serum
Thyroid-Stimulating Hormone,
    Blood

ADDITIONAL CONDITIONS
Adenomas
Amenorrhea
Headaches
Lung Cancer

HYPERSENSITIVITY (ALLERGIC) REACTION
Lymphocyte Transformation Test,
    Blood

ADDITIONAL CONDITIONS
Allergies to Latex Gloves
Dermatitis
Eczema

HYPERTENSION

Aldosterone, Serum and Urine
Angiotensin-Converting Enzyme, Blood
Blood Urea Nitrogen/Creatinine Ratio,
    Blood
Catecholamines, Fractionation-Free,
    Plasma
Catecholamines, Urine
Chemistry Profile, Blood
Complete Blood Count, Blood
Creatinine Clearance, Serum, Urine
Creatinine, Serum
Electrolyte, Blood or Urine
Mean Platelet Volume, Blood
Metanephrines, Total, 24-Hour, Urine
Potassium, Serum
Protein, Quantitative, Urine
Renin, Plasma
Sodium, Plasma, Serum, or Urine
Urea Nitrogen, Plasma or Serum
Uric Acid, Serum
Urinalysis, Urine
Vanillylmandelic Acid, Urine

ADDITIONAL CONDITIONS

Emboli
Emphysema
Encephalopathy
Left Ventricular Heart Disease
Obesity
Oral Contraception Usage
Pericarditis
Pheochromocytoma
Polycythemia
Pregnancy
Renal Disease
Stroke
Vasculitis

HYPERTHERMIA

Blood Culture, Blood
Chest X-Ray, Diagnostic
Chloride, Serum
Complete Blood Count, Blood
Lactic Acid, Blood
Myoglobin, Urine
Potassium, Serum
Sodium, Plasma, Serum, or Urine

ADDITIONAL CONDITIONS

Anesthesia
Fever of Undetermined Origin (FUO)
Liver Abscess
Myocardial Infarction
Pulmonary Emboli
Rheumatic Fever
Sarcoidosis
Seizures
Sepsis
Systemic Lupus Erythematosus (SLE)

HYPERTHYROIDISM
(THYROTOXICOSIS)

Albumin, Serum, Urine, and 24-Hour
    Urine
Calcium, Total, Serum
Chemistry Profile, Blood
Cholesterol, Blood
Hydroxyproline, Total, 24-Hour, Urine
Magnesium, Serum
Mean Platelet Volume, Blood
Thyroid Antimicrosomal Antibody,
    Blood
Thyroid Antithyroglobulin Antibody,
    Serum
Thyroid Function Tests, Blood
Thyroid Scan, Diagnostic
Thyroid-Stimulating Hormone, Blood
Thyroid-Stimulating Hormone,
    Sensitive Assay, Blood
Thyroid-Stimulating Hormone
    Immunoglobulins, Blood
Thyroid Test: Free Thyroxine Index,
    Serum

ADDITIONAL CONDITIONS

Graves' Disease
Hydatidiform Mole
Jodbasedow Disease
Plummer's Disease
Tachycardia

Thyroid Test: Thyroid Hormone
   Binding Ratio, Blood
Thyroid Test: Thyroxine, Blood
Thyroid Test: Thyroxine Free, Serum
Thyroid Test: Triiodothyronine, Blood
Tissue Typing, Blood
Triglycerides, Blood

HYPERVENTILATION
(see Respiratory Alkalosis)

HYPERVOLEMIA
(see Overhydration)

HYPOCALCEMIA
Calcium, Total, Serum
Calcium, Urine
Magnesium, Serum
Parathyroid Hormone, Blood
Phosphorus, Serum

ADDITIONAL CONDITIONS
Burns
Hyperphosphatemia
Hypomagnesemia
Hypoparathyroidism
Liver Failure
Massive Infusion Therapy
Malabsorption
Pancreatitis
Renal Failure
Sepsis
Steroid Use
Thyroid Cancer
Vitamin D Deficiency

HYPOCHROMIC ANEMIA
(see Iron Deficiency Anemia)

HYPOGLYCEMIA
Cortisol, Plasma or Serum
C-Peptide, Serum
Glucagon, Plasma
Glucose, Blood
Glucose-Monitoring Machines,
   Diagnostic
Glucose Tolerance Test, Blood
Insulin Antibody, Blood
Insulin Assay (RIA), Blood
Urinalysis, Urine

ADDITIONAL CONDITIONS
Alcoholism
Bulimia
Following Gastrectomy Surgery
Hyperinsulinism
Pancreatic Cancer

HYPOKALEMIA
Aldosterone, Serum and Urine
Digitoxin, Serum
Digoxin, Serum
Electocardiogram, Diagnostic
Electrolyte, Blood or Urine
pH, Blood
Potassium, Serum
Potassium, Urine
Renin, Plasma

ADDITIONAL CONDITIONS
Alcoholism
Bartter's Syndrome
Burns
Cushing's Syndrome
Diarrhea
Fanconi's Anemia
Hypomagnesemia
Laxative Abuse
Malabsorption
Poisoning
Renal Disease

HYPOMAGNESEMIA
Calcium, Total, Serum
Electrolyte, Blood or Urine
Magnesium, Serum
Magnesium, 24-Hour, Urine
Phosphorus, Serum

ADDITIONAL CONDITIONS
Alcoholism
Aminoglycoside Use
Diabetic Ketoacidosis
Diarrhea
Digitalis Use
Diuretic Use
Hyperaldosteronism
Hypercalcemia
Hyper/Hypothyroidism
Malabsorption
Pancreatitis
Renal Failure

HYPONATREMIA
Cholesterol, Blood
Cortisol, Plasma or Serum
Osmolality, Urine
Sodium, Plasma, Serum, or Urine
Triglycerides, Blood

ADDITIONAL CONDITIONS
Abscess
Adrenocorticoid Deficiency
Burns
Cirrhosis
Congestive Heart Failure
Diuresis
Hypoproteinemia
Hypothyroidism
Nephrosis
Pancreatitis
Peritonitis
Pneumonia
Renal Disease
Syndrome of Inappropriate
    Antidiuretic Hormone Secretion
    (SIADHS)
Tuberculosis

HYPOPARATHYROIDISM
Alkaline Phosphatase, Serum
Calcium, Total, Serum
Calcium, Calculated Ionized, Serum
Calcium, Ionized, Blood
Calcium, 24-Hour, Urine
Chemistry Profile, Blood
Cyclic Adenosine Monophosphate,
    Serum and Urine
Magnesium, Serum
Parathyroid Hormone, Blood
Phosphorus, Serum
Phosphorus, Urine
Uric Acid, Serum
Vitamin D_3, Plasma or Serum

ADDITIONAL CONDITIONS
Addison's Disease
Candidiasis
Diabetes Mellitus
Hypomagnesemia
Pernicious Anemia
Radiation to the Neck
Thyroidectomy

HYPOPHOSPHATEMIA
Calcium, Total, Serum
Chloride, Serum
Magnesium, Serum
Phosphorus, Serum
Sodium, Plasma, Serum, or Urine

ADDITIONAL CONDITIONS
Acromegaly
Chemotherapy Treatment
Hyperglycemia
Hyperparathyroidism
Hypervitaminosis D
Hypokalemia
Hypomagnesemia
Laxative Abuse

Malnutrition
Renal Failure
Steroid Therapy
Stress

HYPOPHYSECTOMY
Complete Blood Count, Blood
Luteinizing Hormone, Blood
Type and Crossmatch, Blood
Urinalysis, Urine

ADDITIONAL CONDITIONS
Acromegaly
Diabetes Mellitus

HYPOPITUITARISM (DWARFISM)
Adrenocorticotropic Hormone,
    Serum
Chromosome Analysis, Blood
Follicle-Stimulating Hormone,
    Serum
Growth Hormone, Blood
Insulin-Like Growth Factor-I, Blood
Luteinizing Hormone, Blood
Zinc, Blood

ADDITIONAL CONDITIONS
Craniopharyngiomas
Headaches
Visual Acuity Loss

HYPOTENSION
Aldosterone, Serum and Urine
Catecholamines, Fractionation-Free,
    Plasma
Catecholamines, Urine
Sodium, Plasma, Serum, or Urine

ADDITIONAL CONDITIONS
Left Ventricular Dysfunction
Myocardial Infarction
Shock

HYPOTHERMIA
Computed Tomography of the Brain,
    Diagnostic
Lactic Acid, Blood
Specific Gravity, Urine
Urea Nitrogen, Plasma or Serum
Urinalysis, Urine

ADDITIONAL CONDITIONS
Alcoholism
Cardiovascular Disease
Frostbite
Hypopituitarism
Malnutrition
Mental Retardation
Myxedema
Raynaud's Disease

HYPOTHYROIDISM (CRETINISM)
(see also Myxedema)
Alkaline Phosphatase, Serum
Chemistry Profile, Blood
Chloride, Sweat, Specimen
Cholesterol, Blood
Complete Blood Count, Blood
Creatine Kinase, Serum
Lactate Dehydrogenase, Blood
Lactate Dehydrogenase Isoenzymes,
    Blood
Lipid Profile, Blood
Red Blood Cell Morphology, Blood
Sodium, Plasma, Serum, or Urine
Thyroid Antimicrosomal Antibody,
    Blood

ADDITIONAL CONDITIONS
Amenorrhea
Constipation
Deafness
Goiter
Myxedema
Thyroiditis
Umbilical Hernia

Thyroid Antithyroglobulin Antibody,
Serum
Thyroid Function Tests, Blood
Thyroid-Stimulating Hormone
(TSH), Blood
Thyroid-Stimulating Hormone, Filter
Paper, Blood
Thyroid-Stimulating Hormone,
Sensitive Assay, Blood
Thyroid Test: Free Thyroxine Index
(FT_4I, T_7), Serum
Thyroid Test: Thyroid Hormone
Binding Ratio, Blood
Thyroid Test: Thyroxin (T_4), Blood
Thyroid Test: Thyroxin (T_4), Free,
Serum

HYPOVOLEMIA

Albumin/Globulin Ratio (A/G Ratio),
Serum
Anion Gap, Blood
Blood Volume, Blood
Complete Blood Count, Blood
Magnesium, Serum
Potassium, Serum
Protein, Total, Serum
Sodium, Plasma, Serum, or Urine
Type and Crossmatch, Blood
Urinalysis, Urine

ADDITIONAL CONDITIONS

Ascites
Bowel Obstruction
Burns
Diabetic Ketosis
Hypotension
Peritonitis
Shock
Tachycardia

HYPOXIA

Bicarbonate, Serum
Blood Gases, Arterial, Blood
Blood Gases, Capillary, Blood
Blood Gases, Venous, Blood
Carbon Dioxide, Partial Pressure,
Blood
Carbon Dioxide, Total Content, Blood
Chest X-Ray, Diagnostic

ADDITIONAL CONDITIONS

Anemia
Carbon Monoxide Poisoning
COPD
Head Trauma
Seizures

HYSTERECTOMY

Complete Blood Count, Blood
Dilation and Curettage, Diagnostic
Hysteroscopy, Diagnostic
Obstetric Sonogram, Diagnostic
Pap Smear, Diagnostic
Potassium, Serum
Prothrombin Time and International
Normalized Ratio, Serum
Sodium, Plasma, Serum, or Urine
Type and Crossmatch, Blood

ADDITIONAL CONDITIONS

Menorrhagia
Uterine Cancer
Uterine Fibroids

IDIOPATHIC THROMBOCYTOPENIA PURPURA (ITP)

Bleeding Time, Duke, Blood
Bleeding Time, Ivy, Blood

ADDITIONAL CONDITIONS

Epistaxis
Hemorrhage
Menorrhagia
Thrombocytopenia

Bone Marrow Biopsy, Diagnostic
Capillary Fragility Test, Diagnostic
Complete Blood Count, Blood
Differential Leukocyte Count,
    Peripheral Blood
Histopathology, Specimen
Mean Platelet Volume, Blood
Platelet Antibody, Blood
Platelet Count, Blood
Red Cell Count, Serum

ILEAL CONDUIT
(see Ostomies)

ILEITIS
(see Crohn's Disease)

IMMUNODEFICIENCY

Acquired Immune Deficiency
    Syndrome (AIDS) Evaluation
    Battery, Diagnostic
Bone Marrow Aspiration Analysis,
    Specimen
Complete Blood Count, Blood
Cytomegalic Inclusion Disease,
    Cytology, Urine
Cytomegalovirus Antibody, Serum
Hepatitis B Core Antibody, Blood
Herpes Cytology, Specimen
Lymph Node Biopsy (Tissue),
    Specimen
Lymphocyte Subset Enumeration,
    Blood
Lymphocyte Transformation Test,
    Blood
Migration Inhibition Test, Blood
Mixed Leukocyte Culture, Specimen
Nocardia Culture, All Sites, Specimen
Oral Cavity Cytology, Specimen
Pneumocystis IFA, Serum
Protein, Electrophoresis, Serum
Rapid Plasma Reagin Test, Blood
T- and B-Lymphocyte Subset Assay,
    Blood
Toxoplasmosis Serology, Serum

ADDITIONAL CONDITIONS

AIDS
Ataxia-Telangiectasia
Cancer
Congenital Immunology Defects
Cytomegalovirus
Diabetes Mellitus
Drugs That Suppress Bone Marrow
Eczema
Hodgkin's Disease
Human Immunodeficiency Virus
Infectious Process
Liver Failure
Post-Transplant
Renal Failure
Sarcoidosis
Sepsis
Silicone Hypersensitivity
Splenectomy
Steroid Use
Thrombocytopenia

IMMUNOGLOBULIN A (IGA) DEFICIENCY

Immunoglobulin A, Serum
Immunoglobulin A Antibodies, Serum

ADDITIONAL CONDITION

Ataxia-Telangiectasia

IMPETIGO

Culture, Skin, Specimen (Bullae for
    Group A Beta-Hemolytic
    Streptococci or Staphylococcus
    aureus)
Gram Stain, Diagnostic

ADDITIONAL CONDITIONS

Fever
Pruritus

IMPOTENCE

Acid Phosphatase, Serum
Alkaline Phosphatase, Serum
Complete Blood Count, Blood
Drug Screen, Blood
Glucose, Blood
Glucose, 2-Hour Postprandial, Serum
Prolactin, Serum
Prostate-Specific Antigen, Serum
Testosterone, Total, Blood

ADDITIONAL CONDITIONS

Acromegaly
Addison's Disease
Arteriosclerosis
Depression
Diabetes Mellitus
Drug Usage
Endocrine Disorders
Hyperthyroidism
Klinefelter's Syndrome
Multiple Sclerosis
Pernicious Anemia
Spinal Cord Injury
Syphilis
Vascular Diseases

INDIGESTION

(see Dyspepsia)

INDUSTRIAL-RELATED DISEASES

Blood Gases, Arterial, Blood
Bronchoscopy, Diagnostic
Chest X-Ray, Diagnostic
Chloride, Serum
Complete Blood Count, Blood
Potassium, Serum
Sedimentation Rate, Erythrocyte, Blood
Sodium, Plasma, Serum, or Urine
Sputum Cytology, Specimen

ADDITIONAL CONDITIONS

Asbestosis
Berylliosis
Byssinosis
Coal Miner's Pneumoconiosis
Siderosis
Silicosis
Talc Pneumoconiosis

INFARCTION

(see Cerebral, Myocardial, or Renal Infarction)

INFECTION

(see Pulmonary, Sepsis, or Urinary Tract Infection)

INFECTIOUS MONONUCLEOSIS

Alkaline Phosphatase, Serum
Antinuclear Antibody, Serum
Aspartate Aminotransferase, Serum
Bilirubin, Total, Serum
Chemistry Profile, Blood
Complete Blood Count, Blood
Cytomegalovirus Antibody, Serum
Differential Leukocyte Count, Peripheral Blood
Epstein-Barr Virus, Serology, Blood
Heterophile Agglutinins, Blood
Lactate Dehydrogenase, Blood
Lactate Dehydrogenase Isoenzymes, Blood
Liver Battery, Serum
Monospot Screen, Blood

ADDITIONAL CONDITIONS

Encephalitis
Epstein-Barr Virus
Fever
Hepatitis
Hyperuricemia
Myocarditis
Splenectomy
Thrombocytopenia

Ornithine Carbamoyltransferase, Blood
Smooth Muscle Antibody, Blood
Tartrate-Resistant Acid Phosphatase,
    Blood
Toxoplasmosis Serology, Serum
Uric Acid, Serum

INFERTILITY
Chromosome Analysis, Blood
Dilation and Curettage, Diagnostic
Estradiol, Serum
Estrogens, Serum and 24-Hour Urine
Histopathology, Specimen
Infertility Screen, Specimen
Laparoscopy, Diagnostic
Luteinizing Hormone, Blood
Progesterone, Serum
Rubin's Test, Diagnostic
Semen Analysis, Specimen
Sims-Huhner Test, Diagnostic

ADDITIONAL CONDITIONS
Amenorrhea
Azoospermia
Endometriosis
Peritubal Adhesions
Sperm Immobilization

INFLAMMATION
Complete Blood Count, Blood
C-Reactive Protein, Serum
Differential Leukocyte Count
    (Neutrophils), Peripheral Blood
Sedimentation Rate, Erythrocyte,
    Blood
Tomography (Site-Specific),
    Diagnostic

ADDITIONAL CONDITIONS
Abscess
Appendicitis
Arthritis
Bronchitis
Cellulitis
Cholecystitis
Conjunctivitis
Diverticulitis
Epiglottitis
Myocarditis
Pelvic Inflammatory Disease
Sinusitis
Spider Bites
Tonsillitis

INFLUENZA
(see also Haemophilus influenzae)
Cold Agglutinin Titer, Serum
Influenza A and B Titer, Blood
Viral Culture, Specimen

ADDITIONAL CONDITIONS
Bronchitis
Fever
Headache
Otitis Media
Pneumonia
Reye's Syndrome
Sinusitis

INSECTICIDE POISONING
Pseudocholinesterase, Plasma

ADDITIONAL CONDITIONS
Convulsions
Dysrhythmias
Seizures

INSOMNIA
Cortisol, Plasma or Serum
Electroencephalogram, Diagnostic
17-Hydroxycorticosteroids, 24-Hour,
    Urine
Oximetry, Diagnostic
Tryptophan, Plasma

ADDITIONAL CONDITIONS
Alcoholism
Depression
Drug Abuse
Rheumatoid Arthritis
Stress

INSULINOMA
Adrenocorticotropic Hormone, Serum
C-Peptide, Serum
Electrolyte, Blood
Gastrin, Serum Glucagon, Plasma
Glucose, Blood
Histopathology, Specimen
Human Chorionic Gonadotropin,
    Beta-Subunit, Serum
Insulin Antibody, Blood
Insulin Assay (RIA), Blood
Vasoactive Intestinal Polypeptide, Blood

ADDITIONAL CONDITIONS
Adenomas
Anxiety
Hypoglycemia
Islet Cell Cancer
Whipple's Disease

INTERMITTENT CLAUDICATION
(see Peripheral Vascular Disease)

INTERVERTEBRAL DISC ABNORMALITIES
Magnetic Resonance Imaging,
    Diagnostic

ADDITIONAL CONDITIONS
Muscle Strain
Neuropathy
Scoliosis
Spinal Cord Compression

INTOXICATION
Alcohol, Blood
Anion Gap, Blood
Bromides, Serum
Cannabinoids, Qualitative, Blood or
    Urine
Drug Screen, Blood
pH, Blood
Toxicology, Drug Screen, Urine
Toxicology, Volatiles Group by GLC,
    Blood or Urine

ADDITIONAL CONDITIONS
Ascites
Ataxia
Delirium Tremens
Encephalopathy
Hepatomegaly

INTRACEREBRAL HEMORRHAGE
(see Hemorrhage)

INTRACRANIAL PRESSURE
Antidiuretic Hormone, Serum
Cerebrospinal Fluid, Routine Analysis,
    Specimen
Computed Tomography of the Brain,
    Diagnostic
Electrolyte, Blood
Specific Gravity, Urine

ADDITIONAL CONDITIONS
Brain Tumor
Cerebral Hemorrhage
Papilledema
Trauma

INTRACRANIAL TUMORS
(see Brain Tumors)

INTRADUCTAL PAPILLOMA (BREAST)
Histopathology, Specimen
Mammography, Diagnostic
Nipple Discharge Cytology, Specimen

ADDITIONAL CONDITIONS
Breast Cancer
Paget's Disease, Breast

INTUSSUSCEPTION
Barium Enema, Diagnostic
Flat Plate X-Ray of Abdomen, Diagnostic
Occult Blood, Stool
Rectal Examination for Mucus and
  Blood, Diagnostic

ADDITIONAL CONDITIONS
Bowel Obstruction
Colon Tumor
Rectal Bleeding

IRON DEFICIENCY ANEMIA (UNCOMPLICATED)
Complete Blood Count, Blood
Ferritin, Serum
Iron, Serum
Mean Platelet Volume, Blood
Total Iron-Binding Capacity, Serum

ADDITIONAL CONDITIONS
Gastrointestinal Bleeding
Hemoglobinuria
Menorrhagia
Pregnancy

ISCHEMIC HEART DISEASE
(see Angina)

ISLET CELL TUMORS
(see Insulinoma)

JAUNDICE
Coombs', Direct, Serum
Coombs', Indirect, Serum
Endoscopic Retrograde Cholangio-
  pancreatography, Diagnostic
Galactose, Screening Test for
  Galactosemia, Urine
Gamma-Glutamyl Transpeptidase, Blood
Hepatitis A Antibody IgM and IgG,
  Blood
Hepatitis B Surface Antigen, Blood
Histopathology, Specimen
Infectious Mononucleosis Screening
  Test, Blood
Leptospira Serodiagnosis, Blood
Leucine Aminopeptidase, Blood
Liver Battery, Serum
Liver Biopsy, Diagnostic
Liver Scan, Diagnostic
Liver Sonogram, Diagnostic
Malaria Smear, Blood
Ornithine Carbamoyltransferase, Blood
Phenobarbital, Plasma or Serum
Red Blood Cell Enzyme Deficiency,
  Screen, Blood
Urobilinogen, Urine

ADDITIONAL CONDITIONS
Alcoholism
Anemia
Cirrhosis
Crigler-Najjar Syndrome
Gilbert's Syndrome
Hepatitis
Infectious Mononucleosis
Liver Cancer
Lymphoma
Pancreatitis
Sarcoidosis
Wilson's Disease

JOCK ITCH
(see Tinea Cruris)

KAPOSI'S SARCOMA
Acquired Immune Deficiency
  Syndrome (AIDS) Evaluation
  Battery, Diagnostic
Biopsy, *Mycobacteria*, Culture

ADDITIONAL CONDITIONS
AIDS
Fever
Gingivitis

Cytomegalovirus Antibody, Serum
Ocular Cytology, Specimen

KERATITIS
Ocular Cytology, Specimen

ADDITIONAL CONDITION
Herpes Simplex Virus

KETOACIDOSIS
Alcohol, Blood
Anion Gap, Blood
Blood Indices (Red Blood Cells), Blood
Chemistry Profile, Blood
Complete Blood Count, Blood
Differential Leukocyte Count,
    Peripheral Blood
Electrolyte, Blood
Glucose, Blood
Ketone Bodies, Blood
Ketone, Semiquantitative, Urine
Magnesium, Serum
Osmolality, Serum
Osmolality, Urine
pH, Blood
Phosphorus, Serum
Potassium, Serum
Red Cell Count, Serum
Salicylate, Blood
Urea Nitrogen, Plasma or Serum
Urinalysis, Urine

ADDITIONAL CONDITIONS
Diabetes Mellitus
Infectious Process
Myocardial Infarction
Trauma

KIDNEY
(see Renal)

KIDNEY STONE
Calcium, Total, Serum
Calcium, Urine
Chemistry Profile, Blood
Creatinine Clearance, Serum, Urine
Cystine, Qualitative, Urine
Electrolyte, Urine
Histopathology, Specimen
Kidney Stone Analysis, Specimen
KUB, Diagnostic
Lithotripsy, Diagnostic
Magnesium, Serum
Magnesium, Urine
Occult Blood, Urine
Oxalate, 24-Hour, Urine
pH, Urine
Phosphorus, Urine
Sodium, Plasma, Serum, or Urine
Uric Acid, Serum
Uric Acid, Urine
Urinalysis, Urine

ADDITIONAL CONDITIONS
de Toni-Franconi Defect
Hyperparathyroidism
Hypervitaminosis D
Metastasis to Bone
Nephritis
Osteoporosis
Renal Tubular Acidosis
Urinary Tract Infection

KIMMELSTIEL-WILSON DISEASE
Creatinine, Serum
Creatinine Clearance, Serum, Urine

ADDITIONAL CONDITIONS
Diabetes Mellitus
Hypertension
Nephrosis

Kidney Biopsy, Specimen
Protein, Urine
Urea Nitrogen, Plasma or Serum

KLINEFELTER'S SYNDROME
Biopsy, Site-Specific (Testes),
  Specimen
Estradiol, Serum
Follicle-Stimulating Hormone, Serum
17-Ketosteroid, Total, 24-Hour, Urine
Luteinizing Hormone, Blood
Oral Cavity Cytology, Specimen
Semen Analysis, Specimen
Testosterone, Total, Blood

ADDITIONAL CONDITIONS
Azoospermia
Gynecomastia
Sterility

KWASHIORKOR
Albumin, Serum, Urine, and 24-Hour
  Urine
Amylase, Serum and Urine
Carotene, Serum
Cholesterol, Blood
Complete Blood Count, Blood
Lipase, Serum
Phospholipids, Serum
Protein, Electrophoresis, Serum
Protein, Total, Serum
Transferrin, Serum
Triglycerides, Blood
Trypsin, Plasma or Serum

ADDITIONAL CONDITIONS
Anorexia Nervosa
Depression
Fistula Draining
Malabsorption
Malnutrition
Nephrosis

LACTOSE INTOLERANCE
d-Xylose Absorption Test, Diagnostic,
  Serum or Urine

ADDITIONAL CONDITION
Malabsorption

LAMBERT EATON SYNDROME
Striational Antibody, Specimen

ADDITIONAL CONDITIONS
Muscle Disease
Oat Cell Carcinoma of Lung

LEAD POISONING
Calcium Disodium EDTA,
  Mobilization Test, 24-Hour, Urine
Coproporphyrin, Urine
Erythrocyte Protopophyrin, Blood
Heavy Metals, Blood and 24-Hour,
  Urine (Urine)
Lead, Blood and Urine
Red Cell Count, Serum
X-Ray of Long Bones (for Increased
  Density), Diagnostic

ADDITIONAL CONDITIONS
Anorexia
Convulsions
Diarrhea
Emphysema
Headache

LEGIONNAIRES' DISEASE
Alkaline Phosphatase, Serum
Brushing Cytology, Specimen,
  Diagnostic
Chest X-Ray, Diagnostic
Histopathology, Specimen

ADDITIONAL CONDITIONS
Emphysema
Endocarditis
Pericarditis

Legionella pneumophila, Culture
Legionella pneumophila, Culture,
   IgM Titer, Blood
Legionella pneumophila, Direct FA
   Smear (Lung), Specimen
Legionnaires' Disease Antibodies,
   Blood
Sputum Cytology, Specimen

LEPROSY (HANSEN'S DISEASE)
Acid-Fast Bacteria, Culture and Stain
Biopsy, Site-Specific, Specimen
Histopathology, Specimen
Immune Complex Assay, Blood
Protein, Total, Serum

ADDITIONAL CONDITIONS
Anemia
Epistaxis
Keratitis
Neuritis
Tattoos

LEPTOSPIROSIS
Alanine Aminotransferase, Serum
Bacterial Serology, Blood
Blood Culture, Blood
Electrolyte, Blood or Urine
Leptospira Culture, Urine
Leptospira Serodiagnosis, Blood

ADDITIONAL CONDITIONS
Fever
Headache
Hypotension
Meningitis
Myocarditis
Renal Failure
Sepsis
Weil's Syndrome

LEUKEMIA
Bone Marrow Biopsy, Diagnostic
Complete Blood Count, Blood
Cryoglobulin, Qualitative, Serum
Immunoelectrophoresis, Serum and
   Urine
Mean Platelet Volume, Blood
Methotrexate, Serum
Muramidase, Serum and Urine
Sudan Black B Stain, Diagnostic
T- and B-Lymphocyte Subset Assay,
   Blood
Tartrate-Resistant Acid Phosphatase,
   Blood
Terminal Deoxynucleotidyl
   Transferase, Diagnostic
Vitamin B_{12}, Serum
Xanthuric Acid, Urine
Zinc, Blood

ADDITIONAL CONDITIONS
Bone Marrow Transplant
Candidiasis
Epistaxis
Fever
Graft-Versus-Host Disease (GVHD)
Joint Pain
Pneumonia
Sepsis

LEUKOCYTOSIS
Bone Marrow Biopsy, Diagnostic
Complete Blood Count, Blood
Differential Leukocyte Count,
   Peripheral Blood
Potassium, Serum

ADDITIONAL CONDITIONS
Infection, Acute
Leukemia
Liver Abscess
Seizure
Sepsis

LEUKOPENIA
Blood Fungus, Culture
Bone Marrow Biopsy, Diagnostic

ADDITIONAL CONDITIONS
Agranulocytosis
Anemia

Complete Blood Count, Blood
Culture (Blood, Ulcerative Lesions,
Urine), Routine, Specimen
Differential Leukocyte Count,
Peripheral Blood
Foreign Body (Catheters or Venous
Access Devices), Routine, Culture
Lymph Node Biopsy, Specimen

Hodgkin's Disease
Malaria
Schistosomiasis
Splenomegaly
Thrombocytopenia
Typhoid
Viral Infections

LEUKORRHEA

Cervical/Vaginal Cytology, Specimen
Complete Blood Count, Blood
Urinalysis, Urine

ADDITIONAL CONDITIONS

Menstruation
Trichomoniasis

LICE

Arthropod Identification, Specimen

ADDITIONAL CONDITIONS

Fever
Typhus

LIVER ABSCESS

Alanine Aminotransferase, Serum
Albumin, Serum, Urine, and 24-Hour
Urine .
Alkaline Phosphatase, Serum
Bilirubin, Direct, Serum
Bilirubin, Total, Serum
Blood Culture, Blood
Liver Battery, Serum
Liver Biopsy, Diagnostic
Liver Scan, Diagnostic
Liver Sonogram, Diagnostic
Prothrombin Time and International
Normalized Ratio, Serum

ADDITIONAL CONDITIONS

Anemia
Diarrhea
Fever
Leukocytosis
Pain, Acute Chest

LIVER CANCER

Alpha-Fetoprotein, Blood
Computed Tomography of the Body
(Liver), Diagnostic
Ki-67 Proliferation Marker, Specimen
Liver Battery, Serum
Liver Biopsy, Diagnostic
Liver Scan, Diagnostic
Liver Sonogram, Diagnostic
5' Nucleotidase, Serum
Ornithine Carbamoyltransferase, Blood

ADDITIONAL CONDITIONS

Ascites
Cachexia
Hepatitis
Hepatomegaly
Jaundice

LIVER DYSFUNCTION

Alanine Aminotransferase, Serum
Alkaline Phosphatase, Serum
Bilirubin, Total, Serum
Gamma-Glutamyl Transpeptidase,
Blood
Leucine Aminopeptidase, Blood
Liver Battery, Serum
Liver Biopsy, Diagnostic
Liver Scan, Diagnostic
Mixing Study (Circulating
Anticoagulants), Plasma
5' Nucleotidase, Serum

ADDITIONAL CONDITIONS

Amyloidosis
Cirrhosis
Galactosemia
Hepatitis
Jaundice
Liver Abscess
Liver Cancer
Sarcoidosis
Schistosomiasis
Syphilis
Tuberculosis
Weil's Syndrome

Ornithine Carbamoyltransferase,
　　Blood
Protein, Urine
Prothrombin Time and International
　　Normalized Ratio, Serum
Striational Antibody, Specimen
Ultrasound, Liver, Diagnostic

LIVER FAILURE
Alanine Aminotransferase, Serum
Albumin, Serum, Urine, and 24-Hour
　　Urine
Albumin/Globulin Ratio, Serum
Alkaline Phosphatase, Serum
Ammonia, Blood
Globulin, Serum
Liver Battery, Serum
5'Nucleotidase, Blood
Paracentesis, Diagnostic
Protein, Total, Serum
Prothrombin Time and International
　　Normalized Ratio, Serum

ADDITIONAL CONDITIONS
Alcoholism
Cancer
Cirrhosis
Hepatitis
Hyperbilirubinemia
Jaundice
Wilson's Disease

LUNG CANCER
Biopsy, Site-Specific (Lung), Specimen
Bone Scan, Diagnostic
Brain Scan, Cerebral Flow and
　　Pathology, Diagnostic
Bronchial Washing, Specimen,
　　Diagnostic
Bronchography, Diagnostic
Bronchoscopy, Diagnostic
Brushing Cytology, Specimen,
　　Diagnostic
CA 15–3, Serum
CA 50, Blood
Chest Tomography, Diagnostic
Chest X-Ray, Diagnostic
Complete Blood Count, Blood
Computed Tomography of the Body
　　(Lung), Diagnostic
Mediastinoscopy, Diagnostic
Mucin-Like Carcinoma-Associated
　　Antigen, Blood
Neuron-Specific Enolase, Serum
Pulmonary Function Test, Diagnostic
Sputum Cytology, Specimen
Striational Antibody, Specimen
Thoracentesis, Diagnostic

ADDITIONAL CONDITIONS
Anemia
Anorexia
COPD
Gynecomastia
Hypercalcemia
Hypoxia
Industrial-Related Diseases
Pleural Effusion
Syndrome of Inappropriate
　　Antidiuretic Hormone Secretion
　　(SIADHS)

LUPOID HEPATITIS
Lupus Panel, Blood

ADDITIONAL CONDITIONS
Chronic Fatigue Syndrome
Liver Disease

LUPUS ERYTHEMATOSUS
Antinuclear Antibody, Serum
Complete Blood Count, Blood

ADDITIONAL CONDITIONS
Leukopenia
Proteinuria

Lupus Panel, Blood
Lupus Test, Blood
Protein, Electrophoresis, Serum
Protein, Total, Serum
Rheumatoid Factor, Blood
Sedimentation Rate, Erythrocyte, Blood

LYME DISEASE
Immunoglobulin G, Serum
Immunoglobulin M, Serum
Lyme Disease Antibody, Blood

ADDITIONAL CONDITIONS
Fever
Headache
Meningitis
Myopericarditis
Pain in Joints
Tick Bite

LYMPHADENITIS
Blood Culture, Blood
Lymph Node Biopsy, Specimen

ADDITIONAL CONDITIONS
Abscess
Cellulitis
Fever

LYMPHANGITIS
Blood Culture, Blood
Wound Culture

ADDITIONAL CONDITIONS
Cat Scratch Disease
Thrombophlebitis

LYMPHOGRANULOMA VENEREUM
Chlamydia Group Titer (Tachoma Titer), Serum
Histopathology, Specimen
Lymphogranuloma Venereum Titer, Blood

ADDITIONAL CONDITIONS
Arthritis
Conjunctivitis
Fever
Headache
Proctitis

LYMPHOMA
Biopsy, Site-Specific, Specimen
Calcium, Total, Serum
Complete Blood Count, Blood
Cytologic Study of Gastrointestinal Tract, Diagnostic
Ki-67 Proliferation Marker, Specimen
Lymph Node Biopsy, Specimen
Mediastinoscopy, Diagnostic
Migration Inhibition Test, Blood
O-Banding (CSF Proteins), Blood
Phosphorus, Serum
Platelet Count, Blood
Potassium, Serum
Proliferation Marker MIB 1–3, Specimen
Tartrate-Resistant Acid Phosphatase, Blood
Uric Acid, Serum
Xanthuric Acid, Urine

ADDITIONAL CONDITIONS
Fever
Lymphadenopathy
Night Sweats

MACROGLOBULINEMIA
(see Waldenström's Macroglobulinemia)

MALABSORPTION
Calcium, Total, Serum
Carotene, Serum
d-Xylose Absorption Test, Diagnostic,
    Serum or Urine
Folic Acid, Serum
Glucose Tolerance Test, Blood
Glucose, 2-Hour Postprandial, Serum
Lipid Profile, Blood
Magnesium, Serum
Phosphorus, Serum
Pyridoxal 5'Phosphate, Plasma
Protein, Total, Serum
Sigmoidoscopy, Diagnostic
Sodium, Plasma, Serum, or Urine
Transferrin, Serum
Trypsin, Plasma or Serum
Trypsin, Stool
Vitamin B_{12}, Serum
Vitamin C, Plasma or Serum

ADDITIONAL CONDITIONS
Anemia
Celiac Sprue
Diarrhea
Hematuria
Hypoalbuminemia
Hypokalemia
Hyponatremia
Malnutrition
Osteomalacia
Tropical Sprue
Ulcerative Colitis
Whipple's Disease

MALARIA
Alanine Aminotransferase, Serum
Alkaline Phosphatase, Serum
Bilirubin, Total, Serum
Blood Indices, Blood
Cold Agglutinin Titer, Serum
Complement, Total, Serum
Complete Blood Count, Blood
Differential Leukocyte Count,
    Peripheral Blood
Liver Battery, Serum
Malaria Smear, Blood
Parasite Screen, Blood
Platelet Count, Blood
Protein, Electrophoresis, Serum
Red Blood Cell Morphology, Blood
Rheumatoid Factor, Blood

ADDITIONAL CONDITIONS
Anemia
Diaphoresis
Fever
Headache
Leukopenia
Mosquito Bite
Urinary Tract Infection

MALIGNANT HYPERTENSION
(see Hypertension)

MALNUTRITION
(see Kwashiorkor and Marasmus)

MANIC-DEPRESSIVE PSYCHOSIS
Cortisol, Plasma or Serum
Lithium, Serum

ADDITIONAL CONDITIONS
Alcoholism
Anorexia Nervosa
Catatonia
Head Injury

MARASMUS
Albumin, Serum, Urine, and 24-Hour
    Urine
Blood Urea Nitrogen/Creatinine
    Ratio, Blood

ADDITIONAL CONDITIONS
Growth Retardation
Hepatomegaly
Hospitalization, Long-Term
Lymphocyte Depletion

Complete Blood Count, Blood
Protein, Electrophoresis, Serum
Protein, Total, Serum
Transferrin, Serum
Vitamin B_6 (Pyridoxine), Plasma

MARFAN'S SYNDROME
Bone Scan, Diagnostic
Echocardiogram, Diagnostic
Hydroxyproline, Total, 24-Hour, Urine
Magnetic Resonance Imaging,
    Diagnostic

ADDITIONAL CONDITIONS
Abortion, Spontaneous
Endocarditis
Kyphoscoliosis
Mitral Valve Prolapse
Myopia

MAROTEAUX-LAMY SYNDROME
Mucopolysaccharides, Qualitative,
    Urine

ADDITIONAL CONDITIONS
Dysrhythmias
Mental Retardation

MEASLES
(see Rubella and Rubeola)

MEGALOBLASTIC ANEMIA
Blood Indices (Red Blood Cells), Blood
Bone Marrow Biopsy, Diagnostic
Complete Blood Count, Blood
Folic Acid, Serum
Folic Acid, Red Blood Cells, Blood
Gastric Analysis, Specimen
Gastric pH, Specimen
Gastrin, Serum
Intrinsic Factor Antibody, Blood
Lactate Dehydrogenase, Blood
Lactate Dehydrogenase Isoenzymes,
    Blood
Parietal Cell Antibody, Blood
Pepsinogen-1 Antibody, Blood
Platelet Count, Blood
Red Blood Cell Morphology, Blood
Reticulocyte Count, Blood
Schilling Test, Diagnostic
Vitamin B_{12}, Serum

ADDITIONAL CONDITIONS
Hyperbilirubinemia
Leukocytosis
Malnutrition
Pernicious Anemia
Vitamin B_{12} Deficiency

MELANOMA
Biopsy, Site-Specific, Specimen
Bone Marrow Aspiration Analysis,
    Specimen
Chest X-Ray, Diagnostic
Computed Tomography of the Body
    (Melanoma Site), Diagnostic
Histopathology, Specimen
Liver Battery, Serum

ADDITIONAL CONDITIONS
Pruritus
Sunburn

MENIERE'S DISEASE
Cerebrospinal Fluid, Protein,
    Specimen
Hearing Test for Loudness-
    Recruitment, Diagnostic

ADDITIONAL CONDITIONS
Head Trauma
Syphilis
Tinnitus
Vertigo

MENINGITIS

Cerebrospinal Fluid, Cytology, Specimen
Cerebrospinal Fluid, Fungus, Culture
Cerebrospinal Fluid, *Mycobacteria,* Culture
Cerebrospinal Fluid, Routine Analysis, Specimen
Computed Tomography of Brain, Diagnostic
Coxsackie A or B Virus Titer, Blood
Cryptococcal Antigen Titer, Serum
Cryptococcal Antigen Titer, Cerebrospinal Fluid (CSF), Specimen
Cryptococcus Antibody Titer, Serum
Gastric Aspirate, Routine, Culture
Herpes Cytology, Specimen
India Ink Preparation, Specimen
Leptospira Serodiagnosis, Blood
Magnetic Resonance Imaging, Diagnostic
O-Banding (CSF Proteins), Plasma
Penicillinase Test, Diagnostic
Sodium, Plasma, Serum, or Urine
Sputum for *Haemophilus* Species, Culture
Toxoplasmosis, Rubella, Cytomegalovirus, Herpes Virus Serology (TORCH), Blood
Viral Culture, Specimen

ADDITIONAL CONDITIONS

AIDS
Arthritis
Convulsions
Fever
Headache
Hydrocephalus
Influenza
Myocarditis
Nephritis
Pneumonia

MENOPAUSE

Biopsy, Site-Specific (Endometrium), Specimen
Bone Scan, Diagnostic
Estradiol, Serum
Estrogens, Serum and 24-Hour Urine
Follicle-Stimulating Hormone, Serum
Hormonal Evaluation, Cytologic, Specimen
17-Ketosteroids, Total, 24-Hour, Urine
Luteinizing Hormone, Blood

ADDITIONAL CONDITIONS

Dyspareunia
Hot Flashes
Night Sweats
Osteoporosis

MENORRHAGIA (HYPERMENORRHEA)

Complete Blood Count, Blood
Cortisol, Plasma or Serum
Estrogens, Serum and 24-Hour Urine
Partial Thromboplastin Time, Plasma
Prothrombin Time and International Normalized Ratio, Serum

ADDITIONAL CONDITIONS

Endometriosis
Hypothyroidism
Menopause
Uterine Cancer

MENSTRUATION

Estrogens, Serum and 24-Hour Urine
Follicle-Stimulating Hormone, Serum
Luteinizing Hormone, Blood

ADDITIONAL CONDITIONS

Anemia
Menorrhagia
Pneumothorax

METABOLIC ACIDOSIS

Blood Gases, Arterial, Blood
Blood Gases, Venous, Blood
Chemistry Profile, Blood
Creatinine, Serum
Dinitrophenylhydrazine Test,
    Diagnostic
Electrolyte, Blood
Glucose, Blood
Salicylate, Blood
Urea Nitrogen, Plasma or Serum
Urinalysis, Urine

ADDITIONAL CONDITIONS

Alcoholic Ketoacidosis
Anoxia
Carbon Monoxide Poisoning
Dehydration
Diabetic Ketoacidosis
Leukemia
Malnutrition
Maple Syrup Urine Disease
Renal Failure
Seizures
Shock

METABOLIC ALKALOSIS

Blood Gases, Arterial, Blood
Electrolyte, Blood
Potassium, Serum
Urinalysis, Urine

ADDITIONAL CONDITIONS

Hypovolemia
Renal Insufficiency
Vomiting

METAL POISONING

Arsenic, Blood
Arsenic, Urine
Cadmium, Serum and 24-Hour
    Urine
Chemistry Profile, Blood
Chromium, Serum
Chromium, Urine
Heavy Metals, Blood and 24-Hour
    Urine
Lead, Blood and Urine
Lithium, Serum
Mercury, Blood
Mercury, 24-Hour Urine
Thallium, Serum or 24-Hour Urine
Urinalysis, Urine
Zinc, Blood

ADDITIONAL CONDITIONS

Ataxia
Coma
Dehydration
Diarrhea
Papilledema
Pulmonary Edema
Renal Failure
Shock
Vomiting

METASTASIS

Acid Phosphatase, Serum
Adrenocorticotropic Hormone,
    Serum
Alkaline Phosphatase, Serum
Alkaline Phosphatase, Heat Stable,
    Serum
Alkaline Phosphatase Isoenzymes,
    Serum
Alpha-Fetoprotein, Blood
Body Fluid Cytology, Specimen
Bone Marrow Biopsy, Diagnostic
Bone Scan, Diagnostic
Bronchial Washing, Specimen,
    Diagnostic
Brushing Cytology, Specimen,
    Diagnostic
CA 15–3, Serum (Breast Metastasis)
Calcium, Total, Serum
Carcinoembryonic Antigen, Serum
Cathepsin-D, Specimen

ADDITIONAL CONDITIONS

Anemia
Ascites
Confusion
Congestive Heart Failure
Dyspnea
Hepatomegaly
Hypercalcemia
Hyperglycemia
Pain, Chronic
Peripheral Edema
Splenomegaly

Cerebrospinal Fluid, Cytology,
  Specimen
Cervical/Vaginal Cytology, Specimen
Chemistry Profile, Blood
Complete Blood Count, Blood
Estradiol Receptor and Progesterone
  Receptor in Breast Cancer,
  Diagnostic
Gamma-Glutamyl Transpeptidase,
  Blood
Gastrin, Serum
Histopathology, Specimen
Human Chorionic Gonadotropin,
  Beta-Subunit, Serum
Magnetic Resonance Imaging,
  Diagnostic
Magnetic Resonance Spectography,
  Diagnostic
Mucin-Like Carcinoma-Associated
  Antigen, Blood
Needle Aspiration, Diagnostic
5'Nucleotidase, Serum
Ocular Cytology, Specimen
Parathyroid Hormone, Blood
Progesterone Receptor Assay, Blood
Serotonin (5-Hydroxytryptamine),
  Plasma
Sputum Cytology, Specimen
Tomography (Site-Specific),
  Diagnostic
Urine Cytology, Urine
Washing Cytology, Specimen

METRORRHAGIA
Cortisol, Plasma or Serum
Estrogens, Serum and 24-Hour
  Urine

MICROCYTIC ANEMIA
Bone Marrow Aspiration Analysis,
  Specimen
Ferritin, Serum
Fetal Hemoglobin, Blood
Heavy Metals, Blood and 24-Hour
  Urine (Urine)
Hemoglobin A_2, Blood
Hemoglobin Electrophoresis, Blood
Iron, Serum
Lead, Blood and Urine
Red Blood Cell Morphology, Blood
Total Iron-Binding Capacity, Serum

MIGRAINE HEADACHES
Arteriogram, Diagnostic
Cerebrospinal Fluid, Glucose,
  Specimen
Cerebrospinal Fluid, Routine
  Analysis, Specimen

ADDITIONAL CONDITIONS
Cervical Cancer
Uterine Cancer

ADDITIONAL CONDITIONS
Dysphagia
Glossitis
Hyperferremia
Thalassemia

ADDITIONAL CONDITIONS
Anorexia
Diplopia
Photophobia
Stress
Vomiting

Cerebrospinal Fluid, Protein,
  Specimen
Computed Tomography of the Brain,
  Diagnostic
Electroencephalogram, Diagnostic
Lumbar Puncture, Diagnostic
Magnetic Resonance Imaging,
  Diagnostic
X-Ray of Skull, Chest, Cervical Spine,
  Diagnostic

MITRAL VALVE REGURGITATION
Echocardiogram, Diagnostic
Transesophageal Sonogram,
  Diagnostic

ADDITIONAL CONDITIONS
Endocarditis
Marfan's Syndrome

MONGOLOIDISM
(see Down Syndrome)

MONILIASIS
(see Vaginitis)

MONONUCLEOSIS
(see Infectious Mononucleosis)

MORQUIO SYNDROME
Mucopolysaccharides, Qualitative,
  Urine

ADDITIONAL CONDITIONS
Dysrhythmias
Mental Retardation

MULTIPLE MYELOMA
Acid Phosphatase, Serum
Albumin, Serum, Urine, and 24-Hour
  Urine
Bence Jones Protein, Urine
Bone Marrow Aspiration Analysis,
  Specimen
Bone Scan, Diagnostic
Calcium, Total, Serum
Complement Components, Serum
Immunoelectrophoresis, Serum and
  Urine
Low-Density Lipoprotein, Blood
Sedimentation Rate, Erythrocyte,
  Blood
T- and B-Lymphocyte Subset Assay,
  Blood
Urinalysis (for Protein), Urine

ADDITIONAL CONDITIONS
Anemia
Hypercalcemia
Osteoporosis
Pathologic Fractures
Renal Failure

MULTIPLE SCLEROSIS
Cerebrospinal Fluid,
  Immunoglobulin G, Specimen
Cerebrospinal Fluid, Myelin Basic
  Protein, Specimen
Cerebrospinal Fluid, Oligoclonal
  Bands, Specimen

ADDITIONAL CONDITIONS
Diplopia
Neuritis
Numbness
Vertigo
Visual Blurring
Weakness

Cerebrospinal Fluid, Protein,
Specimen
Cerebrospinal Fluid, Protein
Electrophoresis, Specimen
Cerebrospinal Fluid, Routine
Analysis, Specimen
Magnetic Resonance Imaging,
Diagnostic
O-Banding (CSF Proteins), Plasma
Somatosensory Evoked Potential,
Diagnostic
Tissue Typing, Blood

MUMPS
Mumps Antibody, Blood

ADDITIONAL CONDITIONS
Meningioencephalitis
Orchiitis
Pancreatitis
Salivary Gland Inflammation

MUSCULAR DYSTROPHY
(see also Duchenne's)
Aldolase, Serum
Aspartate Aminotransferase, Serum
Catecholamines, Fractionation-Free,
Plasma
Creatine, Urine
Creatine Kinase, Serum
Creatine Kinase, Isoenzymes,
Serum
Creatinine, Serum
Electromyogram and Nerve
Conduction Studies, Diagnostic
Lactate Dehydrogenase, Blood
Metanephrines, Total, 24-Hour, Urine
Muscle Biopsy, Specimen
Myoglobin, Serum and Qualitative,
Urine

ADDITIONAL CONDITIONS
Cataracts
Diabetes Mellitus
Dysrhythmias
Myotonia
Testicular Atrophy

MYASTHENIA GRAVIS
Acetylcholine Receptor Antibody,
Serum
Cerebrospinal Fluid,
Immunoglobulin G Ratios and
Immunoglobulin G Index,
Specimen
Electromyogram and Nerve
Conduction Studies, Diagnostic
Electromyogram and Nerve
Conduction (Electromyelogram)
Studies, Diagnostic
Metanephrines, Total, 24-Hour, Urine
Parietal Cell Antibody, Blood
Spirometry, Diagnostic
Striational Antibody, Specimen
Thyroid Antimicrosomal Antibody,
Blood
Thyroid Profile, Blood
Tissue Typing, Blood

ADDITIONAL CONDITIONS
Diplopia
Ptosis
Thyrotoxicosis

MYCOSES

Gastric Cytology, Specimen
Sputum Cytology, Specimen

ADDITIONAL CONDITIONS

Abscess
Dyspnea

MYOCARDIAL CONDUCTION DEFECT

Cardiac Enzymes/Isoenzymes, Blood
Chemistry Profile, Blood
Creatine Kinase, Serum
Creatine Kinase, Isoenzymes, Serum
Digitoxin, Serum
Digoxin, Serum
Electrocardiogram, Diagnostic
Electrophysiologic Study, Diagnostic
Lactate Dehydrogenase, Blood
Lactate Dehydrogenase, Isoenzymes, Blood
Lidocaine, Serum
Procainamide, Serum
Quinidine, Serum
Signal-Averaged Electrocardiography, Diagnostic

ADDITIONAL CONDITIONS

Beta Blockade
Calcium Channel Blockade
Congestive Heart Failure

MYOCARDIAL INFARCTION (MI)

Activated Coagulation Time, Automated, Blood
Anticardiolipin Antibody, Serum
Antimyocardial Antibody, Serum
Aspartate Aminotransferase, Serum
Cardiac Catheterization, Diagnostic
Cardiac Enzymes/Isoenzymes, Blood
Cardiac Output, Diagnostic
Chemistry Profile, Blood
Coronary Intravascular Ultrasound, Diagnostic
C-Reactive Protein, Serum
Creatine Kinase, Serum
Creatine Kinase, Isoenzymes, Serum
D-Dimer Test, Blood
Digitoxin, Serum
Digoxin, Serum
Disopyramide Phosphate, Serum
Echocardiogram, Diagnostic
Electrocardiogram, Diagnostic
Glucose, Blood
Heart Scan, Diagnostic
Hydroxybutyrate Dehydrogenase, Blood
Lactate Dehydrogenase, Blood
Lactate Dehydrogenase Isoenzymes, Blood
Lidocaine, Serum
Low-Density Lipoprotein, Blood
Myoglobin, Qualitative, Urine and Serum
Persantine-Sestamibi Stress Test and Scan, Diagnostic

ADDITIONAL CONDITIONS

Angina Pectoris
Aortic Stenosis
Atherosclerosis
Chest Wall Trauma
Congestive Heart Failure
Diabetes Mellitus
Dissecting Aortic Aneurysm
Duodenal Ulcer
Esophageal Spasm
Esophagitis
Gallbladder Disease
Hiatal Hernia
Hypercholesterolemia
Hypertension
Hypertriglyceridemia
Hyperuricemia
Hypoalbuminemia
Hyponatremia
Metabolic Acidosis
Mitral Valve Prolapse
Muscular Strain
Peptic Ulcer
Pericarditis
Pulmonary Embolus
Shock
Stress
Thrombosis
Vasculitis

Positron Emission Tomography,
    Diagnostic
Procainamide, Serum
Propranolol, Blood
Quinidine, Serum
Signal-Averaged Electrocardiography,
    Diagnostic
Stress Test, Pharmacologic, Diagnostic
Stress/Exercise Test, Diagnostic
Troponin I (cTn-I), Serum
Troponin T (cTn-T), Serum

MYOCARDITIS

Antimyocardial Antibody, Serum
Antinuclear Antibody, Serum
Antistreptolysin-O Titer, Serum
Aspartate Aminotransferase, Serum
Blood Indices (Red Blood Cells, MCV),
    Blood
Cardiac Enzymes/Isoenzymes, Blood
Complete Blood Count, Blood
Coxsackie A or B Virus Titer, Blood
Creatine Kinase, Serum
Creatine Kinase, Isoenzymes, Serum
Differential Leukocyte Count,
    Peripheral Blood
Echocardiogram, Diagnostic
Histopathology, Specimen
Transesophageal Sonogram, Diagnostic

ADDITIONAL CONDITIONS

Congestive Heart Failure
Q Fever
Rocky Mountain Spotted Fever
Toxoplasmosis
Trichinosis
Typhus
Vasculitis

MYOCLONUS

Computed Tomography of the Brain,
    Diagnostic
Electroencephalogram, Diagnostic
Magnetic Resonance Imaging,
    Diagnostic

ADDITIONAL CONDITIONS

Creutzfeldt-Jakob Disease
Encephalopathy
Epilepsy
Ramsay-Hunt Syndrome
Seizures

MYXEDEMA
(HYPOTHYROIDISM)

Alkaline Phosphatase, Serum
Chemistry Profile, Blood
Chloride, Sweat, Specimen
Cholesterol, Blood
Complete Blood Count, Blood
Creatine Kinase, Serum
Creatine, Urine
Electrocardiogram, Diagnostic
Lactate Dehydrogenase, Blood
Lactate Dehydrogenase Isoenzymes,
    Blood
Lipid Profile, Blood
Red Blood Cell Morphology, Blood
Sodium, Plasma, Serum, or Urine
Thyroid Antimicrosomal Antibody,
    Blood
Thyroid Antithyroglobulin Antibody,
    Serum
Thyroid Function Tests, Blood

ADDITIONAL CONDITIONS

Anemia
Bradycardia
Coma
Constipation
Fatigue
Hoarseness
Menorrhagia
Thyroiditis

Thyroid-Stimulating Hormone, Blood
Thyroid-Stimulating Hormone,
    Sensitive Assay, Blood
Thyroid Test: Free Thyroxine Index
    (FT$_4$I, T$_7$), Serum
Thyroid Test: Thyroid Hormone
    Binding Ratio, Blood
Thyroid Test: Thyroxine, Blood
Thyroid Test: Thyroxine, Free, Serum

NARCOTICS
(see Drug Abuse)

NEOPLASIA
(see Tumors)

NEPHRECTOMY
Aspartate Aminotransferase, Serum
Complete Blood Count, Blood
Creatinine, Serum
Erythropoietin, Serum
Lactate Dehydrogenase, Blood
Type and Crossmatch, Blood
Urea Nitrogen, Plasma or Serum
Urinalysis, Urine

ADDITIONAL CONDITIONS
Glomerulonephritis
Kidney Cancer
Pyelonephritis

NEPHRITIS
Anti-DNA, Serum
Kidney Sonogram, Diagnostic

ADDITIONAL CONDITIONS
Dyspnea
Gout
Hemoptysis

NEPHROLITHIASIS
Calcium, Total, Serum
Calcium, Urine
Chemistry Profile, Blood
Creatinine Clearance, Urine
Cystine, Qualitative, Urine
Electrolyte, Blood or Urine
Histopathology, Specimen
Kidney Sonogram, Diagnostic
Kidney Stone Analysis, Specimen
Magnesium, Serum
Magnesium, 24-Hour, Urine
Occult Blood, Urine
Oxalate, Urine
pH, Urine
Phosphorus, Urine
Uric Acid, Serum
Uric Acid, Urine
Urinalysis, Urine

ADDITIONAL CONDITIONS
Fanconi's Syndrome
Gouty Arthritis
Nephrocalcinosis
Osteoporosis
Renal Tubular Acidosis
Sarcoidosis

NEPHROSCLEROSIS
Complete Blood Count, Blood
Creatinine, Serum
Urea Nitrogen, Plasma or Serum
Urinalysis, Urine

ADDITIONAL CONDITIONS
Hypertension
Papilledema
Renal Failure

NEPHROSIS
Albumin, Serum, Urine, and 24-Hour
  Urine
Antinuclear Antibody, Serum
C3 Complement, Serum
C4 Complement, Serum
Creatinine, Serum
Creatinine Clearance, Serum, Urine
Kidney Biopsy, Specimen
Kidney Sonogram, Diagnostic
Protein, Electrophoresis, Serum
Urea Nitrogen, Plasma or Serum
Urinalysis, Urine

ADDITIONAL CONDITIONS
Amyloidosis
Glomerulonephritis

NEPHROTIC SYNDROME
Albumin, Serum, Urine, and 24-Hour
  Urine
Albumin/Globulin Ratio, Serum
Cholesterol, Blood
Creatinine Clearance, Serum, Urine
Electrolyte, Blood or Urine
Fat, Urine
Glucose Tolerance Test, Blood
Glucose, 2-Hour Postprandial, Serum
Kidney Biopsy, Specimen
Kidney Sonogram, Diagnostic
Lipid Profile, Blood
Phosphorus, Serum
Protein, Electrophoresis, Serum
Protein, Electrophoresis, Urine
Protein, Semiquantitative, Urine
Protein, Total, Serum
Sodium, Plasma, Serum, or Urine
Transferrin, Serum
Triglycerides, Blood
Urea Nitrogen, Plasma or Serum
Urinalysis, Urine

ADDITIONAL CONDITIONS
Amyloidosis
Edema
Glomerulonephritis
Heavy Metal Poisoning
Hepatitis B
Hyperlipidemia
Hypoalbuminemia
Syphilis
Systemic Lupus Erythematosus

NEUROBLASTOMA
Bone Scan, Diagnostic
Computed Tomography of the Body
  (Abdomen/Chest), Diagnostic
Homovanillic Acid, 24-Hour, Urine
Magnetic Resonance Imaging,
  Diagnostic
Magnetic Resonance Spectography,
  Diagnostic
Neuron-Specific Enolase, Serum
Vanillylmandelic Acid, Urine

ADDITIONAL CONDITIONS
Diarrhea
Malabsorption
von Recklinghausen's Disease

NEURODEGENERATION
Magnetic Resonance Spectography,
  Diagnostic

ADDITIONAL CONDITIONS
Amyotrophic Lateral Sclerosis (ALS)
Multiple Sclerosis

NEUROFIBROMATOSIS
Biopsy, Site-Specific (Skin, Nerves),
  Specimen

ADDITIONAL CONDITIONS
Bone Cysts
Glioma
Hydrocephalus

Pheochromocytoma
Sarcoma
Scoliosis

NEUROGENIC PULMONARY EDEMA
(see Pulmonary Edema)

NEUROPATHY
Electromyogram and Nerve
    Conduction Studies, Diagnostic
Electron Microscopy, Diagnostic (for
    Nerve Tissue)
Glucose, Blood
Glucose, 2-Hour Postprandial, Serum
Histopathology, Specimen
Lead, Blood and Urine
Nerve Biopsy, Diagnostic
Nerve Conduction Studies,
    Diagnostic
Protoporphyrin, Free Erythrocyte,
    Blood
Vitamin E_1, Serum

ADDITIONAL CONDITIONS
Alcoholism
Amyloidosis
Arthritis, Rheumatoid
Cancer
Charcot-Marie-Tooth Disease
Diabetes Mellitus
Guillain-Barré Syndrome
Leprosy
Multiple Myeloma
Sarcoidosis
Uremia

NEUROSYPHILIS
(see Syphilis)

NIEMANN-PICK DISEASE
Sphingomyelinase, Diagnostic

ADDITIONAL CONDITIONS
Hepatosplenomegaly
Lymphadenopathy

NONTROPICAL SPRUE
(see Celiac Sprue)

OBESITY
Cholesterol, Blood
Glucose, Blood
Insulin-Like Growth Factor-I, Blood
Thyroid Test: Thyroxine, Blood
Thyroid Test: Triiodothyronine, Blood

ADDITIONAL CONDITIONS
Asthma
Cerebrovascular Accident
Diabetes Mellitus
Hypercholesterolemia
Hyperlipidemia
Hypertension

OBSTRUCTION, BOWEL
Alkaline Phosphatase, Serum
Amylase, Serum and Urine
Barium Enema, Diagnostic
Chloride, Serum
Complete Blood Count, Blood
Doppler Ultrasound Flow Studies,
    Diagnostic
KUB, Diagnostic
Occult Blood, Stool
Potassium, Serum
Sigmoidoscopy, Diagnostic
Sodium, Plasma, Serum, or Urine
Urinalysis, Urine

ADDITIONAL CONDITIONS
Colon Cancer
Constipation
Hirschsprung's Disease
Paralytic Ileus

OBSTRUCTIVE JAUNDICE
(see Jaundice)

OCCLUSION, ACUTE ARTERIAL
Arteriogram, Diagnostic
Blood Gases, Arterial, Blood
Complete Blood Count, Blood
Glucose, Blood
Magnetic Resonance Angiography, Diagnostic
Partial Thromboplastin Time, Plasma
Prothrombin Time and International Normalized Ratio, Serum

ADDITIONAL CONDITIONS
Arteriosclerosis
Buerger's Disease
Lymphedema
Raynaud's Disease
Syphilis
Thrombosis
Trauma

ORGANIC BRAIN SYNDROME
Adrenocorticotropic Hormone, Serum
Calcium, Total, Serum
Glucose, Blood
Potassium, Serum
Red Cell Count, Serum
Thyroid-Stimulating Hormone, Blood

ADDITIONAL CONDITIONS
Alzheimer's Disease
Amyotrophic Lateral Sclerosis (ALS)
Anxiety
Cognitive Impairment
Dementia
Depression
Drug Withdrawal
Hydrocephalus
Multiple Sclerosis
Thyrotoxicosis
Wilson's Disease

ORTHOSTATIC HYPOTENSION
Catecholamines, Fractionation-Free, Plasma

ADDITIONAL CONDITIONS
Addison's Disease
Aldosteronism
Diabetes Mellitus
Pheochromocytoma

OSTEOARTHRITIS
(see Arthritis, Osteo)

OSTEOMALACIA
Alkaline Phosphatase, Serum
Bone Scan, Diagnostic
Calcium, Total, Serum
Calcium, Urine
Parathyroid Hormone, Blood
Phosphorus, Serum
Vitamin D_3, Plasma or Serum

ADDITIONAL CONDITIONS
Hyperparathyroidism
Hypocalcemia
Hypokalemia
Renal Tubular Nephrosis
Rickets

OSTEOMYELITIS
Blood Culture, Blood
Complete Blood Count, Blood
Sedimentation Rate, Erythrocyte, Blood

ADDITIONAL CONDITIONS
Drug Abuse
Fever
Pain in Bone
Thrombosis

OSTEOPOROSIS
Bone Scan, Diagnostic
Calcium, Total, Serum

ADDITIONAL CONDITIONS
Anorexia Nervosa
Backache

Cortisol, Plasma or Serum
Estradiol, Serum
Estrogens, Serum and 24-Hour Urine
Glucose, Blood
Phosphorus, Serum
Prolactin, Serum
Protein, Electrophoresis, Urine

Cushing's Syndrome
Hypopituitarism
Leukemia
Malabsorption
Menopause
Multiple Myeloma
Pain in Bone

OSTOMIES
Chloride, Serum
Complete Blood Count, Blood
Potassium, Serum
Sodium, Plasma, Serum, or Urine
Type and Crossmatch, Blood
Urinalysis (from Ileal Conduit), Urine

ADDITIONAL CONDITIONS
Bladder Cancer
Colitis
Colon Cancer
Crohn's Disease
Obstruction, Intestine

OTITIS MEDIA
Biopsy, Anaerobic, Culture
Complete Blood Count, Blood
Ear, Routine, Culture
Gamma Globulin (IgG; Quantitative
    IgG), Plasma
Sputum for *Haemophilus* Species,
    Culture

ADDITIONAL CONDITIONS
Cholesteatoma
Mastoiditis
Meningitis
Upper Respiratory Infection

OVARIAN CANCER
Mucin-Like Carcinoma-Associated
    Antigen, Blood
Obstetric Sonogram, Diagnostic
OCA-125 Antigen, Serum
Urinary Gonadotropin Peptide, Urine

ADDITIONAL CONDITIONS
Ascites
Pain in the Back

OVARIAN FUNCTION TESTS
Androstenedione, Serum
Estradiol, Serum
Estrogens, Serum and 24-Hour Urine
Follicle-Stimulating Hormone, Serum
Hormonal Evaluation, Cytologic,
    Specimen
17-Hydroxyprogesterone, Blood
17-Ketosteroids, Total, 24-Hour, Urine
Luteinizing Hormone, Blood
Pregnanetriol, Urine
Progesterone, Serum

ADDITIONAL CONDITIONS
Abscess, Ovarian
Dysmenorrhea
Hirsutism
Ovarian Cancer

OVERDOSE
(see Poisonings)

OVERHYDRATION
Albumin, Serum, Urine, and 24-Hour
    Urine
Complete Blood Count, Blood
Osmolality, Serum
Osmolality, Urine
Protein, Total, Serum
Sodium, Plasma, Serum, or Urine
Urinalysis, Urine

ADDITIONAL CONDITIONS
Ascites
Congestive Heart Failure
Renal Failure
SIADHS

OVULATION
Progesterone, Serum

ADDITIONAL CONDITION
Infertility

PAGET'S DISEASE, BONE
Acid Phosphatase, Serum
Alkaline Phosphatase, Serum
Bone X-Ray, Diagnostic
Calcium, Total, Serum
Calcium, Urine
Hydroxyproline, Total, 24-Hour, Urine
Phosphorus, Urine

ADDITIONAL CONDITIONS
Fractures
Kyphosis
Pain in Bones

PAGET'S DISEASE, BREAST
Biopsy, Site-Specific (Breast),
    Specimen
Mammography, Diagnostic

ADDITIONAL CONDITIONS
Pruritus
Ulceration

PAIN, ABDOMINAL
Amylase, Serum and Urine
Computed Tomography of the Body
    (Abdomen), Diagnostic
Glucose, Blood
KUB, Diagnostic
Lipase, Serum
Potassium, Serum
Sedimentation Rate, Erythrocyte,
    Blood
Sodium, Plasma, Serum, or Urine
Urinalysis, Urine

ADDITIONAL CONDITIONS
Abscess
Appendicitis
Ascites
Cholelithiasis
Colitis
Colon Cancer
Menstruation
Paralytic Ileus
Pelvic Inflammatory Disease (PID)
Q Fever

PAIN, ACUTE
Complete Blood Count, Blood
Glucose, Blood
Sedimentation Rate, Erythrocyte, Blood
Urinalysis, Urine
X-Ray, Diagnostic

ADDITIONAL CONDITIONS
Aneurysm
Migraine Headache
Trauma
Tumor

PAIN, BACK
Calcium, Total, Serum
Complete Blood Count, Blood
Myelogram, Diagnostic
Phosphorus, Serum
Red Blood Cell Morphology, Blood
Rheumatoid Factor, Blood
Sedimentation Rate, Erythrocyte, Blood
Urinalysis, Urine
X-Ray, Diagnostic

ADDITIONAL CONDITIONS
Arthritis
Disk Degeneration, Spine
Metastasis
Osteomyelitis
Ovarian Cancer
Prostatitis
Vascular Aneurysm

PAIN, CHEST
*(see Angina, Myocardial Infarction,
Pleurisy, or Pneumonia)*

PAIN, CHRONIC
Complete Blood Count, Blood
C-Reactive Protein, Serum
Platelet Count, Blood

ADDITIONAL CONDITIONS
Arthritis
Cancer
Disk Degeneration, Spine

Rheumatoid Factor, Blood
Sedimentation Rate, Erythrocyte,
    Blood
Serotonin, Plasma
Sickle Cell Test, Blood
Thermography, Diagnostic
Urea Nitrogen, Plasma or Serum
Urinalysis, Urine
X-Ray, Diagnostic

Nerve Root Irritation/Compression
Reflex Sympathetic Dystrophy
Sickle Cell Anemia

PAIN, MUSCLE AND BONE
Aspartate Aminotransferase, Serum
Bone Scan, Diagnostic
Calcium, Total, Serum
Complete Blood Count, Blood
Creatine Kinase, Serum
Muscle Biopsy, Specimen
Phosphorus, Serum
Thyroid Test: Thyroxine, Blood
Thyroid Test: Triiodothyronine, Blood
Uric Acid, Serum

ADDITIONAL CONDITIONS
Cerebral Palsy
Hypothyroidism
Muscular Dystrophy
Poliomyelitis
Trichinosis

PAIN, VASCULAR
Cerebrospinal Fluid, Routine Analysis,
    Specimen
Complete Blood Count, Blood
Glucose, Blood
Partial Thromboplastin Time, Plasma
Platelet Count, Blood
Prothrombin Time and International
    Normalized Ratio, Serum
Urinalysis, Urine

ADDITIONAL CONDITIONS
Atherosclerosis
Peripheral Vascular Disease
Thrombosis
Vasculitis

PALPITATIONS, HEART
Alcohol, Blood
Blood Gases, Arterial, Blood
Cardiac Catheterization, Diagnostic
Cholesterol, Blood
Complete Blood Count, Blood
Creatine Kinase, Serum
Echocardiogram, Diagnostic
Electrocardiogram, Diagnostic
Stress Test, Diagnostic
Thyroid Test: Thyroxine, Blood
Thyroid Test: Triiodothyronine, Blood

ADDITIONAL CONDITIONS
Anemia
Anxiety
Cardiomyopathy
Dysrhythmias
Exercise
Syncope
Thyrotoxicosis

PANCREATIC CARCINOMA (OR CANCER)
Amylase, Serum and Urine
CA 19–9, Blood
CA 50, Blood
Computed Tomography of Body
    (Pancreas), Diagnostic
Endoscopic Retrograde
    Cholangiopancreatography,
    Diagnostic
Glucose, Blood

ADDITIONAL CONDITIONS
Diabetes Mellitus
Diarrhea
Jaundice
Pain, Abdominal
Thrombophlebitis

Lipase, Serum
Occult Blood, Stool
Pancreas Sonogram, Diagnostic
Urobilinogen, Urine

PANCREATIC CHOLERA
Amylase, Serum and Urine
Lipase, Serum
Vasoactive Intestinal Polypeptide,
    Blood

ADDITIONAL CONDITIONS
Anemia
Diabetes Mellitus
Hypoaminoacidemia
Skin Rash

PANCREATIC ISLET CELL LESION
Gastrin, Serum
Glucagon, Plasma
Insulin Assay, Blood
Vasoactive Intestinal Polypeptide,
    Blood

ADDITIONAL CONDITIONS
Anemia
Diabetes Mellitus
Hypochlorhydria
Malabsorption

PANCREATIC TRAUMA
Amylase, Serum and Urine
Complete Blood Count, Blood
Glucose, Blood
Lipase, Serum
Peritoneal Fluid Analysis,
Specimen
Urinalysis, Urine

ADDITIONAL CONDITIONS
Anemia
Hyperglycemia
Jaundice

PANCREATITIS
Albumin, Serum, Urine, and 24-Hour
    Urine
Amylase, Serum and Urine
Blood Indices (Red Blood Cells),
    Blood
Body Fluid, Amylase, Specimen
Calcium, Total, Serum
Carotene, Serum
Chemistry Profile, Blood
Complete Blood Count, Blood
Differential Leukocyte Count,
    Peripheral Blood
Endoscopic Retrograde
    Cholangiopancreatography,
    Diagnostic
Gamma-Glutamyl Transpeptidase,
    Blood
Glucose, Blood
Histopathology, Specimen
Leucine Aminopeptidase, Blood
Lipase, Serum
Lipid Profile, Blood
Magnesium, Serum
Methemoglobin, Blood
Protein Electrophoresis, Serum
Triglycerides, Blood
Trypsin, Plasma or Serum
Trypsin, Stool

ADDITIONAL CONDITIONS
Alcoholism
Hypercalcemia
Hyperglycemia
Hyperlipidemia
Hyperuricemia
Hypoalbuminemia
Pleural Effusion
Trauma, Abdominal
Vasculitis

PANIC DISORDER

Computed Tomography of the Brain,
 Diagnostic
Echocardiogram, Diagnostic
Electrocardiogram, Diagnostic
Stress/Exercise Test, Diagnostic
Upper Gastrointestinal Series,
 Diagnostic

ADDITIONAL CONDITIONS

Alcoholism
Depression
Drug Abuse
Mitral Valve Prolapse
Phobias
Tachycardia
Sleep Disorders

PARACENTESIS

Paracentesis, Diagnostic

ADDITIONAL CONDITION

Ascites

PARALYTIC ILEUS

Chloride, Serum
Flat Plate X-Ray of Abdomen,
 Diagnostic
Potassium, Serum
Sodium, Plasma, Serum, or Urine

ADDITIONAL CONDITIONS

Hemorrhage
Pain, Abdominal
Pancreatitis
Peritonitis
Spinal Cord Injury

PARKINSON'S DISEASE

Haloperidol, Serum
Phenothiazines (Chlorpromazine,
 Compazine, Fluphenazine, Mellaril,
 Mesoridazine, Prochlorperazine,
 Prolixin, Serentil, Stelazine,
 Thioridazine, Thorazine,
 Trifluoperazine), Blood
Reserpine, Serum

ADDITIONAL CONDITIONS

Brain Tumor
Carbon Monoxide Poisoning
Seborrhea
Tremors

PAROXYSMAL HYPERTENSION

(see Pheochromocytoma)

PATENT DUCTUS ARTERIOSUS

Blood Gases, Arterial, Blood
Cardiac Catheterization, Diagnostic
Chest X-Ray, Diagnostic
Echocardiogram, Diagnostic
Electrocardiogram, Diagnostic
Transesophageal Sonogram, Diagnostic

ADDITIONAL CONDITIONS

Left Ventricular Failure
Pulmonary Hypertension

PELVIC INFLAMMATORY DISEASE (PID)

Actinomyces, Culture
Biopsy, Anaerobic, Culture
Biopsy, *Mycobacteria,* Culture
Body Fluid, Anaerobic, Culture
Chlamydia Culture
Endometrium, Anaerobic, Culture
Fluorescent Treponemal Antibody-
 Absorbed Double-Stain Test, Serum
Genital, *Candida albicans,* Culture
Genital, *Neisseria gonorrhoeae,*
 Culture
Genital, Routine, Culture

ADDITIONAL CONDITIONS

Abscess
Chlamydia
Dysmenorrhea
Endometriosis
Gonorrhea
Infertility
Pain, Abdomen
Salpingitis

Histopathology, Specimen
Laparoscopy, Diagnostic
Obstetric Sonogram, Diagnostic
Sedimentation Rate, Erythrocyte,
    Blood
Venereal Disease Research Laboratory
    Test, Serum
Wound Culture

PEMPHIGUS

Brushing Cytology, Specimen,
    Diagnostic
Fibroblast Skin Culture
Histopathology, Specimen
Immunofluorescence, Skin Biopsy,
    Specimen
Oral Cavity Cytology, (Scrape)
    Specimen
Pemphigus Antibodies, Blood

ADDITIONAL CONDITIONS

Pneumonia
Septicemia
Shock
Toxemia

PEPTIC ULCER

ABO Group and Rh Type, Blood
Amylase, Serum and Urine
Brushing Cytology, Specimen,
    Diagnostic
Campylobacter-Like-Organism Test,
    Specimen
Complete Blood Count, Blood
Gastric Analysis, Specimen
Gastric pH, Specimen
Gastrin, Serum
Gastroscopy, Diagnostic
Helicobacter pylori, Quick Office
    Serology, Serum
Helicobacter pylori Titer, Blood
Histopathology, Specimen
Occult Blood, Stool
Type and Crossmatch, Blood
Urea Breath Test, Diagnostic
Washing Cytology, Specimen

ADDITIONAL CONDITIONS

Burns
Duodenal Ulcer
Gastric Ulcer
Gastrinoma
Gastritis
Pain, Epigastric
Stress
Zollinger-Ellison Syndrome

PERICARDITIS

Anti-DNA, Serum
Antinuclear Antibody, Serum
Body Fluid, Routine, Culture
Chest X-Ray, Diagnostic
Coxsackie A or B Virus Titer, Blood
C-Reactive Protein, Serum
Echocardiogram, Diagnostic
Electrocardiogram, Diagnostic
Histopathology, Specimen
Pericardiocentesis, Diagnostic
Sedimentation Rate, Erythrocyte, Blood

ADDITIONAL CONDITIONS

Aortic Murmur
Congestive Heart Failure
Dysrhythmias
Infection
Mitral Valve Murmur
Myocardial Infarction
Neoplastic Disease
Radiation Therapy
Tachycardia
Trauma
Uremia

PERIPHERAL NEUROPATHY

Electromyogram and Nerve
    Conduction (Electromyelogram)
    Studies, Diagnostic

ADDITIONAL CONDITIONS

Arteritis
Arthritis, Rheumatoid
Brachial Plexopathy

Glucose, Blood
Glucose, 2-Hour Postprandial, Serum
Glutethimide, Blood
Heavy Metals, Blood and 24-Hour
 Urine (Urine)
Histopathology, Specimen

Brain Tumor
Diabetes Mellitus
Guillain-Barré Syndrome
Leprosy
Sarcoidosis
Uremia

PERIPHERAL VASCULAR DISEASE (PVD)
Ankle-Brachial Index, Diagnostic
Antiphospholipid Antibodies, Serum
Cholesterol, Blood
Doppler Ultrasound Flow Studies,
 Diagnostic
Prothrombin Time and International
 Normalized Ratio, Serum

ADDITIONAL CONDITIONS
Arteriosclerosis
Hypercholesterolemia
Hyperlipidemia
Obesity

PERITONITIS
Abscess, Anaerobic Culture
Body Fluid, Amylase, Specimen
Body Fluid, Anaerobic, Culture
Body Fluid, Fungus, Culture
Body Fluid, *Mycobacteria,* Culture
Body Fluid, Routine, Culture
Body Fluid Analysis, Cell Count,
 Specimen
Body Fluid Cytology, Specimen
Cerebrospinal Fluid, Lactic Acid,
 Specimen
Complete Blood Count, Blood
C-Reactive Protein, Serum
Genital, *Candida albicans,* Culture
Genital, *Neisseria gonorrhoeae,*
 Culture
Genital, Routine, Culture
Histopathology, Specimen
KUB, Diagnostic
Lactic Acid, Blood
Lactate Dehydrogenase, Blood
Magnetic Resonance Imaging,
 Diagnostic
Sedimentation Rate, Erythrocyte,
 Blood
Synovial Fluid Analysis, Diagnostic

ADDITIONAL CONDITIONS
Abscess
Ascites
Burns
Cirrhosis
Diabetic Ketosis
Paralytic Ileus
Sepsis

PERNICIOUS ANEMIA
Blood Indices (Red Blood Cells), Blood
Bone Marrow Biopsy, Diagnostic
Complete Blood Count, Blood
Cytologic Study of Gastrointestinal
 Tract, Diagnostic
Differential Leukocyte Count,
 Peripheral Blood
Folic Acid, Red Blood Cells, Blood
Folic Acid, Serum
Gastrin, Serum
Intrinsic Factor Antibody, Blood
Lactate Dehydrogenase, Blood

ADDITIONAL CONDITIONS
Arthritis, Rheumatoid
Crohn's Disease
Gastrectomy
Gastritis
Graves' Disease
IgA Deficiency

Lactate Dehydrogenase Isoenzymes,
    Blood
Parietal Cell Antibody, Blood
Pepsinogen-1 Antibody, Blood
Platelet Count, Blood
Reticulocyte Count, Blood
Red Blood Cell Morphology, Blood
Schilling Test, Diagnostic
Vitamin B_{12}, Serum
Vitamin B_{12}, Unsaturated Binding
    Capacity, Serum

PHARYNGITIS

Adenovirus Immunofluorescence,
    Diagnostic
Antideoxyribonuclease-B Titer, Serum
Antihyaluronidase Titer, Serum
Antistreptolysin-O Titer, Serum
Complete Blood Count, Blood
Differential Leukocyte Count,
    Peripheral Blood
Infectious Mononucleosis Screening
    Test, Blood
Nose, Routine, Culture
Throat Culture for *Candida albicans,*
    Culture
Throat Culture for *Corynebacterium
    diphtheriae,* Culture
Throat Culture for Group A Beta-
    Hemolytic Streptococci, Culture
Throat Culture for *Neisseria
    gonorrhoeae,* Culture
Throat Culture, Routine, Culture
Viral Culture, Specimen

ADDITIONAL CONDITIONS

AIDS
Diphtheria
Epstein-Barr Virus
Tonsillitis

PHENYLKETONURIA (PKU) DISEASE

Guthrie Test for Phenylketonuria,
    Diagnostic
Phenistix Test, Diagnostic
Phenylalanine, Blood

ADDITIONAL CONDITIONS

Eczema
Mental Retardation
Seizures

PHEOCHROMOCYTOMA

Calcitonin, Plasma or Serum
Catecholamines, Fractionation-Free,
    Plasma
Homovanillic Acid, 24-Hour, Urine
Metanephrines, Total, 24-Hour, Urine
Vanillylmandelic Acid, Urine

ADDITIONAL CONDITIONS

Aortic Aneurysm
Cerebrovascular Accident
Headache
Hyperparathyroidism
Hypertension
Neurofibromatosis
Tachycardia
Thyroid Cancer

PHLEBITIS

(see Thrombophlebitis)

PID

(see Pelvic Inflammatory Disease)

PINWORM
Parasite Screen, Stool

ADDITIONAL CONDITIONS
Enuresis
Insomnia
Pruritus
Urinary Tract Infection

PITUITARY
(see Addison's Disease and Cushing's Syndrome)

PKU DISEASE
(see Phenylketonuria)

PLATELET DENSE GRANULE STORAGE POOL DISEASE OR RELEASE DEFECTS
Lumiaggregometry, Diagnostic

ADDITIONAL CONDITION
Cephalothin Therapy

PLEURAL EFFUSION
(see Effusion, Pleural)

PLEURISY
Biopsy, Routine, Culture
Blood Culture, Blood
Blood Gases, Arterial, Blood
Chest X-Ray, Diagnostic
Complete Blood Count, Blood
Coxsackie A or B Virus Titer, Blood
Histopathology, Specimen
Sputum, Routine, Culture

ADDITIONAL CONDITIONS
Ascites
Congestive Heart Failure
Meningitis
Myocarditis
Pericarditis
Pneumothorax

PNEUMOCONIOSIS
(see Black Lung Disease)

PNEUMONIA
Blood Culture, Blood
Chest X-Ray, Diagnostic
Complete Blood Count, Blood
Legionella pneumophila Culture, IgM Titer, Blood
Pulmonary Function Test, Diagnostic
Sputum, Routine, Culture
Viral Culture, Specimen

ADDITIONAL CONDITIONS
AIDS
Anemia
Aspiration
COPD
Endocarditis
Fever
Hemoptysis
Immunosuppression
Lung Cancer
Pleural Effusion
Right Ventricular Failure
Sepsis

PNEUMOTHORAX
Blood Gases, Arterial, Blood
Chest X-Ray, Diagnostic
Complete Blood Count, Blood
Sputum Cytology, Specimen

ADDITIONAL CONDITIONS
COPD
Cyanosis
Cystic Fibrosis
Dyspnea
Hemothorax
Trauma
Tuberculosis

POISONINGS
Acetaminophen, Serum
Anion Gap, Blood
Blood Gases, Arterial, Blood
Carbon Monoxide, Blood
Cyanide, Blood
Heavy Metals, Blood and 24-Hour Urine
Heavy Metals, Blood and 24-Hour Urine (Urine)
Lead, Blood and Urine
Morphine, Urine
Salicylate, Blood
Toxicology, Drug Screen, Blood or Urine

ADDITIONAL CONDITIONS
Coma
Cyanosis
Depression
Dysrhythmias
Hypertension
Hypotension
Metabolic Acidosis
Seizures
Suicidal Ideation

POLIO
(see Poliomyelitis)

POLIOMYELITIS (POLIO)
Poliomyelitis I, II, III Titer, Blood
Viral Culture, Specimen

ADDITIONAL CONDITIONS
Diarrhea
Fever
Headache
Meningitis
Stiff Neck
Tremors

POLYCYSTIC OVARIAN DISEASE
Luteinizing Hormone, Blood

ADDITIONAL CONDITIONS
Pelvic Inflammatory Disease
Uterine Fibroids

POLYCYTHEMIA VERA
Blood Volume, Blood
Bone Marrow Biopsy, Diagnostic
Complete Blood Count, Blood
Cr-51 (Chromium) Red Cell Survival, Blood
Leukocyte Alkaline Phosphatase, Blood
Red Blood Cell Morphology, Blood
Vitamin B_{12}, Unsaturated Binding Capacity, Serum

ADDITIONAL CONDITIONS
Dizziness
Headache
Hypertension
Obesity
Splenomegaly
Tinnitus

POLYURIA
Glucose, Blood
Glucose, 2-Hour Postprandial, Serum
Urinalysis, Urine

ADDITIONAL CONDITIONS
Diabetes Insipidus
Fanconi's Syndrome
Hypercalcemia
Hyperparathyroidism
Renal Tubular Acidosis

POSTOPERATIVE
(see Surgery)

PRE-ECLAMPSIA
Mean Platelet Volume, Blood

ADDITIONAL CONDITION
Hypertension

PREGNANCY
D-Dimer Test, Blood
Fructosamine, Serum
Glucose Tolerance Test, Blood
Hematocrit, Blood
Hemoglobin, Blood
Human Chorionic Gonadotropin,
   Beta-Subunit, Serum
Pregnancy Test, Routine, Serum
Protein, Urine

ADDITIONAL CONDITIONS
Amenorrhea
Anemia
Gestational Diabetes
Hyperglycemia
Nausea
Rubella
Syphilis

PREOPERATIVE
(see Surgery)

PRIMARY ESSENTIAL HYPERTENSION
(see Hypertension)

PROSTATE CANCER
Acid Phosphatase, Serum
Prostatic Acid Phosphatase by RIA,
   Blood
Prostate-Specific Antigen, Serum

ADDITIONAL CONDITIONS
Anemia
Hematuria
Hydronephrosis
Hyperglycemia
Hypoalbuminemia
Hypophosphatemia
Metastasis to Bone
Uremia
Urinary Tract Infection

PROSTATITIS
Blood Culture, Blood
Complete Blood Count, Blood
Urinalysis, Urine
Urinalysis, Fractional, Urine
Urine Culture, Routine, Clean-Catch,
   Urine

ADDITIONAL CONDITIONS
Chlamydia
Dysuria
Gonorrhea
Tuberculosis
Urinary Tract Infection

PRURITUS
Culture, Skin, Specimen
Toxicology, Drug Screen, Blood or
   Urine (Blood)

ADDITIONAL CONDITIONS
Dermatitis
Iron Deficiency Anemia
Obstructive Biliary Disease
Psychiatric Disturbances
Uremia

PSITTACOSIS
Chlamydia Culture
Chlamydia Group Titer (Tachoma
   Titer), Serum
Cold Agglutinin Screen, Blood
Complement Fixation, Serum
Complete Blood Count, Blood
Protein, Quantitative, Urine
Sedimentation Rate, Erythrocyte,
   Blood

ADDITIONAL CONDITIONS
Epistaxis
Fever
Headache
Pneumonitis

PSORIASIS
Culture, Skin, Specimen
Histopathology, Specimen
Ki-67 Proliferation Marker, Specimen

ADDITIONAL CONDITIONS
Arthritis, Rheumatoid
Candidiasis
Onychomycosis
Streptococcal Infection of the Pharynx

PULMONARY EDEMA
Albumin, Serum, Urine, and
    24-Hour Urine (Urine)
Blood Gases, Arterial, Blood
Blood Urea Nitrogen/Creatinine
    Ratio, Blood
Chest X-Ray, Diagnostic
Complete Blood Count, Blood
Digoxin, Serum
Electrolyte, Blood or Urine
Sputum Cytology, Specimen

ADDITIONAL CONDITIONS
Congestive Heart Failure
Cyanosis
Mitral Valve Stenosis
Myocardial Infarction
Ventricular Septal Defect

PULMONARY EMBOLISM
Antithrombin III Test, Diagnostic
Blood Gases, Arterial, Blood
Chemistry Profile, Blood
Complete Blood Count, Blood
D-Dimer Test, Blood
Electrocardiogram, Diagnostic
Lung Scan, Perfusion and
    Ventilation, Diagnostic
Partial Thromboplastin Time, Plasma
Plasminogen Assay, Blood
Sedimentation Rate, Erythrocyte,
    Blood
Ultrafast Computed Tomography,
    Diagnostic
Venography, Diagnostic

ADDITIONAL CONDITIONS
Atrial Fibrillation
Congestive Heart Failure
Deep Vein Thrombosis
Dyspnea
Fractures of the Hip
Hemoptysis
Hypoxemia
Immobility
Lung Cancer
Myocardial Infarction
Obesity
Pregnancy
Respiratory Alkalosis
Shock
Stroke
Surgery
Syncope
Trauma
Vascular Disease

PULMONARY INFECTION
Blood Culture, Blood
Blood Gases, Arterial, Blood
Chest X-Ray, Diagnostic
Complete Blood Count, Blood
Sputum, Routine, Culture

ADDITIONAL CONDITIONS
COPD
Industrial-Related Diseases
Lung Cancer
Pleural Effusion
Pneumonia
Tuberculosis

PULMONIC STENOSIS
Blood Gases, Arterial, Blood
Cardiac Catheterization, Diagnostic
Chest X-Ray, Diagnostic
Electrocardiogram, Diagnostic

ADDITIONAL CONDITIONS
Atrial Septal Defect
Cardiomyopathy
Dyspnea
Heart Murmur, Systolic

PYELONEPHRITIS
Chemistry Profile, Blood
Complete Blood Count, Blood
Creatinine Clearance, Urine
Nitrite, Bacteria Screen, Urine

ADDITIONAL CONDITIONS
Chlamydia
Cystitis
Gonorrhea
Trichomonas

Urinalysis, Urine
Urine Culture, Routine, Clean-Catch,
  Urine

PYREXIA
Creatine Kinase, Isoenzymes, Serum

Q FEVER
Differential Leukocyte Count,
  Peripheral Blood
Liver Battery, Serum
Weil-Felix Agglutinins, Blood

RABIES
Animals and Rabies Negri Bodies,
  Brain Tissue, Specimen
Fluorescent Rabies Antibody, Brain
  Tissue, Specimen

RAPE TRAUMA
Acid Phosphatase, Vaginal Swab
Blood Group Antigen of Semen,
  Vaginal Swab
Cervical Culture for *Neisseria
  gonorrhoeae,* Culture
Chlamydia Culture
Motile Sperm, Wet Mount, Diagnostic
Pap Smear, Diagnostic (Vulva)
Precipitin Test Against Human Sperm
  and Blood, Vaginal Swab
Pregnancy Test, Routine, Serum
Syphilis, Serum
Trichomonas Preparation, Specimen

RAT-BITE FEVER
Biopsy, Site-Specific (Bite Site),
  Specimen
Differential Leukocyte Count,
  Peripheral Blood
Fluorescent Treponemal Antibody-
  Absorbed Double-Stain Test, Serum

RAYNAUD'S DISEASE
Antinuclear Antibody, Serum
Cold Agglutinin Titer, Serum
Cryoglobulin, Qualitative, Serum
Extractable Nuclear Antigen, Serum

RENAL CALCULI
Calcium, Total, Serum
Kidney Sonogram, Diagnostic
Phosphorus, Serum

Ureteral Obstruction
Urethritis
Urinary Tract Infection

ADDITIONAL CONDITIONS
Leukemia
Pneumonia
Sepsis

ADDITIONAL CONDITIONS
Encephalopathy
Headache
Hepatitis
Pain, Abdominal
Pneumonitis

ADDITIONAL CONDITIONS
Paresthesia
Seizures

ADDITIONAL CONDITIONS
AIDS
Anxiety
Chlamydia
Depression
Gonorrhea
Pregnancy
Trichomoniasis

ADDITIONAL CONDITIONS
Arthritis
Fever
Headache
Lymphangitis
Splenomegaly

ADDITIONAL CONDITIONS
Arthritis, Rheumatoid
Arteriosclerosis
Carpal Tunnel Syndrome
Cyanosis
Gangrene
Systemic Lupus Erythematosus (SLE)

ADDITIONAL CONDITIONS
Gout
Pain, Acute Back
Urinary Tract Infection

Uric Acid, Serum
Urinalysis, Urine

RENAL CELL CANCER
Biopsy, Site-Specific (Kidney), Specimen
Computed Tomography of the Body
    (Kidney), Diagnostic
Intravenous Pyelography, Diagnostic
Kidney Sonogram, Diagnostic
Nephrotomography, Diagnostic
Renal Angiogram, Diagnostic

ADDITIONAL CONDITIONS
Anemia
Fever
Hematuria
Hypercalcemia
Hypoglycemia

RENAL FAILURE
Beta$_2$-Microglobulin, Blood and 24-
    Hour Urine
Bicarbonate, Serum
Chemistry Profile, Blood
Complete Blood Count, Blood
Creatinine, Serum
Creatinine Clearance, Serum, Urine
Electrolyte, Blood or Urine
Globulin, Serum
Immunoelectrophoresis, Serum and
    Urine
Intravenous Pyelography, Diagnostic
Kidney Biopsy, Specimen
Magnesium, Serum
Magnetic Resonance Imaging,
    Diagnostic
Mean Platelet Volume, Blood
Myoglobin, Serum
Myoglobin, Qualitative, Urine
pH, Blood
Phosphorus, Serum
Potassium, Serum
Protein, Semiquantitative, Urine
Technetium-Pentaacetic Acid
    Clearance, Diagnostic
Transferrin, Serum
Urea Nitrogen, Plasma or Serum
Uric Acid, Serum
Urinalysis, Urine

ADDITIONAL CONDITIONS
Aminoglycoside Toxicity
Blood Transfusion Incompatibility
Burns
Dehydration
Disseminated Intravascular
    Coagulation (DIC)
Hypertension
Leptospirosis
Liver Failure
Multiple Myeloma
Myocardial Infarction
Peritonitis
Poisoning
Toxic Shock Syndrome

RENAL HYPERTENSION
Aldosterone, Serum and Urine
Arteriogram, Diagnostic
Chloride, Serum
Intravenous Pyelography, Diagnostic
Potassium, Serum
Renin, Blood
Sodium, Plasma, Serum, or Urine

ADDITIONAL CONDITIONS
Atherosclerosis
Post Transplant Surgery
Renal Stenosis

RENAL INFARCTION
Chemistry Profile, Blood
Creatine Kinase, Serum
Creatine Kinase, Isoenzymes, Serum
Histopathology, Specimen
Kidney Sonogram, Diagnostic

ADDITIONAL CONDITIONS
Abscess
Kidney Cancer
Renal Failure
Renal Hypertension
Trauma

Lactate Dehydrogenase, Blood
Lactate Dehydrogenase Isoenzymes,
    Blood
Urinalysis, Urine

RENIN HYPERTENSION
(see Hypertension)

RESPIRATORY ACIDOSIS
Blood Gases, Arterial, Blood
Chest X-Ray, Diagnostic
Pulmonary Function Test, Diagnostic
Urinalysis, Urine

ADDITIONAL CONDITIONS
Acute Respiratory Distress Syndrome
    (ARDS)
Congestive Heart Failure
COPD
Hypercapnia
Hypoxemia
Kyphoscoliosis
Myocardial Infarction
Shock

RESPIRATORY ALKALOSIS
Blood Gases, Arterial, Blood
Calcium, Total, Serum
Chest X-Ray, Diagnostic
Potassium, Serum
Urinalysis, Urine

ADDITIONAL CONDITIONS
Acute Respiratory Distress Syndrome
Anxiety
Asthma
Congestive Heart Failure
Liver Disease
Pneumonia
Pregnancy
Pulmonary Emboli

RESPIRATORY FAILURE
Alpha$_1$-Antitrypsin, Serum
Blood Culture, Blood
Blood Gases, Arterial, Blood
Chest X-Ray, Diagnostic
Lung Scan, Perfusion and
    Ventilation, Diagnostic
Pulmonary Artery Catheterization,
    Diagnostic
Pulmonary Function Test, Diagnostic
Sputum, Routine, Culture

ADDITIONAL CONDITIONS
Acute Respiratory Distress Syndrome
    (ARDS)
Botulism
Congestive Heart Failure
COPD
Guillain-Barré
Myasthenia Gravis
Pneumonia
Pneumothorax
Poliomyelitis
Pulmonary Edema
Pulmonary Embolus
Spinal Cord Injury

REYE'S SYNDROME
Alanine Aminotransferase, Serum
Ammonia, Blood
Aspartate Aminotransferase, Serum
Bilirubin, Direct, Serum
Creatinine, Serum
Glucose, Random, Blood
Histopathology, Specimen
Liver Biopsy, Diagnostic
Lumbar Puncture, Diagnostic
Partial Thromboplastin Time, Plasma
Prothrombin Time and International
    Normalized Ratio, Serum
Urea Nitrogen, Plasma or Serum

ADDITIONAL CONDITIONS
Bronchitis
Encephalopathy
Hepatic Failure
Hypoglycemia
Myocarditis
Otitis Media
Pericarditis
Pneumonia
Sinusitis
Thrombophlebitis

RHABDOMYOLYSIS
Cocaine, Blood
Creatine Kinase Isoenzymes, Serum
Muscle Biopsy, Specimen
Myoglobin, Serum
Myoglobin, Qualitative, Urine

ADDITIONAL CONDITION
Dermatomyositis

RHEUMATIC FEVER
Antideoxyribonuclease-B Titer, Serum
Antistreptolysin-O Titer, Blood
C-Reactive Protein, Serum
Mean Platelet Volume, Blood

ADDITIONAL CONDITIONS
Cardiomegaly
Congestive Heart Failure
Mitral Valve Stenosis
Pericarditis

RHEUMATOID ARTHRITIS
(see Arthritis)

RHINITIS
Allergen-Specific IgE, Serum
Eosinophil Count, Blood
Sinus X-Rays, Diagnostic

ADDITIONAL CONDITIONS
Nasal Polyps
Osteomyelitis
Sinusitis

RICKETS
(see Osteomalacia)

RINGWORM *(TINEA CAPITIS)*
Culture, Skin (Scalp for *Microsporum audouinii*), Specimen

ADDITIONAL CONDITIONS
Lymphadenopathy
Pruritus

ROCKY MOUNTAIN SPOTTED FEVER
Rocky Mountain Spotted Fever Serology, Serum

ADDITIONAL CONDITIONS
Coma
Fever
Headache
Rash

RUBELLA (GERMAN MEASLES)
Immunoglobulin M, Serum
Rubella Serology, Serum
Toxoplasmosis, Rubella, Cytomegalovirus, Herpes Virus Serology (TORCH), Blood
Viral Culture, Specimen

ADDITIONAL CONDITIONS
Adenitis
Fever
Lymphadenopathy
Pregnancy

RUBEOLA
Differential Leukocyte Count, Peripheral Blood
Histopathology, Specimen
Lymph Node Biopsy, Specimen
Rubeola Serology, Serum

ADDITIONAL CONDITIONS
Fever
Rash

SALMONELLOSIS
Blood Culture, Blood
Complete Blood Count, Blood

ADDITIONAL CONDITIONS
Bacteremia
Enterocolitis

Differential Leukocyte Count,
Peripheral Blood
Febrile Agglutinins, Serum
Methylene Blue Stain, Stool
Salmonella Titer, Blood
Stool Culture, Routine, Stool

Fever
Typhoid

SANFILIPPO'S SYNDROME

Mucopolysaccharides, Qualitative,
Urine
S Mucopolysaccharide Turnover,
Diagnostic

ADDITIONAL CONDITIONS

Dysrhythmias
Mental Retardation

SARCOIDOSIS

Bronchial Washing, Specimen,
Diagnostic
Brushing Cytology, Specimen,
Diagnostic
Chest X-Ray, Diagnostic
Histopathology, Specimen
Ki-67 Proliferation Marker, Specimen
Liver Biopsy, Diagnostic
Liver I-131 Scan, Diagnostic
Mediastinoscopy, Diagnostic
Muramidase (Lysozyme), Serum and
Urine
Nerve Biopsy, Diagnostic
Sputum Cytology, Specimen

ADDITIONAL CONDITIONS

Arthritis
Dyspnea
Fever
Hepatosplenomegaly
Lymphadenopathy
Pleural Effusion
Sinusitis

SARCOMA

Biopsy, Site-Specific (Bone),
Specimen
Bone Scan, Diagnostic
Computed Tomography of the Body
(Bone), Diagnostic
Magnetic Resonance Imaging,
Diagnostic

ADDITIONAL CONDITIONS

Bowel Obstruction
Osteomyelitis
Paralytic Ileus

SCABIES

Culture, Skin (Scrapings for Ova or
Mites), Specimen

ADDITIONAL CONDITIONS

Malnutrition
Pyoderma
Pruritus

SCARLET FEVER

Antistreptolysin-O Titer, Serum
Throat Culture for Group A Beta-
Hemolytic Streptococci,
Culture

ADDITIONAL CONDITIONS

Fever
Tonsillitis
Vomiting

SCHISTOSOMIASIS

Complete Blood Count, Blood
Eosinophil Count, Blood
Liver Battery, Serum
Liver Biopsy, Diagnostic
Liver/Spleen Scan, Diagnostic
Urinalysis, Urine

ADDITIONAL CONDITIONS

Bladder Cancer
Diarrhea
Nephrotic Syndrome
Renal Failure

SCHIZOPHRENIA, CHRONIC
Iron, Serum
Tricyclic Antidepressants, Plasma or
   Serum

ADDITIONAL CONDITIONS
Catatonia
Dementia
Hallucinations
Seizures

SCLERODERMA
Antinuclear Antibody, Serum
d-Xylose Absorption Test, Diagnostic,
   Serum or Urine
Histopathology, Specimen
Scleroderma Antibody, Blood

ADDITIONAL CONDITIONS
Diverticulitis
Dysphagia
Pericarditis
Polyarthralgia
Pulmonary Fibrosis
Pulmonary Hypertension
Raynaud's Phenomenon
Telangiectasia

SCURVY
Capillary Fragility Test, Diagnostic
Vitamin C, Plasma or Serum

ADDITIONAL CONDITIONS
Anemia
Gingivitis
Malnutrition

SECONDARY HYPERTENSION
(see Hypertension)

SEIZURES
Alcohol, Blood
Brain Scan, Cerebral Flow and
   Pathology, Diagnostic
Brain Sonogram, Diagnostic
Calcium, Total, Serum
Carbamazepine, Blood
Carbon Monoxide, Blood
Carboxyhemoglobin, Blood
Cerebral Computed Tomography,
   Diagnostic
Cerebrospinal Fluid, Glucose,
   Specimen
Cerebrospinal Fluid, Protein,
   Specimen
Cerebrospinal Fluid, Routine
   Analysis, Specimen
Chemistry Profile, Blood
Chlordiazepoxide, Blood
Chromium, Serum
Clonazepam, Blood
Cocaine, Blood
Computed Tomography of the Brain,
   Diagnostic
Creatine Kinase, Serum
Diazepam, Serum
Electroencephalogram, Diagnostic
Ethosuximide, Blood
Flurazepam, Serum
Glucose, Blood
Heavy Metals, Blood and 24-Hour,
   Urine (Urine)
Ketone Bodies, Blood

ADDITIONAL CONDITIONS
Alcoholism
Brain Tumor
Carbon Monoxide Poisoning
Cerebrovascular Accident
Drug Abuse
Epilepsy
Hysteria
Poisoning

Ketones, Semiquantitative, Urine
Lidocaine, Serum
Magnesium, Serum
Mephenytoin, Blood
Methsuximide, Serum
Osmolality, Serum
Phenobarbital, Plasma or Serum
Phenytoin, Serum
Primidone, Serum
Pseudocholinesterase, Plasma
Sodium, Plasma, Serum, or Urine
Theophylline, Blood
Thiocyanate, Blood
Thiocyanate, Urine
Toxicology, Drug Screen, Blood or
   Urine (Urine)
Valproic Acid, Blood
Vitamin B_6 (Pyridoxine), Plasma

SENILE DEMENTIA
(see Dementia)

SEPSIS
Abscess, Anaerobic Culture
Blood Culture, Blood
Complete Blood Count, Blood
Electrocardiogram, Diagnostic
Foreign Body, Routine, Culture
Urinalysis, Urine

ADDITIONAL CONDITIONS
Abscess
Arthritis
Bacteremia
Burns
Cancer
Empyema
Immunosuppression
Malnutrition
Pancreatitis
Toxic Shock Syndrome
Urinary Tract Infection

SERUM SICKNESS
C1q Immune Complex Detection,
   Serum
C3 Complement, Serum
C4 Complement, Serum
Heterophile Agglutinins, Blood
Immune Complex Assay, Blood

ADDITIONAL CONDITIONS
Anaphylaxis
Arthritis
Fever
Hepatitis B
Lymphadenopathy
Urticaria

SEXUALLY TRANSMITTED DISEASE
*(see AIDS, Chancroid, Chlamydia,
Gonorrhea, Granuloma Inguinale,
Herpes Hominis II, Human
Papilloma Virus, Lymphogranuloma
venereum, and Syphilis)*

SHINGLES
(see Herpes Zoster)

SHOCK
Aspartate Aminotransferase, Serum
Blood Culture, Blood

ADDITIONAL CONDITIONS
Anaphylaxis
Bacteremias

Blood Gases, Arterial, Blood
Blood Urea Nitrogen/Creatinine Ratio,
    Blood
Cardiac Output, Diagnostic
Complete Blood Count, Blood
Creatinine, Serum
Glucose, Blood
Lactic Acid, Blood
Partial Thromboplastin Time, Plasma
Potassium, Serum
Prothrombin Time and International
    Normalized Ratio, Serum
Pulmonary Artery Catheterization,
    Diagnostic
Urinalysis, Urine

Burns
Coronary Artery Disease
Drug Overdose
Dysrhythmias
Electrolyte Imbalances
Gastrointestinal Bleeding
Hypovolemia
Myocardial Infarction
Myocarditis
Pancreatitis
Post Cardiac Surgery
Post CPR
Pulmonary Hypertension
Sepsis
Toxic Shock Syndrome
Transfusion Reaction
Trauma

SIADHS
*(see Syndrome of Inappropriate
Antidiuretic Hormone Secretion)*

SICKLE CELL ANEMIA
C3 Proactivator, Serum
D-Dimer (for Crisis), Blood
Fetal Hemoglobin, Blood
Hemoglobin Electrophoresis, Blood
Sickle Cell Test, Blood

ADDITIONAL CONDITIONS
Cardiomegaly
Jaundice
Pain, Acute
Splenomegaly

SIGMOIDOSCOPY
Complete Blood Count, Blood
Potassium, Serum
Sodium, Plasma, Serum, or Urine

ADDITIONAL CONDITIONS
Hemorrhage
Polyps in Colon/Rectum
Tumor of Colon/Rectum

SILICOSIS
Chest X-Ray, Diagnostic
Pulmonary Function Test, Diagnostic

ADDITIONAL CONDITIONS
Dyspnea
Tuberculosis

SINUSITIS
Abscess, Anaerobic Culture
Complete Blood Count, Blood
Histopathology, Specimen
Immunoglobulin A, Serum
Nose, Routine, Culture
Sedimentation Rate, Erythrocyte, Blood
Sinus X-Ray, Diagnostic
Tomography Paranasal Sinuses,
    Diagnostic

ADDITIONAL CONDITIONS
Influenza
Pneumonia
Respiratory Infection

SJÖGREN'S SYNDROME
Antinuclear Antibody, Serum
Blood Indices (Red Blood Cells), Blood
Complete Blood Count, Blood
Differential Leukocyte Count,
    Peripheral Blood
Extractable Nuclear Antigen, Serum

ADDITIONAL CONDITIONS
Arthritis, Rheumatoid
Cirrhosis
Hashimoto's Thyroiditis
Polymyositis
Pulmonary Fibrosis
Scleroderma

Histopathology, Specimen
Immune Complex Assay, Blood
Parietal Cell Antibody, Blood
Protein, Electrophoresis, Serum
Red Cell Count, Serum
Rheumatoid Factor, Blood
Sjögren's Antibodies, Blood

Systemic Lupus Erythematosus
  (SLE)
Xerostomia

SPIDER BITES
Arthropod Identification, Specimen
Complete Blood Count, Blood

ADDITIONAL CONDITIONS
Anaphylaxis
Seizures

SPINAL CORD INJURY
Calcium, Total, Serum
Cerebral Computed Tomography,
  Diagnostic
Magnetic Resonance Imaging,
  Diagnostic
Partial Thromboplastin Time, Plasma
Phosphorus, Serum
Prothrombin Time and International
  Normalized Ratio, Serum
Uric Acid, Serum
Urinalysis, Urine

ADDITIONAL CONDITIONS
Brown-Sequard Syndrome
Depression
Hypotension
Hypoxia
Spinal Cord Compression

SPLENOMEGALY
Alanine Aminotransferase, Serum
Aspartate Aminotransferase, Serum
Bone Marrow Biopsy, Diagnostic
Complete Blood Count, Blood
Immunoperoxidase Procedures (for
  Antigens), Diagnostic
Liver Battery, Serum
Mean Platelet Volume, Blood
Platelet Count, Blood
Spleen Scan, Diagnostic
Sputum, Myobacteria, Culture

ADDITIONAL CONDITIONS
Cancer
G-6-PD Deficiency
Histoplasmosis
Infectious Mononucleosis
Leukemia
Metastasis
Polycythemia Vera
Sarcoidosis
Sickle Cell Anemia

STATUS EPILEPTICUS
Cerebral Computed Tomography,
  Diagnostic
Electroencephalogram, Diagnostic
Phenobarbital, Plasma or Serum
Phenytoin, Serum
Valproic Acid, Blood

ADDITIONAL CONDITIONS
Alcoholism
Brain Tumor
Trauma

STEATORRHEA
Fat, Semiquantitative, Stool

ADDITIONAL CONDITION
Whipple's Disease

STERILITY
(see Infertility)

STIMULANT DRUG ABUSE
(see also Drug Abuse)
Amphetamines (Benzedrine,
  Biphetamine, Desoxyn,
  Dexedrine), Blood

ADDITIONAL CONDITIONS
Alcoholism
Depression
Stress

Cocaine, Blood
Methylphenidate, Serum
Phenmetrazine, Blood

STOMATITIS

Differential Leukocyte Count,
  Peripheral Blood
Glucagon, Plasma
T- and B-Lymphocyte Subset Assay,
  Blood
Throat Culture for *Candida albicans*,
  Culture

ADDITIONAL CONDITIONS

AIDS
Cancer
Candidiasis
Herpes Simplex Virus
Malnutrition

STRESS

Adrenocorticotropic Hormone,
  Serum
Aldosterone, Serum and Urine
Cortisol, Plasma or Serum

ADDITIONAL CONDITIONS

Anxiety
Dermatitis
Hypertension
Myocardial Infarction
Stroke

STRESS ULCERS

(see Peptic Ulcers)

STROKE

(see Cerebrovascular Accident)

SUBACUTE BACTERIAL ENDOCARDITIS (SBE)

Blood Culture, Blood
Blood Indices (Red Blood Cells), Blood
C3 Complement, Serum
C4 Complement, Serum
Complement Total, Serum
Complete Blood Count, Blood
C-Reactive Protein, Serum
Echocardiogram, Diagnostic
Sedimentation Rate, Erythrocyte,
  Blood
Teichoic Acid Antibody, Blood
Transesophageal Sonogram,
  Diagnostic
Urinalysis, Urine

ADDITIONAL CONDITIONS

Disseminated Intravascular
  Coagulation (DIC)
Drug Abuse

SUBARACHNOID HEMORRHAGE

Cerebrospinal Fluid, Routine
  Analysis, Specimen
Computed Tomography of the Brain,
  Diagnostic
Lumbar Puncture, Diagnostic
Magnetic Resonance Imaging,
  Diagnostic

ADDITIONAL CONDITIONS

Aneurysm of the Brain
Cerebrovascular Accident (CVA)
Trauma

SUNSTROKE

(see Heat Stroke)

SURGERY, POSTOPERATIVE

- Blood Gases, Arterial, Blood
- Chloride, Serum
- Complete Blood Count, Blood
- D-Dimer Test, Blood
- Glucose, Blood
- Partial Thromboplastin Time, Plasma
- Platelet Count, Blood
- Potassium, Serum
- Prothrombin Time and International Normalized Ratio, Serum
- Sodium, Plasma, Serum or Urine
- Urea Nitrogen, Plasma or Serum
- Urinalysis, Urine

ADDITIONAL CONDITIONS

- Bacteremia
- Emboli
- Hypoxemia
- Pneumonia
- Sepsis
- Thrombosis

SURGERY, PREOPERATIVE

- Carbon Dioxide, Partial Pressure, Blood
- Carbon Dioxide, Total Content, Blood
- Chest X-Ray, Diagnostic
- Chloride, Serum
- Complete Blood Count, Blood
- Creatinine, Serum
- Electrocardiogram, Diagnostic
- Glucose, Blood
- Partial Thromboplastin Time, Plasma
- Platelet Count, Blood
- Potassium, Serum
- Sodium, Plasma, Serum, or Urine
- Type and Crossmatch, Blood
- Urea Nitrogen, Plasma, or Serum
- Urinalysis, Urine

ADDITIONAL CONDITIONS

- Aneurysm
- Appendicitis
- Cancer
- Cholecystitis
- Coronary Artery Disease
- Intestinal Obstruction
- Peripheral Vascular Disease
- Trauma

SYNCOPE

- Carotid Duplex Ultrasonography, Diagnostic
- Carotid Phonoangiography, Diagnostic
- Electrocardiogram, Diagnostic
- Tilt Table Test, Diagnostic

ADDITIONAL CONDITIONS

- Aortic Stenosis
- Atherosclerosis
- Atrioventricular Block
- Cardiomyopathy
- Hypotension
- Neurogenic Syncope
- Pulmonary Stenosis
- Sick Sinus Syndrome
- Vasovagal Syncope

SYNDROME OF INAPPROPRIATE ANTIDIURETIC HORMONE SECRETION (SIADHS)

- Antidiuretic Hormone, Serum
- Electrolyte, Blood or Urine
- Osmolality, Serum
- Osmolality, Urine
- Sodium, Plasma, Serum, or Urine
- Specific Gravity, Urine
- Urea Nitrogen, Plasma or Serum
- Uric Acid, Serum

ADDITIONAL CONDITIONS

- Bronchogenic Cancer
- Hyponatremia
- Leukemia
- Myocardial Infarction
- Myxedema
- Pancreatic Cancer

SYPHILIS

Automated Reagin Testing, Diagnostic
Fluorescent Treponemal Antibody-
  Absorbed Double-Stain, Serum
Hemagglutination Treponemal Test
  for Syphilis (HATTS), Serum
Microhemagglutination-*T. pallidum*
  (MHA-TP) Test, Serum
Rapid Plasma Reagin Test, Blood
Venereal Disease Research Laboratory
  Test, Serum
Venereal Disease Research Laboratory
  Test, Cerebrospinal Fluid,
  Specimen

ADDITIONAL CONDITIONS

AIDS
Aortitis
Hepatitis
Lymphadenopathy
Meningitis
Pregnancy

SYSTEMIC LUPUS ERYTHEMATOSUS (SLE)

Anti-DNA, Serum
Antinuclear Antibody, Serum
C3 Complement, Serum
C4 Complement, Serum
Complete Blood Count, Blood
C-Reactive Protein, Serum
Fluorescent Treponemal Antibody-
  Absorbed Double-Stain Test,
  Serum
Immune Complex Assay, Blood
Lupus Panel, Blood
Lupus Test, Blood
Magnetic Resonance Spectography,
  Diagnostic
Mixing Study (Circulating
  Anticoagulants), Plasma
Platelet Count, Blood
Viscosity, Serum

ADDITIONAL CONDITIONS

Arthritis
Leukopenia
Photosensitivity
Rash
Renal Disease
Stomatitis
Thrombocytopenia

TAY-SACHS DISEASE

Amniocentesis, Diagnostic
Galactose-1-Phosphate, Blood

ADDITIONAL CONDITIONS

Blindness
Dementia
Mental Retardation

TESTICULAR CANCER

Alpha-Fetoprotein, Blood
Biopsy, Site-Specific (Testes),
  Specimen
Computed Tomography of the Body
  (Retroperitoneum), Diagnostic
Human Chorionic Gonadotropin,
  Beta-Subunit, Serum

ADDITIONAL CONDITIONS

Atrophic Testes
Cryptorchid Testes
Gynecomastia
Hydrocele
Leukemia
Virilization

TETANY

Calcium, Total, Serum
Calcium, Urine
Chemistry Profile, Blood
Electrolyte, Blood or Urine
Magnesium, Serum

ADDITIONAL CONDITIONS

Anxiety
Hyperaldosteronism
Hypocalcemia
Hypoparathyroidism
Osteomalacia
Rickets

TETRALOGY OF FALLOT
Blood Gases, Arterial, Blood
Cardiac Catheterization, Diagnostic
Chest X-Ray, Diagnostic
Electrocardiogram, Diagnostic
Hematocrit, Blood
Hemoglobin, Blood
Iron, Serum
Red Cell Count, Serum

ADDITIONAL CONDITIONS
Cyanosis
Emboli
Hypoxia
Polycythemia

THALASSEMIA
Chronic Villi Sampling, Specimen
Complete Blood Count, Blood
Ferritin, Serum
Fetal Hemoglobin, Blood
Hemoglobin Electrophoresis, Blood
Iron and Total Iron-Binding
    Capacity/Transferrin, Serum

ADDITIONAL CONDITIONS
Anemia
Cardiomyopathy
Hypogonadism
Jaundice
Splenomegaly

THORACIC AORTIC ANEURYSM
(see Aneurysm)

THROMBOANGIITIS OBLITERANS
Arteriogram, Diagnostic

ADDITIONAL CONDITIONS
Peripheral Vascular Disease (PVD)
Thrombosis

THROMBOCYTOPENIA
Bone Marrow Biopsy, Diagnostic
Capillary Fragility Test Diagnostic
Complete Blood Count, Blood
Folic Acid, Serum
Liver Battery, Serum
Mean Platelet Volume, Blood
Occult Blood, Urine
Platelet Antibody, Blood
Platelet Count, Blood
Potassium, Serum
Red Blood Cell Morphology, Blood
Vitamin B_{12}, Serum

ADDITIONAL CONDITIONS
AIDS
Alcoholism
Anemia
Cancer
Disseminated Intravascular
    Coagulation (DIC)
Hypersplenism
Idiopathic Thrombocytopenia
    Purpura (ITP)
Leukemia
Sepsis

THROMBOPHLEBITIS
I-125-Labeled Fibrinogen Leg Scan,
    Diagnostic
Partial Thromboplastin Time, Plasma
Prothrombin Time and International
    Normalized Ratio, Serum
Venography, Diagnostic

ADDITIONAL CONDITIONS
Cancer
Congestive Heart Failure
Pulmonary Embolism
Trauma
Varicose Veins

THROMBOSIS
Antiphospholipid Antibodies, Serum
Antithrombin III Test, Diagnostic
D-Dimer Test, Blood
Doppler or Duplex Doppler
    Ultrasound Flow Studies,
    Diagnostic

ADDITIONAL CONDITIONS
Aneurysm
Cancer
Dysfibrinogenemia
Peripheral Vascular Disease (PVD)
Ulcerative Colitis

Fibrinogen, Plasma
Hemoglobin, Blood
I-125-Labeled Fibrinogen Leg Scan,
    Diagnostic
Lung Scan, Perfusion and
    Ventilation, Diagnostic
Magnetic Resonance Angiography,
    Diagnostic
Magnetic Resonance Imaging,
    Diagnsotic
Urinalysis, Urine
Venography, Diagnostic

THRUSH (CANDIDIASIS, MONILIASIS)
Complete Blood Count, Blood
Oral Cavity Cytology, Specimen
Throat Culture for *Candida albicans,*
    Culture
Vaginal Culture

ADDITIONAL CONDITIONS
AIDS
Cancer
Fever
Leukemia
Lymphadenopathy

THYROID
(see Goiter, Hyperthyroidism, Hypothyroidism)

THYROID CANCER
Biopsy, Site-Specific (Thyroid),
    Specimen
Neuron-Specific Enolase, Serum
Thyroid Scan, Diagnostic
Thyroid Sonogram, Diagnostic

ADDITIONAL CONDITIONS
Goiter
Thyroiditis

THYROIDECTOMY
Calcium, Total, Serum
Cholesterol, Blood
Complete Blood Count, Blood
Phosphorus, Serum
Thyroid Test: Thyroxine, Blood
Thyroid Test: Triiodothyronine, Blood
Type and Crossmatch, Blood

ADDITIONAL CONDITION
Hypoparathyroidism

THYROTOXICOSIS
(see Hyperthyroidism)

TIA
(see Transient Ischemic Attack)

TIC DOULOUREUX (TRIGEMINAL NEURALGIA)
Complete Blood Count, Blood
Magnetic Resonance Angiography,
    Diagnostic
Phenytoin, Serum
Platelet Count, Blood
Tegretol, Serum

ADDITIONAL CONDITIONS
Brain Tumor
Multiple Sclerosis
Pain, Acute Facial

TINEA CAPITIS
(see Ringworm)

TINEA CRURIS
Culture, Skin, Specimen

ADDITIONAL CONDITIONS
Candidiasis
Dermatitis
Pruritus

TINNITUS
Cerebral Angiogram, Diagnostic
Cerebral Computed Tomography,
 Diagnostic
Hearing Test for Loudness-
 Recruitment, Diagnostic
Salicylate (Acetylsalicylic Acid),
 Blood
Tuning Fork Test of Weber, Rinne and
 Schwabach Tests, Diagnostic

ADDITIONAL CONDITIONS
Aneurysm
Carotid Occlusion
Otitis Media

TONSILLITIS
Differential Leukocyte Count,
 Peripheral Blood
Throat Culture for Group A Beta-
 Hemolytic Streptococci, Culture

ADDITIONAL CONDITIONS
Esophagitis
Infectious Mononucleosis
Myocarditis
Pharyngitis
Scarlet Fever

TOXEMIA
Chemistry Profile, Blood
Kidney Biopsy, Specimen
Magnesium, Serum
Pregnancy Test, Routine, Serum
Pregnanetriol, Urine
Sodium, Plasma, Serum, or Urine
Urinalysis, Urine

ADDITIONAL CONDITIONS
Diabetes Mellitus
Edema
Hydatidiform Mole
Hypertension
Pregnancy
Renal Disease

TOXIC SHOCK SYNDROME
Bilirubin, Total, Serum
Blood Culture, Blood
Chemistry Profile, Blood
Chloride, Serum
Complete Blood Count, Blood
Creatinine, Serum
Genital, Routine (for *Staphylococcus
 aureus*), Culture
Glucose, Blood
Obstetric Sonogram, Diagnostic
pH, Blood
Potassium, Serum
Prothrombin Time and International
 Normalized Ratio, Serum
Rocky Mountain Spotted Fever
 Serology, Serum
Sodium, Plasma, Serum or Urine
Urea Nitrogen, Plasma or Serum
Urinalysis, Urine
Vaginal Culture (for *Staphylococcus
 aureus*)

ADDITIONAL CONDITIONS
Conjunctivitis
Diarrhea
Erythroderma
Fever
Hypotension
Postpartum
Vomiting

TRANSFUSION REACTION

Antibody Identification, Red Cell, Blood
Blood Culture, Blood
Coombs', Direct, Serum
Coombs', Direct IgG, Serum
Haptoglobin, Serum
Hemoglobin, Plasma and Qualitative, Urine (Urine)
Hemosiderin, Urine
Immunoglobulin A Antibodies, Serum
Occult Blood, Urine
Transfusion Reaction Work-up, Diagnostic

ADDITIONAL CONDITIONS

Chills
Disseminated Intravascular Coagulation (DIC)
Dyspnea
Fever
Graft-Versus-Host Disease
Headache
Hypotension
Renal Failure
Sepsis
Shock

TRANSIENT ISCHEMIC ATTACK (TIA)

Cerebral Angiogram, Diagnostic
Cerebral Computed Tomography, Diagnostic
Cholesterol, Blood
Protein, Electrophoresis, Serum
Triglycerides, Blood
Viscosity, Serum

ADDITIONAL CONDITIONS

Aortic Stenosis
Atherosclerosis
Carotid Stenosis
Diplopia
Dizziness
Hypotension
Stroke

TRANSPLANT REJECTION

Alanine Aminotransferase, Serum
Aspartate Aminotransferase, Serum
Blood Gases, Arterial, Blood
Bone Marrow Biopsy, Diagnostic
Complete Blood Count, Blood
Creatinine, Serum
Ophthalmodynamometry, Diagnostic
Partial Thromboplastin Time, Plasma
Platelet Count, Blood
Prothrombin Time and International Normalized Ratio, Serum
Urea Nitrogen, Plasma or Serum

ADDITIONAL CONDITIONS

Candidiasis
Congestive Heart Failure
Diarrhea
Graft-Versus-Host Disease
Hemorrhage
Renal Failure
Sepsis

TRANSPLANTS (BONE MARROW, CORNEA, HEART, LIVER, LUNG, PANCREAS, RENAL)

Blood Culture, Blood
Blood Gases, Arterial, Blood
Calcium, Total, Serum
Carbon Dioxide, Partial Pressure, Blood
Carbon Dioxide, Total Content, Blood
Chloride, Serum
Complete Blood Count, Blood
Creatinine, Serum
Human Leukocyte Antigen Typing, Blood
Mixed Leukocyte Culture, Specimen
Potassium, Serum
Sodium, Plasma, Serum, or Urine
Type and Crossmatch, Blood
Urea Nitrogen, Plasma or Serum

ADDITIONAL CONDITIONS

Aplastic Anemia
Cancer
Cardiac Failure
Cornea Eye Trauma
Graft-Versus-Host Disease
Insulin Dependent Diabetes
Leukemia
Liver Failure
Lung Failure
Renal Failure

TRANSPOSITION OF THE GREAT ARTERIES
Blood Gases, Arterial, Blood
Cardiac Catheterization, Diagnostic
Chest X-Ray, Diagnostic
Echocardiogram, Diagnostic
Electrocardiogram, Diagnostic
Platelet Count, Blood
Red Cell Count, Serum

ADDITIONAL CONDITIONS
Cardiomegaly
Congestive Heart Failure
Cyanosis

TREMOR
Cerebral Computed Tomography,
    Diagnostic
Electroencephalogram, Diagnostic
Glucose, Blood

ADDITIONAL CONDITIONS
Alzheimer's Disease
Brain Tumor
Encephalopathy
Huntington's Disease
Multiple Sclerosis
Parkinson's Disease
Spinal Cord Trauma
Tourette's Syndrome

TREPONEMA PALLIDUM
(see Syphilis)

TRICHINOSIS
Aldolase, Serum
Eosinophil Count, Blood
Muscle Biopsy, Specimen
Muscle Profile, Specimen
Parasite Screen, Blood
Trichinosis Serology, Serum

ADDITIONAL CONDITIONS
Conjunctivitis
Diarrhea
Dyspnea
Edema
Encephalitis
Fever
Headache
Myocarditis
Nephritis
Pain, Muscle
Photophobia
Pneumonia

TRICHOMONAS
(see Vaginitis)

TRICUSPID ATRESIA
Blood Gases, Arterial, Blood
Cardiac Catheterization, Diagnostic
Chest X-Ray, Diagnostic
Echocardiogram, Diagnostic
Electrocardiogram, Diagnostic

ADDITIONAL CONDITIONS
Cor Pulmonale
Cyanosis
Dyspnea
Polycythemia

TRIGEMINAL NEURALGIA
(see Tic Douloureux)

TRYPANOSOMIASIS
Malaria Smear, Blood
Microfilaria, Peripheral Blood
Parasite Screen, Blood
Trypanosomiasis Serological Test,
    Blood

ADDITIONAL CONDITIONS
Ascites
Edema
Fever
Hepatosplenomegaly
Lymphadenopathy
Myocarditis

TUBAL PREGNANCY
(see Ectopic Pregnancy)

TUBERCULOSIS (TB), PULMONARY
Acid-Fast Bacteria, (Sputum) Culture and Stain
Chest X-Ray, Diagnostic
Liver I-131 Scan, Diagnostic
Mantoux Skin Test, Diagnostic
Muramidase, Serum and Urine
Urinalysis (for Kidney Tuberculosis), Urine

ADDITIONAL CONDITIONS
AIDS
Anorexia
Fever
Pleural Effusion
Urinary Tract Infection

TULAREMIA
Bacterial Serology, Blood
Blood Culture, Blood
Brucellosis Agglutinins, Blood
Complete Blood Count, Blood
Differential Leukocyte Count, Peripheral Blood
Febrile Agglutinins, Serum
Tularemia Agglutinins, Serum
Weil-Felix Agglutinins, Blood

ADDITIONAL CONDITIONS
Enteritis
Fever
Headache
Lymphadenopathy
Ulceration of Lesion

TUMORS
Alkaline Phosphatase, Serum
Alpha-Fetoprotein, Blood
Bone Marrow Biopsy, Diagnostic
CA 15–3, Serum
CA 50, Blood
Carcinoembryonic Antigen, Serum
Cervical/Vaginal Cytology, Specimen
Chest X-Ray, Diagnostic
Chromosome Analysis, Blood
Complete Blood Count, Blood
Estradiol Receptor and Progesterone Receptor in Breast Cancer, Diagnostic
HER-2/Neu Oncogene, Specimen
Histopathology, Specimen
Immunoperoxidase Procedures, Diagnostic (for Antigens)
Magnetic Resonance Imaging, Diagnostic
Mucin-Like Carcinoma-Associated Antigen, Blood
Myelogram, Diagnostic
Needle Aspiration, Diagnostic
Needle Aspiration Cytology, Specimen
Occult Blood, Stool
Proliferation Marker MIB 1–3, Specimen
Sputum, Routine, Culture
Sputum Cytology, Specimen
Urinalysis, Urine
Vanillylmandelic Acid, Urine

ADDITIONAL CONDITIONS
AIDS
Anorexia
Cancer
Dyspnea
Leukemia
Metastasis
Pain, Acute
Pneumonia

TURNER'S SYNDROME
Chromosome Analysis, Blood
Follicle-Stimulating Hormone,
    Serum
Glucose, Blood
Luteinizing Hormone, Blood
Oral Cavity Cytology, Specimen

ADDITIONAL CONDITIONS
Amenorrhea
Coarctation of the Aorta
Diabetes Mellitus
Infertility
Mental Retardation
Osteoporosis
Thyroiditis

TYPHOID
Febrile Agglutinins, Serum
Salmonella Titer, Blood
Stool Culture (for Salmonella),
    Routine, Stool

ADDITIONAL CONDITIONS
Bradycardia
Diarrhea
Headache
Leukopenia
Splenomegaly

TYPHUS
Complement Fixation, Serum
Febrile Agglutinins, Serum
Typhus Titer, Blood
Weil-Felix Agglutinins, Blood

ADDITIONAL CONDITIONS
Chills
Fever
Headache

ULCER
*(see Decubiti, Duodenal, Leg, or
Peptic)*

ULCERATIVE COLITIS
Albumin, Serum, Urine, and 24-Hour
    Urine
Aspartate Aminotransferase, Serum
Barium Enema, Diagnostic
Calcium, Total, Serum
Complete Blood Count, Blood
Creatinine, Serum
Cytologic Study of the
    Gastrointestinal Tract, Diagnostic
Histopathology, Specimen
Lactate Dehydrogenase, Blood
Occult Blood, Stool
Ova and Parasites, Stool
Phosphorus, Serum
Stool, Routine, Culture
Urea Nitrogen, Plasma or Serum
Uric Acid, Serum

ADDITIONAL CONDITIONS
Anemia
Constipation
Diarrhea
Fever
Hemorrhoids
Hypoproteinemia

UNSTABLE ANGINA
(see Angina Pectoris)

UREMIA
Anion Gap, Blood
Creatinine, Serum
Creatinine Clearance, Serum, Urine
Neuron-Specific Enolase, Serum
Platelet Count, Blood
Urea Nitrogen, Plasma or Serum
Urinalysis, Urine

ADDITIONAL CONDITIONS
Anemia
Gastrointestinal Bleeding
Glomerulonephritis
Hypertension
Hyponatremia
Neuropathy
Renal Failure

URETERAL STENTS
Complete Blood Count, Blood
Creatinine, Serum
Urea Nitrogen, Plasma or Serum
Urinalysis, Urine
Urine Culture, Routine, Catheterized,
    Urine

ADDITIONAL CONDITIONS
Bladder Cancer
Prostate Cancer

URETEROSIGMOIDOSTOMY
Calcium, Total, Serum
Chloride, Serum
Complete Blood Count, Blood
Potassium, Serum
Prothrombin Time and International
    Normalized Ratio, Serum
Type and Crossmatch, Blood
Urinalysis, Urine

ADDITIONAL CONDITIONS
Colon Cancer
Metastasis

URINARY TRACT INFECTION
Complete Blood Count, Blood
Foreign Body (Indwelling Catheter),
    Routine, Culture
Nitrite, Bacteria Screen, Urine
Occult Blood, Urine
Urinalysis, Urine
Urine Culture, Routine, Clean-Catch,
    Urine

ADDITIONAL CONDITIONS
Abscess
Cystitis
Diabetes Mellitus
Pregnancy
Prostatitis
Pyelonephritis
Tuberculosis
Urethritis

UTERINE CANCER
Biopsy, Site-Specific (Endometrium,
    Uterus), Specimen
Dilation and Curettage, Diagnostic
Obstetric Sonogram, Diagnostic
Pap Smear, Diagnostic

ADDITIONAL CONDITIONS
Diabetes Mellitus
Menorrhagia
Obesity
Polycystic Ovaries

VAGINAL CANCER
Biopsy, Site-Specific (Vagina),
    Specimen
Colposcopy, Diagnostic
Obstetric Sonogram, Diagnostic
Pap Smear, Diagnostic

ADDITIONAL CONDITIONS
Cervical Cancer
Endometriosis
Polyps
Vaginitis

VAGINITIS
Cervical/Vaginal Cytology, Specimen
Chlamydia Culture
Genital, *Candida albicans,* Culture
Genital, *Neisseria gonorrhoeae,*
    Culture
Glucose, Blood
Herpes Cytology, Specimen
Neisseria gonorrhoeae Smear,
    Specimen
Rapid Plasma Reagin Test, Blood
Trichomonas Preparation, Specimen
Urinalysis, Urine
Venereal Disease Research Laboratory
    Test, Serum

ADDITIONAL CONDITIONS
Candidiasis
Chlamydia
Dysuria
Gonorrhea
Pruritus
Toxic Shock Syndrome
Trichomonas

VARICELLA
(see Chickenpox)

VARICES (ESOPHAGEAL, LEG)
Calcium, Total, Serum
Complete Blood Count, Blood
Esophageal Radiography, Diagnostic
Occult Blood, Stool
Potassium, Serum

ADDITIONAL CONDITIONS
Alcoholism
Edema
Hemorrhage
Pain, Acute

VASCULITIS
Eosinophil Count, Blood
Histopathology, Specimen
Nerve Biopsy, Diagnostic
Raji Cell Assay, Blood
Rheumatoid Factor, Blood
Sedimentation Rate, Erythrocyte,
    Blood

ADDITIONAL CONDITIONS
Alcoholism
Anemia
Hepatitis B
Hypertension
Urticaria

VENOUS STASIS ULCER
(see Ulcer)

VENTRICULAR SEPTAL DEFECT
Blood Gases, Arterial, Blood
Cardiac Catheterization, Diagnostic
Chest X-Ray, Diagnostic
Echocardiogram, Diagnostic
Electrocardiogram, Diagnostic

ADDITIONAL CONDITIONS
Cardiac Murmur
Congestive Heart Failure
Pulmonary Hypertension
Systolic Heart Thrill

VERTIGO
(see also Tinnitus)
Alcohol, Blood
Blood Gases, Arterial, Blood
Carbon Dioxide, Blood
Cerebral Computed Tomography,
    Diagnostic
Magnesium, Serum

ADDITIONAL CONDITIONS
Brain Tumor
Labyrinthitis
Meniere's Disease
Nystagmus
Tinnitus
Trauma to the Head

VIRAL HEPATITIS
(see Hepatitis)

VIRILIZATION
Androstenedione, Serum
Dehydroepiandrosterone Sulfate,
    Serum and 24-Hour Urine (Serum)
Estrogens, Serum and 24-Hour Urine
17-Hydroxycorticosteroids, 24-Hour,
    Urine
17-Hydroxyprogesterone, Serum
17-Ketogenic Steroids, Total, 24-
    Hour, Urine
17-Ketosteroid Fractionation, 24-
    Hour, Urine
Pregnanetriol, Urine
Testosterone, Total, Blood

ADDITIONAL CONDITIONS
Acromegaly
Choriocarcinoma
Hirsutism
Pregnancy

VOMITING
Blood Gases, Arterial, Blood
Chloride, Serum
Potassium, Serum
Sodium, Plasma, Serum, or Urine
Urinalysis, Urine

ADDITIONAL CONDITIONS
Ascites
Bulimia
Cancer
Diabetic Acidosis
Gastroenteritis
Increased Intracranial Pressure
Intestinal Obstruction
Malnutrition
Meniere's Disease
Migraine
Pancreatitis
Paralytic Ileus
Pregnancy
Uremia

VON WILLEBRAND'S DISEASE
Aspirin Tolerance Test, Diagnostic
Bleeding Time, Ivy, Blood
Factor VIII, Blood
Factor VIII R:Ag, Blood
Mixing Study (Circulating
    Anticoagulants), Plasma
Platelet Aggregation, Blood, Platelet
    Aggregation, Hypercoagulable
    State, Blood
von Willebrand Factor Assay, Blood

ADDITIONAL CONDITIONS
Epistaxis
Gastrointestinal Bleeding
Gingivitis
Menorrhagia

WALDENSTRÖM'S MACROGLOBULINEMIA
Bone Marrow Biopsy, Diagnostic
Cryoglobulin, Serum
Immunoelectrophoresis, Serum and
    Urine
Protein, Electrophoresis, Serum
Red Cell Count, Serum

ADDITIONAL CONDITIONS
Anemia
Fatigue
Gastrointestinal Bleeding
Hepatosplenomegaly
Lymphadenopathy
Nausea
Raynaud's Phenomenon
Retinal Hemorrhage
Vertigo

WEIL'S SYNDROME
(see Leptospirosis)

WHIPPLE'S DISEASE
Biopsy, Site-Specific (Pancreas),
    Specimen
Cytologic Study of Gastrointestinal
    Tract, Diagnostic
d-Xylose Absorption Test, Diagnostic,
    Serum or Urine
Electron Microscopy, Diagnostic (for
    Small Bowel Mucosa, Macrophage
    Laden)
Histopathology, Specimen

ADDITIONAL CONDITIONS
Diarrhea
Fever
Gastrointestinal Bleeding
Lymphadenopathy
Malabsorption
Pain, Abdominal
Steatorrhea

WHOOPING COUGH
Bordetella pertussis, Culture

ADDITIONAL CONDITIONS
Anorexia
Lymphocytosis

WILM'S TUMOR
Chromosome Analysis (Deletion of
11p), Blood
Computed Tomography of the Body
(Abdomen), Diagnostic
Histopathology, Specimen
Intravenous Pyelography, Diagnostic

ADDITIONAL CONDITIONS
Anemia
Hematuria
Hypertension
Metastasis
Pain, Abdominal

WILSON'S DISEASE
Ceruloplasmin, Serum
Copper, Serum

ADDITIONAL CONDITIONS
Anemia
Ascites
Cirrhosis
Hepatitis
Jaundice
Splenomegaly

WOUNDS
Abscess, Anaerobic Culture
Biopsy, Anaerobic, Culture
Biopsy, Routine, Culture
Gram Stain (Wound Specimen),
Diagnostic
Nocardia Culture, All Sites, Specimen
Wound Culture
Wound, Fungus, Culture
Wound, *Mycobacteria,* Culture

ADDITIONAL CONDITIONS
Abscess
Burns
Diabetes Mellitus
Fever
Kaposi's Sarcoma
Sepsis
Trauma

XEROSTOMIA
Antinuclear Antibody, Serum
Complete Blood Count, Blood
Differential Leukocyte Count,
Peripheral Blood
Extractable Nuclear Antigen, Serum
Histopathology, Specimen
Immune Complex Assay, Blood
Protein, Electrophoresis, Serum
Rheumatoid Factor, Blood
Sedimentation Rate, Erythrocyte,
Blood
Sjögren's Antibodies, Blood

ADDITIONAL CONDITIONS
Cancer
Dehydration
Postoperative Procedure
Sjögren's Syndrome
Stomatitis

YAWS
Bone Scan, Diagnostic
Culture, Skin, Specimen

ADDITIONAL CONDITIONS
Lymphadenopathy
Rheumatism
Ulcerations of Skin

YELLOW FEVER
Bilirubin, Total, Serum
Bilirubin, Urine
Differential Leukocyte Count,
Peripheral Blood
Electrocardiogram, Diagnostic
Gastric Analysis, Specimen
Urinalysis, Urine
Viral Culture (Group B Arbovirus),
Specimen

ADDITIONAL CONDITIONS
Bradycardia (Late Effect)
Delirium
Gastrointestinal Hemorrhage
Headache
Hypotension
Jaundice
Photophobia
Tachycardia (Initially)

ZOLLINGER-ELLISON SYNDROME

Chloride, Serum
Fat, Semiquantitative, Stool
Gastric Analysis, Specimen
Gastrin, Serum
Pepsinogen-1 Antibody, Blood
Potassium, Serum
Sodium, Plasma, Serum, or Urine

ZOSTER

(see Herpes Zoster)

ADDITIONAL CONDITIONS

Diarrhea
Hemorrhage
Hypercalcemia
Intestinal Obstruction
Pain, Acute Abdominal
Pancreatic Tumor
Peptic Ulcer

PART TWO

Laboratory Tests and Diagnostic Procedures

ABDOMINAL AORTA SONOGRAM (ABDOMINAL AORTA ECHOGRAM), ABDOMINAL AORTA ULTRASOUND, DIAGNOSTIC

Norm: Negative for presence of aneurysm. Normal cross-sectional diameter of adult aorta (maximum internal diameter) varies from 3 cm at the xiphoid to about 1 cm at the bifurcation. Transverse and vertical diameters should be the same. Measurements should be taken at various parts down the length of the aorta. Any significant increase in diameter toward the feet (caudally) is abnormal.

Usage: Localization, measurement, and monitoring of abdominal aortic aneurysm; follow-up evaluation of surgical graft and aortic attachment after surgery for aneurysm; and detection of abdominal aortic atherosclerosis or thrombus. May be indicated in clients with pulsatile abdominal mass, poor circulation of the legs, recent abdominal trauma, and suspected idiopathic aortitis.

Description: Evaluation of the structure, size, and position of the abdominal aorta and branches (celiac trunk; and renal, superior mesenteric, and common iliac arteries) via the creation of an oscilloscopic picture from the echoes of high-frequency sound waves passing over the anterior trunk (acoustic imaging). The time required for the ultrasonic beam to be reflected back to the transducer from differing densities of tissue is converted by a computer to an electrical impulse displayed on an oscilloscopic screen to create a three-dimensional picture of the abdominal aorta and branches. Sonography allows measurement of the luminal diameter of the aorta. A narrowed lumen would indicate atherosclerosis or thrombus, whereas a wider-than-normal lumen with an irregular border may indicate aneurysm. Scattered internal echoes within the aneurysm may indicate an internal clot. A double lumen may indicate a tear in the wall of the abdominal aorta. Surgical grafts from aneurysm repair appear as bright echo reflections.

Professional Considerations:

1. Consent form NOT required.
2. Preparation:
   A. This test should be performed before intestinal barium tests, or else after the barium is cleared from the system (allow several days for clearance).
   B. An enema may be prescribed to be given prior to the sonogram.
   C. The client should wear a gown.
   D. Obtain ultrasonic gel or paste.
3. Procedure:
   A. Client is positioned supine on a procedure table.
   B. The abdomen is covered with conductive gel.
   C. A lubricated transducer is passed slowly along the abdomen at 1-cm intervals along the transverse, then longitudinal lines, covering the area between the xiphoid process and the symphysis pubis. If dissection is suspected, real-time techniques can be used more specifically to locate the site.
   D. Photographs are taken of the oscilloscopic images.
   E. Procedure takes less than 60 minutes.
4. Postprocedure care:
   A. Cleanse skin of ultrasonic gel.
5. Client and family teaching:
   A. Eat a low-residue diet the day before the sonogram, fast from food and fluids after midnight before the test, and refrain from smoking.
   B. Lie as still as possible during the procedure, which is painless and carries no risks.
   C. Results are normally available within 24 hours.
6. Factors that affect results:
   A. Dehydration interferes with adequate contrast between organs and body fluids.
   B. Intestinal barium or gas obscures results by preventing proper transmission and deflection of the high-frequency sound waves.
   C. The more abdominal fat present, the greater the attenuation (reduction in sound wave amplitude and intensity), which interferes with the clarity of the picture.
   D. Aorta may be displaced by scoliosis, a retroperitoneal mass or by para-aortic lymph nodes; in some clients, these can mimic an aneurysm.
7. Other data:
   A. There is some evidence that aneurysms <4 cm diameter may be safely followed by ongoing monitoring and any aneurysm >4 cm diameter should be considered for surgery.

Bibliography:

Breger B, Bruguera C, Gharbi H, Goldberg B, Tan F, Wachira M, Weil F, Palmer PES (eds). Manual of

Diagnostic Ultrasound, USA, WHO, 1995, pp 334, 53–63.

Larcos G, Gruenewald SM, Fletcher JP: Ultrasound screening of families with abdominal aortic aneurysm. Australas Radiol *39*(3):254–256, 1995.

Nguyen D, Hamper UM: False positive dissection of abdominal aortic aneurysm by color Doppler duplex ultrasonography. J Ultrasound Med *14*(6):467–472, 1995.

ABDOMINAL PLAIN FILM
(see Flat Plate X-Ray of Abdomen, Diagnostic)

ABG
(see Blood Gases, Arterial, Blood)

ABI
(see Ankle-Brachial Index, Diagnostic)

ABO GROUP AND RH TYPE, BLOOD

Norm: Specific to each individual.

Usage: Blood transfusion therapy, erythroblastosis fetalis, paternity determinations, pregnancy, and preoperatively.

Description: The ABO blood group is the phenotype of a client's blood resulting from genetic inheritance. The four most common phenotypes are A, B, AB, and O, referring to the type of antigen present on the surface of red blood cells. Rh type refers to whether an Rh antigen is present (Rh-positive) or absent (Rh-negative) on the surface of a client's red blood cells. Routine testing usually tests only for the Rho(D) antigen. If an Rh-negative client receives Rh-positive blood, he or she will develop Rh antibodies, and future Rh-positive transfusions may cause a transfusion reaction. In pregnancy, antibodies from an Rh-negative mother may hemolyze fetal erythrocytes in a fetus who has inherited the Rh-positive antigen from the father (erythroblastosis fetalis/hemolytic disease of the newborn). This test determines the specific ABO phenotype and Rh type by determining which A and B red cell antigens are present as well as whether or not the Rho(D) antigen is present.

Professional Considerations:
1. Consent form NOT required.
2. Preparation:
   A. Assess client for history of recent blood

transfusion reaction, which can result in a positive antibody screen and require further testing. Write affirmative history on blood bank requisition.
   B. Tube: Red-top, red/gray-top, or gold-top, 1–2 tubes.
3. Procedure:
   A. At bedside, ask the client to state full name and compare with the client's name band. Label the sample tube and laboratory requisition with the client's name, identification number, date, time, initials, and sign. Some institutions require additional data.
   B. Draw one or two 10-ml blood samples, depending on institutional requirements.
4. Postprocedure care:
   A. Some institutions require application of a blood band to the client's wrist. The blood bank identification numbers should match the identification numbers on any blood bag used for transfusion for the client.
5. Client and family teaching:
   A. Results are normally available within 24 hours.
6. Factors that affect results:
   A. Hemolyzed specimen invalidates results.
   B. Specimen drawn from extremity into which blood or dextran is infusing invalidates results.
   C. Drugs causing a false-positive Rh test include levodopa, methyldopa, and methyldopate hydrochloride.
   D. Abnormal plasma proteins, cold autoagglutinins, positive direct antiglobulin test, and in some cases bacteremia may interfere with results.
7. Other data:
   A. The test must be performed within 48 hours of specimen collection.

Bibliography:

British Committee for Standards in Haematology, Blood Transfusion Task Force: Recommendations for evaluation, validation and implementation of new techniques for blood grouping, antibody screening and cross-matching. Transfusion Med *5*(2):145–150, 1995.

Garratty G: Problems associated with compatibility testing for patients with autoimmune hemolytic anemia. Southeast Asian J Trop Med Public Health *24* (Suppl 1):76–79, 1993.

Jacobs D, Demott W, Finley P, Horvat R, Kasten B, Tilzer L: Laboratory Test Handbook, 3rd ed. Hudson, OH, Lexi-Comp Inc, 1994, p 1513.

ABSCESS, ANAEROBIC CULTURE
(see Body Fluid, Anaerobic Culture)

ACA
(see Antiphospholipid Antibodies, Serum)

ACCUCHEK, DIAGNOSTIC
(see Glucose Monitoring Machines, Diagnostic)

ACE
(see Angiotensin-Converting Enzyme, Blood)

ACETAMINOPHEN, SERUM

Norm:

		SI Units
Therapeutic level	10–30 µg/ml	66–199 µmol/L
Toxic level	>150 µg/ml	>990 µmol/L
Panic level (hepatotoxicity)	>200 µg/ml	>1320 µmol/L

Overdose Symptoms and Treatment:

Symptoms: Occur in four stages.

Stage I (ingestion to 24 hours) G.I. irritation, pallor, lethargy, diaphoresis, metabolic acidosis and coma (massive ingestions with serum concentration >800 µg/ml have been reported, but coma is usually attributed to a coingestant such as alcohol).

Stage II (24–48 hours) Increased serum hepatic enzymes, right upper quadrant abdominal pain, possible decreased renal function.

Stage III (72–96 hours) Increased AST, increased ALT, nausea, vomiting, jaundice, lethargy, confusion, coma, coagulation disorders, possible decreased renal function.

Stage IV (4 days–2 weeks) Clinical symptoms subside; laboratory values return to baseline.

Treatment:

1. Establish and maintain adequate airway, respiratory, and circulatory function.

2. If client is obtunded or unconscious, appropriate doses of thiamine, dextrose, and naloxone must be considered.

3. Gastric decontamination: In one study, rapid complete bowel lavage with 4G polyethylene glycol electrolyte solution was shown to significantly reduce serum acetaminophen levels. In another, use of activated charcoal prevented acetaminophen absorption when given within 60 minutes of acetaminophen ingestion. Syrup of ipecac may be used to induce emesis for recent ingestion, but must be used with extreme caution.

4. Administration of oral acetylcysteine (Mucomyst by Mead Johnson) for suspected toxic doses (>7.5 g). Mucomyst is most likely to be effective when given within 16 hours after acetaminophen ingestion.

5. Laboratory monitoring: Urine tox screen, hepatic profile q 24 hours × 3–4 days, BUN, Cr, serum electrolytes, serum acetaminophen concentration level 4 hours after ingestion.

6. Coingestion of other substances that delay gastric emptying is an indication for serial measurement to detect late-rising acetaminophen levels.

7. Hemodialysis WILL, but peritoneal dialysis will NOT remove acetaminophen.

Usage: Drug abuse, hepatitis, monitoring for toxicity during acetaminophen therapy, overdose, poisoning, and suicide.

Description: Acetaminophen is a *p*-aminophenol derivative that has antipyretic (direct action on hypothalamus) and moderate analgesic actions. It is absorbed by the GI tract and metabolized by liver microsomes. Half-life is 1–4 hours with peak blood levels reached in 30 minutes to 1 hour. Used for headache, fever, and relief of pain in clients who cannot tolerate aspirin or those with peptic ulcers and/or bleeding disorders. It is the drug of choice (antipyretic/analgesic) in children 13 years of age and younger due to the possible development of Reye's syndrome associated with aspirin.

Professional Considerations:

1. Consent form NOT required.
2. Preparation:
   A. Tube: Red-top, red/gray-top, gold-top, or lavender-top.
   B. Do NOT draw during hemodialysis.
3. Procedure:
   A. Draw a 1-ml blood sample.
4. Postprocedure care:
   A. None.
5. Client and family teaching:
   A. Results are normally available within 24 hours.
   B. If overdose is suspected, prepare client and family for necessary supportive treatment described above.
   C. If activated charcoal was given for elevated levels, client should drink 4–6 glasses of water each day for 2 days to prevent constipation. Activated charcoal will also cause stools to be black for a few days.
6. Factors that affect results:
   A. Cardiovascular, hepatic, gastrointestinal, or renal dysfunction can alter drug absorption and elimination.
7. Other data:
   A. Acetaminophen is present in many medicines: Anacin3, Datril, Liquiprin, Panadoe, Panex, Paracetamol, Phenaphen, Tempra, and Tylenol.

Bibliography:

Chamberlain JM, Gorman RL, Oderda GM, Klein-Schwartz W, Klein BL: Use of activated charcoal in a simulated poisoning with acetaminophen: a new loading dose for N-acetylcysteine? Ann Emerg Med *22*(9):1398–1402, 1993.

Hassig SR, Linscheer WG, Murthy UK, Miller C, Banerjee A, Levine L, Wagner K, Oates RP: Effects of PEG-electrolyte (Colyte) lavage on serum acetaminophen concentrations. A model for treatment of acetaminophen overdose. Dig Dis Sci *38*(8):1395–1401, 1993.

Rose SR: Subtleties of managing acetaminophen poisoning. Am J Hosp Pharm *51*(24):3065–3068, 1994.

Tighe TV, Walter FG: Delayed toxic acetaminophen level after initial four hour nontoxic level. J Toxicol Clin Toxicol *32*(4):431–434, 1994.

Whelpton R, Fernandes K, Wilkinson KA, Goldhill DR: Determination of paracetamol (acetaminophen) in blood and plasma using high performance liquid chromatography with dual electrode coulometric quantification in the redox mode. Biomed Chromatogr *7*(2):90–93, 1993.

ACETONE, SERUM
(see Ketone Bodies, Blood)

ACETONE, URINE

Norm: Keto-Diastix or Multistix: Negative. Quantitative 0.3–2.0 mg/dl.

Usage: Differentiation of diabetic coma and insulin shock; evaluation of glucose control in diabetics; preadmission screening; pregnancy; and screening for ketoacidosis.

Description: Acetone is a byproduct of fat and fatty acid metabolism that provides a source of cellular energy for cells when glucose stores are exhausted or when glucose is prevented from entering cells due to lack of insulin. Acetone entering the bloodstream is almost completely metabolized in the liver. When acetone is formed at a faster-than-normal rate, it is excreted in the urine.

Professional Considerations:

1. Consent form NOT required.
2. Preparation:
   A. Obtain a 50-ml, clean urine container and acetone testing strips or tablets.
   B. Client should empty the bladder 30 minutes prior to specimen collection time and then drink a glass of water.
   C. For specimens obtained from an indwelling urinary catheter, also obtain a catheter clamp, a sterile 10-ml syringe and needle, and an alcohol wipe.
3. Procedure:
   A. Obtain a 20-ml double-voided urine specimen in a clean container.
   B. Specimens from catheter: Clamp the catheter tubing for 15 minutes to allow urine to accumulate above the sample port. Cleanse the sample port with an alcohol wipe and allow to dry. Aspirate 20-ml urine from the sample port, using a sterile syringe and needle. Collect only fresh urine that has accumulated above the sample port. Unclamp the catheter tubing.
   C. Dip the Keto-Diastix, Multistix, or other acetone testing material in fresh urine and hold the strip horizontally for 15 seconds.
   D. Compare the color of the ketone patch on the strip with the color chart on the Keto-Diastix or Multistix container.
   E. Alternate method using Acetest tablets: Place a drop of urine on an Acetest tablet and wait 30 seconds. Compare the color with the Acetest color chart.
4. Postprocedure care:
   A. None.
5. Client and family teaching:
   A. Results are immediately available.
6. Factors that affect results:
   A. Fasting or dieting may cause acetone to appear in the urine.

B. Use of acetone tablets that are darkened invalidates results.

C. Drugs that may cause false-positive results include captopril, levodopa, paraldehyde, and phenazopyridine hydrochloride.

7. Other data:

A. Refrigerate the specimen if the test cannot be performed within 1 hour of collection.

B. In a recent study, ratings on scales of well-being and acute symptoms correlated significantly with the concentration of acetone in urine after acute airborne acetone exposure.

Bibliography:

Kiesswetter E, Blaszkewicz M, Vangala R, Seeber A: Acute exposure to acetone in a factory and ratings of well being. Neurotoxicology 15(3):597–601, 1994.

Kumagai S, Matsunaga: Physiologically based pharmacokinetic model for acetone. Occup Environ Med 52(5):344–352, 1995.

ACETYLCHOLINE RECEPTOR ANTIBODY, SERUM

Norm: ≤0.03 nmol/L.

Usage: Diagnosis and clinical monitoring of myasthenia gravis.

Description: In clients with myasthenia gravis, this antibody interferes with the binding of acetylcholine to receptor sites on the muscle membrane, thus preventing muscle contraction. Assays for acetylcholine receptor antibodies are positive in 85–90% of clients with acute myasthenia gravis and are replacing the Tensilon test as a diagnostic aid for this condition.

Professional Considerations:

1. Consent form NOT required.
2. Preparation:
   A. Tube: Red-top, red/gray-top, or gold-top.
   B. List on the laboratory requisition any recent immunosuppressive drug therapy the client received.
3. Procedure:
   A. Draw a 2-ml blood sample.
4. Postprocedure care:
   A. None.
5. Client and family teaching:
   A. Results may not be available for several days.
6. Factors that affect results:
   A. False-positive results may be caused by D-penicillamine.
7. Other data:
   A. Undetectable titer occurs in clients who have only ocular myasthenia gravis.
   B. *See also Tensilon Test, Diagnostic.*

Bibliography:

Mokhtarian F, Shirazian D, Grob D: Production of anti-acetylcholine receptor-alpha antibody in vitro by peripheral blood lymphocytes of patients with myasthenia gravis: role of immunoregulatory T cells and monocytes. J Lab Clin Med 124(2):231–241, 1994.

Ong BK, Chong PN, Tan SK, Cheah JS, Lui KF: Acetylcholine receptor antibody assay kit: establishment of controls in normals and non-myasthenics and evaluation of sera from patients with thyroid disease. Ann Acad Med Singapore 1993 22(4):567–568, 1993.

ACETYLSALICYLIC ACID
(see Salicylate, Blood)

ACID-FAST BACTERIA, CULTURE AND STAIN

Norm: Negative.

Usage: Acquired immune deficiency syndrome (AIDS); suspected leprosy, mycobacteriosis, or tuberculosis; and differentiation of tuberculosis from carcinoma and bronchiectasis.

Description: *Mycobacterium tuberculosis* is a rod-shaped bacterium that resists decolorizing chemicals after staining, a property termed "acid-fastness." *M. tuberculosis* is transmitted most commonly via the airborne route to the lungs, where it survives well, causes areas of granulomatous inflammation, and, if not dormant, causes cough, fever, and hemoptysis. Acid-fast bacteria *M. avium-intracellulare* is a common cause of infection in clients with AIDS. Culture of sputum is necessary to confirm the diagnosis of tuberculosis and for sensitivity studies for drug therapy.

Professional Considerations:

1. Consent form NOT required.
2. Preparation:
   A. Obtain three small, sterile containers.
   B. *See Client and family teaching.*
3. Procedure:
   A. Aerosolized therapy prior to sputum collection may stimulate sputum production and produce a better specimen.
   B. When tuberculosis is suspected, collect three daily, early-morning sputum, deep-cough specimens in a sterile container.
   C. When leprosy is suspected, obtain smear from nasal scrapings or biopsy from lesions in a sterile container.
4. Postprocedure care:
   A. Provide mouth care.
5. Client and family teaching:
   A. Perform oral hygiene before giving

specimens to reduce chances of contamination.

B. Deep coughs are necessary to produce sputum, rather than saliva. To produce the proper specimen, take several breaths in, without fully exhaling each, then expel sputum with a "cascade cough."

6. Factors that affect results:
   A. Antituberculous drug therapy may cause negative results due to inhibition of growth of *M. tuberculosis*.
   B. A high carbon dioxide atmosphere for growth may increase the number of positive cultures.
   C. Culture medium containing glycerin accelerates growth.

7. Other data:
   A. Culture results may take 3–8 weeks.

Bibliography:

Beaman BL, Beaman L: *Nocardia* species: host-parasite relationships. Clin Microbiol Rev 7(2):213–264, 1994.

Marrie TJ: Pneumonia caused by *Nocardia* species. Semin Respir Infect 9(3):207–213, 1994.

ACID-FAST STAIN, *NOCARDIA* SPECIES, CULTURE

Norm: Negative.

Usage: Aids in diagnosis of mycetoma, *Nocardia brasiliensis*, and nocardiosis.

Description: *Nocardia* is an aerobic, gram-positive, filamentous branching bacteria that segments into reproductive bacillary fragments. It is weakly acid-fast and found outdoors in decayed matter, soil, grass, and straw, and enters the body primarily through inhalation of contaminated dust. The type species, *Nocardia asteroides*, and *N. brasiliensis, N. farcinica, N. otitidiscaviarum, N. nova*, and *N. transvalensis* cause a variety of diseases in both normal and immunocompromised humans and animals. The *N. asteroides* species causes primary skin lesions, visceral infections (most commonly abscesses of the lungs, brain, and subcutaneous tissue), and, sometimes, disseminated infections in humans.

Professional Considerations:

1. Consent form NOT required.
2. Preparation:
   A. Obtain a sterile scalpel or spatula, or a sterile needle and syringe, and aerobic culture media.
3. Procedure:
   A. Obtain a scraping from a skin lesion or an aspirate of an abscess using sterile technique.
   B. Inoculate both aerobic and anaerobic culture media with the specimen.
   C. Aerobic culture media of beef infusion broth or thioglycolate broth may be used.
   D. Initial incubation at temperatures from 38–45°C should be used.
   E. Examine cultures for growth beginning at 48 hours and continue examination daily for 2 weeks.
4. Postprocedure care:
   A. Apply dry sterile dressing to site.
5. Client and family teaching:
   A. Avoid application of creams or lotions to sample site and allow site to remain open to air for healing.
   B. At least 2–3 days are required for growth and results.
6. Factors that affect results:
   A. *Nocardia* growth may be mistaken for nontuberculous *Mycobacterium* when *Mycobacteria* culture media is used.
7. Other data:
   A. Common specimens include pus, tissue, body fluid, and sputum.
   B. Final reports may take 10 days.

Bibliography:

Beaman B, Beaman L: *Nocardia* species: host-parasite relationships. Clin Microbiol Rev 7(2):213–264, 1994.

Boiron P, Provost F: Use of partially purified 54-kilodalton antigen for diagnosis of nocardiosis by Western blot (immunoblot) assay. J Clin Microbiol 28(2):328–331, 1990.

ACIDIFIED SERUM TEST, BLOOD
(see Ham Test, Blood)

ACID PERFUSION (BERNSTEIN) TEST, DIAGNOSTIC

Norm: No burning or pain after saline or acidic infusions.

Usage: Differentiation between chest pain due to cardiac etiology and chest pain due to esophagitis. Not commonly used by cardiologists; more often used by gastroenterologists. Aids diagnosis of gastroesophageal reflux as a cause of nocturnal asthma.

Description: Saline and then acidic solutions are slowly perfused through a nasogastric tube into the stomach. Clients with esophagitis due to relaxation of the lower esophageal sphincter usually experience burning and/or pain after the perfusion of acidic solution, but not after the saline. Gastroesophageal reflux has been found to occur in some clients with nocturnal asthma. Such clients show an exacerbation of asthmatic symptoms when this test is performed.

Professional Considerations:

1. Consent form NOT required.

Risks:

Exacerbation of asthma in asthmatics. Complications of nasogastric tube insertion include bleeding, dysrhythmias, esophageal perforation, laryngospasm, and decreased mean PO_2.

Contraindications:

Cardiac disorders; esophageal varices.

2. Preparation:
   A. Obtain nasogastric tube, tape, gel, glass of water, and a liter each of normal saline solution and 0.1 N hydrochloric acid (HCl) solution.
   B. *See Client and family teaching.*
3. Procedure:
   A. Mark a nasogastric tube at 12 inches from the distal tip.
   B. Insert the nasogastric tube into the stomach and aspirate stomach contents.
   C. Withdraw the nasogastric tube until the 12-inch mark is at the tip of the nares. This ensures that the tube tip is located in the esophagus.
   D. Perfuse normal saline into the nasogastric tube at 60–120 drops per minute. Assess for discomfort after 10 minutes.
   E. Connect 0.1 N HCl solution piggybacked to the normal saline line. Close the clamp on the normal saline and open the line on the HCl solution at a rate of 60–120 drops per minute for 30

minutes or until the client complains of discomfort when asked every 10 minutes or independently.
   F. At the first sign of discomfort, clamp the HCl and open the normal saline until the client experiences no further pain or burning.
   G. Clamp and remove the nasogastric tube.
4. Postprocedure care:
   A. An antacid may be necessary if discomfort continues after the test.
5. Client and family teaching:
   A. Fast and do not smoke for 12 hours prior to the test.
   B. The test may reproduce the pain, but this will help differentiate the cause of the pain, and the discomfort will be temporary.
   C. Antacids should not be ingested within 24 hours prior to the test.
   D. The test involves the insertion of a tube through the nose into the stomach. The insertion may be uncomfortable and cause a pressure-like feeling or cause you to gag and cough. You will be asked to take sips of water and swallow to make the tube insertion easier.
6. Factors that affect results:
   A. None found.
7. Other data:
   A. Has been used in some recent studies to monitor the effect of gastroesphogeal reflux on air exchange.
   B. *See also Esophageal Acidity Test, Diagnostic; and Esophageal Manometry, Diagnostic.*

Bibliography:

Chakrabarti S, Singh K, Singh V, Nain CK, Jindal SK: Airway response to acid instillation in esophagus in bronchial asthma. Indian J Gastroenterol *14*(2):44–47, 1995.

Friesen CA, Streed CJ, Carney LA, Zwick DL, Roberts CC: Esophagitis and modified Bernstein tests in infants with apparent life-threatening events. Pediatrics *94*(4 Pt 1):541–544, 1994.

Ganatra JV, Medow MS, Berezin S, Newman LJ, Glassman M, Bostwick HE, Halata M, Schwarz SM: Esophageal dysmotility elicited by acid perfusion in children with esophagitis. Am J Gastroenterol *90*(7):1080–1083, 1995.

ACID PHOSPHATASE, SERUM

Norm:

Method		SI Units
Bodansky	0.5–2 U/L	2.7–10.7 IU/L
King-Armstrong	0.1–5 U/L	0.2–8.8 IU/L
Bessey-Lowery-Brock	0.1–0.8 U/L	1.7–13.4 IU/L
Gutman	0.1–2 U/L	

Increased: Bone fracture, cancer with bone metastasis, Gaucher's disease, hairy cell leukemia (leukemic reticuloendotheliosis), hepatitis (viral), hyperparathyroidism, idiopathic thrombocytopenic purpura (with bone marrow megakaryocytes), jaundice (obstructive), Laennec's cirrhosis, leukemia (myelogenous), multiple myeloma, osteogenesis imperfecta, Paget's disease (advanced), partial translocation trisomy 21, prostate cancer, prostatic infarction, prostatic surgery or trauma, renal impairment (acute), sickle cell crisis, thrombocythemia, thrombocytosis, thromboembolism, and thrombophlebitis. Drugs include anabolic steroids.

Decreased: Not clinically significant. Drugs include fluorides.

Description: Acid phosphatase is one of a group of enzymes located primarily in the prostate gland and prostatic secretions. Smaller amounts are found in the bone marrow, spleen, liver, kidneys, and blood components such as erythrocytes and platelets. Isoenzymes of acid phosphatase include prostatic isoenzyme and erythrocytic isoenzyme. Used in diagnosing and monitoring treatment response of prostate cancer. Prostatic acid phosphatase (PAP) is less specific and sensitive than prostate-specific antigen (PSA).

Professional Considerations:

1. Consent form NOT required.
2. Preparation:
   A. Tube: Red-top, red/gray-top, or gold-top.
3. Procedure:
   A. Collect a 1-ml blood sample.
4. Postprocedure care:
   A. Send the specimen to the laboratory immediately.

B. Separate the serum, add 0.01 ml of 20% acetic acid per milliliter of serum, and refrigerate if the test is not performed immediately.
5. Client and family teaching:
   A. Results may not be available for several days.
6. Factors that affect results:
   A. Hemolysis or specimens received more than 15 minutes after collection invalidate results.
   B. False-negative results may be due to fluorides, oxalates, or phosphates.
   C. False-positive results may be due to clofibrate.
   D. Elevated levels may be caused by rectal examination, prostatic massage, or urinary catheterization within 2 days prior to the test.
7. Other data:
   A. This test is more helpful for diagnosis in advanced prostate cancer than in early prostate cancer.
   B. Use of prostate-specific acid phosphatase as a tumor marker for prostate cancer is being replaced by *Prostate-Specific Antigen, Serum.*

Bibliography:

Akdas A, Simsek F, Ilker Y, Turkeri L, Ercan H: The value of prostatic acid phosphatase and prostate specific antigen as serum markers in carcinoma of the prostate. Int Urol Nephrol 25(3):271–278, 1993.

Akimoto S, Masai M, Akakura K, Shimazaki J: Tumor marker doubling time in patients with prostate cancer: Determination of prostate-specific antigen and prostatic acid phosphatase doubling time. Eur Urol 27(3):207–212, 1995.

Narayan P, Tewari A, Jacob G, Mahmood I, Gajendran V, Presti J: Differential suppression of serum prostatic acid phosphatase and prostate-specific antigen by 5-alpha-reductase inhibitor. Br J Urol 75(5):642–646, 1995.

ACID PHOSPHATASE, TARTRATE-RESISTANT, BLOOD

(see Tartrate-Resistant Acid Phosphatase, Blood)

ACID PHOSPHATASE, VAGINAL SWAB

Norm: Method: Dilution with a substrate of thymolphthalein monophosphate.

<5:	Normal vaginal secretions.
<7:	Inconclusive.
Between 7 and 50:	Highly suggestive of coitus within the prior 36 hours.
>50:	Confirmation of recent coitus.

Usage: Rape trauma work-up.

Description: Acid phosphatase is one of a group of enzymes located primarily in the prostate gland and prostatic secretions, with smaller amounts

found elsewhere in the body. Normal vaginal secretions contain only low levels of acid phosphatase. Because acid phosphatase is found in such high concentrations in semen, its isolation in high levels from vaginal fluid in cases of suspected rape is strong evidence that coitus occurred recently.

Professional Considerations:

1. Consent form NOT required unless specimen may be used as legal evidence.
2. Preparation:
   A. Obtain speculum, cotton wool swab supplied in a sexual offense kit, and sterile container.
3. Procedure:
   A. If the specimen may be used as legal evidence, have the specimen collection witnessed.
   B. Position the client in the dorsal lithotomy position and drape for privacy and comfort.
   C. Gently scrape the walls of the vagina with a plain cotton wool swab until it is saturated.
   D. Place the swab in a sterile container.
4. Postprocedure care:
   A. Write the client's name, the date, the exact time of collection, and the specimen source on the laboratory requisition. Sign and have the witness sign the laboratory requisition.
   B. Transport the specimen to the laboratory immediately in a sealed plastic bag marked as legal evidence. All clients handling the specimen should sign and mark the time of receipt on the laboratory requisition.
5. Client and family teaching:
   A. Provide repeated and thorough explanation of the purpose and process of specimen collection.
   B. Survivors of sexual assault should be referred to appropriate crisis counseling agencies as well as gynecological follow-up. Facilitate referral if desired by client.
   C. Referral for HIV testing should be reviewed and offered to all sexual assault victims.
   D. Preventive treatment for *Chlamydia*, gonorrhea, and syphilis should be provided to all survivors of sexual assault.
   E. The option of postcoital contraceptive should be reviewed with all survivors of sexual assault.
6. Factors that affect results:
   A. Vaginal swabs for acid phosphatase should be collected as soon as possible

after the rape. Swabs have the highest chance of being positive when collected within 5 hours of the rape and are least likely to be positive after 12 hours. By 48 hours after the rape, normal vaginal levels are usually found.

   B. Negative results may be obtained if the assailant was sexually dysfunctional or has had a vasectomy; or if the woman bathed, douched, or defecated after the rape.
   C. This test cannot identify the perpetrator.
   D. Contamination of the vagina or the specimen with substances other than semen or normal vaginal substances may cause false-positive results.
7. Other data:
   A. Negative results caused by a long time delay between the occurrence of the rape and collection of the vaginal specimen are sometimes used by defense attorneys as evidence that a rape did not occur.
   B. Although swabs may also be taken of other body orifices for evidence of acid phosphatase, they rarely yield positive results when taken more than 5 hours after the sexual assault occurred.
   C. A spot test, intended for field use outside of the lab, is currently being tested. A test swab is covered with the moistened specimen, and characteristic color changes in the swab indicate positive or negative presence of acid phosphatase. Vaginal washings should be evaluated within 24 hours of deposition. Results are independent of sperm count.
   D. *See also Blood Group Antigen of Semen, Vaginal Swab; and Precipitin Test Against Human Sperm and Blood, Vaginal Swab.*

Bibliography:

Hooft PJ, van de Voorde HP: Interference of body products, food and products from daily life with the modified zinc test and the acid phosphatase test. Forensic Sci Int 66(3):187–196, 1994.

Roach BA, Vladutiu AO: Prostatic specific antigen and prostatic acid phosphatase measured by radioimmunoassay in vaginal washings from cases of suspected sexual assault [letter]. Clin Chim Acta 216(1–2):199–201, 1993.

Steinman G: Rapid spot tests for identifying suspected semen specimens. Forensic Sci Int 72(3):191–197, 1995.

ACOUSTIC IMMITTANCE TESTS, DIAGNOSTIC

Norm: Normal acoustic immittance.

Tympanogram: The tympanogram recording shows a symmetrical, shallow upslope and downslope free of notches or peaks with middle ear pressure of –100 daPa to +100 daPa.

Pure Tone Reflex Threshold:

Transbrainstem	70–100 dB HL
Ipsilateral	3–12 dB HL
Reflex decay	<½ baseline/10 seconds

Usage: Assessment of middle ear and tympanic membrane functioning; identification of location of middle ear lesions; and differential diagnosis of brainstem lesions and hearing loss.

Description: The acoustic immittance tests measure middle ear functioning and locates abnormalities via tympanometry and measurement of acoustic reflexes. Tympanometry assesses stiffness of the middle ear by measuring admittance (i.e., how much impedance exists to the flow of sound into the ear). Lower than normal admittance can be caused by cerumen, the presence of fluid in the middle ear, or a perforated tympanic membrane. Higher than normal admittance results when ear scarring is present. Measurement of acoustic reflexes reveals how well the stapedius muscle responds to the delivery of sound against it. Poor or no acoustic reflexes can indicate hearing loss or neurologic or stapedius muscle damage or lesions.

Professional Considerations:

1. Consent form NOT required.

Risks:
Infection.

Contraindications:
May be contraindicated in clients with traumatic head injuries or suspected labyrinthine fistula or in those who have recently undergone ear surgery.

2. Preparation:
   A. Obtain admittance meter, recorder, probe with tips, cuffs and silicone putty, otoscope, and audiometer.
   B. *See Client and family teaching.*
3. Procedure:
   A. The bores of the ear probe are cleansed with wire. The admittance meter is calibrated. The ear canal is inspected, and impacted cerumen is removed.

B. The auricle is lifted up and out, and the admittance meter's cuffed probe is inserted into the external auditory canal until a pressure of –200 daPa is achieved, indicating an adequate seal.
C. Admittance measurement: Admittance recordings are made in response to air pressure changes made by the meter.
D. Acoustic reflex measurement: Acoustic reflexes are then measured by sending a 500-to 4000-Hz tone into either ear. Ipsilateral measurement is performed in the stimulated ear. Contralateral (transbrainstem) measurement may be performed by sending the tone into the opposite ear.
E. Reflex threshold measurement: The reflex threshold is then measured by sending progressively louder tones into the ear in 10-dB increments until a reflex occurs and then decreasing the dB in smaller steps until the lowest level that elicits a reflex is identified.
F. Reflex decay measurement: The reflex decay is measured by sending a 10-second tone equal to the reflex threshold plus 10 dB into the contralateral ear and comparing the degree of initial, 5-second, and 10-second reflexes.
4. Postprocedure care:
   A. Cleanse the ear probe.
5. Client and family teaching:
   A. Avoid moving, talking, or swallowing during the test. The test involves transmitting loud tones into the ear that may be uncomfortable, but will not damage the ear.
6. Factors that affect results:
   A. The most accurate results are obtained when the air seal remains continuous. Silicone putty may be used around the circumference of the canal to help maintain the seal.
   B. Cerumen or silicone putty clogging the probe may cause the tympanogram to show as a flat waveform.
7. Other data:
   A. None.

Bibliography:

Hanks WD, Rose KJ: Middle ear resonance and acoustic immittance measures in children. J Speech Hear Res *36*(1):218–222, 1993.

Sutherland JE, Campbell K: Immittance audiometry. Prim Care *17*(2):233–247, 1990.

Woodford CM: Screening measurements and procedures. Exemplified by an identification audiometry program. Clin Commun Disord *3*(3):36–46, 1993.

ACQUIRED IMMUNE DEFICIENCY SYNDROME EVALUATION BATTERY (AIDS EVALUATION BATTERY), DIAGNOSTIC

Norm: Negative AIDS battery, nonreactive.
Antigen detection by serology: Negative for HIV antigens.
Antibody detection: Negative for HIV antibodies.

LYMPHOCYTE SUBSET ENUMERATION

Total	1500–4000/ml
B cells	65–475/ml
OKT3 cells	875–1900/ml
OKT4 cells (CD4)	450–1400/ml
OKT8 cells	190–725/ml
OKT4:OKT8 ratio	1–3.5
Beta$_2$-microglobulin	<2 mg/ml (<170 nmol/L, SI units)

Usage: Used often in combination with cultures and for confirmation of opportunistic infection to help diagnose acquired immune deficiency syndrome.

Description: Acquired immune deficiency syndrome (AIDS) is caused by human immunodeficiency virus (HIV), a cytoplasmic retrovirus of the human T-cell leukemia/lymphoma virus family that reproduces and infects, even with antibodies against the virus present. There are several strains, and all attack a subgroup of T lymphocytes known as "helper" T cells that are important in cell-mediated immunity. AIDS causes immunosuppression and susceptibility to infection with opportunistic organisms such as *Pneumocystis carinii, Candida albicans, Cryptococcus neoformans, Mycobacterium, Toxoplasma gondii, Herpes simplex,* and *Cryptosporidium.* The predominant modes of transmission of HIV are thought to be (1) direct contact between the blood of an uninfected person and the blood of an infected person, and (2) sexual and body fluid transmission. The incubation period may be as short as 6 days and as long as several years.

HIV is now the leading cause of death in men aged 25–40, the sixth leading cause of death in adolescent males aged 15–24, and the fourth leading cause of death in women aged 25–44. It is estimated that over 1 million U.S. residents are HIV infected— (approximately 1 out of 250). The World Health Organization estimates that by the year 2000 there will be 40 million HIV-infected individuals worldwide.

Persons may be infected with the human immunodeficiency virus for several years without becoming symptomatic when the virus enters a non-replicating latent period. When the virus begins actively replicating, the person may develop AIDS. At 2–6 weeks after infection, clients may develop a viral-like illness consisting of fever, sweats, fatigue, malaise, lymphadenopathy, sore throat, and sometimes splenomegaly. Clients may remain asymptomatic for months to years, depending on the progression of the disease.

In 1993, the CDC expanded the AIDS surveillance case definition to include all HIV infected persons who have <200 CD4 + T lymphocytes/µL or a CD4 + T lymphocyte percentage of total lymphocytes <14. This expansion includes the addition of three clinical conditions: pulmonary tuberculosis, recurrent pneumonia, and invasive cervical cancer. As the number of CD4 + T lymphocytes decreases, the risk and severity of opportunistic illnesses increase. Measures of CD4 + T lymphocytes are used to guide clinical and therapeutic management of HIV infected persons. Antimicrobial prophylaxis and antiretroviral therapies have been shown to be most effective within certain levels of immune dysfunction.

The AIDS evaluation battery results are often considered with other diagnostic tests for opportunistic infection such as body fluid culture and cytology, central nervous system tomography, bronchoscopy, and biopsy to complete the clinical picture description before diagnosis is made. The AIDS evaluation battery is composed of the following tests: blood and body fluid cultures, antigen detection by serology, antibody detection, confirmatory antibody detection methods, and tests for immunologic status evaluation and beta$_2$-microglobulin. No test has yet been developed that by itself confirms HIV infection.

Blood and body fluid cultures have been found to be positive in some persons soon after infection with HIV. Although difficult to do, isolation of HIV has been accomplished in concentrated peripheral blood lymphocytes and body fluids. However, a negative result does not rule out infection (*see Blood Culture, Blood; and Body Fluid, Routine, Culture*).

Antigen detection by serology methods may be positive for the viral antigen (frequently p24 core protein, HIV core antigen) from 1–2 weeks up to about 1 month after infection with the virus. The antigen is detectable during acute (initial) infection, undetectable as the virus becomes latent, and again detectable as the infection progresses. The enzyme-linked immunosorbent assay (ELISA) is used for screening for HIV. Detection of HIV antibody by ELISA must be confirmed by Western blot. Alternate diagnosis may be made by viral culture, antigen detection, or by HIV DNA or RNA polymerase chain reaction (PCR). Quantitative virology using quantitative RNA PCR or branched-chain DNA (bDNA) has become a popular method to access viral load in staging patients or for therapeutic monitoring. Maternal antibodies may be present in infants until 18 months of age; therefore, CD4 counts, viral culture, and/or PCR followed by antibody detection after 18 months must be performed in order to diagnose HIV in infants.

Studies indicate that the frequency of false-positive tests in a low-prevalence population with both the ELISA and Western blot is about 0.0007%, and the frequency of false-negative results in a high-prevalence population is about 0.3%. The usual cause of false-negative tests is testing in the time between transmission and seroconversion, a period that rarely lasts longer than 3 months. It is recommended that repeat testing be done in persons who have positive results, those with no likely risk factors, and those who report positive results from an anonymous test site. Periodic tests are suggested for clients with negative results who continue to practice high-risk behaviors.

Confirmatory antibody detection methods include the Western blot, immunofluorescence, radioimmunoprecipitation, and ELISA tests that detect antibodies to genetically engineered HIV proteins. The Western blot and immunofluorescence methods have similar sensitivities. Immunofluorescence results are obtained more quickly, but are less reliable than the Western blot. Radioimmunofluorescence is more sensitive than the Western blot, but is not widely used due to the technical difficulty of the procedure. Newer ELISA tests are able to pinpoint the specific HIV antibody present in serum by incubating the serum first with specific HIV proteins and then a tagged, anti-immunoglobulin enzyme and measuring the amount of substrate hydrolyzed by the antigen-antibody reaction.

Quantitative testing for HIV p24 antigen may provide a surrogate marker for disease progression: however, this antigen usually disappears from the blood during the asymptomatic phase. The polymerase chain reaction (PCR) for the detection of HIV DNA or RNA has been extensively used in the research setting and has recently proved extremely valuable.

A few alternative detection methods are actively being studied. Two home test kits for HIV detection (Direct Access Diagnostics and ChemTrak) are under review by the FDA. There are currently two FDA-licensed rapid tests: SUDS (Murex) and Recombigen latex agglutination assay (Cambridge Biotech). These tests are attractive for use in areas such as emergency rooms, autopsy rooms, and STD clinics.

Tests for immunologic status evaluation include lymphocyte subset enumeration, T-lymphocyte and B-lymphocyte subset assays, and skin tests with known antigens for the person such as *Candida* or mumps, and often demonstrate normal results until the later stages of infection. As T-lymphocyte helper cells (OKT4 cells) become infected by the human immunodeficiency virus, their numbers decrease. Suppressor T cells (OKT8 cells) may remain normal or increase as virus activity progresses. Lymphocyte counts decrease as immune function decreases. False-negative results to known antigen skin tests indicate that the client's immune function is compromised.

Beta$_2$-microglobulin is an amino acid peptide component of lymphocyte

HLA complexes that increases in the serum in inflammatory conditions and when lymphocyte turnover increases, such as when T-lymphocyte helper (OKT4) cells are attacked by HIV. Rising levels may also be caused by conditions other than HIV. Although beta$_2$-microglobulin levels usually rise with HIV infection, the levels do not always correlate with the stages of the infection (*see Beta$_2$-Microglobulin, Blood and 24-Hour Urine*).

CD4 + T-lymphocyte test results alone should not be used as a surrogate marker for HIV or AIDS. A low CD4 + T-lymphocyte count without a positive HIV test result will not be reportable, since other conditions may be the cause. Health care providers must ensure that persons who have a CD4 + T-lymphocyte count of < 200/μL are HIV infected before initiating treatment for HIV disease.

Professional Considerations:

1. Consent form IS required due to area-specific legal regulations. Testing should be voluntary with appropriate counseling before and after informed consent.
2. Preparation:
   A. Clarify the type of tube needed for lymphocyte subset enumeration if the Becton Dickinson Immunocytology Systems method is not used.
   B. Tube: Red-top, red/gray-top, gold-top, or lavender-top.
3. Procedure:
   A. Antigen detection by serology, antibody detection, and confirmatory antibody detection method: Draw a 5-ml venous blood sample.
   B. Lymphocyte subset enumeration: (Becton Dickinson Immunocytology Systems method). Completely fill two lavender-top tubes with venous blood. Label one tube for complete blood count and the other tube for lymphocyte subset enumeration.
   C. Beta$_2$-microglobulin: Draw a 10-ml venous blood sample in a lavender-top tube.
4. Postprocedure care:
   A. Either leave reusable equipment in the client's room or dispose of the equipment in the room.
5. Client and family teaching:
   A. Explain the purpose of the test, the procedure for collection, and the results to the client.
   B. Two days are required for the Western blot.
   C. Assess client understanding of safe sex practices and provide counseling as needed.

D. CDC National AIDS hotline: 1-800-342-AIDS.
6. Factors that affect results:
   A. Antibody results may be negative up to 35 months after infection due to viral latency.
   B. False-positive ELISA results may be caused by HLA antibody reaction with specific proteins in certain test kits. False-negative ELISA results may occur in a small proportion of clients with AIDS and in some children infected with HIV in utero.
   C. Falsely depressed lymphocyte counts may be caused by steroids and general anesthetics.
   D. Beta$_2$-microglobulin results are invalidated if the person has undergone a scan involving the administration of radioactive dyes within 1 week prior to the test.
7. Other data:
   A. Legal restrictions exist and vary regarding HIV testing and reporting of results.
   B. Demonstration of homogeneous B or T lymphocytes is helpful in prognosis and therapeutic planning of malignant lymphoproliferative disorders.
   C. In a recent study at the National Institute of Allergy and Infectious Diseases, in a small number of HIV-infected clients, infusions of an immune system protein significantly increased levels of the infection-fighting white blood cells normally destroyed during HIV infection.
   D. The Genie assay is faster, is less costly, and yields fewer indeterminate results than the Western blot method in detecting HIV-1 antibodies.
   E. *See also T- and B-Lymphocyte Subset Assay, Blood; and Beta$_2$-Microglobulin, Blood and 24-Hour Urine.*

Bibliography:

Bartlett JG: The Johns Hopkins Hospital guide to medical care of patients with HIV infection, 5th ed. Baltimore, MD, Williams & Wilkins, 1995, pp 1–8.

Castro K, Ward J, Slutsker L, Buehler J, Jaffe H, Berkelman R: 1993 Revised Classification System for HIV infection and expanded surveillance case definition for AIDS among adolescents and adults. Lab Med 24(5):286–294, 1993.

Chan EL, Sidaway F, Horsman GB: A comparison of the Genie and Western Blot assays in confirmatory testing for HIV-1 antibody. J Med Microbiol 44(3):223–225, 1996.

Isada CM, Kasten BL, Goldman M., Gray LD, Aberg JA (eds): Infectious Diseases Handbook. Hudson, OH, Lexi-Comp Inc, 1994, pp 111–114.

Ravel R: Viral and rickettsial infectious diseases. In Clinical Laboratory Medicine, 5th ed. Chicago, Year Book Medical Publishers, 1989, pp 224–275.

Stanley SK, Fauci AS: Aquired Immunodeficiency Syndrome. In Frank M, Austen KF, Claman HN, Unanue ER (eds): Samters Immunologic Diseases, 5th ed. Boston, MA, Little, Brown, 1995, pp 431–455.

ACTH STIMULATION TEST, DIAGNOSTIC

Norm: 17-OHCS levels increase by two to four times between the first and second 24-hour urine collection.

Usage: Definitive diagnosis of Addison's disease.

Description: Adrenocorticotropic hormone (ACTH) is secreted by the pituitary gland and acts on the adrenal cortex to cause release of adrenal hormones. This test measures blood cortisol and urinary 17-hydroxycorticosteroids (17-OHCS) before and after an infusion of ACTH. It is diagnostic of Addison's disease when an infusion of ACTH fails to cause an increase in cortisol or 17-OHCS, urinary metabolites of plasma cortisol.

Professional Considerations:

1. Consent form NOT required.
2. Preparation:
   A. To prevent hypersensitivity reactions when using biologic rather than synthetic ACTH, give 0.5 mg dexamethasone orally before the test.
   B. Obtain a 3-L container with 10 ml of concentrated hydrochloric acid (HCl) preservative.
   C. Write starting time of collection on the laboratory requisition.
3. Procedure:
   A. Discard the first morning urine specimen.
   B. Save all urine voided for 24 hours in a refrigerated, clean, 3-L container to which 10 ml of concentrated HCl have been added. Document the quantity of urine output during the collection period. Include urine voided at the end of the 24-hour period.
   C. Begin a second 24-hour urine collection.
   D. During the second collection, infuse 24 U of ACTH in 500 ml of normal saline intravenously over 8 hours.
4. Postprocedure care:
   A. Record the total 24-hour output on the laboratory requisition and send the entire specimen to the laboratory.
5. Client and family teaching:
   A. Save all urine voided in the 24-hour period, and urinate before defecating to avoid loss of urine. If any urine is accidentally discarded, discard the entire specimen and restart the collection the next day.
6. Factors that affect results:
   A. Maintenance steroids that must be given during the testing period should be in the form of small doses of dexamethasone to avoid falsely elevating 17-OHCS in the urine.

7. Other data:
   A. The test should be repeated in 24 hours if pituitary deficiency is suspected. Pituitary insufficiency would be evident by a gradual but small response to the ACTH stimulation test during the second test.
   B. The ACTH stimulation test is useful for identifying adrenal insufficiency; however, it should not be used for clients suspected of having secondary adrenal insufficiency.

Bibliography:

Bouachour G, Tirot P, Gouello JP, Mathieu E, Vincent JF, Alquier P: Adrenocortical function during septic shock. Intensive Care Med 21(1):57–62, 1995.

Coiro V, Volpi R, Capretti L, Speroni G, Caffarra P, Scaglioni A, et al.: Low-dose ovine corticotropin-releasing hormone stimulation test in diabetes mellitus with or without neuropathy. Metabolism 44(4):538–542, 1995.

Davenport J, Kellerman C, Reiss D, Harrison L: Addison's disease. Am Fam Physician 43(4):1338–1342, 1991.

ACTINOMYCES, CULTURE

Norm: Negative.

Positive: Abscess, actinomycosis, and pelvic inflammatory disease.

Description: A slow-growing, gram-positive, non-acid-fast bacillus that is anaerobic to microaerophilic and shows up in variable lengths and shapes on a gram stain. *Actinomyces israelii* is a part of the normal oral flora in many people. Possibly due to mouth trauma or infection, it sometimes becomes invasive, forms draining sinus tracts, and becomes a chronic, suppurative disease called actinomycosis that spreads by direct extension. The characteristic lesion is a hard, red, nontender nodule that eventually begins draining. Actinomyces is also found in the vaginal smears of a small percentage of women in whom intrauterine devices have been inserted.

Professional Considerations:

1. Consent form NOT required.
2. Preparation:
   A. Obtain a sterile cotton swab and culture media.
3. Procedure:
   A. Swab the drainage (pus from lesion, sinus tract, or fistula; or sputum or tissue biopsy material).
   B. Inoculate the drainage into thioglycolate medium and streak it onto brain-heart infusion agar plates.
   C. Incubate anaerobically for 2 weeks or more.

4. Postprocedure care:
   A. Apply a dry sterile dressing as needed.
   B. Send the specimen to the laboratory immediately.
5. Client and family teaching:
   A. Results will not be available for at least 14 days.
   B. Treatment for actinomycosis usually includes drainage of lesions, and penicillin or tetracycline drug therapy.
6. Factors that affect results:
   A. Do NOT refrigerate or store the specimen.
7. Other data:
   A. Some tissue damage from actinomycosis is not reversible.

Bibliography:

Fiorino AS: Intrauterine contraceptive device-associated actinomycotic abscess and Actinomyces detection on cervical smear.Obstet Gynecol 87(1):142–149, 1996.

Lewis R, McKenzie D, Bagg J, Dickie A: Experience with a novel selective medium for isolation of *Actinomyces* spp. from medical and dental specimens. J Clin Microbiol 33(6):1613–1616, 1995.

ACTIVATED COAGULATION TIME (ACT), AUTOMATED, BLOOD

Norm: Varies, depending on the type of system in use and the type of test reagent or activator. There are currently two commercially available systems for analyzing ACT by automation: ACT II by Medtronic Hemotec Inc., and Hemochron by International Technidyne Corporation.

Hemochron System		
Tube	**Range**	**ACT II**
CA510 FTCA510	105–167 seconds	Multiple methods are available for measuring ACT values; thus, values should be evaluated according to reference levels of the individual machine and test tube used. The ACT II machine has an overall range of 0–999.
K-ACT FTK-ACT	91–151 seconds	
P214/215	110–182 seconds	
S412	186–306 seconds	

Usage: Commonly used for heparin anticoagulation monitoring during bypass surgery, percutaneous transluminal coronary angioplasty (PTCA), interventional radiology, neonatal extracorporeal membrane oxygenation (ECMO), hemofiltration, hemodialysis, and critical and telemetry care.

Increased: Afibrinogenemia, circulating anticoagulants, dysproteinemia, factor deficiency (V, VIII, IX, X, XI, or XII), fibrinolysis, hemophilia, hemorrhagic disease of the newborn, hypofibrinogenemia, hypoprothrombinemia, leukemia, and liver disease. Drugs include heparin calcium and heparin sodium.

Description: Measures the ability of the blood to clot. Fresh whole blood is added to a test tube containing an activator (diatomaceous earth, glass particles, or kaolin) and timed for the formation of a clot. The ACT is more sensitive to the effects of factor VIII deficiency and heparin than is whole-blood clotting time. The ACT test has become a mainstay in monitoring heparin anticoagulation during invasive procedures and is the preferred method for monitoring high-level anticoagulation. The ACT is quick, reliable, easy, and can be performed at the bedside. Disadvantages of the ACT are operator variability and differences between the two commercially available systems.

Professional Considerations:

1. Consent form NOT required.
2. Preparation:
   A. Obtain a tube with a designated activator for the specific ACT test. May be drawn from indwelling venous blood line, extracorporeal blood line port, direct venipuncture, or vacuum draw. Do not obtain blood from a heparinized access line, an indwelling heparin lock, or a hemodialysis line.
   B. Obtain two 5-ml syringes.

3. Procedure: (If using the ACT II system, see instructions below before obtaining client sample.)
   A. *Indwelling venous line sampling:* With the first syringe, withdraw and discard 5 ml of blood. Attach the second syringe and withdraw a 3-ml blood sample.
   Venipuncture sampling: With the first syringe, withdraw and discard 2 ml of blood. Attach the second syringe and withdraw a 3-ml sample.

   Hemochron System:
   B. Dispense exactly 2 ml of blood into the test tube (*note:* tubes P214/P215 require only 0.4 ml of blood). At the same time, depress the start button timer on the machine. Close the tube and agitate it briskly ten times.
   C. Insert the test tube into the Hemochron machine port and rotate clockwise until green light indicator lights. Await the result, which will be displayed in the number of seconds required to obtain coagulation on the Hemochron screen.

   Act II System:
   A. Prewarm the cartridge in the ACT heat block for 3 minutes.
   B. Gently tap or shake the cartridge to resuspend the activator.
   C. Inject the client sample into channel 2, then channel 1 of the cartridge, filling to between the lines (less than 1 ml).
   D. Place the cartridge in the instrument and pull the actuator cover forward. The instrument will sound an audible alert when the endpoint is reached. (*Note:* The instrument has two readout displays. The Channel 1 result is of ACT without heparin; the Channel 2 result is of ACT with the influence of heparin.)

4. Postprocedure care:
   A. If the test is performed at the client's bedside, document on the client's medical record the result of the test, time, date, machine number, tube type or number, site of draw, and rate of infusion in units/hour if the client is receiving IV heparin.
5. Client and family teaching:
   A. Results are normally available within a few minutes.
6. Factors that affect results:
   A. Tests may be affected by hemodilution, poor operator technique, inadequate reagent/specimen mixture, improper storage of test kits, cardioplegic solutions, hypothermia, platelet dysfunction, hypofibrinogenemia, other coagulopathies, and certain medications.
   B. In acute coronary cases, such as unstable angina and acute myocardial infarction, baseline ACTs may be lower and heparin requirements higher, reflecting a thrombogenic state.

7. Other data:
   A. Test cartridges available for the ACT II system: LR ACT, RACT, HR ACT, PT, GPC, and HTC. Test cartridges available for the Hemochron system are listed above under "norms."
   B. Heparin requirements as well as baseline ACTs vary from client to client, so ACT determinations allow a quick titration of the effective heparin dose.
   C. Therapeutic ACT values depend on several factors: type of ACT system, type of test tube and reagent, type of procedure being performed, clinical condition and client, and clinical preference of physician.
   D. HemoTec and Hemochron ACT measurements cannot be used interchangeably.

Bibliography:

Bowers J, Ferguson J III: The use of activated coagulation times to monitor heparin therapy during and after interventional procedures. Clin Cardiol *17*:357–361, 1994.

Ferguson J, Dougherty K, Gaos C, et al.: Relation between procedural activated coagulation time and outcome after percutaneous transluminal coronary angioplasty. J Am Coll Cardiol *23*(5):1061–1065, 1994.

Varga Z, Papp L, Andrassay G: Hemochron versus HemoTec activated coagulation time target values during percutaneous transluminal coronary angioplasty. J Am Coll Cardiol *25*(3): 803–804, 1995.

ACTIVATED PARTIAL THROMBOPLASTIN SUBSTITUTION TEST, DIAGNOSTIC

Norm: Normal factors VIII, IX, X, XI, and XII.

Usage: Helps identify single factor deficiencies causing prolonged PTT, including factors VIII, IX, XI, and XII.

Description: A differential activated partial thromboplastin time (APTT) method that identifies which factor deficiency(ies) is/are present when APTT is prolonged. Known reagents for each factor are systematically added to the client's blood sample. A factor is determined to be deficient when the substitution produces a normal APTT.

Professional Considerations:

1. Consent form NOT required
2. Preparation:
   A. Tubes: Red-top and blue-top.
   B. Preschedule the test with the laboratory.
3. Procedure:
   A. Draw 2–3 ml of blood into a red-top tube and discard. Completely fill a blue-top tube with the blood sample.

4. Postprocedure care:
   A. Hold pressure over the venipuncture site for 5 minutes if the client is receiving heparin therapy. Observe the site closely for development of hematoma.
   B. Write the collection time on the laboratory requisition.
   C. Refrigerate the specimen until the test is completed.
5. Client and family teaching:
   A. Results are normally available within 24 hours.
6. Factors that affect results:
   A. Failure to discard the first few milliliters of blood drawn may contaminate the specimen with tissue thromboplastin, which can activate coagulation.
   B. Failure to completely fill the tube with blood may cause falsely prolonged results.
   C. Hematocrit over 50% may cause falsely prolonged results, and hematocrit under 20% may cause falsely decreased results.
   D. Drawing the sample from a line being kept open with a heparin flush will cause falsely prolonged results.
   E. Reject hemolyzed specimens and specimens received more than 2 hours after collection.
   F. Anticoagulant therapy within 2 weeks prior to the test invalidates results.
7. Other data:
   A. Useful only with single-factor deficiencies.
   B. See also Partial Thromboplastin Time, Plasma.

Bibliography:

Miale JB: Laboratory Medicine: Hematology, 6th ed. St Louis, MO, CV Mosby, 1982, pp 823, 925–926.

Rao LV, Rapaport SI: Factor VIIa-catalyzed activation of factor X independent of tissue factor: Its possible significance for control of hemophilic bleeding by infused factor VIIa. Blood 75(5):1069–1073, 1990.

ACTIVATED PARTIAL THROMBOPLASTIN TIME

(see Partial Thromboplastin Time, Plasma)

ACUTE ABDOMINAL SERIES, DIAGNOSTIC

Norm: Requires interpretation of each test by a radiologist.

Usage: Differential diagnosis of the etiology of acute abdomen. Some examples are abdominal aortic aneurysm dissection, abscess, acute cholecystitis, acute ischemia, acute pancreatitis, appendicitis, bile duct obstruction, bowel strangulation, choledocholithiasis, gastric outlet obstruction, perforated abdominal viscus, peritonitis, pyelonephritis, ruptured ectopic pregnancy, salmonella enterocolitis, and ureteral obstruction.

Description: The acute abdomen is characterized by the abrupt onset of abdominal pain, distention, diminished or absent bowel sounds, and sometimes, guarding. Causes of these symptoms may be many, and pathology within the abdomen is hidden. In addition to a routine external physical assessment, seven routes of diagnostic work-up are used. Less invasive testing is usually performed first.

Laboratory studies include coagulation studies, hemoglobin and hematocrit, and blood volume determinations to rule out internal bleeding, leukocyte differential to determine whether an infectious or inflammatory process is present, amylase level to rule out pancreatic and other pathologies, liver panels to rule out hepatic pathology, blood urea nitrogen and creatinine, urinalysis to rule out urinary tract infection, and stool examination to rule out salmonella. Fine-needle aspiration cytology provides clues to the type of process occurring.

Plain film radiography is a radiograph taken without the use of an injected radiopaque agent. Plain film radiography of the abdomen may identify compression fractures, intestinal obstruction, metastasis, perforated abdominal viscus, pancreatic calcification, and renal calculi.

Contrast radiography involves the injection of a radiopaque agent into the vascular space. The contrast agent enhances the appearance of organ and vascular lumens and thus is more likely to reveal pathology than is plain film radiography. Vascular contrast examinations of the abdominal area such as intravenous pyelography help identify lumbar aortic aneurysms, urinary tract trauma, lesions, or other pathology.

Intestinal contrast examinations such as barium enema, oral cholecystogram, and upper gastrointestinal series may identify colonic lesions or perforation, but should not be performed when obstruction is suspected. They may also rule out appendicitis.

Ultrasound may help diagnose acute abscesses, cholecystitis, Crohn's disease, dilated bile duct, hepatic cancer, hepatic or splenic hematoma, splenomegaly, hydronephrosis, intussusception pancreatitis, pancreatic pseudocyst, pancreatic carcinoma, urinary tract obstruction, and the presence of foreign bodies.

Computed tomography helps identify, differentiate, and evaluate hepatic, pancreatic, renal, and retroperitoneal abscesses, fluid accumulations, masses and cysts, and pancreatitis.

Nuclear medicine studies help identify intra-abdominal abscesses, sites of gastrointestinal bleeding, hematoma, and areas of abnormal tissue metabolism. Nuclear medicine scans may also help to rule out cholecystitis.

In extremely acute situations and when findings from any combination of the above tests are inconclusive, surgical exploration of the abdomen may be required.

Professional Considerations:

1. Consent form NOT required.

Risks:

Allergic reaction to radiographic dye or nuclear medicine radiopharmaceutical for applicable tests (itching, hives, rash, tight feeling in the throat, shortness of breath, bronchospasm, anaphylaxis, death), renal toxicity.

Contraindications:

Previous allergy to x-ray dye, iodine, or seafood or radionuclide for those tests involving injections; renal insufficiency.

2. Preparation:
   A. No preprocedure care is required for plain film radiography.
   B. Intestinal contrast examinations often require clear liquids the day before the test and cathartics and/or cleansing enemas prior to the test. However, this requirement may be waived for a client with acute abdominal symptoms.
   C. Have emergency equipment readily available for tests involving injection of radionuclide or dye.
3. Procedure:
   A. Plain film radiography: The client is positioned in supine, upright, oblique,

and lateral decubitus positions, and radiographic films are taken from various angles. The best results are not obtained from portable films, especially in obese clients. The films should be taken in the radiology department, where the most powerful radiography is available, whenever possible. The lateral decubitus position is used for clients who are unable to stand, and the radiograph is taken horizontally across the table. A "kidneys, ureters, bladder (KUB)" includes the majority of the abdomen and is taken from an anterior to posterior angle. An anterior-posterior scout film is used both prior to an intravenous pyelogram and in combination with an upright abdominal film for suspected intestinal obstruction. Subdiaphragmatic free air from perforated abdominal viscus may be identified with an upright abdominal film or an upright chest film.

B. Vascular contrast examinations: Radiographic dye is injected into an arm vein, and oblique films of the abdomen are taken 15 minutes later. A left posterior oblique position may help identify a lumbar aortic aneurysm because the position enhances visualization by rotating the aorta off of the spine. Arteriography and venography may also help identify blood vessel abnormalities such as aneurysm, hemorrhage, or occlusion.

C. Intestinal contrast examination: The client is placed in a Sims' position. Barium and/or air is instilled into the lower gastrointestinal tract and radiographic films are taken. In upper gastrointestinal series, the client must swallow barium and radiographic films are then taken. Oral cholecystography is a fluoroscopic study in which films of the gallbladder and ducts are taken after administration of a fat stimulus.

D. Ultrasound: The client is positioned on the side or supine, and a series of high-frequency sound waves are transmitted into the abdomen. The echoes reflected from the differing tissue densities are converted by a gel-coated transducer to form patterns of the abdominal structures on an oscilloscope screen.

E. Computed tomography: The client is placed in a supine position on a platform table that moves the client through a circular computed tomography scanner. As several transverse films are taken, differing tissue densities are calculated based on varying absorption of the x-rays. Findings may indicate the need for further computed tomography after the administration of contrast medium.

F. Nuclear medicine studies: At varying time intervals after the intravenous injection of a radioactive tracer, scintigraphic scans, which detect areas of increased concentration of the tracer at sites of pathology, are taken of the abdominal area.

4. Postprocedure care:
   A. Fluids should be encouraged after studies involving the administration of radiopaque dyes or barium.
   B. Cathartics may be prescribed after studies involving the administration of barium.
5. Client and family teaching:
   A. Explain the purpose of each test as appropriate, the procedure for the test, and the results. See individual test listings for specific client teaching.
6. Factors that affect results:
   A. The presence of gastrointestinal barium negates the value of plain film radiography, vascular contrast examinations, ultrasound, computed tomography, and nuclear medicine scintigraphy, and so should be performed last.
   B. Some extra-abdominal conditions that may cause acute abdominal pain include pneumonia, pulmonary or myocardial infarction, and pericarditis. Other conditions that may cause symptoms of acute abdomen include acute intermittent porphyria, diabetic neuropathy, heavy metal poisoning, sickle cell disease, and tabes dorsalis.
7. Other data:
   A. See also Barium Enema, Diagnostic; Flat Plate X-Ray of the Abdomen, Diagnostic; Intravenous Pyelogram, Diagnostic; and Upper Gastrointestinal Series, Diagnostic.
   B. Health care professionals working in a nuclear medicine area must follow federal standards set by the Nuclear Regulatory Commission. These standards include precautions for handling the radioactive material and monitoring of potential radiation exposure.

Bibliography:

de Dombal FT: Acute abdominal pain in the elderly. J Clin Gastroenterol 19(4):331–335, 1994.

Paterson-Brown S, Vipond MN: Modern aids to clinical decision-making in the acute abdomen. Br J Surg 77(1):13–18, 1990.

ADDIS COUNT, 12-HOUR, URINE

Norm:

Erythrocytes	0–5,000/mm^3
Leukocytes	0–500,000/mm^3
Casts	1,000,000/mm^3

Increased: Glomerulonephritis and hematuria.

Description: When subclinical glomerulonephritis is suspected, an Addis count on a 12-hour urine specimen may demonstrate increased erythrocytes and leukocytes and increased rates of cast excretion in amounts too small to be detected in a random urine specimen examined microscopically. The count is performed on the sediment from a portion of the 12-hour collection.

Professional Considerations:

1. Consent form NOT required.
2. Preparation:
   A. Obtain a 1- or a 2-L bottle that has been rinsed in formalin.
3. Procedure:
   A. The clean-catch urine technique must be used to decrease the risk of specimen contamination. See clean-catch collection instructions in "Body Fluid, Routine, Culture."
   B. Keep the specimen container refrigerated during and after specimen collection. For catheterized specimens, keep the drainage bag on ice and empty it into the collection container hourly.
4. Postprocedure care:
   A. Send the entire 12-hour urine specimen to the laboratory.
5. Client and family teaching:
   A. Do not drink any fluids throughout the collection period.
   B. Collect a clean-catch urine sample according to the technique above if this collection method is used.
6. Factors that affect results:
   A. Hematuria, pyuria, and a contaminated specimen will cause falsely elevated results.
7. Other data:
   A. This test is not usually necessary when a thorough history and renal work-up is done.
   B. An approximate Addis count can be performed on a first-morning voided specimen following a 16-hour fast from fluids and food.

Bibliography:

Elder G, Perl S, Yong JL, Fletcher J, Mackie J: Progression from Goodpasture's disease to membranous glomerulonephritis. Pathology 27(3):233–236, 1995.

Jennette JC, Falk RJ: Diagnosis and management of glomerulonephritis and vasculitis presenting as acute renal failure. Med Clin North Am 74(4):893–908, 1990.

ADENOVIRUS ANTIBODY TITER, SERUM

Norm: Negative. Results require interpretation with consideration of the site of the specimen correlated with clinical symptoms.

Current Adenovirus Infection: Fourfold rise in titer.

Increased: Adenovirus infection.

Description: A group of virus types responsible for upper respiratory disease, hemorrhagic cystitis, and epidemic keratoconjunctivitis. The mode of transmission is by direct or indirect contact. Measurement of adenovirus antibody titers is the test of choice for detection of current adenovirus infections. Results are reported as the highest dilution of serum that completely neutralizes the virus.

Professional Considerations:
1. Consent form NOT required.
2. Preparation:
   A. Tube: Red-top, red/gray-top, or gold-top.
3. Procedure:
   A. Draw a 2-ml blood sample no later than 5–7 days after onset of symptoms.
   B. After allowing the specimen to clot at room temperature, centrifuge and separate the serum into a separate vial.
   C. Draw a convalescent sample in 14–21 days.
4. Postprocedure care:
   A. Mark the tube label and laboratory requisition with "acute phase" or "convalescent phase" for the first and second specimens, respectively.
5. Client and family teaching:
   A. Return in 2–3 weeks to have the convalescent sample drawn.
6. Factors that affect results:
   A. Reject hemolyzed or frozen specimens.
   B. Specimens may be stored several weeks at 4–6°C.
   C. Antibody titers for both specimens should be performed by the same laboratory.
7. Other data:
   A. This test is nonspecific for the type of adenovirus present.

Bibliography:

Shimizu T, Sekitani T, Hirata T, Hara H: Serum viral antibody titer in vestibular neuronitis. Acta Otolaryngol Suppl (Stockh) *503*:74–78, 1993.

Sokhandan M, McFadden ER Jr, Huang YT, Mazanec MB: The contribution of respiratory viruses to severe exacerbations of asthma in adults. Chest *107*(6):1570–1574, 1995.

ADENOVIRUS IMMUNOFLUORESCENCE, DIAGNOSTIC

Norm: Negative.

Usage: Adenovirus infection, conjunctivitis, hemorrhagic cystitis, and pharyngitis.

Description: A group of virus types responsible for upper respiratory disease, hemorrhagic cystitis, and epidemic keratoconjunctivitis. The mode of transmission is by direct or indirect contact. Direct immunofluorescence is performed for adenovirus group antigen on a swab or scraping.

Professional Considerations:
1. Consent form NOT required.
2. Preparation:
   A. Obtain a sterile microbiologic swab or scraper and viral transport media. For a tracheal specimen, obtain a sputum trap and a suction cannula.
3. Procedure:
   A. Upper respiratory disease, nasopharyngeal specimen: Advance a curved swab through the nares to the posterior pharyngeal wall and leave it in place for 10 seconds. Remove the swab.
   B. Pharyngeal specimen: In a well-lit location with the client's head tilted back and the mouth open, depress the tongue with a tongue blade. Have the client say "Ah." Swab the posterior pharyngeal wall with a curved wire swab from one side to the other. Swab any lesions or drainage noted. Remove the swab without touching it to any other portions of the oropharynx or mouth.
   C. Tracheal specimen: Obtain a 1- to 3-ml sample of tracheal aspirate via oral or nasotracheal suction directly into a sterile sputum trap.
   D. Hemorrhagic cystitis: Swab or scrape urethral discharge (or a vesicle lesion visualized via cystoscopy). Alternatively, using a small platinum loop, scrape the inside of the anterior urethra.
   E. Keratoconjunctivitis: Do not rinse the eye or apply medication to the conjunctiva prior to specimen collection. Swab or scrape the inflamed surface of the inner, lower conjunctiva or the inner canthus of the eye.
4. Postprocedure care:
   A. Place the swab or scraping in viral transport media or a tightly capped tube containing 2 ml of 1% bovine serum albumin or veal infusion broth.
   B. Refrigerate the specimen.
5. Client and family teaching:
   A. Sampling should be painless.
6. Factors that affect results:
   A. Failure to send the specimen to the laboratory immediately or to chill the sample if the specimen is not sent to the laboratory immediately invalidates the results.
7. Other data:
   A. This test is nonspecific for the type of adenovirus present.

Bibliography:

McDonald JC, Quennec P: Utility of a respiratory virus panel containing a monoclonal antibody pool for screening of respiratory specimens in nonpeak respiratory syncytial virus season. J Clin Microbiol *31*(10):2809–2811, 1993.

Puvion-Dutilleul F, Chelbi-Alix MK, Koken M,

Quignon F, Puvion E, de The H: Adenovirus infection induces rearrangements in the intranuclear distribution of the nuclear body-associated PML protein. Exp Cell Res *218*(1):9–16, 1995.

ADRENOCORTICOTROPIC HORMONE (ACTH, CORTICOTROPIN), SERUM

Norm:

		SI Units
0800 hours, peak	25–100 pg/ml	25–100 ng/L
1800 hours, trough	0–50 pg/ml	0–50 ng/L

Increased: Addison's disease, ectopic ACTH syndrome, pituitary adenoma, pituitary Cushing's syndrome, primary adrenal insufficiency, and stress. Drugs include amphetamine sulfate, calcium gluconate, corticosteroids, estrogens, ethanol, lithium carbonate, and spironolactone.

Decreased: Primary adrenocortical hyperfunction (due to tumor or hyperplasia) and secondary hypoadrenalism.

Description: ACTH is an anterior pituitary hormone that stimulates cortisol and androgen production by the adrenal gland. Diurnal variations of ACTH are typical, with peak levels occurring from 0600 to 0800 and trough levels occurring from 1800 to 2300.

Professional Considerations:

1. Consent form NOT required.
2. Preparation:
   A. Tube: Plastic green-top or plastic lavender-top, and ice-water slush.
   B. *See Client and family teaching.*
3. Procedure:
   A. Draw a 1-ml blood sample at 0600. Repeat the sampling at 1800 if trough levels are needed.
   B. Place the specimen in ice-water slush.
4. Postprocedure care:
   A. Write the collection time on the laboratory requisition.
   B. Transport the specimen to the laboratory immediately. The specimen should be frozen within 15 minutes if it will not be spun and tested within the first hour.
5. Client and family teaching:
   A. Consume a low-carbohydrate diet for 48 hours prior to the test.
   B. Avoid physical and emotional stress for 12 hours prior to the test.
   C. For peak and trough levels, two samples are required at different times of the day because the blood levels fluctuate throughout the day.
   D. Results may take several days.

6. Factors that affect results:
   A. Reject specimens received more than 60 minutes after collection.
   B. Values increase within 90 seconds of traumatic, repeated, or prolonged venipuncture.
   C. Menstrual cycle, pregnancy, and radioactive scanning within 7 days affect ACTH levels.
7. Other data:
   A. The ACTH stimulation test must be performed to confirm the diagnosis of Addison's disease.

Bibliography:

Brown MA, Thou ST, Whitworth JA: Stimulation of aldosterone by ACTH in normal and hypertensive pregnancy. Am J Hypertens *8*(3):260–267, 1995.

Meeran K, Hattersley A, Mould G, Bloom SR: Venipuncture causes rapid rise in plasma ACTH. Br J Clin Pract *47*(5):246–247, 1993.

Terzolo M, Ali A, Pia A, Bollito E, Reimondo G, Paccotti P, Scardapane R, Angeli A: Cyclic Cushing's syndrome due to ectopic ACTH secretion by an adrenal pheochromocytoma. J Endocrinol Invest *17*(11):869–874, 1994.

AFP

(see Alpha-Fetoprotein, Blood)

AFRICAN TRYPANOSOMIASIS, BLOOD

Norm: Negative. No parasites identified.

Positive: African trypanosomiasis (African sleeping sickness).

Description: Also known as sleeping sickness, African trypanosomiasis is a vector-borne parasitic infection endogenous to tropical Africa caused in humans by the bite of a tsetse fly of the genus *Glossina*. Symptoms include a chancre at the site of the bite, progressing to headache, fever, insomnia, anemia, rash, and lymph node swelling. After inoculation, trypanosomes invade all body organs.

CNS symptoms appear in disease stage II. The course of the disease may run months to years and is frequently fatal with treatment and always fatal without treatment.

Professional Considerations:

1. Consent form NOT required.
2. Preparation:
   A. Obtain an alcohol wipe, a lancet, and a capillary tube.
3. Procedure:
   A. Perform this procedure in the early afternoon, again at night, and when the fever spikes occur.
   B. Cleanse the pad of the index or second finger with the alcohol wipe and allow the pad to dry.
   C. Perform a finger stick and fill the capillary tube completely with blood. Quickly seal the capillary tube.
4. Postprocedure care:
   A. Write the name of the parasite suspected and the place(s) and date(s) of recent travel on the laboratory requisition.
5. Client and family teaching:
   A. Results are normally available within 24 hours.
6. Factors that affect results:
   A. Reject clotted specimens.
   B. Transport the capillary tube to the laboratory immediately for thick and thin smears to be performed before blood clots form.
7. Other data:
   A. Person-to-person transmission of African trypanosomiasis is possible either by direct contact with infected blood or from mother to fetus. Pentamidine and Suramin are used for early-stage disease, depending on the causative organism. Melarsoprol is the drug of choice for late-stage treatment.
   B. *See also Trypanosomiasis Serological Test, Blood; and Parasite Screen, Blood.*

Bibliography:

Isharaza WK, Van-Meirvenne N: Variant-specific trypanolytic antibodies in sera from clients infected with Trypanosoma brucei rhodesiense. Bull WHO 68(1):33–37, 1990.

Theodos CM, Mansfield JM: Regulation of B cell responses to the variant surface glycoprotein molecule in trypanosomiasis. J Immunol *144*(10): 4022–4029, 1990.

AIDS EVALUATION BATTERY

(see Acquired Immune Deficiency Syndrome Evaluation Battery, Diagnostic; and T- and B-Lymphocyte Subset Assay, Blood)

ALA

(see Antiphospholipid Antibody, Serum)

ALANINE AMINOTRANSFERASE (ALT, ALANINE TRANSAMINASE, SGPT), SERUM

Norm:

Adult females	4–35 U/L
Adult males	7–46 U/L
Children	
<12 months	≤54 U/L
Age 1–2	3–37 U/L
Age 2–8	3–30 U/L
Age 8–16	3–28 U/L

Increased: Biliary tract obstruction, brain tumor, cerebrovascular accident (increased after 1 week), cirrhosis, congestive heart failure (with liver damage), delirium tremens, dermatomyositis, dysrhythmias, Gaucher's disease, hepatic cancer, hepatic damage, hepatitis (viral, toxic), infectious mononucleosis, intramuscular injections, intestinal infarction, liver passive congestion, local irradiation injury, muscle injury (due to electroshock, infection, seizure, or trauma), muscular dystrophy, myocardial infarction, myoglobinuria, Niemann-Pick disease, obesity, pancreatitis (acute), polymyositis, postoperatively (intestinal surgery), pulmonary infarction, renal infarction, Reye's syndrome, rhabdomyolysis, and shock with liver damage. Drugs include allopurinol, ampicillin, aspirin, barbiturates, bromocriptine mesylate, captopril, chlordiazepoxide, chlorpromazine hydrochloride, cincophen, diphenylhydantoin, fosinopril, and heparin (bovine, porcine).

Decreased: None found.

Description: Alanine aminotransferase (ALT) is an enzyme primarily produced by the liver and found in certain body fluids (e.g., bile, cerebrospinal fluid, plasma, and saliva) and in the heart, liver, kidneys, pancreas, and skeletal muscle. It acts as a catalyst in the transamination reaction that is necessary for amino acid production. This test is most commonly used to evaluate liver injury, where levels may rise to as much as 50 times normal range. The ALT levels are analyzed with aspartate aminotransferase (AST) levels to evaluate the degree of liver injury and to confirm a hepatic cause of AST increase. After the early stage of liver injury, ALT levels surpass AST levels. Serial measurements help track the course of hepatitis. This test may also be used by blood banks to screen for hepatitis in samples of donor blood.

Professional Considerations:

1. Consent form NOT required.
2. Preparation:
   A. Tube: Red-top, red/gray-top, or gold-top.
   B. List medications taken by the client within the last 3 days on the laboratory requisition.
   C. Do NOT draw during hemodialysis.
3. Procedure:
   A. Draw a 1-ml blood sample.
4. Postprocedure care:
   A. The specimen may be refrigerated but not frozen.
5. Client and family teaching:
   A. Results are normally available within 12 hours.
6. Factors that affect results:
   A. Hemolysis causes unreliable results.
   B. Drugs that may cause falsely increased results include erythromycin, opiates, oxacillin sodium (Prostaphlin), and ampicillin (Polycillin).
   C. Falsely decreased results may occur in beriberi, diabetic ketoacidosis, hemodialysis (chronic), liver disease (severe), and uremia.
   D. Serial norms generally vary by less than 10 U/L in the same healthy client.
7. Other data:
   A. The older names for this test were glutamate-pyruvate transaminase and glutamic pyruvic transaminase.

Bibliography:

Kundrotas LW, Clement DJ: Serum alanine aminotransferase (ALT) elevation in asymptomatic US Air Force basic trainee blood donors. Dig Dis Sci *38*(12):2145–2150, 1993.

Sherman KE: Alanine aminotransferase in clinical practice. A review. Arch Intern Med *151*(2):260–265, 1991.

ALBUMIN/GLOBULIN RATIO (A/G RATIO), SERUM

Norm: 1.5:1 to 2.5:1 or ≥1.

Increased: Edema and water intoxication.

Decreased: Burns, cachexia, cirrhosis, collagen diseases, dehydration, glomerulonephritis (chronic), hepatitis, infection, inflammation, nephrotic syndrome, multiple myeloma, renal disease, sarcoidosis, scleroderma, systemic lupus erythematosus, ulcerative colitis, and Waldenström's macroglobulinemia.

Description: An imprecise measurement of the amount of the two major protein factions in the blood. The ratio is derived by subtracting the albumin level from total protein to calculate globulin and then dividing the globulin value into the albumin value. The A/G ratio lacks specificity and has largely been replaced by serum protein electrophoresis.

Professional Considerations:

1. Consent form NOT required.
2. Preparation:
   A. Tube: Red-top, red/gray-top, or gold-top.
   B. Do NOT draw during hemodialysis.
3. Procedure:
   A. Draw a 3-ml blood sample.
4. Postprocedure care:
   A. None.
5. Client and family teaching:
   A. Consume a low-fat diet the day of the test.
   B. Results are normally available within 24 hours.
6. Factors that affect results:
   A. Testing with sulfobromophthalein sodium (Bromsulphalein) within 48 hours prior to specimen collection invalidates the test.
7. Other data:
   A. This test is of little help in diagnosing, as normal ratios can be obtained with abnormal quantities of albumin and/or globulin.

Bibliography:

Beamer N, Coull BM, Sexton G, de Garmo P, Knox R, Seaman G: Fibrinogen and the albumin-globulin ratio in recurrent stroke. Stroke *24*(8):1133–1139, 1993.

ALBUMIN, SERUM, URINE, AND 24-HOUR URINE

Norm: Nephelometric, calorimetric, and nephorimetric.

		SI Units
Serum		
Adult	3.5–5.0 g/dl	35–50 g/L
>Age 60	3.4–4.8 g/dl	34–48 g/L
Average at rest	0.3 g/dl	3 g/L

		SI Units
Urine		
Adult at rest	2–80 mg/24 hours	0.03–0.08 g/day
Adult ambulatory	<150 mg/24 hours	<0.15 g/day
Child <age 10	<100 mg/24 hours	<0.10 g/day

Increased in Serum: Dehydration, diarrhea, meningitis, metastatic carcinomatosis, multiple myeloma, myasthenia, neoplasms, nephrosis, nephrotic syndrome, osteomyelitis, peptic ulcer, pneumonia, polyarteritis nodosa, pregnancy, protein-losing enteropathy, rheumatic fever, rheumatoid arthritis, sarcoidosis, scleroderma, sprue, steatorrhea, stress, systemic lupus erythematosus, trauma, tuberculosis, ulcerative colitis, uremia, vomiting, and water intoxication. Drugs include Bromsulphalein, cytotoxic agents, and oral contraceptives.

Increased in Urine: Acute tubular necrosis, amyloid disease, anemia (severe), Bartter's syndrome, Butler-Albright syndrome, Bright's disease, cardiac disease, central nervous system lesions, cerebrovascular accident, convulsions, cystitis, diabetes insipidus (nephrogenic), diabetic nephropathy, diphtheria, drug reaction, epididymitis, exercise, Fanconi's syndrome, fever, galactosemia, glomerular lesion, glomerulonephritis, glomerulosclerosis, Goodpasture's syndrome, heavy metal poisoning, hyperthyroidism, idiopathic thrombocytopenic purpura, intestinal obstruction, leukemia, liver disease, membranous nephropathy, multiple myeloma, nephritis, nephrosclerosis, nephrotic syndrome, pneumonia, poisoning (arsenic, carbon tetrachloride, ether, lead, mercury, mustard, opiates, phenol, phosphorus, propylene glycol, sulfosalicylic acid, turpentine), polycystic kidney disease, prostatitis, pyelonephritis (bacterial, chronic, with hypertension), renal radiation, renal tubular acidosis, renal vein thrombosis, scarlet fever, septicemia, streptococcal infection, subacute bacterial endocarditis, systemic lupus erythematosus, toxemia of pregnancy, tumor (abdominal, bladder, renal pelvis), typhoid fever, and Wilson's disease. Drugs include amphotericin B, ampicillin, ampicillin sodium, aspirin, bacitracin, barbiturates, cephaloridine, corticosteroids, gentamicin sulfate, gold, kanamycin, mercurial diuretics, neomycin sulfate, phenylbutazone, and polymyxin B.

Decreased in Serum: Ascites, alcoholism, beriberi, brucellosis, burns, cholecystitis, cirrhosis, congenital analbuminemia, congestive heart failure, Crohn's disease, diabetes mellitus, edema, essential hypertension, glomerulonephritis, hemorrhage, hepatitis (viral), Hodgkin's disease, hyperthyroidism, infection, liver diseases, systemic lupus erythematosus (SLE), leukemia (lymphatic, monocytic, and myelogenous), lymphoma, macroglobulinemia, malnutrition, malabsorption syndrome, meningitis, metastatic carcinomatosis, multiple myeloma, myasthenia, neoplasms, nephrosis, nephrotic syndrome, osteomyelitis, peptic ulcer, pneumonia, polyarteritis nodosa, pregnancy, protein-losing enteropathy, rheumatic fever, rheumatoid arthritis, sarcoidosis, scleroderma, sprue, steatorrhea, stress, trauma, tuberculosis, ulcerative colitis, uremia, and water intoxication. Drugs include ampicillin, asparaginase, fluorouracil, and oral contraceptives.

Decreased in Urine: Not clinically significant.

Description: Albumin is one of the two main protein factions of blood. It functions in maintaining oncotic pressure and in transportation of bilirubin, fatty acids, drugs, hormones, and other substances that are insoluble in water. Protein is normally almost completely reabsorbed by the kidneys and undetectable in the urine. Therefore, the presence of detectable albumin, or protein, in urine is indicative of abnormal renal function.

Professional Considerations:
1. Consent form NOT required.
2. Preparation:
   A. Tube: Red-top, red/gray-top, or gold-top for serum albumin.
   B. MAY be drawn during hemodialysis.

C. Obtain a 3-L specimen container without preservative for 24-hour urine albumin and write the beginning time of specimen collection on the container.

D. Obtain a clean specimen container for the spot urine specimen.

E. *See Client and family teaching.*

3. Procedure:

A. Serum: Draw a 1-ml blood sample from an extremity that does not have intravenous fluids infusing into it (to avoid hemodilution and falsely low results). Avoid prolonged application of the tourniquet.

B. 24-hour urine: Collect all urine voided in a 24-hour period and refrigerate. For catheterized clients, keep the collection bag on ice, and empty it hourly into the collection container.

C. Spot urine collection may also be collected.

4. Postprocedure care:

A. Document the quantity of urine output and the ending time for the collection period on the laboratory requisition.

5. Client and family teaching:

A. Consume a low-fat diet the day of the test.

B. Empty the bladder before starting 24-hour urine collection.

C. Save all urine voided in the 24-hour period, and urinate before defecating to avoid loss of urine. If any urine is accidentally discarded, discard the entire specimen and restart the collection the next day.

6. Factors that affect results:

A. The results are invalid if the measurement is performed on plasma rather than serum.

B. Bromsulphalein testing within 2 days prior to specimen collection invalidates serum results.

C. Values are higher when upright or ambulatory.

D. Falsely elevated urine results may be caused by contamination of the specimen with pus, menstrual blood, or vaginal discharge.

E. One study found a diurnal variation in urinary albumin levels in patients with insulin-dependent diabetes. Levels significantly increased between 2400 and 0800.

7. Other data:

A. A 24-hour urine collection for measuring protein loss may be helpful in clients with low serum albumin levels.

Bibliography:

Emerson TE: Unique features of albumin: A brief review. Crit Care Med *17*(7):690–694, 1989.

Hansen PM, Goddijn PP, Kofoed-Enevoldsen A, van Tol KM, Bilo HJ, Deckert T: Diurnal variation in glomerular charge selectivity, urinary albumin excretion and blood pressure in insulin-dependent diabetic patients. Kidney Int *48*(5):1559- 1562, 1995.

Piccoli GB, Quarello F, Salomone M, Iadarola GM, Funaro L, Marciello A, Fidelio T, Ghezzi PM, Cavalli PL, Vercellone A, et al.: Are serum albumin and cholesterol reliable outcome markers in elderly dialysis patients? Nephrol Dial Transplant *10* (Suppl 6):72–77, 1995.

ALCOHOL (ETHANOL), BLOOD

Norm: Negative.

		SI Units
Negative	0 mg/dl	0 mmol/L
Intoxication	>150 mg/dl	32.5 mmol/L
Coma	>300 mg/dl	>65.1 mmol/L
Panic level	350–800 mg/dl	76.0–174.0 mmol/L

Ethanol Poisoning Overdose Symptoms and Treatment:

Ethanol Poisoning Symptoms:

<50 mg/dl	Muscular incoordination
50–100 mg/dl	Worsening incoordination of movement
100–150 mg/dl	Mood and behavior changes
150–200 mg/dl	Delayed reactions
200–300 mg/dl	Ataxia, double vision, nausea, vomiting
300–400 mg/dl	Amnesia, dysarthria, hypothermia
400–700 mg/dl	Respiratory failure, coma, death possible

Ethanol Poisoning Treatment:

Tap water or 3% sodium bicarbonate lavage.
Support oxygenation and breathing.
Hemodialysis WILL remove ethanol, but is seldom necessary unless levels rise above 300 mg/dl. During hemodialysis, levels drop an average of 62 mg%/hour.

Increased: Alcohol ingestion; concomitant use of alcohol and certain drugs (antihistamines, barbiturates, chlordiazepoxide, diazepam, glutethimide, guanethidine, isoniazid, meprobamate, opiates, phenytoin, tranquilizers); ethylene glycol poisoning; and ingestion of liniments, shaving lotion, astringents, elixirs, fluid extracts, tinctures, and cough medicines.

Description: Alcohol (ethanol) is an anesthetic, diuretic, and central nervous system depressant taken orally by clients and sometimes administered intravenously for its inhibitory effects on labor.

Professional Considerations:

1. Consent form NOT required unless the specimen may be used as legal evidence.
2. Preparation:
   A. Tube: Red-top, red/gray-top, gold-top, black-top, or lavender-top.
   B. Do NOT draw during hemodialysis.
   C. If a specific type of alcohol measurement is desired (methanol, isopropanol, ethylene glycol), list the specific alcohol on the laboratory requisition.
3. Procedure:
   A. If the specimen is being collected for legal evidence, have the collection witnessed.
   B. Cleanse the venipuncture site with povidone-iodine solution and allow it to dry.
   C. Draw a 3-ml blood sample.
4. Postprocedure care:
   A. If the specimen may be used for legal evidence, include the exact time of specimen collection on the tube label and sign and have the witness sign the laboratory requisition. Transport the specimen to the laboratory in a sealed plastic bag labeled as legal evidence. Each person handling the specimen should sign and record the time of receipt on the laboratory requisition.
5. Client and family teaching:
   A. Results are normally available within 24 hours.
6. Factors that affect results:
   A. Cleansing the venipuncture site with an alcohol wipe may cause false-positive results.
7. Other data:
   A. Tolerance to alcohol's effects may develop in chronic alcoholics. Therefore, normally lethal levels may not lead to death in these clients.
   B. Only blood alcohol (rather than urine alcohol) levels are acceptable as legal evidence in most countries.
   C. *See also Isopropyl Alcohol, Blood; and Toxicology, Volatiles Group by GLC, Blood or Urine.*

Bibliography:

Cherpitel CJ: Alcohol and casualties: a comparison of emergency room and coroner data. Alcohol *29*(2):211–218, 1994.

Chugh SN, Mittal A, Arora V, Yadav SP, Sood AK: Combined toxicity due to alcohol and aluminium phosphide. J Assoc Physicians India *41*(10):679–680, 1993.

ALDOLASE, SERUM

Norm:

		SI Units
Adult		
Ambulatory	1.0–7.5 U/L (30°C)	0.02–0.13 µKat/L
Bedrest	0.3–3.0 U/L (30°C)	0.005–0.05 µKat/L
Children		
Newborn 10–24 mos.	3.4–11.8 U/L (37°C) or up to 4 times the adult levels.	0.06–0.20 µKat/L
25 mos.–16 yrs.	1.2–8.8 U/L (37°C) or up to 2 times the adult levels	0.02–0.15 µKat/L

Increased: Anemia (megaloblastic, hemolytic), burns, cancer, cirrhosis, congestive heart failure, crushing injury, dermatomyositis, eosinophilic fasciitis, erythroblastosis fetalis, hepatic necrosis, hepatitis (acute viral), hepatoma, jaundice (obstructive), lead intoxication, leukemia (chronic granulocytic), liver metastasis, lymphoma, metastasis, mononucleosis (infectious), muscle trauma, muscular dystrophy, myocardial infarction (acute), myopathy, Niemann-Pick disease, pancreatitis (acute), pericarditis (hemorrhagic), polycythemia vera, polymyositis, prostate cancer, pulmonary infarction, skeletal muscle disease, surgical trauma, and trichinosis. Drugs include aminocaproic acid (large doses), carbenoxolone, chlorinated insecticides, clofibrate, corticotropin, cortisone acetate, labetolol, organophosphorus insecticides, and thiabendazole.

Decreased: Not clinically significant. Drugs include phenothiazines (when aldolase values are initially high in schizophrenics).

Description: An enzyme found throughout the body, but in highest concentrations in skeletal muscle tissue. Because aldolase rises during active skeletal muscle disease, its measurement helps track the progress of diseases such as progressive muscular dystrophy.

Professional Considerations:

1. Consent form NOT required.
2. Preparation:
   A. Tube: Red-top, red/gray-top, or gold-top.
   B. *See Client and family teaching.*
3. Procedure:
   A. Draw a 2-ml blood sample.
4. Postprocedure care:
   A. Place rthe sample on ice for immediate transport to the laboratory.
5. Client and family teaching:
   A. Avoid strenuous exercise for 12 hours prior to sampling.

B. Results are normally available within 24 hours.
6. Factors that affect results:
   A. Reject hemolyzed specimen to avoid falsely elevated results.
   B. Recent intramuscular injections may elevate results.
7. Other data:
   A. While norms are not established for Aldolase isoenzymes A, B, and C, one study (Asaka et al. 1994) found that serum aldolase A/B ratios increased in clients with cancer with normal GPT levels and decreased in clients with liver disease.
   B. Measurement of Aldolase A and gamma-enolase together provides information directly relevant to prognosis in cases of renal cell carcinoma.
   C. May be useful indicator of disease activity in eosinophilic fascitis (EF).

Bibliography:

Asaka M, Kimura T, Meguro T, Kato M, Kudo M, Miyazaki T, Alpert E: Alteration of aldolase isozymes in serum and tissues of patients with cancer and other diseases. J Clin Lab Anal 8(3): 144–148, 1994

Fujimoto M, Sato S, Ihn H, Kikuchi K, Yamada N, Takehara K: Serum aldolase level is a useful indicator of disease activity in eosinophilic fascitis. J Rheumatol 22(3):563–565, 1995.

Karamizrak SO, Ergen E, Tore IR, Akgun N: Changes in serum creatine kinase, lactate dehydrogenase and aldolase activities following supramaximal exercise in athletes. J Sports Med Phys Fitness 34(2):141–146, 1994.

Takashi M, Sakata T, Kato K: Use of serum gamma-enolase and aldolase A in combination as markers for renal cell carcinoma. Jpn J Cancer Res 84(3):304–309, 1993.

ALDOSTERONE, SERUM AND URINE

Norm:

Average-Sodium Diet	Serum	SI Units
Peripheral Blood		
Supine	3–10 ng/dl	0.14–1.9 nmol/L
Upright		
Adult Female		
Pregnant	18–100 ng/dl	0.5–2.8 nmol/L
Nonpregnant	5–30 ng/dl	0.14–0.8 nmol/L
Adult Male	6–22 ng/dl	0.17–0.61 nmol/L
Adrenal Vein	200–800 ng/dl	5.54–2.22 nmol/L
Child		
1 week–12 mos	1–160 ng/dl	0.03–4.43 nmol/L
Age 1–3	5–60 ng/dl	0.14–1.7 nmol/L
Age 3–11	5–70 ng/dl	0.14–1.9 nmol/L
Age 11–15	<5–50 ng/dl	<0.14–1.4 nmol/L

Urinary Aldosterone		SI Units	
Norm urine:	2–26 mg/24 h	5.6–73 nmol/day	

Urinary Sodium	Plasma Renin	µg/day	nmol/day
<30 nmol/day	5–24 Al/ml/h	35–80	97–220
20–50 nmol/day	2–7 Al/ml/h	13–33	36–91
50–100 nmol/day	1–5 Al/ml/h	5–24	14–66
100–150 nmol/day	0.5–4 Al/ml/h	3–19	8–53
150–200 nmol/day		1–16	3–44
200–250 nmol/day		1–13	3–36

Increased in Serum and Urine:
Adrenal tumor (aldosterone-producing adenoma), aldosteronism (primary, secondary), bilateral adrenal hyperplasia, cirrhosis, congestive heart failure, Conn's syndrome, hemorrhage, hyponatremia, hypovolemia, idiopathic cyclic edema, nephrosis (lower nephron), nephrotic syndrome, and renovascular hypertension. Drugs that increase serum levels include estrogens, corticotropin, diuretics that promote sodium excretion, laxatives that are abused, some oral contraceptives, and potassium. Drugs that increase urine levels include angiotensin, deoxycorticosterone, diuretics (loop, thiazide), etiocholanolone, oral contraceptives, and steroids.

Decreased in Serum and Urine:
Addison's disease, primary hypoaldosteronism, salt-wasting syndrome, septicemia, stress, and toxemia of pregnancy. Drugs that decrease serum levels include aminoglutethimide, ACE inhibitors, deoxycorticosterone, etomidate, fludrocortisone, heparin (after several days of continuous therapy), indomethacin, licorice, methyldopa, saralasin. Drugs that decrease urine levels include aminoglutethimide, clonidine, deoxycorticosterone, fludrocortisone, glucocorticoids, labetalol, licorice, heparin, methyldopa, metyrapone, and propranolol.

Description: Aldosterone is a mineralocorticoid secreted by the adrenal cortex that functions in blood pressure and body fluid regulation. It acts on the renal distal tubules, causing increased resorption of sodium and water at the expense of increased excretion of potassium.

Professional Considerations:
1. Consent form NOT required.

2. Preparation:
   A. The client should rest in a supine position for 8–12 hours. The sample should be drawn before noon.
   B. Tube: Red-top, red/gray-top, gold-top; lavender-top, or green-top for serum collection.
   C. For urine test, obtain a 3-L container to which 10 g of boric acid have been added, and a 100-ml specimen container for urinary sample.
   D. *See Client and family teaching.*
3. Procedure:

Serum Test:
A. Collect 2.5-ml blood sample for serum aldosterone.

Urine Test:
A. Discard the first morning urine specimen.
B. Collect all urine voided in a 24-hour period in a refrigerated container to which 10 g of boric acid have been added. Include urine voided at the end of the 24-hour period. For catheterized clients, keep the drainage bag on ice and empty the urine into the collection container hourly.
C. At the end of 24 hours, mix the urine gently and collect a 100-ml aliquot in a clean container.
4. Postprocedure care:
   A. Note total 24-hour urine volume on the laboratory requisition and the aliquot container label.
   B. Transport the samples to the laboratory immediately.
5. Client and family teaching:
   A. Follow a 3 g/day sodium diet for 2 weeks if not contraindicated by medical condition.
   B. Avoid physical or psychological stress throughout the collection period.
   C. Save all urine voided in the 24-hour period, urinate before defecating to avoid loss of urine, and avoid contaminating the specimen with feces or toiled tissue. If any urine is accidentally discarded, discard the entire specimen and restart the collection the next day.
   D. Results may not be available for several days.

6. Factors that affect results:
   A. Radioactive scans within 7 days prior to urine collection invalidate the results.
   B. Hemolysis invalidates the serum results.
   C. Decreased kidney perfusion may cause increased aldosterone and renin values.
   D. Levels may be suppressed in clients with insulin-dependent diabetes mellitus.
   E. An upright client position for serum collection invalidates the results.
7. Other data:
   A. Serum electrolyte and renin levels should be measured prior to this test.

Bibliography:

Brown MA, Thou ST, Whitworth JA: Stimulation of aldosterone by ACTH in normal and hypertensive pregnancy. Am J Hypertens 8(3):260–267, 1995.

Cronin CC, Barry D, Crowley B, Ferriss JB: Reduced plasma aldosterone concentrations in randomly selected patients with insulin-dependent diabetes mellitus. Diabet Med 12(9):809–815, 1995.

Kalhoff H, Rascher W, Diekmann L, Stock GJ, Manz F: Urinary excretion of aldosterone, arginine vasopressin and cortisol in premature infants with maximum renal acid stimulation. Acta Paediatr 84(5):490–494, 1995.

Laragh JH: Renin-angiotensin-aldosterone system for blood pressure and electrolyte homeostasis and its involvement in hypertension, in congestive heart failure and in associated cardiovascular damage (myocardial infarction and stroke). J Hum Hypertens 9(6):385–390, 1995.

Shiah CJ, Wu KD, Tsai DM, Liao ST, Siauw CP, Lee LS: Diagnostic value of plasma aldosterone/potassium ratio in hypoaldosteronism. J Formos Med Assoc 94(5):248–254, 1995.

ALDOSTERONE SUPPRESSION TEST, DIAGNOSTIC

Norm: <5 ng/dl (<0.14 nmol/L SI units).

Primary Aldosteronism: >10 ng/dl (>0.2777 nmol/L SI units).

Usage: Definitive diagnosis of primary aldosteronism.

Description: Aldosterone is a mineralocorticoid secreted by the adrenal cortex that functions in blood pressure and body fluid regulation. It acts on the renal distal tubule, where it increases resorption of sodium and water at the expense of increased potassium excretion. Levels are affected by body position and sodium and potassium levels. The aldosterone suppression test measures aldosterone levels before and after an infusion of saline. In primary aldosteronism, the saline infusion fails to suppress aldosterone levels as much as it suppresses the levels in a normal client.

Professional Considerations:

1. Consent form NOT required.

Risks:

Volume overload, hypertension, myocardial ischemia, congestive heart failure.

Contraindications:

The serum test is contraindicated in clients with congestive heart failure.

2. Preparation:
   A. The client should be positioned upright for 2 hours, then lie in a recumbent position from the onset of the test until second specimen is drawn at the completion of the infusion.
   B. Tubes: Two red-top, red/gray-top, gold-top, green-top, or lavender-top tubes.
   C. Obtain 2 L of 0.9% saline and a 24-hour urine collection container to which 10 g of boric acid have been added.
3. Procedure:

Serum Collection:

A. Draw a 2.5-ml blood sample for the baseline aldosterone level.
B. Infuse 2 L of normal saline intravenously over a 4-hour period to the recumbent client.
C. Draw a final 2.5-ml blood sample for aldosterone level.

Urine Collection:

A. Discard the first morning-urine specimen.
B. Collect all urine voided in a 24-hour period in a refrigerated container to which 10 g of boric acid have been added. Include urine voided at the end of the 24-hour period. For catheterized clients, keep the drainage bag on ice and empty the urine into the collection container hourly.
C. At the end of 24 hours, mix the urine gently and collect a 100-ml aliquot in a clean container.
4. Postprocedure care:
   A. Note the collection site and the time on all laboratory requisitions and blood tubes. For the urine sample, write the total 24-hour urine volume on the laboratory requisition and the aliquot container label.
   B. Transport each specimen to the laboratory immediately after collection.
5. Client and family teaching:
   A. The test takes several hours. Bring reading material or other diversional item.
   B. Results are normally available within 24 hours.

6. Factors that affect results:
   A. Reject hemolyzed specimens.
   B. Radioactive scans within 7 days prior to urine collection invalidate results.
7. Other data:
   A. None.

Bibliography:

Arteaga E, Klein R, Biglieri E: Use of the saline infusion test to diagnose the cause of primary aldosteronism. Am J Med 79(6):722–728, 1985.

Kobayashi S, Seki T, Nonomura K, Gotoh T, Togashi M, Koyanagi T: Clinical experience of incidentally discovered adrenal tumor with particular reference to cortical function. J Urol 150(1):8–12, 1993.

ALKALINE PHOSPHATASE, HEAT STABLE, SERUM

Norm: Interpreted by laboratory. Results are reported in the percentage of alkaline phosphatase that is heat stable. Residual activity >30% favors hepatic origin and <30% favors bone origin *(see Description)*.

Usage: Aids in differentiation of the source of increased alkaline phosphatase activity.

Description: Alkaline phosphatase is an enzyme normally found in bone, liver, intestine, and placenta that rises during periods of bone growth (osteoblastic activity), liver disease, and bile duct obstruction. It is made up of bone, liver, and placental and intestinal isoenzymes that can be separated via heat fractionation. Liver and placental alkaline phosphatase isoenzymes are heat stable, and bone isoenzyme is inactivated by heat. Greater than 30% of the alkaline phosphatase being heat stable suggests activity of liver origin, whereas <30% being heat stable suggests activity of bone origin.

Professional Considerations:

1. Consent form NOT required.
2. Preparation:
   A. Tube: Red-top, red/gray-top, or gold-top.
   B. Do NOT draw during hemodialysis.

3. Procedure:
   A. Draw a 1-ml blood sample.
4. Postprocedure care:
   A. Transport the specimen to the laboratory immediately for testing or for spinning and refrigeration.
5. Client and family teaching:
   A. The client may be asked to fast for 10–12 hours.
   B. Results may take several days.
6. Factors that affect results:
   A. Reject hemolyzed specimens.
   B. Hepatotoxic drugs within 12 hours prior to specimen collection invalidate the test.
   C. Failure to fast prior to the test may result in falsely elevated levels.
   D. Specimens left at room temperature may result in falsely elevated levels.
7. Other data:
   A. Postmenopausal females have slightly increased total alkaline phosphatase and a low percentage of heat-stable fraction, indicating osseous origin.
   B. Recent studies by Patel et al. (1990, 1993) and Rassam et al. (1995) suggest that serum heat stable alkaline phosphatase may be useful in diagnosis and treatment monitoring for breast cancer, squamous cell carcinoma of the head and neck, and leukemia.

Bibliography:

Leroux M, Perry WF: Serum heat-stable alkaline phosphatase in pregnancy. Am J Obstet Gynecol 108(2):235–239, 1990.

Patel P, Baxi B, Adhvaryu S, Balar D: Evaluation of serum sialic acid, heat stable alkaline phosphatase and fucose as markers of breast carcinoma. Anticancer Res 10(4):1071–1074, 1990.

Patel PS, Adhvaryu SG, Balar DB: Clinical significance of serum total and heat-stable alkaline phosphatase in leukemia patients. Tumori 79(5):352–356, 1993.

Rassam MB, al-Bashir NN, al-Salihi AR, Hammash MH, al-Sammerai FT, al-Ubaidi MA, Waheed IN: Heat-stable alkaline phosphatase. A putative tumor marker of head and neck squamous cell carcinoma. Acta Oncol 34(1):49–52, 1995.

ALKALINE PHOSPHATASE, ISOENZYMES, SERUM

(see Alkaline Phosphatase, Serum)

ALKALINE PHOSPHATASE, SERUM

Norm:

Total Alkaline Phosphatase		SI Units
King-Armstrong Method		
Adults age 20–60	4.5–13 U/dl	32–92 U/L
Elderly	Slightly higher	
Newborn	5–15 U/dl	36–107 U/L
Premature newborn	1.5–2 times adult value	

		SI Units
Children: Values remain high until epiphyses close.		
1 month	10–30 U/dl	71–213 U/L
3 years	10–20 U/dl	71–142 U/L
10 years	15–30 U/dl	107–213 U/L
Bodansky Method		
Adults age 20–60	2–4 U/dl	10.7–21.5 U/L
Elderly	Slightly higher	
Children	5–14 U/dl	27–75 U/L
Bessey-Lowrey-Brock Method		
Adults age 20–60	0.8–2.3 U/dl	13.3–38.3 U/L
Elderly	Slightly higher	
Bowers and McComb Method		
Females		
Age 1–12	<350 U/L	<5.95 µKat/L
Puberty: Values may triple.		
Age >15	25–100 U/L	0.43–1.70 µKat/L
Males		
Age 1–12	<350 U/L	<5.95 µKat/L
Age 12–14	<500 U/L	<8.50 µKat/L
Puberty: Values may triple.		
Age >20	25–100 U/L	0.43–1.70 µKat/L

	Isoenzyme Norms	
Heat Inactivation Method	**Percentage of Isoenzyme Inactivated After 16 Minutes at 55°C**	**Fraction of Isoenzyme Inactivated After 16 Minutes at 55°C**
Liver isoenzyme	50–70	0.50–0.70
Bone isoenzyme	90–100	0.90–1.00
Intestinal isoenzyme	50–60	0.50–0.60
Placental isoenzyme		
Trimester 1 to 1 month postpartum	50% of total	

Increased Biliary Isoenzyme: Biliary cirrhosis, biliary duct obstruction, cholangiar obstruction (in hepatitis), and cholestasis.

Increased Bone Isoenzyme: Bone cancer accompanied by bone formation, bone growth or healing, familial hyperphosphatemia, familial osteoectasia, Gaucher's disease, growth hormone overproduction, hyperparathyroidism, hyperthyroidism, leukemia of bone marrow, lymphoma, malabsorption, myositis ossificans, Niemann-Pick disease, osteoblastic metastases, osteogenesis imperfecta, osteomalacia, osteoporosa, osteogenic sarcoma, Paget's disease, polyostotic fibrous dysplasia, renal osteodystrophy, and Rickets.

Increased Intestinal Isoenzyme: Gastrointestinal disease, clients with blood type O or B (some) pancreatic duct obstruction, pancreatic cancer, splenic infarction, steatorrhea (idiopathic), and ulcer (perforated)

Increased Liver I Isoenzyme: Impaired enzyme metabolism, liver congestion, hepatic carcinoma, hepatotoxic drugs, jaundice (obstructive), pregnancy, and vasculitis.

Increased Liver II Isoenzyme: Hepatitis (infectious, viral), parenchymal cell damage.

Increased Placental Isoenzyme: Pregnancy (late).

Increased Total Alkaline Phosphatase: May also be caused by alcoholism, carbohydrate ingestion (large quantities), children, diabetes mellitus, Fanconi's syndrome, fat ingestion, fibrous dysplasia, histiocytosis, Hodgkin's disease, hyperalimentation, hyperparathyroidism (with bone disease), hypophosphatemia, kidney tissue rejection, liver abscess, liver disease, lung cancer, lymphoma, mononucleosis (infectious), multiple myeloma, myocardial infarction, pulmonary infarction, renal infarction, rheumatoid disease, rickets, sarcoidosis, and sickle cell crisis. Drugs include acetohexamide, albumin, allopurinol, aluminum nicotinate, amitriptyline, ampicillin, anabolic steroids, androgens, asparaginase, aspirin, aurothioglucose, azothioprine, baclofen, barbiturates, bromocriptinemesylate, carbamazepine, carmustine, cephaloridine, chlordiazepoxide, chlorpromazine hydrochloride, chlorpropamide, cholestyramine resin, cimetidine, cincophen, clindamycin, clonazepam, colchicine, ergosterol, erythromycin, estrogens, floxuridine, flurazepam, fosinopril, gold sodium, n-hydroxyacetamide, imipramine, imipramine pamoate, indomethacin, isoniazid, lincomycin, meclofenamate sodium, methyldopa, methyldopate hydrochloride, methyltestosterone, metoprolol tartrate, minoxidil, mithramycin, naproxen sodium, niacin, nifedipine, nitrofurantoin, novobiacin, oral contraceptives, oxacillin sodium, oxyphenisatin, papaverine hydrochloride, penicillamine, petrofane, phenobarbital, phenothiazines, phenylbutazone, phenytoin, procainamide hydrochloride, propranolol, propylthiouricil, rifampin, salicylates, sulfamethoxazole sulfisoxazole, sulfisoxazole acetyl, sulfobromophthalein sodium, tetracycline, thiomalate, thiothixene, tolazamide, tolbutamide, tolmetin sodium, valproic acid, and vitamin D.

Decreased: Anemia (pernicious), blood transfusions (massive), celiac disease, cretinism, hypophosphatasia, hypothyroidism, malnutrition, milkalkali syndrome (Burnett's syndrome), nephritis (chronic), osteolytic sarcoma, scurvy, vitamin D intoxication, and zinc depletion. Drugs include edetate disodium, fluorides, oxalates, phosphates, and propranolol.

Description: Alkaline phosphatase is an enzyme found in bone, liver, intes-

tine, and placenta that rises during periods of bone growth (osteoblastic activity), liver disease, and bile duct obstruction. It is made up of bone, liver, placental, biliary, and intestinal isoenzymes that can be separated via electrophoresis. Alkaline phosphatase isoenzymes should be measured for any client who has an elevated alkaline phosphatase level.

Professional Considerations:

1. Consent form NOT required.
2. Preparation:
   A. Tube: Red-top, red/gray-top, or gold-top.
   B. *See Client and family teaching.*
3. Procedure:
   A. Draw a 1-ml blood sample.
4. Postprocedure care:
   A. Transport the specimen to the laboratory for immediate testing or for spinning and refrigeration.
5. Client and family teaching:
   A. Client may be asked to fast for 10–12 hours.
   B. Results are normally available within 24 hours.
6. Factors that affect results:
   A. Reject hemolyzed specimens.
   B. Hepatotoxic drugs within 12 hours prior to collection invalidate the test.
   C. Falsely elevated results may be caused by failure to fast prior to the test or by specimens left at room temperature.
7. Other data:
   A. Isoenzymes are required to interpret the contributing source (liver, bone, placenta) of elevated total alkaline phosphatase.
   B. At least 2 days are required for isoenzyme results.
   C. Differentiation of bone and liver isoenzyme is difficult, because both are derived from a single gene. A monoclonal antibody assay is being tested that may aid in differentiation of liver and bone isoenzyme.

Bibliography:

Gomez B Jr, Ardakani S, Ju J, Jenkins D, Cerelli MJ, Daniloff GY, Kung VT: Monoclonal antibody assay for measuring bone-specific alkaline phosphatase activity in serum. Clin Chem *41*(11):1560–1566, 1995.

Kobayashi T, Kawakubo T: Prospective investigation of tumor markers and risk assessment in early cancer screening. Cancer *73*(7):1946–1953, 1994.

Onwuameze IC: Serum calcium, inorganic phosphate and alkaline phosphatase activity in lactating females. East Afr Med J *72*(6):379–380, 1995.

Price CP, Mitchell CA, Moriarty J, Gray M, Noonan K: Mass versus activity: Validation of an immunometric assay for bone alkaline phosphatase in serum. Ann Clin Biochem *32*(Pt 4):405–412, 1995.

ALLERGEN-SPECIFIC IgE, SERUM

Norm: <2% of serum immunoglobulins.

Adults	<41 U/ml
Children	
Neonate	<12 U/ml
Age 1–3	<10 U/ml
Age 4–6	<24 U/ml
Age 7–8	<46 U/ml
Age 9–12	<116 U/ml
Age 13–14	<63 U/ml

Increased: Allergic rhinitis, asthma (exogenous), anaphylaxis, atopic dermatitis, atopic eczema, echinococcus infestation, eczema, hay fever, hookworm disease, schistosomiasis, and visceral larva migrans. Drugs include aminophenazone, anticonvulsants, asparaginase, hydralazine hydrochloride, oral contraceptives, and phenylbutazone.

Decreased: Asthma (endogenous), pregnancy, and radiation therapy. Drugs include methotrexate.

Description: Immunoglobulin E is a protein produced in the bone marrow that functions as an antibody in response to antigen stimulation in hypersensitivity reactions. IgE levels are influenced by the nature of the allergen, length of exposure to the allergen, symptomatic responses, and hyposensitization treatments. The test is performed by radioimmunoassay.

Professional Considerations:

1. Consent form NOT required.
2. Preparation:
   A. Tube: Red-top, red/gray-top, or gold-top.
   B. List vaccinations, immunizations, and tetanus antitoxin received within the prior 6 months on the laboratory requisition.
   C. List the blood products the client received within 6 weeks prior to the test on the laboratory requisition.
3. Procedure:
   A. Draw a 3-ml blood sample.
4. Postprocedure care:
   A. Transport the specimen to the laboratory immediately.
5. Client and family teaching:
   A. Fast, except for water, 12–14 hours.
   B. Results are normally available within 24 hours.
   C. Refer the client with elevated IgE levels and allergic symptoms to an allergist for more specific testing and guidance on potential treatments and environmental reduction of allergens.
6. Factors that affect results:
   A. A delay in testing invalidates results.
   B. Results are invalidated if the client has undergone a scan using a radioisotope within 1 week prior to the test.
7. Other data:
   A. This test is often used to accompany a negative radioallergosorbent (RAST) test to assess for reactivity to untested allergens.
   B. A newer serum test under investigation to determine its sensitivity is the multiple antigen simultaneous test (MAST), which can simultaneously detect allergies to up to 3.5 allergens in one serum sample.
   C. *See also Allergen-Specific IgE Antibody, Serum and Skin Test for Hypersensitivity, Diagnostic.*

Bibliography:

Costongs GM, Janson PC, Hermans WJ, van Oers RJ, Leerkes B: Evaluation of performance characteristics of automated measurement systems for allergy testing. Eur J Clin Chem Clin Biochem 33(5):295–305, 1995.

Jacquemin MG, Saint-Remy JM: Specific down-regulation of anti-allergen IgE and IgG antibodies in humans associated with injections of allergen-specific antibody complexes. Ther Immunol 2(1):41–52, 1995.

Ogino S, Bessho K, Harada T, Irifune M, Matsunaga T: Evaluation of allergen-specific IgE antibodies by MAST for the diagnosis of nasal allergy. Rhinology 31(1):27–31, 1993.

van der Heijden FL, van Neerven RJ, Kapsenberg ML: Relationship between facilitated allergen presentation and the presence of allergen-specific IgE in serum of atopic patients. Clin Exp Immunol 99(2):289–293, 1995.

ALLERGEN-SPECIFIC IgE ANTIBODY (RAST TEST, RADIOALLERGOSORBENT TEST, ALLERGY SCREEN), SERUM

Norm: Negative.

ImmunoCAP FEIA method: <0.35 kU/L.

Pharmacia CAP System:

	Asymptomatic Clients	Symptomatic Allergy
Perennial allergens	≤10.7 kU/L	>10.7 kU/L
Seasonal allergens	≤8.4 kU/L	>8.4 kU/L
All allergens	≤11.7 kU/L	>11.7 kU/L

Results Reported by Allergen Scores on 0–4 Scale:

0	No IgE detected
1	Borderline
2–4	Increasing levels of IgE

Modified RAST:

Class	Counts	Significance
	0–749	No specific IgE activity
1	750–1600	Borderline activity
2	1601–3600	Low positive
3	3601–8000	Moderate positive
4	8001–18,000	High positive
5	18,001–40,000	Very high positive
6	>40,000	Extreme high positive

Usage: Aids differential diagnosis of allergies (especially food allergies of the immediate type) and monitoring of treatment for specific allergies.

Description: This test measures the amount of IgE directed against specific allergens by binding a specific antigen to a carrier substance and allowing it to react with a specific IgE antibody in the client's blood sample. The amount of bound IgE is then measured. The test is used to identify allergies to foods, grasses, weeds, trees, molds, epidermals, insects, and miscellaneous substances such as house dust, insulin, and silk. An advantage of this test is that the information can be obtained without causing an allergic reaction because the allergen is introduced into the blood sample rather than into the body.

Professional Considerations:

1. Consent form NOT required.
2. Preparation:
   A. Tube: Red-top, red/gray-top, or gold-top.
3. Procedure:
   A. Draw a 2-ml blood sample.
4. Postprocedure care:
   A. Transport the specimen to the laboratory for immediate spinning, serum separation, and refrigeration of serum.
5. Client and family teaching:
   A. Results may take several days.
6. Factors that affect results:
   A. IgE levels are influenced by the nature of the allergen, length of exposure to the allergen, symptomatic responses, and hyposensitization treatments.
   B. Results are invalidated if the client received radioactive dyes within 7 days prior to the test.
   C. False-positive results may be caused by high IgE levels (>3000 U/ml) due to parasitic infection.
7. Other data:
   A. This test correlates 80–85% with subcutaneous skin testing and is more specific.
   B. A total IgE level should also be obtained. If the RAST test is negative but total IgE level is elevated, the allergen may not be one for which the RAST test can be used.
   C. Results may take up to 1 week.
   D. The oral challenge test (OCT) is still the gold standard in the diagnosis of food allergy according to a 1994 study by Roger et al.
   E. *See also Allergen-Specific IgE, Serum and Skin Test for Hypersensitivity, Diagnostic.*

Bibliography:

Costongs GM, Janson PC, Hermans WJ, van Oers RJ, Leerkes B: Evaluation of performance characteristics of automated measurement systems for allergy testing. Eur J Clin Chem Clin Biochem 33(5):295–305, 1995.

Pastorello EA, Incorvaia C, Ortolani C, Bonini S, Canonica GW, Romagnani S, Tursi A, Zanussi C: Studies on the relationship between the level of specific IgE antibodies and the clinical expression of allergy: I. Definition of levels distinguishing patients with symptomatic from patients with asymptomatic allergy to common aeroallergens. J Allergy Clin Immunol *96*(5 Pt 1):580–587, 1995.

Roger A, Pena M, Botey J, Eseverri J, Marin A: The prick test and specific IgE compared with the oral challenge test with milk, eggs and nuts. J Investig Allergol Clin Immunol. *4*(4):178–181, 1994.

ALLERGY SCREEN
(see Allergin-Specific IgE Antibody, Serum)

ALLERGY SKIN TEST
(see Skin Test for Hypersensitivity, Diagnostic)

ALPHA$_1$-ANTITRYPSIN, SERUM

Norm: 80–260 mg/dl (0.8–2.6 g/L, SI units).

Increased: Hepatitis, hyaline membrane disease, infection, inflammation (acute, chronic), liver disease (chronic), neoplasm, pregnancy, and systemic lupus erythematosus (SLE). Drugs include estrogens, oral contraceptives, and steroids.

Decreased: Congenital alpha-antitrypsin deficiency, emphysema, liver disease (chronic), and in newborns (transient).

Description: A major faction of alpha$_1$-globulin protein detected via serum protein immunoelectrophoresis. Alpha$_1$-antitrypsin functions in protection of body fluids by preventing release of protease by dying cells. The test is used to screen for clients at high risk for emphysema and liver disease associated with a congenital absence of the protein. Other uses for this test include nonspecific detection of inflammatory, infectious, and necrotic processes.

Professional Considerations:
1. Consent form NOT required.
2. Preparation:
   A. Tube: Red-top, red/gray-top, or gold-top.
   B. *See Client and family teaching.*
3. Procedure:
   A. Draw a 1-ml blood sample.
4. Postprocedure care:
   A. Freeze the specimen.
5. Client and family teaching:
   A. The client with hypercholesterolemia or hyperlipemia should fast 8–10 hours.
   B. Results are normally available within 24 hours.
6. Factors that affect results:
   A. Reject hemolyzed specimens.
7. Other data:
   A. Levels may also be measured in amniotic fluid.

Bibliography:
Barker AF, Siemsen F, Pasley D, D'Silva R, Buist AS: Replacement therapy for hereditary alpha$_1$-antitrypsin deficiency. A program for long-term administration. Chest *105*(5):1406–1410, 1994.

Deficiency of alpha$_1$-antitrypsin and the liver. Proceedings of a symposium. Bozen/Bolzano, 23 October 1992. Acta Paediatr *393* (Suppl):1–36, 1994.

ALPHA-FETOPROTEIN (AFP), BLOOD

Norm: Tumor marker <8.5 ng/ml

		SI Units
Adult females		
Nonpregnant	0–10 ng/ml	0–10 µg/L
Pregnant		
2 months	<75 ng/ml	<75 µg/L
3 months	<130 ng/ml	<130 µg/L
4 months	<210 ng/ml	<210 µg/L
5 months	<300 ng/ml	<300 µg/L
6 months	<400 ng/ml	<400 µg/L
7 months	<450 ng/ml	<450 µg/L
8 months	<450 ng/ml	<450 µg/L
9 months	<400 ng/ml	<400 µg/L
Immediately postpartum	<375 ng/ml	<375 µg/L
Adult males	0–10 ng/ml	0–10 µg/L
Children	0–30 ng/ml	0–30 µg/L

Increased: Ataxia telangiectasia, cirrhosis, gonadal teratoblastoma, cancer (embryonal, hepatocellular, pancreatic with liver metastases, malignant teratoma of ovary or testes, gastric with liver metastases, biliary system, germ cell tumors), hepatitis (acute, chronic, neonatal), pregnancy (with fetal neural tube defects, multiple fetuses, fetal distress, fetal death), intrauterine death, duodenal atresia, oomphalocele, spontaneous abortion, tetralogy of Fallot (or Turner's syndrome), tyrosinemia, and ulcerative colitis.

Decreased: Has been associated with Down syndrome when less than 0.25 times the normal median.

Description: A globulin protein secreted by liver cells during hepatic cell multiplication and found in high amounts in fetal plasma. Highest adult amounts are found during pregnancy and in primary hepatic cancer. Maternal levels should be measured initially at 15–18 weeks' gestation as a screening method for fetal neural tube defects. Confirmatory testing (for levels greater than 0.5–2.5 times the normal median) should be repeated in 7 days. For positive confirmatory test, ultrasound and amniotic fluid AFP measurement should be performed.

Professional Considerations:

1. Consent form NOT required.
2. Preparation:
   A. Tube: Red-top, red/gray-top, or gold-top.
   B. List on the laboratory requisition: maternal weight, maternal race, week of gestation, and any history of diabetes mellitus.
3. Procedure:
   A. Draw a 1-ml blood sample from the mother.
4. Postprocedure care:
   A. Apply a dry, sterile dressing over the amniocentesis site.
5. Client and family teaching:
   A. Results may take several days.

6. Factors that affect results:
   A. Normal levels are affected by the mother's age, weight, and number of fetuses present.
   B. Reject hemolyzed specimens.
   C. Results are invalid if the client has undergone a radioisotope scan within the prior 2 weeks.
7. Other data:
   A. AFP testing may also be performed on amniotic fluid to detect neurologic congenital defects and Down syndrome. Serum AFP measurement is thought to increase accuracy of antenatal detection of Down syndrome from 35% to 67%, but its accuracy can be affected by maternal weight, smoking history, and diabetes mellitus and by whether the gestational age of the fetus is correctly estimated.
   B. Not a screening test for cancer.
   C. A recent study suggests that the receipt of a negative result on the test does not provide reassurance to the parents.

Bibliography:

Chang TC, Cheng HH: The role of maternal serum alpha-fetoprotein, human chorionic gonadotrophin and oestriol in the antenatal screening of Down syndrome. Med J Malaysia 49(4): 351–354, 1994.

Chen RJ, Chen CK, Chang DY, Chow SN, Huang SC, Hsieh CY, Lin MC, Hsu HC: Immunoelectrophoretic differentiation of alpha-fetoprotein in disorders with elevated serum alpha-fetoprotein levels or during pregnancy. Acta Oncol 34(7): 931–935, 1995.

Goldstein PJ, Sundaram SG, Manimekalai S: Drug interference on alpha-fetoprotein assays. Md Med J 40(6):513–516, 1991.

Kidd J, Cook R, Marteau T: Is routine AFP screening in pregnancy reassuring? J Psychosom Res 37(7): 717–722, 1993.

ALT
(see Alanine Aminotransferase, Serum)

ALTERNATE PATHWAY FACTOR B, SERUM
(see C3 Proactivator, Serum)

AMA
(see Antimitochondrial Antibody, Blood)

AMIKACIN SULFATE, BLOOD

Norm:

		SI Units
Therapeutic peak	20–25 mg/L or µg/ml	34–43 µmol/L
Toxic peak	>35 mg/L or µg/ml	>60 µmol/L
Therapeutic trough	5–10 mg/L or µg/ml	9–17 µmol/L
Toxic trough (adult)	>10 mg/L or µg/ml	>17 µmol/L
Toxic trough (child)	>5 ng/ml	>9 µmol/L

Increased: Aminoglycoside toxicity and impaired renal function.

Decreased: Subtherapeutic levels in client treated with aminoglycoside.

Description: Amikacin is a semisynthetic aminoglycoside antibiotic derived from kanamycin and effective against gram-negative and gram-positive organisms. It is excreted by glomerular filtration, with a half-life of 1.9–2.8 hours. Peak and trough levels should be monitored throughout therapy. Toxicity is possible at trough levels. Steady-state levels are reached after 10–15 hours.

Professional Considerations:
1. Consent form NOT required.
2. Preparation:
   A. Tube: Red-top, red/gray-top, or gold-top.
   B. Do NOT draw during hemodialysis.
   C. Write the time, dose, and route of the most recent dose on the laboratory requisition.
3. Procedure:
   A. Draw a 1-ml blood sample.
4. Postprocedure care:
   A. None.

5. Client and family teaching:
   A. Results are normally available within 24 hours.
6. Factors that affect results:
   A. Cross-reactivity may occur with concomitant antibiotic therapy (cephalosporin, chloramphenicol, clindamcin, kanamycin, penicillin, tetracycline, tobramycin).
7. Other data:
   A. Potentially nephrotoxic, ototoxic, and neurotoxic.
   B. Creatinine clearance should be monitored QD for clients receiving amikacin.
   C. Contreras et al. (1994) found hypoalbuminemia to correlate strongly with amikacin nephrotoxicity.

Bibliography:

Blaser J, Konig C, Fatio R, Follath F, Cometta A, Glauser M: Multicenter quality control study of amikacin assay for monitoring once-daily dosing regimens. International Antimicrobial Therapy Cooperative Group of the European Organization for Research and Treatment of Cancer. Ther Drug Monit 17(2):133–136, 1995.

Contreras AM, Ramirez M, Cueva L, Alvarez S, de Loza R, Gamba G: Low serum albumin and the increased risk of amikacin nephrotoxicity. Rev Invest Clin 46(1):37–43, 1994

Padovani EM, Pistolesi C, Fanos V, Messori A, Martini N: Pharmacokinetics of amikacin in neonates. Dev Pharmacol Ther 20(3–4):167–173, 1993.

Pimentel FL, Abelha F, Trigo MA, Sa LV, Menezes MR: Determination of plasma concentrations of amikacin in patients of an intensive care unit. J Chemother 7(1):45–49, 1995.

AMINO ACID SCREEN, BLOOD
(see Dinitrophenylhydrazine Test, Diagnostic)

AMINOPHYLLINE, BLOOD
(see Theophylline, Blood)

AMIODARONE, PLASMA OR SERUM

Norm: Negative.

		SI Units
Therapeutic level	0.5–2.5 µg/ml	0.8–3.9 µmol/L
Panic level	>2.5 µg/ml	>3.9 µmol/L

For samples tested >24 hours after collection, see also item 6 on the next page.

Panic Level Symptoms and Treatment:

Symptoms: Thyroid dysfunction, impaired hepatic function, jaundice, congestive heart failure, pulmonary fibrosis (irreversible).

Treatment:
Respiratory and hemodynamic support.
Discontinue medication.
Continuous ECG monitoring to identify reappearing dysrhythmias and bradycardia.

Transcutaneous pacemaker
(prophylactically for sinus arrest).
Induce emesis (cautiously) with syrup
of ipecac if soon after ingestion.
Tap water or warm saline lavage
may be added.
Administer activated charcoal, saline
or sorbitol cathartic.
Hemodialysis and peritoneal dialysis
will NOT remove amiodarone.

Usage: Monitoring for therapeutic levels during amiodarone therapy.

Description: Amiodarone is a fat-soluble, Class III antidysrhythmic, with several mechanisms of action, including (weak) negative inotropic activity coupled with compensatory vasodilation, prolongation of cardiac tissue refractory period, depression of sinus node automaticity, and slowing of atrioventricular node conduction. It is used to treat clients with a history of life-threatening dysrhythmias that are not controllable by other drugs. Because amiodarone is fat soluble, with a long half-life, it takes up to 4 weeks to reach steady-state levels and will remain in the fat-storage sites of the body long after it is discontinued. Amiodarone is metabolized and excreted primarily by the liver. This drug's potentially life-threatening side effects necessitate close monitoring of blood levels, as well as clear and specific client teaching about side effects.

Professional Considerations:

1. Consent form NOT required.
2. Preparation:
   A. Tube: Red-top, red/gray-top, or gold-top.
   B. MAY be drawn during hemodialysis.
3. Procedure:
   A. Draw the specimen before the dose, or at least 12 hours after the last dose.
   B. Draw a 1-ml blood sample.
4. Postprocedure care:
   A. None.
5. Client and family teaching:
   A. Results may not be available for several days.
   B. If activated charcoal was given for elevated levels, the client should drink 4–6 glasses of water each day for 2

days to prevent constipation. Activated charcoal will also cause stools to be black for a few days.
6. Factors that affect results:
   A. Height and weight have not been shown to affect plasma concentrations.
   B. Amiodarone levels in stored specimens decrease over time. One study recommends the following correction factors for stored values:

Time Sample Stored Before Testing	Correction Factor
24 hours	Add 8% to obtained value.
48 hours	Add 16% to obtained value.
72 hours	Add 19% to obtained value.
7 days	Add 23% to obtained value.
14 days	Add 32% to obtained value.

7. Other data:
   A. Amiodarone minor side effects include (usually reversible) corneal and skin microdeposits of the drug, causing grayish coloring of the sclera and skin, photosensitivity, and neuromuscular weakness. Side effects may take several months to appear.
   B. Any concurrent digoxin dose should be reduced during amiodarone therapy.
   C. Pollack et al. (1993) found that increases in serum creatinine in client receiving amiodarone may be related to the drug.

Bibliography:

Gumieniczek A, Misztal G, Przyborowski L: Determination of amiodarone in tablets and plasma by high-performance liquid chromatography. Acta Pol Pharm *51*(4–5):325–328, 1994.

Jandreski MA, Vanderslice WE: Clinical measurement of serum amiodarone and desethylamiodarone by using solid-phase extraction followed by HPLC with a high-carbon reversed-phase column. Clin Chem *39*(3):496–500, 1993.

O'Sullivan JJ, McCarthy PT, Wren C: Differences in amiodarone, digoxin, flecainide and sotalol concentrations between antemortem serum and femoral postmortem blood. Hum Exp Toxicol *14*(7):605–608, 1995.

Pollack P, Sharma A, Carruthers S: Creatinine elevation in patients receiving amiodarone correlates with serum amiodarone concentration. Br J Clin Pharmacol *36*(2):125–127,1993.

Vuagnat A, Goedel-Meinen L, Gries E, Hofmann M, Presch A, Blomer H: Stability of amiodarone in serum samples under various storage conditions. Arzneimittelforschung *43*(3):327–330, 1993.

AMITRIPTYLINE

(see Tricyclic Antidepressants, Plasma or Serum)

AMMONIA (NH₃), BLOOD AND URINE

Norm: Norms vary by specific laboratory.

		SI Units
Plasma		
Adult	15–45 µg/dl	11–32 µmol/L
Newborn	90–150 µg/dl	64–107 µmol/L
First 2 weeks	79–129 µg/dl	56–92 µmol/L
Child	40–80 µg/dl	28–57 µmol/L
Urine		
Spot		20–500 µmol/L
24-hour		
Adult	140–1500 mg/N/24h	10–107 mmol/N/24h
Infant	560–2900 mg/N/24h	40–207 mmol/N/24h

Hepatic Encephalopathy Symptoms and Treatment:

Symptoms: (Symptoms do not correlate well with blood levels.) Asterixis, ataxia, coma, confusion, drowsiness, sluggish speech, somnolence, stupor.

Treatment:

Lactulose NG or rectally.
Both hemodialyis and peritoneal dialysis WILL remove NH₃.

Increased: Azotemia, cirrhosis, coma (diabetic, hepatic), congestive heart failure, erythroblastosis fetalis, esophageal varices (hemorrhagic), exercise, hepatic encephalopathy, hepatitis (acute), pneumonia, portacaval shunt, premature infant (with neurologic abnormalities), Reye's syndrome, and shock. Drugs include acetazolamide, ammonium salts, asparaginase, chlorothiazide, heparin calcium, heparin sodium, methicillin sodium, neomycin, thiazide diuretics, and urea.

Decreased: Hypertension (essential, malignant) and renal failure.

Description: Ammonia is a waste product from nitrogen breakdown during protein metabolism. It is metabolized by the liver and excreted by the kidneys as urea. Elevated levels due to hepatic dysfunction may lead to encephalopathy.

Professional Considerations:

1. Consent form NOT required.
2. Preparation:
   A. Tube: Refrigerated gray-top, lavender-top, or heparinized green-top.
   B. Do NOT draw during hemodialysis.
   C. *See Client and family teaching.*
   D. Notify laboratory personnel that a blood sample for ammonia level will be arriving.
3. Procedure: Samples should preferably be taken from arterial or earlobe capillary blood because ammonia metabolism in muscle causes increased levels in venous blood.
   A. *Arterial sampling:* Draw a 1-ml blood specimen.
   B. *Capillary sampling:* Using a lancet, completely fill a capillary tube with blood from the earlobe.
   C. *Venous sampling:* Leaving a tourniquet in place no more than 15 seconds, draw a 1-ml blood specimen. If a syringe is used for blood collection, uncap the tube and transfer the blood into it without using the needle. Tilt the tube back and forth to mix the contents.
4. Postprocedure care:
   A. Place the specimen in an ice-water bath.
   B. Transport the specimen to the laboratory immediately.
5. Client and family teaching:
   A. Fast, except for water, and refrain from smoking for 8–10 hours before sampling.
   B. Avoid stress and strenuous exercise for several hours before sampling.
6. Factors that affect results:
   A. Green-top tubes containing ammonium-heparin should not be used.
   B. Reject hemolyzed specimens.
   C. A delay in processing the specimen may cause falsely elevated results.
   D. A high-protein diet may increase levels.
7. Other data:
   A. Ammonia levels are NOT reliable indicators of impending hepatic coma.

Bibliography:

Huizenga JR, Gips CH, Conn HO, Jansen PL: Determination of ammonia in ear-lobe capillary blood is an alternative to arterial blood ammonia. Clin Chim Acta *239*(1):65–70, 1995.

Huizenga JR, Tangerman A, Gips CH: Determination of ammonia in biological fluids. Ann Clin Biochem *31*(Pt 6):529–543, 1994.

Vanuxem D, Delpierre S, Barlatier A, Vanuxem P: Changes in blood ammonia induced by a maximum effort in trained and untrained subjects. Arch Int Physiol Biochem Biophys *101*(6): 405–409, 1993.

AMNIOCENTESIS AND AMNIOTIC FLUID ANALYSIS, DIAGNOSTIC

Norm:

Routine Analysis:

Color: Colorless, straw-colored, or clear to milky.

		SI Units
Acetylcholinesterase	Negative	
Alpha₁-Fetoprotein		
12 weeks' gestation	≤42 µg/ml	
14 weeks' gestation	≤35 µg/ml	
16 weeks' gestation	≤29 µg/ml	
18 weeks' gestation	≤20 µg/ml	
20 weeks' gestation	≤18 µg/ml	
22 weeks' gestation	≤14 µg/ml	
30 weeks' gestation	≤3 µg/ml	
35 weeks' gestation	≤2 µg/ml	
40 weeks' gestation	≤1 µg/ml	
Normal values may also be reported in multiples of the median (MOM) or 0.5–3.0 MOM.		
Biliribin		
Trimester 1, 2	≤0.074 mg/dl	≤1.2 µmol/L
40 weeks' gestation	≤0.024 mg/dl	≤0.4 µmol/L
Calcium	4 mEq/L	4 mmol/L
Carbon dioxide	16 mEq/L	16 mmol/L
Chloride	102 mEq/L	102 mmol/L
Creatinine		
≤27 weeks' gestation	0.8–1.1 mg/dl	72–99 µmol/L
30–34 weeks' gestation	1.1–1.8 mg/dl	99–162 µmol/L
35–40 weeks' gestation	1.8–4.0 mg/dl	162–360 µmol/L
Estriol		
Trimester 1, 2	≤9 µg/dl	≤309 nmol/L
Term	≤59 µg/dl	≤2023 nmol/L
Glucose	30 mg/dl	2 mmol/L
Lecithin		
<35 weeks' gestation	6–9 mg/dl	
≥35 weeks' gestation	15–20 mg/dl	
Lecithin/sphingomyelin (L/S) Ratio		
Immaturity	≤1.5	
Borderline maturity	1.5–1.5	
Maturity	2.0–4.0	
Postmaturity	≥4.1	
Meconium	Negative	
pH		
Trimester 1, 2	7.12–7.38	7.12–7.38
Term	6.91–7.43	6.91–7.43

		SI Units
Potassium	4.9 mEq/L	4.9 mmol/L
Sodium	133 mEq/L	133 mmol/L
Sphingomyelin	4–6 mg/dl	
Total protein	2.5 g/dl	25 g/L
Urea		
Trimester 1, 2	12–24 mg/dl	
Term	19–42 mg/dl	
Uric acid		
Trimester 1, 2	2.76–4.68 mg/dl	0.17–2.8 mmol/L
Term	7.67–12.13 mg/dl	0.46–0.72 mmol/L

ABNORMALITIES THAT MAY BE FOUND UPON ROUTINE ANALYSIS

Abnormal Color	**Possible Cause**
Yellow	Due to fetal bilirubin, erythroblastosis fetalis
Green	Due to meconium, breech presentation, fetal death, defecation, distress, hypoxia, intrauterine growth retardation, postmaturity, vagal stimulation
Red	Due to presence of blood, intrauterine hemorrhage
Port wine	Acute fetal distress, abruptio placentae
Brown	Oxidized hemoglobin, maternal tissue trauma, fetal death, fetal maceration

Abnormal Bilirubin

			SI Units
Fetal involvement	0.10–0.28 mg/dl	= 1 +	1.6–4.5 μmol/L
Later fetal involvement	0.29–0.36 mg/dl	= 2 +	4.7–5.8 μmol/L
Fetal distress	0.47–0.95 mg/dl	= 3 +	7.6–15.4 μmol/L
Fetal death	>0.95 mg/dl	= 4 +	>15.4 μmol/L

Abnormal Creatinine

35–40 weeks' gestation: Large muscle mass, possible diabetes	>2 mg/dl	>180 μmol/L
Low birthweight	<2 mg/dl	<180 μmol/L

Increased Alpha₁-Fetoprotein: Anencephaly, cystic fibrosis, duodenal atresia, esophageal atresia, fetal bladder neck obstruction with hydronephrosis, fetal death, meningomyelocele, multiple pregnancy, nephrosis (congenital), neural tube defects, spina bifida, oomphalocele, and Turner's syndrome.

Increased Bilirubin: Anencephaly, erythroblastosis fetalis, hemolytic disease of the newborn, hydrops fetalis, intestinal obstruction, and Rh sensitization.

Positive Acetylcholinesterase: Neural tube abnormalities that allow cerebrospinal fluid (which contains acetylcholinesterase) to leak into the amniotic sac.

Positive Meconium: Fetal distress.

Decreased Alpha₁-Fetoprotein: Not applicable.

Decreased Bilirubin: Not clinically significant.

Decreased Creatinine: Fetal lung immaturity.

Chromosome Analysis: Interpretation required.

Description: Detection of fetal jeopardy or genetic disease and determination of fetal maturity. *Amniocentesis* is a 20–30 minute procedure in which an aspiration of amniotic fluid is taken transabdominally and usually performed after week 12 of gestation. In routine analysis, amniotic fluid is examined for levels of calcium, chloride, carbon dioxide, creatinine, estriol, glucose, pH, potassium, sodium, protein, urea, uric acid, culture, and for genetic defects, chromosomal studies, detection of fetal jeopardy or distress (via color, bilirubin) and to measure lung maturity (via L/S ratio) and age (via creatinine) of the fetus. *Alpha$_1$-alpha-fetoprotein* is a globulin protein secreted by the yolk sac and by fetal liver cells during hepatic cell multiplication. Highest amounts are found during pregnancy and in hepatic cancer. Measurement is usually performed from week 16 to 20 to help identify fetal neural abnormalities, gastroesophageal atresia, and nephrosis. *Chromosome analysis* of amniotic fluid cells is performed by examining karyotyped cells for genetic abnormalities such as Down syndrome, Tay-Sachs disease, and other inborn errors of metabolism. Amniotic fluid is examined for color and bilirubin level for purposes of detecting fetal jeopardy or distress due to hemolysis of fetal red blood cells. Erythroblastosis fetalis occurs when maternal antibodies attack fetal red blood cells, causing fetal anemia. This occurs when the mother's blood contains the Rh factor that reacts with fetal erythrocyte antigens. The test is usually performed at gestation week 24 or later and can help determine the need for intrauterine fetal blood transfusion.

Professional Considerations:

1. Consent form IS required.

Risks:
Bleeding, intrauterine death, premature labor, spontaneous abortion.

Contraindications:
Abruptio placentae, incompetent cervix, placenta previa, and a history of premature labor.

2. Preparation:
   A. Obtain an amniocentesis tray, surgical scrub solution, a light-protected container, and povidone-iodine solution. Also obtain RhoGAM for Rh-negative mothers.
   B. Obtain maternal vital signs. Auscultate baseline fetal heart tones.
   C. Note the estimated date of conception and week of gestation on the laboratory requisition.

D. Procedure should be performed in a darkened room if the specimen will be tested for bilirubin.
E. *See Client and family teaching.*

3. Procedure:
   A. The position of the fetus and a pocket of amniotic fluid are determined using ultrasound and palpation, with the mother in a supine position.
   B. The mother's abdominal area is cleansed with surgical scrub solution and povidone-iodine and allowed to dry.
   C. The aspiration site is draped, demarcating a sterile field.
   D. The mother is instructed to place her hands behind her head, and the aspiration site is anesthetized with 1 ml of 1 or 2% lidocaine intradermally and subcutaneously.
   E. A 20- to 22-gauge, 5-inch-long spinal needle with a stylet is inserted through the abdominal wall into the intrauterine cavity, and the stylet is withdrawn.
   F. About 10–15 ml of amniotic fluid is aspirated through the spinal needle into a syringe, and the needle is withdrawn. Use a 20-ml amniotic fluid sample for direct genetic analysis for the four most common mutations responsible for Tay Sach's disease.

4. Postprocedure care:
   A. Apply a dry sterile dressing to the aspiration site.
   B. Inject 5 ml of amniotic fluid into a light-protected (foil-covered or amber) test tube to test for bilirubin. Inject 10 ml of amniotic fluid into a sterile, siliconized glass container or a polystyrene container for culture and genetic and other studies (AFP). Specimens to be transported to another site for testing should be packed in a cool, insulated container to maintain a temperature of 2–5°C. Freezing temperatures should be avoided.
   C. Obtain the mother's vital signs. Auscultate fetal heart tones for changes from the baseline.
   D. The mother should rest on her right side for 15–20 minutes after the procedure.
   E. RhoGAM may be prescribed for Rh-negative mothers.
   F. Transport the amniotic fluid specimen to the laboratory immediately and refrigerate.

5. Client and family teaching:
   A. Empty your bladder immediately prior to the procedure if gestation is 21 weeks or more. You must have a full bladder during the procedure if gestation is 20 weeks or less.
   B. It is important to lie motionless throughout the procedure. You may experience a strong contraction with the needle insertion.
   C. Chromosome analysis results may take up to 4 weeks.

D. Inform the client with abnormal genetic findings of choices regarding pregnancy and pregnancy termination. Also refer the client for genetic counseling prior to future attempts to become pregnant.

E. After the procedure, notify the physician for cramping, abdominal pain, unusual vaginal drainage/fluid loss, fever, chills, dizziness, or more or less than the usual amount of fetal activity.

6. Factors that affect results:

A. Reject frozen or clotted specimens.

B. Inadvertent aspiration of maternal urine can be ruled out by testing the specimen for blood urea nitrogen (BUN) and creatinine. Urine BUN is >100 mg/dl, whereas amniotic fluid is well under 100 mg/dl. Urine creatinine is usually >80 mg/dl, whereas amniotic fluid creatinine is usually ≤4 mg/dl.

C. Nonsiliconized glass containers for routine analysis may result in cell adherence on the sides of the container.

D. Amniotic fluid testing must be performed within 3 days of collection.

E. Amniocentesis should be performed between weeks 24 and 28 when checking for hemolytic disease of the newborn and Rh sensitization.

F. Falsely low bilirubin levels may result from failure to protect the specimen from light.

G. Specimens contaminated with blood should be tested for fetal hemoglobin to determine whether the blood is of maternal or fetal origin. Fetal blood contamination results in falsely high bilirubin levels. Fetal or maternal blood will interfere with measurements of fetal lung maturity and amniotic fluid constituents that are also constituents of plasma, such as protein, potassium, and glucose.

H. Creatinine levels are affected by maternal creatinine clearance and maternal creatinine levels. A concurrent maternal serum creatinine should be drawn. Maternal serum to amniotic fluid creatinine should be about 2:1.

I. Elevated AFP results may be caused by contamination of the specimen with fetal blood.

J. Small and closed neural tube defects may not cause elevated AFP levels.

K. Accurate L/S ratio measurement is not possible if the specimen is contaminated with blood (fetal or maternal) or meconium.

7. Other data:

A. Direct karyotyping of placental villi samples obtained by needle aspiration has been found to yield faster results than amniotic fluid chromosome analysis. *(See Chorionic Villi Sampling, Diagnostic.)*

B. Chromosomal aberration has been found in 4.6% of fetuses in women over 38 years old, the most common being trisomy 21 (62%), Klinefelter's syndrome (11%), and Edward's syndrome (trisomy 18) (11%).

C. For diamniotic twin pregnancies, each amniotic sac should be sampled.

D. A 1995 study by Rousseau et al. suggests that early amniocentesis is feasible from 11 weeks gestation and "can be performed for the usual indications" as an alternative to chorionic villus sampling. In the future, results will be available in less than 1 week using cytogenetic techniques.

E. Prenatal cystic fibrosis profile may be performed by polymerase chain reaction (PCR) for mutations δF508, R553X, g551D, g542X, n1303K, and w1282X.

Bibliography:

Alvarez JG, Ludmir J: Semiautomated multisample analysis of amniotic fluid lipids by high-performance thin-layer chromatography-reflectance spectrodensitometry. J Chromatogr *615*(1):142–147, 1993.

Giorlandino C, Mobili L, Bilancioni E, D'Alessio P, Carcioppolo O, Gentili P, Vizzone A: Transplacental amniocentesis: is it really a higher-risk procedure? Prenat Diagn *14*(9):803–806, 1994.

Rousseau O, Boulot P, Lefort G, Nagy P, Bachelard B, Bonifacj C, Hedon B, Laffargue F, Viala J: Amniocentesis before 15 weeks gestation: Technical aspects and obstetric risks. Eur J Obstet Gynecol Reprod Biol *58*(2):127–130, 1995.

AMNIOTIC FLUID, ALPHA₁-FETOPROTEIN, SPECIMEN

(see Amniocentesis and Amniotic Fluid Analysis, Diagnostic)

AMNIOTIC FLUID, CHROMOSOME ANALYSIS, SPECIMEN

(see Amniocentesis and Amniotic Fluid Analysis, Diagnostic)

AMNIOTIC FLUID, ERYTHROBLASTOSIS FETALIS, SPECIMEN

(see Amniocentesis and Amniotic Fluid Analysis, Diagnostic)

AMNIOTIC FLUID ANALYSIS, SPECIMEN

(see Amniocentesis and Amniotic Fluid Analysis, Diagnostic)

AMOXAPINE

(see Tricyclic Antidepressants, Plasma or Serum)

AMPHETAMINES, BLOOD

Norm: Negative.

Drug	Normal Ranges During Therapy			SI Units nmol/L
	ng/ml	µg/ml	mg/L	
Amphetamine sulfate	20–120	0.02–0.20		150–900
Toxic level	>200		>2	>1500
Chlorphentermine	100–400	0.10–0.40		750–3000
Diethylpropion	1–10	0.001–0.010		7.5–75
Ephedrine	50–100	0.05–0.10		375–750
Fenfluramine	30–300	0.03–0.30		225–2250
Methamphetamine	10–50	0.01–0.05		75–375
Toxic level	>500		>5	>3750
p-Methoxyamphetamine	<200	<0.2		<1500
Methylenedioxy- amphetamine	<400	<0.4		<3000
Toxic level	>400		>4	>3000
Phendimetrazine	30–250	0.03–0.25		225–1875
Phenmetrazine	60–250	0.06–0.25		450–1875
Toxic level	>400		>4	>3000
Phentermine	30–90	0.03–0.09		225–675
Phenylpropanolamine	50–100	0.05–0.10		375–750
Tranylcypromine	10–100	0.01–0.10		75–750

Toxic Levels Symptoms and Treatment:

Symptoms: Psychoses, tremors, convulsions, insomnia, tachycardia, dysrhythmias, impotence, cerebrovascular accident, and respiratory collapse.

Treatment:

Use gastric lavage or induce vomiting (with extreme caution) if within 4 hours of ingestion. (Induction of vomiting is contraindicated in clients with no gag reflex or with central nervous system depression or excitation).

Give a slurry of activated charcoal 1 g/kg (minimum 30 g), followed by a magnesium citrate cathartic.

Amphetamine excretion may be accelerated by acidifying the urine with ammonium chloride 1–2 g intravenously or ascorbic acid 0.5–1.5 g orally every 4–6 hours to keep urine pH <5.5.

Increase fluids to keep urine output 3–6 ml/kg/h.

Consider using mannitol or furosemide to force diuresis (efficacy of acid diuresis has not been clearly established). Both hemodialysis and peritoneal dialysis WILL remove amphetamines.

Barbiturates may counteract amphetamine stimulant effects and chlorpromazine (Thorazine) may help control the symptoms of an overstimulated central nervous system.

Increased: Stimulant drug abuse or use.

Description: Amphetamines are sympathomimetic amines that act on the cortex and reticular activating system of the brain to stimulate the release and block the reabsorption of norepinephrine and dopamine. They cause mood elevation and wakefulness and decrease the perception of fatigue through stimulation of the heart and central nervous system. They are rapidly absorbed from the gastrointestinal tract and reach all tissues, but concentrate in the central nervous system and are excreted by the kidneys. Half-lives vary depending on the individual drug. Synonyms include bennies, crystal, ice, pep pills, speed, uppers, and wake-ups. Blood amphetamine levels are used for monitoring the appropriateness of dosage regime and for detection of amphetamine abuse.

Professional Considerations:

1. Consent form NOT required.
2. Preparation:
   A. Tube: Lavender-top.
   B. Assess for a history of drug abuse.
   C. Do NOT draw during hemodialysis.
3. Procedure:
   A. Draw a 5-ml blood sample.
4. Postprocedure care:
   A. None.
5. Client and family teaching:
   A. Results are normally available within 4 hours.
   B. If activated charcoal was given for elevated levels, drink 4–6 glasses of water each day for 2 days to prevent constipation. Activated charcoal will also cause stools to be black for a few days.
   C. Referrals to appropriate rehabilitation centers and therapeutic community programs should be offered to all addicted clients.
6. Factors that affect results:
   A. High concentrations of beta-phenethylamine, a blood product formed from the decomposition of protein, may mask a low amphetamine level.
7. Other data:
   A. Toxicity in children occurs over a wide range of doses.
   B. Abrupt discontinuation may cause psychotic symptoms.
   C. *See also Toxicology Drug Screen, Blood and Toxicology Drug Screen, Urine.*

Bibliography:

Jacob P 3rd, Tisdale EC, Panganiban K, Cannon D, Zabel K, Mendelson JE, Jones RT: Gas chromatographic determination of methamphetamine and its metabolite amphetamine in human plasma and urine following conversion to N-propyl derivatives. J Chromatogr Biomed Appl *664*(2):449–457, 1995.

Leis HJ, Windischhofer W, Wintersteiger R: Quantitative measurement of amphetamine in human plasma by gas chromatography/negative ion chemical ionization mass spectrometry using (2H$_5$) amphetamine as internal standard. Biol Mass Spectrom *23*(10):637–641, 1993.

AMPHOTERICIN B, BLOOD

Norm: Negative.

Therapeutic levels: 1–2 µg/ml (1–2.2 µmol/L, SI units).
Potential toxicity beyond therapeutic levels.

Toxic Levels Symptoms and Treatment:

Symptoms: Acute tubular necrosis, coagulopathies, hearing loss, hypotension, ventricular fibrillation, coagulopathies.

Treatment:

Treat symptoms and provide supportive therapy as needed until levels decrease.
Prepare the client for the possibility of permanent loss of hearing or renal function.
Hemodialyis and peritoneal dialysis will NOT remove amphotericin significantly.

Usage: Evaluating serum level of amphotericin B and assessing for toxic levels in clients with fever, chills, nausea, or bone marrow suppression.

Description: A potent antifungal antibiotic ineffective against bacteria, viruses, or rickettsiae. Peak levels occur 60–120 minutes after intravenous administration; half-life is 24 hours. Over a 7-day period 40% is excreted in the urine.

Professional Considerations:

1. Consent form NOT required.
2. Preparation:
   A. Tube: Red-top, red/gray-top, or gold-top.
   B. Do NOT draw during hemodialysis.
3. Procedure:
   A. Draw a 5-ml blood sample.
4. Postprocedure care:
   A. None.
5. Client and family teaching:
   A. Results are normally available within 24 hours.
6. Factors that affect results:
   A. Draw the specimen from an extremity that does not have amphotericin B infusing into it.
7. Other data:
   A. None.

Bibliography:

Hulsewede JW, Dermoumi H: Comparison of high-performance liquid chromatography and bioassay of amphotericin B in serum. Mycoses *37*(1–2):17–21, 1994.

Lacroix C, Wojciechowski F, Danger P: Simultaneous determination of itraconazole, hydroxy-itraconazole and amphotericin B in human plasma by HPLC with photodiode array detection. Ann Biol Clin (Paris) *53*(5):293–297, 1995.

AMSLER GRID TEST, DIAGNOSTIC

Norm: The lines are clearly visualized and appear straight. A black dot is visualized in the center of the grid. No distortions of the lines is seen. No blank spots are seen other than within each square.

Usage: Detection of macular edema or macular blind spots.

Description: An optical screening test using a grid of intersecting lines with a black dot in the center. The visual acuity of the macular portion of the retina can be affected by macular edema, causing distortions of the lines, or by scotomas, causing blind spots, which make the grid appear to the client as having blank areas.

Professional Considerations:

1. Consent form NOT required.
2. Preparation:
   A. Obtain an Amsler grid and an eye occluder (eyepatch, handheld, or occluding eyeglasses).
3. Procedure:
   A. With one eye covered, have the client view the Amsler grid at his or her usual reading distance.
   B. Ask whether the black dot is visible, whether the complete square grid is visible when looking at the dot, whether the lines are perfectly straight, and whether any of the lines are blurred or look as though they are moving.
   C. Ask if there are any blank areas on the grid, other than within each square. Have the client draw what he or she sees if the answer to any of the questions is yes.
   D. Repeat the test for the other eye.
4. Postprocedure care:
   A. Refer the client to a specialist if necessary.
5. Client and family teaching:
   A. The test takes less than 30 minutes.
6. Factors that affect results:
   A. Performing this test prior to retinal examination with an ophthalmoscope and fundus exam or refraction test avoids falsely abnormal results due to retinal bleaching from the bright light or loss of focusing ability.
7. Other data:
   A. An abnormal test indicates the need for more specific testing such as fluoroscein angiography.
   B. A study by Schuchard (1993) suggests Amsler grid reports have poor validity and cannot be accurately interpreted for use in the clinical diagnosis of retinal defects.

Bibliography:

Achard OA, Safran AB, Duret FC, Ragama E: Role of the completion phenomenon in the evaluation of Amsler grid results. Am J Ophthalmol 120(3): 322–329, 1995.

Schuchard R: Validity and interpretation of Amsler grid reports. Arch Ophthalmol 111(6):776–780, 1993.

AMYLASE, SERUM AND URINE

Norm Urine	
Mayo clinic method	10–80 amylase U/hour
Somogyi method	26–950 U/24 hours
Beckman method	1–17 U/hour

Norm Serum		SI Units
Somogyi method	50–180 U/dl	92–330 U/L
Beckman method		20–125 U/L
Over age 70		20–160 U/L
Panic level	Three times the upper limit of normal	

Increased: Abdominal aortic aneurysm (ruptured), acute exacerbation of chronic pancreatitis, ampulla of Vater obstruction, cerebral trauma, cholecystitis (acute), choledocholithiasis, common bile duct obstruction, diabetic ketoacidosis, ectopic pregnancy, empyema (gallbladder), hyperthyroidism, intestinal obstruction with strangulation, intra-abdominal abscess, lung cancer, macroamylasemia, mesenteric thrombosis, mumps, pancreatic duct obstruction, pancreatic cancer, pancreatitis (acute), perforated intestine, perforated ulcer, peritonitis, salivary gland disease (acute, duct obstruction, suppurative inflammation), spasm of sphincter of Oddi, surgery (postoperative upper abdominal, peripancreatic), trauma (pancreas, spleen). Drugs include aspirin, opiates, radiographic dyes, and thiazides.

Decreased: Alcoholic liver disease, alcoholism, burns (severe), cachexia, cirrhosis, cystic fibrosis (advanced), hepatic abscess, hepatic cancer, hepatitis, pancreatic cancer, pancreatitis (acute fulminant, advanced chronic), poisoning, renal dysfunction, thyrotoxicosis (severe), and toxemia of pregnancy. Drugs include glucose and fluorides.

Description: An enzyme produced by the pancreas and salivary glands that aids digestion of complex carbohydrates. It is excreted by the kidneys. In acute pancreatitis, serum amylase starts rising at least 2 hours after the onset, peaks at about 24 hours, and returns to normal in 2–3 days after the onset. Urine amylase will be elevated from several hours after the onset until 7–10 days after the onset. Because urine amylase levels remain elevated longer than serum amylase, they are useful for providing evidence of pancreatitis after serum amylase has returned to normal levels.

Professional Considerations:

1. Consent form NOT required.
2. Preparation:
   A. Obtain a urine container without preservatives, including toluene or acetic acid preservatives, in sizes as follows: 1-L size, 2- or 6-hour collection; 2-L size, 8- or 12-hour collection; 3-L size, 24-hour collection.
   B. Tube: Red-top, red/gray-top, or gold-top.
   C. List medications taken in the past 24 hours on the laboratory requisition.
3. Procedure:
   A. Discard the first morning-voided urine specimen.
   B. Collect a timed urine specimen over 2, 6, 8, 12, or 24 hours in a refrigerated or iced container without preservatives or to which toluene or acetic acid has been added. For catheterized clients, keep the drainage bag on ice, and empty the urine into the collection container hourly.
   C. Encourage fluid intake throughout the collection period if not contraindicated.
   D. For serum collection, draw a 1-ml sample at least 2 hours after a meal and before treatment has begun.
4. Postprocedure care:
   A. List the beginning and ending times of urine specimen collection on the laboratory requisition.
   B. Send the urine specimen to the laboratory and refrigerate.
5. Client and family teaching:
   A. For the urine test, save all urine voided in the 2-, 6-, 8-, 12-, or 24-hour period. Urinate before defecating to avoid loss of urine and to avoid contaminating the specimen with feces or toilet tissue. If any urine is accidentally discarded, discard the entire specimen and restart the collection the next day.
   B. Do not drink alcohol for 24 hours before sampling.
6. Factors that affect results:
   A. Urine amylase determinations should not be performed on females during menstruation.
   B. Results reported in U/ml give an inaccurate picture because they are influenced by the varying urine volumes, depending on the length of the collection period.
   C. Reject hemolyzed specimens.
   D. Drugs that may falsely elevate results of serum amylase include aminosalicylic acid, asparaginase, azothioprine, bethanechol, bethanechol chloride, chloride salts, cholinergics, corticosteroids, corticotropin, cyproheptadine hydrochloride, ethacrynic acid, ethyl alcohol (large quantities), fluoride salts, furosemide, indomethacin, loop diuretics, mercaptopurine, methacholine, narcotic analgesics, oral contraceptives, pancreozymin, rifampin, sulfasalazine, and thiazide diuretics.
   E. Falsely decreased results of serum amylase may be caused by citrates and oxalates.
   F. Massive hemorrhagic pancreatic necrosis may cause so much pancreatic cell destruction that amylase cannot be produced, resulting in no elevation in serum amylase.
   G. Contamination of the serum specimen with saliva will cause falsely elevated results.
   H. Serum lipemia may result in falsely low serum amylase results.
   I. Results are invalidated if the specimen is drawn <72 hours after cholecystography with radiopaque dyes.
   J. Falsely high serum amylase results may be caused by renal failure.
   K. Sachdeva et al. (1995) found "marked fluctuation in serum amylase, ranging from 115 to 1160% . . . in patients with macroamylasemia. The reasons for these fluctuations are not clear but may be due to association-dissociation of amylase with serum proteins at variable time intervals. This fluctuation, especially when the amylase becomes normal (as in cases 1 and 3), may lead to confusion in differentiating macroamylasemia from other causes of hyperamylasemia."
7. Other data:
   A. Macroamylassemia causes a high serum but normal urine amylase.
   B. Urine amylase does not produce falsely high results with renal failure as does serum amylase.
   C. Normal serum amylase may occur in pancreatitis, especially chronic pancreatitis.

Bibliography:

Bhayana V, Cohoe S, Ross ML: Analytical evaluation of a newly developed ELISA mass assay for pancreatic amylase. Clin Biochem 28(3):255–261, 1995.

Clave P, Guillaumes S, Blanco I, Nabau N, Merce J, Farre A, Marruecos L, Lluis F: Amylase, lipase, pancreatic isoamylase, and phospholipase A in diagnosis of acute pancreatitis. Clin Chem 41(8 Pt 1):1129–1134, 1995.

Manes G, Rabitti PG, Laccetti M, Pacelli L, Carraturo I,

Uomo G: Early prediction of aetiology and severity of acute pancreatitis by serum amylase and lipase assays. Minerva Gastroenterol Dietol *41*(3): 211–215, 1995.

Recio F, Villamil F: Charge selectivity and urine amylase isoenzymes. Kidney Int (Suppl) *47*:S89–S92, 1994.

Sachdeva CK, Bank S, Greenberg R, Blumstein M, Weissman S: Fluctuations in serum amylase in patients with macroamylasemia. Am J Gastroenterol *90*(5):800–803, 1995.

ANA, SERUM
(see Antinuclear Antibody, Serum)

ANAEROBIC CULTURE
(see Body Fluid, Anaerobic, Culture)

ANDROSTENEDIONE, SERUM

Norm:

		SI Units
Adult female	85–275 ng/dl	3.0–9.6 nmol/L
Postmenopausal	30–140 ng/dl	1.0–4.8 nmol/L
Adult male	70–205 ng/dl	2.6–7.2 nmol/L
Cord blood	30–150 ng/dl	1.0–5.2 nmol/L
Premature newborn	80–446 ng/dl	2.8–15.6 nmol/L
Newborn	20–290 ng/dl	0.7–10.1 nmol/L
Female children		
1–3 months	15–25 ng/dl	0.5–0.9 nmol/L
3–5 months	10–15 ng/dl	0.3–0.5 nmol/L
Male children		
1–3 months	20–45 ng/dl	0.7–1.6 nmol/L
3–5 months	10–40 ng/dl	0.3–1.4 nmol/L
Panic level (all ages)	>1000 ng/dl	>34.9 nmol/L

Usage: Nonspecific evaluation of androgen production in female hirsutism.

Increased: Congenital adrenal hyperplasia, Cushing's syndrome, hirsutism, Stein-Leventhal disease (polycystic ovarian disease), and tumor (adrenal, ovarian).

Decreased: Not clinically significant.

Description: A metabolite of dehydroepiandrosterone sulfate (DHEA-S) produced in the ovaries and the adrenal gland that is converted to testosterone in peripheral tissues. Peak levels occur in the early morning and low levels in the late afternoon. After puberty, levels rise and peak around age 20. Elevation is one of several causes of female hirsutism, which is characterized by a male hair-growth pattern. Very elevated levels suggest the presence of a virilizing tumor.

Professional Considerations:

1. Consent form NOT required.
2. Preparation:
   A. Schedule the test at least 7 days before or after a female client's menstruation.
   B. *See Client and family teaching.*
   C. Tube: Red-top, red/gray-top, or gold-top.
3. Procedure:
   A. Draw a 2-ml blood sample. Draw between 0600 and 0900 for peak levels.
4. Postprocedure care:
   A. Place the specimen on ice.
   B. Transport the specimen to the laboratory immediately for spinning and freezing of serum.
5. Client and family teaching:
   A. Fast for 8 hours before sampling.
   B. Test must be drawn 1 week before or after menstruation to avoid falsely elevated values.
6. Factors that affect results:
   A. Results are invalidated if the client has undergone a scan involving radioactive dyes within 1 week prior to specimen collection.
7. Other data:
   A. Plasma levels do not correlate well with the severity of symptoms.

Bibliography:

Anttila L, Koskinen P, Erkkola R, Irjala K, Ruutiainen K: Serum testosterone, androstenedione and luteinizing hormone levels after short-term medroxyprogesterone acetate treatment in women with polycystic ovarian disease. Acta Obstet Gynecol Scand *73*(8):634–636, 1994.

Castracane VD, Asch RH: Testosterone and androstenedione in premature ovarian failure pregnancies: Evidence for an ovarian source of androgens in early pregnancy. Hum Reprod *10*(3):677–680, 1995.

Gilling-Smith C, Willis DS, Beard RW, Franks S: Hypersecretion of androstenedione by isolated thecal cells from polycystic ovaries. J Clin Endocrinol Metab *79*(4):1158–1165, 1994.

ANGEL DUST
(see Phencyclidine, Qualitative, Urine)

ANGIOCARDIOGRAPHY PROCEDURE, DIAGNOSTIC
(see Cardiac Catheterization, Diagnostic)

ANGIOGRAM (ANGIOGRAPHY), DIAGNOSTIC
(see Arteriogram, Cardiac Catheterization, Cerebral Angiogram, Pulmonary Angiogram, or Renal Angiogram, Diagnostic)

ANGIOGRAPHY, CEREBRAL CORONARY
(see Cerebral Angiogram, Diagnostic)

ANGIOTENSIN-CONVERTING ENZYME (ACE), BLOOD
Norm:

		SI Units
Adults	13–25 kU/L	221–425 µKat/L

Clients under 19 years have higher ACE levels.

Increased: Arthritis (rheumatoid), bronchitis, cervical adenitis, cirrhosis (nonalcoholic), connective tissue disease, fungal diseases, Gaucher's disease, histoplasmosis, Hodgkin's disease, hyperthyroidism (untreated), Langerhans cell histiocytosis, leprosy, myeloma, non-Hodgkin's lymphoma, pulmonary embolus, pulmonary fibrosis, sarcoidosis (active), and scleroderma.

Decreased: Acute respiratory distress syndrome, coccidioidomycosis, diabetes mellitus, farmer's lung, hypothyroidism, pulmonary neoplasm (advanced), severe illness, and tuberculosis. Drugs include estrogen (replacement therapy), L-arginine, and steroids.

Description: An enzyme found mainly in lung epithelial cells and in smaller amounts in blood vessels and renal tissue that converts angiotensin I to angiotensin II, a vasopressor that also stimulates the adrenal cortex to produce aldosterone. High levels of ACE are strongly correlated with pulmonary sarcoidosis.

Professional Considerations:
1. Consent form NOT required.
2. Preparation:
    A. Write the client's age on the laboratory requisition.
    B. Tube: Red-top, red/gray-top, gold-top, or green-top.
    C. *See Client and family teaching.*
3. Procedure:
    A. Draw a 2-ml blood sample.
4. Postprocedure care:
    A. Transport the specimen to the laboratory immediately. Freeze the specimen and store it in dry ice if the test is not performed immediately.
5. Client and family teaching:
    A. Fast for 12 hours before sampling.
6. Factors that affect results:
    A. Reject hemolyzed or lipemic specimens.
    B. A delay in testing or failure to freeze the specimen if not tested immediately may cause falsely low results.
7. Other data:
    A. ACE is useful in evaluating the effectiveness of therapy and in confirming clinical status.

Bibliography:
Higashi Y, Oshima T, Ono N, Hiraga H, Yoshimura M, Watanabe M, Matsuura H, Kambe M, Kajiyama G: Intravenous administration of L-arginine inhibits angiotensin-converting enzyme in humans. J Clin Endocrinol Metab *80*(7):2198–2202, 1995.

Proudler AJ, Ahmed AI, Crook D, Fogelman I, Rymer JM, Stevenson JC: Hormone replacement therapy and serum angiotensin-converting-enzyme activity in postmenopausal women. Lancet *346*(8967):89–90, 1995.

Rosenstein ED, Eskow RN, Lederman DA, Kramer N: Case report: Langerhans cell histiocytosis associated with elevation of angiotensin-converting enzyme levels. Am J Med Sci *310*(2):65–67, 1995.

ANH
(see Atrial Natriuretic Hormone, Plasma)

ANIMALS AND RABIES, SERUM
(see Fluorescent Rabies Antibody [FRA], Specimen)

ANIMALS AND RABIES NEGRI BODIES, BRAIN TISSUE, SPECIMEN

Norm: Negative.

Positive: Rabies.

Description: A postmortem histologic examination of the brain tissue of an animal suspected to have rabies, usually performed after the animal has bitten a human. Rabies produces Negri bodies, a specific and diagnostic lesion of the central nervous system that contains inclusion bodies in the cytoplasm of the nerve cells. Animal specimen examination is the only method to identify rabies because there is no laboratory or diagnostic test to identify the disease in humans until after symptoms appear (listed below). Diagnosis in humans is based on history and symptoms. Symptoms may appear 10 days to a year after the bite, but more commonly appear in humans 2–8 weeks later.

Professional Considerations:

1. Consent form NOT required.
2. Preparation:
   A. Obtain a container and ice or dry ice.
   B. Prepare for the examination by wearing protective clothing, a face shield, and heavy rubber gloves.
3. Procedure:
   A. The animal is killed and decapitated. The head is sealed in a watertight metal container and refrigerated as follows: with regular ice if the specimen will be examined within 24 hours; with dry ice if the specimen will be examined after 24 hours.
   B. Thin-tissue impressions are made from the medulla, the cerebellum, and Ammon's horn of the hippocampus; immersed for 5 seconds in Seller's stain and then in tap water; and examined under high magnification. Negri bodies appear as cherry red, sharply defined, spherical, oval, or elongated bodies containing dark blue-staining granules.

4. Postprocedure care:
   A. Include a detailed history of the date of human exposure, the method of exposure, the names and addresses of the client(s) exposed, the animal's owners, the species and breed of animal, whether it died or was killed, and its vaccination history, if known.
   B. The bitten human should be monitored for the development of signs of rabies, which include laryngeal spasm when drinking water, restless behavior, hyperreactivity or convulsions with increased sensory input, neuromuscular twitching, tachypnea/hyperventilation, and excess salivation.
5. Client and family teaching:
   A. Client and family should observe for signs of rabies (listed above) for the next 12 months. Notify the physician immediately if symptoms appear.
   B. Have pets vaccinated against rabies.
   C. If a bite occurs, clean the wound quickly with a disinfectant to kill any rabies virus in the wound.
   D. The family should follow universal precautions in handling any items from the client that have been contaminated with saliva until a year has passed without symptoms.
6. Factors that affect results:
   A. Inability to obtain animal or brain tissue.
7. Other data:
   A. The likelihood of Negri body development increases with the length of time the animal lives after acquiring rabies. Therefore, Negri bodies may not always be present.
   B. Results should be confirmed by mouse inoculation intracerebrally with the animal's brain tissue.
   C. The only method of preventing rabies is animal vaccination.
   D. Rabies is a reportable disease in most areas, as are animal bites.

Bibliography:

Baer GM, Smith JS: Rabies virus. *In* Lennette EH, Balows A, Hausler WJ, Shadomy HJ (eds): Manual of Clinical Microbiology. Washington DC, American Society for Microbiology, 1985, pp 790–795.

Vodopija I: Current issues in human rabies immunization. Rev Infect Dis *10* (Suppl 4):S758–S763, 1988.

Warrell DA, Warrell MJ: Human rabies and its prevention: An overview. Rev Infect Dis *10* (Suppl 4):S726–S731, 1988.

ANION GAP, BLOOD

Norm:

		SI Units
With K$^+$ in the equation	12–16 mEq/L	12–16 mmol/L
Without K$^+$ in the equation	8–12 mEq/L	8–12 mmol/L

Increased: Carbon monoxide poisoning, cyanide poisoning, dehydration, hypocalcemia, hypomagnesemia, and metabolic acidosis due to diabetic ketoacidosis, ethyl alcohol ketoacidosis, ethylene glycol poisoning, lactic acidosis, methanol poisoning, renal failure, salicylate overdose, and uremia. Drugs include acetaminophen, acetazolamide, ammonium chloride, antihypertensives, carbenicillin, corticosteroids, 5% dextrose in water (prolonged infusion), diazoxide, dimercaprol, ethacrynic acid, ethanol, ethylene glycol, formaldehyde, fructose, furosemide, hippuric acid, hydrogen sulfide, iodine, iron, isoniazid, metformin, methenamine mandelate, methyl alcohol, nalidixic acid, nitrates, nitrites, oxalic acid, paraldehyde, penicillins, phenformin, salbutamol, salicylates, sodium bicarbonate, sodium nitroprusside, sorbitol, streptozotocin, sulfur (elemental), thiazides, ticarcillin, toluene, xylitol, and any drug that may result in hypotension with reduced tissue perfusion or renal failure.

Decreased: Bromism, hyperdilution, hypercalcemia, hypermagnesemia, hypoalbuminemia, hyponatremia, hypophosphatemia, multiple myeloma, polyclonal gammopathy, Waldenstrom's macroglobulinemia. Drugs include alkalis, ammonium chloride, boric acid, bromides, chlorpropamide, cholestyramine, cortisone acetate, corticotropin, hypercalcemia, hyperkalemia, hypermagnesemia, licorice, lithium carbonate, magnesium-containing antacids, phenylbutazone, polymyxin B, oxyphenbutazone, sodium chloride (large amounts intravenously), tromethamine, and vasopressin.

Description: A calculation of the difference between the major cations and the major anions in the blood that helps determine the cause of metabolic acidosis. The two formulas used to determine the anion gap are:

$$\text{Anion Gap} = (Na^+) - (CL^- + HCO_3^-)$$

OR

$$= (Na^+ + K^+) - (CL^- + HCO_3^-)$$

Professional Considerations:
1. Consent form NOT required.
2. Preparation:
   A. Tube: Red-top, red/gray-top, or gold-top.
3. Procedure:
   A. Draw a 10-ml blood sample.
4. Postprocedure care:
   A. None.
5. Client and family teaching:
   A. Not applicable.
6. Factors that affect results:
   A. Metabolic acidosis may exist with a normal anion gap, as when bicarbonate is lost in body fluids and chloride is retained in the following conditions: hyperchloremic acidosis, renal tubular acidosis, biliary or pancreatic fistulas, and ileal loop hypofunctioning.
   B. Iodine absorption from wounds packed with povidone-iodine may cause falsely low results.
   C. Reject hemolyzed specimens.
7. Other data:
   A. Normal anion gap can occur with diarrhea, hyperalimentation, renal tubular acidosis, and ureterostomies.
   B. Treatment for an anion gap acidosis is to correct the cause. Sodium bicarbonate 1–2 mEq/kg has been used in some cases.

Bibliography:

Decaux G, Schlesser M, Coffernils M, Prospert F, Namias B, Brimioulle S, Soupart A: Uric acid, anion gap and urea concentration in the diagnostic approach to hyponatremia. Clin Nephrol 42(2):102–108, 1994.

Slucher B, Levinson SS: Human immunodeficiency virus infection and anion gap. Ann Clin Lab Sci 23(4):249–255, 1993.

Vasuyattakul S, Lertpattanasuwan N, Vareesangthip K, Nimmannit S, Nilwarangkur S: A negative anion gap as a clue to diagnose bromide intoxication. Nephron 69(3):311–313, 1995.

ANKLE-BRACHIAL INDEX (ABI), DIAGNOSTIC

Norm:

Pressure Index	Interpretation
0.85–1.0	Normal
0.75–0.85	Mild occlusive disease
0.50–0.75	Intermittent claudication
0.30–0.50	Severe disease: rest pain may occur; pregangrenous state
<0.30	Poor probability for tissue healing or limb viability unless compensation by collateral blood flow occurs.

Usage: Assessment of arterial blood flow in clients with peripheral vascular disease; monitoring postoperative flow in the lower extremities after vascular surgery such as femoral bypass; assessment of severity of peripheral vascular disease.

Description: The Ankle-Brachial Index (ABI) is a mathematically calculated ratio of the systolic pressure at a pulse point in a lower extremity with peripheral vascular disease as compared to the systolic pressure of the brachial artery. The index provides a quick, noninvasive assessment of how much arterial blood is perfusing the extremity. Typically, an ABI that increases by at least 0.15 (15%) after vascular surgery indicates that the surgery was successful.

Professional Considerations:

1. Consent form NOT required.
2. Preparation:
   A. Obtain a dual-frequency doppler, a marker, two sphygmomanometers, and ultrasonic gel.
3. Procedure:
   A. Client is positioned supine.
   B. The femoral, popliteal, dorsalis pedis, and posterior tibial pulse points in both lower extremities are palpated and identified with a marker.
   C. The sphygmomanometer cuff is placed proximal to the marked site. If the flow is being assessed at the knee, the cuff is placed proximal to the popliteal pulse. If the flow is being assessed at the ankle, the cuff is placed proximal to the ankle.
   D. Ultrasonic gel is placed over the marked site (popliteal or posterior tibial or dorsalis pedis), and the doppler flow signal is identified.
   E. With the doppler in place, the sphygmomanometer cuff is inflated until the doppler flow signal disappears.
   F. The cuff is slowly deflated, and the pressure at which the doppler tone is again audible is noted and recorded.
   G. The brachial systolic blood pressure in both arms is measured using a doppler, and the highest pressure is selected for use in the ABI calculation.
   H. The ABI ratio is calculated with the following equation:

$$ABI = \frac{\text{Lower extremity pressure from step "F"}}{\text{Brachial doppler systolic pressure}}$$

4. Postprocedure care:
   A. Wipe the ultrasonic gel from the skin and remove the sphygmomanometer cuff.
   B. If performing serial ABI measurements

postoperatively, notify the physician for a decrease in ABI of at least 0.15 (15%) or for the loss of a previously palpable pulse or audible doppler tone.

5. Client and family teaching:
   A. This test is painless.
   B. This measurement helps estimate how much blood is flowing to the leg and foot.
6. Factors that affect results:
   A. Values may be inconsistent if the same arm is not used for every brachial pressure measurement.
   B. Immediate postoperative hypotension and low body temperature may necessitate use of a doppler to locate pulse tones because pulses may not be palpable.
7. Other data:
   A. McDermott et al. (1994) found the ankle-brachial index to be a "powerful predictor of survival . . . in patients with peripheral vascular disease." and "Patients with ABIs ≤0.3 have significantly poorer survival than do patients with ABIs 0.31–0.91."
   B. *See also Doppler Ultrasound Flow Studies, Diagnostic.*

Bibliography:

Anderson I: Doppler ultrasound recording of ankle brachial pressure index in the community. J Wound Care *4*(7):325–327, 1995.

de Groote P, Millaire A, Deklunder G, Marache P, Decoulx E, Ducloux G: Comparative diagnostic value of ankle-to-brachial index and transcutaneous oxygen tension at rest and after exercise in patients with intermittent claudication. Angiology *46*(2):115–122, 1995.

McDermott MM, Feinglass J, Slavensky R, Pearce WH: The ankle-brachial index as a predictor of survival in patients with peripheral vascular disease. J Gen Intern Med *9*(8):445–449, 1994.

O'Flynn I: Three methods of taking the brachial systolic pressure to measure the ankle/brachial index: which one is best? J Vasc Nurs *11*(3):71–75, 1993.

Rooke TW, Heser JL, Hallet JW, Gloviczki P, Johnson CM: Hemodynamic changes following the surgical revascularization of lower limbs in patients with arterial occlusive disease: A comparison of six methods. J Vasc Tech *SVII*:27–32, 1993.

ANP

(see Atrial Natriuretic Hormone, Plasma)

ANTEGRADE PYELOGRAPHY, DIAGNOSTIC

Norm: Normal filling of the upper collecting system of the urinary tract. Bladder and bilateral ureters of normal shape, size, and location.

Usage: Antenatal screening for urinary tract dilation; evaluation of upper collecting system status following diversion surgery; identification and localization of ureteral obstruction; measurement of intrarenal pressures; and procedural placement of nephrostomy tube.

Description: Antegrade pyelography is a radiographic contrast examination of the bladder and ureters achieved by injecting radiographic dye percutaneously into the renal pelvis or calyx. It is most commonly performed when retrograde pyelography is contraindicated or when dye injected via retrograde pyelography is prevented from traveling completely through the ureters to the upper collecting system of the urinary tract.

Professional Considerations:

1. Consent form IS required.

Risks:

Allergic reaction to dye (itching, hives, rash, tight feeling in the throat, shortness of breath, bronchospasm, anaphylaxis, death), hematoma, hemorrhage, infection, nephrostomy tube obstruction, pneumothorax, renal toxicity, vasovagal response.

Contraindications:

Bleeding disorders; dehydration, during pregnancy and breast-feeding; previous allergy to iodine, shellfish, or radiographic dye; renal insufficiency; clotting disorders. Sedatives are contraindicated in clients with central nervous system depression.

2. Preparation:
   A. Be aware of the baseline PT/PTT or ACT.
   B. Orders may include a 4-hour fast from food and a sedative.
   C. Obtain povidone-iodine; sterile drapes; 1–2% lidocaine (Xylocaine); a 1.5-inch, 14-gauge needle with stylet; a 20-gauge needle with stylet; tubing; a manometer; sterile specimen containers; a nephrostomy tube, if needed; and a pressure dressing.
   D. Assess baseline vital signs.
   E. The client should disrobe below the waist.
   F. Have emergency equipment readily available.

3. Procedure:
    A. The client is positioned prone on the procedure table.
    B. Ultrasound or fluoroscopy is used to identify the position of the kidney.
    C. A site over the renal pelvis is cleansed with povidone-iodine, allowed to dry, draped, and anesthetized.
    D. Guided by ultrasound or fluoroscopy, a 1.5-inch, 14-gauge needle with a stylet is inserted percutaneously through the chosen site. The needle is removed, leaving the stylet in place. A longer, 20-gauge needle is then inserted through the stylet into the renal pelvis.
    E. The needle is connected to the tubing, and the intrarenal pressure may be measured via a manometer connected to the tubing.
    F. Any urine present is then aspirated. Samples may be sent for culture. Radiopaque contrast medium is injected through the tubing as a series of fluoroscopic images are taken to track the filling of the dye.
    G. Finally, x-rays are taken from several angles to visualize the area.
    H. A nephrostomy tube may be placed at this time.
    I. The needles and stylets are removed and a dry, sterile pressure dressing is applied to the site.

4. Postprocedure care:
    A. Send the urine specimens to the laboratory promptly.
    B. Assess vital signs and the procedure site every 15 minutes × 4, then every 30 minutes × 4, then hourly × 4, then every 4 hours until 24 hours after the procedure.
    C. For hematoma formation or frank bleeding at the site, place pressure on the site and notify the physician immediately.
    D. Be alert for symptoms of infection (fever, tachycardia, tachypnea, chills, hypotension, flank pain), and notify the physician if any of these develop.
    E. Encourage the oral intake of fluids where not contraindicated. Monitor urinary output hourly for quantity and hematuria × 24 hours. Notify the physician for anuria × 8 hours, oliguria, or hematuria.
    F. Assess hourly for patency of the nephrostomy tube, if placed, × 24 hours.
    G. Administer antibiotics and analgesics as prescribed.

5. Client and family teaching:
    A. Remain as motionless as possible during the procedure.
    B. If a nephrostomy tube is placed, save all urine voided after the procedure.
    C. Report chills or pain with urination that occur within 1 week after the procedure.

6. Factors that affect results:
    A. Movement of the client during the

procedure may result in inadvertent puncture of other area structures.

7. Other data:
   A. *See also Retrograde Pyelography, Diagnostic.*

Bibliography:

Bach D, Grutzner G, Kniemeyer HW, Westhoff A, Grabensee B: Diagnostic value of antegrade pyelography in renal transplants: A comparison of imaging modalities. Transplant Proc 25(4):2619, 1993.

Kashi SH, Irving HC, Sadek SA: Does the Whitaker test add to antegrade pyelography in the investigation of collecting system dilatation in renal allografts? Br J Radiol 66(790):877–881, 1993.

ANTIBODY IDENTIFICATION, RED CELL, BLOOD

Norm: Requires interpretation.

Usage: Identification of the specific nature of antibodies detected with more general antibody screens (indirect Coombs' testing).

Description: Irregular antibodies are usually detected in clients who have had prior exposure to foreign antigens through blood transfusions or pregnancy. The presence of these irregular antibodies may cause transfusion reactions and hemolytic disease of the newborn. The exact antibody is identified by combining the client's serum with a panel of red blood cell samples, each containing a known antigen. This test is typically performed in a blood bank.

Professional Considerations:

1. Consent form NOT required.
2. Preparation:
   A. Tube: One lavender-top and one red-top, red/gray-top, or gold-top tube.
   B. Note the client's age, medications, past transfusions of blood products, and number of pregnancies on the laboratory requisition.
3. Procedure:
   A. Draw a 7-ml blood sample in the lavender-top tube.
   B. Draw a 10-ml blood sample in the red-top, red/gray-top, or gold-top tube.
4. Postprocedure care:
   A. None.
5. Client and family teaching:
   A. Results are normally available within 24 hours.
6. Factors that affect results:
   A. Reject hemolyzed specimens.
7. Other data:
   A. Identification of cold-reacting antibodies reactive at ≥30°C may require the use of a blood warmer during transfusion.

Bibliography:

Bromilow IM, Eggington JA, Owen GA, Duguid JK: Red cell antibody screening and identification: A comparison of two column technology methods. Br J Biomed Sci 50(4):329–333, 1993.

Gader A, al-Momen AK, Dahal OK: An evaluation of a new gel system (ID-gel) for antibody screening and identification. Southeast Asian J Trop Med Public Health (Suppl 24) 1:256–258, 1993.

Lamy B, Tissot C, Heyd C, Lamy C: Red cell antibody screening, red cell antibody identification and compatibility testing with the Column Agglutination Technology (CAT). The Bio Vue system. Transfus Clin Biol 1(2):121–127, 1994.

ANTICARDIOLIPIN ANTIBODY
(see Antiphospholipid Antibodies, Serum)

ANTIDEOXYRIBONUCLEASE B TITER (ANTI-DNASE B, STREPTODORNASE), SERUM

Norm:

Adult	<85 Todd U/ml
Child <age 7	<60 Todd U/ml
Child ≥age 7	<170 Todd U/ml

Increased: Glomerulonephritis (poststreptococcal), pharyngitis (streptococcal), pyodermic skin infections, rheumatic fever (acute).

Description: Deoxyribonuclease B is an antigen produced by group A streptococci. The anti-DNase B test detects antibodies to deoxyribonuclease B, which appear when a client has a post-streptococcal infection. The levels increase after a client recovers from a group A streptococcal infection and thus are a reliable indicator of recent hemolytic streptococcal infection.

Professional Considerations:

1. Consent form NOT required.
2. Preparation:
   A. Tube: Red-top, red/gray-top, or gold-top.
   B. List drug therapy and previous vaccinations on the laboratory requisition.
   C. Transport the specimen to the laboratory immediately. Spin and refrigerate the specimen if not tested immediately.
3. Procedure:
   A. Draw a 5-ml blood sample.
4. Postprocedure care:
   A. None.
5. Client and family teaching:
   A. Results are normally available within 48 hours.

6. Factors that affect results:
   A. Reject hemolyzed specimens.
   B. False-negative results may occur in hemorrhagic pancreatitis.
7. Other data:
   A. This test is more sensitive to streptococcal pyoderma than the antistreptolysin-O (ASO) test.

Bibliography:

Gupta R, Prakash K, Kapoor AK: Subclinical group A streptococcal throat infection in school children. Indian Pediatr 29(12):1491–1494, 1992.

Mhalu FS, Matre R: Antistreptolysin O and anti-deoxyribonuclease B titres in blood donors and in patients with features of nonsuppurative sequelae of group A streptococcus infection in Tanzania. East Afr Med J 72(1):33–36, 1995.

ANTIDIURETIC HORMONE (ADH), SERUM

Norm:

Serum Osmolarity	ADH Level	SI Units
270–280 mOsm/kg	<1.5 pg/ml	<1.4 pmol/L
280–285 mOsm/kg	<2.5 pg/ml	<2.3 pmol/L
285–290 mOsm/kg	1–5 pg/ml	0.9–4.6 pmol/L
290–295 mOsm/kg	2–7 pg/ml	1.9–6.5 pmol/L
295–300 mOsm/kg	4–12 pg/ml	3.7–11.1 pmol/L

Increased: Acute intermittent porphyria, cancer (brain, intrathoracic nonpulmonary cancer, gastrointestinal cancer, gynecologic cancer, breast cancer, prostate cancer, sarcoma), cerebrovascular disease, cerebral infection, diabetes insipidus (nephrogenic), ectopic production from neoplasm, Guillain-Barré syndrome, meningitis (tuberculous), pneumonia, syndrome of inappropriate antidiuretic hormone secretion (SIADHS) (caused by malignant tumors, CNS disorders, intrathoracic infections, positive pressure ventilation), and tuberculosis (pulmonary). Drugs include anesthetics, antipsychotics, barbiturates, carbamazepine, chlorothiazide, chlorpropamide, cisplatin, clofibrate, cyclophosphamide, furosemide, estrogens, melphalan, morphine sulfate and other narcotic analgesics, oxytocin citrate, oxytocin injection, psychotropic drugs, thiazides, tolbutamide, tricyclic antidepressants and vidarabine, vinblastine, and vincristine sulfate.

Decreased: Nephrotic syndrome, pituitary diabetes insipidus and psychogenic polydipsia. Drugs include alcohol, demeclocycline, ethanol, lithium carbonate, and phenytoin sodium.

Description: A hormone produced by the hypothalamus and stored and released from the posterior lobe of the pituitary gland in response to increased serum osmolarity. Acts to maintain body water balance through regulation of sodium and potassium and vascular smooth muscle control. Release of ADH is inhibited by decreased serum osmolarity.

Professional Considerations:

1. Consent form NOT required.
2. Preparation:
   A. *See Client and family teaching.*
   B. Tube: Lavender-top made of plastic rather than glass.
   C. Notify laboratory personnel that a specimen for ADH measurement will be arriving shortly.
3. Procedure:
   A. Draw a 5-ml blood sample.
4. Postprocedure care:
   A. Write the collection time on the laboratory requisition.
   B. Transport the specimen to the laboratory for spinning within 10 minutes of collection.
5. Client and family teaching:
   A. Fast and refrain from stress and strenuous activity for 12 hours before the test.
   B. Results are normally available in about 5 days.
6. Factors that affect results:
   A. Reject specimens received more than 10 minutes after collection.
   B. Elevated ADH levels may be caused by physical and psychological stress and positive-pressure mechanical ventilation. Highest levels are obtained at night. Pain, stress, exercise, and elevated blood osmolality will all cause increased secretion.
   C. Decreased ADH levels may be caused by negative-pressure mechanical ventilation, recumbent position, hypo-osmolar blood, and hypertension.
   D. Results are invalidated if the specimen is drawn within 1 week after the client has undergone a scan using radioactive dye.
   E. Glass causes degradation of ADH.

7. Other data:
   A. None.

Bibliography:

Eggert P, Kuhn B: Antidiuretic hormone regulation in patients with primary nocturnal enuresis. Arch Dis Child 73(6):508–511, 1995.

Haycock GB: The syndrome of inappropriate secretion of antidiuretic hormone. Pediatr Nephrol 9(3): 375–381, 1995.

Sorensen JB, Andersen MK, Hansen HH: Syndrome of inappropriate secretion of antidiuretic hormone (SIADH) in malignant disease. J Intern Med 238(2):97–110, 1995.

Spigset O, Hedenmalm K: Hyponatremia and the syndrome of inappropriate antidiuretic hormone secretion (SIADH) induced by psychotropic drugs. Drug Safety 12(3):209–225, 1995.

ANTI-DNA, SERUM

Norm:

Negative: 0–0.9 mg of native DNA/ml of plasma,

or   <70 IU/ml
Borderline SLE   70–200 IU/ml

Increased: Autoimmune disorder (1–2.5 mg/ml), myasthenia gravis, rheumatoid arthritis, sclerosis (systemic), Sjögren's syndrome, systemic lupus erythematosus (SLE) nephritis, and SLE (active = 10–15 mg/ml, remission = 1–2.5 mg/ml).

Description: Detects the presence of antibodies to native deoxyribonuclease that indicate autoimmune activity. The test may be used to monitor the progression (increasing levels) and remission (decreasing levels) of SLE.

Professional Considerations:

1. Consent form NOT required.
2. Preparation:
   A. Tube: Red-top, lavender-top, or gray-top (depending on specific laboratory requirements).
3. Procedure:
   A. Draw a 2-ml blood sample.
4. Postprocedure care:
   A. None.
5. Client and family teaching:
   A. Results may not be available for several days if testing is not performed on site.
6. Factors that affect results:
   A. Results are invalid if the specimen is drawn less than 1 week after the client received a scan using radioactive dye.
   B. Procainamide and hydralazine can induce anti-DNA antibodies.
7. Other data:
   A. In the past it was unnecessary to test clients with negative antinuclear antibodies (ANA). However, there exists a group of ANA-negative lupus clients who have elevated anti-DNA levels.

B. In SLE, immune complexes of anti-DNA may be deposited in the brain, heart, kidneys, and synovial tissue.

Bibliography:

Lorber M, Kra-Oz Z, Guilbrud B, Shoenfeld Y: Natural (antiphospholipid-PDH,-DNA) autoantibodies and their physiologic serum inhibitors. Isr J Med Sci 31(1):31–35, 1995.

Tomer Y, Buskila D, Shoenfeld Y: Pathogenic significance and diagnostic value of lupus autoantibodies. Int Arch Allergy Immunol 100(4):293–306, 1993.

ANTI-DNASE B
(see Antideoxyribonuclease B Titer, Serum)

ANTIHEMOPHILIA FACTOR, BLOOD
(see Factor VIII, Blood)

ANTIHYALURONIDASE (AH) TITER, SERUM

Norm: <128 U/ml.

A fourfold increase between acute and convalescent samples is significant, regardless of the magnitude of the titer.

Increased: Recent group A streptococcal disease, glomerulonephritis (acute), and rheumatic fever (acute).

Description: Hyaluronidase is an extracellular enzyme antigen produced by group A beta-hemolytic streptococci. This test measures levels of antibodies to hyaluronidase which appear in clients who are recovering from group A beta-hemolytic streptococcal infections. Levels increase after a client recovers from a group A beta-hemolytic streptococcal infection (about the second week of infection) and fall 3–5 weeks after infection. Levels are thus a reliable indicator of recent infection due to this etiology.

Professional Considerations:

1. Consent form NOT required.
2. Preparation:
   A. Tube: Red-top, red/gray-top, or gold-top.
   B. List drug therapy and all previous vaccinations on the laboratory requisition.
3. Procedure:
   A. Draw a 5-ml blood sample.
4. Postprocedure care:
   A. Transport the specimen to the laboratory immediately. Spin and refrigerate the specimen if not tested immediately.

5. Client and family teaching:
   A. Return in 1–3 weeks for convalescent samples to be drawn.
6. Factors that affect results:
   A. Reject hemolyzed specimens.
   B. Drugs that may cause falsely suppressed results include antibiotics and corticosteroids.
   C. Falsely elevated results may occur in the presence of hyperlipoproteinemia.
7. Other data:
   A. A better test than the Antistreptolysin-O (ASO) test for detecting antibodies in acute glomerulonephritis, which follows a streptococcal pyoderma.

Bibliography:

Facino RM, Carini M, Stefani R, Aldini G, Saibene L: Anti-elastase and anti-hyaluronidase activities of saponins Sapogenins from Hedera helix, Aesculus hippocastanum, and Ruscus aculeatus: factors contributing to their efficacy in the treatment of venous insufficiency. Arch Pharm (Weinheim), 328(10):720–724, 1995.

ANTI-LA/SS-B TEST, DIAGNOSTIC

Norm: Negative.

Usage: Differential diagnosis of systemic lupus erythematosus (SLE), Sjögren's syndrome, and mixed connective tissue disease.

Positive: Antinuclear antibody (ANA)-negative lupus, neonatal lupus, Sjögren's syndrome.

Description: Anti-LA/SS-B is an autoantibody characteristically found in high titers in clients with primary Sjögren's syndrome or Sjögren's syndrome with (SLE). The SS-B(LA) are antibodies directed against ribonucleic acid (RNA) protein particles that are a cofactor in RNA polymerase III.

Although electrophoresis is the most sensitive method for detecting anti-LA/SS-B, immunodiffusion is the method most commonly used.

Professional Considerations:

1. Consent form NOT required.
2. Preparation:
   A. Tube: Red-top, red/gray-top, or gold-top.
3. Procedure:
   A. Draw a 7-ml blood sample.
4. Postprocedure care:
   A. Transport the specimen to the laboratory for immediate spinning.
5. Client and family teaching:
   A. Results may not be available for several days if testing is not performed on site.
6. Factors that affect results:
   A. None found.
7. Other data:
   A. This test is less sensitive but more specific for primary Sjögren's syndrome than is the anti-Ro/SS-A test.
   B. The presence of both anti-LA/SS-B and anti-Ro/SS-A antibodies is generally associated with milder disease of SLE.
   C. Clients who are positive for antinuclear antibody and who have SS-A but not SS-B are likely to have nephritis.

Bibliography:

Franceschini F, Cretti L, Quinzanini M, Rizzini FL, Cattaneo R: Deforming arthropathy of the hands in systemic lupus erythematosus is associated with antibodies to SSA/Ro and to SSB/La. Lupus 3(5):419-422, 1994.

Garcia Lerma JG, Mendoza AZ, Ramos MJ, Sequi J: Evaluation of recombinant Ro/SSA, La/SSB, Sm, and U1 RNP autoantigens in clinical diagnosis. J Clin Lab Anal 9(1):52–58, 1995.

Jaskowski TD, Schroder C, Martins TB, Mouritsen L, Hill HR: Comparison of three commercially available enzyme immunoassays for the screening of autoantibodies to extractable nuclear antigens. J Clin Lab Anal 9(3):166–172, 1995.

Youinou P, Adler Y, Muller S, Lamour A, Baron D, Humbel RL: Anti-Ro(SSA) and anti-La(SSB) antibodies in autoimmune rheumatic diseases. Clin Rev Allergy 12(3):253–274, 1994.

ANTIMITOCHONDRIAL ANTIBODY (AMA), BLOOD

Norm: Negative at 1:5 to 1:10 dilution.

Suggestive of primary biliary cirrhosis	>1:20
Probable primary biliary cirrhosis	>1:80
Diagnostic of primary biliary cirrhosis	>1:160

Increased: Autoimmune diseases, chronic active hepatitis (20% of clients), cryptogenic cirrhosis, jaundice (drug-induced), myasthenia gravis, and primary biliary cirrhosis.

Decreased or Absent: Drug-induced cholestatic jaundice, extrahepatic obstructive biliary disease, sclerosing cholangitis, and viral hepatitis.

Description: An immunofluorescent test that detects and measures autoimmune immunoglobulins (antibodies) to mitochondria that attack organs which expend large amounts of energy. A majority of clients with primary biliary cirrhosis have antimitochondrial antibodies. This test is usually performed in conjunction with the test for anti–smooth muscle antibodies to aid in differentiating primary biliary cirrhosis and chronic active hepatitis from diffuse, extrahepatic biliary obstruction and other liver diseases.

Professional Considerations:

1. Consent form NOT required.
2. Preparation:
   A. *See Client and family teaching.*
   B. Tube: Red-top, red/gray-top, or gold-top.
3. Procedure:
   A. Draw a 2-ml blood sample.
4. Postprocedure care:
   A. Transport the specimen to the laboratory for immediate spinning.
5. Client and family teaching:
   A. Fast for 8 hours before sampling.
   B. Results may not be available for several days if testing is not performed on site.
6. Factors that affect results:
   A. Reject hemolyzed specimens.
   B. Results are unreliable for clients using oxyphenisatin.
   C. False-positive results may occur in clients with syphilis.
7. Other data:
   A. Although titers over 1:80 are strongly suggestive for primary biliary cirrhosis, liver biopsy is recommended.

Bibliography:

Archimandritis A, Tjivras M, Tsirantonaki M, Hatzis G, Delladetsima I: Sjögren's syndrome with antimitochondrial antibody-negative primary biliary cirrhosis: A case of autoimmune cholangitis. J Clin Gastroenterol *20*(3):268–270, 1995.

Lacerda MA, Ludwig J, Dickson ER, Jorgensen RA, Lindor KD: Antimitochondrial antibody-negative primary biliary cirrhosis. Am J Gastroenterol *90*(2):247–249, 1995.

ANTIMYOCARDIAL ANTIBODY, SERUM

Norm: Negative.

Positive: Cardiomyopathy (idiopathic), Dressler's syndrome, fibrosis (endomyocardial), after myocardial infarction, myocarditis, pericarditis (idiopathic), postpericardiotomy syndrome, post-thoracotomy syndrome, rheumatic fever, rheumatic heart disease, systemic lupus erythematosus, and thoracic injury.

Description: Antimyocardial antibody is an antibody to an organ-specific antigen in myocardial tissue that causes autoimmune damage to the heart and may be detected in serum prior to the appearance of clinical symptoms. The myocardial antigenic determinant is also thought to be a characteristic of streptococci because the antibodies may appear in rheumatic fever or after a streptococcal infection. This test uses an indirect immunofluorescence method by treating extracts of animal cardiac tissue with the client's serum and observing for the development of antigen-antibody immune complexes. Positive results are reported in titers of the lowest dilution at which the immune complexes can be detected, and decreasing titers correlate with response to treatment. This test is used in the detection of an autoimmune etiology for the above-listed conditions and for monitoring therapeutic response to treatment for the above-listed conditions.

Professional Considerations:

1. Consent form NOT required.
2. Preparation:
   A. Tube: Red-top, red/gray-top, or gold-top.
3. Procedure:
   A. Draw a 5-ml blood sample.
4. Postprocedure care:
   A. Transport the specimen to the laboratory for immediate spinning.
5. Client and family teaching:
   A. Results are normally available within 48 hours.
6. Factors that affect results:
   A. No factors known to affect results.
7. Other data:
   A. Myocardial antibodies do not usually occur in clients with coronary insufficiency alone, but do occur in clients who also have had a myocardial infarction.

Bibliography:

Elias JM: Principles and Techniques in Diagnostic Histopathology. Park Ridge, NJ, Noyes Data Corp, 1982.

Turnicky RP, Goodin J, Smialek JE, Herskowitz A, Beschorner WE: Incidental myocarditis with intravenous drug abuse: The pathology, immunopathology, and potential implications for human immunodeficiency virus-associated myocarditis. Hum Pathol *23*(2):138–143, 1992.

ANTINUCLEAR ANTIBODY (ANA), SERUM

Norm: Negative at 1:20 dilution.

Positive: Dermatomyositis, hepatitis (chronic active), mixed connective tissue disease, myasthenia gravis, polymyositis, pulmonary fibrosis (idiopathic), Raynaud's syndrome, rheumatoid arthritis, scleroderma, some healthy older adults, systemic lupus erythematosus (SLE), and Sjögren's syndrome. Drugs include beta-adrenergic blockers, carbamazepine, lovastatin, methyldopa, nitrofurantoin sodium, penicillamine, and tocainide.

Description: Antinuclear antibodies are antibodies the body produces against its own DNA and nuclear material that cause tissue damage and characterize autoimmune diseases. Highest titers occur in SLE. The immunofluorescent procedure results in four characteristic staining patterns, which help differentiate the type of connective tissue disease. These patterns and their specificities include the *homogenous* pattern specific for SLE and other connective diseases; the *peripheral* pattern specific for SLE; the *speckled* pattern specific for mixed connective disease, SLE, Sjögren's syndrome, polymyositis-dermatomyositis, and scleroderma; and the *nucleolar* pattern specific for scleroderma and Sjögren's syndrome. These patterns, however, are not diagnostic of the various diseases. If positive results are obtained, the *anti-DNA* test should be performed to aid differentiation of SLE.

Professional Considerations:

1. Consent form NOT required.
2. Preparation:
   A. Tube: Red-top, red/gray-top, or gold-top.
   B. List drug therapy on the laboratory requisition.
   C. *See Client and family teaching.*
3. Procedure:
   A. Draw a 2-ml blood sample.
4. Postprocedure care:
   A. Transport the specimen to the laboratory for immediate spinning.
5. Client and family teaching:
   A. Fast for 8 hours prior to sampling.
   B. Results may not be available for several days if testing is not performed on site.
6. Factors that affect results:
   A. Reject hemolyzed specimens.
   B. False-negative results may be due to drug therapy with corticosteroids.
   C. Drugs that may cause false-positive results due to a drug-induced syndrome resembling SLE include acetazolamide, aminosalicylic acid, carbidopa, chlorothiazide, chlorpromazine, clofibrate, diphenylhydantoin, ethosuximide, gold salts, griseofulvan microsize, griseofulvan ultramicrosize, hydralazine hydrochloride, hydroxytryptophan, isoniazid, mephenytoin, methlydopa, methyldopate hydrochloride, methylthiouricil, methysergide maleate, oral contraceptives, penicillin, phenylbutazone, phenytoin, primidone, procainamide hydrochloride, propylthiouricil, quinidine gluconate, quinidine polygalacturonate, quinidine sulfate, reserpine, streptomycin sulfate, sulfadimethoxine, sulfonamides, tetracyclines, thiouracil, and trimethadione.
7. Other data:
   A. The peroxidase method may be used, but patterns are not obtained.
   B. Deane et al. (1995) found that in a sample of children with musculoskeletal or dermatologic disease, "the prognosis of children who have positive ANA test results in the absence of autoimmune conditions is usually excellent."

Bibliography:

Deane PM, Liard G, Siegel DM, Baum J: The outcome of children referred to a pediatric rheumatology clinic with a positive antinuclear antibody test but without an autoimmune disease. Pediatrics 95(6):892–895, 1995.

Ichikawa Y, Takaya M, Shimizu H, Uchiyama M, Moriuchi J, Morita K, Hoshina Y, Horiki T: Comparison of antinuclear antibody and other immunohematological profiles among primary Sjögren's syndrome, secondary Sjögren's syndrome associated with rheumatoid arthritis or systemic lupus erythematosus, and corresponding systemic disease. Tokai J Exp Clin Med 18(3–6):133–138, 1993.

Lorber M, Kra-Oz Z, Guilbrud B, Shoenfeld Y: Natural (antiphospholipid-PDH,-DNA) autoantibodies and their physiologic serum inhibitors. Isr J Med Sci 31(1):31–35, 1995.

Zuber M, Miesel R, Brandl B: A patient with a high titer of antinuclear antibody and a functioning adrenal tumour. Clin Rheumatol 14(1):100–103, 1995.

ANTIPHOSPHOLIPID (APA) ANTIBODY, SERUM

Norm: Negative.

Positive: Antiphospholipid/anticardiolipin syndrome(primary, secondary), polymyalgia rheumatica temporal arteritis, thrombosis (systemic venous).

Description: Antiphospholipid antibodies (APA) are a family of immunoglobulins active against phospholipids. Phospholipids are complex triglyceride esters containing long-chain fatty acids, phosphoric acid, and nitrogenous bases. The group includes fatty compounds such as lecithin, found in animal and plant cells. The APA family consists of the anticardiolipin antibodies (ACA), lupus anticoagulant (LA), and antibodies that cause biologic false positive results in syphilis serology. ACA and LA have been described as occurring in thromboses, autoimmune disease, infectious diseases, and neoplastic disease. An APA syndrome that occurs during pregnancy includes loss of the fetus, systemic thromboses, and thrombocytopenia. The pathophysiology of fetal loss is not clearly known, but several theories have been suggested. Clients with APA syndrome are treated with long-term oral anticoagulation.

Professional Considerations:

1. Consent form NOT required.
2. Preparation:
   A. Tube: Red-top, red/gray-top, or gold-top.
3. Procedure:
   A. Draw a 1-ml blood sample.
4. Postprocedure care:
   A. None.
5. Client and family teaching:
   A. Results are normally available within 48 hours.
   B. This test detects antibodies that bind to fatty substances in your body. It helps identify an illness called antiphospholipid syndrome or anticardiolipin syndrome, in which the blood clots faster than normal. It is important to identify and treat this syndrome because it can lead to a greater risk for fetal death and a higher incidence of stroke, heart attack, and blindness.
6. Factors that affect results:
   A. Levels vary, depending on which commercial kit is used for this test, because the assays are not yet standardized.
7. Other data:
   A. In women with previous fetal loss, who have received prophylactic treatment during subsequent pregnancy, the live birth rate is 70%. Treatment has included antiplatelet drugs, immunosuppressives, and/or anticoagulants.

Bibliography:

Brighton TA, Chesterman CN: Antiphospholipid antibodies and thrombosis. Baillieres Clin Haematol 7(3):541–557, 1994.

Chogle AR, Buchanan RR: The clinical associations of lupus anticoagulant and anticardiolipin antibodies. J Assoc Physicians India, 42(7):553–559, 1994.

Harris EN: The antiphospholipid syndrome. Diagnosis, management, and pathogenesis. Clin Rev Allergy Immunol 13(1):39–48, 1995.

Ordi-Ros J, Perez-Peman P, Monasterio J: Clinical and therapeutic aspects associated with phospholipid binding antibodies (lupus anticoagulant and anticardiolipin antibodies). Haemostasis 24(3):165–174, 1994.

Reber G, Arvieux J, Comby E, Degenne D, de Moerloose P, Sanmarco M, Potron G: Multicenter evaluation of nine commercial kits for the quantitation of anticardiolipin antibodies. The Working Group on Methodologies in Haemostasis from the GEHT (Groupe d'Etudes sur l'Hemostase et la Thrombose). Thromb Haemost 73(3):444–452, 1995.

Triplett DA: Antiphospholipid antibodies, lupus anticoagulants and thromboembolic disease. Haematologica 80(Suppl 2):122–126, 1995.

ANTIRIBONUCLEOPROTEIN TEST, DIAGNOSTIC

(see Anti-RNP Test, Diagnostic)

ANTI-RNP TEST (ANTIRIBONUCLEOPROTEIN TEST, EXTRACTABLE NUCLEAR ANTIGEN), DIAGNOSTIC

Norm: Negative.

Usage: Assists in differentiating the type of autoimmune disease occurring. Highest titers ($\geq$1:10,000) are suggestive of mixed connective tissue disease.

Description: An antinuclear antibody present in autoimmune disease detected by an immunofluorescent procedure. Immunofluorescence results in characteristic staining patterns that help differentiate the type of connective tissue disease occurring. Anti-RNP antibodies are associated with a speckled pattern and occur in almost all clients with mixed connective tissue syndrome and about one fourth of clients with scleroderma and discoid and systemic lupus erythematosus. High titers are usually accompanied by clinical symptoms of mixed connective tissue disease.

Professional Considerations:

1. Consent form NOT required.
2. Preparation:
   A. Tube: Red-top, red/gray-top, or gold-top.
   B. *See Client and family teaching.*
3. Procedure:
   A. Draw a 2-ml blood sample.
4. Postprocedure care:
   A. Transport the specimen to the laboratory for immediate spinning.
5. Client and family teaching:
   A. Fast for 8 hours prior to sampling.
   B. Results may not be available for several days if testing is not performed on site.
6. Factors that affect results:
   A. Reject hemolyzed specimens.
   B. False-negative results may be caused by drug therapy with corticosteroids.
   C. Drugs that may cause false-positive results due to a drug-induced syndrome resembling systemic lupus erythemato-

sus (SLE) include acetazolamide, aminosalicylic acid, carbidopa, chlorothiazide, chlorpromazine, clofibrate, diphenylhydantoin, ethosuximide, gold salts, griseofulvan microsize, griseofulvan ultramicrosize, hydralazine, hydrochloride, hydroxytryptophan, isoniazid, mephenytoin, methyldopa, methyldopate hydrochloride, methylthiouricil, methysergide maleate, oral contraceptives, penicillin, phenylbutazone, phenytoin, primidone, procainamide hydrochloride, propylthiouricil, quinidine gluconate, quinidine polygalacturonate, quinidine sulfate, reserpine, streptomycin sulfate, sulfadimethoxine, sulfonamides, tetracyclines, thiouracil, and trimethadione.

7. Other data:
   A. Titer is determined by counterimmunoelectrophoresis (CIE).

Bibliography:

Appelboom T, Kahn MF, Mairesse N: Antibodies to small ribonucleoprotein and to 73-kD heat shock protein: Two distinct markers of mixed connective tissue disease. Clin Exp Immunol 100(3): 486–488, 1995.

Bar-Meir E, Teuber SS, Lin HC, Alosacie I, Goddard G, Terybery J, Barka N, Shen B, Peter JB, Blank M, et al.: Multiple autoantibodies in patients with silicone breast implants. J Autoimmunol 8(2):267–277, 1995.

Jaskowski TD, Schroder C, Martins TB, Mouritsen L, Hill HR: Comparison of three commercially available enzyme immunoassays for the screening of autoantibodies to extractable nuclear antigens. J Clin Lab Anal 9(3):166–172, 1995.

ANTI-RO/SS-A TEST, DIAGNOSTIC

Norm: Negative.

Positive: ANA-negative lupus, neonatal lupus, and Sjögren's syndrome.

Description: Anti-Ro/SS-A is an autoantibody to the cytoplasmic RNA Ro antigen characteristically found in high titers in clients with primary Sjögren's syndrome or Sjögren's syndrome with systemic lupus erythematosus (SLE). Although electrophoresis is the most sensitive testing method for detection of these antibodies, the most common method used is immundiffusion. This test is used in the differential diagnosis of SLE, Sjögren's syndrome, and mixed connective tissue disease.

Professional Considerations:

1. Consent form NOT required.
2. Preparation:
   A. Tube: Red-top, red/gray-top, or gold-top.
3. Procedure:
   A. Draw a 2-ml blood sample.

4. Postprocedure care:
   A. Send the specimen to the laboratory for immediate spinning.
5. Client and family teaching:
   A. Results may not be available for several days if testing is not performed on site.
6. Factors that affect results:
   A. No known factors affect results.
7. Other data:
   A. This test is more sensitive, but less specific, for primary Sjögren's syndrome than is the anti-LA/SS-B test.
   B. The presence of both anti-LA/SS-B and anti-Ro/SS-A antibodies is generally associated with a milder form of SLE.
   C. Clients who are positive for antinuclear antibody and who have SS-A but not SS-B are likely to have nephritis.

Bibliography:

Ben-Chetrit E: The molecular basis of the SSA/Ro antigens and the clinical significance of their autoantibodies. Br J Rheumatol 32(5):396–402, 1993.

Garcia Lerma JG, Mendoza AZ, Ramos MJ, Sequi J: Evaluation of recombinant Ro/SSA, La/SSB, Sm, and U1 RNP autoantigens in clinical diagnosis. J Clin Lab Anal 9(1):52–58, 1995.

Youinou P, Adler Y, Muller S, Lamour A, Baron D, Humbel RL: Anti-Ro(SSA) and anti-La(SSB) antibodies in autoimmune rheumatic diseases. Clin Rev Allergy 12(3):253–274, 1994.

ANTI-SM TEST (EXTRACTABLE NUCLEAR ANTIGEN), DIAGNOSTIC

Norm: Negative.

Usage: Assists in differentiating the type of autoimmune disease occurring. Antibodies specific against Sm strongly suggest systemic lupus erythematosus (SLE).

Description: An antinuclear antibody active against acidic nuclear proteins, present in autoimmune disease detected by an immunofluorescent procedure. Immunofluorescence results in characteristic staining patterns that help differentiate the type of connective tissue disease occurring. Anti-Sm antibodies are associated with a speckled pattern and occur in clients with mixed connective tissue syndrome and in about one fourth of clients with scleroderma, discoid lupus erythematosus, and SLE.

Professional Considerations:

1. Consent form NOT required.
2. Preparation:
   A. Tube: Red-top, red/gray-top, or gold-top.
   B. *See Client and family teaching.*
3. Procedure:
   A. Draw a 2-ml blood sample.

4. Postprocedure care:
   A. Send the specimen to the laboratory for immediate spinning.
5. Client and family teaching:
   A. Fast for 8 hours prior to sampling.
   B. Results may not be available for several days if testing is not performed on site.
6. Factors that affect results:
   A. Reject hemolyzed specimens.
   B. False-negative results may be due to drug therapy with corticosteroids.
   C. Drugs that may cause false-positive results due to a drug-induced syndrome resembling SLE include acetazolamide, aminosalicylic acid, carbidopa, chlorothiazide, chlorpromazine, clofibrate, diphenylhydantoin, ethosuximide, gold salts, griseofulvan microsize, griseofulvan ultramicrosize, hydralazine hydrochloride, hydroxytryptophan, isoniazid, mephenytoin, methyldopa, methyldopate hydrochloride, methylthiouricil, methysergide maleate, oral contraceptives, penicillin, phenylbutazone, phenytoin, primidone, procainamide hydrochloride, propylthiouricil, quinidine gluconate, quinidine polygalacturonate, quinidine sulfate, reserpine, streptomycin sulfate, sulfadimethoxine, sulfonamides, tetracyclines, thiouracil, and trimethadione.
7. Other data:
   A. There is a clinical association of this antibody titer with vasculitis.

Bibliography:

Rahman MA, Isenberg DA: Autoantibodies in systemic lupus erythematosus. Curr Opin Rheumatol 6(5):468–473, 1994.

Vazquez-Abad D, Rothfield NF: Autoantibodies in systemic sclerosis. Int Rev Immunol 12(2–4):145–157, 1995.

ANTI-SMOOTH MUSCLE ANTIBODY, SERUM

Norm: Negative at titer <1:20.

Increased: Asthma (intrinsic) (positive at titer <1:10), biliary cirrhosis (positive at titer 1:10–1:40), chronic active (lupoid) hepatitis (majority of clients) (positive at titers of 1:80–1:320), cryptogenic cirrhosis (rare), malignancies, mononucleosis (infectious with liver damage), tumors (infiltrative), viral hepatitis (acute) (positive at titer <1:10), yellow fever, and in clients aged 50–70 years.

Description: An immunofluorescent test that detects and measures autoimmune immunoglobulins (antibodies) to smooth muscle that appear in chronic active hepatitis and also in response to damaged liver cells. This test is usually performed in conjunction with the test for antimitochondrial antibodies as an aid in differentiating primary biliary cirrhosis and chronic active hepatitis from diffuse, extrahepatic biliary obstruction and other liver diseases.

Professional Considerations:

1. Consent form NOT required.
2. Preparation:
   A. Tube: Red-top, red/gray-top, or gold-top.
   B. *See Client and family teaching.*
3. Procedure:
   A. Draw a 2-ml blood sample.
4. Postprocedure care:
   A. Send the specimen to the laboratory for immediate spinning.
5. Client and family teaching:
   A. Fast for 8 hours prior to sampling.
   B. Results may not be available for several days if testing is not performed on site.
6. Factors that affect results:
   A. Reject hemolyzed specimens.
   B. Antinuclear antibody impairs interpretation of results.
7. Other data:
   A. This test is not diagnostic. A liver biopsy is recommended.
   B. Low titers may occur with infectious mononucleosis, rheumatoid arthritis, liver disease, and malignancies.

Bibliography:

Gutierrez A, Chinchilla V, Espasa A, Perez-Mateo M: Transient detection of antinuclear and anti-smooth muscle antibodies in hepatitis A virus infection [letter]. Am J Gastroenterol 90(1):171, 1995.

Sharpe PC, Dawson JF, O'Kane MJ, Walsh MY, McMillan SA, Nicholls DP: Diffuse plane xanthomatosis associated with a monoclonal band displaying anti-smooth muscle antibody activity. Br J Dermatol 133(6):961–966, 1995.

Takaki A, Sakaguchi K, Ogawa S, Kawamoto H, Tsuji T: Specificities and clinical significance of anti-cytoskeleton antibodies in anti-smooth muscle antibody-positive patients with chronic liver disease. C Acta Med Okayama 48(3):143–149, 1994.

ANTISTREPTOCOCCAL ENZYME

(see Antistreptolysin-O Titer, Serum)

ANTISTREPTOLYSIN-O (ASO) TITER, SERUM

Norm:

Adults	<166 Todd U/ml
Children	
<Age 2	<50 Todd U/ml
Age 2–5	<100 Todd U/ml
Age 5–19	<200 Todd U/ml

A fourfold rise in titer between acute and convalescent specimens is diagnostically significant.

Increased: Acute poststreptococcal endocarditis, acute poststreptococcal glomerulonephritis (500–5000 Todd U/ml), rheumatic fever (inactive < 250 Todd U/ml, active = 500–5000 Todd U/ml), scarlet fever, recent streptococcal disease (small elevations), scarlet fever.

Decreased: Not clinically significant. Levels may decrease with antibiotic therapy.

Description: Antibody to the streptolysin-O enzyme produced by Lancefield group A beta-hemolytic streptococci. These titers rise about 7 days after infection, peak at 3–5 weeks, then gradually return to baseline over the next 6–12 months. Because ASO titers remain elevated in clients with poststreptococcal infections, the test is used to determine whether symptoms such as joint pains, rheumatic fever, or glomerulonephritis are of a poststreptococcal disease origin.

Professional Considerations:

1. Consent form NOT required.
2. Preparation:
   A. Tube: Red-top, red/gray-top, or gold-top.
3. Procedure:
   A. Draw a 1-ml blood sample.
   B. Draw a repeat titer in 10–14 days.
4. Postprocedure care:
   A. Send the specimen to the laboratory for immediate spinning.
5. Client and family teaching:
   A. Repeated ASO titers every 10–14 days are recommended. When poststreptococcal disease occurs, titers begin to rise 1 week after the initial streptococcal infection and peak 2–4 weeks later;

6 months to 1 year is required for postinfection levels to return to the baseline.
   B. Results may not be available for several days if testing is not performed on site.
6. Factors that affect results:
   A. Reject hemolyzed specimens.
   B. Falsely suppressed results may be caused by nephrotic syndromes, antibody deficiency syndromes, or drug therapy with corticosteroids or antibiotics.
   C. Falsely elevated results may be caused by contaminated serum, hyperbetalipoproteinemia, hypercholesterolemia, hyperglobulinemia, lipemic serum, or liver disorders.
   D. The persistent presence of an antibody from a previous, but not recent, infection may mildly increase titers. Only very high titers are indicators of recent infection (e.g., adult, >250 Todd U; child, >333 Todd U).
7. Other data:
   A. Up to 20% of clients with poststreptococcal glomerulonephritis may have normal titers. The anti-DNase-B test is recommended to improve specificity.
   B. *See also Antihyaluronidase Titer, Serum and Streptozyme, Blood.*

Bibliography:

Gray GC, Struewing JP, Hyams KC, Escamilla J, Tupponce AK, Kaplan EL: Interpreting a single antistreptolysin O test: A comparison of the upper limit of normal and likelihood ratio methods. J Clin Epidemiol 46(10):1181–1185, 1993.

Mhalu FS, Matre R: Antistreptolysin O and antideoxyribonuclease B titres in blood donors and in patients with features of nonsuppurative sequelae of group A streptococcus infection in Tanzania. East Afr Med J 72(1):33–36, 1995.

Valtonen JM, Koskimies S, Miettinen A, Valtonen VV: Various rheumatic syndromes in adult patients associated with high antistreptolysin O titres and their differential diagnosis with rheumatic fever. Ann Rheum Dis 52(7):527–530, 1993.

ANTITHROMBIN III (AT-III) TEST, DIAGNOSTIC

Norm:

		SI Units
Plasma	21–30 mg/dl	210–300 mg/L
	85–115% of standard	0.85–1.15
	>50% of control value	
Serum	15–35% lower than plasma values	
Immunologic	17–30 mg/dl	
Functional	80–130%	

Increased: Factor deficiency (V, VII), hemophilia (A, B), hepatitis (acute), inflammation, jaundice (obstructive), menstruation, renal transplant, vitamin K deficiency. Drugs include anabolic steroids, androgens, bishydroxy-coumarin, gemfibrozil, oral contraceptives (progesterone-containing), progesterone, and warfarin sodium.

Decreased: Arteriosclerosis, burns, cardiovascular disease, cerebrovascular accident, carcinoma, cirrhosis, congenital antithrombin III deficiency, deep vein thrombosis, diabetes mellitus (type II), disseminated intravascular coagulation, hepatic disease (abscess, hepatitis), hemocystinuria, hypercoagulation, liver failure (chronic), liver transplant, malignancy (extensive), malnutrition, nephrotic syndrome, post partial hepatectomy, postoperatively, postpartum, pulmonary embolism, septicemia, thromboembolism. Drugs include estrogens, fibrinolytics, gestodene, heparin calcium, heparin sodium, L-asparaginase, and oral contraceptives (estrogen-containing).

Description: A naturally occurring protein IgG immunoglobulin, probably synthesized by the liver, that inhibits coagulation through inactivation of thrombin and other factors. The action of AT-III is catalyzed by heparin. Hereditary AT-III deficiency is an autosomal dominant disease that predisposes clients to venous thrombosis and heparin resistance.

Professional Considerations:

1. Consent form NOT required.
2. Preparation:
   A. Tube: 2.7-ml blue-top or 4.5-ml blue-top.
   B. *See Client and family teaching.*
3. Procedure:
   A. Draw 2.4 ml of blood for a 2.7-ml tube or 4.0 ml of blood for a 4.5-ml tube.
4. Postprocedure care:
   A. Send the specimen to the laboratory for immediate spinning.
5. Client and family teaching:
   A. Fast, except for water, for 10–12 hours before testing.
6. Factors that affect results:
   A. Reject hemolyzed or lipemic specimens.
   B. Results are normally available within 3–5 days.
7. Other data:
   A. Levels of 50–75% indicate moderate risk for thrombosis, whereas levels under 50% indicate significant risk for thrombosis.
   B. A low level in clients taking warfarin indicates that the warfarin is not working effectively.

Bibliography:

Hashimoto K, Yamagishi M, Sasaki T, Nakano M, Kurosawa H: Heparin and antithrombin III levels during cardiopulmonary bypass: Correlation with subclinical plasma coagulation. Ann Thorac Surg 58(3):799–804; discussion 804–805, 1994.

Peddi VR, Kant KS: Catastrophic secondary antiphospholipid syndrome with concomitant antithrombin III deficiency. J Am Soc Nephrol 5(11):1882–1887, 1995.

Schmidt BK: Antithrombin III deficiency in neonatal respiratory distress syndrome. Blood Coagul Fibrinolysis (Suppl 5) 1:S13–S17; discussion S59–S64, 1994.

ANTITHYROGLOBULIN ANTIBODY

(see Thyroid Antithyroglobulin Antibody, Serum)

APEXCARDIOGRAPHY, DIAGNOSTIC

Norm: Normal a wave, c point, e point, o point, rf wave, f point, sf wave, and stasis.

Cardiac Abnormalities	Changes That May Be Found in Apexcardiographic Recording
Aortic valve stenosis	Large a wave, apical impulse occurring late in systole
Atrial fibrillation	Absent a wave, steepened slope of rf wave
Cardiac failure	
Coronary artery disease	Apical impulse occurring late in systole
Mitral regurgitation	Steepened slope of rf wave
Mitral stenosis	Absent a wave, shallow slope of rf wave
Hypertension	Large a wave, apical impulse occurring late in systole
Idiopathic hypertrophic subaortic stenosis	Large a wave
Left ventricular aneurysm	Apical impulse occurring late in systole
Myocardial ischemia or infarction	Apical impulse occurring late in systole
Pericarditis	Steepened slope of rf wave

Usage: Aids in diagnosing heart abnormalities. In conjunction with phonocardiography, helps to identify heart sounds.

Description: Apexcardiography is a method to transfer cardiac movement and pulsations into electrical energy via a transducer and produce a graphic recording of waveforms that characterize the status of the heart. The test takes less than 1/2 hour to perform.

Professional Considerations:

1. Consent form NOT required.
2. Preparation:
   A. Remove jewelry and any metal objects.
   B. The client should disrobe above the waist.
3. Procedure:
   A. The client is placed in a left oblique position, and electrocardiographic limb leads are applied. The transducer tip, covered with electroconductive gel, is strapped in place in contact with the point of maximum impulse at the apex of the heart.
   B. Apexcardiographic recordings are made as the client lies motionless and performs isometric hand-clenching exercises, which increase systemic vascular resistance.
4. Postprocedure care:
   A. Remove transducer and limb leads. Cleanse the electroconductive gel off the transducer and off the client's chest.

5. Client and family teaching:
   A. The test is painless.
   B. Slow, even respirations promote the most accurate test results. You should not talk or move during the procedure.
   C. You will be asked to isometrically clench your fists, which means clenching them and then squeezing them and holding them tightly shut.
6. Factors that affect results:
   A. See above under *Norms*.
   B. Implantable metal devices in the chest wall, such as venous access devices, do not interfere with the test as long as leads are not placed directly over the metal device.
7. Other data:
   A. None.

Bibliography:

Cardoso J, Silva JC, Coutinho J, Campelo M, Simoes L, Maciel MJ, Ramalhao C: Diltiazem effects on left ventricular function: Preliminary results of 12 patients evaluated by calibrated apexcardiogram. Acta Cardiol *50*(1):35–38, 1995.

Dans AL, Bossone EF, Guyatt GH, Fallen EL: Evaluation of the reproducibility and accuracy of apex beat measurement in the detection of echocardiographic left ventricular dilation. Can J Cardiol *11*(6):493–497, 1995.

Manolas J: Accurate noninvasive detection of diastolic dysfunction by current techniques: Fact or fancy? Acta Cardiol *50*(1):7–12, 1995.

Strong A: Apexcardiography. *In* Hamilton HK, Cahill M (eds): Diagnostics, 2nd ed. Springhouse, PA, Springhouse Corporation, 1986, pp 895–897.

APOLIPOPROTEIN A-I (APOPROTEIN-A, APO-A), PLASMA

Norm: Values 5–10% higher in Afro-Americans.

	Male		Female	
Age	**mg/dl**	**SI Units g/L**	**mg/dl**	**SI Units g/L**
Adult				
20–29	81–153	0.81–1.53	80–184	0.80–1.84
30–39	79–155	0.79–1.55	83–187	0.83–1.87
40–49	100–140	1.00–1.40	93–181	0.93–1.81
50–59	81–169	0.81–1.69	76–204	0.76–2.04
60–65	86–166	0.86–1.66	122–214	1.22–2.14
Child				
Birth	41–93	0.41–0.93	38–106	0.38–1.06
0.5–4 yrs	67–163	0.67–1.63	60–148	0.60–1.48
5–7	92–151	0.92–1.51	90–151	0.90–1.51
8–9	96–151	0.96–1.51	94–151	0.94–1.51
10–11	96–151	0.96–1.51	92–151	0.92–1.51
12–13	88–151	0.88–1.51	83–146	0.83–1.46
14–15	85–139	0.85–1.39	96–146	0.96–1.46
16–17	83–146	0.83–1.46	96–151	0.96–1.51

APO A1/B ratio
Female   0.76–3.23
Male   0.85–2.24

Increased: Not clinically significant. Familial hyper-alpha-lipoproteinemia. Drugs include carbamazepine, chlorinated hydrocarbons, clofibrate, estrogen, ethanol, exercise, gemfibrozil, lovastatin, niacin, oral contraceptives (containing estrogen), phenobarbital, phenytoin, pravastatin, simvastatin, weight reduction diet.

Decreased: Cholestasis, coronary artery disease, diabetes mellitus (poorly controlled), hepatocellular abnormalities, hypertriglyceridemia, hypo-alpha-lipoproteinemia, ischemic coronary disease, lipoprotein lipase cofactor deficiency, myocardial infarction, nephrotic syndrome, renal failure (chronic). Drugs include androgens, beta-adrenergic blocking agents, diuretics, probucol, and progestins.

Description: An inherited alpha$_1$-globulin that is the major protein component (70%) of high-density lipoprotein (HDL). It is synthesized in the liver and small intestine and is essential for the transport of peripheral cholesterol to the liver for eventual excretion. Calculation of the ratio of apolipoprotein A-1 to apolipoprotein B is thought to be more useful than HDL cholesterol for identifying clients at risk for coronary artery disease.

Professional Considerations:
1. Consent form NOT required.
2. Preparation:
   A. Tube: Red-top, red/gray-top, or gold-top.

   B. Several testing methods are used to measure apolipoprotein A-1. Clarify the proper blood-drawing procedure with the individual laboratory.
   C. *See Client and family teaching.*
3. Procedure:
   A. Draw a 1-ml blood sample.
4. Postprocedure care:
   A. None.
5. Client and family teaching:
   A. Fast for 12 hours prior to testing.
   B. Refrain from smoking for 4 hours prior to testing.
   C. A ratio of apolipoprotein A to apolipoprotein B is sometimes used to predict coronary heart disease.
6. Factors that affect results:
   A. Reject hemolyzed or lipemic specimens.
   B. Apolipoprotein A-1 levels rise during acute illness.
   C. Levels are decreased in smokers and in clients who consume high-carbohydrate or high-polyunsaturated-fat diets.
7. Other data:
   A. None.

Bibliography:

Brouillette CG, Anantharamaiah GM: Structural models of human apolipoprotein A-I. Biochim Biophys Acta *1256*(2):103–129, 1995.

Fievet C, Igau B, Bresson R, Drouin P, Fruchart JC: Nonenzymatic glycosylation of apolipoprotein A-I and its functional consequences. Diabete Metab *21*(2):95–98, 1995.

Forte TM, McCall MR: The role of apolipoprotein A-I-containing lipoproteins in atherosclerosis. Curr Opin Lipidol *5*(5):354–364, 1994.

Srinivasan SR, Berenson GS: Serum apolipoproteins A-I and B as markers of coronary artery disease risk in early life: the Bogalusa Heart Study. Clin Chem *41*(1):159–166, 1995.

APOLIPOPROTEIN B (APOPROTEIN B, APO B), PLASMA
Norm:

	Male		Female	
Age	mg/dl	SI Units g/L	mg/dl	SI Units g/L
Adult	46–174	0.46–1.74	46–142	0.46–1.42
Child				
Birth	11–31	0.11–0.31	11–31	0.11–0.31
0.5–3 years	23–75	0.23–0.75	23–75	0.23–0.75
5–7	47–106	0.47–1.06	49–110	0.49–1.10
8–9	49–105	0.49–1.05	53–132	0.53–1.32
10–11	52–110	0.52–1.10	54–121	0.54–1.21
12–13	46–113	0.46–1.13	46–110	0.46–1.10
14–15	44–103	0.44–1.03	41–108	0.41–1.08
16–17	48–139	0.48–1.39	41–96	0.41–0.96

APO A1/B ratio
Female 0.76–3.23
Male 0.85–2.24

Increased: Acute illness, angina pectoris, anorexia nervosa, coronary heart disease (premature), Cushing's syndrome, diabetes mellitus, dysglobulinemia, hepatic disease and obstruction, hypercalcemia (infantile), hyperlipemia (familial combined), hypothyroidism, myocardial infarction, nephrotic syndrome, porphyria, pregnancy, renal failure, sexual atelictic dwarfism, sphingolipodystrophies, stress (emotional), and Werner's syndrome.

Decreased: anemia (chronic), alphalipoprotein deficiency, heterozygous hypo-beta-lipoproteinemia, hepatocellular dysfunction, hyperlipoproteinemia (Type I), hyperthyroidism, joint inflammation, lecithin cholesterol acyltransferase deficiency, lipoprotein lipase cofactor deficiency, malabsorption, malnutrition, myeloma, pulmonary disease (chronic), Reye's syndrome, stress (acute physical, weight-reduction diet.

Description: A beta-globulin that is the major protein component of low-density lipoprotein (LDL) and is also found in very low-density lipoprotein (VLDL). Functions in cholesterol synthesis and is required for the secretion into plasma of intestinal and hepatic triglyceride-rich lipoproteins. There are two APO B glycoproteins, APO B-48 and APO B-100, which have different molecular weights. APO B-48 is produced in the small intestine and APO B-100 is produced in the liver. Calculation of the ratio of apolipoprotein A-1 to apolipoprotein B is thought to be more useful than LDL cholesterol for identifying clients at risk for atherosclerosis.

Professional Considerations:
1. Consent form NOT required.
2. Preparation:
   A. Tube: Red-top, red/gray-top, or gold-top.
   B. Several testing methods are used to measure apolipoprotein B. Clarify the proper blood-drawing procedure with the individual laboratory.
   C. *See Client and family teaching.*
3. Procedure:
   A. Draw a 1-ml blood sample.
4. Postprocedure care:
   A. None.
5. Client and family teaching:
   A. Fast for 12 hours prior to testing.
   B. A ratio of apolipoprotein A to apolipoprotein B is sometimes used to predict coronary heart disease.
6. Factors that affect results:
   A. Reject hemolyzed or lipemic specimens.
   B. Apolipoprotein B levels rise during acute illness.
7. Other data:
   A. Desirable reference ranges have not yet been established.

Bibliography:
Humphries SE, Talmud PJ: Hyperlipidaemia associated with genetic variation in the apolipoprotein B gene. Curr Opin Lipidol 6(4):215–222, 1995.

Sehayek E, Eisenberg S: The role of native apolipoprotein B-containing lipoproteins in atherosclerosis: Cellular mechanisms. Curr Opin Lipidol 5(5): 350–353, 1994.

Srinivasan SR, Berenson GS: Serum apolipoproteins A-I and B as markers of coronary artery disease risk in early life: The Bogalusa Heart Study. Clin Chem 41(1):159–166, 1995.

APTT
(see Partial Thromboplastin Time, Plasma)

ARSENIC, BLOOD

Norm:

		SI Units
Whole Blood		
Normal	2–23 µg/L	0.03–0.31 µmol/L
Chronic poisoning	100–500 µg/L	1.33–6.65 µmol/L
Acute poisoning	>600 µg/L	>7.98 µmol/L
Serum	1.7–1.54 µg/L	0.02–0.20 µmol/L

Acute Poisoning Symptoms and Treatment:

Symptoms: Abdominal pain, nausea, vomiting, bloody diarrhea, and thirst progressing to dehydration and fluid and electrolyte imbalance, hematuria, metallic taste, pain (gastrointestinal), renal failure, jaundice, hypoxia, convulsions, coma, and respiratory and cardiovascular collapse. May lead to death.

Treatment:

Induction of emesis.
Lavage GI tract.
Saline cathartic.
Penicillamine chelation.
Dimercaprol (BAL).
Support hemodynamic status.
Replace blood lost to GI hemorrhage.
Both hemodialysis and peritoneal dialysis WILL remove arsenic.

Chronic Poisoning Symptoms and Treatment:

Symptoms: Abnormal erythropoiesis and myelopoiesis, alopecia or thinning of hair, anemia, basophilic stippling, diarrhea, hepatomegaly, hyperkeratosis of palms of hands and soles of feet, leukopenia, Mees lines, peripheral neuropathy, skin pigmentation changes and scaling, and thrombocytopenia.

Treatment:

Avoid exposure to arsenic.
Remove household sources of arsenic (described below).

cides, paints, cosmetics, and antiprotozoal medications. Arsenic inhibits sulfhydryl enzyme systems required for cellular metabolism. Blood specimens are used for rapid confirmation of acute poisoning.

Professional Considerations:

1. Consent form NOT required unless the specimen may be used for legal evidence.
2. Preparation:
   A. Tube: Black-top or green-top (whole blood) or red-top, red/gray-top, or gold-top (serum).
   B. Do NOT draw during hemodialysis.
3. Procedure:
   A. The specimen should be collected and labeled in the presence of a witness if it may be used for legal evidence.
   B. Draw a 20-ml blood sample.
4. Postprocedure care:
   A. Note the exact time of specimen collection, along with the client's name, date, contents, and your signature on the tube label and laboratory requisition.
   B. Have the witness sign the laboratory requisition.
   C. Transport the specimen to the laboratory in a sealed plastic bag labeled as legal evidence if that is the case. Have each person handling the specimen write his or her name and time of receipt of the specimen on the laboratory requisition.
5. Client and family teaching:
   A. For intentional poisoning, refer the client and family for crisis intervention.
   B. For chronic poisoning, the client should be taught to remove household sources of arsenic (described above).
6. Factors that affect results:
   A. A diet rich in seafood may elevate the blood level.
7. Other data:
   A. None.

Increased: Arsenic poisoning and heavy metal poisoning.

Decreased: Not clinically significant.

Description: Arsenic is a trace element found in all human tissues that may become elevated when occupational, environmental, or intentional exposure occurs. It is found environmentally as an ingredient of pesti-

Bibliography:

Bryson PD: Arsenic Comprehensive Review in Toxicology. Rockville, MD, Aspen Publishers, 1989, pp 501–508.

Chen CJ, Hsueh YM, Lai MS, Shyu MP, Chen SY, Wu MM, Kuo TL, Tai TY: Increased prevalence of hypertension and long-term arsenic exposure. Hypertension 25(1):53–60, 1995.

Cullen NM, Wolf LR, St Clair D: Pediatric arsenic ingestion. Am J Emerg Med 13(4):432–435, 1995.

De Kimpe J, Cornelis R, Mees L, Van Lierde S, Vanholder R: More than tenfold increase of arsenic in serum and packed cells of chronic hemodialysis patients. Am J Nephrol 13(6):429–434, 1993.

ARSENIC, HAIR OR TOENAILS, SPECIMEN
Norm:

		SI Units
Hair		
Normal levels	20–60 µg/100 g	<8.7 nmol/g
Chronic poisoning	>100 µg/100 g	<13.4 nmol/g
Nails		
Normal levels	20–60 µg/100 g	<8.7 nmol/g
Chronic poisoning	90–180 µg/100 g	12–24 nmol/g

Poisoning Level Symptoms and Treatment: *See Arsenic, Blood.*

Increased: Arsenic poisoning and industrial or environmental exposure to arsenic.

Decreased: Not clinically significant.

Description: A common heavy metal poison that combines with intracellular proteins and is rapidly removed from the blood. Arsenic, a trace element found in all human tissues, may become elevated when occupational, environmental, or intentional usage occurs. It is found environmentally as an ingredient of pesticides, paints, cosmetics, and antiprotozoal medications. Arsenic inhibits sulfhydryl enzyme systems required for cellular metabolism. Because it can be found in keratin, specimens of hair and nail are used to pinpoint chronic exposure to arsenic.

Professional Considerations:
1. Consent form NOT required.
2. Preparation:
   A. Obtain scissors or nail clippers.
3. Procedure:
   A. *Hair:* Hair samples must contain the root end and distal ends. Collect 0.5 g of hair (preferably pubic hair). Ensure privacy when obtaining a pubic hair sample.
   B. *Nails:* Clip the end of all ten toenails. Collect a total of 0.5 g of nails (prefer-

ably toenails). Place the specimens in a clean, dry envelope or heavy metal-free plastic container.
4. Postprocedure care:
   A. Transport the samples to the laboratory as soon as possible.
5. Client and family teaching:
   A. For chronic poisoning, client should be taught to remove household sources of arsenic (described above).
6. Factors that affect results:
   A. A diet rich in seafood may raise levels.
7. Other data:
   A. Arsenic in toenails represents deposition of arsenic for 6 months.
   B. The earliest detection of excess arsenic in hair is 2 weeks after a dose of arsenic and may persist for months or years.
   C. Following exposure to arsenic, white strips about 1 mm wide extend across the entire base of the nails and contain very high concentrations of arsenic.
   D. Symptoms of chronic toxicity include fatigue, weakness, diarrhea, weight loss, dermatitis, and nausea progressing to paralysis, encephalopathy, renal and hepatic damage, and respiratory tract inflammation.

Bibliography:
Das D, Chatterjee A, Mandal BK, Samanta G, Chakraborti D, Chanda B: Arsenic in ground water in six districts of West Bengal, India: The biggest arsenic calamity in the world. Part 2. Arsenic concentration in drinking water, hair, nails, urine, skin-scale and liver tissue (biopsy) of the affected people. Analyst 120(3):917–924, 1995.
Engel RR, Hopenhayn-Rich C, Receveur O, Smith AH: Vascular effects of chronic arsenic exposure: A review. Epidemiol Rev 15(2):184–209, 1994.
Vienna A, Capucci E, Wolfsperger M, Hauser G: Heavy metal concentration in hair of students in Rome. Anthropol Anz 53(1):27–32, 1995.

ARSENIC, URINE
Norm:

		SI Units
Normal	5–50 µg/24 hours	0.067–0.665 µmol/d
Chronic poisoning	50–5000 µg/L	0.67–66.50 µmol/L
Acute poisoning	>1000 µg/L	>13.3 µmol/L

Poisoning Level Symptoms and Treatment: *See Arsenic, Blood.*

Increased: Arsenic poisoning and metal poisoning.

Decreased: Not clinically significant.

Description: A common heavy metal poison that combines with intracellular proteins and is rapidly removed from the blood. Arsenic, a trace element found in all human tissues, may become elevated when occupational, environmental, or intentional usage occurs. It is found environmentally as an ingredient of pesticides, paints, cosmetics, and antiprotozoal medications. Arsenic inhibits sulfhydryl enzyme systems required for cellular metabolism. Urine specimens are used for rapid confirmation of acute poisoning.

Professional Considerations:

1. Consent form NOT required unless the specimen may be used as legal evidence.
2. Preparation:
   A. Obtain a 3-L container without preservatives.
3. Procedure:
   A. The specimen should be collected and labeled in the presence of a witness if it may be used for legal evidence.
   B. Collect a 24-hour urine sample in a 3-L container without preservatives.
   C. Discard the first morning-urine specimen.
   D. Save all urine voided for 24 hours in a refrigerated, clean, 3-L container without preservatives. Document the quantity of urine output during the collection period. Include urine voided at the end of the 24-hour period. For catheterized clients, keep the drainage bag on ice and empty the urine into the collection container hourly.
4. Postprocedure care:
   A. Note the exact beginning and ending times of urine collection, along with the client's name, date, contents, and your signature on the container and laboratory requisition.
   B. Have a witness sign the laboratory requisition.
   C. Transport the entire specimen to the laboratory in a sealed plastic bag labeled as legal evidence, if that is the case. Have each person handling the specimen write his or her name and the time of receipt of the specimen on the laboratory requisition.

5. Client and family teaching:
   A. Save all urine voided in the 24-hour period, and urinate before defecating to avoid loss of urine. If any urine is accidentally discarded, discard the entire specimen and restart the collection the next day.
   B. For chronic poisoning, the client should be taught to remove household sources of arsenic (described above).
6. Factors that affect results:
   A. A diet rich in seafood may show elevated concentration levels in the urine as high as 500–1500 mg/L with no apparent signs of toxicity.
7. Other data:
   A. None.

Bibliography:

Bryson PD: Arsenic Comprehensive Review in Toxicology. Rockville, MD, Aspen Publishers, 1989, pp 501–508.

Cullen NM, Wolf LR, St Clair D: Pediatric arsenic ingestion. Am J Emerg Med *13*(4):432–435, 1995.

Hakala E, Pyy L: Assessment of exposure to inorganic arsenic by determining the arsenic species excreted in urine. Toxicol Lett *77*(1–3):249–258, 1995.

Moyer TP: Testing for arsenic. Mayo Clin Proc *68*(12):1210–1211, 1993.

ART

(see Automated Reagin Testing, Diagnostic)

ARTERIAL BLOOD GASES

(see Blood Gases, Arterial, Blood)

ARTERIOGRAM, DIAGNOSTIC

Norm: Even filling of the arteries with radiographic dye. The artery walls show progressive narrowing without abrupt occlusions or isolated bulging or narrow areas. No evidence of leakage of the dye into tissues, which would indicate hemorrhage. No evidence of vascular anomalies. No displacement of vessels.

Usage: Aids diagnosis of arterial occlusion, aneurysm, abnormal vascular development, and hemorrhage. Helps identify areas of arterial narrowing due to plaque buildup, tumor, or vascular abnormalities.

Description: An arteriogram is a radiographic examination of arteries through which radiographic contrast medium is flowing. The arteries are assessed for abnormalities in blood flow, such as narrowing or outpouching of the walls, and for collateral circulation.

Professional Considerations:

1. Consent form IS required.

Risks:

Aphasia, cerebrovascular accident, dysrhythmias, embolus, endocarditis, hematoma, hemiplegia, hemorrhage, infection, myocardial infarction, paresthesia, allergic reaction to dye (itching, hives, rash, tight feeling in the throat, shortness of breath, bronchospasm, anaphylaxis, death), renal toxicity.

Contraindications:

Anticoagulant therapy, bleeding disorders, thrombocytopenia, dehydration, uncontrolled hypertension, previous allergy to x-ray dye, iodine, or shellfish, renal insufficiency, during pregnancy or breast-feeding.

---

2. Preparation:
   A. *See Client and family teaching.*
   B. Obtain baseline CBC, PT/PTT, and APTT.
   C. Remove all jewelry and metal objects.
   D. The client should void just prior to the procedure.
   E. Obtain baseline vital signs, and mark peripheral pulses.
   F. Have emergency equipment readily available for anaphylaxis and cardiac arrest.
3. Procedure:
   A. Client is placed supine on the x-ray table.
   B. A maintenance intravenous line is started.
   C. The peripheral pulses are marked, and the extremity is immobilized.
   D. The femoral or brachial artery area is located and cleansed with povidone-iodine and allowed to dry, and the surrounding area is covered with a sterile drape.
   E. A local anesthetic (1–2% Xylocaine) is injected intradermally and subcutaneously over the artery.
   F. The femoral or brachial artery is punctured with a large-bore needle. A wire is passed through the needle and the needle removed over the guidewire.
   G. The catheter is then inserted into the artery over the guidewire, and placement is confirmed via fluoroscopy.
   H. The catheter is advanced under fluoroscopy to a location depending on the area to be examined, and radiographic dye is injected.
   I. Several rapid radiographic pictures are taken of the artery and its branches during and after dye injection.
   J. The catheter is removed and sterile gauze is applied immediately, with pressure, to the site for at least 15 minutes.
4. Postprocedure care:
   A. Apply pressure dressing to arterial puncture site.
   B. The client remains on bedrest with the affected extremity immobilized for 12 hours.
   C. Assess the site and dressing for hematoma or bleeding; the distal pulses for presence and strength; and color, motion, temperature, and sensation of the affected extremity every 15 minutes × 4, every half hour × 4, then every hour × 4, then every 4 hours.
   D. Apply pressure for at least 15 minutes if bleeding occurs.
   E. Encourage oral intake of fluids if not contraindicated.
5. Client and family teaching:
   A. If the abdominal vasculature will be examined, a cathartic may be administered 1 day prior to the test and a tap-water enema may be given on the morning of the test.
   B. Consume clear liquids only for 24 hours and fast from food and fluids for 8 hours prior to the test.
   C. It is normal to experience a brief flushing sensation and possibly nausea when the dye is injected, but the feeling will pass quickly.
   D. It is important to lie still throughout the procedure.
   E. Bedrest and frequent site and extremity checks are performed as standard postprocedure care.
6. Factors that affect results:
   A. Movement of the client during filming may obscure the pictures.
7. Other data:
   A. Clients with cardiomegaly need to be monitored carefully during this procedure or assessed to see if this procedure is fundamentally necessary.
   B. *See also Cardiac Catheterization, Cerebral Angiogram, Pulmonary Angiogram, or Renal Angiogram, Diagnostics.*

Bibliography:

Berger AC, Kleinert JM: Noninvasive vascular studies: A comparison with arteriography and surgical findings in the upper extremity. J Hand Surg [Am] *17*(2):206–210, 1992.

Galt SW, Pearce WH: Preoperative assessment of abdominal aortic aneurysms: Noninvasive imaging versus routine arteriography. Semin Vasc Surg *8*(2):103–107, 1995.

Reagan K, Boxt LM, Katz J: Introduction to coronary arteriography. Radiol Clin North Am *32*(3):419–433, 1994.

ARTHROGRAPHY, DIAGNOSTIC

Norm: Intact soft tissue structures of the joint. Absence of lesions, fractures, or tears.

Usage: Detection of damage to joint connective tissue and structures (i.e., adhesions, tears, fractures).

Description: Arthrography involves fluoroscopic and radiographic examination of a joint after air and/or radiographic dye is injected into it. Arthrography provides better visualization of the connective tissue of joints than routine radiography. It is most commonly used to view the knees and shoulders, but may also be performed on other joints such as the ankle, hip, wrist, or temporomandibular joint.

Professional Considerations:

1. Consent form IS required.

Risks:

Allergic reaction to dye (itching, hives, rash, tight feeling in the throat, shortness of breath, bronchospasm, anaphylaxis, death), renal toxicity; bleeding, hematoma, or infection at injection site.

Contraindications:

Previous allergy to iodine, seafood, or radiographic dye; during pregnancy and in active rheumatoid arthritis; infection of the joint to be studied.

2. Preparation:
    A. Obtain a sterile arthrography tray, povidone-iodine solution, and 1–2% Xylocaine.
    B. Have emergency equipment readily available.
    C. *See Client and family teaching.*
3. Procedure:
    A. The skin is cleansed with povidone-iodine solution and allowed to dry.
    B. A local anesthetic (1–2% Xylocaine) is injected subdermally and subcutaneously around the site to be punctured.
    C. A needle is inserted into the joint space and a small amount of contrast dye injected through it as placement is checked under fluoroscopy.

D. After correct placement is confirmed, the remainder of the dye is injected and the needle withdrawn.
    E. The extremity may be moved briefly through a range of motion, and then several fluoroscopic films are taken of the joint in different positions.
4. Postprocedure care:
    A. Minimize use of the joint for 12 hours.
    B. For knee arthrography, an Ace wrap should be worn over the knee for 3–4 days.
5. Client and family teaching:
    A. Fast from food and fluids for 8 hours prior to the procedure.
    B. Some mild pain and pressure will be felt during the procedure, but local anesthesia will be used to keep these sensations tolerable.
    C. Postarthrography edema and tenderness occur frequently for 1–2 days and may be treated with ice packs and mild analgesia. Symptoms lasting more than 2 days necessitate a physician's assessment.
    D. If air injection was used, it is normal to feel crepitus in the joint for up to 2 days. This is because the air remains in the joint space until it dissolves into the tissues. The air causes a popping or cracking sensation when the joint moves.
6. Factors that affect results:
    A. Fluid in the joint space decreases the quality of the films due to dilution of the dye. If present, it should be aspirated prior to dye injection.
7. Other data:
    A. None.

Bibliography:

Hart DJ, Spector TD: The classification and assessment of osteoarthritis. Baillieres Clin Rheumatol 9(2):407–432, 1995.

Lane NE, Kremer LB: Radiographic indices for osteoarthritis. Rheum Dis Clin North Am 21(2): 379–394, 1995.

ARTHROPOD IDENTIFICATION, SPECIMEN

Norm: Requires interpretation.

Usage: Insect bites.

Description: There are over 1 million species in the phylum Arthropoda, including flies, mosquitos, fleas, lice, scabies, mites, maggots, bed bugs, spiders, cockroaches, termites, ticks, bees, wasps, and scorpions. Specimens are usually presented for identification after a human has been bitten by or infested with them. Arthropod bites may cause a variety of wheals, rashes, or anaphylactic reactions in humans.

Professional Considerations:

1. Consent form NOT required.
2. Preparation:
   A. Obtain alcohol wipes, tweezers, and a container of 70% alcohol.
3. Procedure:
   A. Capture and preserve the arthropod in a sealed container of 70% alcohol. If the arthropod is a tick, rub the tick and site with an alcohol wipe. Then, holding the tick close to the skin with tweezers, pull the tick straight out and apply gentle pulling, without twisting, until the tick lets loose from the skin.
   B. Wash fly larvae in water and then boil for a few minutes before placing in 70% alcohol.
4. Postprocedure care:
   A. Transport the specimen to the laboratory.
5. Client and family teaching:
   A. For arthropod bite or sting, swelling and itching can be controlled by placing a cold washcloth or towel over the site for 20 minutes once per hour. Change to warm washcloths after 1–2 days.
   B. Pain can be reduced by applying a paste of water and baking soda to the site for 5–10 minutes.
   C. Itching can be controlled with calamine lotion.
   D. Use insect repellant whenever venturing into grassy or wooded areas.
   E. The main concern with flea bites is secondary infection. Therefore, keep fingernails short to avoid scratching. Bathe in a tub of water filled with 1 kg starch, apply calamine lotion to skin, and take antihistamines as prescribed. If an infection develops, antibiotics such as neomycin or polymyxin may be prescribed.
6. Factors that affect results:
   A. None.
7. Other data:
   A. Spiders: Two venomous spiders are the brown recluse and the black widow spider, which are more common in the southern United States. The redleg spider of Florida may also produce symptoms of poisoning. Treatment includes slow intravenous administration of 10 ml of 10% calcium gluconate and a muscle relaxant such as diazepam. A commercially prepared antivenom for the black widow, although rarely needed, is available in vials of 6000 U diluted in 2.5 ml of sterile water and given intramuscularly or intravenously.
   B. A generalized systemic reaction to bee, wasp, and ant stings is thought to be IgE mediated. Treatment includes epi-

nephrine hydrochloride 1:1000, 0.3–0.5 ml for an adult and 0.01 ml/kg for a child, prednisone orally to reduce swelling, and diphenhydramine hydrochloride, 25–50 mg orally, to relieve itching.
   C. Lice or scabies frequently found in hair on the head or on the hands, feet, and pubic hair require a thorough application of gamma-benzene hexachloride (Kwell, GBH) cream or lotion. Since GBH is toxic, it is questionable whether it should be used for young children or pregnant mothers.
   D. The puss caterpillar, found in the southeastern United States, especially Texas and Florida, can cause shocklike signs and symptoms. Treatment includes immediate removal of the stinger. This may be followed by slow intravenous administration of 10 ml of 10% calcium gluconate and a muscle relaxant such as diazepam.

Bibliography:

Morsy TA, el Said AM, Salama MM, Arafa MA, Younis TA, Ragheb DA, Abdel Rahman MM: Four species of house dust mites recovered from houses of patients with allergic respiratory diseases. J Egypt Soc Parasitol 25(1):195–206, 1995.

Myers SA, Sexton DJ: Dermatologic manifestations of arthropod-borne diseases. Infect Dis Clin North Am 8(3):689–712, 1994.

Pratt HD, Smith JW: Arthropods affecting humans. In Lennette EH, Balows A, Hausler WJ, Shadomy HJ (eds): Manual of Clinical Microbiology. Washington, DC, American Society for Microbiology, 1985, pp 674–686.

ARTHROSCOPY, DIAGNOSTIC

Norm: Normal muscle, ligament, cartilagenous, synovial, and tendon structures. Absence of tears, degeneration of cartilage, cysts, deposits, or inflammation.

Usage: Carpal tunnel syndrome, joint biopsy, joint surgery, definitive diagnosis of joint disease, and monitoring joint disease progress and response to therapy.

Description: Arthroscopy allows direct visual examination of the interior of a joint via insertion of a fiberoptic endoscope into the joint space. This procedure is most commonly performed on the knee joint, but may also be performed on the ankle, hip, shoulder, temporomandibular, and wrist joints. The knee arthroscopy procedure is described here.

Professional Considerations:

1. Consent form IS required.

Risks:

Hemorrhage, infection, synovial rupture, thrombophlebitis.

Contraindications:

Fibrous ankylosis; infections in the area of the puncture site. Sedatives are contraindicated in clients with central nervous system depression.

2. Preparation:
   A. Shave a 10- to 12-inch radius around the site.
   B. A sedative may be prescribed.
   C. Obtain a sterile arthroscopy tray, povidone-iodine solution, 1–2% Xylocaine, a sterile stockinette, an Ace wrap, a pneumatic thigh cuff, and a compression dressing.
   D. *See Client and family teaching.*
3. Procedure:
   A. The client is positioned supine.
   B. A pneumatic cuff is placed around the thigh.
   C. The leg is cleansed with povidone-iodine solution, allowed to dry, and covered with a stockinette.
   D. After elevating the leg, an Ace wrap is applied distally to proximally.
   E. The pneumatic cuff is inflated to about 300 mmHg (level may vary, depending on client's blood pressure) to act as a tourniquet. The Ace wrap is removed and the leg lowered to bend at the knee.
   F. After the stockinette is opened, the site is anesthetized locally, and a small incision is made in the knee and the synovia transgressed.
   G. The arthroscope is inserted through a cannula, and normal saline and/or epinephrine solutions are injected into the joint to enhance the views of the interior joint. The views may be projected on a video screen and permanent recordings made.
   H. After viewing, biopsy, surgery, or treatment is complete, the arthroscope is removed, the joint is irrigated and drained, and the leg is wrapped with a compression dressing.
   I. The pneumatic cuff is then deflated.
4. Postprocedure care:
   A. The client may resume weight bearing, but should limit activity of the joint for 1–4 days.
   B. An elastic wrap should be worn for 2–4 days.
5. Client and family teaching:
   A. Fast for 8–12 hours prior to the procedure.
   B. It is common for the procedure to cause transient pressure and pain. These will be kept to a tolerable level with local anesthesia.
   C. Elevate the leg as often as possible for 2 days. Use a pillow to raise the leg without causing pain.
   D. An ice pack may help ease postprocedure pain. Use a towel between the ice pack and the joint.
   E. Use crutches for 5–7 days when walking.
   F. Do not exercise the joint more than normal activity for 5–6 weeks after the procedure if surgery was performed.
   G. Call the physician if edema continues more than 3 days or if fever over 101°F (38.3°C) or increased knee pain develops.
6. Factors that affect results:
   A. None.
7. Other data:
   A. None.

Bibliography:

Altchek DW: Arthroscopy of the shoulder. Scand J Med Sci Sports 5(2):71–75, 1995.

Bain GI, Roth JH: The role of arthroscopy in arthritis. Ectomy procedures. Hand Clin 11(1):51–58, 1995.

Boden BP, Kozin SH, Berlet AC: Wrist arthroscopy. Am J Orthop 24(4):310–316, 1995.

Farrell J: In Hamilton HK, Cahill M (eds): Diagnostics, 2nd ed. Springhouse, PA, Springhouse Corporation, 1986, pp 679–682.

Sandmeier RH, Renstrom PA: Ankle arthroscopy. Scand J Med Sci Sports 5(2):64–70, 1995.

ASA

(see Salicylate, Blood)

ASCORBIC ACID, SERUM

(see Vitamin C, Plasma or Serum)

ASM ANTIBODY

(see Anti-Smooth Muscle Antibody, Serum)

ASO TITER, SERUM

(see AntiStreptolysin-O Titer, Serum)

ASPARTATE AMINOTRANSFERASE (AST, ASPARTATE TRANSAMINASE, SGOT), SERUM

Norm

		SI Units
Adult females		
Under age 61	8–20 U/L	0.14–0.34 µKat/L
Over age 60	10–20 U/L	0.17–0.34 µKat/L
Adult males		
Under age 61	8–20 U/L	0.14–0.34 µKat/L
Over age 60	11–26 U/L	0.19–0.44 µKat/L
Children		
Newborn	25–75 U/L	0.43–1.28 µKat/L
Infants	15–60 U/L	0.26–1.02 µKat/L
Age 2–5 months	20–50 U/L	0.34–0.85 µKat/L
Age 1 year	16–35 U/L	0.27–0.60 µKat/L
Age 5 years	19–28 U/L	0.32–0.48 µKat/L
Age 8–12 years	15–40 U/L	0.26–0.68 µKat/L
Age 12–14 years	15–35 U/L	0.26–0.60 µKat/L
Age 14–16 years	15–30 U/L	0.26–0.51 µKat/L

Increased: Acute myocardial infarction (rises 6–12 hours after injury, peaks at 18–24 hours, and returns to normal within 1 week; average increases are about fourfold; large infarcts may cause increases up to fifteenfold), alcoholism, calcium dust inhalation, cerebral infarction, cirrhosis, hepatitis (viral preicteric phase), intestinal injury, intramuscular injections, irradiation injury, lead, lipemia, liver disease, metal poisoning, musculoskeletal diseases, myoglobinuria, pancreatitis (acute), pulmonary infarction, renal infarction, toxic shock syndrome, trauma. Drugs include allopurinol, aluminum nicotinate, amantadine, ampicillin, anabolic steroids, androgens, ascorbic acid, asparaginase, aspirin, azaserine, baclofen, barbiturates, bethanechol chloride, bromocriptine mesylate, captopril, carmustine, carbenicillin, carbon tetrachloride, cardiotonic glycosides, cephalothin sodium, chlordiazepoxide, chloroquine, chlorpromazine hydrochloride, cholinergics, cholestyramine resin, cincophen, clindamycin, clofibrate, cloxacillin, codeine, colchisine, cortisone, cyclacillin, cycloserine, desipramine, dicumarol, digitalis, diphenylhydantoin, disopyramide phosphate, erythromycin, ethionamide, ethyl biscoumacetate, floxuridine, flurazepam, fosinopril, gentamicin sulfate, griseofulvin, guanethidine analogs, hydralazine, n-hydroxyacetamide, ibufenac, isoniazid, lincomycin, lorazepam, meperidine, methotrexate, methyldopa, metoprolol tartrate, mithramycin, morphine, nafcillin, nalidixic acid, narcotics, niacin, nifedipine, nitrofurantoin, oral contraceptives, oxacillin, *para*-aminosalicylic acid, phenothiazines, placebo, polycillin, procainamide hydrochloride, propranolol, propylthiouracil, prostaphlin, pyrantel pamoate, pyrazinamide, pyridoxine, rifampin, salicylates, sulfamethiazole, sulfamethoxypyridazine, theophylline, tetracycline, thiebendazole, thiothixene, thyroid hormone, tolbutamide, tolmetin sodium, troleandomycin, valproic acid, vitamin A, and vitamin B_6.

Decreased: Beriberi, diabetic ketoacidosis, hemodialysis (chronic), liver disease, and uremia (all conditions cause false decreases). Drugs include metronidazole, and trifluoperazine.

Description: A catalytic enzyme found primarily in the heart, liver, and muscle tissue. AST is found in two distinct forms or isoenzymes. c-AST is located in cytoplasm, and m-AST is found in mitochondria. Increases in the serum total AST level occur any time there is serious damage to cells. In addition, AST may be found in complex with IgA in hepatic cancer. AST is also evaluated in comparison with alanine aminotransferase (ALT) to serially monitor liver damage.

Professional Considerations:

1. Consent form NOT required.
2. Preparation:
   A. Tube: Red-top, red/gray-top, or gold-top.
   B. Do NOT draw during hemodialysis.
3. Procedure:
   A. Draw a 1-ml, nontraumatic blood sample.
4. Postprocedure care:
   A. Handle the specimen carefully, avoiding hemolysis.
5. Client and family teaching:
   A. Results are normally available within 12 hours.
6. Factors that affect results:
   A. Hemolysis of the specimen may cause falsely increased values.
7. Other data:
   A. There are no conditions that result in a true decrease in AST. All decreases listed are false decreases.

Bibliography:

Herlong HF: Approach to the patient with abnormal liver enzymes. Hosp Pract [Off] *29*(11):32–38, 1994.

Herrera JL: Abnormal liver enzyme levels. Clinical evaluation in asymptomatic patients. Postgrad Med *93*(2):119–120, 125, 129–132, 1993.

ASPERGILLUS ANTIBODY, SERUM

Norm: Negative <1:8. Suspicious infection: Fourfold rise in paired serum specimens. (Isolation does not prove pathogenesis for opportunistic fungi.)

Increased: Allergic bronchopulmonary aspergillosis, hypersensitivity to *Aspergillus,* immunodeficiency, leukemia, and pulmonary aspergilloma.

Description: *Aspergillus* species are saprophytic, opportunistic fungi that can grow on soil and organic materials and often become airborne in large numbers. Over 200 strains exist and may colonize the human body (respiratory tract, skin, nails, ear canal, burns) and become pathogenic in immunosuppressed clients or when they invade human tissue or when a client becomes sensitized to the organism. In this test, an indirect Coombs' test is performed to identify the presence of *Aspergillus* antibody.

Professional Considerations:

1. Consent form NOT required.
2. Preparation:
   A. Verify whether the client received antifungal skin testing within the last few weeks. Write the dates and names of such tests on the laboratory requisition.
   B. Tube: Red-top, red/gray-top, or gold-top.
3. Procedure:
   A. Collect a 10-ml blood sample as soon as possible after infection is suspected. Label the specimen as the acute sample.
   B. Repeat the test in 2–3 weeks and label the specimen as the convalescent sample.
4. Postprocedure care:
   A. Transport the specimen to the laboratory promptly and refrigerate at 25°C for no longer than 9 hours.
5. Client and family teaching:
   A. Return in 2–3 weeks for the convalescent sampling.
   B. Amphotericin B is used to treat aspergillosis.
6. Factors that affect results:
   A. False-negative results may occur in immunosuppressed clients.
   B. False-positive results may be caused by recent fungal antigen skin tests.
7. Other data:
   A. Five percent of clients without pulmonary aspergillosis or *Aspergillus* allergy will have *Aspergillus* antibodies.
   B. Identification requires that *Aspergillus* be directly identified in body tissues or fluids, be isolated in multiple specimens, and be identified by microscopic observation of characteristic conidial formation.
   C. The lysis-centrifugation method of culturing is the most sensitive method for detecting molds that cause fungemia. Blood cultures for *Aspergillus* are helpful in diagnosing an *Aspergillus* infection only when repeated lysis-centrifugation tests can distinguish between specimen contamination and pathogenesis based on the number of colonies appearing.
   D. A biopsy is required to diagnose invasive aspergillosis.

Bibliography:

Arruda LK, Muir A, Vailes LD, Selden RF, Platts-Mills TA, Chapman MD: Antibody responses to Aspergillus fumigatus allergens in patients with cystic fibrosis. Int Arch Allergy Appl Immunol *107*(1–3):410–411, 1995.

Caballero T, Ferrer A, Diaz-Pena JM, Garcia-Ara C, Pascual C, Martin-Esteban M: Childhood allergic bronchopulmonary aspergillosis. J Allergy Clin Immunol *95*(5 Pt 1):1044–1047, 1995.

Hearn VM, Pinel C, Blachier S, Ambroise-Thomas P, Grillot R: Specific antibody detection in invasive aspergillosis by analytical isoelectrofocusing and immunoblotting methods. J Clin Microbiol *33*(4):982–986, 1995.

Nikolaizik WH, Moser M, Crameri R, Little S, Warner JO, Blaser K, Schoni MH: Identification of allergic bronchopulmonary aspergillosis in cystic fibrosis patients by recombinant Aspergillus fumigatus I/a-specific serology. Am J Respir Crit Care Med *152*(2):634–639, 1995.

ASPIRIN, BLOOD
(see Salicylate, Blood)

ASPIRIN TOLERANCE TEST (ASA TOLERANCE TEST, BLEEDING TIME ASPIRIN TOLERANCE TEST), DIAGNOSTIC

Norm: Requires interpretation. Normal baseline Ivy bleeding time is 2–7 minutes. One study demonstrated bleeding time in normal clients to increase from 2.5 to 4.2 minutes at 2 hours after aspirin ingestion. Bleeding time should return to baseline by 96 hours after aspirin ingestion.

Increased: Bernard-Soulier syndrome, collagen vascular disease, Cushing's disease, disseminated intravascular coagulation, Glanzmann's thrombasthenia, gray platelet syndrome, hypersplenism, thrombocytopenia with immunosuppression, and von Willebrand's disease. Drugs include anticoagulants (oral), aspirin, indomethacin, and phenylbutazone.

Decreased: Drugs include (DDAVP) 1-deamino-8-D-arginine vasopressin.

Description: The Ivy bleeding time test is performed before and after aspirin ingestion for the purpose of evaluating the drug's effect on platelet function. In normal clients, aspirin ingestion has minimal influence on bleeding time.

Professional Considerations:

1. Consent form NOT required for most laboratories.

Risks:
Bleeding, ecchymoses, hematoma.

Contraindications:
In clients who require upper-extremity restraints, have edematous or very cold arms, or are prone to keloid formation. This test should not be performed if there are contraindications to placing or inflating a blood pressure cuff on the arm (casts, rash, A-V fistula). Other contraindications include platelet count <50,000/mm³, severe bleeding disorders, skin infectious diseases,

senile skin changes, or medications containing acetyl groups, such as those containing aspirin, within the prior 5 days.

2. Preparation:
   A. *See Client and family teaching.*
   B. Obtain povidone-iodine, a blood pressure cuff, a lancet, a stopwatch, and filter paper.
3. Procedure:
   A. Cleanse the volar aspect of the forearm with povidone-iodine and allow it to dry completely.
   B. Place the blood pressure cuff on the upper arm and inflate to 40 mmHg.
   C. Make two small incisions 2–3 mm deep on the prepared site. Start timing with the stopwatch.
   D. Remove blood from the wound with filter paper every 15 seconds until bleeding stops. Stop timing with the stopwatch.
   E. If bleeding time is more than 10 minutes, do not proceed further because this test would be contraindicated.
   F. Administer 10 grains (adults) or 5 grains (children weighing less than 32 kg) of aspirin orally.
   G. Repeat steps 3A through 3E after 2 hours.
4. Postprocedure care:
   A. If bleeding time is normal, apply a Band-Aid to the site. If bleeding time is prolonged, apply a pressure bandage to the site.
   B. Assess the site(s) for bleeding every 5 minutes for 1/2 hour. Observe for signs of site infection until healed.
5. Client and family teaching:
   A. Do not take aspirin for 5 days before this test.
   B. Bring reading material or some other diversion because the test takes 2–3 hours.
6. Factors that affect results:
   A. The most sensitive and reproducible measurements may be those taken from a horizontal incision.
7. Other data:
   A. The depth of the puncture with the lancet is difficult to standardize and results in poorly reproducible bleeding times.

Bibliography:

Doutremepuich C, deSeze O, LeRoy D, Lalanne MC, Anne MC: Aspirin at very ultra low dosage in healthy volunteers: Effects on bleeding time, platelet aggregation and coagulation. Haemostasis *20*(2):99–105, 1990.

Israels SJ, McNicol A, Robertson C, Gerrard JM: Platelet storage pool deficiency: Diagnosis in patients with prolonged bleeding times and normal platelet aggregation. Br J Haematol *75*(1):118–121, 1990.

AST
(see Aspartate Aminotransferase, Serum)

AT-III TEST
(see Antithrombin III Test, Diagnostic)

ATRIAL NATRIURETIC HORMONE (ANH, ATRIAL NATRIURETIC PEPTIDE, ANP, ATRIAL NATRIURETIC FACTOR), PLASMA

Norm: 20–77 pg/ml (20–77 ng/L SI units).

Increased: Congestive heart failure (acute), cardiovascular disease accompanied by increased preload, dysrhythmia (paroxysmal atrial tachycardia), pacemaker (atrial), small cell lung cancer, subarachnoid hemorrhage.

Decreased: Congestive heart failure (chronic). Drugs include prazosin, urapidil, and xipamide.

Description: Atrial natriuretic hormone (ANH) is released by cardiac cells in the atria of the heart in response to increased blood volume, which stimulates the volume receptors in the same area. ANH reduces renal reabsorption of sodium, thus having diuretic and antihypertensive effects. It also reduces blood pressure by blocking the secretion of aldosterone and renin and inhibiting the action of angiotensin II. The net effect is reduced preload, after-load, blood volume, and a reduction in systemic hypertension. This test helps identify a shortage of ANH as a cause of chronic congestive heart failure. Other causes of elevations in ANH are still under investigation.

Professional Considerations:
1. Consent form NOT required.
2. Preparation:
   A. Tube: Lavender-top. Also obtain ice.
3. Procedure:
   A. Draw a 5-ml blood sample.
4. Postprocedure care:
   A. Place the specimen immediately on ice and deliver it to the laboratory for immediate spinning.
5. Client and family teaching:
   A. Results are normally available within 24 hours.
6. Factors that affect results:
   A. Results are invalidated if the sample is not kept on ice until it is spun and frozen.
7. Other data:
   A. Secretion of ANH and vasopressin by small cell lung cancer may be a contributing factor to hyponatremia.

Bibliography:
Campling BG, Sarda IR, Baer KA, Pang SC, Baker HM, Lofters WS, Flynn TG: Secretion of atrial natriuretic peptide and vasopressin by small cell lung cancer. Cancer, 75(10):2442–2551, 1995.
Wazna-Wesly JM, Meranda DL, Carey P, Shenker Y: Effect of atrial natriuretic hormone on vasopressin and thirst response to osmotic stimulation in human subjects. J Lab Clin Med 125(6):734–742, 1995.

ATRIAL NATRIURETIC PEPTIDE
(see Atrial Natriuretic Hormone, Plasma)

AUDIOMETRY TEST (PURE TONE AUDIOMETRY AND SPEECH AUDIOMETRY), DIAGNOSTIC

Norm:

Adult	0–25 dB HL hearing sensitivity
Child	0–15 dB HL hearing sensitivity
Word discrimination score	Client is able to repeat list of spoken words with ≥90% accuracy.

Usage: Delineation of type and amount of hearing loss (i.e., conductive, sensorineural, or mixed).

Description: *Pure tone audiometry* is a hearing test using an audiometer that sends tones into the client's ear and vibrations through the bone. It measures the frequencies at which the client is able to hear 50% or more of the tones. The test is able to detect defects in air conduction (conductive hearing loss) through the use of tones and/or defects in air *and* bone conduction (sensorineural hearing loss) through the use of vibrations to help identify the amount and type of hearing loss present. *Speech audiometry* is a hearing test that determines the client's speech reception threshold and word discrimination score by measuring the number of words the client can repeat after hearing them delivered through earphones at precise decibel intensities. Speech audiometry helps differentiate between conductive and sensorineural hearing loss.

Professional Considerations:

1. Consent form NOT required.
2. Preparation:
   A. *See Client and family teaching.*
   B. Ensure that the external auditory canal is free of impacted cerumen.
   C. Obtain an audiometer, earphones, a vibrator for bone conduction testing, and an otoscope.
3. Procedure:
   A. A plastic tube may be inserted into the external auditory canal to maintain the canal's patency during testing with earphones.
   B. The earphones are placed over the ears and fastened in place.
   C. A preliminary tone is demonstrated for the client to become familiar with the test.
   D. The ear not being tested is masked with audiometer noise to prevent crossover interference and subsequent inaccurate estimation of hearing loss.
   E. *Air conduction testing:* The better ear is tested first. The client is instructed to give a signal each time a tone is heard. Starting with 1000 Hz, tones are delivered to the ear, decreasing by increments of 10 dB until a negative response is obtained. Tone levels are then increased in smaller increments, then decreased until the air conduction threshold level is obtained. The air conduction threshold level is the lowest Hz level at which the client is able to hear two out of three tones. This procedure is then repeated several times, starting with a different tone level each time (e.g., 2000, 4000, 8000, 1000, 500, and finally 250 Hz). The second ear is then tested in the same way. Finally, retesting is performed on each ear to determine test/retest reliability. Acceptable variation for retesting for each ear must be within 5 dB above or below the initial test result. Graphic recordings are made of the threshold levels.
   F. *Bone conduction testing:* The better ear is tested first. After removing the earphones, the bone conduction vibrator is held on the mastoid process of the ear. Starting with 250 Hz, tones are delivered to the ear, decreasing by increments at 10 dB until a negative

response is obtained. Tone levels are then increased in smaller increments, then decreased until the bone conduction threshold level is obtained. The bone conduction threshold level is the lowest Hz level at which the client is able to hear two out of three tones. This procedure is then repeated several times, starting with a different tone level each time (500, 1000, 2000, and finally, 4000 Hz). The second ear is then tested in the same way. Finally, retesting is performed on each ear to determine test/retest reliability. Acceptable variation for retesting for each ear must be within 5 dB above or below the initial test result. Graphic recordings are made of the threshold levels.
   G. *Speech reception threshold measurement:* Two-syllable, familiar, spoken words are delivered through the earphones. The client is asked to repeat each word. The speech reception threshold is the decibel level at which the client is able to restate correctly at least half of the words.
   H. *Word discrimination score:* One-syllable, familiar, phonetically balanced words are delivered through the earphones at 30 dB higher than the client's own speech reception threshold. The client is asked to repeat each word. Clients with conductive hearing loss will have a normal word discrimination score. Those with sensorineural hearing loss will have a lower than normal score.
   I. *Amount-of-hearing-loss calculation:* The amount of hearing loss, called the pure tone average (PTA), is calculated by averaging the air conduction threshold levels. Mild hearing loss demonstrates a PTA of 26–40 dB. Moderate hearing loss demonstrates a PTA of 41–55 dB. Moderately severe hearing loss demonstrates a PTA of 56–70 dB. Severe hearing loss demonstrates a PTA of 71–90 dB. Profound hearing loss demonstrates a PTA of over 90 dB.
   J. *Type-of-hearing-loss calculation:* The type of hearing loss is interpreted by examining the relationship between the air conduction threshold levels and the bone conduction threshold levels at the different frequencies. In sensorineural hearing loss, both thresholds are depressed to about the same degree. In conductive hearing loss, only the air conduction thresholds are depressed. In mixed hearing loss, both thresholds are depressed, but air conduction threshold levels are more depressed than bone conduction threshold levels.
4. Postprocedure care:
   A. Cleanse the earphones and otoscope with antiseptic.

5. Client and family teaching:
   A. Stay in an environment free of extremely loud noises for 16 hours prior to the test.
6. Factors that affect results:
   A. Testing should be performed in a very quiet environment for the most accurate results.
   B. The client should not be able to see the examiner as changes in tone level are made. Signals should be delivered in a nonrhythmic pattern.
   C. The client must be able to distinguish between the pure tones and tinnitus or vibrotactile stimulation.
   D. Test/retest differences of more than 10 dB may be due to unreliable equipment.
   E. The use of plastic tubes to maintain external auditory canal patency should be noted on the audiogram.
7. Other data:
   A. *See also Acoustic Immittance Test, Diagnostic.*

Bibliography:

Avan P, Bonfils P, Loth D, Teyssou M, Menguy C: Exploration of cochlear function by otoacoustic emissions: Relationship to pure-tone audiometry. Prog Brain Res *97*:67–75, 1993.

Holtby I, Forster DP: Evaluation of pure tone audiometry and impedance screening in infant school-children. J Epidemiol Community Health *46*(1): 21–25, 1992.

Longinotti C, Fowler CG: Pure tone audiometry. *In* Hamilton HK, Cahill M (eds): Diagnostics, 2nd ed. Springhouse, PA, Springhouse Corporation, 1986, pp 594–597.

Picard M, Ilecki HJ, Baxter JD: Clinical use of BOB-CAT: Testing reliability and validity of computerized pure-tone audiometry with noise-exposed workers, children and the aged. Audiology *32*(1):55–67, 1993.

Pringle MB, Thompson A, Reddy K: A comparison of speech audiometry and pure tone audiometry in patients with secretory otitis media. J Laryngol Otol *107*(9):787–789, 1993.

AUTOERYTHROCYTE SENSITIVITY TEST, DIAGNOSTIC

Norm: Negative.

Usage: Aids differential diagnosis of the etiology of spontaneous bruising and swelling.

Description: The rare autoerythrocyte sensitization syndrome (AESS) (Gardner-Diamond syndrome) is characterized by the appearance of sudden, spontaneous, and severe inflammatory purpura preceded by sensations of pain or burning at the site. It occurs most often in women, often with psychiatric disorders and normal coagulation studies. The bruising characteristically occurs in groups on the extremities and often at times of stress. The syndrome's cause is unknown, but some evidence points to an autoimmune sensitization to erythrocyte stroma because intradermal injection of the client's own RBCs stimulates development of ecchymosis. There is also some evidence for psychogenic etiology. This test helps differentiate self-mutilation from AESS. In a positive test, self-mutilation may be ruled out as the cause of the bruising.

Professional Considerations:

1. Consent form NOT required.

Risks:
Bleeding.

Contraindications:
In clients with known bleeding disorders or abnormal coagulation studies.

---

2. Preparation:
   A. Obtain alcohol wipes, a tourniquet, three needles, and two syringes.
3. Procedure:
   A. Draw a 1-ml blood sample, and place a fresh needle on the syringe.
   B. Cleanse a thigh site that is free of purpura with an alcohol wipe and allow it to dry. Inject 0.1 ml of the client's own whole blood intradermally into the thigh site. Mark the site by drawing a circle around it. A more specific method is to use 0.1 ml of the client's own washed erythrocyte stroma for the injection.
   C. Cleanse a site on the other thigh that is free of purpura with an alcohol wipe and allow it to dry. Inject 0.1 ml of 0.9% saline intradermally into the cleansed site as a control. Mark the site by drawing a circle around it.
   D. A positive reaction consists of the development of painful, edematous erythema at the site of the blood injection, with no reaction at the control site.
4. Postprocedure care:
   A. Assess the sites of injection for reaction, including pain, edema, and erythema.
5. Client and family teaching:
   A. This test helps determine if a process in the body is the cause of bruises for which a reasonable cause can't be found.
6. Factors that affect results:
   A. Uncooperative client.
7. Other data:
   A. None.

Bibliography:

Berman DA, Roenigk HH, Green D: Autoerythrocyte sensitization syndrome (psychogenic purpura). J Am Acad Dermatol 27(5 Pt 2):829–832, 1992.

Gomi H, Miura T: Autoerythrocyte sensitization syn-

drome with thrombocytosis. Dermatology 188(2): 160–162, 1994.

Kossard S, McGrath M, Finley G: Localised recurrent painful bruises. Gardner-Diamond syndrome of autoerythrocyte sensitisation, psychogenic purpura. Australas J Dermatol 34(1):37–38, 1993.

AUTOMATED REAGIN TESTING (ART), DIAGNOSTIC

Norm: Negative.

Titer	Interpretation
Nonreactive	Negative
≤1:8	False-positive
1:9–1:32	Primary stage syphilis(requires interpretation)
>1:32	Secondary stage syphilis

Positive: Syphilis. (*See Factors that affect results* for biologic false-positives.)

Description: A nonspecific, nontreponemal test used for syphilis screening and monitoring of response to therapy in the postchancre period of the primary stage and in the secondary stage when treponemal antibodies are more difficult to detect. When *Treponema pallidum,* the causative agent of syphilis, invades human tissue, reagin is produced and can be isolated from 7 to 21 days after the appearance of the chancre. Results are reported as the highest titer that produces a positive reaction.

Professional Considerations:

1. Consent form NOT required.
2. Preparation:
   A. Tube: Red-top, red/gray-top, or gold-top.
   B. *See Client and family teaching.*
3. Procedure:
   A. Draw a 5-ml blood sample.
4. Postprocedure care:
   A. None.
5. Client and family teaching:
   A. Do not drink alcohol for 24 hours before testing.
   B. Weekly testing for 2 months is recommended before syphilis can be ruled out.
   C. If testing positive:
      i. Notify all sexual contacts from the last 90 days (if early stage) to be tested for syphilis.
      ii. Syphilis can be cured with antibiotics. These may worsen the symptoms for the first 24 hours.
      iii. Do not have sex for 2 months and until after repeat testing has confirmed that the syphilis is cured. Use condoms after that for 2 years.

Return for repeat testing every 3–4 months for the next 2 years to make sure the disease is cured.
      iv. Do not become pregnant for 2 years because syphilis can be transmitted to the fetus.
      v. If left untreated, syphilis can damage many body organs, including the brain, over several years.
6. Factors that affect results:
   A. Reject hemolyzed specimens.
   B. False-negative results may occur prior to the appearance of the chancre in the initial stage of syphilis or during the tertiary stage.
   C. False-negative results may be due to ingestion of alcohol within 24 hours prior to specimen collection.
   D. Biological false-positive results lasting up to 6 months may be due to bejel, chickenpox, DPT immunization, hepatitis (infectious), malaria, measles, mononucleosis (infectious), pneumonia (atypical, pneumococcal), scarlet fever, smallpox vaccination, subacute bacterial endocarditis, or tuberculosis.
   E. Biological false-positive results lasting more than 6 months may be due to hyperglobulinemia, leprosy, leptospirosis, periarteritis nodosa, pinta, rheumatic fever, rheumatoid arthritis, systemic lupus erythematosus (SLE), thyroiditis, vaccinia, or Yaws.
7. Other data:
   A. Suspected false-positive results should be followed by repeat testing at 3, 6, and 9 months.

Bibliography:

Ernst AA, Martin DH: High syphilis rates among cocaine abusers identified in an emergency department. Sex Transm Dis 20(2):66–69, 1993.

Ernst AA, Romolo R, Nick T: Emergency department screening for syphilis in pregnant women without prenatal care. Ann Emerg Med 22(5):781–785, 1993.

Lowhagen GB: Syphilis: Test procedures and therapeutic strategies. Semin Dermatol 9(2):152–159, 1990.

AUTOPSY, DIAGNOSTIC

Norm: Requires interpretation.

Usage: Determination of cause and manner of death, reporting of contagious diseases, quality assurance, teaching and legal purposes.

Description: A postmortem examination and dissection of a corpse. The procedure is usually performed by two pathologists and an assistant.

Professional Considerations:

1. Consent form IS required.
2. Preparation:
   A. After death, determination should be made whether the circumstances of death require that the coroner be notified. Coroner's cases usually include unexpected death, death within 24 hours of admission to a hospital, death while under anesthesia, suspected homicides or suicides, accidental or violent deaths, deaths of clients with contagious disease, or any death occurring under unusual circumstances or involving the public interest. If any of these conditions apply, the coroner should be called by the physician for a determination of the need for an autopsy. If the coroner determines that an autopsy is required, the family should be notified, but next-of-kin permission is not needed.
   B. Autopsy may also be performed without next-of-kin permission when it is necessary to complete the death certificate or when the deceased client has given consent before death.
   C. When the need for an autopsy is determined, other than for coroner's cases, next-of-kin permission must be obtained via signature on the consent form or possibly via a witnessed telephone conversation between the physician and the next of kin. Guidelines vary depending on area laws and institution.
   D. All invasive lines, tubes, and devices should be left intact in the body.
   E. Obtain an autopsy knife with a blade, a scalpel with a disposable blade, toothed forceps, forceps with serrated tips, a medium-long knife with a blade, a long knife with a blade, scissors with one pointed and one blunt blade, scissors with two blunt blades, scissors for cutting bones, intestinal scissors (enterotome), scissors with long curved blades, a 1-mm probe, a metal metric rule, a costatome, rib shears, intestinal clamps, a vibratory saw with large blades, an amputating saw, a band saw, a hammer with a hook, a chisel, bone-cutting forceps, a meter stick, a body scale, an organ scale, balances, a ladle, a graduate, sea sponges, pans with fixative, pan and pail containers, a large container for fixation of gross organs in solution, fixing solution, string, needles, abrasive hand stone and oil, and a slicing machine.
   F. Obtain containers for the samples for toxicologic studies, culture, or cytology.
   G. Make sure that the autopsy permit name and identification number correspond to the name and identification number on the client's body. If there are no tags on the body, have the nurse, physician, or relative identify the body.
   H. Wear a mask, an eye or face shield, gloves, and a plastic apron.
3. Procedure:
   A. *Recording:* The sequence of events and findings of autopsy are recorded either by concurrently written notes or by a foot-operated dictation machine. Descriptions of the body and organs, including condition, arrangement, and weight of the organs, are made and recorded as the dissection is performed.
   B. *Sequence:* The sequence of the autopsy may vary. In cases in which a specific cause of death is suspected, the appropriate body cavity for that cause may be opened first. A usual autopsy proceeds in the following order: external examination; incision of the skin, ribs, and sternoclavicular joints; examination of thoracic and abdominal cavities; removal and examination of the organs of the trunk (thymus, heart, lungs, mediastinal lymph nodes, spleen, intestines, diaphragm, liver, gallbladder, pancreas, stomach, duodenum, rectum, spermatic cords, testes, adrenals, uterus, ovarian tubes, ovaries, bone marrow [sternal, vertebral, femoral], neck organs, bones, joints, and muscles); and removal and examination of the organs of the cranium and spine (brain, eyes, ears, paranasal sinuses, pituitary gland, spinal cord, and spinal root ganglia).
   C. *Content of assessment:* In the external examination, the body is observed and palpated, and the length, size, and weight are measured. Rigor mortis, edema, or jaundice are noted. The head, lymph nodes, and genitalia are assessed. A "Y" incision is then made on the torso, and the thoracic and abdominal cavities are assessed. The arrangement and status of the organs and the presence of adhesions, excess fluid, or gas is noted. As they are excised, the weight, size, and contents of the organs and blood vessels are as-

sessed. Biopsies, sections, and smears may be taken throughout the process. The organs of the cranium and spine are then assessed. An incision is made from ear to ear over the vertex of the cranium, and the scalp is separated from the skull with a scalpel. The anterior portion of the scalp is pulled down over the forehead and face. After the skull is opened with a saw and the top portion removed, the brain is removed and placed in 10% formalin. Biopsies of the brain are taken if a virus is suspected. The remainder of the head organs are removed and examined. Formalin is injected into the eyes before removal. The spinal cord is then removed and examined for lesions. Complete organs or portions of organs may be fixed in solution for later reference. An alternative method is to remove the trunk organs in one block, with examination of organs on a dissecting table.

4. Postprocedure care:
   A. The body is cleansed and the incisions are sewn. The body may or may not be embalmed at this point.

5. Client and family teaching:
   A. Autopsy incisions will not be visible should an open-casket wake be held.
   B. Durable Power of Attorney for Health Care does NOT apply after death.
6. Factors that affect results:
   A. A routine hospital autopsy should be interrupted and the coroner notified if any unexpected findings that may be of traumatic origin are encountered.
7. Other data:
   A. The order of authority for granting permission for an autopsy is normally spouse, adult child, parent, adult sibling, other relative, and any other person accepting responsibility for burial of the body. This order may vary by area laws.
   B. Be aware of religious considerations concerning autopsy.

Bibliography:

Powers JM: Practice guidelines for autopsy pathology. Autopsy procedures for brain, spinal cord, and neuromuscular system. Autopsy Committee of the College of American Pathologists. Arch Pathol Lab Med *119*(9):777–783, 1995.

Veress B, Alafuzoff I: Clinical diagnostic accuracy audited by autopsy in a university hospital in two eras. Qual Assur Health Care *5*(4):281–286, 1993.

BACTERIAL SEROLOGY, BLOOD

Norm: Requires interpretation.

Usage: Suspected bacterial infections. Most commonly, legionellosis, leptospirosis, *Mycoplasma, Rickettsia* (typhus fever, spotted fever, scrub typhus, trench fever, and Q fever), staphylococcal, streptococcal, and *Yersinia.*

Description: An indirect method of identifying blood bacterial infections by assessing the host response (antibody production) to the invading microorganism. Results may be reported qualitatively (positive, negative) or quantitatively (titers) and should be interpreted in consideration of the predictive value of the specific test. Bacterial serology produces faster results than cultures of some organisms that take several weeks to grow.

Professional Considerations:

1. Consent form NOT required.
2. Preparation:
   A. Tube: Red-top, red/gray-top, or gold-top.
   B. *See Client and family teaching.*
3. Procedure:
   A. Two blood samples, 1 week apart, should be drawn. The first specimen should be drawn as soon as possible after the onset of symptoms and then frozen. The second specimen should be drawn at least 1 week later, and then both specimens should be assayed at the same time.
   B. Draw a 10-ml blood sample.
4. Postprocedure care:
   A. None.
5. Client and family teaching:
   A. Fast for 8 hours prior to testing.
   B. Return in 1 week for follow-up testing.
6. Factors that affect results:
   A. Reject hemolyzed or grossly lipemic specimens.
   B. False-negative results may be due to immunosuppression or antibiotic therapy.
7. Other data:
   A. A single positive antibody is insufficient to support a diagnosis because low persistent levels are common.

Bibliography:

Leinonen M: Serological diagnosis of pneumococcal pneumonia—will it ever become a clinical reality? Semin Respir Infect *9*(3):189–191, 1994.

Stein A, Raoult D: Q fever endocarditis. Eur Heart J *16* (Suppl B):19–23, 1995.

BAEP

(see Brainstem Auditory Evoked Potential, Diagnostic)

BANDING IN GENETIC DISORDERS, DIAGNOSTIC

Norm: Cytogenic techniques with numerical designations map each chromosome for abnormalities.

Female   44 autosomes + 2X chromosomes
         karyotype: 46,XX
Male   44 autosomes + 1X and 1Y chromosomes
         karyotype: 46,XY

Usage: Assists in the diagnosis of genetic and neoplastic disorders.

Description: Banding techniques are used for chromosome identification. Human chromosomes are numbered in 23 pairs. Each chromosome pair has a unique pattern with intricate detail produced by different distributions of DNA in the chromosomes. Banding helps detect different regions of the same chromosome for use in identification of both the chromosome and chromosomal abnormalities. R banding uses a reverse Giemsa stain called acridine orange, which produces reverse contrast to the light Q bands detected by quinacrine mustard and dark and light crossband G bands detected with trypsin and Giemsa stain. R dark bands are useful for observing the very dark ends of chromosomes. The chromosome count per cell and banded karyotype with interpretation is included in the testing.

Professional Considerations:
1. Consent form NOT required.
2. Preparation:
   A. Tube: Green-top.
3. Procedure:
   A. Draw a 4-ml blood sample.
4. Postprocedure care:
   A. None.
5. Client and family teaching:
   A. Results are normally available in 1–2 weeks.
   B. Refer the client with abnormal results for genetic counseling.
6. Factors that affect results:
   A. Heparin in the specimen collection tube must be sodium heparin.
7. Other data:
   A. This method is used widely in European countries, especially France.

Bibliography:

Delach JA, Rosengren SS, Kaplan L, Greenstein RM, Cassidy SB, Benn PA: Comparison of high resolution chromosome banding and fluorescence in situ hybridization (FISH) for the laboratory evaluation of Prader-Willi syndrome and Angelman syndrome [see comments]. Am J Med Genet 52(1):85–91, 1994.

Fletcher J: Immortalized cell lines. Chromosome preparation and banding. Methods Mol Biol 29:51–57, 1994.

Huang B, Meyer JM, Jackson-Cook CK: Heritability and heteromorphic distributions of AluI chromosome banding variants in twins. Am J Med Genet 57(3):429–436, 1995.

Imai HT: A theoretical approach to chromosome banding pattern analysis. Jpn J Genet 68(2):97–118, 1993.

BANDS, BLOOD
(see Differential Leukocyte Count, Peripheral Blood)

BARBITURATES, QUANTITATIVE, BLOOD

Norm: Negative.

Levels During Barbiturate Therapy		SI Units
Amobarbital		
Therapeutic	1–5 µg/ml	4.4–22.1 µmol/L
Toxic	>10 µg/ml	>44.2 µmol/L
Panic	>70 µg/ml	>309.4 µmol/L
Butabarbital		
Therapeutic	1–2 µg/ml	4.4–8.4 µmol/L
Toxic	10–40 µg/ml	44.2–176.8µmol/L
Pentobarbital		
Therapeutic	1–5 µg/ml	4.4–22.1 µmol/L
Therapeutic coma	20–50 µg/ml	88.4–221 µmol/L
Toxic	>10 µg/ml	>44.2 µmol/L
Panic	>60 µg/ml	>265.2 µmol/L
Phenobarbital		
Therapeutic	15–40 µg/ml	66.3–176.8 µmol/L
Toxic	35–80 µg/ml	154.7–353.6 µmol/L
Panic	>100 µg/ml	>442 µmol/L

Levels during Barbiturate Therapy (continued)		SI Units
Secobarbital		
Therapeutic	1–2 µg/ml	4.2–8.4 µmol/L
Toxic	3–40 µg/ml	13.3–176.8 µmol/L
Panic	>50 µg/ml	>221 µmol/L

Panic Level Symptoms and Treatment:

Symptoms: Central nervous system depression (ataxia, confusion, drowsiness) progressing to respiratory depression, hypotension, and coma. Death may occur with ingestion of 1 g of pentobarbital or with 1.5 g of phenobarbital or 2 g of secobarbital.

Treatment:
Protect airway and provide oxygen.
Gastric lavage with tap water or saline up to 24 hours after ingestion.
Do NOT induce emesis.
Administer activated charcoal.
Diurese with urea if hemodynamically stable and adequate renal function is present.
Alkalinize urine.
Delay absorption by subcutaneous or intramuscular routes by packing sites with ice or using tourniquets.

	Removed by Hemodialysis	Removed by Hemoperfusion	Removed by Peritoneal Dialysis
Amobarbital	Yes	Yes	No
Pentobarbital	No	Yes	
Phenobarbital	Yes	Yes	Yes
Secobarbital	No		No

Usage: Drug abuse, overdose, suicide attempt, and monitoring blood levels during barbiturate therapy.

Description: Barbiturates are a group of central nervous system depressants used as hypnotics, anticonvulsants, sedatives, and preoperatively. They are thought to act at the level of the reticular activating system. Barbiturates are metabolized in the liver and excreted by the kidneys. Overdose may lead to coma and death from respiratory arrest.

Professional Considerations:
1. Consent form NOT required unless the specimen may be used as legal evidence.
2. Preparation:
   A. Tube: Red-top, red/gray-top, gold-top, lavender-top, or black-top.
   B. Do NOT draw the sample for amobarbital or phenobarbital level during hemodialysis.
   C. Sample for pentobarbital MAY be drawn during hemodialysis.
3. Procedure:
   A. Collection should be witnessed if the specimen may be used as legal evidence.
   B. Draw a 2-ml blood sample.

4. Postprocedure care:
   A. If the specimen may be used as legal evidence, write the client's name, the exact time of the blood draw, and the contents of the tube on the tube label and the laboratory requisition. Sign and have the witness sign the laboratory requisition. Transport the specimen to the laboratory in a sealed plastic bag labeled as legal evidence.
   B. Refrigerate the specimen if not tested immediately.
5. Client and family teaching:
   A. For intentional overdose, refer the client and family for crisis intervention.
   B. Client with panic level symptoms will require intensive care for at least 24 hours. If a lethal dose was ingested, death is possible.
   C. Physical and psychological addiction occur in clients taking barbiturates over a long period of time. Serious withdrawal symptoms that may occur include severe headache, body pains, numbness or burning in the arms and legs, seizures, hallucinations, chest pain, sweating, and breathing difficulties. Seek medical treatment if any of these symptoms occur.
   D. If activated charcoal was given for elevated levels, the client should drink 4–6 glasses of water each day for 2

days to prevent constipation. Activated charcoal will also cause stools to be black for a few days.

6. Factors that affect results:
   A. Reject hemolyzed specimens to avoid falsely decreased results.
   B. Drugs that may cause falsely elevated results include atropine sulfate, dexochlorpheniramine, ethotoin, glutethimide, meperidine hydrochloride, phenytoin, salicylamide, and theophylline.
   C. Amobarbital cross-reactivity may occur with any of the other barbiturates. Pentobarbital cross-reactivity may occur with secobarbital or phenobarbital.

7. Other data:
   A. Panic level symptoms may occur with smaller doses if alcohol is also ingested.

Bibliography:

Ferslew KE, Hagardorn AN, McCormick WF: Application of micellar electrokinetic capillary chromatography to forensic analysis of barbiturates in biological fluids. J Forensic Sci *40*(2):245–249, 1995.

Kojima T, Taniguchi T, Yashiki M, Miyazaki T, Iwasaki Y, Mikami T, Ohtani M: A rapid method for detecting barbiturates in serum using EI-SIM. Int J Legal Med *107*(1):21–24, 1994.

BARIUM ENEMA (BE), DIAGNOSTIC

Norm: Requires interpretation. Characteristics examined include filling, passage pattern of barium, and the contour, patency, position, and mucosal pattern of the colon.

Usage: Part of the diagnostic work-up for bowel obstruction, celiac sprue, colorectal cancer, diverticulitis, diverticulosis, gastroenteritis, Hirschsprung's disease, intestinal cancer, intestinal polyps, intussusception, irritable bowel syndrome, and ulcerative colitis.

Description: A fluoroscopic and radiographic examination of the large intestine after rectal instillation of barium sulfate with or without air for the purpose of identifying structural abnormalities or slowing of normal intestinal activity.

Professional Considerations:

1. Consent form NOT required.

Risks:

Constipation, dizziness, infection, intestinal impaction, rectal or bowel perforation, recto/vaginal perforation, and vasovagal reaction.

Contraindications:

Severe active ulcerative colitis accompanied by toxicity and megacolon, perforated intestine, toxic megacolon, tachycardia.

2. Preparation:
   A. Laxatives and/or cathartic suppositories are usually indicated the day prior to and on the morning of the test to facilitate complete emptying of the intestines. However, they may be contraindicated for certain clients with conditions such as ulcerative colitis or intestinal obstruction.
   B. If the client is pregnant, notify the physician prior to exam preparation.
   C. *See Client and family teaching.*

3. Procedure:
   A. After baseline abdominal radiographs are taken, the client lies in a Sims' position on a tilt table and receives a slow administration of barium sulfate or barium sulfate with air insufflation via a rectal tube.
   B. As the client assumes different positions, the filling is monitored by fluoroscopy.
   C. Spot films are taken during and at the completion of the filling.
   D. The rectal tube is withdrawn and the barium expelled, after which another film is taken to examine the pattern of the intestinal mucosa and determine how well emptying has occurred.

4. Postprocedure care:
   A. Where not contraindicated, the client should increase fluid intake for 24–48 hours.
   B. Where not contraindicated, a mild cathartic may be prescribed to facilitate emptying of the barium from the intestine.
   C. Stools should be inspected by the client or the health care professional for passage of barium for 48 hours. Barium stools will look chalky white in color.
   D. Failure to have a bowel movement within 2 days after the test should be reported to the physician.

5. Client and family teaching:
   A. It is important to have the bowel emptied of stool before the procedure. A low-residue diet may be prescribed for 1–3 days prior to the test. (Kember et al., 1995 found that a low-residue diet did not offer any advantage over a normal diet in preparation for the test if purgatives were used.)
   B. A clear liquid diet is usually prescribed for 1 day prior to and on the morning of the test. A normal diet may be resumed after the procedure.
   C. A laxative may be prescribed prior to and after the procedure.

D. The procedure takes about 60 minutes. It is important to hold your breath when you are asked to do so during the procedure.

E. Make sure all of the barium empties from the intestinal tract after the procedure. Drinking fluids and taking laxatives or enemas after the procedure may be prescribed for this purpose.

F. *See Postprocedure care.*

G. Call the physician if stomach or lower abdominal pain is experienced or if stools are much smaller than the normal diameter.

6. Factors that affect results:
   A. Failure to achieve complete emptying of the intestinal tract prior to the test may necessitate a repeated barium enema.

7. Other data:
   A. The barium enema should be performed before a barium swallow.

Bibliography:

Hough DM, Malone DE, Rawlinson J, De Gara CJ, Moote DJ, Irvine EJ, Somers S, Stevenson GW: Colon cancer detection: an algorithm using endoscopy and barium enema. Clin Radiol 49(3): 170–175, 1994.

Kember PG, McBride KD, Tweed CS, Collins MC: A blinded prospective trial of low-residue versus normal diet in preparation for barium enema. Br J Radiol 68(806):128–129, 1995.

Kewenter J, Brevinge H, Engaras B, Haglind E: The yield of flexible sigmoidoscopy and double-contrast barium enema in the diagnosis of neoplasms in the large bowel in patients with a positive Hemoccult test [see comments]. Endoscopy 27(2): 159–163, 1995.

Paulfrey ME: Barium enema. Lower gastrointestinal examination. In Hamilton HK, Cahill M (eds): Diagnostics, 2nd ed. Springhouse, PA, Springhouse Corporation, 1986, pp 723–825.

Scullion DA, Wetton CW, Davies C, Whitaker L, Shorvon PJ: The use of air or CO_2 as insufflation agents for double contrast barium enema (DCBE): Is there a qualitative difference? Clin Radiol 50(8):558–561, 1995.

BARIUM SWALLOW, DIAGNOSTIC

Norm: Requires interpretation. Characteristics examined include filling of the pharynx and esophagus, mucosal patterns, and esophageal size, contour, and peristaltic motion.

Usage: Part of the diagnostic workup for achalasia, duodenal ulcer, esophageal diverticula, esophageal varices, head and neck cancer, hiatal hernia, pharyngeal muscle disorders, polyps, strictures, stomach cancer, and ulcers.

Description: A fluoroscopic and radiographic examination of the pharynx and esophagus as mixtures of barium sulfate are swallowed. The test takes 20–30 minutes.

Professional Considerations:

1. Consent form NOT required.

Risks:

Constipation, dizziness, intestinal impaction, vasovagal reaction.

Contraindications:

During pregnancy; clients with upper tract dysphagia, due to the risk of barium aspiration; and in clients with intestinal obstruction.

2. Preparation:
   A. *See Client and family teaching.*

3. Procedure:
   A. The client is positioned on a tilt table.
   B. After baseline fluoroscopic examinations of the heart, lungs, and abdomen, the client takes one swallow of a thick barium mixture while cineradiographic films are taken.
   C. The client then takes several swallows of a thin barium mixture while its passage is recorded via fluoroscopy and radiography.
   D. The process is repeated with the table tilted to various positions.
   E. About 350–450 ml of barium is swallowed during the entire procedure.

4. Postprocedure care:
   A. Where not contraindicated, the client should increase fluid intake for 24–48 hours after the test.
   B. Where not contraindicated, a mild cathartic may be prescribed to facilitate emptying of barium from the gastrointestinal tract.
   C. Failure to have a bowel movement within 2 days should be reported to the physician.

5. Client and family teaching:
   A. Fast for 8 hours prior to the procedure.
   B. This procedure lasts approximately 15 minutes.
   C. Make sure all of the barium empties from the intestinal tract after the procedure. Drinking fluids and taking laxatives or enemas after the procedure may be prescribed for this purpose.
   D. *See Postprocedure care.*
   E. Call the physician if stomach or lower abdominal pain is experienced or if stools are much smaller than the normal diameter.

6. Factors that affect results:
   A. None.

7. Other data:
   A. None.

Bibliography:

Ginai AZ, van Buuren HR, Hop WC, Schalm SW: Oesophageal varices: How reliable is a barium swallow? Br J Radiol 66(784):322–326, 1993.

Paulfrey ME: Barium swallow. Esophagography. In

Hamilton HK, Cahill M (eds): Diagnostics, 2nd ed. Springhouse, PA, Springhouse Corporation, 1986, pp 723–785.

Penington GR: Severe complications following a barium swallow investigation for dysphagia [see comments]. Med J Aust 159(11–12):764–765, 1993.

BARR BODY ANALYSIS BUCCAL SMEAR FOR STAINING SEX CHROMATIN MASS, DIAGNOSTIC

Norm:

	Number of Barr Bodies
Normal female (XX)	1
Normal male (XO)	0
Turner syndrome (female) (XO)	0
Klinefelter syndrome (male) (XXY)	1
Klinefelter syndrome (male) (48 XXXY)	2
Klinefelter syndrome (male) (49 XXXYY)	2
Klinefelter syndrome (male) (49XXXXY)	3

Usage: Screening for sex chromosome abnormalities.

Description: A Barr body, or sex chromatin body, is a tightly coiled, X chromosome lying against the nuclear membrane of female cells or any cell with more than one X chromosome. It shows up as a dark-staining body in the shape of a half-moon and is absent in male cells. Barr bodies are believed to function in early embryonic development and later become inactivated to maintain gene balance of Xs to autosomes. The number of Barr bodies in a client is one less than the number of Xs.

Professional Considerations:

1. Consent form NOT required.
2. Preparation:
   A. Rinse the mouth with mouthwash.
   B. Obtain a metal spatula, saline, two slides, and preservative.
3. Procedure:
   A. Gently scrape the buccal mucosa with the metal spatula dipped in saline.
   B. Clean the spatula and repeat the procedure gently but firmly.
   C. Smear the material on the two slides and place them in the preservative.
4. Postprocedure care:
   A. Label the container of the slides with the client's name, the date, and the contents.
5. Client and family teaching:
   A. Refer the client with abnormal results for genetic counseling.
6. Factors that affect results:
   A. None known.
7. Other data:
   A. Barr bodies do not give any information about Y chromosomes.

B. Human chromosome analysis, rather than buccal smears, should be used for evaluations of newborns with ambiguous genitalia.

Bibliography:

Danso AP, Tobani C: Cytogenetics in urology. Cent Afr J Med 40(10):281–286, 1994.

Simpson JL, Ljungqvist A, de la Chapelle A, Ferguson-Smith MA, Genel M, Carlson AS, Ehrhardt AA, Ferris E: Gender verification in competitive sports. Sports Med 16(5):305–315, 1993.

BASAL GASTRIC SECRETION TEST

(see Hollander Test, Diagnostic)

BASAL METABOLIC RATE (BMR), DIAGNOSTIC

Norm: −20% to +5% of standardized norms.

Increased: Anemia, congestive heart failure, hyperthyroidism, intercurrent serious illness, and presence of stimulating drugs.

Decreased: Adrenalin imbalance, female athletes (Dahlstron 1995), hypothyroidism, obesity, and sedation.

Description: A rarely used indirect method of measuring the body's response to circulating thyroid hormone in the resting state. The BMR was the most reliable method for this purpose before the development of T_3 and T_4 assays. The major form of energy expenditure in the resting client is body heat, which consumes oxygen. The amount of oxygen consumed by the client can be used to estimate heat production and, therefore, basal metabolism. The test has poor reliability in mild thyroid disorders because the BMR is affected by many variables, including obesity, adrenal dysfunction, and anxiety.

Professional Considerations:

1. Consent form NOT required.
2. Preparation:
   A. The client should be in a resting state when evaluated. The test is usually performed in the early morning.
   B. Ensure that the client completely understands the procedure and the necessity to remain relaxed and calm throughout the test.
   C. *See Client and family teaching.*
3. Procedure:
   A. The client breathes in and out through the mouthpiece of a closed-circuit spirometer for 2–6 minutes.
   B. Oxygen consumption values are compared to a table of standardized normals for clients of the same sex and age and with the same body surface area.
4. Postprocedure care:
   A. Normal diet and activity may be resumed.
5. Client and family teaching:
   A. Fast from food and fluids for 12 hours before testing.
   B. Plan to be relaxed and rested when tested. It is important to remain in this state throughout the test.
6. Factors that affect results:
   A. Medications or caffeine before testing will increase the BMR.
   B. The presence of any anxiety will prevent a true basal reading.
7. Other data:
   A. After age 50, the BMR drops 10–15% due to loss of lean body mass.

Bibliography:

Dahlstrom M, Jansson E, Ekman M, Kaijser L: Do highly physically active females have a lowered basal metabolic rate? Scand J Med Sci Sports 5(2):81–87, 1995.

Hayter JE, Henry CJ: A re-examination of basal metabolic rate predictive equations: The importance of geographic origin of subjects in sample selection. Eur J Clin Nutr 48(10):702–707, 1994.

Pannemans DL, Westerterp KR: Energy expenditure, physical activity and basal metabolic rate of elderly subjects. Br J Nutr 73(4):571–581, 1995

Taaffe DR, Pruitt L, Reim J, Butterfield G, Marcus R: Effect of sustained resistance training on basal metabolic rate in older women. J Am Geriatr Soc 43(5):465–471, 1995.

Yoshida T, Sakane N, Umekawa T, Kondo M: Relationship between basal metabolic rate, thermogenic response to caffeine, and body weight loss following combined low calorie and exercise treatment in obese women. Int J Obes Relat Metab Disord 18(5):345–350, 1994.

BASOPHILS
(see Differential Leukocyte Count, Peripheral Blood)

BASOS
(see Differential Leukocyte Count, Peripheral Blood)

BE
(see Barium Enema, Diagnostic)

BENCE JONES PROTEIN, URINE

Norm: Negative.

Positive: Amyloidosis (primary), benign monoclonal gammopathy, cryoglobulinemia, Fanconi's syndrome (adult), hyperparathyroidism, multiple myeloma, osteomalacia, and Waldenstrom's macroglobulinemia.

Description: A low-molecular weight, light-chain immunoglobulin synthesized by malignant plasma cells in the bone marrow and initially broken down and reabsorbed by the kidneys. In multiple myeloma, such a large amount of these proteins are produced that they exceed the kidneys' capacity to metabolize them. This causes them to spill into the urine. Prolonged production of Bence Jones protein eventually causes degeneration of the renal tubular cells, and the protein accumulates in the tubules, causing inclusions that may lead to renal failure. Subsequently, increasing amounts of the protein spill into the urine and can be detected by thermal coagulation and acid tests and confirmed by immunoelectrophoresis.

Professional Considerations:

1. Consent form NOT required.
2. Preparation:
   A. Obtain a clean specimen container without preservatives.
3. Procedure:
   A. Obtain a 25-ml first morning-voided, random urine specimen in a clean container. A fresh specimen may be taken from a urinary drainage bag.
4. Postprocedure care:
   A. Send the specimen to the laboratory and refrigerate.
5. Client and family teaching:
   A. Results are normally available within 24 hours.

6. Factors that affect results:
   A. Failure to refrigerate the specimen may result in false-negative results.
   B. False-positive results may be caused by chronic renal insufficiency, connective tissue diseases (such as rheumatoid arthritis, systemic lupus erythematosus (SLE), scleroderma, polymyositis, or Wegener's granulomatosis), and other malignancies (lymphoma; leukemia; and metastatic cancer of the lung, or of the gastrointestinal or genitourinary tracts).
   C. Drugs that may cause false-positive results include aminosalicylic acid, cephaloridine, chlorpromazine, penicillin (high doses), promazine hydrochloride, sulfisoxazole, and tolbutamide.
   D. False-negative results may be caused by very alkaline urine and severe urinary tract infections in which urea splitting occurs.
7. Other data:
   A. In light-chain disease, pancytopenia is absent.

Bibliography:

Aguzzi F, Gasparro C, Bergami MR, Merlini M: High-sensitivity electrophoretic method for the detection of Bence Jones protein and for the study of proteinuria in unconcentrated urines. Ann Clin Biochem.*30*(Pt 3):287–292, 1993.

Macart M, Forzy G, Gerbaut L, Vekich AJ, Guilbaud JC: Measuring urinary protein with the new BioRad reagent kit: Evaluation and comparison with five other methods. Ann Biol Clin (Paris) *52*(5):355–360, 1994.

BENEDICT'S TEST, DIAGNOSTIC

Norm: Blue or negative.

Usage: Screening for disorders of glucose or amino acid metabolism.

Positive: Congenital deficiency of homogentisic acid, hyperglycemia, and melituria.

Description: A copper-reduction test that detects sugars, reducing substances, and homogentisic acid in the urine. Clients with a hereditary absence of homogentisic acid oxidase are unable to metabolize homogentisic acid, a by-product of phenylalanine and tyrosine metabolism. Some of the unmetabolized homogentisic acid is excreted in the urine, and the remainder causes ochronosis, a condition characterized by joint deposition of homogentisic acid that eventually causes joint degeneration. Benedict's solution is made of quantitative and qualitative reagent, each containing cupric sulfate dissolved in sodium sulfate, but in different concentrations. When Benedict's solution is heated in the presence of sugar, homogentisic acid, or other reducing substances, the cupric sulfate is reduced and a yellow to red precipitate forms.

Professional Considerations:

1. Consent form NOT required.
2. Preparation:
   A. Obtain a clean container, two Pyrex test tubes, a wooden test-tube holder, a beaker, a Bunsen burner, a pipette, a dropper, and Benedict's solution.
3. Procedure:
   A. Obtain a 10-ml random urine specimen in a clean container without preservative. A fresh specimen may be taken from a urinary drainage bag.
   B. Pipette 5 ml of Benedict's solution into a Pyrex test tube.
   C. Add 8 drops of urine.
   D. Mix the test tube gently.
   E. Using the wooden test-tube holder, boil the mixture over a Bunsen burner for 2 minutes, then cool to room temperature.
   F. Observe the color of the test-tube mixture and interpret the results as noted in the table below.
4. Postprocedure care:
   A. Refrigerate the specimen if the test is not performed immediately.
5. Client and family teaching:
   A. The specimen must be free of stool and toilet tissue.
   B. Results are normally available within 24 hours.
6. Factors that affect results:
   A. Results are most accurate on a freshly voided specimen.
   B. Glycosuria will cause a false-positive

Color	Glucose Quantitative	Glucose Qualitative
Blue	0 mmol/L	Negative
Green	14 mmol/L	Trace
Green + yellow precipitate	28 mmol/L	1+
Yellow-green	56 mmol/L	2+
Brown	83 mmol/L	3+
Orange-red	>110 mmol/L	4+

result when Benedict's solution is used for detection of homogentisic acid.

C. Drugs and reducing substances that may cause false-positive results include ampicillin, ampicillin sodium, aminosalicylic acid, ascorbic acid, camphor, carbamazepine, cefaclor, cefadroxil monohydrate, cefamandole nafate, cefazolin sodium, cefonicid sodium, cefoperazone sodium, ceforanide, cefotaxime sodium, cefotetan disodium, cefoxitin sodium, ceftazidime, ceftizoxime sodium, ceftriaxone, cefuroxime axetil, cephalexin, cephaloridine, cephalothin sodium, cephradine, cephapirin sodium, chloral hydrate, chloramphenicol, chloroform, cimetidine, formaldehyde, fructose, galactose, glucosamine, glucuronic acid, homogentisic acid, levodopa, metaxalone, moxalactam disodium, nalidixic acid, nitrofurantoin, nitrofurantoin sodium, paraldehyde, penicillin G benzathine, penicillin G potassium, penicillin G procaine, phenol, probenecid, salicylates, streptomycin sulfate, sulfonamides, tetracyclines, turpentine, and uric acid.

7. Other data:

A. Any reducing substance found in the urine may cause false-positive results.

B. Use other methods of glucose measurement to help differentiate glucosuria from urine containing homogentisic acid.

Bibliography:

Hegedus ZL, Nayak U: Homogentisic acid and structurally related compounds as intermediates in plasma soluble melanin formation and in tissue toxicities. Arch Int Physiol Biochim Biophys *102*(3):175–181, 1994.

BENTIROMIDE TEST

(see Chymex Test for Pancreatic Function, Diagnostic)

BENZODIAZEPINES, PLASMA AND URINE

Norm: Blood and urine: Negative.

Urine Panic Level: >200 ng/ml.

Therapeutic Plasma Values		SI Units
Chlordiazepoxide	700–1000 ng/ml	2.34–3.34 µmol/L
Panic level	>5000 ng/ml	>16.70 µmol/L
Clonazepam	15–60 ng/ml	48–190 nmol/L
Panic level	>80 ng/ml	>254 nmol/L
Diazepam	100–1000 ng/ml	0.35–3.51 µmol/L
Panic level	>5000 ng/ml	>17.55 µmol/L
Flurazepam	Information not available	
Panic level	>0.2 µg/ml	>0.5 µmol/L
Lorazepam	50–240 ng/ml	156–746 nmol/L
Midazolam	Information not available	
Oxazepam	Information not available	
Prazepam	0.12–1.0 µg/ml	0.4–3.1 µmol/L
Temazepam	Information not available	
Triazolam	Information not available	

Panic Level Symptoms and Treatment:

Symptoms: Somnolence, confusion, ataxia, diminished reflexes, vertigo, slurred speech, respiratory depression, and coma.

Treatment:

Gastric lavage within warm tap water or 0.9% saline if within 2 hours of ingestion.

Administer activated charcoal.

Monitor for central nervous system depression.

Protect airway. Support breathing with oxygen and mechanical ventilation if necessary.

Do NOT induce emesis.

Implement seizure precautions.

Flumazenil has been used as a competitive antagonist to reverse the profound effects of benzodiazepine overdose. Use of Flumazenil is contraindicated if concomitant tricyclic antidepressants were taken.

Do NOT use barbiturates.

Forced diuresis and/or hemodialysis will NOT remove benzodiazepines. No information was found on whether peritoneal dialysis will remove these drugs.

Positive: Drugs include chlorazepate dipotassium, chlordiazepoxide, clonazepam, diazepam, flurazepam hydrochloride, lorazepam, midazolam, oxazepam, prazepam, temazepam, and triazolam.

Usage: Suspected drug overdose and drug-use screening.

Description: Benzodiazepines are nonbarbiturate, sedative hypnotic, and anticonvulsant schedule-IV drugs used to treat anxiety and insomnia. They are strongly protein bound, metabolized in the liver, and excreted in urine and feces. Benzodiazepines have long half-lives of 30–200 hours. Overdose may lead to coma and death from respiratory arrest. Serum levels are used to determine therapeutic and toxic levels and the full range of benzodiazepines, but are not generally helpful in gauging the effects of overdose. Detection of the presence, but not the levels, of only those benzodiazepines that are excreted as oxazepam (above) is performed via urine assay.

Professional Considerations:

1. Consent form NOT required.
2. Preparation:
   A. *Blood test:* Tube: Lavender-top. MAY be drawn during hemodialysis.
   B. *Urine test:* Obtain a clean specimen container.
3. Procedure:
   A. *Blood test:* Draw a 3-ml blood sample.
   B. *Urine test:* Collect a 30-ml, clean, voided urine sample. A fresh specimen may be taken from a urinary drainage bag.
4. Postprocedure care:
   A. Refrigerate the urine specimen until tested.
5. Client and family teaching:
   A. Offer substance abuse and/or crisis intervention counseling if applicable.
   B. Referrals to appropriate rehabilitation centers and therapeutic community programs should be offered to all addicted clients who may be interested.
   C. Results are normally available within 24 hours.
   D. If activated charcoal was given for elevated levels, the client should drink 4–6 glasses of water each day for 2 days to prevent constipation. Activated charcoal will also cause stools to be black for a few days.
6. Factors that affect results:
   A. False-positive urine test results are seen with oxaprozin.
7. Other data:
   A. The positive predictive value for detecting benzodiazepines in urine using the Triage visual panel was 77%.
   B. Withdrawal symptoms may occur after even a single large dose of benzodiazepines.

Bibliography:

Matuch-Hite T, Jones P Jr, Moriarity J: Interference of oxaprozin with benzodiazepines via enzyme immunoassay technique [letter]. J Anal Toxicol *19*(2):130, 1995.

Needleman SB, Porvaznik M: Identification of parent benzodiazepines by gas chromatography/mass spectroscopy (GC/MS) from urinary extracts treated with B-glucuronidase. Forensic Sci Int *73*(1):49–60, 1995.

Schenck CH, Mahowald MW: Long-term, nightly benzodiazepine treatment of injurious parasomnias and other disorders of disrupted nocturnal sleep in 170 adults. Am J Med *100*(3):333–337, 1996.

Valentine JL, Komoroski EM: Use of visual panel detection method for drugs of abuse: Clinical and laboratory experience with children and adolescents. J Pediatr *126*(1):135–140, 1995.

BERNSTEIN TEST
(see Acid Perfusion Test, Diagnostic)

BETA-1C, SERUM
(see C3 Complement, Serum)

BETA-GLUCOSIDASE, DIAGNOSTIC

Norm: Positive.

Usage: Screening for Gaucher's disease, a sphingolipid storage disease.

Description: Beta-glucosidase deficiency is an autosomal recessive disease resulting in a gangliosidosis called Gaucher's disease, which is quickly fatal in infants but progresses more slowly in older children. Beta-glucosidase is an enzyme found in peripheral blood leukocytes that normally metabolizes the glycolipid glucocerebroside. In Gaucher's disease, glucocerebroside accumulates and causes splenomegaly, hepatomegaly, anemia, thrombocytopenia, erosion of long bones and pelvic bones, and mental retardation (in infantile form).

Professional Considerations:

1. Consent form NOT required.
2. Preparation:
   A. Tube: Green-top and container of ice.
   B. If the specimen must be sent to an outside laboratory for processing, notify the in-house laboratory that a specimen will be drawn.
3. Procedure:
   A. Draw a 7-ml blood sample.
   B. Place the specimen on ice.

4. Postprocedure care:
   A. Transport the specimen to the laboratory immediately.
   B. For transport to an outside laboratory, the specimen must be transported in an ice bath the same day.
5. Client and family teaching:
   A. Results are normally available within 72 hours.
6. Factors that affect results:
   A. Results are invalid for specimens not placed on ice.
7. Other data:
   A. Anemia can be severe enough to cause respiratory difficulty.
   B. Enzyme infusion therapy is recommended treatment in type 3 Gaucher's disease.

Bibliography:

Corssmit EP, Hollak CE, Endert E, van Oers MH, Sauerwein HP, Romijn JA: Increased basal glucose production in type I Gaucher's disease. J Clin Endocrinol Metab *80*(9):2653–2657, 1995.

Erikson A, Astrom M, Mansson JE: Enzyme infusion therapy in the Norrbottnian (type 3) Gaucher disease. Neuropediatrics *26*(4):203–207, 1995.

Niederau C, Holderer A, Heintges T, Strohmeyer G: Glucocerebrosidase for treatment of Gaucher's disease: First German long-term results. J Hepatol *21*(4):610–617, 1994.

BETA-LACTAMASE PRODUCTION TEST, DIAGNOSTIC
(see Penicillinase Test, Diagnostic)

BETA₂-MICROGLOBULIN, BLOOD AND 24-HOUR URINE

Norm:

		SI units
Blood	<2 µg/ml	<170 nmol/L
Urine	<120 µg/24 hours	<10 mmol/day

Increased: AIDS, aminoglycoside toxicity, Crohn's disease, hepatitis, leukemia (chronic lymphocytic), malignancies (some), multiple myeloma, renal disease (glomerular), sarcoidosis, and vasculitis.

Description: An amino acid peptide component of lymphocytes that increases in inflammatory conditions and when lymphocyte turnover increases, such as in lymphocytic leukemia or when T-lymphocyte helper (OKT4) cells are attacked by human immunodeficiency virus. Beta₂-microglobulin is metabolized by the renal tubules, with over 99% being reabsorbed. Blood beta₂-microglobulin becomes elevated with malfunctioning glomeruli, but drops with malfunctioning tubules. The test (both blood and urine) is most often used for evaluation of renal disease, chronic lymphocytic leukemia, and AIDS. Although beta₂-microglobulin levels rise with HIV infection, the levels do not always correlate with the stages of the infection.

Professional Considerations:

1. Consent form NOT required.
2. Preparation:
   A. Tube: Lavender-top or 3-L urine collection container and toluene preservative.
   B. Follow protective isolation precautions for clients with AIDS.
   C. Write the exact beginning time of the 24-hour urine collection on the laboratory requisition.
3. Procedure:
   A. Draw a 2-ml blood sample.
   B. For 24-hour urine, discard the first morning-urine specimen. Save all urine voided for 24 hours in a refrigerated, clean, 3-L container to which toluene preservative has been added. Document the quantity of urine output during the specimen collection period. Include voiding at the end of the 24-hour period. For catheterized clients, keep the drainage bag on ice and empty the urine into the collection container hourly.
4. Postprocedure care:
   A. Compare the quantity of urine in the specimen container with urinary output records. If the specimen contains less urine than was recorded as output, some of the sample may have been discarded, thus invalidating the results.
   B. Document the quantity of urine output and the ending time for the 24-hour collection period on the laboratory requisition.
5. Client and family teaching:
   A. Offer support and referrals for AIDS, cancer, or Crohn's disease as appropriate. The national AIDS Hotline is (800)342-AIDS. AIDS Clinical Trials Information Services, National Institutes of Health: (301)496–8210.
   B. Save all urine voided in the 24-hour period. Urinate before defecating to avoid loss of urine. If any urine is acci-

dentally discarded, discard the entire specimen and restart the collection the next day.
C. Results are normally available within 24 hours.
6. Factors that affect results:
    A. Results are invalidated if the client has received radioactive dyes within 1 week prior to the test.
7. Other data:
    A. Results can be normal in HIV infection.
    B. *See also Acquired Immune Deficiency Syndrome (AIDS) Evaluation Battery, Diagnostic.*

Bibliography:

Honkanen E, Pettersson T, Teppo AM: Urinary alpha 1- and beta 2-microglobulin in light chain protein- uria. Clin Nephrol *44*(1):22–27, 1995.

Ricci G, D'Ambrosi A, Resca D, Masotti M, Alvisi V: Comparison of serum total sialic acid, C-reactive protein, alpha 1-acid glycoprotein and beta 2-mi- croglobulin in patients with non-malignant bowel disease. Biomed Pharmacother *49*(5):259–262, 1995.

Saito A, Takagi T, Sugiura K, Ono M, Minakuchi K, Teroaka S, Ota K: Maintaining low concentra- tions of plasma beta-2-microglobulin through continuous slow haemofiltration. Nephrol Dial Transplant *10* (Suppl 3):52–56, 1995.

BETKE-KLEIHAUER STAIN (FETAL HEMOGLOBIN STAIN, KLEIHAUER-BETKE STAIN, K-B), DIAGNOSTIC

Norm:

	HbF Cells
Adults	< 2%
Children	
Newborn	60–90%
6 months	<5%
1 year	<2%

Usage: Assessment of fetal-maternal hemorrhage in the newborn for deter- mination of the amount of Rh im- mune globulin (RhoGAM) needed.

Increased: Anemia (aplastic, congen- ital hemolytic, myeloblastic, myeloph- thisic, untreated pernicious, refractory, sickle cell, sideroblastic, spherocytic), diabetes, erythroleukemia, Fanconi's anemia, hereditary persistence of fetal hemoglobin (HPFH), hyperthyroidism, hypothyroidism, infants (small-for-ges-

tational-age, with chronic intrauterine anoxia, with developmental abnormali- ties), leakage of fetal hemoglobin into maternal bloodstream, leukemia (all types, acute, chronic), myelofibrosis, paroxysmal nocturnal hemoglobin- uria, pregnancy, thalassemia, thyrotox- icosis, and trisomy D syndrome. Drugs include anticonvulsants.

Description: This test measures the amount of hemoglobin present in the fetal form (HbF) compared to the adult form (HbA). When blood is pre- sent in the stool, emesis, or mucus of a newborn, this test differentiates "swallowed blood syndrome" as a re- sult of maternal bleeding from infant gastrointestinal hemorrhage.

Professional Considerations:
1. Consent form NOT required.
2. Preparation:
    A. Tube: Lavender-top, or obtain a clean container for the mucus specimen.
3. Procedure:
    A. Draw a 2-ml blood sample.
    B. For gastrointestinal or mucus speci- mens from an infant, use a clean glass or plastic container to collect a small amount of emesis, stool, or mucus.
4. Postprocedure care:
    A. None.
5. Client and family teaching:
    A. Cord blood may be sent as a positive control.
    B. Results are normally available within 24 hours.
6. Factors that affect results:
    A. Reject hemolyzed specimens or speci- mens received more than 6 hours after collection.
    B. Smears must be fixed within 1 hour after preparation.
7. Other data:
    A. A newborn cord blood specimen is rec- ommended as a source of fetal blood to be used as a positive control.

Bibliography:

Bruner JP, Rosemond RL: Twin-to-twin transfusion syndrome: A subset of the twin oligohydramnios- polyhydramnios sequence. Am J Obstet Gynecol *169*(4):925–930, 1993.

Saade GR, Moise KJ, Belfort MA, Hesketh DE, Carpen- ter RJ: Fetal and neonatal hematologic parame- ters in red cell alloimmunization: Predicting the need for late neonatal transfusions. Fetal Diagn Ther *8*(3):161–164, 1993.

BICARBONATE (HCO₃), PLASMA

Norm:

		SI Units
Adult		
Normal venous range	22–29 mEq/L	22–29 mmol/L
Normal arterial range	21–28 mEq/L	21–28 mmol/L
Newborn		
Normal venous range	16–24 mEq/L	16–24 mmol/L
Panic venous range	<15 mEq/L	<15 mmol/L
	or >35 mEq/L	or >35 mmol/L

Increased: Anoxia, burns (extensive), compensated respiratory acidosis, gastric lavage, fat embolism, gastric suction, hypokalemia, metabolic alkalosis, and vomiting. Drugs include barbiturates (causing respiratory depression), corticosteroids (chronic use), diuretics, laxative (abuse), opiates (causing respiratory depression), oral glutamine, and alkaline salts.

Decreased: Compensated respiratory alkalosis, diabetes mellitus, diarrhea, ethylene glycol poisoning, metabolic acidosis, and renal failure. Drugs include acid salts, ammonium chloride, acetazolamide, cholestyramine, cyclosporine, methanol, and salicylate toxicity.

Description: Bicarbonate is part of the bicarbonate-carbonic acid buffering system and is mainly responsible for regulating the pH of body fluids. It also facilitates the transport of carbon dioxide from the body tissues to the lungs. In the digestive tract, bicarbonate is secreted by the pancreas and liver into the duodenum to neutralize the acid chyme entering from the stomach. Serum bicarbonate levels are approximated from the serum carbon dioxide level minus 1.2 mmol (the average concentration of carbonic acid). More accurate diagnoses regarding the buffering system can be determined by obtaining an arterial blood sample for blood gas analysis.

Professional Considerations:

1. Consent form NOT required.
2. Preparation:
   A. Tube: Green-top.
3. Procedure:
   A. Draw a 1-ml blood sample anaerobically.
4. Postprocedure care:
   A. None.
5. Client and family teaching:
   A. Results are normally available within 2 hours.
   B. Treatment may require intravenous access.
6. Factors that affect results:
   A. Ingestion of acidic or alkaline solutions may cause increased or decreased results respectively.
7. Other data:
   A. Bicarbonate does not improve the hemodynamic condition of critically ill clients with lactic acidosis.
   B. Prolonged tourniquet application before phlebotomy does not lower serum bicarbonate.

Bibliography:

Bany-Mohammed FM, Macknin ML, van Lente F, Medendorp SV: The effect of prolonged tourniquet application on serum bicarbonate. Cleve Clin J Med 62(1):68–70, 1995.

Cooper DJ, Walley KR, Wiggs BR, Russell JA: Bicarbonate does not improve hemodynamics in critically ill patients who have lactic acidosis: A prospective controlled clinical study. Ann Intern Med 112(7):492–498, 1990.

Welbourne TC: Increased plasma bicarbonate and growth hormone after oral glutamine load. Am J Clin Nutr 61(5):1058–1061, 1995.

BILE, URINE

Norm:

Reagent screening test: negative.

Quantitative: <0.2mg/dl.

Increased or Positive: Biliary tract obstruction, cirrhosis, hepatitis (acute, alcoholic, chronic, drug-induced), hyperthyroidism, infectious mononucleosis, septicemia, and tumor (biliary tract, liver).

Description: This is a routine test used to detect unsuspected liver disease where jaundice is absent. The test is also used in the differential diagnosis of jaundice because plasma bilirubin present as a result of hemolytic disorders exists in a water-soluble form that cannot be filtered by the kidneys. Bilirubinuria is detected by a yellow foam that forms in a shaken specimen or by a yellow-orange to brown urine color. Serial levels can guide clinical management of liver and biliary disorders.

Professional Considerations:

1. Consent form NOT required.
2. Preparation:
   A. Obtain a clean container and a paper bag.
3. Procedure:
   A. Obtain a 50-ml random urine specimen in a clean glass or plastic container. A fresh specimen may be taken from a urinary drainage bag.
4. Postprocedure care:
   A. Write the collection time on the laboratory requisition.
   B. Place the specimen in the paper bag and transport it to the laboratory immediately.
   C. Refrigerate the specimen if the test will not be performed within 1 hour of collection.
5. Client and family teaching:
   A. Inform the nurse immediately after the specimen has been obtained.
   B. Do not contaminate the urine specimen with stool.
   C. Results are normally available within 24 hours.
6. Factors that affect results:
   A. Reject specimens received more than 1 hour after collection.
   B. Drugs that may cause false-positive results include chlorpromazine, mefenamic acid, phenothiazines, and salicylates.
   C. Drugs that may cause false-negative results include ascorbic acid, ethoxazene hydrochloride, and phenazopyridine.
   D. False-positive results may be caused by contamination of the specimen with stool.
   E. False-negative results may be caused by prolonged exposure of the specimen to room temperature or to light.
7. Other data:
   A. Bilirubinuria is an insensitive indicator of liver disease.
   B. Urinary bile acids are higher in formula-fed infants compared to breast-fed infants.

Bibliography:

Clayton PT, Castells M, Mieli-Vergani G, Lawson AM: Familial giant cell hepatitis with low bile acid concentrations and increased urinary excretion of specific bile alcohols: A new inborn error of bile acid synthesis? Pediatr Res *37*(4 Pt 1):424–431, 1995.

Inoue T: Developmental pattern of urinary ketonic bile acids during the neonatal period. Kurume Med J *42*(2):79–86, 1995.

Wahlen E, Strandvik B: Effects of different formula feeds on the developmental pattern of urinary bile acid excretion in infants. J Pediatr Gastroenterol Nutr *18*(1):9–19, 1994.

BILE FLUID EXAMINATION, DIAGNOSTIC

Norm: Absent or rare cholesterol and calcium bilirubinate crystals. More than 10 crystals per glass slide is considered positive.

Positive: Carcinoma, cholelithiasis, cholecystitis, idiopathic pancreatitis, and parasitism.

Negative: Not applicable.

Description: Bile fluid is examined for cholesterol monohydrate, calcium bilirubinate, and calcium carbonate crystals in order to identify cholelithiasis and cholecystitis when the usual tests (including imaging) are negative.

Professional Considerations:

1. Consent form IS required. See individual procedure listings for procedure-specific risks and contraindications.
2. Preparation:
   A. *See Client and family teaching.*
   B. Obtain specimen traps, suction tubing, cholecystokinin, and a gastroduodenal tube.
   C. Establish patent IV access.
3. Procedure:
   A. A double-lumen gastroduodenal tube is inserted into the duodenum and the position is confirmed by fluoroscopy. Alternatively, an upper gastrointestinal endoscope may be inserted into the duodenum.
   B. A 100-U dose of cholecystokinin is given intravenously over 1 minute to induce gallbladder contraction.
   C. Bile is then aspirated over 10–30 minutes in sequence according to its color (yellow from the common bile duct, green and more viscous bile from the gallbladder, and pale yellow from the liver and/or hepatic ducts).
4. Postprocedure care:
   A. Assess for pain or intestinal discomfort.
5. Client and family teaching:
   A. Fast for 8–12 hours prior to the test.
   B. The procedure takes 45 minutes.
   C. Results are normally available within 24 hours.

6. Factors that affect results:
   A. A specimen pH <4.5 may produce false-positive bilirubin precipitate, which may be confused with calcium bilirubinate.
7. Other data:
   A. Imaging studies may show negative results for gallbladder disease.
   B. Three or more of the following cytologic criteria are observed in carcinoma cases more often than in non-carcinoma cases: loss of honeycomb arrangement, enlarged nuclei, loss of polarity, bloody background, flat nuclei, and cell-in-cell arrangement.

Bibliography:

Nakajima T, Tajima Y, Sugano I, Nagao K, Sakuma A, Koyama Y, Kondo Y: Multivariate statistical analysis of bile cytology. Acta Cytol *38*(1):51–55, 1995.

Stolk MF, van Erpecum KJ, Renooij W, Portincasa P, van de Heij-Henegouwen GP: Gallbladder emptying in vivo, bile composition, and nucleation of patients with cholesterol gallstones. Gastroenterology *108*(6):1882–1888, 1995.

BILE SALT ABSORPTION TEST (BILE SALT BREATH TEST, C-14 CHOLATE BREATH TEST), DIAGNOSTIC

Norm: Negative breath test and negative stool specimen.

Usage: Assessment of bacterial overgrowth in the digestive tract, disease of the ileum, and malabsorption of bile salts.

Description: A screening test for disorders of bile acid malabsorption. This test measures both fecal fat excretion and exhaled radioactive carbon dioxide released after C-14 triolein ingestion. In the normal client, bile salts are completely reabsorbed in the intestinal tract before reaching the colon. In the presence of ileal disease or dysfunction, some unabsorbed bile salts reach the colon and are oxidized by colonic bacteria. In GI tract bacterial overgrowth, bacteria act on bile salts before they can be reabsorbed. Abnormal fecal fat excretion indicates fat malabsorption due to impaired synthesis and/or secretion of bile salts.

Professional Considerations:

1. Consent form NOT required.

2. Preparation:
   A. Antibiotics are usually discontinued 4 weeks prior to the test.
   B. *See Client and family teaching.*
   C. Obtain a special commode and a 24-hour stool collection container from the gastrointestinal laboratory.
3. Procedure:
   A. A baseline breath sample is taken.
   B. The client ingests a C-14 triolein test meal containing 60 g of fat.
   C. Hourly breath samples are obtained and measured for $14\text{-}CO_2$ for 2–7 hours.
   D. A 72-hour stool specimen is collected.
   E. An increase in $14\text{-}CO_2$ of more than 50% in the breath test or an increase in fecal fat of more than 12% is a positive test.
4. Postprocedure care:
   A. None.
5. Client and family teaching:
   A. Fast for 8 hours prior to the test.
   B. Results are normally available 24 hours after the 72-hour stool collection is completed.
6. Factors that affect results:
   A. Results are questionable in diabetes mellitus, gross obesity, hyperlipidemia, pyrexial illness, thyroid disorders, and chronic lung disease because metabolic changes in these conditions may affect $14\text{-}CO_2$ excretion independently of fat absorption.
   B. H_2-receptor antagonists have increased bile acid deconjugation due to bacterial overgrowth.
7. Other data:
   A. Results are difficult to interpret in the presence of liver disease because of altered hepatic lipid metabolism.

Bibliography:

O'Brien S, Mulcahy H, Fenlon H, O'Broin A, Casey M, Burke A, FitzGerald MX, Hegarty JE: Intestinal bile acid malabsorption in cystic fibrosis. Gut *34*(8):1137–1141, 1993.

Shindo K, Fukumura M: Effect of H_2-receptor antagonists on bile acid metabolism. J Investig Med *43*(2):170–177, 1995.

BILIRUBIN, DIRECT (CONJUGATED), SERUM

(see Bilirubin, Serum)

BILIRUBIN, INDIRECT (UNCONJUGATED, FREE), SERUM

(see Bilirubin, Serum)

BILIRUBIN (TOTAL, DIRECT [CONJUGATED] AND INDIRECT [UNCONJUGATED]), SERUM

Norm:

		SI Units
Total bilirubin		
1 month–adult	<1.5 mg/dl	1.7–20.5 µmol/L
Premature infant		
Cord	<2.8 mg/dl	<48 µmol/L
24 hours	1–6 mg/dl	17–103 µmol/L
48 hours	6–8 mg/dl	103–137 µmol/L
3–5 days	10–12 mg/dl	171–205 µmol/L
Full-term infant		
Cord	<2.8 mg/dl	<48 µmol/L
24 hours	2–6 mg/dl	34–103 µmol/L
48 hours	6–7 mg/dl	103–120 µmol/L
3–5 days	4–6 mg/dl	68–103 µmol/L
Direct bilirubin	0.0–0.3 mg/dl	1.7–5.1 µmol/L
Indirect bilirubin	0.1–1.0 mg/dl	1.7–17.1 µmol/L

Increased Total Bilirubin: Alcoholism, anemia (pernicious), biliary calculi, biliary obstruction, biliary scar tissue, carcinoma of pancreas head, cholangitis, cirrhosis, Crigler-Najjar syndrome, Dubin-Johnson syndrome, erythroblastosis fetalis, fasting (prolonged), Gilbert's disease, hemolysis (autoimmune), hemorrhage, hepatitis (alcoholic, infectious, toxic, viral, obstructive), hereditary spherocytosis, impaired liver function, malaria, mononucleosis (infectious), myocardial infarction, pancreatitis (biliary tract origin), pulmonary embolism, sickle cell anemia, toxic shock syndrome, transfusion reactions, and tumor. Drugs include acetazolamide, aminophenol, androgens, antimalarials, ascorbic acid, asparaginase, aspirin, barbiturates, carmustine, cholinergics, chlordiazepoxide, chloroquine hydrochloride, chloroquine phosphate, chlorothiazide sodium, chlorpromazine hydrochloride, cholinergics, clindamycin, dextran, diazoxide, dicoumarol, dicumarol, epinephrine bitartrate, epinephrine borate, epinephrine hydrochloride, erythromycin, ethanol, ethoxazene hydrochloride, floxuridine, flurazepam, fosinopril, histidine, hydroxychloroquine sulfate, imipramine, indican, indomethacin, iproniazid, iron, isoniazid, isoproterenol hydrochloride, levodopa, lincomycin, meclofamate, methanol, methyldopa, methyltestosterone, morphine sulfate, niacin, novobiocin, novobiocin sodium, oral contraceptives, penicillin, phenazopyridine, phenelzine sulfate, phenothiazines, phenprocoumon, phenylbutazone, primaquine phosphate, procainamide hydrochloride, protein, pyrazinamide, pyrimethamine, quinacrine hydrochloride, quinidine gluconate, quinidine polygalacturonate, quinidine sulfate, radiographic dyes, rifampin, streptomycin sulfate, tetracyclines, theophylline, thiazide diuretics, tyrosine, vitamin A, and warfarin sodium.

Increased Direct Bilirubin: Biliary obstruction, carcinoma of head of the pancreas, cirrhosis, Dubin-Johnson syndrome, hepatitis (acute, alcoholic, infectious, viral, toxic), and rotor syndrome. Also, drugs that increase total bilirubin levels.

Increased Indirect Bilirubin: Anemia (pernicious), autoimmune hemolysis, Bartter's syndrome, cirrhosis (acute, alcoholic, nonalcoholic), Crigler-Najjar syndrome, erythroblastosis fetalis, Gilbert's disease, hepatitis (all types), hereditary spherocytosis, intracavitary and soft tissue hemorrhage, malaria, myocardial infarction, septicemia, sickle cell disease, and transfusion reaction (hemolytic). Also, drugs that increase total bilirubin levels.

Decreased Total, Direct, and Indirect Bilirubin: Not clinically significant. Drugs include barbiturates, caffeine, chlorine, citrate, corticosteroids, dicophane, ethanol penicillin, protein, salicylates, sulfonamides, thioridazine, and urea.

Description: Bilirubin is produced in the liver, spleen, and bone marrow and is also a by-product of hemoglobin breakdown. Total bilirubin levels can be broken down into direct (conjugated) bilirubin, which is primarily excreted via the intestinal tract, and indirect (free) bilirubin, which circulates primarily in the bloodstream. Total bilirubin levels rise with any type of jaundice, whereas direct and indirect levels rise depending on the etiology of the jaundice. Direct (conjugated) bilirubin is that portion of bilirubin which is normally excreted primarily by the gastrointestinal tract, with only small amounts entering the bloodstream. When obstructive or hepatic jaundice occurs, increasing amounts of conjugated bilirubin enter the bloodstream, rather than the gastrointestinal tract, and they are filtered and excreted by the kidneys. Indirect bilirubin (free or unconjugated bilirubin) is the portion of bilirubin that normally circulates in the bloodstream. When hemolytic jaundice occurs, increasing amounts of free bilirubin accumulate in the bloodstream as a result of increased hemoglobin breakdown. There is no direct laboratory test for indirect bilirubin; rather, it is a calculation of total bilirubin minus direct bilirubin.

Professional Considerations:

1. Consent form NOT required.
2. Preparation:
   A. *See Client and family teaching.*
   B. Tube: Red-top, red/gray-top, or gold-top or a lancet and capillary tube for heelstick specimens. Also obtain foil.
   C. Do NOT draw blood during hemodialysis.
3. Procedure:
   A. Draw a 1-ml blood sample.
   B. For babies, collect heelstick blood in a capillary tube. Prewarming the heel is not necessary. Cleanse the lateral curvature of the heel with an alcohol wipe and allow it to dry. Puncture the lateral curvature of the heel with a lancet and collect blood in a capillary tube. Avoid puncturing the posterior curvature of the heel.
4. Postprocedure care:
   A. Leave the heelstick site open to air.
   B. Protect the sample from light. Wrap it

in foil or place it in a darkened refrigerator if the test will not be run immediately.
5. Client and family teaching:
   A. Eat a diet low in yellow foods (e.g., carrots, yams, yellow beans, pumpkin) for 3–4 days before sampling.
   B. Fast for 4 hours before sampling.
   C. Serum levels will be elevated with the use of alcohol, morphine, theophylline, ascorbic acid, and aspirin.
   D. Results are normally available within 24 hours.
6. Factors that affect results:
   A. Reject hemolyzed or grossly lipemic specimens.
   B. Results are invalidated if the client received a radioactive scan within 24 hours prior to the test.
   C. Cord blood values may be elevated.
   D. Drugs that may cause falsely elevated values include acetazolamide, androgens, chlordiazepoxide, chlordiazepoxide hydrochloride, chlorpromazine, erythromycin, erythromycin ethylsuccinate, indomethacin, isoniazid, methanol, nitrofurantoin, nitrofurantoin sodium, oxacillin sodium, oxyphenbutazone, phenothiazines, phenylbutazone, salicylates, sulfinpyrazone, sulfonylureas, sulfonamides, and vitamin A.
7. Other data:
   A. Indirect bilirubin levels may increase in hemolytic disease in the newborn to >20 mg/dl.
   B. Neonate treatment for serum bilirubin >15 mg/dl may include exchange transfusion or phototherapy. Phototherapy converts bilirubin into a colorless compound that has no effects on the neonate.
   C. Biliary atresia can be differentiated from infantile hepatitis using bilirubin conjugates with Micronex chromatography.

Bibliography:

Ito F, Ando H, Watanabe Y, Ito T: Serum bilirubin fractions in cholestatic pediatric patients: Determination with Micronex high-performance liquid chromatography. J Pediatr Surg *30*(4):596–599, 1995.

Lott JA, Doumas BT: Direct and total bilirubin tests: Contemporary problems. Clin Chem *39*(4):641–647, 1993.

Sykes E, Epstein E: Laboratory measurement of bilirubin. Clin Perinatol *17*(2):397–416, 1990.

BILIRUBIN, TOTAL, SERUM
(see Bilirubin, Serum)

BILIRUBIN, URINE

Norm: Negative ≤0.02 mg/dl (≤0.34 µmol/L, SI units).

Positive or Increased: Cirrhosis, hepatitis (alcoholic, chronic, acute, drug-induced), hyperthyroidism, malignancy (hepatic or biliary tract), mononucleosis (infectious), and septicemia.

Description: Screens for the presence of conjugated bilirubin in the urine. Bilirubin is a by-product of hemoglobin breakdown that is normally excreted by the gastrointestinal tract. When obstructive or hepatic jaundice occurs, conjugated bilirubin enters the bloodstream, rather than the gastrointestinal tract, and is filtered and excreted by the kidneys.

Professional Considerations:

1. Consent form NOT required.
2. Preparation:
   A. Obtain Icotest tablets, N-Multistix, or Chemstrips for urine samples, and a clean container.
3. Procedure:
   A. Collect a 20-ml fresh random urine sample in a clean container.
   B. Follow package directions exactly for either Icotest tablets, N-Multistix, or Chemstrips for urine samples.
4. Postprocedure care:
   A. None.
5. Client and family teaching:
   A. Phenothiazines and ascorbic acid may affect results.
   B. Results are normally available within 24 hours.
6. Factors that affect results:
   A. Drugs that may cause false-positive results with Icotest tablets include salicylates.
   B. Drugs that may cause false-negative results with Icotest tablets include ascorbic acid.
   C. Drugs that may cause false-positive N-Multistix or Chemstrip bilirubin results include phenazopyridine and phenothiazines.
   D. A delay in performing the test may result in false-negative results.
7. Other data:
   A. Even trace amounts of bilirubin in the urine require further diagnostic investigation.
   B. Pruritus associated with hepatic cholestasis can be improved with the use of phototherapy.
   C. There is good agreement between the use of Multistix and Clinitek 200+ analyzer.

Bibliography:

Gallagher EJ, Schwartz E, Weinstein RS: Performance characteristics of urine dipsticks stored in open containers. Am J Emerg Med 8(2):121–123, 1990.

Lott JA, Johnson WR, Luke KE: Evaluation of an automated urine chemistry reagent-strip analyzer. J Clin Lab Anal 9(3):212–217, 1995.

Rosenthal E, Diamond E, Benderly A, Etziono A: Cholestatic pruritus: Effect on phototherapy on pruritus and excretion of bile acids in urine. Acta Paediatr 83(8):888–891, 1994.

BIOPSY, ANAEROBIC, CULTURE

Norm: No growth.

Positive: Cellulitis, decubiti, gangrenous or inflamed tissues and wounds caused by *Actinomyces, Arachnia, Bacteroides fragilis, Bacteroides melaninogenicus, Bifidobacterium, Clostridium, Eubacterium, Fusobacterium, Lactobacillus, Peptostreptococcus, Propionibacterium, Veillonella,* and others.

Description: Many anaerobic bacteria are present as part of the normal flora in humans. They obtain energy for growth and metabolism from fermentation reactions, rather than from oxygen. When displaced from their location into other body tissues or spaces, they become pathogenic. Anaerobes of clinical importance in humans most commonly cause infections in the skin, intestinal tract, vagina, brain, upper respiratory tract, lungs, and peritoneum. Special collection methods are necessary for the isolation of anaerobes. Anaerobic cultures are grown on complex media, and identification is made using colony morphology, pigmentation, fluorescence, and gas-liquid chromatography.

Professional Considerations:

1. Consent form IS required for the biopsy.

Risks:
See Biopsy, Site-Specific, Specimen.

Contraindications:
See Biopsy, Site-Specific, Specimen.

2. Preparation:
   A. Obtain the baseline PT/PTT.
   B. Alert laboratory personnel that an anaerobic specimen will be arriving shortly.
   C. Obtain povidone-iodine, sterile drapes, a biopsy tray, and a sterile specimen container or Petri dish.
3. Procedure:
   A. The site is prepared with povidone-iodine, allowed to dry, and then draped.
   B. Ultrasound may be helpful for needle

guidance in obtaining internal organ needle biopsies.

C. A biopsy of the tissue is obtained by the physician, taking care to avoid contamination of the specimen with other area organisms and to minimize exposure of the specimen to air.

D. After it is obtained, the biopsied material is quickly placed on premoistened sterile gauze in a sterile, 100-mm Petri dish or in a sterile container with the cap loosened.

E. An anaerobic transport container such as the Bio-Bag type A Anaerobic Culture Set (Marion) may be used. It consists of a gas-impermeable plastic bag and two ampules: one that generates hydrogen and the other that releases resazurin indicator.

F. Place the container or Petri dish inside the plastic bag with both ampules and seal the bag with a heat sealer.

G. Crush the gas-generator ampule. Hydrogen from the gas-generator ampule should combine with oxygen in the presence of a catalyst to produce water vapor condensation inside the bag. *(See Anaerobic Culture for instructions for liquid specimens.)*

4. Postprocedure care:
   A. Write the collection time on the laboratory requisition.
   B. Transport the sample to the laboratory immediately.
   C. Apply a dry, sterile dressing to the biopsy site.
   D. Observe the site for drainage, redness, edema, or pain until it is healed.

5. Client and family teaching:
   A. Report signs of infection at the operative site to the physician: increasing pain, redness, swelling, purulent drainage, or fever >101°F (38.3°C).
   B. Results are normally available within 4 days.

6. Factors that affect results:
   A. Overexposure to air may cause the anaerobe to die.
   B. Do not refrigerate the specimen.

7. Other data:
   A. The use of swabs to obtain anaerobic cultures is not recommended. When necessary, commercial anaerobic swab sets consisting of two containers must be used.
   B. Cultures of an unwashed small-intestinal mucosal biopsy specimen are as useful as a culture of small-intestinal aspirate for bacterial overgrowth analysis.

Bibliography:

Allen SD, Siders JA, Marler LM: Current issues and problems in dealing with anaerobes in the clinical laboratory. Clin Lab Med *15*(2):333–364, 1995.

Allen SD, Siders JA, Marler LM: Isolation and examination of anaerobic bacteria. *In* Lennette EH, Balows A, Hausler WJ, Shadomy HJ (eds): Manual of Clinical Microbiology. Washington DC, American Society for Microbiology, 1985, pp 413–433.

Riordan SM, McIver CJ, Duncombe VM, Bolin TD: Bacteriologic analysis of mucosal biopsy specimens for detecting small-intestinal bacterial overgrowth. Scand J Gastroenterol *30*(7):681–685, 1995.

BIOPSY, FUNGUS, CULTURE

Norm: No growth.

Positive: *Blastomyces dermatitidis, Coccidioides immitis, Cryptococcus neoformans, Histoplasma capsulatum, Sporothrixschenckii, Candida albicans, Candida tropicalis, Aspergillus fumigatus, Aspergillus flavus,* and others.

Description: Fungi are slow-growing, eukaryotic organisms that can grow on living and nonliving organic materials and are subdivided into yeasts and molds. Only a few fungi species infect humans. Normal host defense mechanisms limit the damage they cause superficially. Factors that predispose persons to fungal infections by lowering the normal host defense mechanisms include administration of broad-spectrum antibiotics and/or cancer chemotherapy, invasive lines, poor nutritional status, parenteral nutrition, surgery, trauma, and long-term use of steroids. Some fungi can be inhaled or introduced by traumatic inoculation into deep tissue spaces and cause serious infections. Although tentative identification of fungi can be made quickly with staining techniques, culture of the organism on special fungal culture media is required to confirm a diagnosis of a fungal infection.

Professional Considerations:

1. Consent form IS required.

Risks:
See Biopsy, Site-Specific, Specimen.

Contraindications:
See Biopsy, Site-Specific, Specimen.

---

2. Preparation:
   A. Obtain the baseline PT/PTT or ACT.
   B. Obtain a sterile container, a culture dish, or an appropriate tube. See procedure on next page for other site-specific supplies needed.

3. Procedure:

A. *Hair:* Examine the scalp with a Wood's lamp and remove fluorescent, fractured, or distorted hairs, and place them in a dry, sterile culture dish.

B. *Skin:* Cleanse the skin with an alcohol wipe. Remove any scales at the circumference of the lesion with a sterile scalpel. Obtain a scalpel or punch biopsy and place the tissue in a dry, sterile culture dish.

C. *Nails:* Cleanse the nails with an alcohol wipe. Scrape off the outermost layer and/or scrapings from beneath the edge of the nails with a scalpel and place them in a dry, sterile culture dish.

D. *Bone marrow:* Cleanse the skin over the aspiration site with povidone-iodine and allow it to dry completely. A physician performs an aspiration of enough bone marrow for two inoculations of media and either leaves it in the sterile syringe or injects it into a green-top tube containing heparin. The specimen can be refrigerated no longer than 12 hours before culturing.

E. *Tissues:* Biopsied material obtained during surgery should be placed in a sterile cup containing a small amount of saline without preservatives. For abscess drainage, a portion of the abscess wall should be submitted. The specimen can be refrigerated no longer than 10 hours before culturing.

4. Postprocedure care:
   A. Write the exact time of the specimen collection on the laboratory requisition.
   B. Write any current antifungal therapy on the laboratory requisition.
   C. Transport the specimen to the laboratory immediately.
   D. Apply a dry, sterile dressing to the bone marrow aspiration or biopsy site. Observe the site for redness, tenderness, edema, or drainage until healed.

5. Client and family teaching:
   A. Preliminary results are normally available within 5 days, the final results in 6 weeks.
   B. If fungus is suspected, treatment is started as a life-saving measure before the final results are obtained.
   C. Report signs of infection at the operative site to the physician: increasing pain, redness, swelling, purulent drainage, or fever >101°F (38.3°C).

6. Factors that affect results:
   A. Do not refrigerate hair, skin, or nail specimens.
   B. Best results are obtained if cultures are inoculated immediately. Other than noted above, the maximum time allowed between specimen collection and inoculation is 3 hours.

7. Other data:
   A. No growth for 4–6 weeks is required for fungal culture results to be confirmed as negative.
   B. Open lung biopsy provides a better yield than broncho-alveolar lavage in immunocompromised clients.
   C. Ultrasound-guided, fine-needle aspiration is recommended in clients with pulmonary or pleural aspergillosis.

Bibliography:

Ellis ME, Apence D, Bouchama A, Antonius J, Bazarbashi M, Khougeer F, De Vol EB: Open lung biopsy provides a higher and more specific diagnostic yield compared to broncho-alveolar lavage in immunocompromised patients. Fungal Study Group, Scand J Infect Dis *27*(2):157–162, 1995.

Tikkakoski T, Lohela P, Paivansalo M, Kerola T: Pleuropulmonary aspergillosis: US and US-guided biopsy as an aid to diagnosis. Acta Radiol *36*(2):122–126, 1995.

BIOPSY, MYCOBACTERIA, CULTURE

Norm: No growth.

Positive: *M. ulcerans, M. tuberculosis, M. bovis, M. marinum, M. kansasii, M. simiae, M. asiaticum, M. scrofulaceum, M. szulgai, M. gordonae, M. flavescens, M. xenopi, M. avium, M. intracellulare, M. gastri, M. malmoense, M. haemohilum, M. nonchromogenicum, M. terrae, M. triviale, M. fortuitum, M. chelonei, M. phlei, M. smegmatis,* and *M. vaccae.*

Description: *Mycobacteria* are rod-shaped, aerobic bacteria that resist decolorizing chemicals after staining, properties termed acid-fastness and alcohol-fastness. Nineteen *Mycobacteria* species are capable of producing human disease characterized by destructive granulomas that can necrose, ulcerate, and cavitate. *Mycobacterium tuberculosis* is transmitted via the airborne route most commonly to the lungs, where it survives well, causes areas of granulomatous inflammation, and if not dormant causes cough, fever, and hemoptysis. Mycobacterial infections can also occur in superficial body parts and internal organs.

Professional Considerations:

1. Consent form IS required for the biopsy.

Risks:
See Biopsy, Site-Specific, Specimen.

Contraindications:
See Biopsy, Site-Specific, Specimen.

2. Preparation:
   A. Obtain the baseline PT/PTT or ACT.
   B. Obtain a sterile container large enough to hold the tissue biopsy.
3. Procedure:
   A. Place a large (pea-sized) amount of biopsied material in a sterile container and transport it to the laboratory immediately.
4. Postprocedure care:
   A. Specific to site and surgery.
   B. Write the exact time of the specimen collection on the laboratory requisition.
5. Client and family teaching:
   A. If tuberculosis is suspected, wear a mask until no longer infectious, and cough only into the mask. Do not cough into the air outside the mask because this can spread the disease.
   B. Results may take up to 2 months, but treatment is started prior to results if tuberculosis is suspected.
   C. Report signs of infection at the operative site to the physician: increasing pain, redness, swelling, purulent drainage, or fever >101°F (38.3°C).
6. Factors that affect results:
   A. Do not refrigerate the specimen.
   B. The maximum time allowed between specimen collection and inoculation is 3 hours.
   C. Antituberculous drug therapy may cause negative results because of the inhibition of the growth of *M. tuberculosis*.
   D. A high carbon dioxide atmosphere for growth may increase the number of positive cultures.
   E. A culture medium containing glycerin accelerates growth.
7. Other data:
   A. Cultures for *M. tuberculosis* may take 3–8 weeks to grow.
   B. Bone marrow biopsy for *Mycobacteria* should be performed only on severely immunocompromised clients.
   C. Liver biopsy can be performed to diagnose infection in HIV-infected clients who have unexplained fever and abnormal liver function test results.

Bibliography:

Cavicchi M, Pialoux G, Carnot F, Offredo C, Romana C, Deslandes P, Dupont B, Berthelot P, Pol S: Value of liver biopsy for the rapid diagnosis of infection in human immunodeficiency virus-infected patients who have unexplained fever and elevated serum levels of alkaline phosphatase or gamma-glutamyl transferase. Clin Infect Dis 20(3):606–610, 1995.
Riley UB, Crawford S, Barrett SP, Abdulla SH: Detection of mycobacteria in bone marrow biopsy specimens taken to investigate pyrexia of unknown origin. J Clin Pathol 48(8): 706–709, 1995.

BIOPSY, ROUTINE, CULTURE

Norm: No growth.

Usage: Cellulitis, decubiti, inflamed tissues and wounds, and internal organs.

Description: An excision or a needle-punch sample of tissue suspected to be infected is taken and inoculated on bacterial culture media.

Professional Considerations:
1. Consent form IS required for the biopsy.

Risks:
See Biopsy, Site-Specific, Specimen.

Contraindications:
See Biopsy, Site-Specific, Specimen.

2. Preparation:
   A. Obtain the baseline PT/PTT or ACT.
   B. Obtain a sterile container large enough to hold the tissue biopsy.
3. Procedure:
   A. Decubiti should be debrided prior to the biopsy.
   B. Surface wounds, skin, nails, and mucosal surfaces should be cleansed with an alcohol wipe and allowed to dry just prior to the biopsy.
   C. Obtain 20–500 mg of tissue via excision with a scalpel or with a needle punch using an aseptic technique. Take care not to contaminate the specimen with surrounding tissue.
   D. Place the biopsied material in a sterile container and transport it to the laboratory immediately.
4. Postprocedure care:
   A. Specific to site and surgery.
   B. Write the collection time on the laboratory requisition.
5. Client and family teaching:
   A. Final results may take up to a week, but treatment may occur following biopsy culture.
   B. Report signs of infection at the operative site to the physician: increasing pain, redness, swelling, purulent drainage, or fever >101°F (38.3°C).
6. Factors that affect results:
   A. Do not refrigerate the specimen.
   B. The maximum amount of time allowed between specimen collection and inoculation is 3 hours.
7. Other data:
   A. Final results may take up to 7 days.
   B. Cultures of the prostate are to be interpreted with pathologic characterization of locations contiguous to the cultures tissue.

Bibliography:

Moyer MP: Tumor cell culture. Methods Enzymol 254:153–165, 1995.
Peterson CA: Cell culture systems as tools for studying age-related changes in skeletal muscle. J Gerontol Biol Sci Med Sci 50 (Spec No):142–144, 1995.
Pretlow TG, Yang B, Pretlow TP: Organ culture of benign, aging, and hyperplastic human prostate. Microsc Res Tech 30(4):271–281, 1995.

Wreghitt TG, Smyth RL, Scott JP, Higenbottam T, Gray JJ, Stewart S, Wallwork J: Value of culture of biopsy material in diagnosis of viral infections in heart-lung transplant recipients. Transplant Proc *22*(4):1809–1810, 1990.

BIOPSY, SITE-SPECIFIC, SPECIMEN

Norm: Interpreted by pathologist.

Usage: Abscess (abscess wall), acute interstitial nephritis (kidney), adrenal feminization (testis), alcoholic myopathy (muscle), alveolar proteinosis (lung), amebiasis (rectum), amyloidosis (tissue), amyotrophic lateral sclerosis (muscle), arthritis (joint), bronchogenic carcinoma (lung, lymph node, pleura), brucellosis (spleen, tissue), carcinoma of pancreas head (pancreas), cat scratch disease (lymph node), Chagas' disease (lung, lymph node), chancroid (lymph node), celiac disease (small intestine), cholesterol ester storage disease (liver), chromoblastomycosis (tissue), chronic inflammatory splenomegaly (spleen), cirrhosis (liver), coccidioidomycosis (joint), coccidiosis (small intestine), colon cancer (colon), de Quervain's thyroiditis (thyroid), Dubin-Johnson syndrome (liver), farmer's lung (lung), fatty liver (liver), female infertility, filariasis (lymph node), galactosemia (liver), Gaucher's disease (skin), germinal aplasia (testis), glucuronyl-transferase deficiency (liver), goiter (thyroid, Goodpasture's syndrome (kidney), glycogenesis (liver), gonorrhea (rectum), Hamman-Rich syndrome (lung), Hashimoto's thyroiditis (thyroid), hemochromatosis (liver), hepatitis (liver), Hirschsprung's disease (rectum), histiocytosis (spleen), Hurler's syndrome (skin), Hodgkin's disease (lymph node, spleen), hypophosphatemia (bone), hyperthyroidism (muscle), hypertension (endomyocardium), immunodeficiency (lymph node), infectious mononucleosis (lymph node), jaundice (liver), kidney transplant rejection (kidney), Kimmelstiel-Wilson syndrome (kidney), Klinefelter's syndrome (testis), legionnaire's disease (lung), leprosy (nasal scrapings, lepromatous lesion), leukemia (spleen), lymphangitis (lymph node), lymphatic leukemia (lymph node), lymphogranuloma venereum (lymph node), lymphoma (lymph node), malabsorption (small intestine), male infertility (testicle), McArdle syndrome (muscle), menstrual irregularities (endometrium), metabolic diseases (muscle, skin), metachromatic leukodystrophy (nerve), metastasis (liver, lymph node), mitochondrial myopathy (muscle), muscular dystrophy (muscle), myasthenia gravis (muscle), myotonia congenital (muscle), myotubular myopathy (muscle), narcotic addiction (liver), nemaline myopathy (muscle), Niemann-Pick disease (rectum, skin), osteomalacia (bone), osteopenia (bone), parasitic infections (spleen), pelvic inflammatory disease (endometrium), pleural tumor (pleura), pneumoconiosis (lung, lymph node), pneumocystis pneumonia (lung), polyarteritis nodosa (tissue), polymyalgia rheumatica (muscle, temporal artery), polymyositis (muscle), poststreptococcal glomerulonephritis (kidney), proctitis (rectum), rat-bite fever (joint fluid), renal disease (kidney tissue), Reye's syndrome (liver), rheumatoid pleurisy (pleura), Riedel's thyroiditis (thyroid), Rocky Mountain spotted fever (skin), sarcoidosis (lung, lymph node, tissue), schistosomiasis (bladder, rectum), scleroderma (tissue), septic pylephlebitis (liver), Sjögren's syndrome (kidney), Stein-Leventhal syndrome (ovary), stiff-man syndrome (muscle), stomach carcinoma (bone marrow, liver, lymph node), systemic lupus erythematosus (full-thickness skin, tissue), temporal arteritis (temporal artery), toxemia of pregnancy (kidney), trichinosis (muscle), tuberculosis (bone marrow, lung, lymph node, spleen), tularemia (lymph node), Turner's syndrome (ovary, testis), ulcerative colitis (liver, rectum), villous adenoma (rectum), visceral larva migrans (liver), Wegener's granulomatosis (kidney), Whipple's disease (lymph node, small intestine), Wilson's disease (liver), and yellow fever (liver).

Description: An excision or a needle-punch sample of body tissue taken under sterile technique and examined microscopically for cell morphology and tissue abnormalities. The procedure takes 15–30 minutes.

Professional Considerations:

1. Consent form IS required for most specimens and is specific to the institution.

Risks:

Allergic reaction to local anesthetic (itching, hives, rash, tight feeling in the throat, shortness of breath, bronchospasm, anaphylaxis, death). Infection, hematoma, mild to severe bleeding, organ damage, and hemorrhage. Death is possible from biopsies of internal organs.

Contraindications:

Previous allergy to local anesthetic. Biopsy may be contraindicated in clients with coagulation defects.

2. Preparation:
   A. Obtain the baseline PT/PTT or ACT.
   B. Type and crossmatch may be pre-scribed 24 hours prior to the biopsy.
   C. Obtain sterile containers, one with 10% formaldehyde, the other with sterile saline.
3. Procedure:
   A. Decubiti should be debrided prior to the biopsy.
   B. Surface wounds, skin, and mucosal surfaces should be cleansed with an alcohol wipe and allowed to dry just prior to the biopsy.
   C. Obtain 20–500 mg of tissue via needle aspiration, excision, or needle-punch using an aseptic technique. Do not contaminate the specimen with other tissue in the area.
   D. Place the biopsied material in a sterile container of 10% formaldehyde and in another with sterile saline. Transport the specimens to the laboratory immediately.
4. Postprocedure care:
   A. Specific to site and surgery. A dry, sterile dressing or a Band-Aid dressing is required.
   B. Write the collection time on the laboratory requisition.
   C. Assess vital signs and the site for bleeding or hematoma formation every 15 minutes × 4, then every 30 minutes × 2.
   D. Observe for signs of infection (fever, chills, hypotension, tachycardia) × 24–48 hours.
5. Client and family teaching:
   A. Fast from food, and drink only clear liquids after midnight and before the biopsy.
   B. Report signs of infection at the operative site to the physician: increasing pain, redness, swelling, purulent drainage, or fever >101°F (38.3°C).
   C. Check temperature every 6 hours × 24 hours, and notify the physician if fever, chills, faintness, weakness, or dizziness

occurs. Place pressure over the site × 10 minutes if bleeding is noted.
   D. Results are normally available within 72 hours.
6. Factors that affect results:
   A. Do not refrigerate the specimen.
7. Other data:
   A. The full report may take up to 5 days.

Bibliography:

Noguchi M, Kumaki T, Taniya T, Miyazaki I: Bilateral cervical lymph node metastases in well-differentiated thyroid cancer. Arch Surg *125*(6):804–806, 1990.

Wu YX, Kawabe K: Primary culture of smooth muscle cells from benign prostatic hyperplasia. J Smooth Muscle Res *30*(2):51–56, 1994.

BLASTOMYCOSIS (GILCHRIST'S) SKIN TEST, DIAGNOSTIC

Norm: Negative.

Usage: Diagnosis of *Blastomyces dermatitidis.*

Description: Blastomycosis, a chronic granulomatous and suppurative fungal disease of the lungs and skin, occurs primarily in 20-to 40-year-old males in rural areas throughout the world. There is no evidence of transmission from one client to another, and there is usually no epidemic. The mode of transmission is thought to be inhalation of spores from soil. The spores then disseminate by invading the blood and lymphatic systems. Blastomycosis skin lesions may be erythematous nodes or papular lesions, which can break down, ulcerate, drain, and spread.

Professional Considerations:

1. Consent form NOT required.
2. Preparation:
   A. Obtain a sterile container for the biopsy specimen.
3. Procedure:
   A. Using a sterile technique, a biopsy is taken from the periphery of a skin lesion where pus and yeast cells are found. A wet mount of the specimen shows broadly attached buds on thick-walled cells.
4. Postprocedure care:
   A. Apply a dry, sterile dressing to the site if bleeding occurs.
5. Client and family teaching:
   A. Report signs of infection at the biopsy site to the physician: increasing pain, redness, swelling, purulent drainage, or fever >101°F (38.3°C).
   B. Results are normally available within 72 hours.

6. Factors that affect results:
   A. Treatment with amphotericin B may cause false-negative results.
7. Other data:
   A. Blastomycosis is a general term used in parts of the world to refer to any infection caused by budding yeasts in the tissue.

Bibliography:

Abuodeh RO, Scalarone GM: Comparative studies on the detection of delayed dermal hypersensitivity in experimental animals with lysate and infiltrate antigens of Blastomyces dermatitidis. Mycoses 37(5–6):149–153, 1994.

BLEEDING TIME, DUKE, BLOOD

Norm: 1–5 minutes.

Increased: Anemia (aplastic, pernicious), collagen diseases, congenital heart disease, disseminated intravascular coagulopathy, drug sensitivity, ethyl alcohol ingestion along with aspirin ingestion, factor deficiency (I, II, V, VII, VIII, IX, XI), fibrinolytic activity, Glanzmann's disease, hemorrhagic disease of the newborn, Hodgkin's disease, hypothyroidism, idiopathic thrombocytopenic purpura, infections (measles, mumps, streptococcal), leukemia (acute), liver disease (severe), mononucleosis (infectious), multiple myeloma, purpura hemorrhagica, scurvy, thrombasthenia, thrombocytopathy, thrombocytopenia purpura (secondary due to allergy), von Willebrand's disease, and uremia. Drugs include anticoagulants (oral), aspirin, indomethacin, and phenylbutazone.

Decreased: Not clinically significant.

Description: The duration of active bleeding from a standardized superficial puncture wound of the skin is measured. It is most helpful as an indicator of platelet abnormality, either in their number or function.

Professional Considerations:

1. Consent form NOT required.

Risks:

Bleeding, hematoma, infection, ecchymoses.

Contraindications:

This test is contraindicated in clients with a platelet count <50,000/mm^3, in clients with severe bleeding disorders, or in clients who have taken medications containing aspirin within 7 days prior to the test.

2. Preparation:
   A. Obtain alcohol wipes, a lancet, a stopwatch, and filter paper.
3. Procedure:
   A. Cleanse the site for puncture with an alcohol wipe and allow it to dry completely.
   B. Make a small lancet puncture in the fingertip or ear lobe and simultaneously start the stopwatch.
   C. Remove blood from the wound by gently blotting with filter paper, without exerting pressure on the wound, every 30 seconds.
   D. When blood flow ceases, stop timing with the stopwatch. If bleeding continues for more than 20 minutes, discontinue the test and apply pressure to the site.
4. Postprocedure care:
   A. Apply a dry, sterile dressing to the site after bleeding stops.
5. Client and family teaching:
   A. Do not take aspirin for 7 days prior to the test.
   B. Call the physician if there are signs of infection at the test site: increasing pain, bleeding, redness, swelling, purulent drainage, or fever >101°F (38.3°C).
   C. Results are normally available within 24 hours.
6. Factors that affect results:
   A. A uniform incision is difficult to make without considerable skill.
   B. Pressing too hard on the blood with the filter paper disturbs the platelet plug and prolongs bleeding time.
7. Other data:
   A. The depth of the puncture with the lancet is difficult to standardize and results in difficulty reproducing bleeding times.
   B. Daily administration of 75 mg of aspirin for 2 weeks in healthy pregnant women yielded results of Duke's bleeding time within normal limits.

Bibliography:

Blake JC, Sprengers D, Grech P, McCormick PA, McIntyre N, Burroughs AK: Bleeding time in patients with hepatic cirrhosis. Br Med J Clin Res 301 (6742):12–15, 1990.

Doutremepuich C, deSeze O, LeRoy D, Lelanne MC, Anne MC: Aspirin at very ultra low dosage in healthy volunteers: Effects on bleeding time, platelet aggregation and coagulation. Haemostasis 20(2):99–105, 1990.

Rymark P, Berntorp E, Nordsjo P, Liedholm H, Melander A, Gennser G: Low-dose aspirin to pregnant women: Single pharmacokinetics and influence of short term treatment on bleeding time. J Perinat Med 22(3):205–211, 1994.

BLEEDING TIME, IVY, BLOOD

Norm: 1–9 minutes. Panic range: >15 minutes. Shorter in men than in women, and shorter in clients over 50 years of age.

Increased: Anemia (aplastic, pernicious), collagen diseases, congenital heart disease, disseminated intravascular coagulopathy, drug sensitivity, ethyl alcohol ingestion along with aspirin ingestion, factor deficiency (I, II, V, VII, VIII, IX, XI), fibrinolytic activity, Glanzmann's disease, hemorrhagic disease of the newborn, Hodgkin's disease, hypothyroidism, idiopathic thrombocytopenic purpura, infections (measles, mumps, streptococcal), leukemia (acute), liver disease (severe), mononucleosis (infectious), multiple myeloma, purpura hemorrhagica, scurvy, thrombasthenia, thrombocytopathy, thrombocytopenia purpura (secondary due to allergy), von Willebrand's disease, and uremia. Drugs include anticoagulants (oral), aspirin, indomethacin, and phenylbutazone.

Decreased: Not clinically significant.

Description: The duration of active bleeding from superficial incisions of the skin is measured. It is most helpful as an indicator of platelet abnormality, either in their number or function. This method is more sensitive than the Duke bleeding time because a blood pressure cuff is used to increase venous pressure and ensure capillary filling without interfering with venous return.

Professional Considerations:

1. Consent form NOT required for most labs.

Risks:

Bleeding, hematoma, infection, ecchymoses, scar, or keloid formation.

Contraindications:

This test is contraindicated in clients who require upper-extremity restraints, have edematous or very cold arms, or are prone to keloid formation. It should not be performed if there are contraindications to placing or inflating a blood pressure cuff on the arm (casts, rash, dressings, A-V fistula). Other contraindications include platelet count <50,000/mm^3, severe bleeding disorders, skin infectious diseases, and senile skin changes or if the client has taken medications containing acetyl groups within 7 days prior to the test.

2. Preparation:
   A. *See Client and family teaching.*
   B. Obtain a blood pressure cuff, a manometer, alcohol wipes, a stopwatch, a lancet, and filter paper.
3. Procedure:
   A. Cleanse the volar aspect of the forearm with an alcohol wipe and allow it to dry completely. Choose a site with no superficial veins.
   B. Place the blood pressure cuff on the upper arm and inflate it to 40 mmHg.
   C. Make two small incisions or puncture wounds 2–3 mm deep with the lancet on the site that was cleansed with alcohol. Start timing with the stopwatch.
   D. Remove blood from the wounds by gently blotting with filter paper, without exerting pressure on the wound, every 30 seconds.
   E. When the blood flow ceases, stop timing with the stopwatch. If bleeding continues for more than 20 minutes, discontinue the test and apply pressure to the site.
   F. Calculate the bleeding time by averaging the bleeding time of both incisions.
4. Postprocedure care:
   A. If the bleeding time is normal, apply a dry dressing to the site. If the bleeding time is prolonged, apply a pressure bandage to the site.
5. Client and family teaching:
   A. Do not take aspirin for 7 days prior to the test.
   B. Call the physician if there are signs of infection at the test site: increasing pain, bleeding, redness, swelling, purulent drainage, or fever >101°F (38.3°C).
   C. Results are normally available within 24 hours.
6. Factors that affect results:
   A. A uniform incision is difficult to make without considerable skill.
   B. Pressing too hard on the blood with the filter paper disturbs the platelet plug and prolongs bleeding time.
7. Other data:
   A. The depth of the puncture with the lancet is difficult to standardize and results in difficulty reproducing bleeding times.

B. Healthy pregnant women given 75 mg of aspirin for 2 weeks have an increased bleeding time by Ivy tests.

Bibliography:

Doutremepuich C, deSeze O, LeRoy D, Lalanne MC, Anne MC: Aspirin at very ultra low dosage in healthy volunteers: Effects on bleeding time, platelet aggregation and coagulation. Haemostasis 20(2):99–105, 1990.

Israels SJ, McNicol A, Robertson C, Gerrard JM: Platelet storage pool deficiency: Diagnosis in patients with prolonged bleeding times and normal platelet aggregation. Br J Haematol 75(1):118–121, 1990.

Rymark P, Berntorp E, Nordsjo P, Liedholm H, Melander A, Gennser G: Low-dose aspirin to pregnant women: single dose pharmacokinetics and influence of short term treatment on bleeding time. J Perinat Med 22(3):205–211, 1994.

BLEEDING TIME, MIELKE, BLOOD

Norm: 2.5–10 minutes.

Increased: Anemia (aplastic, pernicious), collagen diseases, congenital heart disease, disseminated intravascular coagulopathy, drug sensitivity, ethyl alcohol ingestion along with aspirin, factor deficiency (I, II, V, VII, VIII, IX, XI), fibrinolytic activity, Glanzmann's disease, hemorrhagic disease of the newborn, Hodgkin's disease, hypothyroidism, idiopathic thrombocytopenic purpura, infections (measles, mumps, streptococcal), leukemia (acute), liver disease (severe), mononucleosis (infectious), multiple myeloma, purpura hemorrhagica, scurvy, thrombasthenia, thrombocytopathy, thromboctyopenia purpura (secondary due to allergy), von Willebrand's disease, and uremia. Drugs include anticoagulants (oral), aspirin, indomethacin, and phenylbutazone.

Decreased: Not clinically significant.

Description: The duration of active bleeding from a standardized superficial incision of the skin is measured. It is particularly helpful as an indicator of platelet abnormality, either in the number or function of the platelets. This method is more sensitive than the Duke bleeding time because a blood pressure cuff is used to increase venous pressure and ensure capillary filling without interfering with venous return. Because the template standardizes the length and depth of the incision, this is the most accurate manual method for measuring bleeding time. An automated Surgicutt instrument is available to further standardize the incision.

Professional Considerations:

1. Consent form NOT usually required.

Risks:

Bleeding, hematoma, infection, ecchymoses, scar, or keloid formation.

Contraindications:

In clients who require upper-extremity restraints, have edematous or very cold arms, or are prone to keloid formation. The test should not be performed if there are contraindications to placing or inflating a blood pressure cuff on the arm (casts, rash, dressings, A-V fistula). Other contraindications include platelet count <50,000/mm^3, severe bleeding disorders, skin infectious diseases, and senile skin changes, or if the client has taken medications containing acetyl groups within 7 days prior to the test.

2. Preparation:
   A. *See Client and family teaching.*
   B. Obtain a blood pressure cuff and a manometer, alcohol wipes, a stopwatch, a template, and filter paper.

3. Procedure:
   A. Cleanse the volar aspect of the forearm with an alcohol wipe and allow it to dry completely. Choose a site with no superficial veins.
   B. Place the blood pressure cuff on the upper arm and inflate to 40 mmHg.
   C. *Manual incision:* Using a specially calibrated template to pass the blade through, make two incisions 9 mm long and 1 mm deep on the site that was cleansed with alcohol. Start timing with the stopwatch.
   D. *Automated incision:* Place the Surgicutt instrument on the site that was cleansed with alcohol and start the stopwatch at the same time as the device is triggered. The device will make a standardized 5 mm long × 1 mm deep puncture incision. Repeat at a second site.
   E. Remove the blood from the wound by gently blotting with the filter paper, without exerting pressure on the wound, every 30 seconds.

F. When the blood flow ceases, stop timing with the stopwatch. If bleeding continues for more than 20 minutes, discontinue the test and apply pressure to the site.

G. Calculate the bleeding time by averaging the bleeding time of both incisions.

4. Postprocedure care:
   A. If the bleeding time is normal, apply the dressing to the site. If the bleeding time is prolonged, apply a pressure bandage to the site.
   B. A butterfly closure may be required for 24 hours.

5. Client and family teaching:
   A. Do not take aspirin for 7 days prior to the test.
   B. Call the physician if there are signs of infection at the test site: increasing pain, bleeding, redness, swelling, purulent drainage, or fever >101°F (38.3°C).
   C. Results are normally available within 24 hours.

6. Factors that affect results:
   A. With standardized incisions, one incision yields as much information as two nonstandardized incisions.
   B. Pressing too hard on the blood with the filter paper disturbs the platelet plug and prolongs the bleeding time.

7. Other data:
   A. None.

Bibliography:

Israels SJ, McNicol A, Robertson C, Gerrald JM: Platelet storage pool deficiency: Diagnosis in patients with prolonged bleeding times and normal platelet aggregation. Br J Haematol 75(1):118–121, 1990.

Mielke CH: Measurement of the bleeding time. International committee communications. Thromb Haemost 52:210–211, 1984.

BLEEDING TIME ASPIRIN TOLERANCE TEST

(see Aspirin Tolerance Test, Diagnostic)

BLOOD CULTURE, BLOOD

Norm: Negative or no growth.

Positive: Bacteremia and septicemia.

Description: Blood is inoculated in aerobic and anaerobic laboratory culture media and observed for growth of pathogenic organisms. Blood cultures may be positive in either bacteremia or septicemia. Bacteremia is a localized infection, such as in a particular organ or area of tissue, in which a small portion of the infectious bacteria escapes into the bloodstream. It may occur transiently, without infection after tooth brushing or specialized procedures such as dental surgery, bronchoscopy, tonsillectomy, endoscopy, cystoscopy, and transurethral resection. Septicemia occurs when a large amount of pathogenic micro-organisms are dispersed throughout the bloodstream, and is usually accompanied by systemic shock symptoms. Blood cultures are generally drawn as the fever is spiking, from two different sites at the same time (one immediately after the other) and again 3 hours later. The number and frequency may vary by institution and practitioner. For clients in whom antimicrobial therapy has preceded blood cultures, the number of times cultured may be doubled (i.e., double cultures drawn four different times). Results are reported as the amount of growth after a specific number of days.

Professional Considerations:

1. Consent form NOT required.
2. Preparation:
   A. Obtain alcohol, a sterile gauze, povidone-iodine, two needles, two 30-ml syringes, and two anaerobic and two aerobic culture bottles.
   B. MAY be drawn during hemodialysis.
3. Procedure:
   A. Palpate the vein to determine location. Do not touch the site after cleansing.
   B. Cleanse the site for culture with an alcohol wipe and allow it to dry.
   C. Cleanse the site with povidone-iodine and allow it to dry completely or for at least 1 minute.
   D. Draw 10–20 ml of blood into a syringe. Avoid aspirating air into the syringe. If bacteremia is suspected, increase the volume of blood drawn to 30 ml.
   E. Place a fresh needle on the syringe.
   F. Remove the caps from the vacuum culture bottles and inject 5–10 ml into a vacuum bottle containing an anaerobic culture medium and 5–10 ml into a vacuum bottle containing an aerobic culture medium. If bacteremia is suspected, inject at least 15 ml into each bottle. Depending on the size of the bottle, more blood may be required to obtain at least a 1:10 dilution. Mix both bottles gently.
   G. Immediately repeat the above procedure at a different site.
4. Postprocedure care:
   A. Cleanse the puncture site with antiseptic and apply pressure.
   B. Write the collection time on the laboratory requisition.
   C. Write the presumptive diagnosis and

the recent antimicrobial therapy on the laboratory requisition.

D. Transport the specimens to the laboratory for incubation within 1 hour.

5. Client and family teaching:
   A. Call the physician if there are signs of infection at the culture site: increasing pain, redness, swelling, purulent drainage, or fever >101°F (38.3°C).
   B. Antibiotic or antifungal treatment will begin after the cultures are taken and prior to the final results.
   C. The first results are normally available in 24 hours and continue for up to 2 weeks.

6. Factors that affect results:
   A. Reject specimens received more than 1 hour after collection.
   B. Increasing the volume of blood cultured in suspected bacteremia may yield more positive cultures.
   C. False-negative results or delayed growth may be obtained when blood cultures are drawn after antimicrobial therapy has begun.
   D. Some common skin flora that may contaminate blood cultures include *Staphylococcus epidermis,* diphtheroids, and *Propioni* bacterium.
   E. Hirakata et al. (1996) found a higher incidence of positive blood cultures in clients receiving hyperalimentation.

7. Other data:
   A. Pathogenic species most often cultured include *Actinobacter, Bacteroides, Brucella, Citrobacter, Clostridium, Enterobacter, Escherichia coli, Francisella, Haemophilus, Klebsiella, Leptospira, Listeria, Mycobacterium, Neisseria, Nocardia, Pseudomonas, Salmonella, Serratia, Staphylococcus, Streptococcus,* and *Vibrio.*
   B. The contamination rate for blood cultures collected using iodophor (povidone-iodine) is greater than when using iodine tincture.
   C. Clients on antimicrobial therapy have an enhanced yield for staphylococci using a FAN bottle compared to the standard aerobic BacT/Alert bottle.

Bibliography:

Hirakata Y, Furuya N, Iwata M, Kashitani F, et al: Assessment of clinical significance of positive blood cultures of relatively low-virulence isolates. J Micro Micro Biol *44*(3):195–198, 1996.

Prego V, Glatt AE, Roy V, Thelmo W, Dincsoy H, Raufman JP: Comparative yield of blood culture for fungi and myobacteria, liver biopsy, and bone marrow biopsy in the diagnosis of fever of undetermined origin in human immunodeficiency virus-infected patients. Arch Intern Med *150*(2): 333–336, 1990.

Strand CL, Wajsbort RR, Sturmann K: Effect of iodophor vs iodine tincture skin preparation on blood culture contamination rate. JAMA *269*(8): 1004–1006, 1993.

Weinstein MP, Mirrett S, Reimer LG, Wilson ML, Smith-Elekes S, Chuard CR, Joho KL, Reller LB: Controlled evaluation of BacT/Alert standard aerobic and FAN aerobic blood culture bottles for detection of bacteremia and fungemia. J Clin Microbiol *33*(4):978–981, 1995.

BLOOD CULTURE WITH ANTIMICROBIAL REMOVAL DEVICE (ARD), CULTURE

Norm: Negative or no growth.

Positive: Bacteremia and septicemia.

Description: The Antimicrobial Removal Device (ARD) (Marion Scientific, Kansas City, Missouri) is a vial containing adsorbent resins designed to remove antibiotics from blood before it is cultured. The device is intended to help remove the inhibitory effects of antibiotics on blood-borne micro-organisms so that faster growth may be obtained in culture and more timely diagnoses may be made. Methods designed to lessen the influence of antimicrobial activity in conventional blood cultures include adding sodium polyanetholsulfonate to the culture medium, adding beta-lactamase to the medium, and diluting the blood in the culture medium. While the ARD method is estimated to be several times more expensive than conventional blood cultures, studies have found conflicting results as to its value in increasing the yield of positive cultures and increasing the speed of confirmation of positive cultures.

Professional Considerations:

1. Consent form NOT required.
2. Preparation:
   A. Obtain alcohol, sterile gauze, povidone-iodine, two needles, two 30-ml syringes, and two ARD vials.
3. Procedure:
   A. Palpate the vein to determine the location. Do not touch the site after cleansing.
   B. Cleanse the site for culture with an alcohol wipe and allow it to dry.
   C. Cleanse the site with povidone-iodine and allow it to dry completely or for at least 1 minute.
   D. Draw 15–20 ml of blood into a syringe. Avoid aspirating air into the syringe.
   E. Place a fresh needle on the syringe.
   F. Inject 10 ml of blood into an ARD vial.
   G. Immediately repeat the above procedure at a different site.
4. Postprocedure care:
   A. Write the exact time of the specimen collection on the laboratory requisition.
   B. Write the presumptive diagnosis and

recent antimicrobial therapy on the laboratory requisition.

C. Transport the specimens to the laboratory within 2 hours. Upon arrival in the laboratory, the vials should be shaken on a rotator for 15 minutes. The contents should then be removed and each inoculated into a brain-heart infusion medium and incubated at 35°C. They should be subcultured at 3 hours, 24 hours, 48 hours, 1 week, and 2 weeks.

5. Client and family teaching:
A. Preliminary results will be available within 24 hours and final results in 2 weeks.
B. Therapy will be initiated before the final results.

6. Factors that affect results:
A. Reject specimens received more than 2 hours after collection.

7. Other data:
A. *See also Blood Culture, Blood.*

Bibliography:

Doern GV: Manual blood culture systems and the antimicrobial removal device. Clin Lab Med *14*(1): 133–147, 1994.

BLOOD FUNGUS, CULTURE

Norm: Negative or no growth.

Usage: Definitive diagnosis of systemic fungal infections.

Description: Fungi are slow-growing, eukaryotic organisms that can grow on living and nonliving organic materials, and are subdivided into yeasts and molds. Factors that predispose clients to fungal infections by lowering the normal host defense mechanisms include administration of broad-spectrum antibiotics or chemotherapy, invasive lines, poor nutritional status, parenteral nutrition, surgery, trauma, and long-term use of steroids. Some fungi may be inhaled or introduced by traumatic inoculation into deep tissue spaces and cause serious infections. Although tentative identification of fungi can be made quickly with staining techniques, culture of the organism in special fungal culture media is required to confirm a diagnosis of a fungal infection. Fungal cultures are generally inoculated on at least three media to facilitate recovery of all etiologic agents.

Professional Considerations:

1. Consent form NOT required.
2. Preparation:
A. Obtain alcohol wipes, sterile gauze, povidone-iodine, two needles, two 20-ml syringes, and two fungal culture bottles.

3. Procedure:
A. Palpate the vein to determine the location. Do not touch the site after cleansing.
B. Cleanse the site for culture with an alcohol wipe and allow it to dry.
C. Cleanse the site with povidone-iodine and allow it to dry completely or for at least 1 minute.
D. Remove the caps from two fungal culture vacuum bottles, cleanse the rubber stoppers with an alcohol wipe and 2% iodine, and allow them to dry.
E. Draw a 10-ml blood sample into a syringe.
F. Place a fresh needle on the syringe and inject the 10 ml of blood into a vacuum bottle containing a blood culture medium specific for fungi. Mix the bottle gently.
G. Immediately repeat the above procedure at a different site.

4. Postprocedure care:
A. Wipe the venipuncture site with an antimicrobial agent.
B. Write the collection time on the laboratory requisition.
C. Write the presumptive diagnosis and recent antifungal therapy on the laboratory requisition.
D. Incubate the culture bottles at 25–30°C in the laboratory.

5. Client and family teaching:
A. Preliminary results will be available within 72 hours and final results in 30 days.
B. Treatment for potential infection will begin prior to obtaining results.

6. Factors that affect results:
A. Some common skin flora that may contaminate blood cultures include *Staphylococcus epidermidis,* diphtheroids, and *Propioni* bacterium.

7. Other data:
A. Fungal cultures of blood must be incubated at least 30 days before being reported as negative.
B. Fungi most often cultured from blood include *Blastomyces dermatitidis, Coccidioides immitis, Cryptococcus neoformans, Histoplasma capsulatum, Histoplasma duboisii, Paracoccidioides brasiliensis, Candida albicans, Aspergillus fumigatus,* and *Pseudallescheria boydii.*
C. The BacT/Alert system may miss some fungi growth. This problem can be overcome by prolonged incubation and terminal subculture when fungal infection is considered to be likely.
D. Detection of amphotericin B resistance of yeast isolates (*Candida species, Torulopsis glabrata, Saccharomyces cerevisiae, Cryptococcus neoformans*) within 12–14 hours after inoculation of the test medium is possible.

Bibliography:

Breathnach A, Evans J: Growth and detection of filamentous fungi in the BacT/Alert blood culture system. J Clin Pathol *48*(7):670–672, 1995.

Hazen KC, Chery MP, Han Y: Potential use of BacT/Alert automated blood culture system for antifungal susceptibility testing. J Clin Microbiol *32*(3):848–850, 1994.

BLOOD GASES, ARTERIAL (ABG), BLOOD

Norm: Must be corrected for body temperature.

		SI Units
pH		
Adults	7.35–7.45	7.35–7.45
Panic values	≤7.2 and >7.6	≤7.2 and >7.6
Children		
Birth–2 months	7.32–7.49	7.32–7.49
2 months–2 years	7.34–7.46	7.34–7.46
Over 2 years	7.35–7.45	7.35–7.45
$PaCO_2$	35–45 mmHg	4.7–6.0 kPa
Panic values	≤20 mmHg	<2.7 kPa
	>70 mmHg	>9.4 kPa
PaO_2	75–100 mmHg	10.0–13.3 kPa
Panic values	≤40 mmHg	<5.3 kPa
HCO_3	22–26 mEq/L	22–26 mmol/L
Panic values	≤10 mEq/L	<10 mmol/L
	>40 mEq/L	>40 mmol/L
O_2 Saturation	96–100%	0.96–1.00
Panic value	≤60%	<0.60
Oxyhemoglobin Dissociation Curve	No shift	

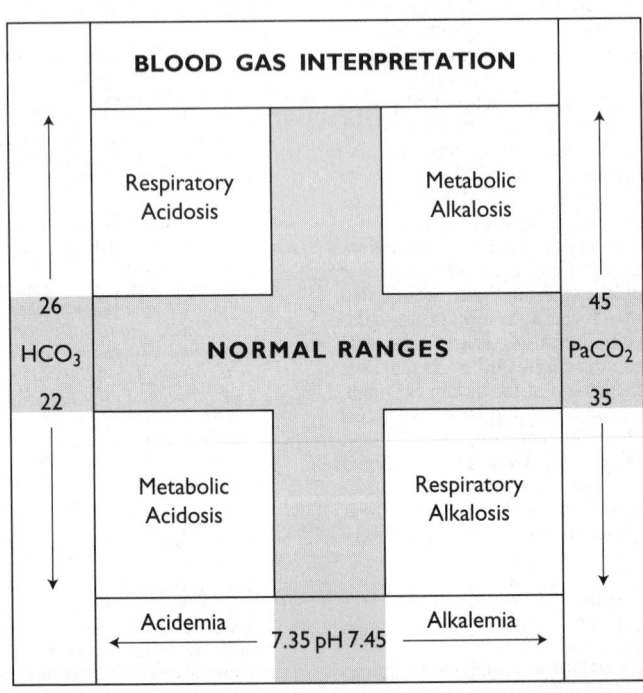

Increased pH: Alkali ingestion, Cushing's disease, diarrhea, fever, high altitude, hyperventilation, hysteria, intestinal obstruction (pyloric, duodenal), metabolic alkalosis, peptic ulcer therapy, renal disease, respiratory alkalosis, salicylate intoxication, and vomiting (excessive). Drugs include sodium bicarbonate.

Increased $PaCO_2$: Acute intermittent porphyria, aminoglycoside toxicity, asthma (late stage), brain death, coarctation of the aorta, congestive heart failure, electrolyte disturbance (severe), emphysema, empyema, hyaline membrane disease, hyperemesis, hypothyroidism (severe), hypoventilation (alveolar), metabolic alkalosis, near drowning, pleural effusion, pleurisy, pneumonia, pneumothorax, poisoning, pulmonary edema, pulmonary infection, renal disorders, respiratory acidosis, respiratory failure, shock, tetralogy of Fallot, transposition of the great vessels, and vomiting. Drugs include aldosterone, ethacrynic acid, metolazone, prednisone, sodium bicarbonate, and thiazides.

Increased PaO_2: Hyperbaric oxygenation and hyperventilation.

Increased HCO_3: Anoxia, metabolic alkalosis, and respiratory acidosis.

Increased O_2 Saturation: High altitudes, hypocapnia, hypothermia, increased cardiac output, hyperbaric oxygenation, increased oxygen affinity for hemoglobin, oxygen therapy, positive end expiratory pressure (PEEP) added to mechanical ventilation, respiratory alkalosis.

Decreased pH: Addison's disease, asthma, cardiac disease, diabetic ketoacidosis, diarrhea, emphysema, dysrhythmias, hepatic disease, hypercapnia, hypoventilation, malignant hyperthermia, metabolic acidosis, myocardial infarction, nephritis, nephrosis, pneumonia, pulmonary edema, pulmonary embolism, pulmonary infection, pulmonary malignancy, pulmonary obstructive disease, renal disease, respiratory acidosis, respiratory failure, sepsis, and shock.

Decreased $PaCO_2$: Dysrhythmias, asthma (early stage), diabetic ketoacidosis, diabetes mellitus, fever, high altitude, hyperventilation, metabolic

acidosis, respiratory alkalosis, and salicylate intoxication. Drugs include acetazolamide, dimercaprol, methicillin sodium, nitrofurantoin, nitrofurantoin sodium, tetracycline, and triamterene.

Decreased PaO_2: Acute respiratory distress syndrome, anoxia, anesthesia, aortic valve stenosis, arteriovenous shunt, asthma, atelectasis, atrial septal defect, berylliosis, carbon monoxide poisoning, cerebrovascular accident, coarctation of the aorta, emphysema, flail chest, Hamman-Rich syndrome, head injury, hyaline membrane disease, hypercapnia, hypoventilation, lung resection, lymphangitic carcinomatosis, near drowning, phrenic nerve paralysis, pickwickian syndrome, pain causing restricted diaphragmatic breathing, pleural effusion, pneumonia, pneumothorax, poisoning, poliomyelitis (acute), pulmonary adenomatosis, pulmonary embolism, pulmonary infection, pulmonary hemangioma, pulmonic stenosis, respiratory failure, sarcoidosis, shock, smoke inhalation, status epilepticus, tetanus, transposition of the great vessels, tricuspid atresia, and ventricular septal defect.

Decreased HCO_3: Hypocapnia, metabolic acidosis, and respiratory alkalosis.

Decreased O_2 Saturation: Acute respiratory distress syndrome, anesthesia, anoxia, anorexia, aortic valve stenosis, arteriovenous shunt, asthma, atelectasis, atrial septal defect, berylliosis, carbon monoxide poisoning, cerebrovascular accident, coarctation of the aorta, congenital heart defects, decreased cardiac output, decreased oxygen affinity for hemoglobin, emphysema, fever, flail chest, Hamman-Rich syndrome, head injury, hyaline membrane disease, hypercapnia, hypoventilation, hypoxia, lung resection, lymphangitic carcinomatosis, near drowning, phrenic nerve paralysis, pickwickian syndrome, pain causing restricted diaphragmatic breathing, pleural effusion, pneumonia, pneumothorax, poisoning, poliomyelitis (acute), pulmonary adenomatosis, pulmonary embolism, pulmonary infection, pulmonary hemangioma, pulmonic stenosis, respiratory acidosis, respiratory failure, sarcoidosis, shock, smoke inhalation, status epilepticus,

NORMAL OXYHEMOGLOBIN DISSOCIATION CURVE

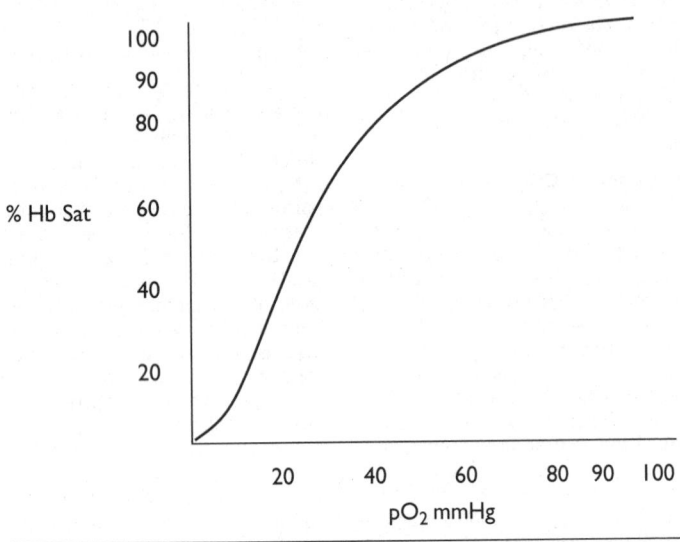

tetanus, transposition of the great vessels, tricuspid atresia, and ventricular septal defect.

Oxyhemoglobin Dissociation Curve

See diagram above.

Shift to Left: 2,3,-DPG deficiency, high altitudes, hypocapnia, hypothermia, increased oxygen affinity for hemoglobin, and respiratory alkalosis.

Shift to Right: Cluster headaches, decreased oxygen affinity for hemoglobin, emphysema, fever, hypercapnia, increased production of 2,3-DPG, and respiratory acidosis.

Description: The arterial blood gas test measures the dissolved oxygen and carbon dioxide in the arterial blood and reveals the acid-base state and how well the oxygen is being carried to the body. The *pH* is the measurement of free H+ ion concentration in circulating blood. Intracellular metabolism results in the continuous production of hydrogen ions, which are buffered as either an acid (HCO_3) or base (H_2CO_3). The body demands that pH remain constant. The kidneys and lungs regulate pH by preserving the ratio of acid to base. Any alteration in the ratio between bicarbonate and carbonic acid will cause a

reciprocal change in release or uptake of free H+, thereby altering pH value. Significant deviations in pH can be life threatening. *Bicarbonate* (HCO_3^-) and carbonic acid (H_2CO_3) are both components of the body's acid-base system that influence pH. The *partial pressure of carbon dioxide* (pCO₂, PaCO₂) is the amount of carbon dioxide in the blood based on the pressure it exerts in the bloodstream and represents the degree of alveolar ventilation occurring. When pH decreases, more CO₂ dissociates from carbonic acid and is exhaled through the lungs, counteracting the pH reduction and increasing the breathing rate. The *partial pressure of oxygen* (pO₂, PaO₂) is the amount of oxygen dissolved in plasma and represents the status of alveolar gas exchange with inspired air. *Oxygen saturation* (O₂ Sat) is the amount of oxygen actually bound to hemoglobin (as a percentage of the maximum amount that could be bound) and available for transport throughout the body. SaO₂ applies to arterial hemoglobin saturation:

Oxygen saturation = Oxygen content × [100/Oxygen capacity]

The oxyhemoglobin dissociation curve represents the affinity of hemoglobin for oxygen by demonstrating the normal levels of arterial oxygen saturation (O_2 Sat, SaO_2) of hemoglobin at varying partial pressures of oxygen. *P-50* is the partial pressure of oxygen at which the given hemoglobin sample is 50% saturated. The Hem-O-Scan machine analyzes and plots the hemoglobin-oxygen dissociation on a curve. When the curve is shifted to the left, more oxygen is delivered to the tissues for a given partial pressure of oxygen; when the shift is to the right, less oxygen is delivered to the tissues. Generally, decreased oxygen saturation to <90–92% must be addressed by thorough assessment of the client and clinical status.

Professional Considerations:

1. Consent form NOT required.

Risks:

Prolonged bleeding, hematoma, infection or nerve damage near puncture site.

Contraindications/Precautions:

In clients with bleeding disorders or anticoagulated states, repeated sampling from an invasive arterial catheter is preferred over arterial punctures.

2. Preparation:
   A. An Allen's test should be performed on both wrists prior to drawing radial artery specimens. Occlude both the ulnar and radial arteries in the wrist with two fingers for 10 seconds, then release the finger over the radial artery and look for the return of pink coloring into the hand above the wrist. If the coloring returns, the radial artery is not occluded and blood gases may be drawn from that site. Select the wrist with the swiftest return of pink coloring.
   B. Obtain a blood gas syringe, a 23-gauge needle, a povidone-iodine swab, alcohol wipes, sterile gloves, sterile gauze, and a container of ice.
   C. The client should rest for 30 minutes prior to specimen collection.
3. Procedure:
   A. The site for arterial puncture may be anesthetized with 1–2% Xylocaine.
   B. Attach a 1-inch long, 23-gauge needle to a plastic or glass blood gas syringe containing 0.5 ml of lithium heparin (1000 U/ml). Rotate the syringe to coat the inside surface with heparin (1000

U/ml) and eject the heparin through the needle into the sterile gauze.
   C. Cleanse the site for puncture with povidone-iodine and then with alcohol and allow it to dry.
   D. While wearing a sterile glove, palpate the artery and puncture the skin at a 30–45-degree angle (for radial artery), a 45–60-degree angle (for brachial artery), or a 45–90-degree angle (for femoral artery) with the bevel of the needle turned up.
   E. Advance the needle until the artery is punctured, and allow the syringe to autofill with at least 0.6 ml of arterial blood.
   F. Remove the syringe and needle and apply pressure to the sterile gauze over the site while discarding the needle, expelling the air from the syringe, and quickly capping the syringe with a rubber stopper and gently mixing the specimen.
   G. Immediately place the specimen in an ice bath.
4. Postprocedure care:
   A. Record the client's body temperature and the mode and amount of oxygen delivery on the laboratory requisition.
   B. Transport the specimen to the laboratory for processing within 15 minutes.
   C. If the specimen was obtained via direct arterial puncture, hold pressure over the site for 5–10 minutes.
5. Client and family teaching:
   A. Results are normally available within 30 minutes.
   B. The client's temperature is necessary in order to calculate and interpret the results.
   C. Results are interpreted according to disease/condition and compared to previous blood gas results.
6. Factors that affect results:
   A. Reject clotted specimens.
   B. If the client is receiving endotracheal suctioning or respiratory therapy treatments, the specimen should be drawn at least 20 minutes after either procedure.
   C. Failure to expel all air from the blood gas syringe will result in a falsely elevated PaO_2 and a falsely decreased $PaCO_2$.
   D. Failure to place the specimen in an ice bath may result in a decreased pH, PaO_2, and oxygen saturation.
   E. Failure to expel the heparin from the syringe prior to specimen collection may result in decreased pH, $PaCO_2$, and PaO_2.
   F. Specimen storage at room temperature accelerates the fall in pH.
   G. Elevated body temperature decreases the oxygen saturation result.
   H Clients with a history of cigarette smoking can have decreased arterial oxygen saturation after anesthesia.
   I. Elevated WBC causes a rapid pH drop.

J. Sodium fluoride can cause either an increase or a decrease in pH.

K. A prolonged time lapse between collection and testing may result in a decreased pH.

7. Other data:

A. If arterial blood is not practical to obtain, venous blood may be obtained by venipuncture, but accuracy is evident only for monitoring pH, $PaCO_2$, and base excess.

B. Evaluation of pH should take into consideration alterations in electrolyte, carbon dioxide, oxygen, and bicarbonate levels.

C. Samples of cord blood stored in heparinized syringes for >30 minutes result in significant changes in pH and PCO_2.

D. Earlobe gas analysis is an accurate substitute for arterial sampling.

E. In anemia, oxygen saturation may be normal, but hypoxia may still be present due to decreased oxygen-carrying capacity.

F. Continuous oxygen saturation monitoring via pulse oximetry is useful during cardiac catheterization in conjunction with intracardiac pressure measurement in detecting intracardiac abnormalities.

G. See also Pulse Oximetry, Diagnostic.

Bibliography:

Anderson S: ABG's. Six easy steps to interpreting blood gases. Am J Nurs 90(8):42–45, 1990.

Owen P, Farrell TA, Steyn W: Umbilical cord blood gas analysis; a comparison of two simple methods of sample storage. Early Hum Dev 42(1):67–71, 1995.

Pandit JJ: Sampling for analyzing blood gas pressures. Arterial samples are better [letter; comment]. Br Med J 310(9686):1071–1072, 1995.

Pitkin AD, Roberts CM, Wedzicha JA: Arterialised earlobe blood gas analysis: An underused technique. Thorax 49(4):364–366, 1994.

Pretto JJ, Rochford PD: Effects of sample storage time, temperature and syringe type on blood gas tensions in samples with high oxygen partial pressures. Thorax 49(6):610–612, 1994.

BLOOD GASES, CAPILLARY, BLOOD

Norm: Must be corrected for body temperature.

		SI Units
pH		
Adults	7.35–7.45	7.35–7.45
Panic values	<7.2 or >7.6	<7.2 or >7.6
Children (arterialized capillary sample)		
Birth–2 months	7.32–7.49	7.32–7.49
2 months–2 years	7.34–7.46	7.34–7.46
Over 2 years	7.35–7.45	7.35–7.45
pCO_2	26.4–41.2 mmHg	3.5–5.4 kPa
Panic values	<20 mmHg	<2.7 kPa
	>70 mmHg	>9.4 kPa
pO_2	75–100 mmHg	10.0–13.3 kPa
Panic values	<40 mmHg	<5.3 kPa
HCO_3	22–26 mEq/L	22–26 mmol/L
Panic values	<10 mEq/L	<10 mmol/L
	>40 mEq/L	>40 mmol/L
O_2 Saturation	96–100%	0.96–1.00
Panic value	<60%	<0.60

Increased pH: See Blood Gases, Arterial, Blood.

Increased pCO₂: See Blood Gases, Arterial, Blood.

Increased pO₂: See Blood Gases, Arterial, Blood.

Increased HCO₃: See Blood Gases, Arterial, Blood.

Increased O₂ Saturation: See Blood Gases, Arterial, Blood.

Decreased pH: See Blood Gases, Arterial, Blood.

Decreased pCO₂: See Blood Gases, Arterial, Blood.

Decreased pO₂: Capillary pO_2 interpretation is limited to assessment for hypoxia.

Decreased HCO₃: See Blood Gases, Arterial, Blood.

Decreased O₂ Saturation: *See Blood Gases, Arterial, Blood.*

Description: A method for determining acid-base status from a heel-stick for capillary blood. Used mostly in infants to assess pH and pCO_2. *(See Blood Gases, Arterial, for complete description of the test components.)*

Professional Considerations:

1. Consent form NOT required.
2. Preparation:
   A. Warmth may be applied to the heel for 15 minutes prior to collection, but is not necessary.
   B. Obtain alcohol wipes, a lancet, sterile gauze, two capillary tubes with a metal stirrer, and a magnet.
3. Procedure:
   A. Cleanse an area on the medial or lateral plantar surface of the heel with an alcohol wipe and allow it to dry.
   B. Using a 2.5-mm lancet, puncture the heel until a free flow of blood is obtained.
   C. Wipe away the first drop of blood.
   D. Completely fill two heparinized, 250-ml capillary tubes without air bubbles and add a heparinized metal stirrer. Quickly seal them and mix well by maneuvering a magnet around the tubes.
4. Postprocedure care:
   A. Place the capillary tubes in an ice bath.
   B. Write the client's temperature, mode and amount of oxygen delivery, and the type and site of the specimen collection on the laboratory requisition.
   C. Place pressure on the heel for 5–10 minutes and leave the site open to air to heal.
   D. Transport the specimens to the laboratory within 15 minutes.

5. Client and family teaching:
   A. The client's temperature is important in evaluating results.
   B. Results are normally available within 30 minutes.
   C. Results are interpreted according to disease/condition and compared to previous gases.
6. Factors that affect results:
   A. Avoid milking the heel.
   B. Reject hemolyzed or clotted specimens.
   C. Storage at room temperature accelerates the fall in pH.
   D. Elevated white blood counts cause a rapid pH drop.
   E. Sodium fluoride can cause either an increase or a decrease in pH.
   F. A prolonged time lapse between collection and testing may result in decreased pH.
   G. Capillary blood gas specimens are contraindicated in low cardiac output, vasoconstriction, shock, and hypotension because the results will not be valid.
7. Other data:
   A. Avoid puncturing over previous puncture sites.
   B. Avoid puncturing the posterior curvature of the heel.
   C. Specimens may also be taken from the earlobe in adults.
   D. Evaluation of pH should take into consideration alterations in electrolyte, carbon dioxide, oxygen, and bicarbonate levels.

Bibliography:

Courtney SE, Weber KR, Breakie LA, Malin SW, Bender CV, Guo SM, Siervogel RM: Capillary blood gases in the neonate. A reassessment and review of the literature. Am J Dis Child *144*(2):168–172, 1990.

Dar K, Williams T, Aitken R, Woods KL, Fletcher S: Arterial versus capillary sampling for analysing blood gas pressures. Br Med J *310*(6971):24–25, 1995.

BLOOD GASES, VENOUS, BLOOD

Norm: Must be corrected for body temperature.

		SI Units
pH	7.32–7.43	7.32–7.43
Panic value	<7.2 or >7.6	<7.2 or >7.6
pCO_2	38–50 mmHg	5.0–6.7 kPa
pO_2	20–49 mmHg	2.6–6.5 kPa
HCO_3	22–26 mEq/L	22–26 mmol/L
Panic value	<10 mEq/L	<10 mmol/L
	>40 mEq/L	>40 mmol/L
O_2 saturation	60–80%	0.60–0.80

Increased pH: *See Blood Gases, Arterial, Blood.*

Increased pCO_2: *See Blood Gases, Arterial, Blood.*

Increased pO$_2$: Interpretation of oxygen levels is not appropriate on venous blood specimens.

Increased HCO$_3$: *See Blood Gases, Arterial, Blood.*

Increased O$_2$ Saturation: Interpretation of oxygen saturation is not appropriate on venous blood specimens.

Decreased pH: *See Blood Gases, Arterial, Blood.*

Decreased pCO$_2$: *See Blood Gases, Arterial, Blood.*

Decreased pO$_2$: Interpretation of oxygen levels is not appropriate on venous blood specimens.

Decreased HCO$_3$: *See Blood Gases, Arterial, Blood.*

Decreased O$_2$ Saturation: Interpretation of oxygen saturation is not appropriate on venous blood specimens.

Description: A method for assessing acid-base status and for cellular hypoxia without performing an arterial puncture. Venous blood gases may be used in situations where assessment of oxygenation is unnecessary. *(See Blood Gases, Arterial, for complete descriptions of the test components.)*

Professional Considerations:

1. Consent form NOT required.
2. Preparation:
   A. The client should rest quietly for 30 minutes prior to specimen collection.
   B. Obtain alcohol wipes, a tourniquet, a needle, a syringe or Vacutainer, heparin, and a green-top tube.
3. Procedure:
   A. Draw 1 ml of heparin (1000 U/ml) into a 3-ml syringe and coat the inside of the syringe with heparin. Eject the heparin.
   B. Draw a 2-ml venous blood sample into the syringe, taking care to avoid getting air bubbles mixed with the blood.
   C. Inject blood from the syringe into the tube.
   D. Alternately, perform a Vacutainer collection directly into a heparinized, green-top tube and remove the tube from the Vacutainer before removing the needle from the vein.
   E. The specimen may be obtained from cord blood.
4. Postprocedure care:
   A. Place the specimen on ice.
   B. Write the client's temperature and the type of specimen on the laboratory requisition.

C. Write the mode and amount of oxygen delivery on the laboratory requisition.
5. Client and family teaching:
   A. Do not pump your fist during collection.
   B. The client's temperature is needed to interpret results.
   C. Results are normally available within 30 minutes.
   D. Results require interpretation depending on disease/condition and compared to previous gases.
6. Factors that affect results:
   A. Avoid using a tourniquet, if possible. If one is used, it should be left in place while drawing the sample.
   B. Reject clotted specimens or specimens not received on ice.
   C. Storage at room temperature accelerates the fall in pH.
   D. Elevated white blood counts cause a rapid pH drop.
   E. Sodium fluoride can cause either an increase or a decrease in pH.
   F. A prolonged time lapse between collection and testing may result in decreased pH.
7. Other data:
   A. For data on oxygenation, arterial blood is required.
   B. Evaluation of pH should take into consideration alterations in electrolyte, carbon dioxide, oxygen, and bicarbonate levels.

Bibliography:

Barry PW, Mason NP, Collier D: Sampling for analysing blood gas pressures. Mount Everest study supports use of capillary samples [letter]. Br Med J *310*(6986):1072, 1995.

Gregg AR, Weiner CP: Normal umbilical arterial and venous acid-base and blood gas values. Clin Obstet Gynecol *36*(1):24–32, 1993.

BLOOD GROUP ANTIGEN OF SEMEN, VAGINAL SWAB

Norm: Blood group antigens may be identified in 80% of the population. Blood group matches the victim's where coitus has not occurred or where the perpetrator's blood group matches that of the victim. Blood group differs from the victim's where coitus has occurred with a perpetrator of a different ABO blood group.

Usage: Rape trauma investigation.

Description: Approximately 80% of the population (both males and females) are classified as having a dominant secretor gene that causes them to secrete their ABO blood group antigen in their body fluids. Samples of vaginal fluid are analyzed for soluble A, B, and

H blood group substances for the purpose of identifying the blood group of the perpetrator of a sexual assault. Although the results can be compared with the blood group antigen obtained from body fluid of the suspected assailant, this test cannot confirm this client as the perpetrator. However, it can rule out a suspect if the blood group antigens are different.

Professional Considerations:

1. Consent form NOT required unless results may be used for legal evidence.
2. Preparation:
   A. Obtain a speculum, a cotton wool swab supplied in a sexual offense kit, glass slides, and a Coplin jar of 95% ethanol.
3. Procedure:
   A. If the specimen may be used as legal evidence, have the specimen collection witnessed.
   B. Position the woman in a lithotomy position and drape her for privacy and comfort.
   C. Gently scrape the walls of the vagina with a plain cotton wool swab until it is saturated.
   D. Roll the swab onto two glass slides and place the slides in a Coplin jar of 95% ethanol.
4. Postprocedure care:
   A. Write the client's name, the date, the exact time of collection, and the specimen source on the laboratory requisition. Sign and have the witness sign the laboratory requisition.
   B. Transport the specimen to the laboratory immediately in a sealed plastic bag marked as legal evidence. All persons handling the specimen should sign and mark the time of receipt on the laboratory requisition.
5. Client and family teaching:
   A. Offer the client and family immediate counseling/crisis intervention and support. Survivors of sexual assault should be referred to appropriate crisis-counseling agencies as well as gynecological follow-up. Facilitate the connection if desired by the client.
   B. Referral for HIV testing should be reviewed and offered to all sexual assault victims.
   C. Preventive treatment for chlamydia, gonorrhea, and syphilis should be provided to all survivors of sexual assault.
   D. The option of postcoital contraceptive should be reviewed with all survivors of sexual assault.
   E. Results will be available within 5 days.
   F. National Coalition Against Sexual Assault phone number is (202) 483-7165.
6. Factors that affect results:
   A. Results are inconclusive if the victim's and the suspect's blood group are the same.
   B. Vaginal swabs for blood group antigen detection should be collected as soon as possible after the rape. Semen is rarely detected in the vagina more than 72 hours after coitus.
   C. Negative results may be obtained if the assailant was sexually dysfunctional or has had a vasectomy or if the woman bathed, douched, or defecated after the rape.
7. Other data:
   A. *See also Acid Phosphatase, Vaginal Swab, and Precipitin Test Against Human Sperm and Blood, Vaginal Swab.*

Bibliography:

Nakazato M: Human prostate acid phosphatase is carrier protein for ABH blood group antigens of semen. Tohoku J Exp Med *172*(4):155–165, 1994.

Tucker S, Claire E, Ledray LE, Werner JS, Claire E: Sexual assault evidence collection. Wis Med J *89*(7):407–411, 1990.

Wee KP: Disputed paternity: the historical perspectives. Ann Acad Med Singapore *22*(1):33–36, 1993.

BLOOD INDICES, BLOOD

Norm:

		SI Units
Mean Corpuscular Hemoglobin (MCH)		
Adults	26–34 pg	1.61–2.11 fmol
Children		
Newborn		
Day 1	1–38 pg	2.36 fmol
Days 2–3	37 pg	2.30 fmol
Days 4–8	36 pg	2.23 fmol
Days 9–13	33 pg	2.05 fmol
2–8 weeks	30 pg	1.86 fmol

		SI Units
3 months	28 pg	1.73 fmol
4–5 months	27 pg	1.67 fmol
6–11 months	26 pg	1.61 fmol
1–2 years	25 pg	1.55 fmol
3 years	26 pg	1.61 fmol
4–10 years	27 pg	1.67 fmol
11–15 years	28 pg	1.73 fmol

Mean Corpuscular Hemoglobin Concentration (MCHC)

Adults	31–38%	19.2–23.58 mmol/l
Children		
Newborn		
Days 1–3	36%	22.34 mmol/l
Days 2–8	35%	21.72 mmol/l
Days 9–13	34%	21.10 mmol/l
2–8 weeks	33%	20.48 mmol/l
3–5 months	34%	21.10 mmol/l
6–11 months	33%	20.48 mmol/l
1–2 years	32%	19.86 mmol/l
3 years	35%	21.72 mmol/l
4–15 years	34%	21.10 mmol/l

Mean Corpuscular Volume (MCV)

Adults	82–98 m^3	82–98 fl
Children		
Newborn	106 μ^3	106 fl
Day 1		
Days 2–3	105 μ^3	105 fl
Days 4–8	103 μ^3	103 fl
Days 9–13	98 μ^3	98 fl
2–8 weeks	90 μ^3	90 fl
3 months	82 μ^3	82 fl
4–5 months	80 μ^3	80 fl
6–11 months	77 μ^3	77 fl
1 year	78 μ^3	78 fl
2 years	77 μ^3	77 fl
3 years	79 μ^3	79 fl
4–10 years	80 μ^3	80 fl
11–15 years	82 μ^3	82 fl

Increased MCV: Alcoholism (chronic), anemia (acquired hemolytic, aplastic, immune hemolytic, macrocytic induced by megaloblastic anemias, pernicious [early]), cirrhosis, chronic lymphocytic leukemia, cytomegalovirus, diabetic ketoacidosis, diabetes mellitus, DNA synthesis disorders (inherited), folate deficiency, hepatic disease, infants, leukocytosis (marked), methanol poisoning, newborns, pancreatitis, preleukemia, reticulocytosis, sprue, and vitamin B$_{12}$ deficiency.

Increased MCH: Anemia (macrocytic, pernicious), cold agglutinin conditions, dysproteinemia, infants, newborns, and presence of monoclonal blood proteins. Drugs include heparin calcium and heparin sodium.

Increased MCHC: High titer of cold agglutinins, hereditary spherocytosis, infants, intravascular hemolysis, lipemia, and newborns. Drugs include heparin calcium and heparin sodium.

Decreased MCV: Anemia (chronic, dyserythropoietic, iron deficiency, microcytic, pyridoxine responsive, sickle cell), alpha- or beta-thalassemia, chlorasis, chronic disease, diverticulitis, diverticulosis, endocarditis, G-6-PD deficiency, gangrene, hemoglobin H, leukocytosis (marked), malaria, myocarditis, radiation therapy, red cell fragmentation, subacute bacterial endocarditis, and warm autoantibodies.

Decreased MCH: Anemia (iron deficiency, microcytic, normocytic).

Decreased MCHC: Anemia (iron deficiency, chronic, megaloblastic, microcytic, sideroblastic).

Description: Blood indices encompasses a group of six different blood tests, the MCH, MCHC, MCV, RBC, Hct, and Hgb, that are used to establish the characteristics and hemoglobin content of the red blood cells. *(See Red Blood Cell; Hematocrit; and Hemoglobin.)* They assist in the diagnosis and differentiation of compensated and uncompensated anemias. A stained blood smear is prepared to study the shape and size of the red blood cell. Combined with staining, the indices assist in determinations of red blood cell morphology. This visual or electronic counting of erythrocytes is regarded as the most reliable index for distinguishing and differentiating erythrocyte morphology. MCH is the average weight of the hemoglobin of each red blood cell, expressed in picograms. MCHC is a calculated value of the amount of hemoglobin present in the red blood cell compared to its size. A ratio of weight to volume is expressed as a percentage. MCV is a calculated value, expressed in cubic microns, of the average volume of an erythrocyte.

Professional Considerations:

1. Consent form NOT required.
2. Preparation:
   A. Tube: Lavender-top.
3. Procedure:
   A. Draw a 7-ml blood sample. A stained blood smear is prepared.
4. Postprocedure care:
   A. The collection tube should be filled completely, inverted, and gently rotated to thoroughly mix the anticoagulant.
   B. The serum sample is stable at room temperature for 10 hours, may be refrigerated for up to 18 hours, and should not be frozen.
5. Client and family teaching:
   A. Results are normally available within 24 hours.

B. All results must be available to make an accurate interpretation associated with diagnosis/condition.
6. Factors that affect results:
   A. Reject hemolyzed specimens.
   B. High altitude affects MCV (standard deviation [SD] =.810 fl), MCH (SD = .583 pg), and MCHC (SD = .630 g/dl).
7. Other data:
   A. Bone marrow suppression in the chronically ill can be a frequent cause of anemia.
   B. Production of macroreticulocytes is an early sign of engraftment post bone marrow transplant.
   C. *See also Red Blood Cell Morphology, Blood.*

Bibliography:

d'Onofrio G, Chirillo R, Zini G, Caenaro G, Tommasi M, Micciulli G: Simultaneous measurement of reticulocyte and red blood cell indices in healthy subjects and patients with microcytic and macrocytic anemia. Blood 85(3):818–823, 1995.

Piedras J, Loria A, Galvan I: Red blood cell indices in a high altitude hospital population. Arch Med Res 26(1):65–68, 1995.

BLOOD UREA NITROGEN
(see Urea Nitrogen, Plasma or Serum)

BLOOD UREA NITROGEN/CREATININE RATIO, BLOOD

Norm:

Normal = 10:1–15:1.
Diminished urea concentration: <10:1.
Inadequate renal function: >15:1.

Increased: Azotemia, burns, cachexia, catabolic states, Cushing's disease, dehydration, excessive protein intake, fever, gastrointestinal bleeding, glomerular disease, heart failure, hemorrhage, hypercalcemia, hypertension, impaired renal blood flow, ileal conduit, infection, muscle or tissue destruction, prerenal azotemia, shock, surgery, swallowing of food into the upper airway, thyrotoxicosis, urinary reabsorption (ureterocolostomy), and urinary tract obstruction (rare). Drugs include tetracyclines and steroids.

Decreased: Diarrhea, diet (inadequate protein intake), hemodialysis, hepatic insufficiency, hyperammonemias (genetic), intravenous therapy (prolonged), ketosis, marasmus, malnutrition, pregnancy, renal failure (muscular people, chronic), rhabdomyolysis, syndrome of inappropriate antidiuretic hormone secretion (SIADHS), and vomiting. Drugs include phenacemide. Drugs that increase only the creatinine and not the blood urea nitrogen (BUN) include cephalosporins, cimetidine, tetracyclines, and trimethoprim.

Description: The BUN/creatinine ratio assists in the interpretation of laboratory values in assessing renal failure and in the evaluation of an elevated BUN level. This test is a more sensitive indicator of the relationship between BUN and creatinine than each separate test because BUN rises at a greater rate than creatinine in renal disease.

Professional Considerations:
1. Consent form NOT required.
2. Preparation:
   A. Tube: Red-top, red/gray-top, or gold-top.

3. Procedure:
   A. Draw a 5-ml blood sample.
4. Postprocedure care:
   A. None.
5. Client and family teaching:
   A. Assess knowledge and provide information about adequate dietary protein.
6. Factors that affect results:
   A. Low-protein diet lowers BUN value.
7. Other data:
   A. Before a change in BUN is significant, there exists approximately 60% renal impairment.

Bibliography:

Boeniger MF, Lowry LK, Rosenberg J: Interpretation of urine results used to assess chemical exposure with emphasis on creatinine adjustments: A review. Am Ind Hyg Assoc J *54*(10): 615–627, 1993.

Ducharme MP, Smythe M, Strohs G: Drug-induced alterations in serum creatinine concentrations. Ann Pharmacother *27*(5):622–633, 1993.

Jackson AA: Salvage of urea-nitrogen and protein requirements. Proc Nutr Soc *54*(2):535–547.

BLOOD VOLUME, BLOOD .

Norm:

Blood volume	8.5–9% of body weight
Adult female	54.01–63.89 ml/kg
Adult male	52.95–70.13 ml/kg
Erythrocyte volume	
Adult female	21.65–26.83 ml/kg
Adult male	24.16–32.38 ml/kg
Plasma volume	
Adult female	31.53–38.01 ml/kg
Adult male	28.27–38.63 ml/kg

Usage: Anemia, differentiation of relative polycythemia from absolute polycythemia, preoperative or postoperative evaluation to estimate need for replacement blood, and unexplained hypotension.

Description: Blood volume is comprised of plasma and cellular components and varies with body weight, muscle mass, height, age, sex, environment, and physical activity. This nuclear medicine test uses a dilution technique that measures blood volume after radiolabeled albumin and radiolabeled red blood cells are injected intravenously. A tagged sample of the client's blood is then measured for blood volume, erythrocyte volume, and plasma volume with a scinticounter. This test is based on the principle of adding a known quantity of tracer substance to an unknown quantity of diluent (blood). The final tracer concentration should be inversely proportional to the volume of blood. Radiolabeled albumin is used to measure plasma volume, and the radiolabeled red blood cells are used to measure volume of the cellular component of blood. This test is helpful in differentiating between fluid shifts or other causes of decreased plasma volume (relative polycythemia) and increased red blood cell mass (absolute polycythemia).

Professional Considerations:
1. Consent form NOT required.

Risks:

Allergic reaction to radiolabeled albumin (itching, hives, rash, tight feeling in the throat, shortness of breath, bronchospasm, anaphylaxis, death), hematoma or infection at injection site.

Contraindications:

Previous allergy to radioactive dyes, iodine, or shellfish; during pregnancy; while breast-feeding; hypersensitivity to iodine; extended clotting times; in edematous or hemorrhaging clients.

2. Preparation:
   A. Have emergency equipment readily available.
   B. Obtain alcohol wipes, a tourniquet, a 19-gauge needle, five syringes, one glass green-top tube, two plastic green-top tubes, a centrifuge bag, a sterile glass beaker of 3 ml Strumia formula solution, chilled sterile 0.9% saline solution, and centrifuge.
   C. Draw a 25-ml blood sample and inject into a sterile centrifuge bag to which 3-ml of Strumia formula solution has been added. Add 50–100 mCi of Cr-51 (sodium chromate) to the container and gently agitate it for 3 minutes. Then fill the bag with sterile, chilled 0.9% saline and centrifuge it at a 45-degree angle for 7 minutes. Remove the supernatant fluid and resuspend the cells in 10 ml of sterile 0.9% saline solution.
   D. Obtain a mixture of 5 ml of I-125 albumin in 20 ml of sterile normal saline solution for plasma volume measurement.
   E. Lugol's solution may be used to prevent uptake of I-125 albumin by the thyroid gland.
3. Procedure:
   A. Draw an 8-ml blood sample in a heparinized green-top tube and label it as the baseline sample.
   B. *Injection for red blood cell volume measurement:* Draw 2–3 ml of the CR-51-labeled red blood cell solution into a syringe with a 19-gauge needle. Note the exact amount in the syringe. Inject the mixture directly into a vein in the right arm of the client.
   C. *Injection for plasma volume measurement:* Draw 2–3 ml of the I-125 albumin 2 mCi/ml into a syringe. Note the exact amount in the syringe. Inject the mixture directly into a vein in the right arm of the client.
   D. *Recovery of tagged blood for blood volume determination:* At 10 and 20 minutes after the two tracer injections, draw an 8-ml blood sample from the left arm in a heparinized plastic, rather

than glass, green-top tube. Label each sample with the time drawn.
   E. Using the multidose vials from which the Cr-51-tagged red blood cells and I-125 albumin were drawn as controls, measure blood volume, red blood cell volume, and plasma volume of the samples with a scintillation well counter.
4. Postprocedure care:
   A. None.
5. Client and family teaching:
   A. This test involves injection of a nuclear medicine tracer, followed by two timed blood sample collections. Total test time is less than 1 hour.
   B. Results are normally available within 24 hours.
6. Factors that affect results:
   A. Blood volume is usually highest in the morning.
   B. Glass tubes used for the tagged sample may cause falsely low plasma volume results because glass absorbs energy from I-125 albumin.
   C. The Cr-51 rate of tagging red blood cells varies with pH, type of anticoagulant, and body temperature. In general, tagging should be complete by 5 minutes after injection.
   D. If the client has recently taken polyvitamins or antibiotics, Cr-51 may not label the client's own red blood cells. Blood bank Cr-51-labeled O-Rh-negative blood should be substituted.
   E. Injection through intravenous tubing or tissue extravasation of tracer will cause falsely decreased results.
   F. Two post-tracer-injection blood samples are required both to establish that mixing of Cr-51-labeled red blood cells is complete and to determine the rate of loss of the I-125 albumin tracer.
   G. If the 10- and 20-minute sample results vary by more than 3%, a third sample should be drawn 60–90 minutes after the initial injection.
7. Other data:
   A. No isolation of the client is necessary.

Bibliography:

Ferrant A: What clinical and laboratory data are indicative of polycythemia and when are blood volume studies needed? Nouv Rev Fr Hematol *36*(2):151–154, 1994.

BLOOD VOLUME DETERMINATION STUDIES, DIAGNOSTIC

Norm: Requires interpretation.

Usage: Differential diagnosis of pericardial effusion from pericardial cysts or tumors, diagnosis of peripheral vascular disease, and thrombophlebitis.

Description: A nuclear medicine study of circulation dynamics in which a tracer is circulated in the blood for a period of time. Measures of diluted radioactivity are used to calculate the volume distribution of compartments and regions of the circulation. Pericardial effusions are detected by examining the blood volumes in and around the heart. Peripheral vascular disease and thrombophlebitis are detected by examining the rates at which the venous pools of the legs change in volume with exercise and posture changes.

Professional Considerations:

1.   Consent form IS required.

Risks:

Allergic reaction to radiolabeled albumin (itching, hives, rash, tight feeling in the throat, shortness of breath, bronchospasm, anaphylaxis, death), hematoma or infection at injection site.

Contraindications:

Previous allergy to iodine, x-ray dye, seafood, or a nuclear medicine radiolabeled albumin tracer.

2.   Preparation:
     A.   Have emergency equipment readily available.

B.   Establish intravenous access in an arm vein.
3.   Procedure:
     A.   A tracer of labeled albumin, red blood cells, or substances bound by plasma proteins is injected intravenously and allowed to circulate. The circulatory compartment to be studied is scanned, and a well counter is used to compare the diluted radioactivity of the compartment with a standard. This is followed by calculation of the volume distribution of the compartment.
4.   Postprocedure care:
     A.   Encourage the oral intake of fluids.
5.   Client and family teaching:
     A.   The risk of radioactivity from this test is less than that of a regular x-ray.
6.   Factors that affect results:
     A.   Blood volume is highest in the morning.
7.   Other data:
     A.   No isolation of the client is necessary.
     B.   Health care professionals working in a nuclear medicine area must follow federal standards set by the Nuclear Regulatory Commission. These standards include precautions for handling the radioactive material and monitoring of potential radiation exposure.

Bibliography:

Carlsen O, Bruun P: A method for determination of normal or abnormal blood volume in patients subjected to radionuclide cardiography. Scand J Clin Lab Invest *50*(1):63–67, 1990.

Vissing SF, Nielsen SL: Regional blood volume in man determined by radiolabeled erythrocytes. Clin Physiol *8*(3):303–308, 1988.

B-LYMPHOCYTES, BLOOD

Norm:

		SI Units
Adults	270–640/mm³ or 270–640/μL	270–640 cells × 10⁶/L
	5–15% of circulating lymphocytes	
	or 25–35% of total lymphocytes	0.25–0.35
Children		
Newborn	61% of total lymphocytes	0.61
Infants	60% of total lymphocytes	0.60
Age 6	42% of total lymphocytes	0.42
Age 12	38% of total lymphocytes	0.38

Increased: Active antibody formation in young children, agranulocytosis, bacterial infections (acute, chronic), brucellosis, Burkitt's lymphoma, carcinoma, chickenpox, cytomegalovirus, DiGeorge syndrome, hepatitis (viral), hyperthyroidism, influenza, leukemia (lymphocytic), leukosarcoma, lymphocytosis (infectious), lymphoma (non-Hodgkin's), measles, malnutrition, mononucleosis (infectious), multiple myeloma, mumps, parathyroid fever, pertussis, pneumonia (viral), scurvy, syphilis, thyrotoxicosis, tuberculosis, tularemia, typhoid fever, typhus, and Waldenstrom's macroglobulinemia.

Decreased: Anemia (aplastic), burns, cardiac failure, Cushing's disease, Hodgkin's disease, immunoglobulin deficiency, leukemia (chronic granulocytic, monocytic), lymphatic irradiation, stress reactions, systemic lupus erythematosus (SLE), terminal carcinoma, thymic hypoplasia (children), trauma, and uremia. Drugs include corticotropin, cortisone acetate, epinephrine bitartrate, epinephrine borate, epinephrine hydrochloride, and nitrogen mustard.

Description: B-lymphocytes are white blood cells with a short lifespan that are produced by bone marrow and are responsible for humoral immunity and production of immunoglobulin and specific antibodies. They are found in the lymph nodes, spleen, bone marrow, and blood and are a primary defense against virulent, encapsulated, bacterial pathogens. When stimulated by an antigen, they transform themselves into plasma cells that rapidly secrete antibodies. These antibodies neutralize viruses, interfere with the absorption of foreign proteins, and detoxify other proteins.

Professional Considerations:

1. Consent form NOT required.
2. Preparation:
   A. Tube: Green-top.
3. Procedure:
   A. Draw a 5-ml blood sample.
4. Postprocedure care:
   A. None.
5. Client and family teaching:
   A. Inform the physician of past (6-month) history of colds and infections.
6. Factors that affect results:
   A. Medications containing epinephrine cause unreliable results.
7. Other data:
   A. Plasma cells seldom appear in the blood, but they may appear in increased numbers in severe infections, especially in children, to reinforce immunity when sufficient antibodies are not available.

Bibliography:

Kyle RA: Prognostic factors in multiple myeloma. Stem Cells (Dayt) *13* (Suppl 2):56–63, 1995.

Pacheco SE, Shearer WT: Laboratory aspects of immunology. Pediatr Clin North Am *41*(4):623–655, 1994.

BMR

(see Basal Metabolic Rate, Diagnostic)

BODY FLUID, AMYLASE, SPECIMEN

Norm: Negative.

Positive: Benign ovarian cyst fluid, esophageal rupture, necrotic bowel, pancreatic ascites, pancreatic duct trauma, pancreatitis (with or without pseudocyst), perforated peptic ulcer, and malignant pleural effusions in the presence of cancer of the lung, breast, gastrointestinal tract, ovary, and lymphoma.

Description: Amylase is produced in large quantities by the pancreas, salivary glands, and certain malignant tumors. It is produced in lesser quantities by the fallopian tubes and lungs. Amylase from the pancreas and salivary glands is normally contained in the gastrointestinal tract. The presence of a significant amount of amylase in a body fluid specimen indicates a pathological process.

Professional Considerations:

1. Consent form NOT required. See individual procedures for procedure-specific risks and contraindications.
2. Preparation:
   A. Obtain a pleural or peritoneal aspiration tray and a clean container or red-top tube. Sterile 0.9% saline is needed for peritoneal lavage.
3. Procedure:
   A. Obtain a body fluid specimen via needle aspiration of pleural or peritoneal fluid, or by catheter irrigation and aspiration of the peritoneum, and inject it into a clean container or red-top tube.
4. Postprocedure care:
   A. Apply a dry, sterile dressing to the site.
5. Client and family teaching:
   A. Results are normally available within 72 hours.
6. Factors that affect results:
   A. When collecting ascitic fluid, the location of the collection site or of the catheter tip will likely affect the level of amylase that may be present. For example, a catheter directed to the left upper quadrant may produce a false-negative specimen.
7. Other data:
   A. A common finding of lung carcinoma with pleural effusion.
   B. Amylase levels indicative of saliva can be obtained on penile swabs, vaginal swabs, and breast swabs in sexual assault cases.

Bibliography:

Hammel P, Levy P, Voitot H, Levy M, Vilgrain V, Zins M, et al.: Preoperative cyst fluid analysis is useful for the differential diagnosis of cystic lesions of the pancreas. Gastroenterology *108*(4):1230–1235, 1995.

Keating SM, Higgs DF: The detection of amylase on swabs from sexual assault cases. J Forensic Sci Soc *34*(2):89–93, 1994.

BODY FLUID, ANAEROBIC CULTURE

Norm: Negative. No growth.

Positive: Aspiration pneumonia, biliary tract infections, bite wounds, bronchiectasis, chronic osteomyelitis, chronic sinus infection, dental and mouth infections, deep tissue infection or necrosis, gastrointestinal infections (especially of the colon), gynecologic intra-abdominal or extra-abdominal infections, immunodeficiency states, immunosuppressive therapy, infections caused by *Actinomyces, Arachnia, Bacteroides fragilis, Bacteroides melaninogenicus, Bifidobacterium, Clostridium, Coccidioides, Eubacterium, Fusobacterium, Lactobacillus, Peptostreptococcus, Propioni bacterium, Veillonella,* and others; malignancy, and trauma (accidental, surgical). Drugs include aminoglycosides.

Description: The test identifies anaerobic bacterial infections in body fluids, including ascitic fluid, bile, cerebrospinal fluid, pleural fluid, and synovial fluid, and from wounds and abscesses. Anaerobes live and grow where there is no free oxygen and obtain energy for growth and metabolism from fermentation reactions rather than from oxygen. Anaerobes are part of the normal flora of the skin, oral cavity, lower gastrointestinal tract, urethra, and the female external genital tract. When displaced from their location into other body tissues or spaces, they become pathogenic, causing localized abscesses in oxygen-poor body cavities and specific body organs. Untreated anaerobic infections may lead to bacteremia. Special collection methods are necessary for isolation of anaerobes. Anaerobic cultures are grown on complex media, and identification is made using colony morphology, pigmentation, fluorescence, and gas-liquid chromatography.

Professional Considerations:

1. Consent form IS required for some of the procedures used to obtain the specimen.

See specific procedures for risks and contraindications.

2. Preparation:
   A. Notify laboratory personnel that an anaerobic specimen will be arriving.
   B. For the needle and syringe method, obtain a needle, a syringe, a sterile "gassed-out" tube (a tube flushed with oxygen-free carbon dioxide or nitrogen gas), and a double stopper.
   C. For the two-tube swab method, obtain several sterile swabs prepared and stored in oxygen-free carbon dioxide tubes and tubes containing prereduced transport media with a methylene blue indicator as needed.

3. Procedure:
   A. *Needle and syringe method:* Expel all air from the syringe. Aspirate the specimen directly into the syringe. Carefully expel any air from the syringe. Immediately inject the specimen into a sterile "gassed-out" tube, preferably with a double stopper to prevent the introduction of air when the specimen is injected. If this anaerobic transport tube is not available, the needle can be tightly capped or imbedded in a sterile rubber stopper. Since the specimen must be centrifuged, the volume should be over 2 ml. In the presence of extensive wounds involving large amounts of tissue or multiple lesions, several samples should be taken.
   B. *Two-tube swab method:* Collect the specimen on at least two sterile swabs that have been prepared and stored in oxygen-free tubes. Expose the swabs to air as briefly as possible. Keeping the methylene blue transport tube upright, quickly place the swabs in the tubes and close them tightly. Never let the swab samples dry out.
   C. Alternatively, an anaerobic transport container may be used.

4. Postprocedure care:
   A. Apply a sterile dressing over the aspiration site.
   B. Keep the specimen at room temperature and transport it to the laboratory within 30 minutes for immediate processing. Some anaerobes survive for only a short time after collection.
   C. Write the specimen source, any recent antibiotic therapy, and the client's diagnosis and symptoms on the laboratory requisition.

5. Client and family teaching:
   A. Results are normally available within 72 hours.
   B. Report signs of infection at the aspiration site to the physician: increasing pain, redness, swelling, purulent drainage, or fever >101°F (38.3°C).
   C. Treatment of the condition may begin before the results are obtained.

6. Factors that affect results:
   A. Reject small specimens (a few drops)

in a syringe received more than 10 minutes after collection.

B. Reject larger specimens (>1 ml) in a syringe received more than 1 hour after collection.

C. Reject specimens in anaerobic oxygen-free vials or tubes received more than 3 hours after collection.

D. Exposure of the specimen to air may cause false-negative results.

E. Failure to use anaerobic transport specimen containers may cause false-negative results.

F. Do not use methylene blue indicator tubes if the ring of blue extends beyond the top surface of the tube.

G. Letting the specimens dry out invalidates the results.

H. The client's symptoms, condition, and type of organism suspected determine the specific type of anaerobic culture medium selected.

7. Other data:
   A. Malignancy, immunosuppressive deficiency states, immunosuppressive therapy, and some types of antibiotic therapy favor the multiplication of endogenous anaerobes.
   B. The use of swabs to obtain anaerobic cultures is not recommended. When necessary, commercial anaerobic swab sets consisting of two containers must be used.

Bibliography:

Bannister ER, Woods GL: Evaluation of routine anaerobic blood cultures in the BacT/Alert blood culture system. Am J Clin Pathol *104*(3):279– 282, 1995.

Kelloff JA, Bankert DA, Manzella JP, Parsey KS, Scott SL, Cavanaugh SH: Clinical comparison of isolator and thiol broth with ESP aerobic and anaerobic bottles for recovery of pathogens from blood. J Clin Microbiol *32*(9):2050–2055, 1994.

Mermel LA, Maki DG: Detection of bacteremia in adults: Consequences of culturing an inadequate volume of blood. Ann Intern Med *119*(4):270–272, 1993.

Paisley JW, Lauer BA: Pediatric blood cultures. Clin Lab Med *14*(1):17–30, 1994.

BODY FLUID, FUNGUS, CULTURE

Norm: Negative. No growth.

Positive: *Blastomyces dermatitidis, Coccidioides immitis, Cryptococcus neoformans, Histoplasma capsulatum, Sporothrix schenckii, Candida albicans, Candida tropicalis, Aspergillus fumigatus, Aspergillus flavus,* and others.

Description: Fungi are slow-growing, eukaryotic organisms that can grow on living and nonliving organic materials and are subdivided into yeasts and molds. Normal human host defense mechanisms limit the damage they cause superficially. Some fungi can be inhaled or introduced by traumatic inoculation into deep tissue spaces and cause serious infections. Factors that predispose a client to a fungal infection include immunosuppression, treatment with corticosteroids or broad-spectrum antibiotics, or debilitated states. Although tentative identification of fungi can be made quickly with staining techniques, culture of the organism on special fungal culture media is required to confirm a diagnosis of a fungal infection.

Professional Considerations:

1. Consent form NOT required for the culture, but may be required for the procedure used to obtain the specimen.

2. Preparation:
   A. Obtain a sterile specimen container, sterile gloves, a needle, a syringe, and any necessary aspiration trays, depending on the site to be cultured.
   B. For urine collection, obtain a sterile container and povidone-iodine wipes. If the client will be collecting the specimen independently, instructions should include a demonstration.
   C. Obtain the specimen early in the day so that it may be processed promptly.

3. Procedure:
   A. Use an aseptic technique to collect a specimen of the body fluid to be cultured.
   B. The specimen should be examined for yeast cells at the bedside whenever possible or placed in a sterile container and transported promptly to the laboratory.
   C. Urine collection:
      i. Instruct the client to void and discard the urine.
      ii. Thirty minutes later, while holding the labia open or foreskin back, cleanse the urethral meatus in an outward circular motion with each of three povidone-iodine wipes. Allow the iodine to dry while protecting the urethral meatus from contamination.
      iii. Instruct the client to void a small amount and then stop the stream of urine.
      iv. Place the sterile specimen container under the urethral meatus and have the client void into it, filling it no more than halfway, before again stopping the stream of urine. Cap the specimen container.

4. Postprocedure care:
   A. Apply an appropriate dressing as needed.

B. Write the collection date and time, specimen source, suspected disease, and any recent antibiotic or antifungal therapy on the laboratory requisition.

C. Transport the specimen to the laboratory immediately.

D. Do not refrigerate.

5. Client and family teaching:

A. Preliminary results are normally available within 72 hours, final results in about 30 days.

B. Treatment is usually begun prior to final results.

6. Factors that affect results:

A. Best results are obtained if cultures are inoculated immediately. Other than noted above, the maximum time allowed between specimen collection and inoculation is 3 hours.

7. Other data:

A. Four to 6 weeks are required for fungal culture results.

B. More yeast is acquired using Fan bottles.

Bibliography:

Breathnach A, Evans J: Growth and detection of filamentous fungi in the BacT/Alert blood culture system. J Clin Pathol 48(7):670–672, 1995.

Weinstein MP, Mirrett S, Reimer LG, Wilson ML, Smith-Elekes S, Chaurd CR, Joho KL, Reller LB: Controlled evaluation of BacT/Alert standard aerobic and FAN aerobic blood culture bottles for detection of bacteremia and fungemia. J Clin Microbiol 33(4):978–981, 1995.

BODY FLUID, GLUCOSE, SPECIMEN

Norm: See below.

		SI Units
Cerebrospinal fluid: Lags behind blood glucose levels by 2–4 hours. Fasting to 4 hours postprandially 50–80% of serum glucose:		
Adult	40–80 mg/dl	2.2–4.4 mmol/L
Premature infant	24–63 mg/dl	1.3–3.5 mmol/L
Full-term infant	34–119 mg/dl	1.9–6.6 mmol/L
Child	35–75 mg/dl	1.9–4.1 mmol/L
Peritoneal fluid	70–100 mg/dl	3.8–5.5 mmol/L
Pleural fluid	Same as blood glucose level, with a time lag of 2–4 hours or no less than 40 mg/dl (2.2 mmol/L) below blood glucose	
Fasting	60–110 mg/dl	3.3–6.1 mmol/L
Synovial fluid	No more than 10 mg/dl (0.6 mmol/L, SI units) lower than blood glucose level	

Increased CSF Glucose: Brain tumor, cerebral hemorrhage, cerebral trauma, diabetic coma, hyperglycemia, hypothalamic lesions, increased intracranial pressure, and uremia.

Increased Peritoneal, Pleural, or Synovial Fluid Glucose: Hyperglycemia and primary and symptomatic diabetes.

Decreased CSF Glucose: Brain abscess, brain tumor, cancer, central nervous system sarcoidosis, choroid plexus tumor, coccidioidomycosis, increased intracranial pressure, encephalitis (mumps or herpes simplex origin), hypoglycemia, leukemic infiltration, lupus myelopathy, lymphocytic choriomeningitis, lymphoma, melanomatosis, meningeal carcinomatosis, meningitis (acute pyogenic, aseptic, chemical, cryptococcal, fungal, granulomatous, pyogenic, rheumatoid, tuberculous, viral), neurosyphilis, rheumatoid arthritis, subarachnoid hemorrhage, toxoplasmosis, and tuberculoma of brain.

Decreased Peritoneal Fluid Glucose: Peritoneal carcinomatosis, peritonitis (tuberculous), and hypoglycemia.

Decreased Pleural Fluid Glucose: Infection (bacterial), effusion (malignant, neoplastic, rheumatoid, septic, tuberculous), and hypoglycemia.

Decreased Synovial Fluid Glucose: Arthritis (inflammatory, noninflammatory, rheumatoid, septic, tuberculous) and hypoglycemia.

Description: Body fluid glucose content is similar to blood serum glucose content. Most abnormalities result in a decreased body fluid glucose due to increased utilization of glucose by the pathogenic process. This test is interpreted by comparing a blood glucose level to the body fluid glucose level.

Professional Considerations:

1. Consent form IS required for the procedure used to obtain the specimen. See specific procedures for risks and contraindications.
2. Preparation:
   A. Tube: Red-top, red/gray-top, or gold-top for blood glucose specimen.
   B. Obtain a sterile specimen container, a tube, or an evacuated glass bottle, and a sterile tray (arthrocentesis, lumbar puncture, paracentesis, thoracentesis) depending on the procedure being performed.
3. Procedure:
   A. Draw a 5-ml blood sample for glucose in a red-top tube.
   B. Collect the appropriate specimen as follows:
      i. *Cerebrospinal fluid (CSF):* Collect 3–5 ml of cerebrospinal fluid in a sterile glass tube via a spinal tap no more than 4 hours postprandially.
      ii. *Peritoneal fluid:* Collect 5 ml of peritoneal fluid in a sterile glass tube via a paracentesis immediately after blood glucose specimen collection.
      iii. *Pleural fluid:* Collect 5 ml of pleural fluid in a sterile glass tube via thoracentesis 2–4 hours after blood glucose specimen collection.
      iv. *Synovial fluid:* Collect 3–5 ml of synovial fluid in a sterile gray-top tube containing sodium fluoride via arthrocentesis immediately after blood glucose specimen collection.
4. Postprocedure care:
   A. Apply a sterile dressing to the sites.
   B. Write the specimen source and collection time on the laboratory requisition.
   C. Transport the specimens to the laboratory immediately. Analysis must be performed promptly on freshly collected specimens to avoid erroneous results due to glycolysis.
   D. For CSF collection, the client should lie flat or with the head of the bed elevated no higher than 30 degrees for up to 8 hours, and oral intake of fluids should be increased.

5. Client and family teaching:
   A. Report to the physician if there are signs of infection at the collection site: increasing pain, redness, swelling, purulent drainage, or fever >101°F (38.3°C).
   B. Results are normally available within 24 hours.
6. Factors that affect results:
   A. This method provides the least reliable diagnosis of bacterial peritonitis.
7. Other data:
   A. None.

Bibliography:

Rodriguez-Panadero F, Mejias JL: Low glucose and pH levels in malignant pleural effusion: Diagnostic significance and prognostic value in respect to pleurodesis. Am Rev Respir Dis *139*(1):663–667, 1989.

Slovis CM, Negus RA, Amerson SM, Kutner MH: Bedside cerebrospinal fluid glucose analysis. Ann Emerg Med *18*(9):931–933, 1989.

BODY FLUID, *MYCOBACTERIA* CULTURE

Norm: No growth after 8 weeks.

Usage: Diagnose the presence of *Mycobacterium* in body fluid.

Description: *Mycobacteria* are nonmotile, nonsporeforming, straight, or slightly curved rods that resist staining by Gram's method or by acid solutions because of their high-lipid-containing cell walls. They grow slowly, with colonies developing after 2 days to 8 weeks of incubation. Some species are found in soil and water. Others are obligate parasites. The most common *Mycobacteria* causing human disease are *M. asiaticum, M. avium-scrofulaceum complex, M. fortuitum, M. haemophilum, M. kansasii, M. leprae, M. malmoense, M. marinum, M. simiae, M. szulgai, M. tuberculosis complex, M. ulcerans,* and *M. xenopi.* These organisms may attack any organ, but the primary site of infection is usually the lungs. Tubercle bacillus is the most common *Mycobacterium* infection in the United States, except in clients with AIDS. The bacilli are usually inhaled and are small enough to be carried into the alveoli without being expelled.

Professional Considerations:

1. Consent form NOT required for the culture, but may be required for the procedure used to obtain the specimen.

Risks:
Complications of nasogastric tube insertion include bleeding, dysrhythmias, esophageal perforation, laryngospasm, and decreased mean PO_2.

Contraindications:
For nasogastric tube insertion: esophageal varices.

2. Preparation:
   A. Obtain a sterile specimen container.
   B. For gastric lavage, obtain a nasogastric tube, lubricant, sterile water, a sterile 50-ml syringe, and a sterile specimen container.
   C. For paracentesis, thoracentesis, pericardiocentesis, or arthrocentesis obtain the appropriate sterile procedure tray.
3. Procedure:
   A. *Sputum specimen:* Collect an early-morning sputum specimen of 5–10 ml on three separate days. Label the specimens sequentially.
   B. *Gastric lavage:* Used for clients who cannot produce sputum. The specimen should be obtained in the early morning after an 8-hour fast from food and fluids. Insert a nasogastric tube into the stomach. Instill 20–50 ml of sterile water into the stomach through the nasogastric tube with a sterile syringe; then aspirate the fluid out of the stomach with the syringe. Remove the nasogastric tube.
   C. *Peritoneal fluid:* Collect 5–10 ml of peritoneal fluid in a sterile syringe via paracentesis using an aseptic technique.
   D. *Pleural fluid:* Collect 5–10 ml of pleural fluid in a sterile syringe via thoracentesis using an aseptic technique.
   E. *Pericardial fluid:* Collect 5–10 ml of pericardial fluid in a sterile syringe via pericardiocentesis using an aseptic technique.
   F. *Synovial fluid:* Collect 5–10 ml of synovial fluid in a sterile syringe via arthrocentesis using an aseptic technique.
   G. *Urine:* Collect first morning-voided specimens via the clean-catch technique or via aspiration from an indwelling urinary catheter or suprapubic puncture on 3 separate days. Label the specimens sequentially. *See clean-catch collection instructions in the test "Body Fluid, Routine, Culture."*
4. Postprocedure care:
   A. Apply a dry sterile dressing to the aspiration site. Observe the site for drainage or bleeding hourly × 4.
   B. For specimens obtained via pericardiocentesis or thoracentesis, assess vital signs every 15 minutes × 4, then every 30 minutes × 2, then hourly × 4. Observe for dysrhythmias × 24 hours.
   C. Write the specimen source, collection time, current antibiotic or antifungal therapy, and clinical diagnosis on the laboratory requisition. The request to culture the specimen for *Mycobacteria* must be specified on the laboratory requisition.
   D. Transport the specimen to the laboratory promptly. Refrigerate urine specimens if not cultured immediately.
5. Client and family teaching:
   A. *Needle aspiration:* Call the physician if there are signs of infection at the procedure site: increasing pain, redness, swelling, purulent drainage, or fever >101°F (38.3°C).
   B. *Sputum:* Deep coughs are necessary to produce sputum rather than saliva. To produce the proper specimen, take in several breaths without fully exhaling each, then expel sputum with a "cascade cough."
   C. Results are normally available within 72 hours.
6. Factors that affect results:
   A. Specimens are best if collected in the early morning upon arising and before eating or drinking.
7. Other data:
   A. Sputum induction by respiratory therapy may be required.

Bibliography:
Levy H, Feldman C, Kallengbach JM: The diagnostic yield of prebronchoscopy sputa and bronchial washings in patients with biopsy-proven pulmonary tuberculosis. S Afr Med J 75(11):527–528, 1989.

Radhika S, Gupta SK, Chakrabarti A, Rajwanshi A, Joshi K: Role of culture for *mycobacteria* in fine-needle aspiration diagnosis of tuberculous lymphadenitis. Diagn Cytopathol 5(3):260–262, 1989.

BODY FLUID, ROUTINE, CULTURE

Norm: No growth.

Usage: Identification and isolation of aerobic infectious organisms.

Positive Urine Culture: Titers >100,000/ml indicate urinary tract infection (viral [cytomegalovirus] or bacterial [frequently *Escherichia coli, Klebsiella, Proteus, Staphylococcus,* or *Streptococcus*]).

Negative Urine Culture: Titers <1000/ml are not considered clinically significant, but more likely result from contamination due to poor collection technique.

Description: Routine body fluid culture is an aseptic collection of an aerobic culture that may be performed on ascitic, pericardial, pleural, or synovial fluids and on bone marrow or urine. For urine specimens collected via suprapubic puncture, anaerobic culture may be performed.

Professional Considerations:

1. Consent form NOT required for the culture, but may be required for the procedure used to obtain the specimen.
2. Preparation:
   A. Obtain povidone-iodine, sterile towels, and an appropriate sterile tray (paracentesis, thoracentesis, arthrocentesis, bone marrow aspiration).
   B. For the clean-catch urine culture, obtain povidone-iodine wipes and a sterile specimen container.
   C. For the urine culture for indwelling urinary catheter, obtain alcohol wipes, a needle, and a 10-ml syringe.
   D. For the urine culture from suprapubic puncture, force fluids (200 ml/hour × 6 hours), and instruct the client not to void. The bladder must be full and distended for puncture. Obtain a sterile red-top tube (or an anaerobic culture container for recovery of anaerobic organisms), povidone-iodine, and an aspiration tray.
   E. Cultures should be obtained before starting antibiotic or antifungal therapy whenever possible.
3. Procedure:
   A. *Ascitic, pericardial, pleural, or synovial fluid:*
      i. Cleanse the collection site with povidone-iodine and allow it to dry.
      ii. The physician uses an aseptic technique to collect a minimum of 2 ml of fluid via paracentesis, pericardiocentesis, thoracentesis, or arthrocentesis and transfers it into a closed, sterile container or Petri dish that is free of preservative.
   B. *Bone marrow:*
      i. The physician uses an aseptic technique to collect a small amount of bone marrow via bone marrow aspiration and transfers it into a Petri dish that is free of any preservative.
      ii. *See Bone Marrow Aspiration Analysis, Specimen* for procedural details.
   C. *Urine culture from clean-catch specimen* (also known as *urine culture, routine, specimen*): The clean-catch urine technique must be used to decrease the risk of specimen contamination.
      i. Have the client void to empty the bladder of longstanding urine. Thirty minutes later, obtain a 10-ml clean-catch urine specimen or sample from a straight or indwelling catheter in a sterile container.
      ii. *Male:* Retract the foreskin and cleanse the glans of the penis with soap and water. Then cleanse the glans with antiseptic-moistened cotton balls, using a circular motion from the urethral meatus outward and discarding each cotton ball after one use.
      Female: While holding the labia minora apart, cleanse the mucous membranes surrounding the periphery of the urethral meatus by using antiseptic-moistened cotton balls. Use the first cotton ball to wipe from front to back on one side, followed by the same procedure with the second cotton ball on the opposite side; then cleanse directly over the meatus with the third cotton ball. Discard each cotton ball after one use.
      iii. Have the client void a small amount of urine and discard. Then stop the stream and place the specimen container in the urine path and void 30–90 ml (1–3 ounces) of urine into the container. Avoid contaminating the container by touching the inside of the container to the body.
   D. *Urine culture from indwelling catheter:*
      i. Clamp the tubing for 15 minutes to allow the urine to accumulate in the upper portion of the tubing.
      ii. Cleanse the needle port of the rubber catheter with an alcohol wipe and allow it to dry.
      iii. Insert a sterile needle attached to a syringe through the port, and withdraw 10 ml of urine. Collect only fresh urine as it drains. Do not collect urine that has already passed the collection point.
      iv. Remove the syringe and discard the needle. Expel the syringe contents into a sterile specimen cup and cap tightly. Remove the clamp from the tubing.
   E. *Urine culture from suprapubic puncture:*
      i. Cleanse the skin around the aspiration site with povidone-iodine and allow it to dry.
      ii. Drape the aspiration site with sterile towels.
      iii. The physician performs the suprapubic puncture into the bladder and withdraws at least 10 ml of urine.
      iv. For aerobic culture, the needle is removed from the syringe after withdrawal, and the urine is expelled into a sterile container.
      v. For anaerobic culture, a fresh needle is placed on the syringe, and the urine is quickly injected into an anaerobic culture container.

F. Body fluids and bone marrow aspirates may be inoculated into blood culture media.

4. Postprocedure care:
   A. Apply a dry, sterile dressing to the aspiration site. Observe the site for drainage or bleeding hourly × 4.
   B. For specimens obtained via pericardiocentesis or thoracentesis, assess vital signs every 15 minutes × 4, then every 30 minutes × 2, then hourly × 4. Observe for dysrhythmias × 24 hours.
   C. Write the specific collection site, date, time, client's age, diagnosis, and recent antibiotic or antifungal therapy on the laboratory requisition. Requests for anaerobic culture must be specified on the requisition.
   D. Send the specimen to the laboratory immediately. Urine specimens should be refrigerated if not cultured immediately. Specimens from other sites should not be refrigerated.

5. Client and family teaching:
   A. Call the physician if signs of infection appear at the procedure site: increasing pain, redness, swelling, purulent drainage, or fever >101°F (38.3°C).
   B. Results are usually available within 5 to 30 days.
   C. Treatment may begin prior to culture results.

6. Factors that affect results:
   A. Reject specimens not tightly sealed.
   B. Refrigeration decreases the accuracy of results for all except urine specimens.
   C. Antibiotic or antifungal therapy initiated before specimen collection may produce false-negative results.
   D. The most frequent interference with urine culture results is improper collection technique, which results in specimen contamination.
   E. An early-morning urine specimen yields the highest concentration of microorganisms.

7. Other data:
   A. Preliminary results are reported in 24 hours. At least 48 hours is required for the isolation of organisms in the presence of pathogens. Fungi and *Mycobacteria* may take several weeks. Gram stains should be available within 1 hour.
   B. *Mycobacteria* and *Chlamydia* infections of the urinary tract are not diagnosed by this test.
   C. If cytomegalovirus is suspected, several urine specimens are recommended because the virus is shed intermittently.

Bibliography:

el-Touny M, Osman L, Abd-el-Hamid T, Sabbour MS: Re-evaluation of the value of ascitic fluid pH lactate dehydrogenase and total proteins in the diagnosis of spontaneous bacterial peritonitis (SBP). J Trop Med Hyg *92*(1):6–9, 1989.

Jacobs DF, Kasten BL, DeMott WR, Wolfson WL: Laboratory Test Handbook, 2nd ed. Cleveland, OH, Lexi-Comp, 1990, pp 672–762.

Stamm WE, Hooten TM, Johnson JR, Johnson C, Stapleton A, Roberts PL, Moseley SL, Fihn SD: Urinary tract infections: From pathogenesis to treatment. J Infect Dis *159*(3):400–406, 1989.

BODY FLUID ANALYSIS, SPECIMEN

Norms:

Pericardial Fluid	SI Units
Appearance	Clear to pale yellow
Glucose	
Transudate	Approximates whole blood levels (Whole blood adult norm 60–89 mg/dl, Whole blood child norm 51–85 mg/dl)
Exudate	Lower than whole blood levels
Lactate dehydrogenase	
Transudate	≤Client's serum LD (serum adult norm 45–90 U/L, serum child norm 60–170 U/L)

Peritoneal Fluid:	SI Units
Appearance	Clear or pale yellow
Albumin	Negative

Peritoneal Fluid *(continued)*		SI Units
Alkaline phosphatase		
Adult female	76–250 U/L	
Adult male	90–239 U/L	
Ammonia	<50 g/L	
Cholesterol		
Transudate	<46 mg/dl	<1.19 mmol/L
Exudate	>46 mg/dl	>1.19 mmol/L
Glucose		
Transudate	60–110 mg/dl	3.3–6.1 mmol/L
Exudate	Lower than whole blood levels (whole blood adult norm 60–89 mg/dl, child norm 51–85 mg/dl)	
Lactic acid	10–20 mg/dl	1.1–2.3 mmol/L
Lactate dehydrogenase		
Transudate	≤ Client's serum LD (serum adult norm 45–90 U/L, child norm 60–170 U/L)	
Exudate	>Client's serum LD	
pH	7.4	7.4
Specific gravity		
Transudate	<1.016	<1.016
Exudate	>1.016	>1.016
Total protein		
Transudate	<2.5 g/dl	<25 g/L
Exudate	>3 g/dl	>30 g/L
Volume	<100 ml	
White blood cells		
Transudate	<100/mm^3	<100 × 10^9/L
Exudate	>1000/mm^3	>1000 × 10^9/L

Pleural Fluid		SI Units
Appearance	Clear, slightly amber	
Cholesterol		
Transudate	<60 mg/dl	<1.55 mmol/L
Exudate	>60 mg/dl	>1.55 mmol/L
Glucose		
Transudate	Approximates whole blood levels (whole blood adult norm 60–89 mg/dl, child norm 51–85 mg/dl)	
Exudate	Lower than whole blood levels	
Lactate dehydrogenase		
Transudate	≤Client's serum LD (serum adult norm 45–90 U/L, child norm 60–170 U/L)	
Exudate	>Client's serum LD	
pH	7.4	
Specific gravity		
Transudate	<1.016	<1.016
Exudate	>1.016	>1.016

Pleural Fluid *(continued)*		SI Units
Total protein		
Transudate	<2.5 g/dl	<25 g/L
Exudate	>3 g/dl	>30 g/L
Volume	<25 ml	
White blood cells		
Transudate	<100/mm³	<100 × 10⁹/L
Exudate	>1000/mm³	>1000 × 10⁹/L

Synovial Fluid		SI Units
Appearance	Clear or colorless to pale yellow	
Crystals	Absent	
Glucose		
Transudate	≤10 mg/dl lower than blood glucose (whole blood adult norm 60–89 mg/dl, child norm 51–85 mg/dl)	
Exudate	Lower than whole blood levels	
Lactate dehydrogenase		
Transudate	≤ Client's serum LD (serum adult norm 45–90 U/L, child norm 60–170 U/L)	
Exudate	>Client's serum LD	
pH	7.4	
Specific gravity		
Transudate	<1.016	<1.016
Exudate	>1.016	>1.016
Total protein		
Transudate	1–3 g/dl	10–30 g/dl
Exudate	>3 g/dl	>30 g/dl
Volume	<4 ml	
Viscosity	High	
White blood cells		
Transudate	<100/mm³	<100 × 10⁹/L
Exudate	>1000/mm³	>1000 × 10⁹/L

Increased Volume

Pericardial Fluid	**Peritoneal Fluid**
Cardiac tamponade	Abscess
Constrictive pericarditis	Ascites
Pericardial effusion	Hepatic disease
	Peritonitis
	Portal hypertension

Pleural Fluid	**Synovial Fluid**
Bacterial pneumonia	Amyloidosis
Bronchogenic carcinoma	Aseptic necrosis
Chronic hepatic disease	Bacterial infection
Congestive heart failure	Charcot's joint

Increased Volume *(continued)*

Pleural Fluid *(continued)*

Constrictive pericarditis
Hypertrophic pulmonary osteoarthropathy
Hypoproteinemia
Lymphoma
Metastatic carcinoma
Neoplasm
Nephrotic syndrome
Pulmonary infarct
Rheumatoid disease
Systemic lupus erythematosus
Trauma
Tuberculosis
Viral pneumonia

Synovial Fluid *(continued)*

Connective tissue disease
Crystal-induced arthritis
Epiphyseal dysplasia
Gout
Hemochromatosis
Osteoarthritis
Osteochondritis dissecans
Paget's disease
Polymyositis
Psoriasis
Regional enteritis
Reiter's disease
Rheumatic fever
Rheumatic arthritis
Sarcoidosis
Scleroderma
Sickle cell disease
Subacute bacterial endocarditis
Systemic lupus erythematosus
Traumatic arthritis
Ulcerative colitis
Villonodular synovitis

Causes of Turbidity

Pericardial Fluid

Abscess

Peritoneal Fluid

Abscess

Pleural Fluid

Abscess
Bacterial infection
Rheumatic fever
Rheumatoid disease
Tuberculosis

Synovial Fluid

Abscess
Floating cartilage fragments
Inflammation
Leukocytes
Pseudogout
Rheumatoid arthritis
Septic arthritis
Systemic lupus erythematosus
Tuberculous arthritis

Causes of Milky Color

Synovial Fluid

Gouty arthritis
Lymphatic drainage
Rheumatoid arthritis
Systemic lupus erythematosus
Tuberculous arthritis

Pink or Red Color

Pericardial Fluid	**Peritoneal Fluid**
Hemorrhage	Hemorrhage
Trauma	Trauma
Traumatic tap	Traumatic tap

Pleural Fluid	**Synovial Fluid**
Congestive heart failure	Hemophilic arthritis
Hemorrhage	Hemorrhage
Pancreatitis	Joint fracture
Pneumonia	Neurogenic arthropathy
Postmyocardial infarction syndrome	Osteoarthritis
Pulmonary infarction	Pigmented villonodular synovitis
Trauma	Recent hemarthrosis
Traumatic tap	Rheumatoid arthritis
Tumor	Septic arthritis
	Trauma
	Traumatic arthritis
	Traumatic tap
	Tumor

Increased lactic acid Infection (pleural, peritoneal), and malignancy.

Decreased Glucose

Pericardial Fluid	**Peritoneal Fluid**
(Not applicable)	Rheumatoid effusion

Pleural Fluid	**Synovial Fluid**
Bacterial infection	Inflammatory arthritis
Malignancy	Noninflammatory arthritis
Neoplastic effusion	Rheumatoid arthritis
Septic effusion	Rheumatoid effusion
Tuberculous effusion	Septic arthritis
	Tuberculous arthritis

Decreased pH

Pleural Fluid	**Peritoneal Fluid**
Empyema	Peritoneal effusion
Esophageal rupture	
Loculated effusion	
Parapneumonic effusion	
Tuberculous effusion	

Decreased Synovial Fluid Viscosity: Gout, inflammatory joint disease, rheumatic fever, rheumatoid arthritis, sepsis, septic arthritis, and trauma.

Description: A sample of body fluid is obtained for analysis of its various components and for detection of the presence of abnormal constituents that may be caused by pathogenic processes. Some conditions that may cause abnormalities include neoplasm, infection, inflammation, leakage of gastrointestinal tract contents or secretions, trauma, and hemorrhage.

Professional Considerations:

1. Consent form IS required for the procedure used to obtain the specimen. See specific procedures for risks and contraindications.

2. Preparation:
   A. Obtain sterile tubes or evacuated glass bottles for the specimens.
   B. Obtain a sterile specimen container, a tube, or an evacuated glass bottle, and a sterile tray (arthrocentesis, pericardiocentesis, paracentesis, thoracentesis) depending on the procedure being performed.
   C. Obtain alcohol wipes, a tourniquet, a needle, a syringe, and a gray-top tube for blood glucose, and a red-top tube for lactate dehydrogenase comparisons to body fluid levels.
3. Procedure:
   A. A sample of body fluid is obtained by needle aspiration under sterile conditions.
   B. The amount collected varies based on the purpose of the procedure and type of specimen.
   C. Draw a 7-ml blood sample in the gray-top tube for whole blood glucose and a 7-ml blood sample in the red-top tube for lactate dehydrogenase levels.
4. Postprocedure care:
   A. Apply a sterile dressing to site.
5. Client and family teaching:
   A. Report signs of infection at the collection site to the physician: increasing pain, redness, swelling, purulent drainage, or fever >101°F (38.3°C).
   B. Results are normally available within 72 hours.
6. Factors that affect results:
   A. None.
7. Other data:
   A. Ascitic fluid collection versus fluid from an overdistended bladder can be differentiated with a urea nitrogen analysis. Urine urea nitrogen should be greater than 12 g/dl, whereas ascitic fluid should be less.
   B. *See also Body Fluid, Glucose, Specimen; Body Fluid Analysis, Cell Count, Specimen; and Body Fluid, Amylase, Specimen.*

Bibliography:

Ben-Ezra J, Stastny JF, Harris AC, Bork L, Frable WJ: Comparison of the clinic microscopy laboratory with the cytopathology laboratory in the detection of malignant cells in body fluid. Am J Clin Pathol 102(4):439–442, 1994.

Hammel P, Levy P, Voitot H, Levy M, Vilgrain V, Zins M, Flejou JF, Molas G, Ruszniewski P, Bernades P: Perioperative cyst fluid analysis is useful for the differential diagnosis of cystic lesions of the pancreas. Gastroenterology 108(4):1230–1235, 1995.

BODY FLUID ANALYSIS, CELL COUNT, SPECIMEN

Norm:

		SI Units
Pericardial Fluid		
Red blood cells	None	
White blood cells	<500/mm^3	
Polys	0–25%	0–0.25
Peritoneal Fluid		
Cell count	<500/mm^3	
Red blood cells	None	
Transudate	Few	
Exudate	Variable	
White blood cells	<300/μl	0–0.30 × 10^9/L
Polys	0–25%	0–0.25
Pleural Fluid		
Cell count	<1000/mm^3	
White blood cells		
Transudate	Few	
Exudate	Many	
Eosinophils	0–10%	0–0.10
Lymphocytes	0–50%	0–0.50
Neutrophils	0–50%	0–0.50
Polys	0–25%	0–0.25
Synovial Fluid		
Red blood cells	None	

Synovial Fluid (continued)

		SI Units
White blood cells	0–200/µl	0–0.20×10^9/L
Polys	0–25%	0–0.25
Neutrophils	0–25%	0–0.25
Lymphocytes	0–78%	0–0.78
Monocytes	0–71%	0–0.71
Clasmatocytes	0–26%	0–0.26
Macrophages	0–26%	0–0.26
Synovial cells	0–12%	0–0.12
Unclassified	0–21%	0–0.21

Increased Leukocytes: Acute gouty arthritis, carcinoma (pleural fluid), chylothorax (pleural fluid), congestive heart failure (pleural fluid), empyema (pleural fluid), gonorrheal arthritis, inflammation (pleural fluid), lymphatic leukemia, lymphocytic leukemia (pleural fluid), lymphomas (pleural fluid), parapneumonic effusion (pleural fluid), postpneumonic effusion (pleural fluid), rheumatic fever, rheumatoid arthritis, septic arthritis, tuberculosis (pleural fluid), tumors, and uremia (pleural fluid).

Increased Polymorphonuclear Cells: Bacterial inflammation, bacterial peritonitis, and infectious processes (acute).

Increased Eosinophils: Infarcts, parasites, pneumothorax, postpneumonic effusions, rheumatic fever, rheumatoid arthritis, and tumors.

Increased Plasma Cells: Chronic inflammation, Hodgkin's disease, and lymphoma. Atypical plasma cells may be associated with multiple myeloma.

Decreased Glucose: Rheumatoid effusion (synovial fluid).

Description: The specific body fluid is tested for white blood count and differential, total red blood cell count, protein, lactic acid dehydrogenase, and other tests. The various cell counts of body fluids assist in the differentiation of exudate from transudate. Body fluid analysis may be performed on the following body fluids: ascitic, cyst, joint, pericardial, peritoneal, pleural, and synovial.

Professional Considerations:

1. Consent form IS required for the procedure used to obtain the specimen. See specific procedures for risks and contraindications.
2. Preparation:
   A. The client should be properly positioned and the specimen site cleaned and prepped.
   B. Obtain heparin 1000 U/ml concentration.
   C. Obtain a sterile specimen container, a tube or an evacuated glass bottle, and a sterile tray (arthrocentesis, pericardiocentesis, paracentesis, thoracentesis) depending on the procedure being performed.
3. Procedure:
   A. A sample of body fluid is obtained by needle aspiration under sterile conditions.
   B. The amount collected varies based on the purpose of the procedure and the type of specimen.
4. Postprocedure care:
   A. Apply a small dressing to the aspiration site.
   B. To each 100 ml of body fluid add 1 ml of 1000 U of heparin/ml concentration. Additional heparin will not alter results.
   C. Write the specimen source on the laboratory requisition.
   D. Transport the specimen to the laboratory immediately.
5. Client and family teaching:
   A. Report signs of infection at the operative site to the physician: increasing pain, redness, swelling, purulent drainage, or fever >101°F (38.3°C).
   B. See individual procedure listings for procedure-specific teaching.
   C. Results are normally available within 72 hours.
6. Factors that affect results:
   A. Reject contaminated or hemolyzed specimens.
7. Other data:
   A. Ascitic fluid collection versus fluid from an overdistended bladder can be differentiated with a urea nitrogen analysis. Urine urea nitrogen should be greater than 12 g/dl, whereas ascitic fluid should be less.

Bibliography:

Jacobs DF, Kasten BL, DeMott WR, Wolfson WL: Laboratory Test Handbook, 2nd ed. Cleveland, OH, Lexi-Comp, 1990, pp 465–466.

Ratjen F, Bredendiek M, Zheng L, Brendel M, Costabel U: Lymphocyte subsets in bronchoalveolar lavage fluids of children without bronchopulmonary disease. Am J Resp Crit Care Med 152(1):174–178, 1995.

BODY FLUID CYTOLOGY, SPECIMEN
(see Brushings Cytology, Specimen; Bronchial Washings, Specimen, Diagnostic; Cerebrospinal Fluid, Cytology, Specimen; Cytologic Study of Breast Cyst, Effusions, Nipple Discharge, Respiratory Tract or Urine, Diagnostic; Needle Aspiration Cytology, Specimen; and Oral Cavity Cytology, Specimen)

BONE MARROW ASPIRATION ANALYSIS, SPECIMEN (BONE MARROW BIOPSY, BONE MARROW IRON STAIN, IRON STAIN, BONE MARROW)

Norm: Red marrow contains connective tissue, fat cells, and hematopoietic cells. Yellow marrow contains connective tissue and fat cells. Interpretation of cell count and histopathology by a hematologist, pathologist, or oncologist is required.

Response to Staining: Iron stain for hemosiderin: 2+.

Periodic Acid-Schiff (PAS) Glycogen Reactions: Negative.

Sudan Black B (SBB) Granulocyte: Negative.

DIFFERENTIAL CELL COUNT

	Adult (%)	Child (%)	Infant (%)
Basophils	0.1	0.06	0.07
Eosinophils	3.1	3.6	2.6
Hemocytoblasts	0.1–1.0		
Lymphocytes (all stages)	2.7–24	16	49
Megakaryocytes	0.03–0.5	0.1	0.05
Plasmacytes	0.1–1.5	0.4	0.02
Promyelocytes	0.5–8.0	1.4	0.76
Reticulum cells	0.1–2.0		
Undifferentiated cells	0.0–0.1		
Neutrophils, total	56.5	57.1	32.4
Metamyelocytes	9.6–24.6	23.3	11.3
Neutrophilic	10–32		
Eosinophilic	0.3–3.7		
Basophilic	0–0.3		
Monocytes (all stages)	0–2.7		
Myeloblasts	0.1–5.0	1.2	0.62
Myelocytes	4.2–15	18.4	2.5
Neutrophilic	5.0–20		
Eosinophilic	0.1–3.0		
Basophilic	0–0.5		
Segmented granulocyte	6.0–12.0	12.9	3.6
Neutrophilic	7.0–30		
Eosinophilic	0.2–4.0		
Basophilic	0–0.7		
Band cells	9.5–15.3	0	14.1
Neutrophilic	10–35		
Eosinophilic	0.2–2.0		
Basophilic	0–0.3		

	Adult (%)	Child (%)	Infant (%)
Erythroid series			
Normoblasts, total	25.6	23.1	8.0
Pronormoblasts	0.2–4.0	0.5	0.1
Basophilic normoblasts	1.5–5.8	1.7	0.34
Polychromatophilic normoblasts	5.0–26.4	18.2	6.9
Orthochromic normoblasts	3.6–21	2.7	0.54
Promegaloblasts	0		
Basophilic megaloblasts	0		
Polychromatic megaloblasts	0		
Orthochromic megaloblasts	0		

M:E Ratio: (Myeloid:Erythroid is the ratio of white blood cells to nucleated red blood cells.)

Adult	6:1–2:1
Birth	1.85:1
2 weeks	11:1
1–2 months	5.5:1
1–20 years	2.95:1

Usage: Helps to distinguish primary and metastatic tumors. Assists in the identification, classification, and staging of neoplasias. Aids evaluation of the progress and/or response to the treatment of neoplasias. Assists in the definitive diagnosis of blood disorders. Culture of an aspirated sample can aid in the identification of infections such as histoplasmosis or tuberculosis. Histologic examination aids in the diagnosis of carcinoma, granulomas, lymphoma, or myelofibrosis. Iron stain showing decreased hemosiderin levels may indicate iron deficiency and SBB stain differentiates acute granulocytic leukemia from acute lymphocytic leukemia.

Increased Eosinophils: Bone marrow carcinoma, eosinophilic leukemia, lymphadenoma, myeloid leukemia, and pernicious anemia (relapse).

Increased Lymphocytes: Aplastic anemia, hypoplasia of the bone marrow, infectious lymphocytosis or mononucleosis, lymphatic leukemoid reactions, lymphocytic leukemia (B-cell and T-cell), lymphoma, macroglobulinemia, myelofibrosis, and viral infections.

Increased Megakaryocytes: Acute hemorrhage, aging, chronic myeloid leukemia, hypersplenism, idiopathic thrombocytopenia, infection, megakaryocytic myelosis, myelofibrosis, pneumonia, polycythemia vera, and thrombocytopenia.

Increased Plasma Cells: Agranulocytosis, amyloidosis, aplastic anemia, carcinomatosis, collagen disease, hepatic cirrhosis, Hodgkin's disease, hypersensitivity reactions, infection, irradiation, macroglobulinemia, malignant tumor, multiple myeloma, rheumatic fever (acute), rheumatoid arthritis, serum sickness, syphilis, and ulcerative colitis.

Increased Granulocyte: Hypoplasia of the bone marrow, infections, myelocytic leukemia, myelocytic leukemoid reaction, and myeloproliferative syndrome.

Increased Normoblasts: Anemia (iron deficiency, hemolytic, megaloblastic), blood loss (chronic), erythema, erythroid-type myeloproliferative disorders, hypoplasia of the bone marrow, and polycythemia vera.

Increased M:E Ratio above 7:1: Decreased hematopoiesis, erythroid hypoplasia, infection, leukemoid reactions, and myeloid leukemia.

Increased Diffuse Bone Marrow Hyperplasia: Myeloprolifer-ative syndromes and pancytopenia reactions.

Decreased Megakaryocytes: Anemia (aplastic, pernicious), bone marrow hyperplasia (with carcinomatous or leukemic deposits), cirrhosis, irradiation (excessive), and thrombocytopenia purpura. Drugs include benzene, chlorothiazides, and cytotoxic drugs.

Decreased Granulocyte: Agranulocytosis, hyperplasia of the bone marrow, and ionizing radiation.

Decreased Normoblasts: Anemia (aplastic, hypoplastic), folic acid or vitamin B_{12} deficiency.

Decreased M:E Ratio below 2:1: Agranulocytosis, anemia (iron deficiency, normoblastic, pernicious, posthemolytic, posthemorrhagic), erythroid activity (increased), hepatic disease, myeloid formation (decreased), polycythemia vera, sprue, and steatorrhea.

Decreased Diffuse Bone Marrow Hypoplasia: Aging, cellular infiltrations, dengue fever, myelofibrosis, myelosclerosis, myelotoxic agents, osteoporosis, rubella, and viral infections.

Description: Bone marrow is the soft, organic, spongelike material contained in the medullary cavities, long bones, some haversian canals, and within the spaces between trabeculae of cancellous bone. It is composed of red and yellow marrow, with the chief function being production of erythrocytes, leukocytes, and platelets. Only the rusty, red marrow produces blood cells. The yellow marrow is formed of connective tissue and fat cells, which are inactive. During infancy and childhood, bone marrow is primarily red marrow, and in the adult, 50% is red marrow. The bone marrow aspiration procedure obtains a sample of bone marrow by needle. A stained blood smear of the sample is evaluated for bone marrow morphology and examination of blood cell erythropoiesis, cellularity, differential cell count, bone marrow iron stores, and M:E ratios.

Professional Considerations:

1. Consent form IS required.

Risks:

Bleeding, heart damage (with sternal biopsy), hemorrhage, infection, meningitis.

Contraindications:

Bone marrow aspiration is contraindicated in hemophilia, hemostasis, and coagulation defects.

2. Preparation:
   A. Obtain a bone marrow aspiration tray, laboratory slides and stains, and a lavender-top or green-top tube.
   B. Obtain a sterile container of Zenker's acetic acid solution if a bone marrow biopsy will be performed.
   C. Pain medication may be given to lessen procedure discomfort.
3. Procedure:
   A. The most common sites for bone marrow aspiration include the sternum (preferred for bone marrow biopsy), the posterior, superior iliac spine (for needle biopsy), and the anterior iliac crest and vertebral spinous in the adult. For infants under 18 months, the anterior tibia site is used, and for children, the iliac crest is preferred.
   B. The designated site is prepped, shaved, and draped. After a local anesthetic is injected and under sterile technique, a 1/8-inch stab wound is made. A Jamshidi needle with the stylet in place is inserted until the outer surface of the bone is impinged. The needle guard is engaged and the outer needle is inserted with a boring motion, about 3 mm deep, into the bone marrow cavity.
   C. *For bone marrow aspiration:* The stylet is removed and a 10-ml syringe is attached to the needle. When aspiration of 0.2 to 0.5 ml of bone marrow has entered the syringe, it is removed and given to a technician for preparation of a stained blood smear. A second syringe may be attached and a 2-ml sample of bone marrow withdrawn and placed into a lavender-top tube containing EDTA or a heparinized green-top tube.
   D. *For bone marrow biopsy:* The stylet is removed and a biopsy or inner needle with a trephine tip is inserted. A tissue plug is removed and placed into a container of Zenker's acetic acid solution.
   E. The needle is withdrawn.
4. Postprocedure care:
   A. Apply a pressure dressing to the bone marrow aspiration site.
   B. Observe the aspiration site for bleeding.
5. Client and family teaching:
   A. Bone marrow aspiration is painful, but only for a few moments. Preprocedure pain medicine may be used to lessen the discomfort. It is also normal to experience a deep pressure feeling as the bone marrow is withdrawn.
   B. It is important to lie very still during the procedure.
   C. Results are normally available within 24–72 hours.
   D. Call the physician if there are signs of infection at the procedure site: increasing pain, redness, swelling, purulent drainage, or for fever >101°F (38.3°C).
6. Factors that affect results:
   A. Cytotoxic drugs, folic acid, iron, liver or vitamin B_{12} agents, and recent blood transfusions should be noted before the biopsy.
   B. Send the specimen to the laboratory immediately.

7. Other data:
   A. The presence of normal bone marrow at one site does not eliminate the possibility of disease elsewhere in the bone marrow.
   B. Normal M:E ratio may be associated with aplastic anemia, myeloma, and myelosclerosis.

Bibliography:

Cervantes F, Rozman C, Feliu E: Prognostic evaluation of initial bone marrow histopathologic features in chronic granulocytic leukemia. Acta Haematol 82(1):12–15, 1989.

Federico M, Magin RL, Swartz HM, Wright RM, Silingardi V: Detection of bone marrow involvement in patients with cancer. Tumori 75(2):90–96, 1989.

BONE MARROW BIOPSY, DIAGNOSTIC

(see Bone Marrow Aspiration Analysis, Specimen)

BONE MARROW IRON STAIN

(see Bone Marrow Aspiration Analysis, Specimen)

BONE MARROW SCAN, DIAGNOSTIC

Norm: Even concentration of the radionuclide throughout the reticuloendothelial system, red blood cells, and bone marrow.

Usage: Assists in the diagnosis of defects in bone marrow, bone marrow depression following chemotherapy or radiation, and in the differential determinations of myeloproliferative disorders. Differentiates acute from chronic hemolysis and bone infarction from osteomyelitis in sickle cell disease. Aids in the selection of bone marrow biopsy sites and in the staging of Hodgkin's disease, lymphomas, and metastatic diseases of the bone marrow. Assists in evaluation of hyperplasia of the bone marrow associated with chronic hemolytic anemia and polycythemia vera.

Description: The bone marrow scan is a nuclear medicine study in which the radionuclide, indium chloride, is administered intravenously and followed by radiographic imaging of the entire body. This scan can be nonspecific in conditions of diffuse disease such as osteomyelitis and tumor. However, areas of increased vascularity and hyperproliferation of bone marrow can be demonstrated much earlier with a bone marrow scan than with conventional radiography.

Professional Considerations:

1. Consent form IS required.

Risks:

Hematoma at injection site.

Contraindications:

Pregnancy or during breast-feeding.

---

2. Preparation:
   A. The client should void before the procedure.
   B. Have emergency equipment readily available.
3. Procedure:
   A. The radionuclide, indium chloride, is administered intravenously.
   B. Whole-body imaging is planned for 48 hours after intravenous injection.
   C. If the radioisotope Tc-99m sulfur colloid is given, the scan can be completed 1 hour after the intravenous injection.
4. Postprocedure care:
   A. None.
5. Client and family teaching:
   A. Notify the physician for previous reaction to radionuclide.
   B. An IV may be inserted for the scan and removed after the scan is complete. Some technicians may use direct venipuncture for the injection.
   C. Results are normally available within 24 hours.
6. Factors that affect results:
   A. None found.
7. Other data:
   A. Health care professionals working in a nuclear medicine area must follow federal standards set by the Nuclear Regulatory Commission. These standards include precautions for handling the radioactive material and monitoring of potential radiation exposure.

Bibliography:

Juweid M, Sharkey RM, Siegel JA, Behr T, Goldenberg DM: Estimates of red marrow dose by sacral scintigraphy in radioimmunotherapy patients having non-Hodgkin's lymphoma and diffuse bone marrow uptake. Cancer Res 55(Suppl 23):5827s–5831s, 1995.

Patel S, Pearson D, Hosking DJ: Quantitative bone scintigraphy in the management of monostatic Paget's disease of bone. Arthritis Rheum 38(10):1506–1512, 1995.

Todorovic-Tirnamic M, Obradovic V, Han R, Goldner B, Stankovic D, Sekulic D, Lazic T, Djordjevic B: Diagnostic approach to reflex sympathetic dystrophy after fracture: radiography or bone scintigraphy? Eur J Nucl Med 22(10):1187–1193, 1995.

BONE SCAN (BONE SCINTIGRAPHY), DIAGNOSTIC

Norm: Even concentration of radioactive isotope throughout the osseous tissues.

Usage: Detection, staging, and evaluation of osseous metastatic disease. Detection of pathologic conditions that cause increased uptake, including aseptic necrosis, bone fractures, bone infarction, bone infection, bone metastasis, bone necrosis, bone tumors, bone trauma, osseous metastatic disease, osteoarthritis, osteomyelitis, Paget's disease, renal osteodystrophy, and soft tissue calcification. Differentiation of cellulitis from osteomyelitis. Monitoring of degenerative bone disorders, bone grafts, and prosthetic joint replacements. Aids in the selection of a biopsy site in the abnormal bone, in the evaluation of the effectiveness of arthritides, and in suspected abuse of a child.

Description: A nuclear medicine radioactive isotope study that will show bone changes from a few weeks up to 6 months before conventional radiographs. The radioactive isotope, Tc-99m diphosphonate (technetium disphosphate), is administered intravenously. As the entire body is scanned, images from the low-level radioactive isotope in the bony tissues are recorded on paper or film, creating two-dimensional images of the skeletal outlines. The epiphyses of growing bones or new bone formation show up as areas of high metabolism, or concentration, and are called "hot spots." Conversely, areas of low concentration, associated with ischemia or tumor displacement, are referred to as "cold spots." Increased uptake of the isotope by bone tissue indicates an abnormality in that area. Bone scintigraphy is especially important in detecting metastatic tumors and fractures not immediately seen on x-ray, especially in the spine, ribs, face, and small bones of the hands and feet. This test is invaluable in evaluating clients with osteomyelitis. Its disadvantage is that when showing an abnormality, it is nonspecific as to the pathologic process present.

Professional Considerations:
1. Consent form NOT required.

Risks:
Hematoma at injection site.

Contraindications:
During pregnancy, breast-feeding, and for clients who cannot lie still for an extended period of time.

2. Preparation:
   A. The client should not drink unnecessary fluids for 2–4 hours.
   B. Obtain an alcohol wipe, a tourniquet, a needle, a syringe, and radioactive isotope.
   C. Remove all jewelry and metal objects.
   D. Sedatives are used only if the client is unable to lie still for the scan.
   E. The client should void prior to the intravenous radioisotope being administered.
3. Procedure:
   A. Tc-99m diphosphonate (technetium diphosphate) is administered intravenously into a vein of the arm.
   B. During the next 2–3 hours, the client must drink 32 ounces of water to promote renal filtering of excess tracer.
   C. The client should void just prior to the scan to remove any tracer not picked up by bone that was filtered by the kidney.
   D. 1–3 hours after the injection, the client is placed in a supine position on the scanning table and instructed to lie still while the entire body is scanned and two-dimensional images of the skeleton are recorded.
4. Postprocedure care:
   A. If deep sedation was used, follow institutional protocol for postsedation monitoring. Typical monitoring includes continuous ECG monitoring and pulse oximetry, with continual assessments (q 5–15 minutes) of airway, vital signs, and neurologic status until the client is lying quietly awake, is breathing independently, and responds appropriately to commands spoken in a normal tone. The client should not operate a motor vehicle for 24 hours after receiving sedation.
   B. Check the injection site for redness or swelling. If a hematoma is present, apply warm soaks.
   C. Encourage oral fluid intake.
5. Client and family teaching:
   A. The radioisotope delivers less radiation than a regular radiograph and the scanning machine is detecting the injected isotope, rather than exposing him or her to radiation.
   B. Do not drink fluids for 4 hours prior to the scan.

C. The radioisotope will be injected intravenously before the scan.

D. Most of the radioactive material will be excreted from the body through urine and stool within 48 hours and it is not harmful to other people nearby.

E. Results are normally available within 24 hours.

6. Factors that affect results:

A. Failure to void prior to the test may cause an overdistended urinary bladder that can interfere with pelvic imaging.

7. Other data:

A. Health care professionals working in a nuclear medicine area must follow federal standards set by the Nuclear Regulatory Commission. These standards include precautions for handling the radioactive material and monitoring of potential radiation exposure.

Bibliography:

Calgar M, Tokgozoglu AM, Ercan MT, Aras T, Bekdik CF: The value of Tc-99m citrate scintigraphy in chronic osteomyelitis. An indicator of the involved bone. Clin Nucl Med *20*(8):712–716, 1995.

Lin WY, Wang SJ, Lan JL: Evaluation of arthritis in Reiter's disease by bone scintigraphy and radiography. Clin Rheumatol *14*(4):441–444, 1995.

Patel S, Pearson D, Hosking DJ: Quantitative bone scintigraphy in the management of monostotic Paget's disease of the bone. Arthritis Rheum *38*(10):1506–1512, 1995.

BONE SCINTIGRAPHY, DIAGNOSTIC

(see Bone Scan, Diagnostic)

BONE X-RAY, DIAGNOSTIC

Norm: Negative.

Usage: Identification of abnormal growth patterns by serial radiography. Detection of ankylosing spondylitis, congenital abnormalities, fractures, healing fractures, infection, joint destruction, osteomyelitis, the presence of joint fluid, and tumors.

Description: Specific bones are radiographed in several positions in order to visualize the bone from all angles.

Professional Considerations:

1. Consent form NOT required.
2. Preparation:
   A. Handle injured parts carefully.
   B. Shield the client's testes, ovaries, or pregnant abdomen.
3. Procedure:
   A. The client is placed on the radiography table in several positions, with a radiograph taken in each position.

B. The client must lie still for the radiograph.

4. Postprocedure care:

A. The client remains in the radiology department until it is determined that the films are satisfactory.

5. Client and family teaching:

A. The amount of exposure to radiation is minimal and not dangerous.

B. It is important to stay still during the radiograph.

C. Results are normally available within 24 hours.

6. Factors that affect results:

A. Movement results in an unsatisfactory radiograph.

B. Too little or too much exposure results in a radiograph that is too light or too dark and may need to be repeated for interpretation.

7. Other data:

A. Wear a lead apron if remaining in the room with the client during radiography.

Bibliography:

Lin WY, Wang SJ, Lan JL: Evaluation of arthritis in Reiter's disease by bone scintigraphy and radiography. Clin Rheumatol *14*(4):441–444, 1995.

Ohba T, Ogawa Y, Shinohara Y, Hiromatsu T, Uchida A, Toyoda Y: Limitations of panoramic radiography in the detection of bone defects in the posterior wall of the maxillary sinus: an experimental study. Dentomaxillofac Radiol *23*(3):149–153, 1994.

Ryan PJ, Fogelman I: Osteoporotic vertebral fractures: diagnosis with radiography and bone scintigraphy. Radiology *190*(3):669–672, 1994.

Suei Y, Tanimoto K, Wada T: Simple bone cyst. Evaluation of contents with conventional radiography and computed tomography. Oral Surg Oral Med Oral Pathol *77*(3):296–301, 1994.

BORDETELLA PERTUSSIS, CULTURE

Norm: No growth.

Usage: Diagnosis of pertussis (whooping cough).

Description: Pertussis is a highly communicable, acute bacterial infection of the tracheobronchial tree caused by *Bordetella pertussis,* a gram-negative coccobacilli. The disease occurs commonly in children throughout the world. Mode of transmission is thought to be either direct contact with the respiratory discharges of infected clients or by inhalation of airborne droplets. It is most communicable in the early stages, before the paroxysmal cough appears. Pertussis is characterized by an explosive cough, followed by a "whooping" sound on inspiration.

Professional Considerations:

1. Consent form NOT required.
2. Preparation:
   A. Wear mask and gloves when collecting the specimen.
   B. Obtain a culture tube, flexible wire swab, penlight, and tongue blade or "cough plate."
3. Procedure:
   A. Obtain a sterile swab of the nasopharynx or have the client cough onto a cough plate held in front of his or her mouth.
   B. To obtain nasopharyngeal swab:
      i. With the client's head tilted back, use a penlight and tongue depressor to visualize the nasopharynx.
      ii. Gently pass the swab through the nostril and into the nasopharynx, keeping the swab near the septum and floor of the nose.
      iii. Rotate the swab quickly and remove it carefully, making sure it does not touch the tongue or the sides of the nostril.
4. Postprocedure care:
   A. Hand-deliver the specimen to the laboratory immediately.
   B. Inform laboratory personnel if pertussis is suspected, because a special growth medium is required.
5. Client and family teaching:
   A. Observe for signs of pertussis in other children who were in contact with the infected child and who were not immunized.
   B. Therapy may begin prior to culture results.
   C. In the absence of antibiotic therapy, the period of communicability is considered to be from 7 days after exposure to 3 weeks after the paroxysmal cough appears. With erythromycin treatment, the period of communicability extends 7 days after the treatment is initiated.
   D. Results are normally available within 72 hours.
6. Factors that affect results:
   A. An insufficient specimen or current antibiotic therapy may cause false-negative results.
7. Other data:
   A. Immunization is available for pertussis prevention.
   B. A preliminary report should be available in 24 hours.

Bibliography:

Bejuk D, Begovac J, Bace A, Kuzmanovic-Sterk N, Aleraj B: Culture of *Bordella pertussis* from three upper respiratory tract specimens. Pediatr Infect Dis J *14*(1):64–65, 1995.

Deville JG, Cherry JD, Christenson PD, Pineda E, Leach CT, Kuhls TL, Viker S: Frequency of unrecognized *Bordetella pertussis* infections in adults. Clin Infect Dis *21*(3):639–642, 1995.

Doebbeling BN, Feilmeier ML, Herwaldt LA: Pertussis

in an adult man infected with the human immunodeficiency virus. J Infect Dis *161*(6):1296–1298, 1990.

BOTULISM, DIAGNOSTIC PROCEDURES, STOOL

Norm: Negative culture.

Usage: To diagnose the presence of *Clostridium botulinum* in the culture of feces.

Botulism Symptoms and Emergency Treatment:

Symptoms: diarrhea, dizziness, double-vision, fatigue, gastrointestinal pain, headache, nausea, weakness, vomiting. Cardiac and respiratory paralysis is possible.

Treatment:
1. Establish IV access.
2. Administer trivalent botulism antitoxin (Connaught Laboratories, LTD) (Note: Anaphylaxis is possible if the antitoxin is given to clients with asthma, hay fever, horse or horse serum allergies, or past exposure to horse serum.)
3. Follow package insert instructions for sensitivity testing prior to antitoxin administration.
4. Induce vomiting (with extreme caution) with syrup of ipecac, if the syrup can be given soon after the ingestion of the contaminated food. (Induction of emesis is contraindicated in clients with no gag reflex, or with central nervous system depression or excitation.)
5. Use gastric lavage if emesis does not produce the contaminated food.
6. Give activated charcoal slurry.
7. Give saline cathartic if no ileus is present.
8. Monitor for respiratory decompensation, which may occur suddenly in clients with botulism. Elective intubation is advisable for large ingestions.
9. Notify the state health department and the Centers for Disease Control (CDC) (404)639–2206. The medical emergency number is (404)639–2888.

Description: Botulism is a severe food poisoning resulting from the ingestion of the bacterial endotoxins of *Clostridium botulinum*. The exotoxin from *C. botulinum* exerts central nervous system actions and may lead quickly to death if an antidote is not administered prior to the onset of neurologic symptoms. Botulism most frequently occurs in home-canned food that has not been sufficiently heated during the canning process.

Professional Considerations:

1. Consent form NOT required.
2. Preparation:
   A. Obtain a sterile specimen container.
3. Procedure:
   A. Collect a stool specimen directly into a sterile, wide-mouthed, waxed container with a tight-fitting lid. Be sure there is no urine or paper in the specimen.
   B. If a stool specimen is not readily available, a rectal swab may be substituted. Insert a sterile microbiologic swab into the rectum and leave in place for 10 seconds. Remove the swab and send it to the laboratory in a culture container.
4. Postprocedure care:
   A. Properly seal the container to avoid leakage and contamination of others.
   B. Refrigerate the specimen if it cannot be sent immediately to the laboratory.
5. Client and family teaching:
   A. Avoid contaminating the stool with urine or toilet paper.
   B. Botulism may be prevented by cooking foods sufficiently to inactivate the toxins.
   C. An antitoxin is available for botulism.
   D. If activated charcoal was given for elevated levels, the client should drink 4–6 glasses of water each day for 2 days to prevent constipation. The activated charcoal will also cause stools to be black for a few days.
   E. Results are normally available within 72 hours.
6. Factors that affect results:
   A. Specimens not refrigerated invalidate the results.
7. Other data:
   A. In infant botulism, the organism and the toxin can be found in bowel contents, but not in serum. The presence of the toxin can be demonstrated by injecting mice with 0.4 ml of the suspected food, the client's fecal extract, and his or her serum. The presence of toxin results in flaccid paralysis within 24 hours and death within 3 days.
   B. The treatment for botulism is to give an antitoxin. However, the antitoxin only inactivates unbound toxins.
   C. Botulism is reportable to the CDC, Atlanta, Georgia.
   D. *See also Clostridial Toxin, Serum.*

Bibliography:

Centers for Disease Control and Prevention: foodborne botulism—Oklahoma, 1994. JAMA *273*(15):1167, 1995.

Gutierrez AR, Bondensteiner J, Gutmann L: Electrodiagnosis of infantile botulism. J Child Neurol *9*(4):362–365, 1994.

Hathway CL: Botulism: the present status of the disease. Curr Top Microbiol Immunol *195*:55–75, 1995.

BRAIN BIOPSY, DIAGNOSTIC

Norm: Normal tissue.

Usage: Identification and classification of tumors of the brain.

Description: Specimens of brain tissue are obtained during a craniotomy and sent to the pathology laboratory. The electron microscope is used to identify and classify tumors for more accurate diagnosis, upon which proper therapy and prognosis depend. The pathologist may also examine the specimen for antigen localization, which identifies the cell of origin of the antigen. This identifies the origin of metastatic carcinoma.

Professional Considerations:

1. Consent form IS required.

Risks:

Blindness, cerebrovascular accident, headache, infection, meningitis, paralysis.

Contraindications:

Anticoagulant therapy, bleeding disorders, increased intracranial pressure.

2. Preparation:
   A. Obtain a specimen container.
   B. Arrange for immediate handling of the specimen in pathology.
3. Procedure:
   A. A fresh specimen of brain tissue is placed in a plastic container with saline-moistened, sterile gauze and given to the pathologist who is in the operating room or waiting in the laboratory for the immediate delivery of the specimen.
   B. If immediate preparation of the specimen by the pathologist is not possible, the specimen is immediately cut into 1-mm cubes and placed in a vial of 2–4% phosphate, cacodylate-buffered glutaraldehyde, paraformaldehyde, or other fixative, according to the policy of the institution.

4. Postprocedure care:
   A. Tailor care to the procedure used to gain access to the brain tissue.
5. Client and family teaching:
   A. Results are normally available within 24 hours.
6. Factors that affect results:
   A. The specimen must be fresh.
   B. Placing the specimen in formalin, in the wrong fixative, or taking more than 2–3 minutes to place it in the fixative after collection invalidates the results.
   C. If antigen localization is done, the antisera must be available.
7. Other data:
   A. Brain scans are usually performed prior to surgery to assist in specific localization of the tumor for biopsy.

Bibliography:

Lunardi P, Acqui M, Maleci A, Di Lorenzo N, Fortuna A: Ultrasound-guided brain biopsy: a cliental experience with emphasis on its indication. Surg Neurol *39*(2):148-151, 1993.

Nielsen CJ, Gjerris F, Pedersen H, Jensen FK, Wagn P: Brain biopsy in AIDS. Diagnostic value and consequence. Acta Neurochir (Wien) *127*(1–2):99–102, 1994.

Vinters HV, Secor DL, Read SL, Frazee JG, Tomiyasu U, Stanley TM, Ferreiro JA, Akers MA: Microvasculature in brain biopsy specimens from patients with Alzheimer's disease: an immunohistochemical and ultrastructural study. Ultrastruc Pathol *18*(3):333–348, 1994.

BRAIN ECHOGRAM
(see Brain Sonogram, Diagnostic)

BRAIN SCAN, CEREBRAL FLOW AND PATHOLOGY, DIAGNOSTIC

Norm: Negative.

Usage: Abscess of the brain, brain tumors, contusions, cerebral vascular accidents, and hematomas.

Description: A nuclear medicine scan of the brain after the intravenous injection of a radioactive isotope. An immediate scan after the injection will show changes in the cerebral blood flow from one side of the brain compared to the other side. A later scan will show pathogenic tissue, which has a greater concentration of the isotope present than has normal tissue. This method of brain scanning has largely been replaced by newer, faster, and better quality SPECT scanning.

Professional Considerations:
1. Consent form IS required.

Risks:
Infection.

Contraindications:
Pregnancy and in clients who cannot lie still for an extended length of time.

2. Preparation:
   A. Potassium chloride capsules are given 2 hours before the isotope injection to prevent an inordinate amount of the isotope uptake in the choroid plexus. Too much uptake in the choroid plexus would simulate a pathologic condition in the cerebrum.
3. Procedure:
   A. The client is placed in a supine position on the scanning table with the isotope scanner in position over the head.
   B. The radioactive isotope is injected into a vein in the arm, and the scan is started immediately for the study of cervical flow.
   C. The scan is repeated 1 hour later to detect the presence of pathogenic tissue.
4. Postprocedure care:
   A. Encourage the oral intake of fluids.
5. Client and family teaching:
   A. Most of the radioactive material will be excreted from the body through urine and stool within 48 hours and is not harmful to other persons nearby.
   B. Venous access will be necessary.
   C. Results are normally available within 24 hours.
6. Factors that affect results:
   A. None found.
7. Other data:
   A. Health care professionals working in a nuclear medicine area must follow federal standards set by the Nuclear Regulatory Commission. These standards include precautions for handling the radioactive material and monitoring of potential radiation exposure.
   B. *See also Single Photon Emission Computed Tomography (SPECT Scan), Brain, Diagnostic.*

Bibliography:

Gean AD, Kates RS, Lee S: Neuroimaging in head injury. New Horiz *3*(3):549–561, 1995.

Otsubo H, Hwang PA, Hoffman HJ, Becker LE, Gilday DL, Chuang SH, Harwood-Nash D: Neuroimaging studies in children with temporal lobectomy. Child Nerv Syst *11*(5):281–287, 1995.

Mena I, Giombetti RJ, Miller BL, Garrett K, Villanueva-Meyer J, Mody C, Goldberg MA: Cerebral blood flow changes with acute cocaine intoxication: clinical correlations with SPECT, CT and MRI. NIDA Res Monogr *138*:161–173, 1994.

Shiminski-Maher T, Shields M: Pediatric brain tumors: diagnosis and management. J Pediatr Oncol Nurs 12(4):188–198, 1995.

BRAIN SONOGRAM (BRAIN ECHOGRAM, BRAIN ULTRASOUND, ECHOENCEPHALOGRAM), DIAGNOSTIC

Norm: Normal position of the brain's midline structures and normal blood flow velocity.

Usage: Diagnosis of brain deformities in newborns and infants, space-occupying lesions, structural shifts due to cerebral edema, subdural hematoma, or extradural hematoma. Determination of viability of brain tissue based on the sequential measurement of blood flow velocity. Brain sonograms can also be used for early detection of cerebral ischemia during a carotid endarterectomy while cerebral blood flow is interrupted.

Description: An ultrasound beam is transmitted through the skull. The time required for the beam to be reflected back to the transducer is converted to an electrical impulse displayed on an oscilloscope screen and measured to determine the structure, position, and blood flow of the brain. A shift in the third ventricle of more than 3 mm from midline is abnormal. An enlargement of the third ventricle of more than 10 mm in the adult or of more than 7 mm in the child is abnormal.

Professional Considerations:

1. Consent form NOT required.
2. Preparation:
   A. Remove jewelry and metal objects from the client's head and neck.
   B. Obtain ultrasonic gel or paste.
3. Procedure:
   A. The client is placed in a supine position.
   B. A small transducer, with water-soluble paste applied to it, is placed on the side of the head over the temporoparietal region.
   C. Ultrasonic beams are sent into the head and their reflection is recorded on the oscilloscope and photographed.
4. Postprocedure care:
   A. Cleanse the paste from the scalp.
5. Client and family teaching:
   A. Do not drink hot or cold caffeine-containing beverages on the morning of the test.
   B. It is normal to hear an echo that sounds like repetitious humming or a musical note as the brain structures reflect the ultrasonic beam.
   C. This procedure takes approximately 1 hour.
   D. Results are normally available within 24 hours.
6. Factors that affect results:
   A. Failure to remove jewelry and metal objects from the head and neck will interfere with the clarity of the oscilloscope pictures.
7. Other data:
   A. Follow-up studies using computed tomography scan or radionucleotides may be indicated.

Bibliography:

Babcock DS: Sonography of the brain in infants: role in evaluating neurologic abnormalities. Am J Roentgenol 165(2):417–423, 1995.

Becker G, Krone A, Koulis D, Lindner A, Hofmann E, Roggendorf W, Bogdahn U: Reliability of transcranial colour-coded real-time sonography in assessment of brain tumours: correlation of ultrasound, computed tomography and biopsy findings. Neuroradiology 36(8):585–590, 1994.

Larsen FS, Pott F, Hansen BA, Ejlersen E, Knudsen GM, Clemmesen JD, Secher NH: Transcranial Doppler sonography may predict brain death in patients with fulminant hepatic failure. Transplant Proc 27(6):3510–3511, 1995.

BRAIN ULTRASOUND

(see Brain Sonogram, Diagnostic)

BRAINSTEM AUDITORY-EVOKED POTENTIAL (BAEP), DIAGNOSTIC

Norm: Normal waveform.

Usage: Primarily used to evaluate brainstem function. Aids in evaluation of coma. Used in screening of high-risk infants for sudden death syndrome and for hearing impairment. The presence of waveforms in the absence of cephalic reflexes, spontaneous respirations, and isopotential electroencephalogram (EEG) suggest reversibility of the coma. The absence of all waveforms except wave I in the same clinical setting suggests extensive structural brainstem damage and implies brain death.

Adults: May be prescribed to test the time required for nerve signals to travel from the ear to the brainstem.

Description: Waveforms that are conducted to the surface of the brain measure the electrical potential that originates in the subcortical auditory pathways in response to acoustic stimuli. Since this electrical potential is not altered by metabolic factors or by most central nervous system depressants and is present even when EEG activity is absent due to a drug overdose, its presence suggests reversibility of the coma. In the absence of clinical signs and radiologic abnormalities, a BAEP abnormality may indicate an infratentorial neoplasm such as an acoustic neuroma related to damaged nerve cells in the brainstem that transmit balance information to the brain. It is also helpful in diagnosing brainstem lesions in multiple sclerosis.

Professional Considerations:

1. Consent form NOT required.
2. Preparation:
   A. Remove earrings.
3. Procedure:
   A. An electrode is placed on the scalp at the vertex and a reference electrode is placed on the ear lobe.
   B. Headphones are applied, which mask the auditory responses of the outer ear.
   C. A series of square-wave clicks of varying intensities and frequencies are presented to the ear and the waveforms are recorded.
4. Postprocedure care:
   A. None.
5. Client and family teaching:
   A. Radiologic examinations usually accompany this test.
   B. Results are normally available within 24 hours.
6. Factors that affect results:
   A. None.
7. Other data:
   A. This test can be conducted on alert or comatose clients.

Bibliography:

Hickey, JV: Clinical Practice of Neurological and Neurosurgical Nursing. Philadelphia, JB Lippincott, 1992, p 108.
Philip PA, Philip M: Evoked potentials in the prognosis of traumatic lesions of the central nervous system. Phys Med Rehab Clin North Amer 5(3):643–656, 1994.

BRAZELTON NEONATAL BEHAVIORAL ASSESSMENT SCALE, DIAGNOSTIC

Norm: Normal reflexes for gestational age and a median or above grade score for each neurologic and/or psychosocial response.

Usage: Evaluation of newborns to determine neurologic deficits. Used mainly to evaluate preterm infants and to compare results with later development.

Description: A series of observations of the newborn with 29 criteria, each having several grades. These include observation of the baby while awake and asleep, noting his or her alertness, eye-following, response to sound, irritability, social interest in the examiner, consolability, and response to 20 primitive reflexes.

Professional Considerations:

1. Consent form NOT required.
2. Preparation:
   A. None.
3. Procedure:
   A. The baby is evaluated and given a score in each area that is tested.
4. Postprocedure care:
   A. None.
5. Client and family teaching:
   A. The parent may be asked to stay with the infant throughout the test.
   B. The assessment takes 25–35 minutes to complete.
   C. The test should be repeated periodically throughout the child's development for comparison and analysis of any deficits.
6. Factors that affect results:
   A. Assessment cannot be completed accurately if the infant is crying.
7. Other data:
   A. None.

Bibliography:

Davis M, Emory E: Sex differences in neonatal stress reactivity. Child Dev 66(1):14–27, 1995.
Gatts JD, Fernbach SA, Wallace DH, Singra TS: Reducing crying and irritability in neonates using a continuously controlled early environment. J Perinatol 15(3):215–221, 1995.
Oyemade UJ, Cole OJ, Johnson AA, Knight EM, Westney OE, Laryea H, Hill G, Cannon E, Fomufod A, Westney LS, et al.: Prenatal predictors of performance on the Brazelton Neonatal Behavioral Assessment Scale. J Nutr 124(Suppl 6):1000S–1005S, 1994.

BREAST SONOGRAM (BREAST ECHOGRAM, BREAST ULTRASOUND), DIAGNOSTIC

Norm: Normal breast tissue boundaries demonstrate bright echo reflections. The nipple and skin reflections are higher than the areola echo reflection. Fat demonstrates low reflectivity, with a mixture of low and strong echoes, whereas connective tissue and ligaments are bright. Tumors and cysts are absent. Younger breasts have less fatty tissue than older breasts.

Usage: Detection of tiny breast tumors, differentiation of breast cysts from breast tumors less than ¼ inch in diameter; screening for breast abnormalities in low-risk clients or where mammography is not readily available; helpful for clients with radiographic dense breasts or breast prostheses; and evaluation of symptomatic clients who are pregnant or lactating.

Description: A noninvasive test in which a picture of breast tissue is produced on a screen by beaming high-frequency sound waves into the breast and computer-processing the signals received back through a transducer. The time required for the ultrasonic beam to be reflected back to the transducer from differing densities of tissue is converted by a computer to an electrical impulse displayed on an oscilloscopic screen to create a three-dimensional picture of the breast. An advantage of this test is that it can display all breast tissue, whereas radiography cannot. In clients with fibrocystic breast disease, the water path method of sonography may be used.

Professional Considerations:

1. Consent form NOT required.
2. Preparation:
   A. Obtain ultrasonic gel or paste.
3. Procedure:
   A. The client is positioned supine-oblique and rolled 35 degrees toward the side of the breast that will be examined. A sponge, blanket roll, or folded towel may be used to support the shoulders and hips. The client's arm on the same side to be examined should be placed behind the head.
   B. A greasy, conductive paste is applied to the 5.0- or 7.5-MHz, small-diameter, high-frequency, transducer.
   C. The transducer is passed methodically over all of the skin of the breast. Any known breast mass is identified, and the surrounding area in a 3-cm square is marked on the breast. The breast and marked area are scanned transversely from the inferior margin toward the head in small intervals, followed by sagittal scans moving medially to laterally. Scanning is performed with light pressure.

D. Photographs are taken of the oscilloscopic display.
E. Dedicated water path breast instrumentation:
   i. The client is positioned either prone on a special bed, with the breast suspended over and into water, or supine with a bag of water overlying the breast.
   ii. Scanning is performed in 1- to 2-mm intervals through the water path with a transducer. Any lesions are identified in two axes.
4. Postprocedure care:
   A. Cleanse the skin of the ultrasonic paste.
5. Client and family teaching:
   A. Wear a two-piece outfit to facilitate breast exposure for exam (if the test is performed on an outpatient basis).
   B. Some facilities request that no deodorants, powders, or perfumes be worn the day of the test.
   C. The procedure will take approximately 30 minutes.
   D. A breast sonogram may improve the accuracy of the diagnosis when used as an adjunct to mammography.
   E. Results are normally available in 1–2 days.
6. Factors that affect results:
   A. Compression of the breast may be used to eliminate nipple shadows, enable the use of higher frequency transducers, and improve delineation of the tissue. However, compression causes a misrepresentation of the breast anatomy.
7. Other data:
   A. Negative sonographic results should not be used to conclude a lesion is benign.

Bibliography:
DiVito J, Rossmann MD: Breast sonography: technique to mimic mammographic position. J Ultrasound Med *13*(1):33–36, 1994.
Richter K: Techniques for detecting and evaluating breast lesions. J Ultrasound Med *13*(10):797–802, 1994.

BREATH HYDROGEN ANALYSIS, DIAGNOSTIC

Norm: <20 ppm elevation over fasting level.

Usage: Assessment of orocaecal transit time; determination of lactose intolerance; screening for early diagnosis of necrotizing enterocolitis; and evaluation of peptic ulcer disease before and during treatment with ranitidine.

Description: This test measures the hydrogen exhaled at specific time intervals during the first 3 hours after ingestion of the carbohydrate (such as lactose, lactulose, fructose, or sucrose) being studied. In the normal client, hydrogen is produced exclusively by the bacterial metabolism of carbohydrates. Clients who are unable to digest or absorb carbohydrates in the small intestine have an increased volume of carbohydrates reaching the colon. These carbohydrates are metabolized in the colon, producing hydrogen, which is absorbed in the colon and exhaled by the lungs. The hydrogen breath test detects higher than normal levels and abnormal timing of peak releases of exhaled hydrogen. Ranitidine inhibits the action of histamine on the H_2-receptors of the parietal cells of the stomach, thus reducing hydrochloric acid production. The breath test can be used to evaluate hydrogen release after administration of the ranitidine.

Professional Considerations:

1. Consent form NOT required.
2. Preparation:
   A. *See Client and family teaching.*
   B. Obtain a syringe or balloon.
3. Procedure:
   A. After measuring a basal breath hydrogen level, an oral dose of lactose, 1 g/kg of body weight, is given.
   B. End-alveolar air is expired into a 30-ml glass syringe or a special plastic balloon.
   C. The breath sample is injected into an analyzer to determine H_2 and CO_2 concentration.
   D. A rise of 720 ppm in exhaled hydrogen is diagnostic for lactose malabsorption.
   E. Clients with bacterial overgrowth of the small intestine will have an in-

creased production of hydrogen, with an early peak (within 3 hours) of hydrogen release after carbohydrate ingestion.
   F. Clients with disease of the small intestine and carbohydrate malabsorption have a later peak of hydrogen release.
4. Postprocedure care:
   A. Resume normal diet.
5. Client and family teaching:
   A. Fast from midnight prior to the test. A carbohydrate-controlled diet the day before the test affects the fasting breath hydrogen levels and may improve the test accuracy.
   B. Do not use laxatives or enemas for 3 days before testing.
   C. Do not smoke for at least 15 minutes before testing.
6. Factors that affect results:
   A. Diarrhea within 3 days prior to the test invalidates the results.
   B. Storage of the samples allows for leakage of the gases. A glass syringe stored on its side with the barrel lubricated with mineral oil will have negligible leakage over a 2-week period. Upright storage may result in leakage of mineral oil and loss of the barrel seal.
7. Other data:
   A. Hydrogen content increases as carbohydrate malabsorption increases.

Bibliography:

Sleisenger M, Fordtran J: Gastrointestinal Disease: Pathophysiology, Diagnosis, Management. Philadelphia, WB Saunders, 1989, p 276.

Bruun E, Meyer JN, Rumessen JJ, Gudmand-Hoyer E: Breath hydrogen analysis in patients with ileoanal pouch anastomosis. Gut *37*(2):256–259, 1995.

BREATH TEST (CARBON-13 OR CARBON-14 UREA BREATH TEST)

(see Urea Breath Test, Diagnostic)

BROMIDES, SERUM

Norm: Negative.

		SI Units
Reference range	0–5 mg/dl	0–0.6 mmol/L
Panic levels		
Bromide ion	>120 mg/dl	>15 mmol/L
Sodium bromide	>150 mg/dl	>15 mmol/L
	>15 mEq/L	>15 mmol/L

Panic Levels Symptoms and Treatment:

Symptoms: Abdominal pain, ataxia, central nervous system depression (coma), cyanosis, eye irritation (if inhaled), gastrointestinal tract corrosion (if swallowed), increased cerebrospinal fluid pressure, mental disturbance (confusion, hallucinations, irritability, mania), rash, tachycardia, respiratory irritation (if inhaled), shock, vertigo, vomiting.

Treatment:

For bromide poisoning due to inhalation:
Give oxygen.
Maintain patent airway and support breathing.
Monitor for and treat pulmonary edema.

For bromide poisoning from ingestion:
Induce vomiting with syrup of ipecac. (Induction of vomiting is contraindicated in clients with no gag reflex, or with central nervous system depression or excitation.)
Perform gastric lavage.

General intervention:
Administer 1 g NaCl in water orally q 1 hour until serum bromide level is less than 50 mg/dl.
Monitor for and treat shock symptoms.
Monitor liver and kidney function.
Hydrate and provide mild diuresis.
Both hemodialysis and peritoneal dialysis WILL remove bromides.

Usage: Screening for bromide toxicity.

Increased: Exposure to vapors in photography and chemical industries, exposure to bromides in pesticides, and ingestion of over-the-counter medications such as Bromo-Seltzer.

Description: Bromide is a reddish-brown, nonvolatile liquid that gives off suffocating vapors that are highly toxic and severely irritating to the skin. Bromide replaces chloride in the body tissues, resulting in sedation and depression of the central nervous system. For this reason, it was used in the past as a medication to sedate clients until more effective, less toxic medications became available.

Professional Considerations:

1. Consent form NOT required.
2. Preparation:
   A. Tube: Red-top, red/gray-top, gold-top, or green-top.
   B. Do NOT draw during hemodialysis.
3. Procedure:
   A. Draw a 5-ml blood sample.
4. Postprocedure care:
   A. Monitor closely for signs of bromide toxicity.
5. Client and family teaching:
   A. Bromide poisoning rarely causes death.
6. Factors that affect results:
   A. Falsely elevated levels may occur in clients receiving iodine therapy.
7. Other data:
   A. Alcoholics are especially susceptible to bromide intoxication.

Bibliography:

Littleton P, Midgley J, Mode N, Carter N, Smith A: Serum bromide measurements in infants below 1000 g, for determination of corrected bromide space. Br J Biomed Sci *50*(4):355–357, 1993.

BRONCHIAL ASPIRATE, FUNGUS, CULTURE

Norm: Negative. No growth.

Usage: Diagnosis of the presence and type of potentially pathogenic fungi in the bronchi.

Positive: *Aspergillus fumigatus, Aspergillus flavus, Blastomyces dermatitides, Candida albicans, Candida tropicalis, Coccidioides immitis, Cryptococcus neoformans, Histoplasma capsulatum,* and *Sporothrix schenckii.*

Description: Fungi are slow-growing, eukaryotic organisms that can grow on living and nonliving organic materials and are subdivided into yeasts and molds. Normal human host defense mechanisms limit the damage they cause superficially. Some fungi can be inhaled or introduced by traumatic inoculation into deep tissue spaces and cause serious infections. Although tentative identification of fungi can be made quickly with staining techniques, culture of the organism on special fungal culture media is required to confirm a diagnosis of a fungal infection.

Professional Considerations:

1. Consent form is NOT required unless a bronchoscopy is used to obtain the specimen.
2. Preparation:
   A. Obtain a sterile container or suction trap, suction tubing, sterile suction catheter, and gloves.
   B. Prepare a suction machine or a wall suction.
   C. *See Bronchoscopy, Diagnostic (Preparation)* if this method is used.
3. Procedure:
   A. A specimen trap is inserted into the suctioning line of a flexible, fiberoptic bronchoscope or between the suctioning catheter and a regular suctioning line. When the bronchoscope is in place or the suction catheter is completely inserted into the bronchi, suction is applied and a specimen is obtained while holding the suction trap upright.
   B. Specimens obtained by expectoration should be collected early in the morning after the client has removed any dentures and gargled and rinsed the mouth with water. A deep cough is required to deliver a good specimen and the specimen should be expectorated directly into a sterile cup.
4. Postprocedure care:
   A. Write the collection time on the laboratory requisition.
   B. Write any current antibiotic or antifungal therapy on the laboratory requisition.
   C. Transport the specimen to the laboratory immediately.
   D. *See Bronchoscopy, Diagnostic* if this method is used.
5. Client and family teaching:
   A. *See Bronchoscopy, Diagnostic* if this method is used.
   B. To produce a specimen by coughing, take several breaths in, without fully exhaling in-between. When you feel you cannot breathe any more air in, cough out forcefully and catch the sputum in a specimen cup.
   C. 4–6 weeks are required for a final fungal culture report.
6. Factors that affect results:
   A. The specimen should be obtained with the first suctioning.
   B. A break in the sterile technique invalidates the results.
   C. The best results are obtained if the cultures are inoculated immediately. The maximum time allowed between specimen collection and inoculation is 3 hours.
7. Other data:
   A. None.

Bibliography:

McElvein RB: Procedures in the evaluation of chest disease. Clin Chest Med, *13*(1): 1–9, 1992.

Weinberger SE: Recent advances in pulmonary medicine (1). New Engl J Med *328*(19):1389–1397, 1993.

Weinberger SE: Recent advances in pulmonary medicine (2). New Engl J Med *328* (20):1462–1470, 1993.

BRONCHIAL ASPIRATE, ROUTINE, CULTURE

Norm: No growth or growth of only normal upper respiratory flora.

Usage: Diagnosis of infections of the tracheobronchial tree.

Description: Sputum obtained via bronchoscopy, routine tracheal suctioning, or coughing is cultured and Gram stained. Suctioned samples may be obtained nasotracheally, endotracheally, or through a tracheostomy.

Professional Considerations:

1. Consent form NOT required.
2. Preparation:
   A. Obtain a sterile container or suction trap, suction tubing, a sterile suction catheter, and gloves.
   B. Prepare the suction machine or wall suction.
   C. *See Bronchoscopy, Diagnostic (Preparation)* if this method is used.
3. Procedure:
   A. A specimen trap is inserted into the suctioning line of a flexible, fiberoptic bronchoscope or between the suctioning catheter and a regular suctioning line. When the bronchoscope is in place or the suction catheter is completely inserted into the bronchi, suction is applied and a specimen is obtained while holding the suction trap upright.
   B. Specimens obtained by expectoration should be collected early in the morning after the client has removed any dentures and gargled and rinsed the mouth with water. A deep cough is required to deliver a good specimen and the specimen should be expectorated directly into a sterile cup.
4. Postprocedure care:
   A. Write the collection time on the laboratory requisition.
   B. Write any current antibiotic or antifungal therapy for the client on laboratory requisition.
   C. *See Bronchoscopy, Diagnostic* if this method is used.
5. Client and family teaching:
   A. To produce a specimen by coughing, take several breaths in, without fully exhaling in-between. When you feel you cannot breathe any more air in, cough out forcefully and catch sputum in a specimen cup.

B. *See Bronchoscopy, Diagnostic* if this method is used.

C. Cultures with no growth can be reported in 48 hours. Final results take up to 10 days.

6. Factors that affect results:

A. The specimen should be obtained with the first suctioning.

B. Reject specimens more than 4 hours old.

7. Other data:

A. None.

Bibliography:

Baselski VS, Wunderlind RG: Diagnosis of pneumonia [review]. Clin Microbiol Rev 7(4):533–558, 1994.

Chastre J, Fagon JY, Bornet-Lesco M, Calvat S, Dombret MC, al Khani R, Basset F, Gibert C: Evaluation of bronchoscopic techniques for the diagnosis of nosocomial pneumonia. Amer J Resp Crit Care Med 152(1):231–240, 1995.

BRONCHIAL CHALLENGE TEST

(see Methacholine Challenge Test, Diagnostic)

BRONCHIAL CULTURE

Norm: No growth.

Usage: Diagnosis of infections of the bronchi.

Description: To prevent contamination of the specimen by the upper respiratory tract, endotracheal tube, tracheostomy tube, or the insertion of the bronchoscope, the culture is obtained by a protected specimen brush that touches only the specimen site.

Professional Considerations:

1. Consent form NOT required for the test, but IS required for the bronchoscopy procedure used to obtain the specimen. See *Bronchoscopy, Diagnostic* for risks and contraindications.

2. Preparation:

A. *See Bronchoscopy, Diagnostic.*

B. Obtain a sterile specimen container.

3. Procedure:

A. A protected specimen brush is used to obtain a specimen of the specific area visualized via bronchoscopy (*see Bronchoscopy, Diagnostic*).

B. A protected specimen brush may also be inserted via an endotracheal tube or a tracheostomy tube for a blind local culture.

C. The disposable brush end can be smeared on a slide and then cut off and placed in a sterile container.

4. Postprocedure care:

A. Write current antibiotic or antifungal therapy on the laboratory requisition.

B. *See Bronchoscopy, Diagnostic.*

5. Client and family teaching:

A. *See Bronchoscopy, Diagnostic.*

6. Factors that affect results:

A. *See Bronchoscopy, Diagnostic.*

7. Other data:

A. *See Bronchoscopy, Diagnostic.*

Bibliography:

Haglund LA, et al.: Invasive pneumococcal disease in central Oklahoma: emergence of high level penicillin resistance and multiple antibiotic resistance. J Infect Dis 10(8):1532, 1993.

Limper AH, Allen RM: Diagnosing ventilator-associated pneumonia: the role of bronchoscopy [review]. Mayo Clinic Proc 69(10):962–968, 1994.

BRONCHIAL WASHING (BRONCHO-ALVEOLAR LAVAGE), SPECIMEN, DIAGNOSTIC

Norm: Negative for culture and cytology.

Usage: Diagnosis of infections and pathologic processes in the lungs.

Description: Procedure useful to obtain respiratory tract specimens for culture and cytology when very few secretions are present. Specimens are obtained from a normal saline wash, which is instilled into the bronchi and then suctioned out. Saline may be instilled via a bronchoscope, an endotracheal tube, or a tracheal tube. A bronchoalveolar wash will provide a specimen from the alveoli and is done by inserting the flexible fiberoptic bronchoscope as far into the bronchiole as possible and instilling the saline at that point. This procedure is used when adequate deep sputum specimens cannot be obtained and is often helpful in diagnosing pneumocystic pneumonia.

Professional Considerations:

1. Consent form NOT required unless the washing is done via bronchoscopy. See *Bronchoscopy, Diagnostic* for risks and contraindications if bronchoscopy is used to obtain the specimen.

2. Preparation:

A. Obtain a specimen trap, suction tubing, a sterile suction catheter, and sterile gloves.

B. Prepare a wall suction or a suction machine.

C. If the washing is performed during bronchoscopy, obtain sterile specimen containers for the bronchoscope.

D. *See Bronchoscopy, Diagnostic* if this procedure is used.

3. Procedure:

A. A specimen trap is inserted into the

suctioning line from the broncho-scope, or between the suctioning catheter and the suctioning line.

B. Up to 20 ml of normal saline is in-stilled into the respiratory tract via the bronchoscope, the endotracheal, or the tracheal tube, and the specimen is obtained when suction is applied to the bronchoscope catheter or suction catheter.

4. Postprocedure care:
   A. Write the time of specimen collection and any current antibiotic or antifun-gal therapy on the laboratory requisi-tion.
   B. *See Bronchoscopy, Diagnostic* if this procedure is used.
5. Client and family teaching:
   A. *See Bronchoscopy, Diagnostic* if this procedure is used.
   B. Results are normally available within 1–2 days.
6. Factors that affect results:
   A. Bronchial washing specimens must be collected using a sterile technique.
7. Other data:
   A. May be used to diagnose *Pneumocystis carinii* in client with AIDS.

Bibliography:

Bajwa MK, Henein S, Kamholz SL: Fiberoptic bron-choscopy in the presence of space-occupying in-tracranial lesions. Chest *104*(1):101–103, 1993.

Inzumi TV, Myers JL: Clinical and histologic spectrum of bronchiolitis. Seminar Respir Med *13*(1): 191–195, 1992.

BRONCHO-ALVEOLAR LAVAGE, SPECIMEN

(see Bronchial Washing, Specimen, Diagnostic)

BRONCHOGRAPHY, DIAGNOSTIC

Norm: Normal tracheobronchial tree. The left bronchus is longer, nar-rower, and less vertical than the right mainstem bronchus. The bronchi are free of lesions or narrowing.

Usage: Diagnosis of bronchocuta-neous fistulas, bronchial obstruction, chronic bronchitis, chronic pneumo-nia, lesions, cysts, and cavities in the bronchial tree, pulmonary tumors, and bronchiectasis-producing hemoptysis.

Description: A radiographic exami-nation of the tracheobronchial tree using contrast media. A radiopaque io-dine contrast solution, usually with an oil base, is instilled into the trachea and bronchi through a catheter or bronchoscope. Abnormalities may be visualized on x-ray after the dye coats the bronchial trees. The test may be performed under local or general anesthesia. This test is used less fre-quently now because of the increased availability of tomography.

Professional Considerations:

1. Consent form IS required.

Risks:

Dizziness, dyspnea, allergic reaction to dye (itching, hives, rash, tight feeling in the throat, shortness of breath, bronchospasm, anaphylaxis, death), renal toxicity. *See also risks for Bronchoscopy, Diagnostic,* if this procedure is used.

Contraindications:

Previous allergic reaction to dye; pregnancy, acute respiratory infections, and respiratory insufficiency. *See also contraindications for Bronchoscopy, Diagnostic,* if this procedure is used.

---

2. Preparation:
   A. *See Client and family teaching.*
   B. Sedation may be prescribed prior to the procedure if general anesthesia will be used.
   C. Ephedrine or Atropine may be pre-scribed to decrease secretions and minimize vagally induced bradycardia.
   D. Meticulous mouth care should be per-formed to minimize the number of bacteria introduced into the bronchi.
   E. Remove any dentures or eyeglasses.
   F. Have emergency resuscitation equip-ment readily available.
3. Procedure:
   A. A local anesthetic is applied in the nose and mouth to suppress the gag reflex.
   B. After the client has assumed a sitting position, a catheter or bronchoscope is passed into the trachea.
   C. The pharynx, larynx, and major bronchi are anesthetized.
   D. Radiopaque dye is instilled. Laryn-gospasms are possible at this time.
   E. The client and the catheter or bron-choscope are rotated on a tilt table so that the dye will coat all portions of the area to be studied.
   F. The procedure is usually performed on only one lung at a time to maintain good gas exchange and as a precaution for a possible allergic reaction to the dye.

G. It is important that the client not cough so that there is adequate dye retained to reach and fill the alveoli. Rapid shallow breathing helps to suppress the urge to cough.

H. Observe closely for impaired breathing.

4. Postprocedure care:

A. Use postural drainage to promote the removal of mucus and exudate from the lungs. Aerosol therapy may also be used.

B. Continue the assessment of the respiratory status. If deep sedation was used, follow institutional protocol for postsedation monitoring. Typical monitoring includes continuous ECG monitoring and pulse oximetry, with continual assessments (q 5–15 minutes) of airway, vital signs, and neurologic status until the client is lying quietly awake, is breathing independently, and responds appropriately to commands spoken in a normal tone.

C. Observe closely for postprocedure complications, which may include pneumonia, delayed hypersensitivity reaction, laryngospasms, hoarseness, and stridor.

D. Expectorant may be prescribed to help remove secretions and contrast media.

5. Client and family teaching:

A. Fast for 8–12 hours before the procedure.

B. The test will take approximately 1 hour.

C. Make arrangements for someone else to drive you home, as you will not be permitted to drive if sedation or anesthesia is used.

D. Do not eat or drink until the gag reflex has returned, about 2 hours after the procedure.

E. A sore throat and slight fever for 2–3 days after the test is not unusual.

F. Normal activity, including driving, may be resumed 24 hours after the procedure.

6. Factors that affect results:

A. The procedure should be stopped if the client becomes uncooperative or if impaired respiratory function is noted.

B. Bronchial secretions may interfere with dye passage into all areas of the bronchial tree.

7. Other data:

A. None.

Bibliography:

Koyama H, Nishimura K, Mio T, Izumi T: Emphysematous changes assessed by selective alveolobronchography and bronchodilator response in chronic airflow obstruction. Lung *172*(2):103–112, 1994.

Marcos SK, Anderson PB: Pediatric bronchography performed through the flexible bronchoscope. Eur J Radiol *17*(2):134–136, 1993.

Pagana K, Pagana T (eds): Diagnostic Testing and Nursing Implications: A Case Study Approach, 2nd ed. St. Louis, MO, CV Mosby, 1990, pp 161–163.

BRONCHOSCOPY, DIAGNOSTIC

Norm: Normal larynx, trachea, and bronchi.

Usage: Used to examine the bronchi for abscesses, aspiration pneumonia, hemoptysis and unresolved pneumonias, strictures, tumors, removal of foreign objects, and to obtain deep sputum specimens and tissue biopsies.

Description: Direct visual examination of the larynx, trachea, and bronchi with a rigid bronchoscope or a flexible fiberoptic bronchoscope.

Professional Considerations:

1. Consent form IS required.

Risks:

Bleeding, bronchospasm, cardiopulmonary arrest, dysrhythmias, hypotension, hypoxia, pneumothorax.

Contraindications:

Pregnancy; clients with severe shortness of breath who cannot tolerate interruption of high flow oxygen. Such clients may be intubated for the procedure to ensure optimal oxygenation. Sedatives are contraindicated in clients with central nervous system depression.

---

2. Preparation:

A. Obtain vital signs, activated partial thromboplastin time, platelet count, and prothrombin time.

B. Remove any dentures or eyeglasses.

C. Sedation may be prescribed.

D. Prepare suctioning equipment.

E. Have emergency resuscitation equipment readily available.

3. Procedure:

A. The nasopharynx and oropharynx are anesthetized with a local anesthetic.

B. The client is placed in a sitting or supine position.

C. After the tube is passed through the mouth or nose into the larynx, more local anesthetic is sprayed into the trachea to inhibit the cough reflex.

D. If the client has a large endotracheal tube in place, the flexible bronchoscope can be inserted through it.

E. The trachea and bronchi are visually examined for abnormal color, structure, or lesions.

F. Mucus is then suctioned until clear, bronchial washings are performed and the specimens collected, and biopsies are obtained if the flexible tube is used.

G. The rigid bronchoscope is used to retrieve foreign bodies and excise lesions.

H. The client is observed for impaired respirations or laryngospasms throughout the procedure.

4. Postprocedure care:

A. No food or fluids are given until the gag reflex has returned, about 2 hours after the procedure.

B. The client should not attempt to swallow saliva until the gag reflex has returned. Saliva should be expectorated into an emesis basin. Observe the client's sputum for blood if a biopsy was performed. If a tumor is suspected, collect postbronchoscopy sputum specimens for cytology.

C. Observe postanesthesia precautions if a sedative was given. If deep sedation was used, follow institutional protocol for postsedation monitoring. Typical monitoring includes continuous ECG monitoring and pulse oximetry, with continual assessments (q 5–15 minutes) of airway, vital signs, and neurologic status until the client is lying quietly awake, is breathing independently, and responds appropriately to commands spoken in a normal tone.

D. Observe closely for postprocedure complications, including bronchospasm, bacteremia, bronchial perforation (indicated by facial or neck crepitus), cardiac dysrhythmias, fever, hemorrhage from the biopsy site, hypoxemia, laryngospasm, pneumonia, and pneumothorax.

5. Client and family teaching:

A. Fast from the midnight prior to the procedure. Your diet will be restarted a few hours after the procedure.

B. Arrange for transportation home after an ambulatory procedure, as you will not be permitted to drive for 24 hours after receiving sedation.

C. Notify the physician if experiencing fever or difficulty in breathing during the next 48–72 hours.

D. Begin drinking or eating approximately 2 hours after the procedure.

6. Factors that affect results:

A. The procedure should be stopped if the client becomes uncooperative or if impaired respiratory function is noted.

7. Other data:

A. None.

Bibliography:

Allen RM, Dunn WF, Limper AH: Diagnosing ventilator-associated pneumonia: the role of bronchoscopy [review]. Mayo Clinic Proc 69(10):962–968, 1994.

Lanser K: Bronchoscopy in respiratory tract diseases [review]. Internist 23(6):564–568, 1995.

Pagana K, Pagana T (eds): Diagnostic Testing and Nursing Implications: A Case Study Approach, 2nd ed. St. Louis, MO, CV Mosby, 1990, pp 122–124.

BRUCELLOSIS AGGLUTININS, BLOOD

Norm: Negative. Titers of 1:20–1:80 are normal in farmers with cattle, swine, goats, or sheep, or in endemic areas without clinical manifestations.

Positive: Brucellosis due to *Brucella abortus, Brucella canis,* or *Brucella melitensis.* Titers >160 indicate past or present infection. A fourfold increase in the titer within 2 weeks indicates an acute infection.

Description: Brucellosis (Bang's disease, Malta fever, Mediterranean fever, undulant fever) is a systemic disease acquired from animals that lasts days to years. It is found with greatest frequency in Europe, North Africa, Asia, Mexico, and South America. *Brucella* is an obligate parasite on animals. The mode of transmission to humans is through direct body tissue contact with fluids, milk, and dairy products of infected animals. Onset may be acute or insidious and symptoms may include arthralgia, body aches, chills, diaphoresis, depression, fever(s), headache, weakness, pneumonitis, and nonpurulent meningitis. In this test, *Brucella* antigens are mixed with a client's serum and observed for an agglutination reaction. A positive reaction is followed by serial dilutions of serum and retesting. The results are expressed as the highest titer showing agglutination. Agglutination indicates the presence of antibodies generated by any of three closely related *Brucella* species and is used in the indirect diagnosis of human brucellosis.

Professional Considerations:

1. Consent form NOT required.

2. Preparation:

A. Tube: Red-top, red/gray-top, or gold-top.

3. Procedure:

A. Draw a 5-ml venous blood sample.

4. Postprocedure care:

A. Send the specimen to the laboratory for immediate testing.

5. Client and family teaching:

A. Serial testing is recommended for clients with positive titers. Titers usually begin rising 5–30 days after exposure and peak in 1–2 months.

6. Factors that affect results:
    A. Reject hemolyzed specimens.
    B. Falsely elevated titers may occur in clients who have received *Brucella* skin testing.
    C. Falsely elevated titers may occur with cross-reactions of the *Brucella* test antigens with agglutinins produced by clients with tularemia, cholera, and *Proteus* Ox-19 infections, and in clients recently vaccinated against cholera.
    D. Falsely depressed titers may occur in immunosuppressed clients or clients receiving antibiotic therapy.
7. Other data:
    A. Isolation of the organism is necessary to confirm the diagnosis.
    B. Brucellosis is a reportable disease in most areas.

Bibliography:
Burnett JW: Brucellosis. Cutis *56*(1):28, 1995.
Rowen JI, Englund JA: Brucellosis presenting with cough. Pediatr Infect Dis J *14*(8):721–722, 1995.
Young EJ: Brucellosis: current epidemiology, diagnosis, and management. Curr Clin Top Infect Dis *15*:115–128, 1995.

BRUCELLOSIS SKIN TEST, DIAGNOSTIC

Norm: No reaction.

Usage: Screening for Brucellosis caused by *Brucella abortus, Brucella canis,* or *Brucella melitensis.*

Description: Brucellosis is a systemic disease acquired from animals that lasts days to years, causing symptoms of arthralgia, body aches, chills, diaphoresis, depression, fever(s), headache, weakness, pneumonitis, and nonpurulent meningitis. This test uses a *Brucella* derivative injected under the skin to detect the presence of antibodies generated by any of three closely related *Brucella* species, and is used in the indirect diagnosis of human brucellosis.

Professional Considerations:

1. Consent form NOT required.
2. Preparation:
    A. Obtain a 25-gauge, 1-inch needle, marking pen, and 0.1 ml of Brucellergen or protein *Brucella* extract.
3. Procedure:
    A. Cleanse the volar aspect of the forearm with an alcohol wipe and allow it to dry completely.
    B. Inject 0.1 ml of Brucellergen or a protein *Brucella* extract intradermally.
    C. Circle the area of injection with a pen.

4. Postprocedure care:
    A. Note the appearance of the site after 24 and 48 hours. If a reaction is present (edema, redness, induration), measure the diameter.
5. Client and family teaching:
    A. Do not wash off circular marking until the test is read.
6. Factors that affect results:
    A. In infected clients, local reaction may be accompanied by exacerbation of symptoms.
    B. A hypersensitive client may have both a local and a systemic reaction.
7. Other data:
    A. This test is unreliable and seldom used. It may stimulate the agglutination titer.
    B. Like the tuberculosis skin test, the brucellosis skin test only reveals prior exposure to the organism and is of no value in the diagnosis of clinical brucellosis.
    C. *See also Brucellosis Agglutinins, Blood.*

Bibliography:
Burnett JW: Brucellosis. Cutis *56*(1):28, 1995.
Fischbach FT: A Manual of Laboratory and Diagnostic Tests. Philadelphia, JB Lippincott, 1988.
Rowen JI, Englund JA: Brucellosis presenting with cough. Pediatr Infect Dis J*14*(8):721–722, 1995.
Ryan KJ (ed): Sherris Medical Microbiology: An Introduction to infectious Diseases. Norwalk, CT, Appleton and Lange, 1994.
Young EJ: Brucellosis: current epidemiology, diagnosis, and management. Curr Clin Top Infect Dis *15*:115–128, 1995.

BRUSHING CYTOLOGY, SPECIMEN, DIAGNOSTIC

Norm: Negative. Requires interpretation.

Positive: Allergic reaction, asbestosis, Barrett's esophagus, cryptosporidiosis, echinococcosis, Goodpasture's syndrome, infection (herpes virus, cytomegalovirus, measles virus, fungal), Legionnaire's disease, neoplasm (primary or metastatic), paragonimiasis, pneumonia (lipoid, *Pneumocystic carinii*), pulmonary infection (anaerobic), and strongyloidiasis.

Description: A brushing is taken (usually via endoscopy, bronchoscopy, cystoscopy, or gastroscopy) from a particular body site, smeared onto a slide and stained, examined microscopically, and possibly cultured. The specimens may be examined for bacterial and tumor antigens. Possible sites may be the bronchus, colon, esophagus, stomach, oropharynx, small bowel, trachea, or urethra.

Professional Considerations:

1. Consent form NOT required.
2. Preparation:
   A. Obtain a brush, a glass slide, and fixative container.
   B. Label the slide with the client's name.
3. Procedure:
   A. Obtain a brushing from a body site or a lesion.
   B. Gently roll the brush over the slide and immediately fix in 95% ethyl alcohol.
   C. For bronchial brushings, omit the slide and transport the disposable brush immediately to the laboratory.
   D. The specimens for the culture require a double-sheathed brush sealed with the sheath after specimen collection.
4. Postprocedure care:
   A. Write on the laboratory requisition the date, the site brushed, and the client's diagnosis, age, and history pertinent to this test.
   B. Transport the fixative container or brush to the laboratory.
5. Client and family teaching:
   A. The test is painless.
   B. Results are normally available within 24 hours.
6. Factors that affect results:
   A. Do NOT allow the slide to dry before fixing in alcohol.
7. Other data:
   A. May be used to diagnose *Pneumocystis carinii* in clients with AIDS.

Bibliography:

Akosa AB, Barker F, Desa L, Benjamin I, Krausz T: Cytologic diagnosis in the management of gallbladder carcinoma. Acta Cytol *39*(3):494–498, 1995.

Cohen MB, Wittchow RJ, Johlin FC, Bottles K, Raab SS: Brush cytology of the extrahepatic biliary tract: comparison of cytologic features of adenocarcinoma and benign biliary strictures. Mod Pathol *8*(5):498–502, 1995.

Danel C, Erzurum SC, McElvaney NG, Crystal RG: Quantitative assessment of the epithelial and inflammatory cell populations in large airways of normals and individuals with cystic fibrosis. Am J Respir Crit Care Med *153*(1):362–368, 1996.

Koss LG: Cytologic diagnosis of oral, esophageal, and peripheral lung cancer. J Cell Biochem (Suppl *17*F):66–81, 1993.

BUCCAL SMEAR FOR SEX CHROMATIN EVALUATION, DIAGNOSTIC

(see Barr Body Analysis Buccal Smear for Staining Sex Chromatin Mass, Diagnostic)

BUN

(see Urea Nitrogen, Plasma or Serum)

BUN/CREATININE RATIO, BLOOD

(see Blood Urea Nitrogen/Creatinine Ratio, Blood)

C1q IMMUNE COMPLEX DETECTION, SERUM

Norm: None detected.

Increased or Positive: Arthritis, glomeruloneophritis (acute), hepatitis (serum), infectious disease, inflammatory bowel disease, neoplasms, primary biliary cirrhosis, rheumatic disease, subacute bacterial endocarditis, systemic lupus erythematosus, thrombotic thrombocytopenic purpura, and vasculitis.

Description: *Complement* is a term describing 20 specific serum globulin proteins that, in combination with antigen-antibody complexes, cause lysis of erythrocytes sensitized to the antibody contained in the complex. The nine major complement components are labeled C1 to C9. C1q immune complex is a component of C1 complement that is bound into a circulating immune complex (CIC) when foreign antigens react with IgG or IgM antibodies in the body. It is very important because immune complex reactions involving the C1q component activate the classical pathway of the complement cascade. Many tests for circulating immune complexes are based on C1q binding properties. Exacerbations of immune complex disease cause elevated CICs because the lymphoreticular system is unable to clear the immune complex effectively. This test is used in serial monitoring of the progress of immune complex disease that activates the classical pathway of the complement cascade.

Professional Considerations:

1. Consent form NOT required.
2. Preparation:
   A. Tube: Red-top, red/gray-top, or gold-top.

3. Procedure:
   A. Draw a 3-ml venous blood sample.
4. Postprocedure care:
   A. Send the specimen to the laboratory immediately, as complement is very unstable.
5. Client and family teaching:
   A. Serial measurements are recommended.
   B. Results are normally available within 24 hours.
6. Factors that affect results:
   A. The presence of serum cryoglobulins may cause false-positive results.
   B. Recent heparin therapy may interfere with accurate results.
   C. Reject hemolyzed specimens.
7. Other data:
   A. False-negative results occur about 10% of the time; therefore, a negative result does not rule out disease.
   B. *See also Complement Components, Serum; Complement Fixation, Serum; and Complement Total, Serum.*

Bibliography:

Borque L, Olivan V, Iguaz F: Development and validation of an automated particle-enhanced nephelometric immunoassay method for the measurement of human plasma C1q. J Clin Lab Anal *9*(5):302–307, 1995.

Ruiz S, Henschen-Edman AH, Tenner AJ: Localization of the site on the complement component C1q required for the stimulation of neutrophil superoxide production. J Biol Chem *270*(51):30627–30634, 1995.

C3 ACTIVATOR, SERUM
(see C3 Proactivator, Serum)

C3 COMPLEMENT (BETA-1C GLOBULIN), SERUM
Norm:

		SI Units
Adult	83–177 mg/dl	0.83–1.77 g/L
Cord blood	65–111.8 mg/dl	0.65–1.12 g/L
Child	86.6–135.8 mg/dl	0.87–1.36 g/L

Increased: Acute-phase plasma protein response such as infection, inflammation, malignancy with metastasis, necrotizing disorders, rheumatic fever, and rheumatoid arthritis.

Decreased: Anemia (pernicious, folic acid deficiency), anorexia nervosa, arthralgias, celiac disease, cirrhosis, congenital C3 deficiency, disseminated intravascular coagulation, glomerulonephritis (acute), membranoproliferative, poststreptococcal hepatitis (chronic active), hypocomplementeric nephritis, immune complex disease, infection (recurrent pyogenic), liver disease (chronic), malnutrition (protein), multiple myeloma, multiple sclerosis, real transplant rejection, septicemia (gram-negative), serum sickness, subacute bacterial endocarditis, systemic lupus erythematosus (active, with renal involvement), and uremia.

Description: *Complement* is a term describing 20 specific serum globulin proteins that, in combination with antigen-antibody complexes, cause lysis of erythrocytes sensitized to the antibody contained in the complex. The nine major complement components are labeled C1 to C9. C3 complement is one of the nine major components of total complement protein and is involved in both the classical and alternate pathways of the complement cascade that function in humoral immunologic responses. Activation of the complement cascade functions in phagocytic activity, destruction of foreign bacteria, and the inflammatory response. This test evaluates the integrity of the cascade and is increased during acute-phase responses and inflammatory processes. Serial C3 levels may reflect the progress of such conditions based on the return of values to normal levels.

Professional Considerations:

1. Consent form NOT required.
2. Preparation:
   A. Tube: Red-top, red/gray-top, or gold-top.
3. Procedure:
   A. Draw a 3-ml venous blood sample.
4. Postprocedure care:
   A. None.
5. Client and family teaching:
   A. Serial measurements are recommended.
   B. Results are normally available within 24 hours.
6. Factors that affect results:
   A. Complement is heat sensitive and de-

teriorates rapidly. Send the specimen to the laboratory immediately.

B. Reject hemolyzed specimens or specimens received more than 1–2 hours after collection.

C. Freeze serum if not tested within 2 hours.

7. Other data:

A. *See also C3 Proactivator, Serum; Complement Components, Serum; Complement Fixation, Serum; and Complement Total, Serum.*

Bibliography:

Matveevskaya NS, Alyoshkin VA, Rozina MN: Isolation of the C3 complement component and its C3d subunit from IY-1 fraction of Cohn's fractionation of human plasma. J Chromatogr B Biomed Appl *664*(1):261–266, 1995.

Singer L, Whitehead WT, Akama H, Katz Y, Fishelson Z, Wetsel RA: Inherited human complement C3 deficiency. An amino acid substitution in the beta-chain (ASP549 to ASN) impairs C3 secretion. J Biol Chem *269*(45):28494–28499, 1994.

Zwirner J, Dobos G, Gotze O: A novel ELISA for the assessment of classical pathway of complement activation in vivo by measurement of C4-C3 complexes. J Immunol Methods *186*(1):55–63, 1995.

C3 PROACTIVATOR (ALTERNATE PATHWAY FACTOR B, C3 ACTIVATOR), SERUM

Norm: 20–42 mg/dl or 0.20–0.42 g/l (2.16–4.54 mmol/l, SI units)

Increased: Diffuse intravascular coagulation, inflammation, subacute bacterial endocarditis, bacteremia (with shock symptoms), paroxysmal nocturnal hemoglobinuria, and sickle cell disease.

Decreased: Chronic liver disease, glomerulonephritis (acute), and systemic lupus erythematosus.

Description: Used in serial monitoring of the progress of immune complex diseases. A factor involved in the alternate pathway of the complement cascade, which is involved in the humoral immune response. Polysaccharides, bacterial endotoxins, or aggregated IgA or IgG immunoglobulins reacting with factor B produce an enzyme that activates the C3 component of complement and initiation of the alternate pathway of the complement cascade.

Professional Considerations:

1. Consent form NOT required.
2. Preparation:
   A. Tube: Red-top, red/gray-top, or gold-top.
3. Procedure:
   A. Draw a 3-ml venous blood sample.
   B. Allow the specimen to clot at room temperature for 30 minutes.
   C. Refrigerate the specimen at 4°C for 1 hour.
   D. Remove the specimen from the refrigerator.
4. Postprocedure care:
   A. Send the specimen to the laboratory after refrigerating, as described above.
5. Client and family teaching:
   A. Serial measurements are recommended.
6. Factors that affect results:
   A. Reject hemolyzed specimens or specimens received more than 2 hours after collection.
   B. Freeze the serum if the test cannot be performed within 2 hours after collection.
7. Other data:
   A. *See also C3 Complement, Serum; Complement Components, Serum; Complement Fixation, Serum; and Complement Total, Serum.*

Bibliography

Holme ER, Whaley K: Complement and related clinical disorders. Blood *3*(2):120–129, 1989.

Muscari A, Bozzoli C, Massarelli G, Puddu GM, Palareti G, Legnani C, D'Atena T, Mazzuca A, Miniero R, Toscano V, et al.: Complement components and fibrinogen: correlations and association with previous myocardial infarction. Cardiology *86*(3):232–237, 1995.

C4 COMPLEMENT, SERUM

Norm:

		SI Units
Female	15–52 mg/dl	0.73–2.53 µmol/L
Male	15–60 mg/dl	0.73–2.91 µmol/L

Increased: Cancer, juvenile rheumatoid arthritis, and rheumatoid spondylitis.

Decreased: Congenital C4 complement deficiency, cryoglobulinemia, glomerulonephritis, Henoch-Schonlein purpura, hepatitis (chronic active), hereditary angioedema, hypergammaglobulinemic state, immune complex disease, lupus nephritis, renal transplant rejection, serum sickness, subacute bacterial endocarditis, and systemic lupus erythematosus (active).

Description: *Complement* is a term describing 20 specific serum globulin proteins that, in combination with antigen-antibody complexes, cause lysis of erythrocytes sensitized to the antibody contained in the complex. The nine major complement components are labeled C1 to C9. C4 complement is one of the nine components of total complement protein and is involved in only the classical pathway of the complement cascade that functions in humoral immunologic responses. C4 complement deficiency is an inherited autosomal recessive trait and results in decreased resistance to infection. Activation of the complement cascade functions in phagocytic activity, destruction of foreign bacteria, and the inflammatory response. C3 and C4 levels are helpful in distinguishing the etiology of glomerulonephritis, as C3 is decreased, but C4 is usually normal when the cause is poststreptococcal.

Professional Considerations:

1. Consent form NOT required.
2. Preparation:
   A. Tube: Red-top, red/gray-top, or gold-top.
3. Procedure:
   A. Draw a 3-ml blood sample.
4. Postprocedure care:
   A. Allow the specimen to clot for 15–30 minutes at room temperature, then refrigerate.
   B. Freeze the serum if not processed immediately.
5. Client and family teaching:
   A. Serial measurements are recommended.
6. Factors that affect results:
   A. Complement is heat sensitive and deteriorates rapidly. Send the specimen to the laboratory immediately.
   B. Reject hemolyzed specimens or specimens received more than 1–2 hours after collection.
7. Other data:
   A. *See also C3 Complement, Serum; Complement Components, Serum; Complement Fixation, Serum; and Complement Total, Serum.*

Bibliography:

Dodds AW, Ren XD, Willis AC, Law SK: The reaction mechanism of the internal thioester in the human complement component C4. Nature *379*(6561):177–179, 1996.

Kramer J, Srivastava LM, Ferenczy E, Fust G: Complement C4, factor B and C3 polymorphism in north India. Acta Microbiol Immunol Hung *42*(3): 315–319, 1995.

C-14 CHOLATE BREATH TEST

(see Bile Salt Absorption Test, Diagnostic)

CA 15-3 (CARCINOGENIC ANTIGEN 15-3), SERUM

Norm: <22 U/ml.

Increased: Adenoma of salivary gland; breast cancer; benign breast disease; breast cancer metastasis; lung cancer; ovarian benign disease; recurrence after remission in breast cancer with bone metastasis.

Decreased: Positive response to therapy.

Description: A tumor marker that detects the membrane antigen against human milk globules and the antigens from human breast carcinoma. This test is not specific enough to be used in screening but rather correlates with tumor progression.

Professional Considerations:

1. Consent form NOT required.
2. Preparation:
   A. Tube: Red-top, red/gray-top, or gold-top.
3. Procedure:
   A. Collect a 2-ml blood sample.
4. Postprocedure care:
   A. Evaluate other antigen tests and breast biopsy results.
5. Client and family teaching:
   A. Elevated levels correlate positively to recurrence of disease.
   B. Results are normally available within 7 days.
6. Factors that affect results:
   A. Persons with benign breast or ovarian disease may have elevated levels.
7. Other data:
   A. Results >25 U/ml are found in women with metastatic breast carcinoma.
   B. CA 15-3 when used in conjunction with CA 125 can improve the management of women presenting with a pelvic mass.

Bibliography:

Asai S, Tang X, Ohta Y, Tsutsumi Y: Myoepithelial carcinoma in pleomorphic adenoma of salivary gland type, occurring in the mandible of an infant. Pathol Int *45*(9):677–683, 1995.

Devine PL, Duroux MA, Quin RJ, McGuckin MA, Joy GJ, Ward BG, Pollard CW: CA 15-3, CASA, MSA, and TPS as diagnostic serum markers in breast cancer. Breast Can Res Treat *34*(3): 245–251, 1995.

Hou MF, Huang TJ, Hsieh JS, Huang YS, Huang CJ, Chan HM, Wang JY, Chen YL, Jong SB, Yang CC: Comparison of serum CA 15-3 and CEA in breast cancer. Kao Hsiung I Hsueh Ko Hsueh Tsa Chih (KAO) *11*(12):660–666, 1995.

Iwase H, Kobayashi S, Itoh Y, Fukuoka H, Kuzushima I, Iwata H, Yamashita I, Naitoh A, Itoh K, Masaoka A: Evaluation of serum tumor markers

in patients with advanced or recurrent breast cancer. Breast Cancer Res Treat *33*(1): 83–88, 1995.

Tomlinson IP, Whyman A, Barrett JA, Kremer JK: Tumour marker CA 15-3: possible uses in the routine management of breast cancer. Eur J Cancer (ARV) *31A*(6):899–902, 1995.

Woolas RP, Conaway MR, Xu F, Jacobs IJ, Yu Y, Daly L, Davies AP, et al.: Combinations of multiple serum markers are superior to individual assays for discriminating malignant from benign pelvic masses. Gynecol Oncol *59*(1):111–116, 1995.

CA 19-9 (CARBOHYDRATE AG 19-9, GICA, GASTROINTESTINAL CANCER ANTIGEN), BLOOD

Norm: This value is arbitrary and statistically derived. One AU equals 0.59 ng/ml of antigen.

		SI Units
Norm	<37 AU/ml	<37 kU/L
Metastasis	>1000 AU/ml	>1000 kU/L

Usage: Tumor marker antigen that is helpful in post-therapeutic monitoring to determine the success of therapy or the presence of cancer recurrence. Useful for monitoring gastrointestinal cancers, head and neck tumors, and gynecologic tumors. Predicts the recurrence of stomach, pancreatic, liver, and colorectal malignancies. Is used in combination with other tumor markers to measure the effectiveness of treatment or earlier detection of recurrence and development of metastases. Most effective for monitoring pancreatic cancer.

Increased: Intra-abdominal carcinoma, pancreatic carcinoma (most frequently elevated marker; elevated levels found in 80% of clients with pancreatic cancer), and possibly with other adenocarcinomas such as lung, gastric, biliary, and colonic. Also cholangitis, cirrhosis, and pancreatitis (acute).

Description: A carbohydrate antigen, related to the Lewis blood group antigen. CA 19-9 is a carbohydrate antigen that has been shown to be elevated in the sera of some clients with gastrointestinal tumors. Elevated levels can indicate recurrence of cancer before radiographic or clinical findings by 1 to 7 months.

Professional Considerations:

1. Consent form NOT required.
2. Preparation:
   A. Tube: Red-top, red/gray-top, or gold-top.
   B. MAY be drawn during hemodialysis.
3. Procedure:
   A. Draw a 2-ml venous blood sample.
   B. The sample can be frozen for shipping.
4. Postprocedure care:
   A. None.
5. Client and family teaching:
   A. Results may be delayed if the sample is sent off-site for testing.
6. Factors that affect results:
   A. False-positive results may occur with no disease or with benign disease, particularly inflammatory disease of the bowel.
7. Other data:
   A. Elevated levels are found in cystic fibrosis and in human seminal fluid.
   B. Individuals who are Lewis (a-b) phenotype (6% of the population) cannot synthesize cancer antigen CA 19-9, CA 50, and CA 195 and this may account for the lesser diagnostic value of these markers.
   C. CA 19-9 with CEA is useful when monitoring patients for possible recurrence of gastric carcinoma.

Bibliography:

Guadagni F, Roselli M, Cosimelli M, et al.: CA 72-4 serum marker—a new tool in the management of carcinoma patients. Cancer Invest *13*(2):227–238, 1995.

Hakomou BI: Tumor associated carbohydrate markers: in serological cancer markers. *In:* Serological Cancer Markers: S. Sell (ed). Totowa, NJ: Humana Press, pp 207–232, 1992.

Jacobs EL, Haskell CM: Clinical use of tumor markers in oncology. Curr Probl Cancer *15*(6):324–326, 1991.

Ng WW, Tong KJ, Tam TN, Lee SD: Clinical values of CA 19-9, CA 125 and CEA in malignant obstructive jaundice. Chinese Med J *55*(6):438–446, 1995.

Nicolini A, Caciagli M, et al.: Usefulness of CEA, PA, ICA, A72.4, and CA 195 in the diagnosis of primary colorectal cancer and its relapse. Cancer Detect Prev *19*(2):183–195, 1995.

Ramage JK, Donaghy A, Farrant JM, et al.: Serum

tumor markers for the diagnosis of cholangiocarcinoma in primary sclerosing cholangitis. Gastroenterology 108(3):865–869, 1995.

CA 50 (CARBOHYDRATE ANTIGEN 50), BLOOD

Norm: <17 U/ml.

Increased: Colorectal adenocarcinomas, digestive tract carcinoma, esophageal squamous cell carcinoma, non-small cell lung carcinoma, pancreatic cancer, transitional cell bladder carcinoma.

Decreased: Positive response to therapy.

Description: A tumor marker that increases with many malignancies, particularly those of the digestive tract. This test is not specific enough for screening and correlates more with tumor progression than with tumor regression.

Professional Considerations:

1. Consent form NOT required.
2. Preparation:
   A. Tube: Red-top, red/gray top, or gold-top.
3. Procedure:
   A. Collect a 7-ml blood sample.
4. Postprocedure care:
   A. Evaluate other antigen tests and the liver function studies.
5. Client and family teaching:
   A. Results are normally available within 7 days.
6. Factors that affect results:
   A. False-positive results occur in benign liver disease.
7. Other data:
   A. CA 50 is higher for more undifferentiated and advanced stage bladder tumors.
   B. CA 50 cannot be used as a tumor marker in cirrhotic patients, as cytolysis increases this test result.

Bibliography:

Alvarea JA: Sensitivity of monoclonal antibodies to carcinoembryonic antigen, tissue polypeptide antigen, alpha-fetoprotein, carbohydrate antigen 50, and carbohydrate antigen 19-9 in the diagnosis of colorectal adenocarcinoma. Dis Colon Rectum 38(5):535–542, 1995.

Collazos J: Study of the tumor marker carbohydrate 50 in liver cirrhosis. Pathogenetic considerations. Clin Nucl Med 18(1):56–59, 1993.

Moreno SJ: The usefulness of the carbohydrate antigen CA 50 in the prognosis of transitional-cell bladder carcinomas. Arch Esp Urol 46(9):775–778, 1993.

Niklinski J, Furman M: Clinical tumour markers in lung cancer. Eur J Cancer Prev 4(2):129–138, 1995.

Pasanen PA: A prospective study of serum tumor markers carcinoembryonic antigen, carbohydrate

antigens 50 and 242, tissue polypeptide antigen and tissue polypeptide specific antigen in the diagnosis of pancreatic cancer with special reference to multivariate diagnostic scores. Br J Cancer 69(3):562–565, 1994.

CA 125 (CANCER ANTIGEN 125), BLOOD

Norm: <35 U/ml. (<35 kU/L, SI units).

Increased: Endometriosis, menses, nonmucinous ovarian epithelial neoplasms, neoplasms (breast, cervix, colon, endometrium, liver, lung, lymphoma, ovary, pancreas, liver, colon), pancreatitis (acute), pelvic inflammatory disease, peritonitis (acute), pregnancy (first trimester), and ovarian abscess.

Description: Cancer antigen 125 is a glycoprotein present in normal endometrial tissue and in mucinous uterine fluid. It enters the circulation only when natural barriers are destroyed. In the presence of endometrial or ovarian malignancy, a persistently rising CA 125 level may be associated with progression of the disease and poor therapeutic response. Normal levels do not rule out extensive tumor presence or recurrence. CA 125 is also expressed by neoplasms of the pancreas, liver, colon, breast, and lung in smaller percentages.

Professional Considerations:

1. Consent form NOT required.
2. Preparation:
   A. Tube: Red-top, red/gray-top, or gold-top.
3. Procedure:
   A. Draw a 1-ml blood sample.
4. Postprocedure care:
   A. None.
5. Client and family teaching:
   A. Due to a high incidence of false-negatives and false-positives, this test is useful only to monitor for a change from normal to abnormal or a rising titer. The test should not be used for screening.
6. Factors that affect results:
   A. Antineoplastic therapy may lower results.
7. Other data:
   A. Sensitivity of this test to ovarian cancer is 75–80%.

Bibliography:

Blaakaer J, Hogdall CK, Micic S, Toftager-Larsen K, Hording U, Bennett P, Bock J: Ovarian carcinoma serum markers and ovarian steroid activity—is there a link in ovarian cancer? A correlation of inhibin, tetranectin and CA 125 to ovarian activity and the gonadotropin levels. Eur J Obstet Gynecol Reprod Biol 59(1):53–56, 1995.

Kaminska JA, Kowalska MM, Sablinska B, Pietrzak P: Usefulness of determination of CA 125 in monitoring patients with ovarian carcinoma. Eur J Gynaecol Oncol 14 (Suppl):128–132, 1995.

Mozas J, Castilla JA, Jimena P, Gil T, Acebal M, Herruzo AJL: Serum CA 125 in the diagnosis of acute pelvic inflammatory disease. Int J Gynaecol Obstet 44(1):53–57, 1994.

Pittaway DE, Rondinone D, Miller KA, Barnes K: Clinical evaluation of CA 125 concentrations as a prognostic factor for pregnancy in infertile women with surgically treated endometriosis. Fertil Steril 64(2):321–324, 1995.

CAC, BLOOD
(see Circulating Anticoagulant, Blood)

CADMIUM, SERUM AND 24-HOUR URINE
Norm:

		SI Units
Serum		
Nonsmoker	0.1–0.50 µg/dl	0.89–4.45 nmol/L
Excess exposure	>10 µg/dl	>89 nmol/L
Panic level	>41 µg/dl	>365 nmol/L
Urine		
Nonsmoker	0.5–4.7 µg/L	4.4–41.8 nmol/L
Excess exposure	>10 µg/L	>88.97 nmol/L

Panic Level Symptoms and Treatment:

Symptoms: Abdominal cramps, acute renal failure, diarrhea, exhaustion, headache, nausea, pulmonary edema (when cadmium dust or fumes are inhaled), shock, vertigo, vomiting.

Treatment:

Give demulcents.

Use gastric lavage with milk or water.

Induce vomiting with a saline cathartic or a syrup of ipecac if within ½ hour of exposure. (Induction of vomiting is contraindicated in clients with no gag reflex, or with central nervous system depression or excitation.)

Give saline or sorbitol cathartic.

Closely monitor and support respiratory and hemodynamic status.

Activated charcoal is NOT helpful.

Monitor for liver and kidney damage.

CaNa$_2$ EDTA will enhance cadmium removal for acute exposure only.

Description: Cadmium is a heavy metal obtained from zinc ores and is used in the manufacture of alloys, in storage batteries, and in electroplating. The general population is exposed to small amounts daily through food, water, air, and cigarette smoke. Cadmium is a respiratory tract irritant that can produce fatal pulmonary edema, proliferative interstitial pneumonia, and cardiovascular collapse if inhaled as dust or fumes. Cadmium ingestion poisoning produces a sudden onset of severe gastrointestinal symptoms within 30 minutes. Chronic exposure can produce osteomalacia, and renal and hepatic disorders, and can also cause severe gastroenteritis. Cadmium is not metabolized in the body. It accumulates in tissue, concentrating primarily in the kidneys and the liver. More than 95% of the blood cadmium is contained in the erythrocytes. Serum levels are used for diagnosis of acute cadmium intoxication. Urine cadmium levels are measured to detect chronic exposure. It is believed that urine cadmium levels >10 mg/L (>88.97 nmol/L, SI units) are indicative of renal tubular damage.

Increased: Industrial exposure to cadmium dust and fumes, and ingestion of contaminated water or food stored in cadmium-plated containers.

Decreased: Not clinically significant.

Professional Considerations:
1. Consent form NOT required.
2. Preparation:
   A. *Serum:* Tube: Green-top or black-top.
   B. *Urine:* Obtain a 3-L, metal-free container without a preservative.

3. Procedure:
   A. *Serum:* Draw a 5-ml blood specimen in a metal-free tube.
   B. *Urine:*
      i. Discard the first morning urine specimen.
      ii. Save all the urine voided for 24 hours in a refrigerated, clean, metal-free, 3-L container without preservatives. Include the urine voided at the end of the 24-hour period. For catheterized clients, keep the drainage bag on ice and empty urine into the collection container hourly.
4. Postprocedure care:
   A. Send the serum specimen to the laboratory immediately.
   B. *Urine:*
      i. Compare urine quantity in the specimen container with the urinary output record for the test. If the specimen contains less urine than was recorded as output, some urine may have been discarded, thus invalidating the test.
      ii. Document the quantity of urine output for the collection period on the laboratory requisition.
      iii. It is best to send the entire specimen to the laboratory so that it can be measured and mixed well before being tested.

5. Client and family teaching:
   A. *Urine:* Save all the urine voided in the 24-hour period and urinate before defecating to avoid loss of urine. If any urine is accidentally discarded, discard the entire specimen and restart the collection the next day.
   B. A client with elevated levels should identify and reduce sources of cadmium exposure and see the physician regularly for monitoring of the effects of chronic cadmium exposure.
6. Factors that affect results:
   A. Reject hemolyzed specimens.
   B. Urine levels increase with aging.
   C. Cadmium levels normally increase with aging.
7. Other data:
   A. Death may occur if pulmonary edema, shock, or renal failure is caused by cadmium poisoning.

Bibliography:

Basun H, Lind B, Nordberg M, Nordstrom M, Bjorksten KS, Winblad B: Cadmium in blood in Alzheimer's disease and non-demented subjects: results from a population-based study. Biometals 7(2):130–134, 1994.

Berglund M, Akesson A, Nermell B, Vahter M: Intestinal absorption of dietary cadmium in women depends on body iron stores and fiber intake. Environ Health Perspect 102(12):1058–1066, 1994.

CALCITONIN (THYROCALCITONIN), PLASMA OR SERUM

Norm:

		SI Units
Serum		
Adult female	<25 pg/ml	<25 ng/L
Adult male	<40 pg/ml	<40 ng/L
Term newborn, cord blood	30–240 pg/ml	30–240 ng/L
Neonate, 2 days old	91–580 pg/ml	91–580 ng/L
Neonate, 7 days old	77–293 pg/ml	77–293 ng/L
Plasma		
Basal		
Female	≤0.105 ng/ml	
Male	≤0.155 ng/ml	

Increased: Anemia (pernicious), cancer (breast, lung, thyroid), chronic renal failure, Cushing's disease (type II), ectopic calcitonin production, hypercalcemia, islet cell tumors, medullary cancer of the thyroid, parathyroid adenoma or hyperplasia, pheochromocytoma, renal failure (chronic), thyroiditis, uremia, and Zollinger-Ellison syndrome.

Decreased: Not clinically significant.

Description: Calcitonin (thyrocalcitonin), is a thyroid gland polypeptide hormone that helps maintain normal serum calcium and phosphorus levels. It is secreted in response to hypercalcemia. Its functions include inhibition of calcium absorption from the gastrointestinal tract, inhibition of calcium resorption from the bone and soft tissues by osteoclasts and osteocytes, and increasing the amount of renal calcium excretion. Calcitonin functions in calcium homeostasis by antagonizing parathyroid hormone and vitamin D to lower serum calcium levels.

Professional Considerations:

1. Consent form NOT required.
2. Preparation:
   A. *See Client and family teaching.*
   B. Tube: Green-top tube, or chilled red-top or chilled red/gray-top, or gold-top tube.
   C. Notify laboratory personnel that a specimen for calcitonin measurement will be delivered.
3. Procedure:
   A. Draw a 3-ml venous blood sample.
4. Postprocedure care:
   A. Send the specimen to the laboratory immediately for immediate serum separation into a plastic tube, followed by freezing.
5. Client and family teaching:
   A. Fast (except for sips of water) for 8 hours before sampling.
   B. A few days are required for completion of this test in the laboratory.
6. Factors that affect results:
   A. Reject hemolyzed specimens.
7. Other data:
   A. None.

Bibliography

Bucht E, Rong H, Sjoberg HE, Sjostedt U, Granberg B, Torring L: Serum calcitonin forms and concentrations in young and elderly healthy females. Calcif Tissue Int 56(1):32–37, 1995.

Wimalawansa SJ, Bailey F: Validation, role in perioperative assessment, and clinical applications of an immunoradiometric assay for human calcitonin. Peptides 16(2):307–312, 1995.

Zofkova I, Kancheva RL: The effect of nifedipine on serum parathyroid hormone and calcitonin in postmenopausal women. Life Sci 57(11):1087–1096, 1995.

CALCIUM, CALCULATED IONIZED, SERUM

Norm: 46–50% of total calcium.

Increased: *See Calcium, Ionized, Blood.*

Decreased: *See Calcium, Ionized, Blood.*

Description: Calculated ionized calcium is an indirect method for calculating the amount of ionized (biologically active) calcium based on serum protein levels. Normally, 46–50% of total calcium is ionized and most of the remainder (40%) is bound to proteins. The remaining 8–10% is complexed with anions such as bicarbonate and lactate and is biologically inactive. Of the portion bound to proteins, 80% is bound to albumin and 20% is bound to globulin. Calculated ionized calcium is also called protein-corrected total calcium, as a formula is used to calculate the amount of protein-bound calcium and deduct that from the total calcium level to derive an estimate of the biologically active ionized calcium. This method is often imprecise and unreliable, especially in clients with low or high protein levels, and is being replaced by newer laboratory methodologies for ionized calcium measurement.

Professional Considerations:

1. Consent form NOT required.
2. Preparation:
   A. *See Calcium, Total, Serum; Albumin Serum, Urine and 24-Hour Urine; and Protein, Serum* for instructions on drawing the blood for the results needed for the calculation.
3. Procedure:
   A. Obtain total calcium, albumin, and globulin levels and calculate the amount of ionized calcium with the following formulas:
   Step 1. % of protein-bound Ca^{++} = 8(albumin g/dl) + 2(globulin g/dL) + 3.
   Step 2. % of ionized Ca^{++} = total calcium mg/dl – % of protein-bound Ca^{++}.
4. Postprocedure care:
   A. Not applicable.
5. Client and family teaching:
   A. None.
6. Factors that affect results:
   A. Results are unreliable for hypoproteinemic or hyperproteinemic states. The ion-selective electrode procedure should be used for these clients.
7. Other data:
   A. Other formulas exist for calculation of ionized calcium. Many of these formulas have been disputed, which makes the reliability of this calculation questionable.
   B. See also *Calcium, Ionized, Blood,* and *Calcium, Total, Serum.*

Bibliography:

June CH, Rabinovitch PS: Intracellular ionized calcium. Methods Cell Biol 41:149–174, 1994.

Sorva A, Valimaki M, Risteli J, Risteli L, Elfving S, Takkunen H, Tilvis R: Serum ionized calcium, intact PTH and novel markers of bone turnover in bedridden elderly patients. Eur J Clin Invest 24(12):806–812, 1994.

Toffaletti J: Physiology and regulation. Ionized calcium, magnesium and lactate measurements in critical care settings. Am J Clin Pathol 104(4 Suppl 1):S88–S94, 1995.

CALCIUM, IONIZED (FREE CALCIUM, DIALYZABLE CALCIUM), BLOOD

Norm: 46–56% of total serum calcium.

		SI Units
Serum		
Adults	4.64–5.28 mg/dl	1.16–1.32 mmol/L
Newborn	2.24–2.46 mEq/L	
Cord blood	5.2–6.40 mg/dl	1.30–1.60 mmol/L
2 hours old	4.84–5.84 mg/dl	1.21–1.46 mmol/L
1 day old	4.40–5.44 mg/dl	1.10–1.36 mmol/L
3 days old	4.60–5.68 mg/dl	1.15–1.42 mmol/L
5 days old	4.88–5.92 mg/dl	1.22–1.48 mmol/L
Children, teens	4.80–5.52 mg/dl	1.20–1.38 mmol/L
Capillary Blood		
6–36 hours old	4.20–5.48 mg/dl	1.05–1.37 mmol/L
60–84 hours old	4.40–5.68 mg/dl	1.10–1.42 mmol/L
108–132 hours old	4.80–5.92 mg/dl	1.20–1.48 mmol/L
Whole Blood		
Adults		
Age 18–60 years	4.60–5.08 mg/dl	1.15–1.27 mmol/L
Age 60–90 years	4.64–5.16 mg/dl	1.16–1.29 mmol/L
Age >90 years	4.48–5.28 mg/dl	1.12–1.32 mmol/L
Plasma		
Adults	4.12–4.92 mg/dl	1.03–1.23 mmol/L

Increased: Acidemia, hypervitaminosis D, malignancy, hyperaparathyroidism (primary), and tumors that produce or elevate parathyroid hormone. Drugs include hydrochlorothiazide (chronic use), and lithium.

Decreased: Alkalemia; burns; following citrate-containing blood transfusions; hyperosmolar states; hypoparathyroidism (primary); magnesium deficiency; multiple organ failure; pancreatitis; postoperatively; pseudohypoparathyroidism; sepsis, trauma; and Vitamin D deficiency. Drugs include anticonvulsants, danazol, foscarnet, furosemide, and hyperosmolar solutions.

Description: Ionized calcium is a cation that circulates freely in the bloodstream and comprises 46–50% of all circulating calcium. Levels increase and decrease directly with increases and decreases in blood pH. For every 0.1 pH unit decrease, ionized calcium increases 1.5–2.5%. Ionized calcium is sometimes considered a more sensitive and reliable indicator of primary hyperparathyroidism for clients with low albumin than is total serum calcium, as ionized calcium is not affected by changes in serum albumin concentrations.

Professional Considerations:
1. Consent form NOT required.
2. Preparation:
   A. The client should lie supine for 30 minutes.
   B. Tube: Red-top, red/gray-top, gold-top, or green-top tube that does not contain zinc heparin. Also obtain ice.
   C. Do NOT draw during hemodialysis.
3. Procedure:
   A. Completely fill the tube with blood, without using a tourniquet. Use a Vacutainer to collect the specimen directly into the tube without removing the tube stopper.
   B. Capillary tubes from heelstick specimens are also acceptable.
   C. Place the specimen immediately on ice.
4. Postprocedure care:
   A. Deliver the specimen to the laboratory immediately and refrigerate.
5. Client and family teaching:
   A. Results are normally available within 4 hours.
   B. For chronic hypocalcemia, food sources high in calcium include milk, egg yolks, cheese, beans, cauliflower, chard, kale, and rhubarb.

6. Factors that affect results:
   A. Prolonged exposure of the serum to air causes an increase in pH that, in turn, causes an increased ionized calcium level. Collect the specimens anaerobically.
   B. The test must be performed within 48 hours of specimen collection.
   C. A diurnal variation exists, with the lowest values occurring in the early morning hours (0200–0400) and the highest values occurring at mid-evening.
7. Other data:
   A. This is the most reliable test for diagnosing hyperparathyroidism in clients with low albumin.
   B. *See also Calcium, Total, Serum,* and *Calcium, Calculated Ionized, Serum.*

Bibliography:

Hristova EN, Cecco S, Niemela JE, Rehak NN, Elin RJ: Analyzer-dependent differences in results for ionized calcium, ionized magnesium, sodium, and pH. Clin Chem *41*(11):1649–1653, 1995.

June CH, Rabinovitch PS: Intracellular ionized calcium. Methods Cell Biol *41*:149–174, 1994.

Koch SM, Mehlhorn U, McKinley BA, Irby SL, Warters RD, Allen SJ: Arterial blood sampling devices influence ionized calcium measurements. Crit Care Med *23*(11):1825–1828, 1995.

Lyon ME, Guajardo M, Laha T, Malik S, Henderson PJ, Kenny MA: Zinc heparin introduces a preanalytical error in the measurement of ionized calcium concentration. Scand J Clin Lab Invest *55*(1):61–65, 1995.

Minisola S, Pacitti MT, Scarda A, Rosso R, Romagnoli E, Carnevale V, Scarnecchia L, Mazzuoli GF: Serum ionized calcium, parathyroid hormone and related variables: effect of age and sex. Bone Miner *23*(3):183–193, 1993.

CALCIUM, TOTAL, SERUM

Norm:

		SI Units
Adults		
18–60 years	8.6–10.0 mg/dl	2.15–2.50 mmol/L
60–90 years	8.8–10.2 mg/dl	2.20–2.55 mmol/L
>90 years	8.2–9.6 mg/dl	2.05–2.40 mmol/L
Children		
Cord blood	8.2–11.2 mg/dl	2.05–2.80 mmol/L
Premature infant	6.2–11.0 mg/dl	1.55–2.75 mmol/L
≤10 days	7.6–10.4 mg/dl	1.90–2.60 mmol/L
10 days–2 years	9.0–11.0 mg/dl	2.25–2.75 mmol/L
2–12 years	8.8–10.8 mg/dl	2.20–2.70 mmol/L
12–18 years	8.4–10.2 mg/dl	2.10–2.55 mmol/L
Panic levels		
Tetany	<7 mg/dl	<1.75 mmol/L
Coma	>12 mg/dl	>2.99 mmol/L
Possible death	≤6 mg/dl	≤1.50 mmol/L
	≥14 mg/dl	≥3.49 mmol/L

Panic Levels Symptoms and Treatment:

Symptoms of Hypercalcemia: Constipation, ECG changes (shortened ST-segment), lethargy, muscle weakness, nausea, neurologic depression (headache, apathy, reduced level of consciousness) progressing to coma, vomiting.

Treatment of Hypercalcemia Panic Levels:

Correct the cause.
Give normal saline and diuretics to speed renal calcium excretion.
Give calcitonin or steroids to move calcium intracellularly.
Hemodialysis WILL remove calcium.

Symptoms of Hypocalcemia: Convulsions, carpopedal spasm (positive Trousseau's sign), dysrhythmias, ECG changes (prolonged ST-segment and QT interval), facial spasm (positive Chvostek's sign), muscle cramps, numbness, tetany, tingling, and muscle twitching, spasms of the larynx.

Treatment of Hypocalcemia Panic Levels:

Implement seizure precautions.
Maintain continuous ECG monitoring.
Correct the cause.
Give calcium, magnesium, and vitamin D replacement.

IV calcium chloride or calcium gluconate 100 mg of elemental calcium or 4–7 ml of 10% calcium chloride mixed in 50–100 ml of solution over 20 minutes. Follow with calcium infusion at 1–2 mg/kg/hour.

Increased: Acidosis (respiratory), acromegaly, acute tubular necrosis (recovery phase), Addison's disease, berylliosis, bacteremia, coccidioidomycosis, diet (high-calcium), ectopic neoplasms that produce parathyroid hormone, familial hypocalciuric hypercalcemia, hepatic disease (chronic advanced), histoplasmosis, hyperparathyroidism (primary, tertiary-renal), hyperthyroidism, hypervitaminosis (vitamin D or A intoxication), immobility (prolonged), infants (idiopathic), leukemia, lymphoma, malignancy (bladder, breast, kidney, lung), metastatic bone cancer, milk-alkali (Burnett's) syndrome, multiple endocrine neoplasia, multiple myeloma, mycoses, osteoporosis, Paget's disease, peptic ulcer diet, pheochromocytoma, polycythemia vera, porphyria, renal calculi, renal osteomalacia (induced by aluminum), renal transplantation, respiratory disease, rhabdomyolysis, sarcoidosis, and tuberculosis. Drugs include anabolic steroids, androgens, antacids (alkaline), calcium gluconate, calciferol, calcium salts, calusterone, chlorothiazide sodium, chlorthalidone, danazol, diethylstilbestrol, dihydrotachysterol, diuretics, ergocalciferol, estrogens, indomethacin, isotretinoin, lithium carbonate, parathyroid hormone, progesterone, secretin, tamoxifen, testolactone, theophylline (toxicity), thiazide diuretics, thyroid hormones, vitamin A, and vitamin D.

Decreased: Alkalosis, bacteremia, blood transfusions (excessive without replacement of calcium), burns, cachexia, celiac disease, chronic renal disease, cystic fibrosis of pancreas, diarrhea, Fanconi's syndrome (with renal tubular acidosis), hypomagnesemia, hypoparathyroidism, hypoproteinemia, infection (severe), malabsorption, Milkman's syndrome, nephritis, nephrosis, nephrotic syndrome, obstructive jaundice, osteomalacia, pancreatitis (acute), parathyroidectomy, pregnancy (late), pseudohypoparathyroidism, renal failure, renal insufficiency, renal tubular acidosis, rickets, sprue, starvation, toxic shock syndrome, thyroidectomy with accidental removal of parathyroid gland, and vitamin D deficiency. Drugs include acetazolamide, albuterol, alprostadil, aminoglycosides, antacids, anticonvulsants, asparaginase, aspirin, barbiturates (in elderly), calcitonin, carbamazepine, carbenoxolone, carboplatin, corticosteroids, cholestyramine resin, fluorides, furosemide, gastrin, gentamicin, glucagon, glucose, heparin, hydrocortisone, indapamide, insulin, iron, isoniazid, laxatives (excessive), magnesium salts, mercurial diuretics, mestranol, mithramycin, methicillin, phenobarbital, phenytoin, phosphates, plicamycin, and saline (in hypercalcemic state) tetracycline (during pregnancy).

Description: Calcium is a cation that is absorbed into the bloodstream from dietary sources and functions in bone formation, nerve impulse transmission, contraction of myocardial and skeletal muscles, and in blood clotting by converting prothrombin to thrombin. Calcium is stored in the teeth and bones, and circulating calcium is filtered by the kidneys, with most being reabsorbed when serum calcium levels are normal. In order to maintain a normal calcium balance and counteract any excreted calcium, at least 1 g of calcium must be ingested daily. Normally, 46–50% of total calcium is ionized and most of the remainder (40%) is bound to proteins. Only ionized calcium can be used by the body. The remaining 8–10% is complexed with anions such as bicarbonate and lactate and is biologically inactive. Total serum calcium values increase and decrease directly with serum albumin levels, but ionized calcium levels do not. For every 1 g/dl decrease in albumin, total serum calcium decreases by 0.8 mg/dl. When acidosis is present, more calcium is ionized. In alkalosis, most is bound to protein and cannot be used by the body.

Professional Considerations:
1. Consent form NOT required.
2. Preparation:
   A. Tube: Red-top, red/gray-top, or gold-top.
   B. Do NOT draw during hemodialysis.

3. Procedure:
   A. Leaving the tourniquet in place less than 1 minute, draw a 1-ml venous blood sample.
4. Postprocedure care:
   A. Send the specimen to the laboratory for spinning within 1 hour.
5. Client and family teaching:
   A. Eat a diet with normal calcium levels, 800 mg/day (15–20 mmol/day, SI units), for 3 days before sampling.
   B. Fast, except for water, for 8 hours (only for multichannel tests).
   C. For elevated levels, avoid foods high in calcium, ambulate when possible, and increase fluid intake unless contraindicated.
6. Factors that affect results:
   A. Reject hemolyzed specimens.
   B. Falsely elevated values may be caused by hemolysis, dehydration, or hyperproteinemia.
   C. Falsely decreased values may be caused by dilutional hypervolemia, adminis-
   tration of intravenous sodium chloride, or by the administration of sulfobromosulphalein sodium (Bromsulphalein) dye within 2 days prior to specimen collection.
   D. Serum calcium should be corrected for the serum albumin. For every gram below 4 mg/dl, add 0.8 to the calcium level.
7. Other data:
   A. Hypercalcemia can induce digoxin toxicity and decreased neuronal permeability.
   B. *See also Calcium, Calculated Ionized, Serum,* and *Calcium, Ionized, Blood.*

Bibliography:

June CH, Rabinovitch PS: Intracellular ionized calcium [review]. Methods in Cell Biol *41*:149–174, 1994.

Rose MB: Clinical Laboratory Tests: Values and Implications. Springhouse, PA, Springhouse Corporation, 1995.

Treseler KM: Clinical Laboratory and Diagnostic Tests: Significance and Nursing Implications, 3rd ed. Norwalk, CT, Appleton and Lange, 1995.

CALCIUM, URINE

Norm: Semiquantitative Sulkowitch test: 1+ to 2+.

Quantitative Tests		SI Units
Random specimen	<40 mg/dl	<1.0 mmol/L
24-hour specimen		
Low-calcium diet	<150 mg/day	<3.7 mmol/day
Normal-calcium diet	100–250 mg/day	2.5–6.2 mmol/day
High-calcium diet	250–300 mg/day	6.2–7.5 mmol/day

Increased: Acromegaly, amyotrophic lateral sclerosis, bone metastasis, cancer (primary) of the breast or lung, Fanconi's syndrome (with renal tubular acidosis), Crohn's disease, diabetes mellitus, diet (high-calcium), ectopic hyperparathyroidism, glucocorticoid excess, hypercalcemia, hyperparathyroidism, hyperthyroidism, hypervitaminosis D, idiopathic hypercalciuria, immobility (long-term), leukemia, lymphoma, metastasis, medullary sponge kidney, multiple myeloma, nephrolithiasis, osteoporosis, Paget's disease, renal tubular acidosis, sarcoidosis, ulcerative colitis, and Wilson's disease. Drugs include ammonium chloride, androgens, anabolic steroids, antacids, cholestyramine, furosemide, mercurial diuretics, parathyroid hormone, and vitamin D.

Decreased: Chronic renal failure, familial hypocalciuric hypercalcemia, hypocalcemia, hypoparathyroidism, malabsorption, milk-alkali syndrome, metastatic carcinoma of the prostate, nephrosis, osteomalacia, preeclampsia, pseudohypoparathyroidism, renal insufficiency, renal osteodystrophy, rickets (vitamin-D-resistant), steatorrhea, and vitamin D deficiency. Drugs include aspirin, indomethacin, oral contraceptives, sodium phytate, thiazide diuretics, and viomycin.

Description: A cation that is absorbed into the bloodstream from dietary sources and that functions in bone formation, nerve impulse transmission, contractility of muscles, and blood clotting. Calcium is stored in the bones and circulating calcium is filtered by the kidneys, with most being reabsorbed when serum calcium levels are normal. When serum calcium levels rise above normal, the kidneys reabsorb less calcium, and elevated levels of calcium appear in the urine. Whereas quantitative tests must be performed by a laboratory, the Sulkowitch test is a semiquantitative test suitable for home use.

Professional Considerations:

1. Consent form NOT required.
2. Preparation:
   A. Note daily dietary level of calcium intake for the prior 3 days on the laboratory requisition.
   B. Obtain a 3-L container with hydrochloric acid (HCl) additive or an acid-washed glass bottle for 24-hour collection. Write the starting date and the time on the container.
   C. Obtain a small container to collect a random sample.
3. Procedure:
   A. *24-hour collection (quantitative):*
      i. Discard the first morning urine specimen.
      ii. Begin to time a 24-hour urine collection.
      iii. Save all the urine voided for 24 hours in a clean, plastic, 3-L container to which 10 ml of 6N HCl has been added, or an acid-washed glass bottle. Include the urine voided at the end of the 24-hour period.
   B. *Random specimen collection (quantitative):*
      i. When evaluating for hypocalciuria, collect a postprandial specimen. When evaluating for hypercalciuria, collect an early-morning specimen before breakfast. Obtain a 100-ml random urine specimen in a clean container. A fresh specimen may be taken from a urinary drainage bag.
   C. *Sulkowitch test (semiquantitative):*
      i. Obtain a 20-ml random urine specimen.
      ii. Follow the package instructions.
4. Postprocedure care:
   A. Compare the urine quantity in the specimen container with the urinary output record for the test. If the specimen contains less urine than was recorded as output, some urine may have been discarded, thus invalidating the test.
   B. Document the quantity of urine output for the collection period on the laboratory requisition.
   C. Send the specimen to the laboratory within 1 hour.
5. Client and family teaching:
   A. The client should consume a diet with normal calcium levels, 600–800 mg/day (15–20 mmol/day, SI units), for 3 days.
   B. Save all the urine voided in the 24-hour period and urinate before defecating to avoid loss of urine. If any urine is accidentally discarded, discard the entire specimen and restart the collection the next day.
   C. Clients with elevated levels should be told to notify the physician for symptoms of renal calculi (flank or abdominal pain, severe dysuria).
6. Factors that affect results:
   A. Failure to add HCl to the collection container prior to starting the collection will result in falsely decreased results.
   B. All the urine voided for the 24-hour period must be included to avoid a falsely low result.
   C. For a random specimen, a delay in processing may cause falsely decreased results.
   D. Elevated urine phosphate may caused decreased results.
7. Other data:
   A. 20–25% of clients who form calcium stones have hyperuricosuria.
   B. *See also Calcium, Total, Serum.*

Bibliography:

McKane WR, Khosla S, Burritt MF, Kao PC, Wilson DM, Ory SJ, Riggs BL: Mechanism of renal calcium conservation with estrogen replacement therapy in women in early postmenopause—a clinical research center study. J Clin Endocrinol Metab *80*(12):3458–3464, 1995.

Ozcan T, Kaleli B, Ozeren M, Turan C, Zorlu G: Urinary calcium to creatinine ratio for predicting preeclampsia. Am J Perinatol *12*(5):349–351, 1995.

Rodgers A, Hibbert B, Probyn T: Determination of urinary calcium oxalate crystallization mechanisms and kinetics using flow cytometry. Urol Int *55*(2):93–100, 1995.

CALCIUM DISODIUM EDTA MOBILIZATION TEST, 24-HOUR, URINE

(see Lead Mobilization Test, 24-Hour, Urine)

CALIFORNIA ENCEPHALITIS VIRUS TITER (LA CROSSE VIRUS TITER), SERUM

Norm: Less than a fourfold increase in titer in paired sera (acute and convalescent sera).

Usage: Supports the diagnosis of viral encephalitis.

Description: The California encephalitis virus commonly produces aseptic meningitis, which occurs in the summer and is clinically indistinguishable from enteroviral disease. Encephalitis is an inflammation of the brain caused by an arbovirus infection transmitted by infected mosquitoes and tics. It causes an abrupt onset of severe frontal headache, fever of 38–40°C, stiff neck, sore throat, and sometimes lethargy, convulsions, and coma. Incidence is highest in children and in the inhabitants of the north central states of the United States.

Professional Considerations:

1. Consent form NOT required.
2. Preparation:
   A. Tube: Red top, red/gray-top, or gold-top.
   B. MAY be drawn during hemodialysis.
3. Procedure:
   A. Draw a 15-ml venous blood sample.
   B. Repeat the test for a convalescent serum specimen in 10–14 days.
4. Postprocedure care:
   A. Send the specimen to the laboratory within 2 hours.
5. Client and family teaching:
   A. Return in 10 days to 2 weeks for repeat testing.
6. Factors that affect results:
   A. Reject hemolyzed specimens.
   B. The serum should be separated from the clot within 2–3 hours.
7. Other data:
   A. The virus can rarely be isolated from blood or spinal fluid in the acute phase.
   B. Serologic diagnosis can be made by demonstrating rising antibody titers between the acute and convalescent specimens.
   C. Specific serologic diagnosis may be complicated by cross-reactions in clients with prior exposure to dengue or other flaviviruses.

Bibliography:

Leber SM, Brunberg JA, Pavkovic IM: Infarction of basal ganglia associated with California encephalitis virus. Pediatr Neurol 12(4):346–349, 1995.

Reisen WK, Hardy JL, Lothrop HD: Landscape ecology of arboviruses in southern California: patterns in the epizootic dissemination of western equine encephalomyelitis and St. Louis encephalitis viruses in Coachella Valley, 1991–1992. J Med Entomol 32(3):267–275, 1995.

Sherrie's Medical Microbiology: An Introduction to Infectious Diseases: Ryan, K (ed). Norwalk, CT, Appleton and Lange, 1994.

cAMP

(see Cyclic Adenosine Monophosphate, Serum and Urine)

CAMPYLOBACTER-LIKE-ORGANISM (CLO) TEST (RAPID UREASE TEST), SPECIMEN

Norm: Negative (CLO test gel turns yellow 24 hours after specimen insertion).

Positive: Presence of *Helicobacter pylori* (amount present is decided by deepening in color of the specimen).

Description: This is a simple test used to determine the presence of *H. pylori* in gastric mucosal biopsies. *H. pylori* has been implicated as a primary etiologic factor in duodenal ulcer disease, gastric ulcer and non-ulcer dyspepsia. By causing chronic inflammation, *H. pylori* may weaken mucosal defenses and allow acid and pepsin to disrupt the epithelium. *H. pylori* produces large amounts of urease enzyme. Although urease primarily allows *H. pylori* to utilize urea as a nitrogen source; the breakdown of urea also produces high local concentrations of ammonia that enable the organism to tolerate a low pH. Simple tests such as the CLO test enable a rapid diagnosis. The CLO test is a sealed plastic slide holding an agar gel that contains urea, a pH indicator, phenol red, buffers and bacteriostatic agents that help prevent false color changes that could lead to false-positive readings. If the urease enzyme of *H. pylori* is present in an inserted tissue sample, the resulting degradation of urea causes the pH to rise and the color of the gel turns from yellow to a bright magenta color.

Professional Considerations:

1. Consent form NOT required, but IS required for the endoscopy procedure used to obtain the specimen. *See Gastro-Esophago-Duodenoscopy, Diagnostic* for risks and contraindications.
2. Preparation:
   A. *See Client and family teaching.*
   B. Inspect the CLO test slide to make sure that the well is full and is a yellow color. If a CLO test slide has an orange color, it should be used with caution, as it may give a false-positive result.
   C. *See also Esophagogastroduodenoscopy, Diagnostic.*
3. Procedure:
   A. Immediately before endoscopy, place the CLO test on a warming plate at 30–40°C. Warming helps to speed the chemical reaction.
   B. Obtain a tissue sample from the gastric mucosa via endoscopy. Place the sample immediately in the well of the CLO test slide.
4. Postprocedure care:
   A. Be certain that the tissue specimen is completely immersed so that it will have maximum contact with the urea and bacteriostat in the gel.
   B. Reseal the CLO test container.
   C. Keep the CLO test in a warm place for the next 3 hours.

D. *See also Esophagogastroduodenoscopy, Diagnostic.*

5. Client and family teaching:
   A. Do not take antibiotics or bismuth salts for at least 3 weeks prior to the test.
   B. This test will help identify whether the *H. pylori* bacteria is present in your stomach. This bacteria is thought to be a cause of ulcers and gastritis.
   C. Since *H. pylori* therapy is only 50–75% effective, it is important that you return for retesting 28 days after completing therapy to confirm complete eradication of *H. pylori.*
   D. *See also Esophagogastroduodenoscopy, Diagnostic.*
6. Factors that affect results:
   A. False-negative results may occur when very low numbers of *H. pylori* are present or when the bacterium has a patchy distribution.
   B. The CLO test will be less sensitive if the client has recently been taking antibiotics or bismuth.
7. Other data:
   A. The CLO test has proven to be an accurate test with few false-negative results (Lee 1994).

Bibliography:

Crantock L, Willett I: Sensitivity of CLO test not affected by pre-immersion of biopsy forceps in formalin (letter). Gastrointest Endosc *39*(6):858, 1993.

DeCross AJ, Peura DA: Role of *H. pylori* in peptic ulcer disease. Contemporary Gastroenterology, (5):18–26, 1992.

Lee N, Lee TT, Fang KM: Assessment of four rapid urease test systems for detection of *Helicobacter pylori* in gastric biopsy specimens. Diagn Microbiol Infect Dis *18*(2):69–74, 1994.

Qurechi H, Ahmed W, Lodi TZ, Zubers SJ: Comparison of commercially available CLO test with the locally prepared test. JPMS Pak Med Assoc *43*(7):139–140, 1993.

CAMPYLOBACTER PYLORI

(see Helicobacter Pylori, Quick Office Serology, Serum and Titer, Blood)

CANNABINOIDS, QUALITATIVE, BLOOD OR URINE

Norm: None present. Negative.

Usage: Testing for use of marijuana.

Description: Marijuana is derived from an Asiatic herb, Cannabis sativa, and contains many biologically active chemicals, with most of the pharmacologic effects resulting from 9-tetrahydrocannabinol (THC). THC has an unusually high lipid solubility, so it is widely distributed in the body, with a high affinity for brain tissue. THC affects mood, memory, motor coordination, cognitive ability, sensorium, time sense, and self-perception. The effects are dose-related and are three to four times more potent when smoked than when ingested or injected. THC is metabolized to numerous active and inactive metabolites called cannabinoids. Seventy percent of the dose from smoking THC is excreted within 72 hours in the urine and feces. Because of slow release of THC from tissue storage sites, urine may test positive for 2–5 days after marijuana use by infrequent smokers. The primary psychoactive metabolite, which is also the most abundant and inactive, is 11-hydroxy-THC. Most immunoassay tests use antibodies directed at 11-hydroxy-THC. Immunoassays are also available to measure the drug, THC, which can be used in the treatment of persistent nausea and vomiting associated with cancer chemotherapy or to decrease the pain of glaucoma.

Professional Considerations:

1. Consent form NOT required but is usually obtained for pre-employment testing or for medicolegal specimens.
2. Preparation:
   A. Tube: Red-top, red/gray-top, or gold-top. Also obtain a sterile plastic urine collection container.
   B. Do NOT draw during hemodialysis.
3. Procedure:
   A. If specimens are being obtained for medicolegal purposes, the collection, transportation, and processing should be performed in the presence of a witness.
   B. Draw a 5-ml venous blood sample.
   C. Obtain a random 50-ml urine specimen in a sterile plastic container.
4. Postprocedure care:
   A. Write the exact time of the specimen collection and the source, date, and client's name on the laboratory requisition.
   B. If the specimen may be used as legal evidence, sign and have the witness sign the laboratory requisition. Transport the specimen to the laboratory in a sealed plastic bag labeled as legal evidence. Each client handling the specimen should sign and write the time of specimen receipt on the laboratory requisition.
5. Client and family teaching:
   A. The long-term effects of marijuana use include impaired lung structure, chromosomal mutation, higher incidence of birth defects, mononucleic white

blood cells, memory impairment, flashbacks, and impairment of fertility.

B. Offer substance abuse counseling referral to all clients using cannabinoids without a medical prescription.

6. Factors that affect results:
   A. Serum levels of THC peak within 10–30 minutes of inhalation and within 3 hours of ingestion depending on the dosage.
   B. Urine levels peak from 2 to 6 hours after THC has entered the system.
   C. Urine levels are detectable for 4–6 days in acute users and for 20–77 days in chronic users.

7. Other data:
   A. Because of the cardiac stimulant effects, cannabinoids may pose a threat to clients with cardiovascular disease.
   B. Marijuana is the most widely used illicit drug in the United States.
   C. The signs and symptoms of cannabis intoxication are tachycardia; conjunctival infection; hypotension; muscle weakness; tremors; unsteadiness; increased deep tendon reflexes; psychological and cognitive impairments; hallucinations; loss of consciousness; and, rarely, death.
   D. Common street names for marijuana include Acapulco gold, Colombian, grass, hash, herb, J, jay, joint, Mary Jane, Panama red, pot, reefer, smoke, tea, and weed.

Bibliography:

Cone EJ, Huestis MA: Relating blood concentrations of tetrahydrocannibinal and metabolites to pharmacologic effects and time of marijuana usage [review]. Thera Drug Monitoring: 15(6):527–532, 1993.

Heustis MA, Simpson AH, Holicky BJ, Henningfield JE, Cone EJ: Characterization of the absorption phase of marijuana smoking. Clin Pharm Ther 52(1):31–41,1992.

Mikkelsen SL, Delaney RA, Paoli C: Effects of heating urine prior to assay for drugs of abuse. Lab Med 23(1):41–43, 1992.

CAPILLARY FRAGILITY TEST (RUMPEL-LEEDE TOURNIQUET TEST), DIAGNOSTIC

Norm: Negative or 1+.
Within a radius of 2.5 cm:

Females = 10 or less petechiae

Males = 5 or less petechiae

Increased: Aplastic anemia, acute leukemia, chronic nephritis, decreased estrogen level in postmenopausal female, disseminated intravascular coagulation, dysproteinemia, factor VII deficiency, fibrinogen deficiency, Glanzmann's disease, influenza, idiopathic thrombocytopenia purpura, liver disease, long-term steroid use, measles, polycythemia vera, prothrombin deficiency, scarlet fever, thrombocytopenia, scurvy, vascular purpura, vitamin K deficiency, and von Willebrand's disease, hereditary telangiectasia.

Decreased: Drugs include glucocorticoids.

Description: This test, also known as the tourniquet test, is a nonspecific evaluation to measure capillary wall weakness and deficiencies in platelet number and function. An inflated blood pressure cuff at a specific pressure for a fixed period of time produces increased pressure and hypoxia in the capillaries distal to the cuff. Decreased capillary resistance causes the capillaries to rupture, which leads to bleeding and the formation of petechiae.

Professional Considerations:
1. Consent form NOT required.

Risks:
Bleeding, infection, hematoma, ecchymosis.

Contraindications:
The test is contraindicated if routine tourniquet use for drawing blood specimens produces petechiae. This test is contraindicated in clients who have edematous or very cold arms or if there are contraindications to placing or inflating a blood pressure cuff on the arm (e.g., casts, rash, dressings, A-V fistula). Other contraindications include platelet count <50,000/mm^3, severe bleeding disorders, anticoagulant therapy, senile skin changes, or if the client has taken medications containing aspirin within 7 days prior to the test.

2. Preparation:
   A. Obtain a blood pressure cuff, manometer, and watch.
   B. Inspect the arm carefully for the presence of pre-existing petechiae.

3. Procedure:
   A. Apply a blood pressure cuff to the arm and inflate to a level midway between the client's systolic and diastolic pressures, but not higher than 100 mmHg.

B. Leave the cuff inflated for 5 minutes and observe the arm at least 1 inch distal to the cuff for the formation of petechiae.

C. The test results are reported in a range from negative to +4, depending on the number of petechiae appearing in a 5-cm diameter circle:

Negative = No petechiae
+1 = 1–10 petechiae
+2 = 11–20 petechiae
+3 = 21–50 petechiae
+4 = >50 petechiae

If pre-existing petechiae are present, count the number of additional petechiae formed during the test.

4. Postprocedure care:
A. Deflate and remove the blood pressure cuff.
B. Client should open and close the hand to hasten blood return to the distal extremity.

5. Client and family teaching:
A. A good explanation of the test procedure is essential, as the test may cause discomfort to the client.

6. Factors that affect results:
A. Failure to keep the cuff inflated for 5 minutes.

7. Other data:
A. A positive test in women over age 40 may not be pathogenic.
B. A variation of this positive-pressure test is the negative-pressure test, in which a small suction cup is applied for 1 minute to the skin, and the number of resulting petechiae are counted.
C. The test should not be repeated on the same extremity for at least 1 week.

Bibliography:

Bennington J (ed): Saunders Dictionary and Encyclopedia of Laboratory Medicine and Technology. Philadelphia, WB Saunders, 1984, p 251.

Byrne CJ, Saxton DF, Pelikan PK, Nugent PM: Laboratory Tests: Implications for Nursing Care. Menlo Park, CA, Addison-Wesley, 1986, pp 546–547.

Ravel R: Clinical Application of Laboratory, 5th ed. Chicago, London, Year Book Medical Publishers, 1989, p 91.

CARBAMAZEPINE, BLOOD

Norm: Negative.

		SI Units
Therapeutic value	4–12 µg/ml	17–51 µmol/L
Panic level	>20 µg/ml	>84 µmol/L

Panic Level Symptoms and Treatment:

Symptoms:

Stage I: (Levels >25 µg/ml)—stupor, coma up to 24 hours, seizures, respiratory depression.

Stage II: (Levels >15–25 µg/ml)—adventitial choreiform movements, combativeness, hallucinations, moderate stupor.

Stage III: (Levels 11–15 µg/ml)—mild drowsiness

Stage IV: (Levels <11 µg/ml)—ataxia and nystagmus with otherwise normal neurologic status. Relapse to earlier stages may recur unexpectedly. Ataxia, blurred vision, CNS depression, coma, diplopia, dizziness, drowsiness, dysrhythmias (conduction defects, sinus tachycardia), dystonic reaction, hallucination, hypotension, nystagmus, reduced myocardial contractility, pulmonary edema, respiratory depression, seizures (when levels exceed 20 µg/ml), vomiting.

Treatment:
Do NOT induce emesis.
Perform gastric lavage if the drug has been recently ingested (most effective mechanism to reduce absorption).
Maintain/protect airway.
Give activated charcoal unless ileus is present.
Treat hypotension with fluids and vasopressors.
Treat seizures with diazepam, phenobarbital or phenytoin.

Monitor for cardiovascular toxicity (ECG, vital signs, renal function, electrolytes, CBC).
Carbamazepine CANNOT be hemodialyzed out of the body.
Hemoperfusion for at least 4 hours WILL remove 50 mg to 2.4 grams of carbamazepine in most clients.

Increased: Drug abuse, glossopharyngeal neuralgia, renal failure (increases metabolite 10,11-epoxide), tic douloureux, and trigeminal neuralgia. Drugs include cimetidine, erythromycin, isoniazid, propoxyphene, verapamil, and calcium channel blockers.

Decreased: Convulsions, epilepsy, and seizures. Drugs include phenobarbital, primidone, and phenytoin.

Description: Carbamazepine is an anticonvulsant, anticholinergic sedative, antidepressant, and muscle relaxant that is used alone or with other anticonvulsants to treat seizures. This drug is metabolized in the liver, with a half-life of 10–30 hours in adults and 8–19 hours in children. Steady-state levels occur in 2–6 days. Carbamazepine crosses the placenta and appears in breast milk.

Professional Considerations:
1. Consent form NOT required.
2. Preparation:
   A. Serum should be drawn before the morning dose is given.
   B. Tube: Green-top, red-top, red/gray-top, or gold-top.
   C. MAY be drawn during hemodialysis.
3. Procedure:
   A. Draw a 7-ml venous blood sample.
4. Postprocedure care:
   A. Reject hemolyzed specimens.
5. Client and family teaching:
   A. Early toxic signs include fever, sore throat, oral ulcers, easy bruising, unusual bleeding, and joint pain.
   B. Levels should be checked weekly × 12

during initiation of therapy, then monthly for 2–3 years.
   C. If activated charcoal was given for elevated levels, the client should drink 4–6 glasses of water each day for 2 days to prevent constipation. Activated charcoal will also cause stools to be black for a few days.
6. Factors that affect results:
   A. Absorption of the drug is enhanced with the eating of food.
   B. Therapeutic values should be toward the lower norms when both carbamazepine and other anticonvulsants are taken.
   C. Peak levels occur 2–4 hours after oral dosage.
7. Other data:
   A. Side effects include bone marrow depression, eosinophilia, hepatic dysfunction, and urticaria.
   B. The trade name for carbamazepine is Tegretol.

Bibliography:

Matsuda Y, Akazawa R, Teraoka R, Otsuka M: Pharmaceutical evaluation of carbamazepine modifications: comparative study for photostability of carbamazepine polymorphs by using fourier transformed reflection absorption infrared spectroscopy and colorimetric measurement. J Pharm Pharmacol 46(3):162–167, 1994.

Spigset O, Carleberg L, Mjoindua T, Norstron A: Carbamezepine interference in a high-performance liquid chromatography analysis for perphenazine. Ther Drug Mon 16(3):332–333, 1994.

Weaver DF, Camfield P, Fraser A: Massive carbamazepine overdose: Clinical and pharmacologic observations in five episodes. Neurology 38:755–759, 1988.

CARBOHYDRATE AG 19-9, BLOOD
(see CA 19-9, Blood)

CARBOHYDRATE ANTIGEN 50, BLOOD
(see CA 50, Blood)

CARBON-13 OR CARBON-14 UREA BREATH TEST
(see Urea Breath Test, Diagnostic)

CARBON DIOXIDE, PARTIAL PRESSURE (pCO_2), BLOOD
Norm:

		SI Units
Arterial sample	35–45 mmHg	4.7–6.0 kPa
Panic level	<20 mmHg	<2.6 kPa
	>70 mmHg	>9.2 kPa
Arterialized capillary sample (<age 2)	26.4–41.2 mmHg	3.5–5.4 kPa
Venous sample	38–50 mmHg	5.0–6.7 kPa

Increased: Acute intermittent porphyria, aminoglycoside toxicity, asthma (late stage), brain death, coarctation of the aorta, congestive heart failure, electrolyte disturbance (severe), emphysema, empyema, hyaline membrane disease, hyperemesis, hypothyroidism (severe), hypoventilation (alveolar), metabolic alkalosis, near drowning, pleural effusion, pleurisy, pneumonia, pneumothorax, poisoning, pulmonary edema, pulmonary infection, renal disorders, respiratory acidosis, respiratory failure, shock, tetralogy of Fallot, transposition of the great vessels, and vomiting. Drugs include aldosterone, bicarbonate (HCO_3), ethacrynic acid, hydrocortisone, laxatives, metolazone, prednisone, thiazides, thromethamine, and viomycin.

Decreased: Dysrhythmias, asthma (early stage), diabetic ketoacidosis, diabetes mellitus, fever, high altitude, hyperventilation, metabolic acidosis, respiratory alkalosis, and salicylate intoxication. Drugs include acetazolamide, dimercaprol, dimethadione, methicillin sodium, nitrofurantoin, nitrofurantoin sodium, phenformin, tetracycline, and triamterene.

Description: Carbon dioxide gas present in air and also occurring as a nutritional metabolite is essential to the body's regulation of acid-base buffer system. This test measures the partial pressure exerted by carbon dioxide (pCO_2) dissolved in the blood, and reflects the body's ability to produce carbonic acid and the efficiency of lung alveoli to excrete carbon dioxide. Laboratory measurement of pCO_2 assists in differentiating respiratory from metabolic causes of acidosis and alkalosis.

Professional Considerations:

1. Consent form NOT required.
2. Preparation:
   A. The client should rest for 30 minutes prior to specimen collection.
   B. Obtain a 22-gauge needle, a green-top tube, a glass syringe, heparin, 2% lidocaine, sterile gauze, and ice.
   C. Do NOT draw during hemodialysis.
3. Procedure:
   A. Brachial, femoral, and radial arteries are choice sites for obtaining blood specimens. If an arterial site is selected, anesthetize surrounding tissue.
   B. Draw a 5-ml anaerobic arterial or mixed venous blood sample into a heparinized, green-top tube or glass syringe.
   C. To maintain the blood specimen anaerobically, completely fill syringe or green-top tube with blood. If using a syringe, place the needle in a rubber stopper or apply a rubber cap immediately. Avoid pulling back on the syringe plunger. When using a green-top vacuum tube, remove it from the adaptor before removing the needle from the artery or vein and do not remove the stopper from the tube.
   D. Place the specimen immediately in an ice bath and send the specimen to the laboratory while maintaining anaerobic integrity.
4. Postprocedure care:
   A. Hold direct pressure over the site for 3–5 minutes.
   B. Write the time of collection on the requisition.
5. Client and family teaching:
   A. Results are normally available within 4 hours.
6. Factors that affect results:
   A. Reject specimens containing air bubbles, not packed in ice, or received more than 15 minutes after collection. Test results are more accurate if performed within 15–20 minutes after specimen collection.
7. Other data:
   A. The pCO_2 level must be analyzed with consideration given to electrolyte and pH levels.
   B. *See also Carbon Dioxide, Total Content, Blood*, as pCO_2 is only a measure of the pressure exerted by carbon dioxide present in the blood.

Bibliography:

Barton CW, Wang EJ: Correlation of end-tidal CO_2 measurements to arterial $PaCo_2$ in nonintubated patients. Ann Emer Med 23(3):560–563, 1994.

Lind L: Veno-arterial carbon dioxide and pH gradient and survival in critical illness. Eur J Clin Investigation 25(3): 201–205, 1995.

CARBON DIOXIDE (CO₂) TOTAL CONTENT, BLOOD

Norm:

		SI Units
Adult	22–30 mEq/L	22–30 mmol/L
	38–50 mmHg	
Panic level	<15 mEq/L	<15 mmol/L
	>50 mEq/L	>50 mmol/L
Neonates–2 years	32–44 mmHg	
Child >2 years	22–26 mEq/L	22–26 mmol/L

Increased: Adrenal cortex hormone imbalance, airway obstruction, alcoholism, aldosteronism, bradycardia, cardiac disorders, emphysema, fat embolism, hypoventilation, metabolic alkalosis, pneumonia, pulmonary dysfunction, prolonged nasogastric tube drainage, pyloric obstruction, renal disorders, respiratory acidosis, respiratory disease, and vomiting (severe). Drugs include antacids, corticotropin, cortisone acetate, mercurial diuretics, sodium bicarbonate, and thiazide diuretics.

Decreased: Alcoholic ketosis, dehydration, diabetic ketoacidosis, diarrhea (severe), drainage of intestinal fluid (gastric suction), head trauma, high fever, hepatic disorders, hyperventilation, lactic acidosis, malabsorption syndrome, metabolic acidosis, renal disorders, renal failure (acute), respiratory alkalosis (compensated), salicylate intoxication, starvation, and uremia. Drugs include acetazolamide, ammonium chloride, aspirin, chlorothiazide diuretics, dimercaprol, methicillin, nitrofurantoin, paraldehyde, and tetracycline.

Description: Carbon dioxide (CO₂) gas is present in air and also occurs as a nutritional metabolite. Total carbon dioxide level reflects the total amount of carbon dioxide in the body (i.e., in solution bound to proteins and bound as bicarbonate, carbonate, and carbonic acid) and is a general guide to the body's buffering capacity. Total CO₂ content is a bicarbonate and base solution that is regulated by the kidneys. CO₂ gas is acidic and is regulated by the lungs. Since over 80% of CO₂ is present in the form of bicarbonate, this test is a good reflection of bicarbonate level. Elevated or decreased levels indicate an acid-base imbalance and are related to hyperventilation or hypoventilation due to a variety of causes, as well as metabolic etiology. Total CO₂ is generally measured with electrolytes in the SMA-6 test, but may be measured alone.

Professional Considerations:
1. Consent form NOT required.
2. Preparation:
   A. Tube: Green-top. Obtain a container of ice for the arterial samples.
   B. Do not allow the client to clench/unclench the hand prior to blood drawing.
   C. Do NOT draw during hemodialysis.
3. Procedure:
   A. Collect the specimen without a tourniquet, or quickly after tourniquet application, to prevent stasis.
   B. Completely fill a heparinized green-top tube with venous blood to prevent diffusion of CO₂ into the tube. Collect the specimen directly into the tube, without exposing to the air.
   C. In the newborn, blood may be drawn from the heel, fingertips, or toes.
   D. Write the body temperature on the laboratory requisition.
4. Postprocedure care:
   A. Place the arterial sample on ice immediately.
   B. Transport the specimen to the laboratory within 15 minutes.
5. Client and family teaching:
   A. Results are normally available within 4 hours.
6. Factors that affect results:
   A. Pumping the fist prior to venipuncture may cause falsely elevated results.
   B. High altitudes require a decrease in values of 5 mmHg/mile (3 mmHg/km).
   C. A clotted sample or air bubbles in the sample invalidate the results.
   D. Hyperthermia causes an increased CO₂ level. Values must be corrected for temperature abnormalities.
7. Other data:
   A. *See also Carbon Dioxide, Partial Pressure, Blood.*

Bibliography:

Gasman JD, Fisherman RS, Raffin TA: Monitoring cardiopulmonary resuscitation role of blood and end tidal carbon dioxide tension. Crit Care Med 23(5):799–800, 1995.

LaValle TL, Perry AG: Capnography: assessing end-tidal CO2 levels. Dimen Crit Care Nurs 14(2): 70–77, 1995.

CARBON MONOXIDE (CO), BLOOD

Norm:

	% of Total Hemoglobin
Rural environment, nonsmoker	0.05–2.5
Heavy smoker	5–10
Acute toxicity	>25
Newborn	10–12

Panic Level Symptoms and Treatment:

Symptoms: Symptoms correlate poorly with blood levels. Levels over 10% cause dizziness, headache, dyspnea on exertion, and impaired judgment. Levels over 30% additionally cause nausea, syncope, tachycardia, tachypnea, and vomiting. Deep coma, convulsions, respiratory failure and death may occur at levels over 50%.

Treatment:

Continuous ECG monitoring.
Laboratory work: arterial blood gas, electrolytes, creatine kinase, urinalysis. Repeat blood carbon monoxide measurements q 2–4 hours until results are <15%.
100% oxygen via high-flow mask.
Treat metabolic acidosis.
Observe for and treat seizures with diazepam, phenobarbital, or phenytoin.
Treat cerebral edema with hyperventilation via mechanical ventilation and osmotic diuresis.
Hyperbaric oxygen for severely elevated levels.
Both hemodialysis and peritoneal dialysis WILL remove carbon monoxide.

Increased: Accidental or intentional inhalation of fumes from combustion of carbon-containing fuels (due to smoking or exposure to passive smoke, automobile exhaust fumes, or gas-burning appliances).

Decreased: Not clinically significant.

Description: Carbon monoxide (CO) is a chemical asphyxiant found in the fumes of automobile exhaust, improperly functioning furnaces, and defective gas-burning appliances. When inhaled, it combines with the hemoglobin in the red blood cells with an affinity 200 times greater than oxygen. This produces a hemoglobin derivative, carboxyhemoglobin, which is unable to transport or release oxygen throughout the body, resulting in hypoxia.

Professional Considerations:

1. Consent form NOT required.
2. Preparation:
   A. Tube: Lavender-top or green-top.
   B. Do NOT draw during hemodialysis.
3. Procedure:
   A. If specimen will be tested immediately, draw a 5- to 10-ml blood sample as soon as possible after exposure. Prevent contamination of the specimen with room air.
   B. If specimen will not be tested immediately, draw a specimen as above, but completely fill a heparinized, green-top tube.
4. Postprocedure care:
   A. Deliver the specimen to the blood gas laboratory immediately.
5. Client and family teaching:
   A. For accidental inhalation, refer the client and/or family for crisis intervention.
   B. Carbon monoxide cannot be seen, tasted, or smelled. It can be emitted by gas fireplaces, poorly vented gas clothes dryers, charcoal, wood, gas or coal stoves, cars, and kerosene heaters. An in-home CO detector is an inexpensive safety essential that can provide early warning of rising levels.
6. Factors that affect results:
   A. Draw a sample before administering oxygen, if possible.
   B. Newborn levels are higher than adult levels because of an immature respiratory system combined with a more rapid turnover of hemoglobin.

7. Other data:
   A. The results are most accurate if tested immediately, but the specimen may be stored in the refrigerator for several hours if the tube is completely filled and tightly stoppered.

Bibliography:

LeFever Kee J: Handbook of Laboratory and Diagnostic Tests with Nursing Implications, 2nd ed. Norwalk, CT, Appleton and Lange, 1994.

Ruth-Sahd L: Treating carbon monoxide poisoning. Nursing 22(1):33, 1992.

Stewart P et al.: Sources of CO in biological systems and applications of CO detection technologies. Sem Perinatol 18(1):2–10, 1994.

CARBOXYHEMOGLOBIN, BLOOD

(see Carbon Monoxide, Blood)

CARCINOEMBRYONIC ANTIGEN (CEA), SERUM

Norm:

		SI Units
Nonsmoker	<2.5 ng/ml	<2.5 mg/L
Smoker	<5.0 ng/ml	<5.0 mg/L

Increased: Cancer (breast, esophageal, gastrointestinal, ovarian, pancreatic, prostate, pulmonary), chronic ischemic heart disease, cirrhosis, hypothyroidism, inflammatory bowel disease, inflammatory processes, leukemia, neuroblastoma, pancreatitis (acute), pneumonia (bacterial), pulmonary emphysema, radiation therapy (recent), renal failure (acute), tobacco smokers (chronic), and trauma. Drugs include antineoplastics and hepatotoxic drugs.

Decreased: Not clinically significant.

Description: CEA is a glycoprotein produced by the fetus from age 2–6 months and secreted by gastrointestinal cells. It is an antigen that can be found in trace amounts in healthy adults, but is secreted in greater amounts during rapid multiplication of epithelial cells, especially of the gastrointestinal tract. This test is not diagnostic, but because levels are increased in malignancies, CEA provides a guide to management and helps evaluate the success of surgery and other forms of cancer treatment. This test is most valuable in the early detection of recurrent colorectal cancer because blood levels may rise 3 months before clinical symptoms of the recurrent disease are present. CEA levels may be measured every 1–3 months to monitor response to and direct therapy for colorectal cancer. Normal levels occur within 4–6 weeks after effective therapy.

Professional Considerations:

1. Consent form NOT required.
2. Preparation:
   A. Tube: Red-top, red/gray-top, or gold-top.
   B. MAY be drawn during hemodialysis.
3. Procedure:
   A. Draw a 1-ml venous blood sample without hemolysis.
4. Factors that affect results:
   A. Reject hemolyzed specimens.
   B. Results are invalid if client has undergone a radioactive scan within 2 weeks prior to the test if a radioimmunoassay method is used.
   C. CEA results obtained with a different assay method and different specimen typed cannot be used interchangeably. It is recommended that only one assay method and specimen type be utilized consistently.
7. Other data:
   A. Cells must be separated from the serum or plasma within 6 hours. The specimen is then stable at room temperature for 3 days or in a refrigerator for 1 week.
   B. Levels may exceed 10 ng/ml (10 mg/L, SI units) in acute inflammatory disorders and 12 ng/ml (12 mg/L, SI units) in the presence of neoplasm.

Bibliography:

Imamiua M, Jamarichi H, Mamake T: Resected case of carcinoid tumor of the liver metastatic from the breast. Gastroenterol 30(3):398–402, 1995.

Rodriquez dePaterna L, Arnaiz F, Estenoz J, Ortuno B, Lanzos E: Study of serum tumor markers CEA, CA 15.3 and CA 27.29 as diagnostic parameters in patients with breast carcinoma. Int J Biol Markers 10(1):24–29, 1995.

CARCINOGENIC ANTIGEN 15-3

(see CA 15-3, Serum)

CARDIAC CATHETERIZATION (ANGIOCARDIOGRAPHY, CARDIOANGIOGRAPHY, CARDIAC CATHETERIZATION, AND CORONARY ANGIOGRAPHY), DIAGNOSTIC

Norm: Normal heart anatomy with normal chamber volumes and pressures, normal wall and valve motion, and patent coronary arteries. Normal cardiac output and chamber pressures are listed below:

	Normal Pressures
Cardiac output (CO): 4–8 L/min	
Right heart catheterization	
Right atrial (RA)	3–11 mmHg
Right atrial mean	6 mmHg
Right ventricular systolic	20–30 mmHg
Right ventricular end-diastolic	<5 mmHg
Pulmonary artery systolic (PAS)	20–30 mmHg
Pulmonary artery end-diastolic (PAEDP)	8–15 mmHg
Pulmonary artery mean (PAM)	<20 mmHg
Pulmonary artery wedge pressure (PAWP) or pulmonary capillary wedge pressure(PCWP)	4–12 mmHg
Left heart catheterization	
Ascending aorta systolic	140 mmHg
Ascending aorta diastolic	90 mmHg
Ascending aorta mean	105 mmHg
Left ventricle (LV) systolic	140 mmHg
Left ventricular end-diastolic	8–12 mmHg
Left atrium mean	12 mmHg

Usage: Identification, documentation, and quantitation of congenital disorders of the heart and diseases and disorders of the greater vessels of the heart; evaluation of cardiac muscle function; evaluation of coronary artery patency; identification of ventricular aneurysms; and identification and quantitation of the severity of acquired or congenital cardiac valve disease.

Description: Cardiac catheterization involves passing a catheter through the brachial or femoral artery or antecubital or femoral vein into the left or right side of the heart via the aorta or vena cava, respectively. Angiographic films can be taken after radiopaque dye is injected from the catheter tip. The dye makes it possible to visualize chamber function, valve function, and chamber size. Measurements of oxygen content and pressure, and flow rate of blood, can be obtained in each chamber, along with the cardiac output and perfusion of the coronary arteries.

Professional Considerations:

1. Consent form IS required.

Risks:
Air embolism, allergic reaction to dye (itching, hives, rash, tight feeling in the throat, shortness of breath, bronchospasm, anaphylaxis, death), asystole, cardiac tamponade, cerebrovascular accident (left heart catheterization), congestive heart failure, cerebrovascular accident, dysrhythmias, embolus (left heart catheterization), endocarditis, hematoma, hemorrhage, hemothorax, hypovolemia, infection, myocardial infarction, pneumothorax, pulmonary edema, pulmonary embolism (right heart catheterization), renal toxicity, retroperitoneal bleed, thrombophlebitis (right heart catheterization with antecubital site), thrombus (left heart catheterization), and vagal response (right heart catheterization). This invasive procedure poses a 2% risk of complications.

Contraindications/Precautions:

Pregnancy, severe cardiomyopathy, severe dysrhythmias, uncontrolled congestive heart failure. This procedure should be performed with extreme caution on clients allergic to local anesthetics, iodine, shellfish, or radiopaque contrast material. Steroids and diphenhydramine should be given preprocedure to these clients.

2. Preparation:
   A. *See Client and family teaching.*
   B. Routine cardiac medications may be given with a small sip of water.
   C. Record the baseline height and weight for the calculation of dye dosage.
   D. Sedation is usually prescribed for relaxation, but the client remains awake.
   E. Assess peripheral pulses and mark them for easy location.
   F. Assess baseline ECG and arterial blood pressure and monitor continuously due to the potential for occurrence of cardiac dysrhythmias during the procedure.
   G. Have emergency cardiac medications and emergency equipment readily available.

3. Procedure:
   A. *Left heart catheterization:* In a cardiac catheterization laboratory under fluoroscopy, a long catheter is inserted through a percutaneously inserted sheath into the brachial or femoral artery retrograde via the aorta into the left ventricle or to the beginning of the coronary arteries. Radiopaque dye is then injected from the catheter tip, and the patency of the coronary arteries (coronary angiography, coronary arteriography, cineangiography, or angiocardiography), left ventricular function (contrast ventriculography), and bicuspid and aortic valve function are assessed and recorded radiographically.
   B. *Right heart catheterization:* In a cardiac catheterization laboratory under fluoroscopy, a long catheter is inserted through a percutaneously inserted sheath into an antecubital or femoral vein through the vena cava, right atrium, and right ventricle, and into the pulmonary artery. Heart chamber and pulmonary artery pressures may be measured, as well as cardiac output, tricuspid and pulmonary valve function, and right ventricular function. Radiographic films of the procedure are made.

4. Postprocedure care:
   A. Maintain bedrest for 4–6 hours.

B. Apply a pressure dressing to the arterial catheter insertion site and immobilize the extremity for 4–6 hours. A sandbag may be placed over an arterial site. Check the dressing and site for bleeding and hematoma formation along with vital sign and pulse checks. Bedrest and extremity immobilization may be extended in clients receiving heparin.
   C. Check vital signs and peripheral pulses, color, skin temperature, and sensation of the procedural extremity every 15 minutes × 4, then every 30 minutes × 2, then hourly × 8–12 hours. Also check for low back or flank pain, which may indicate a retroperitoneal bleed.
   D. Assess for dysrhythmias, chest pain, or symptoms of cardiac tamponade.
   E. An analgesic may be prescribed for catheterization site discomfort.
   F. Encourage the oral intake of fluids if not contraindicated.
   G. Resume diet.

5. Client and family teaching:
   A. Fast from food for 8 hours and from fluids for 3 hours before the procedure.
   B. The procedure lasts 1–3 hours.
   C. A momentary warm flush and metallic taste or racing pulse may be experienced when the dye is injected. It is also normal to feel a few skipped beats when the catheter is in the ventricle.
   D. If coronary angiography will be performed, you might experience momentary chest pain while the dye is injected into the arteries, but no damage will result.
   E. It is important to lie motionless throughout the procedure. Symptoms of more than momentary chest pain should be verbalized immediately.
   F. Vital signs, pulse checks, and assessments for pain will be taken postprocedure at frequent intervals.
   G. Report any difficulty breathing during and after the procedure.

6. Factors that affect results:
   A. Atherosclerosis of peripheral vessels prohibits easy passage of the catheter.

7. Other data:
   A. The procedure should be stopped for severe chest pain, neurological symptoms of a cerebrovascular accident, cardiac dysrhythmias, or hemodynamic changes.
   B. Due to the risk of complete coronary artery occlusion from plaque disruption or coronary artery perforation, it is advisable (and legally required in many states) to have backup cardiothoracic surgery availability whenever performing a cardiac catheterization.

Bibliography:

Aliabadi D, Icenagle M, Samaan S, Roldan C, Holland M: Transesophageal echocardiographically guided angiography of an anomalous coronary artery. Amer Heart J *129*(1):193–195, 1995.

Goldsmith MF: Realizing potential of MR coronary angiography may ease patients' test load and diagnosis costs. JAMA 271(4):256, 1994.

Hill JA: Single-stage coronary angiography and angioplasty: a new standard? Amer J Cardiol 75(1):75–76, 1995.

CARDIAC ENZYMES/ISOENZYMES (CK, LD, ALT, AST), BLOOD

Norm: Results are method dependent and should be compared with the reference values of the laboratory performing the test.

		SI Units
Creatine Kinase (CK)		
Adult female	<80 U/L	<1.33 mkat/L
Adult male	<90 U/L	<1.50 mkat/L
Newborn	<200 U/L	<3.33 mkat/L
CK Isoenzymes	**% of Total CK**	**Fraction of Total CK**
CK_1BB (brain)	0–3	0-0.03
CK_2MB (heart)	0–6	0–0.06
CK_3MM (muscle)	90–97	0.90–0.97

		SI Units
Lactate Dehydrogenase (LD)		
Wroblewski method 30°C	150–450 U	72–217 IU/L
Adult		
≤Age 60	45–90 U/L	45–90 U/L
>Age 60	55–102 U/L	55–102 U/L
Child		
Newborn	160–500 U/L	160–500 U/L
Neonate	300–1500 U/L	300–1500 U/L
Infant	100–250 U/L	100–250 U/L
Child	60–170 U/L	60–170 U/L

Lactate Dehydrogenase Isoenzymes (Agarose, Electrophoresis)

	% of Total LD	Fraction of Total CK
Fraction LD_1	14–26	0.14–0.26
Fraction LD_2	29–39	0.29–0.39
Fraction LD_3	20–26	0.20–0.26
Fraction LD_4	8–16	0.08-0.16
Fraction LD_5	6–16	0.06-0.16

		SI Units
Aspartate Aminotransferase (AST, SGOT)		
Adult female		
≤Age 60	8–20 U/L	8–20 U/L
>Age 60	10–20 U/L	10–20 U/L
Adult male		
≤Age 60	8–20 U/L	8–20 U/L
>Age 60	11–26 U/L	11–26 U/L
Children		
Newborn	16–72 U/L	16–72 U/L
Infant	15–60 U/L	15–60 U/L
Age 1 year	16–35 U/L	16–35 U/L
Age 5 years	19–28 U/L	19–28 U/L

Alanine Aminotransferase (ALT, SGPT)		SI Units
Adult female		
≤Age 60	8–20 U/L	8–20 U/L
>Age 60	7–16 U/L	7–16 U/L
Adult male		
≤Age 60	8–20 U/L	8–20 U/L
>Age 60	6–24 U/L	6–24 U/L
Children		
Newborn	5–28 U/L	5–28 U/L
Infant	5–28 U/L	5–28 U/L

Increased: Patterns in myocardial infarction are generally as follows:

CK: Total CK levels may be normal in acute myocardial infarction, even when the CK-MB isoenzyme is elevated. CK levels begin rising before LD and AST levels. In general, CK begins rising at 4–8 hours, peaks at 12–24 hours, and returns to baseline by 3–4 days after the onset of myocardial damage.

CK Isoenzymes: CK_2MB begins rising at 6 hours, peak at 18 hours, and returns to baseline by 72 hours after the onset of myocardial damage.

LD: Total LD levels begin rising at 24 hours, peak at 3–4 days, and return to baseline in 8–12 days.

LD Isoenzymes: LD_1 peaks with an LD_1:LD_2 ratio inversion 48 hours after onset of damage.

AST: AST initially rises at 6–10 hours, peaks at 12–48 hours, and returns to baseline by 4–6 days after the onset of myocardial damage.

AST/ALT Ratio: ≥3.1, or double that of the baseline after myocardial damage.

Increases in Selected Other Conditions: Cardiomyopathy (total CK, CK_1BB, CK_2MB, total LD), congestive heart failure (CK_2MB [rare], total LD, AST, ALT), myocardial infarction (total CK, CK_2MB, CK_3MM, total LD, LD_1, LD_2 LD_1:LD_2 inversion, AST [marked], ALT [slight], AST/ALT ratio), myocarditis (total CK, CK_2MB), pericarditis (AST), pulmonary infarction (total CK, AST, total LD, LD_2, LD_3), and severe angina (total CK [rare], CK_2MB).

Decreased: See individual test listings. Decreases not applicable for myocardial infarction.

Description: Cardiac enzymes are a group of enzymes released by the heart as a result of myocardial injury. They aid in the differential diagnosis of myocardial infarction from congestive heart failure, pericarditis, pulmonary infarction, angina, and other conditions. Creatine kinase (CK) is an enzyme found in specific body tissues, and lactate dehydrogenase is an enzyme present in many tissues. Both are comprised of subcomponent isoenzymes that are released in fairly consistent patterns when myocardial injury occurs. Isoenzyme CK_2MB (found mainly in the heart) is normally absent in the serum, but becomes present and increases in a specific pattern when released from damaged myocardial cells. Isoenzymes LD_1 and LD_2 (found mainly in the heart and red blood cells) are normally present in a fairly constant ratio of about 1:2 in the serum, but begin rising after myocardial damage until the ratio reverses. Serial levels of CK and LD and isoenzymes of both are evaluated for demonstration of characteristic patterns of rise and fall when differentiating suspected acute myocardial infarction from other disorders that may cause similar symptoms. Serum aspartate aminotransferase (AST) is an enzyme found in several body organs, including large amounts in the heart, but is nonspecific for myocardial injury. It is sometimes compared to serum alanine aminotransferase (ALT) levels, which are found mainly in the liver, with only small amounts in the heart and other organs. An AST level that rises much more than an ALT level can help identify whether the etiology is due to cardiac injury. *See also Creatine Kinase, Serum; Lactate Dehydrogenase, Blood; Alanine Aminotransferase, Serum; and*

Aspartate Aminotransferase, Serum for discussion of abnormalities caused by etiologies other than cardiac.

Professional Considerations:

1. Consent form NOT required.
2. Preparation:
   A. Tube: Red-top, red/gray-top, or gold-top.
   B. MAY be drawn during hemodialysis.
3. Procedure:
   A. Draw a 5-ml venous blood sample without hemolysis.
   B. Samples are drawn immediately with suspected myocardial infarction and serially at 12, 24, and 48 hours or every 8 hours for three samples.
4. Postprocedure care:
   A. The serum should be separated and left at room temperature for LD and ALT measurement; the CK serum should be frozen if not tested within 24 hours of specimen collection.
5. Client and family teaching:
   A. Samples will be drawn in a set sequence to evaluate changes in laboratory results to facilitate the plan of care.
6. Factors that affect results:
   A. Reject hemolyzed specimens, which invalidate several values.
   B. Drugs that may cause falsely elevated LD, AST, and ALT levels include heparin (porcine, bovine). See individual tests for a more detailed listing of drugs that affect the results.
   C. Alcohol ingestion within 24 hours of specimen collection causes increased values.
   D. If intramuscular injections must be given, they should be given after or at least 1 hour before this test.
7. Other data:
   A. Previous terminology used for aspartate aminotransferase includes serum glutamic oxaloacetic transaminase (SGOT). Previous terminology for alanine aminotransferase includes serum glutamic pyruvic transaminase (SGPT) and glutamic pyruvate transaminase (GPT). Previous terminology used for lactate dehydrogenase includes lactic acid dehydrogenase (LDH).

Bibliography:

Baral R, Luo X, Watanabe H. Yamasawa I, Ibukiyama C: Role of MB isoforms in the early diagnosis of acute myocardial infarction. Int Med *33*(4):210–215, 1994.

Dorogy ML, Hooks GC, Cameron RW, Davis RC: Clinical and angiographic correlates of normal creatine kinase with elevated MB isoenzymes possible in acute myocardial infarction. Amer Heart J *130*(2):211–217, 1995.

Kee Lefever J: Handbook of Laboratory and Diagnostic Tests, 2nd ed. Norwalk, CT, Appleton and Lange, 1994.

Laurino JP, Fischberg-Bender E, Galligan S, Chang J: An immunochemical mass assay for the direct measurement of creatine kinase MB2. Ann Clin Lab Science *25*(3):252–263, 1995.

Tierney LM, McPhee SL, Papdakis MD: Current Medical Diagnosis and Treatment. Norwalk, CT, Appleton and Lange, 1995.

CARDIAC OUTPUT, THERMODILUTION, DIAGNOSTIC

Norm: 4–8 L/minute.

Usage: Evaluation of hemodynamic instability, shock states; determination of optimal myocardial function preoperatively via Starling curve; evaluation of response to fluid administration and inotropic drugs. Cardiac output is performed to determine the amount of blood being propelled forward by the heart.

Description: Cardiac output is the product of heart rate and stroke volume. It is the volume of blood ejected from the heart over the time period of 1 minute. The determinants of cardiac output are preload, afterload, and heart rate in beats per minute and stroke volume in milliliters per beat ($CO = HR \times SV$). Stroke volume is the volume of blood ejected with each ventricular contraction and is the difference between the volume of the left ventricle at end diastole and the volume remaining in the ventricle at end systole. In an average-sized adult at rest, cardiac output is approximately 4–8 L/min. In diseased states, cardiac output is usually found to be less than normal and may be so low that an adequate blood supply to the body's tissues cannot be delivered. A low cardiac output may be the result of poor filling of the ventricle (reduced preload) or poor forward emptying of the ventricle (increased afterload). Some causes of low resting cardiac output are diminished myocardial function resulting from myocardial infarction, aortic stenosis, arterial hypertension, and cardiomyopathy. The thermodilution method of cardiac output determination measures the change in core temperature in the pulmonary artery before and after injection of a specific quantity of injectate of a known temperature. The change in temperature reflects the cardiac output in an inverse manner and is used to plot a cardiac output thermodilution curve. A low cardiac output produces a greater change in temperature for a longer period of time than does a high cardiac output.

Professional Considerations:

1. Consent form IS required for insertion of pulmonary artery catheter.

Risks:

Pulmonary embolus from dislodgment of clot on catheter. *See Pulmonary Artery Catheterization, Diagnostic,* for catheter-specific risks and contraindications.

Contraindications:

None. Injections should be kept to the minimum volume needed for clients who are fluid overloaded.

2. Preparation:
   A. Client must have a pulmonary artery catheter in place.
   B. Obtain a cardiac output tubing, a 10-ml syringe, and injectate. Also obtain ice if injectate is less than 10° cooler than the client's core temperature. Iced injectate should also be used for hemodynamically unstable clients and hypothermic clients.
3. Procedure:
   A. The client may be positioned up to 60 degrees head-of-bed elevation, but should be positioned similarly for each cardiac output measurement. Hemodynamically unstable clients should be positioned supine.
   B. Cardiac output is performed through a 2- or 3-lumen pulmonary artery catheter. A 3-lumen catheter contains two lumens that exit in the right atrium for measurements of central venous pressure, cardiac output injection, and fluid infusions, and one lumen that exits in the pulmonary artery plus a thermistor at the distal catheter tip in the pulmonary artery for measurement of core blood temperature.
   C. A computation constant is selected for the specific injectate temperature and quantity, and the catheter in use is entered into the computer that will calculate cardiac output. The injectate used must be at least 10° cooler than the client's core temperature for the most accurate thermodilution curve.
   D. After the catheter placement has been verified, a bolus of 5 ml or 10 ml of iced or room temperature intravenous fluid (D5W or NS) is injected into the external catheter port that exits in the right atrium. The injection should begin as the client begins exhalation and should be completed within 4 seconds.

E. As the fluid exits into the right atrium, it cools the blood that is in the right atrium. This volume of cooled blood moves into the right ventricle and then into the pulmonary artery.

F. In the pulmonary artery, the catheter thermistor senses the temperature change as the cooled blood passes over it. The thermistor will record a decrease in temperature followed by a gradual return to body temperature as the cold solution flows distally. The resulting temperature change is plotted on a temperature-time curve by the cardiac output computer.

G. Generally, three (3) cardiac output readings are obtained and averaged to calculate cardiac output. However, the procedure may be stopped and the cardiac output calculated if the second measurement is within 10% of the first measurement.

4. Postprocedure care:
   A. Resume slow flush infusion to maintain patency of cardiac output lumen, if used before injection.
5. Client and family teaching:
   A. The client will not feel injections.
6. Factors that affect results:
   A. Too much/too little of injectate solution injected will produce erroneous values.
   B. Injection not completed within 4 seconds will produce a falsely high value.
   C. If the catheter is kinked, the cardiac output value will be falsely high.
   D. If the catheter is not inserted far enough for the cardiac output port to be distal to the tip of the cordis (introducer), retrograde injection into the cordis will produce a falsely high cardiac output.
   E. Changes in stroke volume resulting from dysrhythmias or changing heart rates can produce wide variations in serial cardiac output readings.
   F. An incorrect catheter computation constant entered into the cardiac output calculation will produce an erroneous value.
7. Other data.
   A. None.

Bibliography:

Daily EK, Schroeder JS: Techniques in Hemodynamic Monitoring, 5th ed. St. Louis, MO, CV Mosby, 1994.

Guillrani ER, Fuster V, Gersch BJ, McGoon MD, McGoon DC: Cardiology Fundamentals and Practice, Vols. I, II. St. Louis, MO, Mosby Year Book, 1991.

Medley RS, DeLapp TD, Fisher DG: Comparability of the thermodilution cardiac output method proximal injectate versus proximal infusion lumens. Heart Lung *21*(1):12, 1992.

Rubini A, DelMonte D, Catena V, Atta I, Cesaro M, Soranzo D, Rattazzi G, Alati GL: Cardiac output measurement by the thermodilution method: an in vitro test of accuracy of three commercially available automatic cardiac output computers. Inten Care Med *21*(2):154–158, 1995.

CARDIAC RADIOGRAPHY, DIAGNOSTIC

Norm: Normal size, shape, and appearance of the heart and lungs. Posterior-anterior and lateral views should demonstrate no enlargement or bulging of the right ventricle, right ventricular outflow tract, left ventricle, or pulmonary veins; and no aortic abnormalities. The left cardiac border should be convex, rather than straight.

Usage: Congestive heart failure, abnormalities of the aortic arch (calcifications); some aneurysms; transposition; evaluation of the appearance, size, and shape of the heart and lungs; and verification of invasive line placement and position.

Description: A radiograph of the thoracic area and subsequent examination of the film for abnormalities. The procedure of choice is that carried out in the radiology department with the client in a standing or erect sitting position for posterior-anterior and left-lateral views of the chest. The posterior-anterior position provides the most realistic view of cardiac size and shape. In this position, the heart is closer to the film than in an anterior-posterior view, resulting in less distortion of cardiac size and shape due to shadows created by distance.

Professional Considerations:

1. Consent form NOT required.

Risks:

Hypotension while holding breath; fetal damage during first trimester of pregnancy.

Contraindications:

First trimester of pregnancy. Assess for contraindications to performing the Valsalva maneuver (recent myocardial infarction, bradycardia). If these conditions are present, teach the client how to hold the breath without bearing down.

---

2. Preparation:
   A. Remove radiopaque objects above the waist such as jewelry and clothing with snaps. Also remove electrocardiographic patches with snaps when not contraindicated.
   B. The abdomen and pelvis should be shielded by lead during pregnancy.
3. Procedure:
   A. For the posterior-anterior view, position the client standing or sitting erect with arms held slightly out from the sides, chest expanded, and shoulders pressed forward. The radiographic film is placed against the anterior chest.
   B. For left lateral views, the client stands with his or her arms elevated from the shoulders and forearms resting on the arm of the radiographic equipment, if necessary. The radiographic film is placed against the left side of the chest.
   C. The client must take a deep breath and hold it while the radiograph is taken.
   D. For clients unable to stand or sit erect, an anterior-posterior view is taken with the client sitting in as high a Fowler's position as possible and the radiographic plate positioned behind the back and chest.
4. Postprocedure care:
   A. Replace the electrocardiographic monitoring patches and leads, if removed.
5. Client and family teaching:
   A. You must breathe in and hold your breath and lie very still during the procedure.
6. Factors that affect results:
   A. Radiopaque objects such as jewelry and wires create shadows on the film.
   B. The cardiac size and shape appear larger in an anterior-posterior radiograph than in a posterior-anterior radiograph.
   C. Cardiopulmonary congestion requires an increase in exposure.
   D. Inadequate films result when the client is unable to hold a deep inspiration during exposure.
   E. Movement obscures the clarity of the picture.
   F. Thoracic deformity such as scoliosis affects radiographic interpretation.
7. Other data:
   A. Although contraindicated during the first trimester, this is the procedure of choice when necessitated during pregnancy, as the amount of radiation delivered is up to 20 times less than that of the nuclear medicine cardiac series.

Bibliography:

Shub C: Stable angina pectoris: Cardiac evaluation and diagnostic testing. Mayo Clin Proc 65(92):243–255, 1990.

Stanford W, Galvin JR, Skorton DJ, Marcus ML: The evaluation of coronary bypass graft patency: Direct and indirect techniques other than coronary arteriography. Am J Roentgenol 156(1):15–22, 1991.

CARDIOANGIOGRAPHY, DIAGNOSTIC

(see Cardiac Catheterization, Diagnostic)

CAROTENE, SERUM

Norm:

		SI Units
Adult	50–200 µg/dl	0.74–3.72 µmol/L
	50–300 IU/l	
Child	40–130 µg/dl	0.7–2.3 µmol/L
Infant	0–40 µg/dl	0.0–0.7 µmol/L

Increased: Amenorrhea, anorexia nervosa, diarrhea, diabetes mellitus, excessive dietary carotene intake, hypercholesterolemia, hyperlipidemia, hypervitaminosis A, hypothyroidism, myxedema, nephritis (chronic), nephrotic syndrome, and pancreatitis.

Decreased: Celiac disease, cystic fibrosis, fever, infectious hepatitis, jaundice (obstructive), kwashiorkor, liver disease, low-fat diet, malabsorption, pancreatic insufficiency, poor dietary intake, pregnancy, and steatorrhea.

Description: Carotene is a fat-soluble precursor of vitamin A that exists in green and yellow vegetables. A small portion of carotene is absorbed from the intestines, and contributes to the yellow serum color. With the aid of fats and bile salts, however, the majority of carotene is normally converted to retinol in the intestines, then absorbed into the bloodstream and stored in the liver. Since low values indicate poor dietary intake or malabsorption, this test is most commonly used as a screening test for malabsorption syndrome. Carotenemia, or elevated carotene levels, is characterized by yellow skin pigmentation with no scleral color change. The client may also have malaise, itching, or weight loss. The condition is usually benign and treated with changes in diet.

Professional Considerations:

1. Consent form NOT required.
2. Preparation:
   A. Tube: Red-top, red/gray-top, or gold-top; and a paper bag.
   B. *See Client and family teaching.*
3. Procedure:
   A. Draw a 6-ml venous blood sample.
   B. Place the specimen in a paper bag or otherwise protect it from light.
4. Postprocedure care:
   A. Transport the specimen to the laboratory for immediate spinning and freezing in a plastic vial until carotene can be measured.

B. If results are low due to poor dietary intake, institute diet teaching.
5. Client and family teaching:
   A. You may have to eliminate carotene-rich foods for 2–3 days. A high-carotene diet may be prescribed for several days if the test purpose is to evaluate ability to absorb carotene.
   B. Fast for 8 hours before sampling.
6. Factors that affect results:
   A. Reject hemolyzed specimens.
7. Other data:
   A. This is a nonspecific test. There may be an overlap between carotene levels of normal clients and those with malabsorption syndromes. Dietary intake must be considered when interpreting results.

Bibliography:

Johnson EJ, Suter PM, Sahyoun N, Ribaya-Mercado JD, Russell RM: Relation between beta-carotene intake and plasma and adipose tissue concentrations of carotenoids and retinoids. Am J Clin Nutr *62*(3):598–603, 1995.

Mastroiacovo P, Pace V: Plasmatic values of some antioxidant vitamins on healthy children. Panminerva Medica *36*(4):192–194, 1994.

Torun M, Yardim S, Sargin H, Simsek B: Evaluation of serum beta-carotene levels in patients with cardiovascular diseases. J Clin Pharm Ther *19*(1): 61–63, 1994.

CAROTID DOPPLER (CAROTID ARTERY ECHOGRAM, CAROTID ARTERY ULTRASOUND), DIAGNOSTIC

Norm: 100% bloodflow throughout carotid arteries.

Usage: Noninvasive study performed to assess the presence, location, and severity of atherothrombotic disease. Study aids in detection of turbulent arterial blood flow and anatomic changes in the carotid vasculature such as stenosis or occlusion of the carotid arteries.

Description: A Doppler ultrasonic probe (which sends high-frequency sound waves) is placed on the neck over the carotid artery. The Doppler senses the reflection of moving red blood cells. The velocity of the blood flow influences the reflection of the ultrasound waves. These data are amplified and graphic recordings of the waveforms common to each vessel, along with sound recordings of the blood flow, are produced.

Professional Considerations:
1. Consent form NOT required.
2. Preparation
   A. Test is noninvasive, painless, and accurate, requiring no preprocedure preparation or postprocedure management.
   B. Obtain ultrasonic gel.
3. Procedure
   A. The client lies in a supine position.
   B. Ultrasonic gel is placed on the client's neck.
   C. The Doppler instrument is placed over the neck in the area of the carotid artery. The instrument is moved over the common carotid artery to the bifurcation of the internal and external carotid arteries.
   D. As the Doppler instrument receives reflected ultrasound waves, an audible sound is heard, and the blood flow velocity is measured and reflected as a series of images. These images allow for visualization of the vessels and vessel size.
4. Postprocedure care:
   A. Wipe the gel from the client's skin.
5. Client and family teaching:
   A. The test is painless and lasts 15 minutes or less.
6. Factors that affect results:
   A. The client must be able to lie motionless during the test.
7. Other data:
   A. None.

Bibliography:
Chang YJ, Lin DSK, Ryu SJ, Wai YY: Common carotid artery occlusion: evaluation with duplex sonography. AJNR *12*(5):1099–1105, 1995.

Urabe T, Shioya-Morikawa N: Differentiation of embolic and thrombotic middle cerebral artery occlusion using ultrasonic carotid flow velocity analysis. J Neuro Sci *1282*:181–187, 1995.

Weinstein R: Noninvasive carotid duplex ultrasound imaging for the evaluation and management of carotid atherosclerotic disease. Hematol Oncol Clin North Amer *6*(5):1131–1139, 1992.

CAROTID PHONOANGIOGRAPHY (CPA), DIAGNOSTIC

Norm: Normal graph of sound of carotid artery blood flow. Absence of bruits.

Usage: Evaluation of circulation to the brain; diagnosis of etiology of syncope, ataxia, transient ischemic attack, or other neurologic symptoms; evaluation of bruit noted on clinical physical examination.

Description: Carotid phonoangiography (CPA) is an oscillographic recording of the blood flow through the carotid arteries that provides a noninvasive study of bruits during systole and diastole. Turbulent blood flow caused by plaque, stenosis, and/or partial occlusion of the artery emits sound variations that can be recorded and appear as disruptions to the oscillographic pattern. Severity and location of the occlusion can be diagnosed quickly with this noninvasive test. CPA is about 85% accurate for detection of significant (>40%) stenosis of the carotid, and for localization of stenosis. It may be completed in conjunction with Doppler ultrasound or invasive study of carotid circulation.

Professional Considerations:
1. Consent form NOT required.
2. Preparation:
   A. Obtain special phonoangiographic equipment, transducer, recorder, and film, and/or magnetic tape for storage or recordings.
   B. *See Client and family teaching.*
3. Procedure:
   A. The client is placed in a supine position.
   B. The transducer is first placed directly over the clavicle (common carotid artery); then midway up the neck (carotid bifurcation); and, finally, directly below the mandible (internal carotid artery).
   C. At each point, soundings are made.
   D. The client is asked to hold his or her breath during each oscillographic recording.
   E. Recordings are obtained and stored on film and/or magnetic tape for study.
   F. The test may be repeated on the ipsilateral side for comparison.
4. Postprocedure care:
   A. None.
5. Client and family teaching:
   A. It is important to lie motionless and cooperate with breath-holding.
   B. Remove any jewelry and clothing from the upper chest and neck area.
6. Factors that affect results:
   A. The client must be able to cooperate with the test.
   B. Complete occlusion of the carotid will emit no flow sound to be picked up by the phono transducer.
7. Other data:
   A. None.

Bibliography:

Friedman DP: What constitutes a routine angio-graphic examination for a patient presenting with transischemic attacks or other less specific symptoms of extracranial cerebral vascular disease? Am J Roentgenol *165*(2):482–483, 1995.

Hickey JV: The Clinical Practice of Neurological and Neurosurgical Nursing. Philadelphia, JB Lippincott, 1992.

of the Body, Diagnostic; and Tomography Paranasal Sinuses, Diagnostic)

CATECHOLAMINES, FRACTIONATION, PLASMA
(see Catecholamines, Plasma)

CAT SCAN
(see Cerebral Computed Tomography, Diagnostic; Chest Tomography, Diagnostic; Computed Tomography

CATECHOLAMINES, FRACTIONATION FREE, PLASMA
(see Catecholamines, Plasma)

CATECHOLAMINES, PLASMA

Norm: Values vary by laboratory.

		SI Units
Fractionation		
Standing		
Epinephrine	0–140 pg/ml	0–762 pmol/L
Norepinephrine	200–1700 pg/ml	1088–9256 pmol/L
Dopamine	0–30 pg/ml	0–163 pmol/L
Supine		
Epinephrine	0–110 pg/ml	0–599 pmol/L
Norepinephrine	70–750 pg/ml	381–4083 pmol/L
Dopamine	0–30 pg/ml	0–163 pmol/L
Fractionation Free		
Total	150–650 pg/ml	886–3843 pmol/L

Increased Epinephrine: Anger, electroconvulsive therapy, exercise (extreme), fear, ganglioblastoma (slight increase), ganglioneuroma (slight increase), hypoglycemia, hypotension, hypothyroidism, ketoacidosis (diabetic), kidney disease, myocardial infarction (acute), neuroblastoma (slight increase), paragangliomas (slight increase), pheochromocytoma (continuous or intermittent increase), postoperatively, prolonged exposure to cold, shock, stress, thyrotoxicosis, and volume depletion. Drugs include epinephrine bitartrate, epinephrine borate, epinephrine hydrochloride, and ethanol (in large amounts).

Increased Norepinephrine: Anxiety, burns, exercise (extreme), ganglioblastoma (large increase), ganglioneuroma (large increase), hypoglycemia, hypotension, hypothyroidism, ketoacidosis (diabetic), kidney disease, myasthenia gravis, myocardial infarction (acute), neuroblastoma (large increase), paragangliomas (large in crease),

pheochromocytoma (slight increase), postoperatively, progressive muscular dystrophy, shock, thyroid disease, thyrotoxicosis, and volume depletion. Drugs include ethanol (in large amounts) and norepinephrine bitartrate.

Increased Dopamine: Ganglioneuroma and neuroblastoma. Drugs include dopamine hydrochloride.

Increased Catecholamines (Any): Drugs include aspirin, decongestants, sympathomimetics, and tricyclics.

Decreased Epinephrine: Not applicable.

Decreased Norepinephrine: Anorexia nervosa, autonomic nervous system dysfunction, and orthostatic hypotension.

Decreased Dopamine: Parkinson's disease.

Decreased Catecholamines (Any): Drugs include barbiturates and reserpine.

Description: The catecholamines (epinephrine, norepinephrine, and dopamine) are found in the adrenal medulla, neurons, and the brain. This test is used to help rule out the presence of catecholamine-secreting tumors such as pheochromocytoma.

Epinephrine is a hormone and neurotransmitter synthesized from tyrosine and secreted after the splanchnic nerve is stimulated due to hypoglycemia, stress, fear, or anger. Epinephrine acts during the body's fight-or-flight response to dilate the bronchioles, increase the heart rate, increase glycogenolysis to provide more glucose for body fuel, and decrease peripheral resistance and blood flow to the skin and kidneys.

Norepinephrine is the predominant catecholamine hormone and neurotransmitter secreted by the adrenal medulla in response to splanchnic nerve stimulation and is also secreted by certain neurons in the peripheral nervous system. Synthesized from dopamine and in the presence of tyramine, norepinephrine acts to increase blood pressure through constriction of the peripheral vasculature, dilate the pupils, and relax the gastrointestinal system. It also functions as an intermediary in epinephrine synthesis.

Dopamine is a neurotransmitter found in the brain, sympathetic ganglia, liver, lungs, intestines, and retina. A product of dopa decarboxylation, dopamine acts to dilate renal arteries, increase the heart rate, and constrict the peripheral vasculature.

In a fractionated test, total catecholamines are differentiated into the portions comprised by epinephrine, norepinephrine, and dopamine. Plasma levels reveal the balance between synthesis, release, uptake, catabolism, and excretion of catecholamines. In pheochromocytoma, the tumor secretes increased amounts of catecholamines, causing paroxysmal or persistent hypertension. Therefore, catecholamine levels are most helpful when drawn during or just after a hypertensive episode. Total catecholamine levels exceeding 1000 pg/ml are suggestive of pheochromocytoma, and levels over 2000 pg/ml are presumptive of this condition. In normal clients, epinephrine and norepinephrine results should be higher when the clients are standing than when they are supine. Absence of this difference may indicate autonomic nervous system dysfunction.

Professional Considerations:

1. Consent form NOT required.
2. Preparation:
   A. *See Client and family teaching.*
   B. Insert heparin lock 24 hours prior to the test.
   C. Tubes: Two chilled lavender-top or green-top.
   D. Notify laboratory personnel that a specimen for plasma catecholamine levels will be drawn and must be spun and frozen immediately upon arrival in the laboratory.
3. Procedure: Baseline level specimens should be collected between 0600 (6 A.M.) and 0800 (8 A.M.) as follows:
   A. The client should relax in a recumbent position prior to the procedure for 40–60 minutes.
   B. Withdraw and discard 3 ml of heparin and blood from the heparin lock. Draw a 10-ml venous blood sample from the heparin lock and inject it into a chilled, green-top or lavender-top tube, depending on laboratory requirements. Once the specimen is collected, relock the site according to institutional protocol.
   C. Follow postprocedure care instructions and have the specimen transported to the laboratory immediately.
   D. Have the client stand for 10 minutes and draw a second specimen as in step 3B. Remove or flush the heparin lock according to institutional protocol.
4. Postprocedure care:
   A. Mix the specimen well by gently inverting several times, but avoid agitation. Place the specimen in an ice bath and transport it to the laboratory immediately. Write the body position (supine or standing) and the collection time on the laboratory requisition.
5. Client and family teaching:
   A. Explain test and guidelines thoroughly, since without the client's compliance, the results are unreliable.
   B. Do not eat foods high in amines for 48 hours. These foods include avocados, bananas, beer, cheese, chocolate, cocoa, coffee, fava beans, grains, tea, vanilla, walnuts, and wine.
   C. Medications that increase catecholamines may be prescribed withheld for 48 hours. Diuretics, antihypertensives, and sympathomimetics (including nonprescriptive cold and allergy medications) must be withheld for 5–14 days.
   D. Follow a normal-sodium diet for 3 days and fast from food and fluids for 10–12 hours before sampling.

E. Avoid strenuous exercise and tobacco smoking immediately prior to testing.

F. Evaluate the client's understanding of the importance of following pretest instructions to ensure accuracy of the results.

G. Results may not be available for at least 1 week.

6. Factors that affect results:

A. Reject specimens received in the laboratory more than 5 minutes after collection. Plasma catecholamine levels drop quickly if the red blood cells are not separated within 5 minutes of specimen collection. The specimen should be spun in a refrigerated centrifuge or chilled carrier. Plasma should be separated from the red blood cells and frozen upright in a plastic vial at –70°C.

B. The trauma of direct venipuncture may increase the amount of catecholamines in the specimen.

C. Stressors such as a cold or hypoglycemia may cause elevated results.

D. The results may be invalid if the client has undergone a radioactive scan within 1 month prior to specimen collection.

E. The results of this test are unreliable in clients taking ascorbic acid, chloral hydrate, chlorpromazine, decongestants, hydralazine, isuprel, levodopa, methenamine mandelate, methyldopa, phenothiazines, quinine, quinidine, theophylline, or tricyclic antidepressants.

F. Drugs that may cause falsely elevated results include amphetamines, bronchodilators, isoproterenol hydrochloride, and vasodilators.

G. Drugs that may cause falsely decreased results include anticonvulsants, antidysrhythmics, and barbiturates.

H. A diet high in amines may elevate the results.

7. Other data:

A. Because plasma catecholamine levels are difficult to measure, urine catecholamine measurements are more often used.

B. This test is often used in conjunction with urinary levels and VMA determinations to diagnose pheochromocytoma or neuroblastoma.

C. The complete analysis may take up to 1 week.

Bibliography:

Lenders JW, Eisenhofer G, Armando I, Keiser HR, Goldstein DS, Kopin IJ: Determination of metanephrines in plasma by liquid chromatography with electrochemical detection. Clin Chem *39*(1):97–103, 1993.

Nanda AS, Feldman A, Liang CS: Acute reversal of pheochromocytoma-induced catecholamine cardiomyopathy. Clin Cardiol *18*(7):421–423, 1995.

Tietz NW (ed): Clinical Guide to Laboratory Tests, 2nd ed. Philadelphia, WB Saunders, 1990.

CATECHOLAMINES, URINE

Norms:

		SI Units
Random Urine		
Total catecholamines	0–18 µg/dl	0–103 nmol/dl
Daytime Specimen		
Total catecholamines	1.4–7.3 µg/h	8–43 nmol/h
24-Hour Urine		
Total catecholamines	0–135 µg/M^2/D^2	0–796 nmol/m^2/D^2
Panic level	>200 µg/M^2/D^2	>1180 nmol/m^2/D^2
Epinephrine		
Adult	0–15 µg	0–82 nmol/D
Children		
Age 1–4	0–6 µg/D	0–33 nmol/D
Age 4–10	0–10 µg/D	0–55 nmol/D
Age 10–15	0.5–20 µg/D	2.7–110 nmol/D
Epinephrine panic level	>50 µg/D	>295 nmol/D
Norepinephrine		
Adult	0–100 µg/D	0–590 nmol/D
Children		
Age 1–4	0–29 µg/D	0–170 nmol/D
Age 4–10	8–65 µg/D	47–380 nmol/D
Age 10–15	15–80 µg/D	89–470 nmol/D

24-Hour Urine (continued)   **SI Units**

Dopamine

Age 4 years to adult	65–400 µg/D	384-2364 nmol/D
Age 4 years or less	40–260 µg/D	236–1535 nmol/D

Increased: Burns, exercise (strenuous), ganglioneuroma, neuroblastoma, pheochromocytoma and other catecholamine-secreting tumors and stress (severe anger, anxiety). Drugs include caffeine, ethanol (large amounts), reserpine (short-term use), and sympathomimetics.

Decreased: Anorexia nervosa, familial dystonia, and idiopathic orthostatic hypotension. Drugs include guanethidine sulfate, phenothiazines, and reserpine (chronic use).

Description: Catecholamines are a group of hormones that are secreted from the adrenal medulla (epinephrine and norepinephrine) and are also released from nerve endings (epinephrine, norepinephrine, and dopamine). These hormones function in the fight-or-flight response, sympathetic nervous system functioning, blood pressure and hemodynamic controls, and response to stressors. Catecholamines are degraded and excreted by the kidneys and can be measured in random urine samples. In pheochromocytoma, the tumor secretes increased amounts of catecholamines, causing paroxysmal or persistent hypertension. Therefore, 24-hour urine catecholamine levels are helpful in detecting paroxysmal secretion that occurs throughout the day and may be missed by random plasma levels.

Professional Considerations:

1. Consent form NOT required.
2. Preparation:
   A. Obtain a clean container for random urine.
   B. For 24-hour collections, obtain a clean, 3-L container to which hydrochloric acid (HCl) preservative has been added.
3. Procedure: Random or 24-hour urine.
   A. *Random collection:* Collect a 50-ml random urine specimen in a clean container.
   B. *24-hour collections:*
      i. Discard the first morning urine specimen.
      ii. Begin to time a 24-hour urine collection.
      iii. Save all the urine voided for 24 hours in a refrigerated, 3-L container to which HCl preservative has been added. Include the urine voided at the end of the 24-hour period.
      iv. For catheterized clients, keep the drainage bag on ice and empty the urine into the acidified collection container hourly.
4. Postprocedure care:
   A. Compare the urine quantity in the specimen container with the urinary output record for the test. If the specimen contains less urine than was recorded as output, some of the sample may have been discarded, invalidating the test.
   B. Document the 24-hour urine quantity on the laboratory requisition.
   C. Keep the specimen chilled until testing.
5. Client and family teaching:
   A. Save all the urine voided in the 24-hour period, and urinate before defecating to avoid loss of urine.
6. Factors that affect results:
   A. All the urine voided for the 24-hour period must be included to avoid a falsely low result.
   B. The client should have a quiet environment and avoid strenuous exercise throughout the specimen collection period.
   C. Foods that may cause falsely elevated levels include bananas, beer, Chianti wines, cheese, walnuts, and coffee.
   D. Hypoglycemia may cause falsely elevated levels.
   E. Drugs that may cause unreliable results due to interference with the laboratory fluorescence testing method include ascorbic acid, ampicillin, ampicillin sodium, chloral hydrate, epinephrine bitartrate, epinephrine borate, epinephrine hydrochloride, erythromycin, erythromycin ethylsuccinate, hydralazine hydrochloride, methenamine mandelate, methyldopa, methyldopate hydrochloride, niacin, quinidine gluconate, quinidine polygalacturonate, quinidine sulfate, riboflavin, salicylates, tetracyclines, and vitamin B complex.
7. Other data:
   A. A random urine sample may be prescribed just following a hypertensive episode for pheochromocytoma diagnosis.
   B. Urine samples are easier to study than plasma catecholamines and so are more frequently used for diagnosis.

C. Urine levels of vanillylmandelic acid (VMA) (urinary metabolite of epinephrine), metanephrine (urinary metabolite of epinephrine and norepinephrine), and homovanillic acid (urinary metabolite of dopamine) are often prescribed in conjunction with this test.

D. 24-hour urine catecholamines are more reliable than plasma catecholamines.

Bibliography:

Ross GA, Newbould EL, Thomas J, Bouloux PM, Besser GM, Perrett D, Grossman A: Plasma and 24-hour urinary catecholamine concentrations in normal patient populations. Ann Clin Biochem *301*:38–44, 1993.

Tormey WB, Fitzgerald RJ: Lack of uniformity in the clinical approach to the interpretation of urinary catecholamines and chemical metabolites. Irish J Med Sci *164*(2): 146–150, 1995.

CATHEPSIN-D, SPECIMEN

Norm:

Normal reference range	<30 pmol/mg CP
Borderline-positive	30–70 pmol/mg CP
Positive (high-risk)	>70 pmol/mg CP

Increased: Increased total antigen amounts of Cathepsin D in breast tissue have been associated with increased disease recurrence, more frequent metastasis, and increased mortality in breast cancer clients.

Decreased: Not clinically significant.

Description: Cathepsin D is an independent prognostic factor associated with high risk for metastasis in breast cancer. It is an estrogen-inducible lysosomal protease that is believed to have a role in tumor invasion and metastasis. The overexpression of Cathepsin D is associated with visceral and increased soft tissue metastases and decreased overall survival.

Professional Considerations:

1. Consent NOT required, but IS required for the procedure used to obtain the specimen. See the specific procedure for risks and contraindications.

2. Preparation:
   A. Obtain biopsy equipment.

3. Procedure:
   A. Specimen requirement: 0.5–1.0 g of solid tumor, trimmed of excess fat.
   B. The tissue is cut into small pieces, then quick-frozen on dry ice in a cryostat or in liquid nitrogen within 20 minutes of excision.
   C. The specimen is placed in a 60-ml biopsy bottle without formalin, with the cap secured.
   D. Label the specimen bottle with the client's name, the date collected, and the client's identification number.
   E. The tissue must remain frozen.

4. Postprocedure care:
   A. Apply a dry, sterile dressing to the biopsy site.
   B. Use a mild analgesic for site tenderness.

5. Client and family teaching:
   A. Use a mild analgesic for site tenderness.
   B. Notify the physician for increased/purulent drainage, redness, or increasing tenderness at the site.
   C. This test is investigational.

6. Factors that affect results:
   A. None found.

7. Other data:
   A. Cathepsin D may be prescribed in combination with other prognostic tests. The test has been recommended for investigative use only and should not be used as a diagnostic procedure without confirmation of the diagnosis by another medically established diagnostic product or procedure.

Bibliography:

Armes OA, Gerald WL, et al.: Immunohistochemical detection of Cathepsin D in T2 No Mo breast carcinoma. Am J Surg Pathol *18*:158, 1994.

Schulz DC, Bagel S, Wright LM, Tucker S, Lange MK, Tachowsky T, Longo S, Meedbala S, Alhadeff JA: Western blotting and enzymatic activity analysis of Cathepsin D in breast tissue and sera of patients with breast cancer and benign breast disease of normal controls. Cancer Res *54*(1): 48–54, 1994.

CBC

(see Complete Blood Count, Blood)

CD4

(see Acquired Immune Deficiency Syndrome Evaluation Battery, Diagnostic)

CEA

(see Carcinoembryonic Antigen, Serum)

CELL WALL–DEFECTIVE BACTERIA (L-FORM CULTURE, L-PHASE ORGANISM CULTURE STUDIES), CULTURE

Norm: Negative. No growth.

Positive: : Indicates infection by bacteria that has developed strains with cell wall variances, which makes differential diagnosis difficult by normal culture studies. Examples are *Haemophilus influenza, Enterobacteriaceae, Staphylococcus aureus,* and Cat Scratch disease.

Description: Cell wall–defective bacteria culture is a specific culture method used to detect and study bacteria that have developed a genetic strain with a different (i.e., defective) cell wall. The strain develops as an adaptation to survive antibiotic therapy or other stressors in the bacterial environment, such as phazes, amino acids, hyperimmune disease, muralytic enzymes, or lysoenzymes. This method uses hyperosmolar or hypertonic culture matter, which allows some replication to the parental type for identification.

Professional Considerations:

1. Consent form NOT required.
2. Preparation:
   A. Obtain a hypertonic culture medium container for blood cultures.
   B. Obtain the routine equipment needed according to the site to be cultured.
3. Procedure:
   A. *Blood culture:* Draw a 10-ml blood sample in a special hypertonic culture media container.
   B. *Sites other than blood:* Culture the suspected infection site by routine methods and notify the laboratory of the special culture test required. *(See Culture, Routine, Specimen.)*
4. Postprocedure care:
   A. Write the study requested, recent antibiotic therapy, specimen source, date, and clinical symptoms on the laboratory requisition.
5. Client and family teaching:
   A. Results may take up to 4 weeks.
6. Factors that affect results:
   A. Cell wall–defective bacteria cultures are very sensitive to contamination. Strict aseptic technique is important.
7. Other data:
   A. None.

Bibliography:

Balows A (ed): Manual of Clinical Microbiology, 5th ed. Washington, DC, American Society for Microbiology, 1290–1292, 1991.

Ivanova E, Andreeva S, Veljanov D, Raspopova A: Radiometric study on the invasion capability of Streptococcus pyogenes A49 L-forms in tissue cultures. Acta Microbiol Bulg, *29:*73–78, 1993.

Shimokawa O, Ikeda M, Umeda A, Nakayama H: Serum inhibits penicillin-induced L-form growth in Staphylococcus aureus: a note of caution on the use of serum in cultivation of bacterial L-forms. J Bacteriol *176*(9):2751–2753, 1994.

C-ERB-2

(see HER-2 Neu Oncogene, Specimen)

CEREBRAL ANGIOGRAM (CEREBRAL ANGIOGRAPHY), DIAGNOSTIC

Norm: Symmetrical pattern of vascular circulation to the brain with no areas of absent vessels. The vessels are smooth and there are no areas of pooling of the contrast dye (which would indicate bleeding from the vessels or aneurysm).

Usage: Suspected cerebral aneurysm or other cerebral vascular disease such as fistulas, spasms, atherosclerosis, or arteriovenous malformations; tumors of the brain; and work-up for transient ischemic attack or other neurologic signs and symptoms. The need for angiography may be suggested by brain scan findings.

Description: Cerebral angiogram is a procedure performed in the radiology department using a special radiographic machine with a rapid biplane cassette changer. It involves a series of radiographic views of the cerebral circulation obtained after intra-arterial injection of a contrast medium showing the patterns of circulation, any interruptions to circulation, or changes in vessel wall appearance.

Professional Considerations:

1. Consent form IS required.

Risks:

Allergy to contrast medium, aphasia, embolus, hematoma, hemiplegia, hemorrhage, infection, loss of consciousness, renal toxicity, transient ischemic attack.

Contraindications:

Atherosclerosis; coagulopathy, dehydration; previous allergy to iodine, shellfish, or contrast medium; renal disease, hepatic disease; thyroid disease; or allergy to contrast medium; during pregnancy or breast-feeding.

2. Preparation:
   A. *See Client and family teaching.*
   B. Have emergency equipment readily available.
   C. Remove all jewelry and metal objects such as hairpins from the client's head area.
   D. Obtain sterile gauze, tape, alcohol, or other skin-cleansing agent, arterial catheter, razor, contrast medium, normal saline or heparinized normal saline, syringes, and automatic contrast injector.
   E. For clients who are unable to cooperate, and especially for children, a general anesthetic may be administered by an anesthesia professional.

3. Procedure:
   A. The client is placed supine on a special radiographic table.
   B. A site for intra-arterial injection is selected and prepared by cleansing the skin with 70% alcohol or povidone-iodine and injecting a local anesthetic.
      i. *Carotid artery:* The client's neck must be hyperextended by placing a rolled towel under the shoulders, and his or her head must be immobilized with tape.
      ii. *Femoral artery:* The area must be shaved prior to cleansing. A long catheter is threaded through the femoral artery to the aortic arch.
      iii. *Brachial artery:* The area may require shaving prior to cleansing. The brachial artery is the least common injection site. A blood pressure cuff is applied distal to the injection site and inflated before the injection to prevent contrast medium flow to the lower arm.
   C. Needle/catheter placement appropriate to the site is performed by the physician and verified by fluoroscopy.
   D. Contrast medium (xenon-133 or technetium-99m pertechnetate) is injected and the client is carefully observed for signs of an allergic reaction such as hives, flushing, or stridor.
   E. A series of radiographs of the head, both of the anterior and lateral views, are taken during the 5–15 seconds after the injection. Approximately another 6 seconds after the arteries appear, capillary and venous blood flow may be studied by radiographs.
   F. The contrast injection may be repeated and the views varied to complete the study, as indicated by the suspected abnormalities.
   G. The artery catheter is kept open with continuous or intermittent flushing or with heparinized normal saline.

4. Postprocedure care:
   A. The catheter is withdrawn and pressure is applied to the artery for at least 15 minutes.
   B. Apply a dry, sterile or pressure dressing to the site and observe for bleeding or hematoma formation at the catheter insertion site.
   C. Maintain bedrest for 12–24 hours.
   D. Assess neurologic status and vital signs hourly × 4 hours, then every 4 hours for 20 hours.
   E. For femoral or brachial approaches, immobilize the leg or arm straight for 12 hours. Check color, motion, temperature, sensation, and distal pulses of the immobilized extremity every 15 minutes × 4 hours, then every 30 minutes × 2 hours, then every 1 hour × 4 hours, then every 4 hours × 12 hours.
   F. For the carotid approach, observe for respiratory distress, dysphagia, or hoarseness, which may indicate extravasation of the dye.
   G. If general anesthesia was used, continue the assessment of respiratory status and follow institutional protocol for postsedation monitoring. Typical monitoring includes continuous ECG monitoring and pulse oximetry, with continual assessments (q 5–15 minutes) of the airway, vital signs, and neurologic status until the client is lying quietly awake, is breathing independently, and responds appropriately to commands spoken in a normal tone.

5. Client and family teaching:
   A. Fast from food and fluids for 4–8 hours prior to the procedure.
   B. It is important to lie still for this test. A sensation of burning may be felt due to the injection of the contrast medium, but this feeling lasts for only a few moments.

6. Factors that affect results:
   A. Head movement during the study obscures the clarity of the radiographs.
   B. Radiopaque objects such as earrings obstruct the view of the internal vasculature.

7. Other data:
   A. The femoral artery approach has the advantage of providing visualization of both carotid arteries and both vertebral arteries, extending the study to the supply vessels.

Bibliography:

Friedman DP: What constitutes a routine angiographic examination for a patient presenting with TIA or other less specific symptoms of extracranial cerebral vascular disease? Am J Roentgenol *165*(2):482, 1995.

Heiserman JE, Dean BL, Hodak JA, Flom RA, Bird CR, Drayer BP, Fram EK: Neurologic complications of cerebral angiography. AJNR *15*(8):1401–1407, 1994.

Hoff DJ, Wallace MC, Brugge KG, Gentile F: Rotational angiography assessment of cerebral aneurysms. AJNR *15*(10):1945–1948, 1994.

CEREBRAL ANGIOGRAPHY
(see Cerebral Angiogram, Diagnostic)

CEREBRAL COMPUTED TOMOGRAPHY, DIAGNOSTIC

Norm: Normal appearing skull and symmetry, and size of cerebral or other brain tissue. Cerebrum appears with black-gray shadings, and bone or other very dense tissues appear white. There is normally no evidence of tumor, high density to whitish hematoma, edema, or congenital abnormalities such as hydrocephalus.

Usage: Brain tumor (astrocytoma, meningioma, metastatic, or primary lesions); cerebral atrophy or infarction; cerebral edema; cerebrovascular accident (CVA); evaluation of neurologic symptomatology; evaluation of effects of surgery, radiation, or chemotherapeutic treatment of intracranial tumors; head injury; hematoma (epidural, subdural); hydrocephalus; and other acute hemorrhage.

Description: Computed tomography (CT) utilizes special radiographic equipment and computers to produce a series of images (or tomographs) of cross sections of the brain tissues. Images may be "slices" taken of the skull and brain across anterior-posterior, horizontal, sagittal, or coronal planes. Although contrast medium may be used, the test is often noninvasive and therefore provides a safe, effective diagnostic tool for the study of tumors of the brain, evaluating neurologic clinical changes, evaluating CVA or intracranial bleeds, and assessing clients with possible head injury for hematoma before symptoms are evident.

Professional Considerations:

1. Consent form IS required when contrast medium is injected as part of the study.

Risks:
Allergic reaction to contrast media (itching, hives, rash, tight feeling in the throat, shortness of breath, bronchospasm, anaphylaxis, death), dehydration, renal toxicity, vomiting.

Contraindications:
Claustrophobia. Dehydration, severe liver or kidney disease, previous allergy to contrast medium, iodine or shellfish, pregnancy and renal insufficiency, if CT with contrast will be performed. Weight >136 kg or >300 pounds may exceed the capabilities of some equipment.

2. Preparation:
   A. Remove all jewelry, hairpins, wigs, and/or dentures.
   B. Establish intravenous access and have emergency equipment readily available if contrast medium will be used.
   C. Have emergency equipment readily available for CT with contrast.

3. Procedure:
   A. The client is placed on a movable radiographic table in a supine position. The table has a specialized headrest with straps that are positioned to immobilize the head.
   B. The table head is moved into a circular CT scanner, which moves around the client's head, taking an extensive series of radiographs at each degree of a 180-degree arch.
   C. The automated computer then produces a reconstruction of the images, which shows slices through the skull and the brain.
   D. The study may then continue to include intravenous administration of 50–100 ml xenon or other preparation. A second series of views is completed. The client is observed for rash or respiratory difficulty, which may indicate reaction to the contrast medium. Reactions develop within 30 minutes.

4. Postprocedure care:
   A. None for CT without contrast.
   B. For CT with contrast, observe for side effects such as headache, nausea, and vomiting and delayed hypersensitivity reaction.
   C. Resume previous diet.

5. Client and family teaching:
   A. You must lie very still for this test.
   B. If a contrast medium will be used, fast from midnight before the test.
   C. Results are normally available the same day.
   D. Inform CT personnel if you feel claustrophobic in enclosed spaces.

6. Factors that affect results:
   A. Movement of the client's head interferes with the quality of the films.
   B. Metal objects such as jewelry or hairpins interfere with complete visualization.

7. Other data:
   A. Computed tomography is an expensive, highly technical study.

B. Because this is a noninvasive study with rapidly improving technology, it is growing in importance as a screening for head trauma or suspected head trauma and as part of a general neurologic work-up.

C. Contrast medium is often needed for visualization of tumors and subdural hematomas.

D. *See Computed Tomography of the Body, Diagnostic.*

Bibliography:

Awadalla S, Doster SK, Yamada KA: Neurologic emergencies in internal medicine. *In* Ewald GA, McKenzie CR (eds): Manual of Medical Therapeutics, 28th ed. Department of Medicine, Washington University School of Medicine, St. Louis, MO, pp 535–541, 1995.

Hossain Naheedy M: Normal CT and MRI anatomy of the brain. *In* Haaga JR, Lanzieri CF, Sartoris DJ, Zerbouni EA (eds): Computed Tomography and Magnetic Resonance Imaging of the Whole Body, 3rd ed, Vol 1. St. Louis, MO, Mosby Year Book, pp 75–102, 1994.

CEREBROSPINAL FLUID, CYTOLOGY, SPECIMEN
(see Cerebrospinal Fluid, Routine, Culture and Cytology)

CEREBROSPINAL FLUID, FUNGUS, CULTURE
(see Cerebrospinal Fluid, Routine, Culture and Cytology)

CEREBROSPINAL FLUID, GLUCOSE, SPECIMEN

Norm: (Fasting) 50–80% of serum glucose.

		SI Units
Adult	40–80 mg/dl	2.2–4.4 mmol/L
Premature infant	24–63 mg/dl	1.3–3.5 mmol/L
Full-term infant	34–119 mg/dl	1.9–6.6 mmol/L
Child	35–75 mg/dl	1.9–4.1 mmol/L

Increased: Brain tumor, cerebral hemorrhage, cerebral trauma, diabetic coma, hyperglycemia, hypothalamic lesions, increased intracranial pressure, and uremia.

Decreased: Brain abscess, brain tumor, cancer, central nervous system sarcoidosis, choroid plexus tumor, coccidioidomycosis, encephalitis (mumps or herpes simplex origin), hypoglycemia, increased intracranial pressure, leukemic infiltration, lupus myelopathy, lymphocytic choriomeningitis, lymphoma, melanomatosis, meningeal carcinomatosis, meningitis (acute pyogenic, aseptic, chemical, cryptococcal, fungal, granulomatous, pyogenic, rheumatoid, tuberculous, viral), neurosyphilis, rheumatoid arthritis, subarachnoid hemorrhage, toxoplasmosis, and tuberculoma of brain.

Description: Cerebrospinal fluid (CSF) glucose content is related to the blood serum glucose content of 1-4 hours earlier. Most abnormalities result in a decreased CSF glucose due to increased utilization of glucose by the pathogenic process. This test is interpreted by comparing a blood glucose level to CSF glucose level.

Professional Considerations:

1. Consent form IS required for the lumbar puncture, which is necessary to obtain the specimen. *See Lumbar Puncture, Diagnostic* for procedure risks and contraindications.

2. Preparation:
   A. Obtain a lumbar puncture tray, sterile drapes, and 1–2% Xylocaine.
   B. Tube: Red-top, red/gray-top, or gold-top.

3. Procedure:
   A. Draw a 1-ml blood sample.
   B. 3–10 ml of CSF is collected by a physician in sequentially numbered sterile glass tubes via a spinal tap between L3-4 or L4-5, or from the ventricles of the brain during special procedures.

4. Postprocedure care:
   A. Transport the specimens to the laboratory immediately. Analysis must be performed on a freshly collected specimen to avoid erroneous results due to glycolysis.
   B. Refrigerate the CSF if it is not analyzed promptly.

5. Client and family teaching:
   A. *See Lumbar Puncture, Diagnostic.*

6. Factors that affect results:
   A. Falsely decreased levels may be caused by cellular and bacterial utilization if the test is not performed immediately.
   B. *See Lumbar Puncture, Diagnostic.*

7. Other data:
   A. *See Lumbar Puncture, Diagnostic.*

Bibliography:

Kjeldsberg CR, Knight JA (eds): Body Fluids: Laboratory Examination of Amniotic, Cerebrospinal, Seminal, Serous & Synovial Fluids, 3rd ed. Chicago: ASCP Press, 1993, pp 65–157.

Sunderland PM: The neurologic system: structure and function of the nervous system. In: McCance KL, Huether SE (eds): Pathophysiology: the Biologic Basis for Disease in Adults and Children, 2nd ed. St. Louis, MO: Mosby Year Book, 1994.

CEREBROSPINAL FLUID, IMMUNOGLOBULIN G (IgG), IMMUNOGLOBULIN G RATIOS AND IMMUNOGLOBULIN G INDEX, IMMUNOGLOBULIN G SYNTHESIS RATE, SPECIMEN

Norm:

IgG:	0.5–5 mg/dl (5–50 mg/L, SI units), or <12% of CSF total protein.
IgG/albumin ratio:	22–28% of serum IgG/albumin ratio.
IgG index:	0.3–0.7.
Immunoglobulin G synthesis rate:	–9.9 to +3.3 mg/day or 0.14 ± 1.8 mg/day.

Increased: Brain tissue destruction, CNS infection (chronic), CNS lupus erythematosus, CNS vasculitis, Guillain-Barré syndrome, multiple sclerosis, neurosyphilis, and Sjögren's syndrome (primary with CNS involvement).

Decreased Immunoglobulin G: Not applicable.

Decreased Immunoglobulin G Index: Contamination of cerebrospinal fluid (CSF) with blood from spinal tap, intracerebral hemorrhage, or disturbance of the blood-brain barrier.

Decreased Immunoglobulin G Synthesis Rate: Not applicable.

Description: *IgG antibodies* comprise a portion of immunoglobulin proteins secreted by beta-lymphocytes. They act as antibacterial and antiviral neutralizers of toxins produced by bacteria and viruses by activating phagocytic cells. Although slow to develop, they remain present in CSF long after the bacteria and viruses have disappeared and reappear rapidly on subsequent exposure to the antigens. IgG antibodies are identified by electrophoretic testing of the CSF that separates the protein into its component factors.

The *IgG ratio and IgG index* help rule out the possibility that blood has entered the CSF, bringing with it increased amounts of IgG antibodies. If this is the case, IgG and albumin will be present in about the same proportion in which they are present in the bloodstream, as evidenced by the IgG/albumin ratio of CSF compared to the IgG/albumin ratio of serum.

The *IgG index* measures CSF production of IgG by the following formula:

$$\text{(CSF IgG/CSF albumin)} \div \text{(serum IgG/serum albumin)}$$

The elevation of either measure indicates the presence of CNS disease.

The *IgG synthesis rate* helps rule out the possibility that blood has entered the CSF, bringing with it increased amounts of IgG antibodies. If this is the case, IgG synthesis will be greater in CSF than in serum, indicating the presence of CNS disease. The rate is calculated according to the "formula of Tourtellote":

$$\text{IgG synthesis (mg/day)} = [(IgG_{CSF} - IgG_{serum}/369) - (Alb_{CSF} - Alb_{serum}/230) \times (IgG_{serum}/Alb_{serum})\,0.43] \times 5$$

Professional Considerations:

1. Consent form IS required for the lumbar puncture, which is necessary to obtain CSF. *See Lumbar Puncture, Diagnostic* for procedure risks and contraindications.
2. Preparation:
   A. A CT scan is typically performed to rule out increased intracranial pressure prior to lumbar puncture in critically ill clients or those with changed mental status.
   B. Obtain a lumbar puncture tray, sterile drapes, and 1–2% Xylocaine.
   C. Tube: Red-top, red/gray-top, or gold-top.
3. Procedure:
   A. 3–10 ml of CSF is collected by a physician in sequentially numbered sterile glass tubes via a spinal tap between L3-

4 or L4-5, or from the ventricles of the brain during special procedures.

B. Draw a 2-ml blood sample for IgG/albumin ratio (also known as IgG/albumin index) and comparison of the serum and CSF IgG.

4. Postprocedure care:

A. See also Lumbar Puncture, Diagnostic.

B. Transport the specimens to the laboratory immediately.

C. Refrigerate the CSF if it is not analyzed promptly.

5. Client and family teaching:

A. See Lumbar Puncture, Diagnostic.

6. Factors that affect results:

A. This test should be performed on tube 2 or higher to lessen the chance of contamination of the specimen with blood from a traumatic spinal tap.

B. The results are invalidated if the client has recently undergone a myelogram.

C. Immunoglobulin G synthesis rate norms vary by laboratory.

D. Protein >100 mg/dl results in yellow-tinged CSF.

7. Other data:

A. The possibility exists that CSF IgG may be elevated due to leakage of serum into the spinal canal during disruption of the blood-brain barrier. The CSF IgG ratios and IgG index test should be performed to rule out this possibility.

B. The IgG synthesis rate sensitivity is 70–96%, which is slightly less sensitive and reproducible than the IgG index.

C. In one study, 55% of clients with multiple sclerosis had an elevated IgG synthesis rate.

D. See also Lumbar Puncture, Diagnostic.

Bibliography:

Kjeldsberg CR, Knight JA (eds): Body Fluids: Laboratory Examination of Amniotic, Cerebrospinal, Seminal, Serous & Synovial Fluids, 3rd ed. Chicago: ASP Press, 1993, pp 65–157.

Tourtellotte WW, Potvin AR, Fleming JO, et al.: Multiple sclerosis: Measurement and validation of central nervous system IgG synthesis rate. Neurology 30:240–244, 1980.

CEREBROSPINAL FLUID, LACTIC ACID, SPECIMEN

Norm:

	SI Units
9–26 mg/dl	1.13–3.23 mmol/L

Increased: Brain abscess, central nervous system carcinoma, cerebral infarct, cerebral ischemia, cerebral trauma, hydrocephalus, hypotension, increased cerebrospinal fluid (CSF), white blood cells, intracranial hemorrhage, low CSF glucose, meningitis (bacterial, fungal, tuberculous), multiple sclerosis, respiratory alkalosis, and seizures.

Decreased: Not clinically significant.

Description: Elevated cerebrospinal fluid (CSF) lactic acid levels indicate increased glucose utilization and anaerobic metabolism associated with decreased oxygenation of the brain and/or increased intracranial pressure. This test aids in the differentiation of meningitis and in identification of central nervous system disease processes.

Professional Considerations:

1. Consent form IS required for the lumbar puncture, which is necessary to obtain CSF. See Lumbar Puncture, Diagnostic for procedure risks and contraindications.

2. Preparation:

A. A CT scan is typically performed to rule out increased intracranial pressure prior to the lumbar puncture in critically ill clients or those with changed mental status.

B. See also Lumbar Puncture, Diagnostic.

C. Obtain a lumbar puncture tray, sterile drapes, and 1-2% Xylocaine.

3. Procedure:

A. 3–10 ml of CSF is collected by a physician in sequentially numbered sterile glass tubes via a spinal tap between L3-4 or L4-5, or from the ventricles of the brain during special procedures.

4. Postprocedure care:

A. See Lumbar Puncture, Diagnostic.

5. Client and family teaching:

A. See Lumbar Puncture, Diagnostic.

6. Factors that affect results:

A. Discard the first specimen because it is most likely to be contaminated with blood.

B. Lactic acid determination should be performed on tube 2 or higher to lessen the chance of blood contamination.

C. Refrigerate the CSF if it is not analyzed promptly.

7. Other data:

A. Cell counts and other chemical and serologic studies may also be performed on this sample.

B. See also Lumbar Puncture, Diagnostic.

Bibliography:

Dager SR, Kenny MA, Artru AA, Metzger HD, Bowden DM, Rainey JM: Effects of sodium lactate infusion on cisternal lactate and carbon dioxide levels. Am J Psychiatry 150(10):1568, 1993.

Travlos A, Anton HA, Wing P: Cerebrospinal fluid cell count following spinal cord injury. Arch Phys Med Rehabil 75(3):293–296, 1994.

Wevers RA, Engelke U, Wendel U, de Jong JG, Gabreels FJ, Heerschap A: Standardized method for high-resolution 1H-NMR of cerebrospinal fluid. Clin Chem *41*(5):744-751, 1995.

CEREBROSPINAL FLUID, MYCOBACTERIA, CULTURE
(see Cerebrospinal Fluid, Routine, Culture and Cytology, Specimen)

CEREBROSPINAL FLUID, MYELIN BASIC PROTEIN, OLIGOCLONAL BANDS, PROTEIN, AND PROTEIN ELECTROPHORESIS, SPECIMEN

Norm:

		SI Units
Myelin Basic Protein		
Negative	<4 ng/ml	<4 mg/L
Active demyelination	>6 ng/ml	>6 mg/L
Oligoclonal Bands	Absent	
Total Protein		
Adults		
20–40 years		
Lumbar	15–45 mg/dl	150–450 mg/L
Cisternal	15–25 mg/dl	150–250 mg/L
Ventricular	5–15 mg/dl	50–150 mg/L
40–50 years	20–50 mg/dl	200–500 mg/L
50–60 years	20–55 mg/dl	200–550 mg/L
>60 years	30–60 mg/dl	300–600 mg/L
Children		
Premature infant	400 mg/dl	400 mg/L
Full-term newborn	20–170 mg/dl	200–1700 mg/L
1–4 weeks	30–150 mg/dl	300–1500 mg/L
4–12 weeks	20–100 mg/dl	200–1000 mg/L
3–6 months	15–50 mg/dl	150–500 mg/L
6 months–10 years	10–30 mg/dl	100–300 mg/L
10–20 years	15–45 mg/dl	150–450 mg/L

Protein Electrophoresis		Fraction of Total CSF Protein
Prealbumin	2–7%	0.02–0.07
Albumin	45–76%	0.45–0.76
Alpha$_1$ globulin	1.1–7%	0.01–0.07
Alpha$_2$ globulin	3–12%	0.03–0.12
Beta globulin	7.5–18%	0.07–0.18
Gamma globulin	3–13%	0.03–0.13

Increased Myelin Basic Protein: Cerebral infarcts, demyelinating diseases, and multiple sclerosis (acute).

Increased Oligoclonal Bands: CNS lesions (destructive), CNS lupus erythematosus, CNS vasculitis, diabetes mellitus, Guillain-Barré syndrome, multiple sclerosis, neurosyphilis, panencephalitis (progressive rubella, subacute sclerosing), polyneuropathy, and Sjögren's syndrome (primary involving the CNS).

Increased Protein: Anesthetics (spinal), arteriosclerosis (cerebral), aseptic meningeal reaction, brain abscess, brain tumor, cerebral aneurysm (ruptured), coccidioidomycosis, cord tumor, diabetic neuropathy, encephalitis (postinfectious), Froin's syndrome, Guillain-Barré syndrome, head trauma (bloody), heavy metal poisoning, hemorrhage (intracerebral, subarachnoid), herpes zoster, hyperproteinemia, infections (acute, coxsackie virus, echovirus), lead encephalopathy, measles, meningitis (acute pyogenic, bacterial, cryptococcal, fungal, tuberculous, viral), meningoencephalitis (bacterial, mycotic), multiple sclerosis, mumps, myxedema, neuropathy (retrobulbar), poliomyelitis (acute anterior), polyneuritis (ascending), sarcoidosis, syphilis (tabes dorsalis, general paresis, meningovascular), systemic lupus erythematosus, thrombosis (cerebral), and toxoplasmosis (congenital). Drugs that increase cerebrospinal fluid (CSF) protein at toxic levels include ethanol, isopropanol, phenytoin, and phenytoin sodium.

Protein Electrophoresis:

Increased Beta-Globulin: Cerebrovascular disease, meningitis (acute), neoplasms.

Increased Gamma Globulin: Multiple sclerosis, neurosyphilis, and subacute sclerosing leukoencephalitis.

Increased IgG: Guillain-Barré syndrome, meningoencephalitis (viral), multiple sclerosis, neurosyphilis, subacute sclerosing panencephalitis, and systemic lupus erythematosus of the CNS.

Decreased Myelin Basic Protein: Not applicable.

Decreased Oligoclonal Bands: Not applicable.

Decreased Protein: Not applicable.

Description: *Myelin basic protein* is a part of the myelin protein that comprises the sheath surrounding myelinated nerves. The myelin sheath surrounds and insulates nerve axons and functions to speed nerve impulse conduction. In demyelinating diseases, the myelin sheath is broken down, resulting in the release of myelin basic protein into the CSF. The detection of myelin basic protein in CSF aids in the diagnosis and staging of demyelinating diseases.

Oligoclonal bands are identified via protein electrophoresis, which separates CSF protein into its component factors. They are present only in certain CNS diseases that cause the normally homogenous gamma globulin to break up into specific bands called oligoclonal bands. This signifies the presence of antibodies produced in the CNS. Oligoclonal bands help differen-

tiate CNS diseases that produce similar signs and symptoms.

Elevated CSF *protein* levels provide a nonspecific indicator of serious disease. Protein levels normally remain constant and are elevated in CSF only during increased tissue catabolism or by a disturbance in the normal capillary impermeability to plasma proteins.

Electrophoretic testing of CSF separates the protein into its component factors. Synthesis of the immunocompetent cells contained in the CNS and small amounts of protein that diffuse from the bloodstream account for the protein content of the CSF. Under normal circumstances, CSF contains minute amounts of protein. Inflammation and infection increase the permeability of blood vessels, allowing all proteins to more easily cross the blood-brain barrier. Certain disease states produce characteristic changes in specific types of CSF protein, such as albumin, alpha globulin, beta globulin, and gamma globulin. Electrophoresis is a measurement of proteins, which under the influence of an electrical field, at a pH of 8.6, separate by charge, size, and shape. This separation produces homogeneous bands that are plotted on specially treated paper. IgG immunoglobulin is the principle immunoglobulin represented with protein electrophoresis.

Professional Considerations:

1. Consent form IS required for the lumbar puncture, which is necessary to obtain CSF. *See Lumbar Puncture, Diagnostic* for procedure risks and contraindications.
2. Preparation:
   A. A CT scan is typically performed to rule out increased intracranial pressure prior to the lumbar puncture in critically ill clients or those with changed mental status.
   B. *See Lumbar Puncture, Diagnostic.*
3. Procedure:
   A. 3–10 ml of CSF is collected by a physician in sequentially numbered sterile glass tubes via a spinal tap between L3-4 or L4-5, or from the ventricles of the brain during special procedures.
4. Postprocedure care:
   A. Apply a Band-Aid over the spinal tap site.
   B. *See also Lumbar Puncture, Diagnostic.*
   C. Refrigerate the CSF if it is not analyzed promptly.
   D. Monitor for headaches, dizziness, or change in level of consciousness.

5. Client and family teaching:
   A. *See also Lumbar Puncture, Diagnostic.*
6. Factors that affect results:
   A. Discard the first specimen.
   B. Myelin basic protein determination should be performed on tube 2.
   C. Cell counts and other chemical and serologic studies may also be performed on this specimen.
   D. Transport the specimens to the laboratory immediately. Analysis must be performed promptly on freshly collected specimens to avoid erroneous results due to cell lysis and disintegration.
   E. Falsely elevated protein levels may result from a traumatic spinal puncture.
   F. Drugs that may cause falsely elevated CSF protein results include aspirin, chlorpromazine, phenacetin, salicylates, streptomycin sulfate, and sulfonamides.
7. Other data:
   A. Serum electrophoresis should be performed if oligoclonal bands are found in the CSF. Oligoclonal bands would be considered abnormal only if they are absent in the serum.
   B. Protein >100 mg/dl results in yellow-tinged CSF.
   C. *See also Lumbar Puncture, Diagnostic.*

Bibliography:

Bergquist J, Gilman SD, Ewing AG, Ekman R: Analysis of human cerebrospinal fluid by capillary electrophoresis with laser-induced fluorescence detection. Anal Chem 66(20):3512–3518, 1994.

Norris FH, Burns W, U KS, Mukai E, Norris H: Spinal fluid cells and protein in amyotrophic lateral sclerosis. Arch Neurol 50(5):489–491, 1993.

Sellebjerg FT, Frederiksen JL, Olsson T: Anti-myelin basic protein and anti-proteolipid protein antibody-secreting cells in the cerebrospinal fluid of patients with acute optic neuritis. Arch Neurol 51(10):1032–1036, 1994.

Travlos A, Anton HA, Wing P: Cerebrospinal fluid cell count following spinal cord injury. Arch Phys Med Rehabil 75(3):293–296, 1994.

Watson MA, Scott MG: Clinical utility of biochemical analysis of cerebrospinal fluid. Clin Chem 41(3):343–360, 1995.

CEREBROSPINAL FLUID, OLIGOCLONAL BANDS, SPECIMEN

(see Cerebrospinal Fluid; Myelin Basic Protein; Oligoclonal Bands; Protein, and Protein Electrophoresis, Specimen)

CEREBROSPINAL FLUID, PROTEIN, SPECIMEN

(see Cerebrospinal Fluid; Myelin Basic Protein; Oligoclonal Bands; Protein, and Protein Electrophoresis, Specimen)

CEREBROSPINAL FLUID, PROTEIN ELECTROPHORESIS, SPECIMEN

(see Cerebrospinal Fluid; Myelin Basic Protein; Oligoclonal Bands; Protein, and Protein Electrophoresis, Specimen)

CEREBROSPINAL FLUID, ROUTINE, CULTURE AND CYTOLOGY

Norm:

Routine Culture: No growth.

Fungus Culture: No growth after several weeks.

Mycobacteria Culture: No growth after 8 weeks.

Cytology: Cerebrospinal fluid free of abnormal cells.

		SI Units
Adults and children	0–5 cells/μL	$0–5 \times 10^6$/L
Newborn	0–30 cells/μL	$0–30 \times 10^6$/L
Adults		
Neoplastic cells	Negative	Negative
Erythrocytes	0–10/μL	$0–10 \times 10^6$/L
Leukocytes	0–10/μL	$0–10 \times 10^6$/L
Differential lymphocytes	63–99%	
Beta-lymphocytes	0–4%	
T-lymphocytes	89–97%	
Monocytes	3–37%	
Neutrophils	Absent	
Eosinophils	0–5%	

		SI Units
Children		
Neoplastic cells	Negative	Negative
Erythrocytes		
Newborn	0–675/μL	0–675 $\times$ 10^6/L
Leukocytes		
Infants	0–30/μL	0–30 $\times$ 10^6/L
1–4 years	0–20/μL	0–20 $\times$ 10^6/L
5–20 years	0–10/μL	0–20 $\times$ 10^6/L

Cytology Usage: Establish the presence of primary or metastatic neoplasm; diagnosis of cryptococcal meningitis, bacterial meningitis, or cerebral hemorrhage, brain abscess, encephalitis (postinfection), lead encephalopathy, neurosyphilis, sarcoidosis (meningeal), and study of CNS changes related to acquired immune deficiency syndrome.

Positive Routine Culture: CNS infections, encephalitis, meningitis, and sepsis neonatorum.

Negative Routine Culture: Normal finding.

Positive Fungus Culture: Brain abscess, meningitis, and systemic fungal infections.

Negative Fungus Culture: Normal finding.

Positive Mycobacteria Culture: Mycobacterial meningitis. The most common *Mycobacteria* causing human disease are *M. asiaticum, M. aviumscrofulaceum* complex, *M. fortuitum, M. haemophilum, M. kansasii, M. leprae, M. malmoense, M. marinum, M. simiae, M. szulgai, M. tuberculosis* complex, *M. ulcerans,* and *M. xenopi.*

Negative Mycobacteria Culture: Normal finding.

Description: This test includes cultures for anaerobic, aerobic, and acid-fast organisms, bacteria, protozoa, fungi, or viruses. A culture of cerebrospinal fluid (CSF) for fungus is performed to detect systemic fungal infections and normally harmless fungi that become pathogenic in the presence of immunosuppressive conditions. Although tentative identification of fungi can be made quickly with staining techniques, a culture of the organism on special fungal culture media is required to confirm a diagnosis of a fungal infection. Cell count and cytologic examination (the number and character of cells) is performed to identify the presence of abnormal cells, infective organisms, or variations in the usually low numbers of red and white blood cells. Abnormalities include increases in the numbers of normal cells and/or the presence of neoplastic cells.

Professional Considerations:

1. Consent form IS required for the lumbar puncture, which is necessary to obtain CSF. *See Lumbar Puncture, Diagnostic* for procedure risks and contraindications.
2. Preparation:
   A. A CT scan is typically performed to rule out increased intracranial pressure prior to the lumbar puncture in critically ill clients or those with changed mental status.
   B. *See also Lumbar Puncture, Diagnostic.*
3. Procedure:
   A. 3–10 ml of CSF is collected by a physician in sequentially numbered sterile glass tubes via a spinal tap between L3–4 or L4–5, or from the ventricles of the brain during special procedures.
4. Postprocedure care:
   A. Write the specimen source, collection time, current antibiotic or antifungal therapy, and clinical diagnosis on the laboratory requisition.
   B. *See also Lumbar Puncture, Diagnostic.*
   C. Transport the specimens to microbiology immediately. Analysis must be performed promptly on freshly collected specimens.
   D. Monitor for headaches, dizziness, or change in level of consciousness.
5. Client and family teaching:
   A. *See Lumbar Puncture, Diagnostic.*
   B. Growth of fungi may take several weeks.
6. Factors that affect results:
   A. The results are invalid when the specimen stands over 1 hour at room temperature.
   B. Previous radiation, intrathecal therapy, myelogram, or pneumoencephalogram

may cause cytologic changes that produce false results.

C. Microbiologic studies should be performed on tube 3 or higher to lessen the chance of skin contamination.

D. At least 5 ml is necessary to detect fungal and mycobacterial infections.

7. Other data:

A. Glucose and protein determinations may also be performed on this specimen.

B. If CNS infection is strongly suspected, but initial cell counts are normal, the test should be repeated a few hours later to detect rising white cell counts.

C. Store CSF for culture in a bacteriologic incubator when not tested promptly.

D. A portion of the sample should be frozen at –20°C when viral meningitis is suspected.

E. For positive CSF cultures, sensitivity = 92%, specificity = 95%, false-positive = 5%, and false-negative = 8%. The results are most accurate when samples are obtained prior to the initiation of antibiotic therapy.

F. *See also Lumbar Puncture, Diagnostic.*

Bibliography:

Kappel TJ, Manivel JC, Gosivitz JJ: Atypical lymphocytes in spinal fluid resembling posttransplant lymphoma in a cardiac transplant recipient. Acta Cytol *38*(3):470–474, 1994.

Oschmann P, Kaps M, Volker J, Dorndorf W: Meningeal carcinomatosis: CSF cytology, immunocytochemistry and biochemical tumor markers. Acta Neurol Scand *89*(5):395–399, 1994.

Sindern E, Malin J: Phenotypic analysis of cerebrospinal fluid cells over the course of Lyme meningoradiculitis. Acta Cytol *39*(1):73–75, 1995.

CEREBROSPINAL FLUID, ROUTINE ANALYSIS, SPECIMEN

Norms:

		SI Units
Appearance	Clear, colorless	
Specific gravity	1.006–1.008	1.006–1.008
Pressure	50–175 mmH$_2$O	50–175 mmH$_2$O
pH	7.30–7.40	
AST	0–19 U	
Bicarbonate	22.9 mEq/L	
Calcium	2.1–2.7 mEq/L	1.05–1.35 mmol/L
	4.2–5.4 mg/dl	1.05–1.35 mmol/L
Chloride	118–132 mEq/L	118–132 mmol/L
Cholesterol	0.2–0.6 mg/dl	
pCO$_2$	42–52 mmHg	
Creatinine	0.4–1.5 mg/dl	
Glucose (fasting)	40–80 mg/dl	2.2–4.4 mmol/L
Glutamine	6–16 mg/dl	
Iron	1–2 mg/dl	
Lactate	10–18 mg/dl	
LD	1/10 of serum level	
Magnesium	2.0–3.1 mEq/L	
Phosphorus	1.2–2.1 mEq/L	
Potassium	2.7–3.9 mEq/L	0.15–0.45 g/L
Protein	15–45 mg/dl	150–450 mg/L
Sodium	138–154 mEq/L	
Urea	6–28 mg/dl	
Uric acid	0.5–4.5 mg/dl	
WBC	0–10 mg/L	

Increased: Acute anterior poliomyelitis *(protein, WBC)*, alcoholism *(pressure [possibly])*, aseptic meningeal reaction *(protein, WBC)*, brain abscess *(protein, neutrophils)*, brain tumor *(pressure, protein, glucose)*, cerebral hemorrhage *(RBC, pressure, protein)*, cerebral thrombosis *(protein, lymphocytes)*, cerebral trauma *(pressure, glucose)*, coccidioidomycosis *(pressure, protein, WBC)*, coma (diabetic) *(glucose)*, cord tumor *(protein, WBC)*, diabetes mellitus *(protein)*, encephalitis (postinfectious) *(pressure,* protein, lymphocytes), Guillain Barré (protein), head trauma (pressure, protein), herpes zoster (protein, WBC), infections (protein), hyperglycemia (glucose), hypothalamic lesions (glucose), lead encephalopathy (pressure, protein, WBC), meningitis (acute pyogenic) (pressure, protein, neutrophils), meningitis (aseptic) (pressure, protein, WBC), meningitis (cryptococcal, fungal, tuberculous, viral) (pressure, protein, lymphocytes), meningoencephalitis (primary amebic) (pressure, protein, WBC), measles (pressure [possibly], protein, WBC), multiple sclerosis (protein, lymphocytes), mumps (pressure [possibly], protein, WBC), polyneuritis (protein, lymphocytes), pseudotumor cerebri (pressure), subarachnoid hemorrhage (pressure, protein), subdural hematoma (pressure, protein, lymphocytes), syphilis (protein, lymphocytes), uremia (pressure, protein, glucose), and viral infections (coxsackie and echovirus) (neutrophils).

Decreased: Only decreased glucose is significant. See Cerebrospinal Fluid, Glucose, Specimen.

Description: Analysis of cerebrospinal fluid (CSF) components is performed to aid diagnosis of a wide variety of CNS diseases, including infectious diseases.

Professional Considerations:

1. Consent form IS required for the lumbar puncture, which is necessary to obtain CSF. See Lumbar Puncture, Diagnostic for procedure risks and contraindications.
2. Preparation:
   A. A CT scan is typically performed to rule out increased intracranial pressure prior to the lumbar puncture in critically ill clients or those with changed mental status.
   B. See Lumbar Puncture, Diagnostic.
3. Procedure:
   A. 3–10 ml of CSF is collected by a physician in sequentially numbered sterile

glass tubes via a spinal tap between L3-4 or L4-5, or from the ventricles of the brain during special procedures.
4. Postprocedure care:
   A. Apply a Band-Aid over the spinal tap site.
   B. See also Lumbar Puncture, Diagnostic.
   C. Transport specimens to the laboratory immediately.
   D. Monitor for headaches, dizziness, or change in level of consciousness.
5. Client and family teaching:
   A. See Lumbar Puncture, Diagnostic.
6. Factors that affect results:
   A. Discard the first specimen.
   B. Cell counts, chemistry, and serology should be performed on tube 2.
   C. Microbiologic studies should be performed on tube 3 or higher to lessen the chance of skin contamination.
   D. The analysis must be performed promptly on freshly collected specimens to avoid erroneous results due to cell lysis, disintegration, and continued glycolysis.
   E. Colored or very cloudy spinal fluid requires additional mixing with 0.5 ml sterile sodium citrate per 5 ml of CSF to prevent clotting. This item is not applicable if tuberculous meningitis is suspected.
7. Other data:
   A. Handle specimens cautiously to prevent self-contamination.
   B. Refrigerate the CSF if it is not analyzed promptly.
   C. Cloudy specimens may be caused by elevated white blood cells. Yellow specimens may be caused by elevated protein. Pink or red specimens may be caused by red blood cells.
   D. See also Lumbar Puncture, Diagnostic.

Bibliography:

Barry E, Hauser WA: Pleocytosis after status epilepticus. Arch Neurol 51(2):190–193, 1994.

Tessler MJ, Wiesel S, Wahba RM, Quance DR: A comparison of simple identification tests to distinguish cerebrospinal fluid from local anaesthetic solution. Anaesthesia 49(9):821–822, 1994.

Travlos A, Anton HA, Wing P: Cerebrospinal fluid cell count following spinal cord injury. Arch Phys Med Rehabil 75(3):293–296, 1994.

Watson MA, Scott MG: Clinical utility of biochemical analysis of cerebrospinal fluid. Clin Chem 41(3):343–360, 1995.

CERULOPLASMIN (CP), SERUM

Norm:

		SI Units
Adult	14–40 mg/dl	0.93–2.65 μmol/L
Newborn	1–30 mg/dl	0.06–1.99 μmol/L
Age 6–12 months	15–50 mg/dl	0.99–3.31 μmol/L
Age 1–12 years	30–65 mg/dl	1.99–4.30 μmol/L

Increased: Cancer, cirrhosis, infection, pregnancy, primary sclerosing cholangitis, rheumatoid arthritis, hepatitis, myocardial infarction, and thyrotoxicosis. Drugs include oral contraceptives, estrogens, dilantin, and methadone.

Decreased: Hepatic disease, kwashiorkor, malabsorption (such as sprue), nephrosis, nephrotic syndrome, in early infancy, and Wilson's disease.

Description: Ceruloplasmin is an alpha$_2$-globulin transport protein that transports copper and aids in mobilizing iron stores. It is an acute-phase reactant that becomes elevated during stress, pregnancy, and infection. This test is most often used to aid diagnosis of Wilson's disease, in which subnormal quantities of ceruloplasmin are manufactured by the liver. The resulting tissue deposition of copper causes brain and liver damage.

Professional Considerations:

1. Consent form NOT required.
2. Preparation:
   A. Tube: Red-top, red/gray-top, or gold-top.
3. Procedure:
   A. Draw a 1-ml blood sample.
4. Postprocedure care:
   A. None.
5. Client and family teaching:
   A. Results may not be available for several days.
6. Factors that affect results:
   A. Hemolysis invalidates the results.
   B. The results are unreliable in infants under 3 months of age.
7. Other data:
   A. The serum level of ceruloplasmin is determined via electrophoresis.

Bibliography:

Kiyosawa I, Matsuyama J, Nyui S, Fukuda A: Ceruloplasmin concentration in human colostrum and mature mold. Biosci Biotechnol Biochem 59(4): 713–714, 1995.

Ogihara H, Ogihara T, Miki M, Yasuda H, Mino M:. Plasma copper and antioxidant status in Wilson's disease. Pediatr Res 37(2):219–226, 1995.

Thomas GR, Jensson O, Gudmundsson G, Thorsteinsson L, Cox D: Wilson disease in Iceland: a clinical and genetic study. Am J Hum Genet 56(5):1140–1146, 1995.

Yamazaki M, Ito S, Ysami A, Tani N, Hanyu O, Nakagawa O, Nakamura H, Shibata A: Urinary excretion rate of ceruloplasmin in non-insulin-dependent diabetic patients with different stages of nephropathy. Eur J Endocrinol 132(6):681–687, 1995.

CERVICAL CULTURE

Norm: Negative for pathogenic vaginal microorganisms.

Positive: The most common organisms recovered in positive cervical cultures include *Actinomyces, Candida, Chlamydia, Mobiluncus, Gardenella, Herpes, Neisseria gonorrhoeae,* and *Trichomonas.*

Description: A cervical culture is included in routine gynecologic examinations or in cases of cervicitis, leukorrhea, vaginitis, suspected infection, and/or rape. A smear is usually included as well. The specimen is obtained via a vaginal examination.

Professional Considerations:

1. Consent form NOT required.
2. Preparation:
   A. The client must disrobe below the waist.
   B. Obtain a speculum, a sterile Culturette, glass slides, two spatuli, potassium hydroxide, and a sterile 0.9% saline.
3. Procedure:
   A. Position the client in the dorsal lithotomy position and drape for privacy and comfort.
   B. Insert a speculum into the vagina and expose the cervix and vaginal walls.
   C. Collect exudate from the cervix and/or vagina on a sterile Culturette. The exudate may be expressed from the cervix by gently pressing it between two spatuli. Smear exudate onto two glass slides. Place one slide in the potassium hydroxide fixative, and the other in the sterile 0.9% saline.
4. Postprocedure care:
   A. Write the clinical data, specimen source, and any recent antibiotic therapy on the laboratory requisition.
   B. Send the specimen to the laboratory within 2 hours. Do not refrigerate the specimen.
5. Client and family teaching:
   A. Do not douche for 24 hours before the test.
   B. Several days may be required for growth in the culture. Empiric therapy is often begun while the client awaits culture results.
   C. Instruct the client with a positive culture on the preventive measures appropriate to the grown organism, where applicable.
   D. The client with a positive test for a sexually transmitted organism should inform all sexual partners of the infection, return for a follow-up culture 7–10 days after finishing the medication prescribed for the infection, and refrain from sexual activity with another person until negative follow-up cultures are received.
6. Factors that affect results:
   A. The test must be repeated if the Culturette is contaminated by touching

the speculum or walls of the labia or if other contamination occurs during the procedure.

B. If *Actinomyces* is suspected, a special anaerobic culture container with a theocolate broth must be obtained.

C. *Chlamydia* is difficult to culture with this method.

7. Other data:

A. A fish odor from a fresh slide treated with potassium hydroxide is a positive indication for *Gardenella.*

B. Yeast vaginal infections, especially *Candida,* are easily noted microscopically when spores are stained by potassium hydroxide.

C. On saline-treated culture slides, the *Trichomonas* organism has a typical pear shape and flagella.

Bibliography:

Beatty WL, Byrne GI, Morrison RP: Repeated and persistent infection with *Chlamydia* and the development of chronic inflammation and disease. Trends Microbiol *2*(3):94–98, 1994.

Dean D, Oudens E, Bolan G, Padian N, Schachter J: Major outer membrane protein variants of *Chlamydia trachomatis* are associated with severe upper genital tract infections and histopathology in San Francisco. J Infec Dis *172*(4): 1013–1022, 1995.

Hori S, Tsutsumi Y: Histological differentiation between *Chlamydial* and bacterial epididymitis: Nondestructive and proliferative versus destructive and abscess forming—immunohistochemical and clinicopathological findings. Hum Pathol *26*(4):402–407, 1995.

CERVICAL CULTURE FOR *NEISSERIA GONORRHOEAE,* CULTURE

Norm: No *Neisseria gonorrhoeae* is isolated.

Positive: Gonorrheal infection of the female genitalia.

Negative: No infection is detected.

Description: *N. gonorrhoeae* is a pyogenic, gram-negative, oxidase-positive cocci that is an obligate parasite of humans. It is the causative organism of the sexually transmitted infection gonorrhea. *N. gonorrhoeae* inhabits the mucous membranes of the genital tract and may also be found in the oral mucosa of clients who engage in oral sex. The symptoms include dysuria, purulent urethral discharge, proctitis, and pharyngitis. Females are often asymptomatic. Left untreated, gonorrhea leads to skin lesions, arthritis, meningitis, and reproductive problems. The cervix is the best site for obtaining accurate culture specimens in females.

Professional Considerations:

1. Consent form NOT required.
2. Preparation:

   A. The client should disrobe below the waist.

   B. Obtain a special packaged culture swab with culture medium, a speculum, and warm water.

3. Procedure:

   A. Place the client in the dorsal lithotomy position.

   B. Lubricate the speculum with warm water and insert it into the vagina to expose the cervix.

   C. Clean off any mucus with a dry cotton swab.

   D. Insert a sterile cotton-tipped swab into the endocervical canal and move the swab from side to side.

   E. Hold the swab in place for several seconds and then withdraw it and place it in a special culture medium (Jembec or Mager-Martin).

   F. Alternatively, gently compress the cervix between the speculum blades to express exudate onto the swab.

   G. Cultures of the throat and the anus may also be taken to test for *N. gonorrhoeae.*

4. Postprocedure care:

   A. Send the specimen to the laboratory immediately. Do not refrigerate the specimen.

5. Client and family teaching:

   A. Do not douche for 24 hours before the test.

   B. Gonorrhea is a reportable disease.

   C. If your test is positive, you should inform all your sexual partners of the infection, return for follow-up culture 7–10 days after finishing antibiotics, and refrain from sexual activity with another person until negative follow-up cultures are received.

   D. Instruct the client with a positive culture on the preventive measures appropriate to a grown organism, where applicable.

6. Factors that affect results:

   A. A lubricant gel should not be used.

   B. Care must be taken not to contaminate the culture tip by touching the sides of the vagina during the procedure.

7. Other data:

   A. This test is often included in a rape-trauma work-up.

   B. *See also Neisseria Gonorrhoeae Smear, Specimen.*

   C. For positive results, the client should also be serologically tested for syphilis.

Bibliography:

Blake MS, Blake CM, Apicella MA, Mandrell RE: Gonococcal opacity: lectin-like interactions between opa proteins and Lipooligosaccharide. Infect Immun *63*(4):1434–1439, 1995.

Gorby G: Digital confocal microscopy allows measurement and three-dimensional multiple spectral reconstruction of Neisseria Gonorrhoeae/epithelial cell interactions in the human fallopian tube organ culture model. J Histochem Cytochem 42(3):297–306, 1994.

CERVICAL/VAGINAL CYTOLOGY, SPECIMEN
(see Pap Smear, Diagnostic)

CHAGAS' DISEASE SEROLOGICAL TEST
(see Trypanosomiasis Serological Test, Blood)

CHEM-6, –7, –12, –20
(see SMA–6, –7, –12, 20, Blood)

CHEMISTRY PROFILE, BLOOD

Norm:

		SI Units
Albumin (Nephelometric, Colorimetric)		
Adults	3.5–5.5 g/dl	35–55 g/L
>Age 60	3.4–4.8 g/dl	34–48 g/L
Average at rest	0.3 g/dl	3 g/L
Alkaline Phosphatase		
Adults		
Age 20–60		
Bodansky	2–4 U/dl	10.7–21.5 IU/L
King-Armstrong	4–13 U/dl	28.4–92.3 IU/L
Bessey-Lowrey-Brock	0.8–2.3 U/dl	13.3–38.3 IU/L
Elderly	Slightly higher	
Newborn	1–4 times adult values	
Children: Values remain high until epiphyses close.		
Females		
Age 2–10	100–350 U/L	
Age 10–13	110–400 U/L	
Males		
Age 2–13	100–350 U/L	
Age 13–15	125–500 U/L	
Aspartate Aminotransferase		
Adult females		
<Age 60	8–20 U/L	8–20 U/L
≥Age 60	10–20 U/L	10–20 U/L
Adult males		
<Age 60	8–20 U/L	8–20 U/L
≥Age 60	11–26 U/L	11–26 U/L
Children		
Newborn	16–72 U/L	16–72 U/L
Infant	15–60 U/L	15–60 U/L
Age 1 year	16–35 U/L	16–35 U/L
Age 5 years	19–28 U/L	19–28 U/L
Bilirubin		
1 month–adult	<1.5 mg/dl	1.7–20.5 µmol/L
Premature infant		
Cord	<2.8 mg/dl	<48 µmol/L
24 hours	1–6 mg/dl	17–103 µmol/L
48 hours	6–8 mg/dl	103–137 µmol/L
3–5 days	10–12 mg/dl	171–205 µmol/L

Bilirubin *(continued)*		**SI Units**
Full–term infant		
Cord	<2.8 mg/dl	<48 µmol/L
24 hours	2–6 mg/dl	34–103 µmol/L
48 hours	6–7 mg/dl	103–120 µmol/L
3–5 days	4–6 mg/dl	68–103 µmol/L

Calcium

Adult	4.5–5.5 mEq/L	
	8.2–10.2 mg/dl	2.05–2.54 mmol/L
Child	4.5–5. 8 mEq/L	
	9.0–11.5 mg/dl	2.24–2.86 mmol/L
Infant	5.0–6.0 mEq/L	
	8.6–11.2 mg/dl	2.15–2.79 mmol/L
Newborn	3.7–7.0 mEq/L	
	7.0–11.5 mg/dl	1.75–2.87 mmol/L
Panic levels	≤10 mEq/L	
	≥13 mEq/L	
Tetany	<7 mg/dl	<1.75 mmol/L
Coma	>12 mg/dl	>2.99 mmol/L
Possible death	≤ 6 mg/dl	≤1.50 mmol/L
	≤14 mg/dl	≤3.49 mmol/L

Creatinine

Jaffe, manual method	0.8–1.5 mg/dl	70–133 µmol/day
Jaffe, kinetic or enzymatic method		
Adults		
Female	0.5–1.1 mg/dl	44–97 µmol/L
Male	0.6–1.2 mg/dl	53–106 µmol/L
Elderly	May be lower	May be lower
Children		
Cord blood	0.6–1.2 mg/dl	53–106 µmol/L
Newborn	0.8–1.4 mg/dl	71–124 µmol/L
Infant	0.7–1.7 mg/dl	62–150 µmol/L
Age 1 female	≤0.5 mg/dl	≤44 µmol/L
Age 1 male	≤0.6 mg/dl	≤53 µmol/L
Age 2–3 female	≤0.6 mg/dl	≤53 µmol/L
Age 2–3 male	≤0.7 mg/dl	≤62 µmol/L
Age 4–7 female	≤0.7 mg/dl	≤62 µmol/L
Age 4–7 male	≤0.8 mg/dl	≤71 µmol/L
Age 8–10 female	≤0.8 mg/dl	≤71 µmol/L
Age 8–10 male	≤0.9 mg/dl	≤80 µmol/L
Age 11–12 female	≤0.9 mg/dl	≤80 µmol/L
Age 11–12 male	≤1.0 mg/dl	≤88 µmol/L
Age 13–17 female	≤1.1 mg/dl	≤97 µmol/L
Age 13–17 male	≤1.2 mg/dl	≤106 µmol/L
Age 18–20 female	≤1.2 mg/dl	≤106 µmol/L
Age 18–20 male	≤1.3 mg/dl	≤115 µmol/L

Lactate Dehydrogenase

Wroblewski method	150–450 U	72–217 IU/L
30°C		
Adult		
<Age 60	45–90 U/L	45–90 U/L
≥Age 60	55–102 U/L	55–102 U/L

Lactate Dehydrogenase *(continued)*		**SI Units**
Newborn	160–500 U/L	160–500 U/L
Neonate	300–1500 U/L	300–1500 U/L
Infant	100–250 U/L	100–250 U/L
Child	60–170 U/L	60–170 U/L
Phosphorus		
Adults <age 60	3.0–4.5 mg/dl	0.97–1.45 mmol/L
Females ≥age 60	2.8–4.1 mg/dl	0.90–1.30 mmol/L
Males ≥age 60	2.3–3.7 mg/dl	0.74–1.20 mmol/L
Children		
Cord blood	3.7–8.1 mg/dl	1.19–2.62 mmol/L
Premature infant	5.4–10.9 mg/dl	1.74–3.52 mmol/L
Newborn	3.5–8.6 mg/dl	1.13–2.78 mmol/L
Infant	4.5–6.7 mg/dl	1.45–2.16 mmol/L
Child	4.5–5.5 mg/dl	1.45–1.78 mmol/L
Protein, Total		
Adults	6.0–8.0 g/dl	60–80 g/L
Children		
Premature infant	4.3–7.6 g/dl	43–76 g/L
Newborn	4.6–7.4 g/dl	46–74 g/L
Infant	6.0–6.7 g/dl	60–67 g/L
Child	6.2–8.0 g/dl	62–80 g/L
Urea Nitrogen		
Young adults (<40)	5–18 mg/dl	1.8–6.5 mmol/L
Adults	5–20 mg/dl	1.8–7.1 mmol/L
Elderly (>60)	8–21 mg/dl	2.9–7.5 mmol/L
Mild azotemia	20–50 mg/dl	7.1–17.7 mmol/L
Panic level	>100 mg/dl	>35.7 mmol/L
Children		
Cord blood	21–40 mg/dl	7.5–14.3 mmol/L
Premature infant, first 7 days	3–25 mg/dl	0.1–0.9 mmol/L
Full-term newborn	4–18 mg/dl	1.4–6.4 mmol/L
Infant	5–18 mg/dl	1.8–6.4 mmol/L
Child	5–18 mg/dl	1.8–6.4 mmol/L
Uric Acid		
Adult females	2.4–6.0 mg/dl	143–357 µmol/L
		0.17–0.45 mmol/L
Adult males	3.4–7.0 mg/dl	202–416 µmol/L
		0.21–0.51 mmol/L
Children	2.5–5.5 mg/dl	119–327 µmol/L
		0.15–0.33 mmol/L
Elderly	3.5–8.5 mg/dl	204–550 µmol/L
		0.21–0.51 mmol/L
Panic level	>12 mg/dl	>714 µmol/L

Increased: See individual test listings.

Decreased: See individual test listings.

Description: A chemistry profile is a group of several laboratory tests performed on one blood sample and measured on an automated instrument. It can be performed for routine screening on healthy populations or for the purpose of detecting specific changes for a client. This profile generally includes the following tests: *Albumin, Serum; Alkaline Phosphatase, Serum; Aspartate Aminotransferase, Serum; Bilirubin, Serum; Calcium, Serum;*

Creatinine, Serum; Lactate Dehydrogenase, Blood; Phosphorus, Serum; Protein, Total, Serum; Urea Nitrogen, Plasma or Serum; and Uric Acid, Serum. See individual test listings for individual test descriptions.

Professional Considerations:

1. Consent form NOT required.
2. Preparation:
   A. Tube: Red-top, red/gray-top, or gold-top.
   B. Do NOT draw during hemodialysis.
3. Procedure:
   A. Draw a 5-ml blood sample.
4. Postprocedure care:
   A. None.
5. Client and family teaching:
   A. See individual test listings.
   B. Results are normally available within 24 hours.
6. Factors that affect results:
   A. See individual test listings.
7. Other data:
   A. See individual test listings.

Bibliography:

Labeur C, Rosseneu M, Henderson O: International Lp(a) standardization. Chem Phys Lipids *67–68*: 265–270, 1994.

Muros M, Lopez T, Leon C, Merino M, Calvo M: Analytical interferences from calcium dobesilate in five serum assays. Clin Chem *39*(2):371, 1993.

Preshaw LE: The reference range as a control. Clin Chem *39*(2):367, 1993.

CHEST TOMOGRAPHY, DIAGNOSTIC

Norm: Normal structures and organ content of the chest, including the chest wall, the lungs, the heart, and the diaphragm; absence of neoplasm, infective process, or structural changes.

Usage: Metastatic tumor of lung or thoracic skeleton; primary tumors of the thoracic skeleton; chondrosarcoma, myeloma, or Ewing's sarcoma in children; osteomyelitis of the spine, sternum, or ribs; work-up following chest trauma for dislocations of the sternoclavicular joint; diagnosis and evaluation of the extent and involvement of soft tissue sarcomas or lymphomas, hemangiomas, and nerve sheath tumors; examination of mediastinal injury, infection, and sternal involvement; axillary space study of lymph node abnormalities for evidence of metastatic processes, infection, or axillary vein thrombosis. Although the mammogram is more widely used, cancer of the breast with other breast abnormalities may be seen on chest tomography to diagnose or aid in the diagnosis of breast tissue diseases. Pleura are examined for lung effusions, extent and location of infection, empyemas, plaques typical of asbestos disease, bulbous emphysema, and fibrotic pleural disease. The diaphragm is examined for hernias or tumors. The heart may be examined for cardiomyopathy, pericardial effusion, location and extent of congenital anomalies, tumor, or calcifications. Also, great vessel abnormalities and aortic aneurysms can be noted.

Description: Tomographic scanning is special radiographic scanning using scintillation detectors that can produce transverse sectional views of the chest area, providing a two-dimensional image. With computed tomography (CT or CAT scan) of the lung, the specialized computers produce a series of cross-sectional or transverse views of the whole thoracic area. The test aids diagnostic study of the chest wall, breast tissue, axillary space, lungs, pleural space, diaphragm, spinal cord and spine at the thoracic level rib structure, sternum, and mediastinal space.

Professional Considerations:

1. Consent form NOT required.

Risks:
None.

Contraindications:
Screen client for contraindications to performing the Valsalva maneuver (recent myocardial infarction, bradycardia). If present, teach the client how to hold breath without bearing down.

2. Preparation:
   A. The client must disrobe above the waist and remove all jewelry and metal objects.
   B. Shield the uterus if the client is a pregnant female.
3. Procedure:
   A. The test is performed with a specialized x-ray scintillator and computer in a radiology laboratory with specialized personnel.
   B. The client is placed in a supine position on the CT radiographic table, which moves into the x-ray scintillography

machine for a series of views. The client will be asked to take a deep breath and hold it for some views. The automated computer then produces reconstructed images that show "slices" of the chest.

C. The test takes approximately 15 minutes for all views, transverse and oblique.

4. Postprocedure care:
   A. None.

5. Client and family teaching:
   A. The procedure may be frightening for the client, who must cooperate for the best results. Fear usually stems from fear of enclosed spaces. Good explanations and preparation are necessary.
   B. This test is noninvasive and carries no risk.

6. Factors that affect results:
   A. Movement of the client interferes with the accuracy of the films.
   B. Jewelry and metal objects obstruct the views.

7. Other data:
   A. Because it is a noninvasive study with rapidly improving technology, computed tomography is growing in importance as a diagnostic tool.
   B. Tomography is expensive.
   C. *See also Computed Tomography of the Body, Diagnostic.*

Bibliography:

Dajczman E, Hanley J, Lisbona A, Wolkove N, Kreisman H: Comparison of response evaluation in small cell lung cancer using computerized tomography and chest radiography. Lung Cancer 11(1–2): 51–60, 1994.

Kuhlman JL: Parenchymal lung disease. *In* Haaga JR, Lanzier CF, Sartoris DJ, Zerbouni EA (eds): Computed Tomography and Magnetic Resonance Imaging of the Whole Body, 3rd ed., Vol. St. Louis, MO, Mosby Year Book, pp 647–712, 1994.

CHEST X-RAY (CXR), DIAGNOSTIC

Norm: Normal anatomy and no pathologic changes evident.

Usage: Chest x-ray may be used as a general screening tool preoperatively or for general physical examinations or may be prescribed for a specific diagnostic purpose. Provides information regarding the anatomic location and abnormalities of the heart, great vessels, lungs, soft tissue of the chest and mediastinum, and the bones. A number of pulmonary, cardiac, and orthopedic abnormalities may be seen on chest x-ray, particularly if serial films are available for study. Pulmonary uses include abscess, acute respiratory distress syndrome (ARDS), atelectasis, bronchitis, cystic fibrosis, emphysema, fibrosis bullae, hemothorax, malignancies of the lung, pleural effusion, pneumonia, pneumothorax, pulmonary edema, and tuberculosis calcific changes. Cardiac uses include congestive heart failure and determination of heart size. Uses in the great vessels include abnormalities of aortic arch (calcification), some aneurysms, and transposition. Orthopedic uses include bone tumors, fracture of clavicles, kyphosis, rib fractures, scoliosis, and spinal fractures. General uses include placement of central lines, endotracheal tubes, tracheostomy tubes, chest tubes, nasogastric tubes, pacemaker wires and intra-aortic balloon pumps, foreign bodies, lymph node enlargement, mediastinal changes, and pulmonary artery catheter placement.

Description: X-rays are passed through the chest and react on a special photographic plate. Normally, the lungs are radiolucent. Bones, and fluid-containing bodies such as the heart, the aorta, and any tumor or infiltrate are more dense than the lungs and can be easily visualized. Chest x-rays can be performed with the client standing or sitting upright, during inhalation, and in anterior-posterior, posterior-anterior, and lateral views. Portable, in-bed, anterior-posterior chest x-rays can be performed for clients too ill to transport to the radiology department.

Professional Considerations:

1. Consent form NOT required.

Risks:
Fetal teratogenicity, vasovagal response (hypotension, bradycardia) to breath-holding.

Contraindications/Precautions:
Chest x-rays may be contraindicated in pregnancy, unless the benefits of performing them outweigh the risks to the fetus. Screen the client for contraindications to performing the Valsalva maneuver (recent myocardial infarction, bradycardia). If these conditions are present, teach the client how to hold breath without bearing down.

2. Preparation:
   A. Remove all jewelry, clothing with snaps, electrocardiographic patches (if not contraindicated), and other metal objects from the chest area that may interfere with the interpretation of the results.
   B. Females should be asked if they are pregnant or if there is any possibility that they may be pregnant.
3. Procedure:
   A. The client is positioned sitting or standing upright in front of the x-ray machine, with arms held slightly out from the sides, chest expanded, and shoulders pressed forward. The radiographic film is placed against the anterior chest.
   B. For lateral views, the client stands with his or her arms elevated from the shoulders, and with the forearms resting on the arm of the radiographic equipment, if necessary. The radiographic film is placed flush against the right or left side of the chest.
   C. As the client holds very still and takes in a deep breath and holds it, one or more radiographs are taken.
   D. For portable radiographs, the client is positioned sitting in a high Fowler's position and the portable x-ray machine is moved into place in front of the chest for the radiographic exposure onto the plate positioned behind the back and chest.
4. Postprocedure care:
   A. Replace the electrocardiographic patches and wires, if they have been removed.
   B. Return personal belongings to the client and help him or her dress.
   C. In the event of portable x-ray, help the client return to a comfortable position.
5. Client and family teaching:
   A. It is important to breathe in deeply, hold your breath, and remain motionless while the x-ray is taken.
   B. An x-ray takes approximately 15 minutes to complete and verify that the images are properly exposed.
   C. No restrictions are necessary on food or fluid intake.
   D. No sedation is used for this procedure.
   E. Views are taken in various positions on the table or chair.
6. Factors that affect results:
   A. "Vascular structures that can simulate neoplasms include normal structures such as the subclavian artery and left brachiocephalic, azygos, and pulmonary veins and abnormal structures such as congenital and acquired anomalies of the thoracic aorta and its branches, pulmonary arteries and veins, superior and inferior venae cavae, and azygos and hemizygous veins. Other entities such as postoperative changes,

massive pulmonary embolism, false ventricular aneurysm, and esophageal varices can also be misinterpreted. Important radiographic features that help distinguish these vascular structures from true neoplasms include proximity to known vascular structures, smooth margination, mural calcification, round or oval configuration, poor or nonvisualization in one of two orthogonal views, and absence or altered position of normal vascular structures. Knowledge of patient history and a detailed understanding of normal mediastinal anatomic structures and common variants help in making the correct diagnosis. Familiarity with these entities will result in the proper, most cost-efficient evaluation" (Cole et al. 1995).
   B. Clothing, jewelry, and metal objects cause shadows on the film.
   C. Movement obscures the clarity of the picture.
   D. Improper positioning makes radiographs difficult to interpret.
   E. Portable radiographs are not as reliable as those performed in radiology departments. The anterior-posterior position may cause the heart to appear larger than it is.
   F. Overexposure or underexposure results in inadequate visualization.
   G. The experience of the physician interpreting the films affects the accuracy of the findings.
7. Other data:
   A. Chest x-ray is not suggested as a first-line screening tool for tuberculosis or cancer because of possible dangers from frequent radiographic exposure.
   B. Health care workers in areas near frequent x-rays should wear an x-ray badge to track exposure level. They should wear a lead apron when remaining in the room with the client during exposure. For portable radiographs, health care workers should stand at least 5 feet from the x-ray source during exposure.

Bibliography:

Bearcroft PW, Small JH, Flower CD: Chest radiography guidelines for general practitioners: a practical approach. Clin Radiol 49(1):56–58, 1994.

Cole TJ, Henry DA, Jolles H, Proto AV: Normal and abnormal vascular structures that simulate neoplasms on chest radiographs: clues to the diagnosis. Radiographics 15(4):867–891, 1995.

Dajczman E, Hanley J, Lisbona A, Wolkove N, Kreisman H: Comparison of response evaluation in small cell lung cancer using computerized tomography and chest radiography. Lung Cancer 11(1–2):51–60, 1994.

CHLAMYDIA CULTURE

Norm: No *Chlamydia* are isolated.

Positive: *Chlamydia* infection.

Negative: No *Chlamydia* are isolated.

Description: *Chlamydia* are intracellular parasites with the characteristics of bacteria and of viruses that cause psittacosis, pneumonia, eye infections, and lymphogranuloma venereum. The mode of transmission for *C. psittaci* is thought to be inhalation of the agent from the droppings of, or direct contact with, infected birds. The mode of transmission for *C. trachomatis* is direct contact of the infant with the mother's cervix during birth or direct contact through sexual activity. The culture method is more widely used for diagnosis of *C. trachomatis* than *C. psittaci*. *C. trachomatis* diseases include (1) lymphogranuloma venereum venereal disease characterized by edema and infection of the lymph nodes of the inguinal, perirectal, and intra-abdominal areas; (2) a less serious, often asymptomatic genital infection; (3) trachoma—a serious eye infection; and (4) neonatal infections—usually conjunctivitis and pneumonia in babies of infected mothers. This test is seldom performed when *C. psittaci* is suspected, because there is danger of transmission of the disease to laboratory workers from inhalation of the parasite from the sample sent for testing. The serum test *Chlamydia Group Titer, Serum* is the most common test used to diagnose this infection.

Professional Considerations:

1. Consent form NOT required.
2. Preparation:
   A. Obtain sterile cotton-tipped culture swabs, a cytobrush, and a culture medium.
   B. Where *Chlamydia psittaci* is suspected, health care workers should wear a mask when obtaining a specimen to avoid inhalation of the microorganism.
3. Procedure:
   A. The specimens for culture are obtained by vigorous scraping or swabbing of suspected sites. A cytobrush may be used. Purulent drainage does not provide accurate or adequate results.
   B. *Eye culture:*
      i. Cleanse any mucus or purulent drainage from the eye with a dry cotton swab.
      ii. Using a sterile cotton-tipped swab or cytobrush, firmly swab or scrape the inner canthus or lower conjunctiva. Withdraw the swab and place it in a sucrose-phosphate-glutamate (SPG)

medium or other special culture medium approved for *Chlamydia* cultures by the specific laboratory.
   C. *Cervical culture (for* C. trachomatis):
      i. The client should disrobe below the waist.
      ii. Position the client in the dorsal lithotomy position and drape her for comfort and privacy.
      iii. Lubricate the speculum with warm water and insert it into the vagina to expose the cervix.
      iv. Cleanse any mucus or purulent drainage with a dry cotton swab.
      v. Insert a sterile cotton-tipped swab or a cytobrush into the endocervical canal within the os and swab or scrape vigorously. Hold the swab or brush in place for several seconds and then withdraw the swab.
   D. *Urethral culture (for* C. trachomatis):
      i. Aspirate secretions and obtain scraping from the urethra. For males, a wire loop may be inserted into the urethra to obtain the specimen.
   E. *Respiratory culture (for* C. psittaci):
      i. Obtain a biopsy or brushings of lung tissue via bronchoscopy, aspirate of lung secretions, a throat swab, or a sputum sample.
4. Postprocedure care:
   A. Place the specimen in an SPG medium or other special culture medium approved for *Chlamydia* cultures by the specific lab.
   B. Write the specimen source, site, collection time, and suspected diagnosis on the laboratory requisition.
   C. Send the specimen to the laboratory and refrigerate.
   D. The specimen must be cultured within 24 hours.
5. Client and family teaching:
   A. Several days may be required for culture results. Empiric therapy is often started while the client awaits culture results.
   B. For a positive cervical *Chlamydia* culture, your sexual partners should subsequently be tested.
6. Factors that affect results:
   A. Reject specimens received more than 24 hours after collection.
   B. The use of a cytobrush is recommended.
   C. Two specimens are recommended, as *Chlamydia* lives inside normal cells and thus is difficult to diagnose.
7. Other data:
   A. Diagnosis of *C. psittaci* is rarely made by culture.

Bibliography:

Carroll JC: *Chlamydia trachomatis* during pregnancy. To screen or not to screen. Can Fam Physician *39*:97–102, 1995.

Sellors JW: Screening for Chlamydial infection: Taking stock. Can Fam Physician *41*:188–192, 1995.

CHLAMYDIA GROUP TITER, SERUM

Norm:

>   <1:16 = Normal titer.
>   >1:16 = Previous exposure to *Chlamydia*.
>   1:32 in babies = Positive for *Chlamydia trachomatis*.
>   1:16 in adults = Positive for *Chlamydia psittaci*.

Usage: Suspected *Chlamydia psittaci* or *C. trachomatis* infections, including lymphogranuloma venereum or trachoma eye infection.

Description: *See under Chlamydia Culture* for a description of *Chlamydia*. This test uses complement fixation or microimmunofluorescence to measure the amount of IgG antibodies to *Chlamydia*. It is a nonspecific, in vitro, antigen-antibody study that detects previous exposure to *Chlamydia* organisms. *Chlamydia* infection is confirmed by a fourfold increase in serial titers.

Professional Considerations:

1. Consent form NOT required.
2. Preparation:
   A. Tube: Red-top, red/gray-top, gold-top, or SST.
3. Procedure:
   A. Draw a 5-ml blood sample.
4. Postprocedure care:
   A. Transport the specimen to the laboratory immediately.
5. Client and family teaching:
   A. Several days may be required for titer results. Empiric therapy is often started while you await the results. *Chlamydia* is curable with medication.

   B. For elevated titer, your sexual partner(s) should subsequently be tested.
   C. *Chlamydia* infection may cause difficulties with conception in the future and, in pregnancy, may cause premature labor.
6. Factors that affect results:
   A. Reject hemolyzed specimens.
   B. Serious illness, immune disorders, and immunosuppressive therapy may interfere with antigen-antibody reaction and show false-negative results.
   C. Antibiotic therapy may cause false-negative results.
7. Other data:
   A. *Chlamydia* titer is not used in neonatal infection diagnosis because the mother's autoantibodies to *Chlamydia* are present in the neonate for up to 9 months.

Bibliography:

Corcoran GD, Ridgway GL: Antibiotic chemotherapy of bacterial sexually transmitted diseases in adults: a review. Int J STD AIDS 5(3):165–171, 1994.

Dean D, Oudens E, Bolan G, Padian N, Schachter J: Major outer membrane protein variants of *Chlamydia trachomatis* are associated with severe upper genital tract infections and histopathology in San Francisco. J Infect Dis *172*(4):1013–1022, 1995.

Klepser ME, Quintiliani R, Nightingale CH: Treatment of uncomplicated infects caused by *Chlamydia trachomatis* and *Neisseria gonorrhoeae.* Connecticut Medicine *58*(8):489–494, 1994.

CHLORAMPHENICOL, BLOOD

Norm: Negative.

		SI Units
Therapeutic level	10–25 µg/ml	31–77 µmol/L
Trough level	<5 µg/ml	<15 µmol/L
Gray baby syndrome	40–100 µg/ml	124–309 µmol/L
Panic level	>50 µg/ml	>154 µmol/L

Panic Level Symptoms and Treatment:

Symptoms: Hematopoietic toxicity, including reversible bone-marrow suppression and irreversible aplasia, may occur; hemolysis; allergic reaction; and peripheral neuritis.

Treatment:
Monitor closely.
Maintain peak serum levels below 25 µg/ml by dose adjustments.
Hemodialysis WILL remove the drug.
Peritoneal dialysis will NOT remove chloramphenicol.

Usage: Evaluation for appropriate dosing when Chloramphenicol is used for treatment of *Chlamydia;* infants with severe anaerobic infections; *Haemophilus influenza;* meningitis; *Mycoplasma;* rickettsias; *Salmonella;* or typhoid.

Description: Chloramphenicol is a potent, broad-spectrum, synthetic antibiotic used for gram-negative, gram-positive, and anaerobic microorganisms when other antibiotics cannot be used or are ineffective. It is metabolized by the liver and excreted by the kidneys, with a half-life of 2.5–3.0 hours in clients with normal hepatic and renal function. Chloramphenicol levels, complete blood counts, and reticulocyte levels must be closely monitored during therapy due to the risk of bone marrow depression side effects.

Professional Considerations:

1. Consent form NOT required.
2. Preparation:
   A. Tube: Red-top, red/gray-top, gold-top, or green-top or lavender-top.
   B. Do NOT draw during hemodialysis.
3. Procedure:
   A. Draw a 1-ml blood sample. For a trough level, draw the specimen just prior to the next dose. For a peak level, draw the specimen 15 minutes after completion of the dose.
4. Postprocedure care:
   A. Send the specimen to the laboratory for immediate separation of test sample. Freeze the sample after separation if not tested immediately.

5. Client and family teaching:
   A. Results are normally available within 24 hours.
6. Factors that affect results:
   A. Concurrent use of phenobarbital may reduce chloramphenicol levels.
   B. Toxic levels are more likely to occur in clients with impaired renal or hepatic function.
   C. Therapeutic levels may last for up to 8 hours after administration.
7. Other data:
   A. Bone marrow suppression is most commonly dose related, but may occur up to 2 months after completion of any dose of therapy and be irreversible.
   B. Can cause gray baby syndrome in premature infants with impaired hepatic function, and in newborns less than 3 weeks old, resulting in cardiovascular collapse and death.

Bibliography:

Acharya G, Butler T, Ho M, Sharma PR, Tiwari M, Adhikari RK, Khagda JB, Pokhrel B, Pathak UN: Treatment of typhoid fever: randomized trial of a three-day course of ceftriaxone versus a fourteen-day course of chloramphenicol. Am J Tropical Med Hygiene 52(2):162–165, 1995.

Dalton MJ, Clarke MJ, Holman RC, Krebs JW, Fishbein DB, Olson JG, Childs JE: National surveillance for Rocky Mountain spotted fever, 1981–1992: Epidemiologic summary and evaluation of risk factors for fatal outcome. Am J Tropical Med Hygiene 52(5):405–413, 1995.

Holt DE, Hurley R, Harvey D: A reappraisal of chloramphenicol metabolism: detection and quantification of metabolites in the sera of children. J Antimicrobial Chemother 35(1):115–127, 1995.

CHLORAZEPATE DIPOTASSIUM

(see Benzodiazepines, Plasma and Urine)

CHLORDIAZEPOXIDE, BLOOD

Norm: Negative.

		SI Units
Therapeutic levels	700–100 ng/ml	2.34–3.34 µmol/L
Panic level	>5000 ng/ml	>16.7 µmol/L

Panic Level Symptoms and Treatment:

Symptoms: Drowsiness, dysarthria, ataxia, and confusion.

Treatment:

Give activated charcoal.
Administer syrup of ipecac. (*Note:* Induction of vomiting is contraindicated in clients with no gag reflex, or with central nervous system depression or excitation.)
Perform neurologic checks q 1 hour.
Perform gastric emptying.
Monitor and protect airway.
Flumazenil has been used as a competitive antagonist to reverse the profound effects of benzodiazepine overdose. Use of Flumazenil is contraindicated if concomitant tricyclic antidepressants were taken.

Do NOT use barbiturates.
Forced diuresis and/or hemodialysis will NOT remove benzodiazepines. No information was found on whether peritoneal dialysis will remove these drugs.

Usage: Drug abuse, ongoing monitoring for therapeutic dosage, and overdose.

Description: Chlordiazepoxide is a mild benzodiazepine used for relief of mild to severe anxiety and tension; withdrawal symptoms of acute alcoholism, preoperative apprehension, and anxiety. It is also used for the short-term treatment of insomnia, acute treatment for seizures, and management of alcohol withdrawal symptoms. Chlordiazepoxide is metabolized by the liver and excreted by the kidneys, with a half-life of 5–30 hours. Overdosage may lead to respiratory depression and coma. Levels chronically over the therapeutic range may cause renal dysfunction.

Professional Considerations:

1. Consent form NOT required.
2. Preparation:
   A. Tube: Red-top, red/gray-top, or gold-top.
   B. Do NOT draw during hemodialysis.
3. Procedure:
   A. Collect a 3-ml blood sample.
4. Postprocedure care:
   A. None.

5. Client and family teaching:
   A. For the client who takes chlordiazepoxide regularly, watch for, and call the physician in the event of, early signs of overdose: drowsiness, unsteady gait, and/or confusion.
   B. For an intentional overdose, refer the client and his or her family for crisis intervention.
   C. Referrals to appropriate rehabilitation centers and therapeutic community programs should be offered to all addicted clients who may be interested.
   D. If activated charcoal was given for elevated levels, the client should drink 4–6 glasses of water each day for 2 days to prevent constipation. The activated charcoal will also cause stools to be black for a few days.
6. Factors that affect results:
   A. Kidney disease elevates blood levels.
7. Other data:
   A. The drug should be tapered, rather than abruptly withdrawn.
   B. *See also Benzodiazepines, Plasma and Urine.*

Bibliography:

Closser MH, Brower KJ: Treatment of alprazolam withdrawal with chlordiazepoxide substitution and taper. J Substance Abuse Treatment *11*(4): 319–323, 1994.

Hoey LL, Nahum A, Vance-Bryan K: A retrospective review and assessment of benzodiazepines in the treatment of alcohol withdrawal in hospitalized patients. Pharmacotherapy *14*(5):572–578, 1994.

Newman JP, Terris DJ, Moore M: Trends in the management of alcohol withdrawal syndromes. Laryngoscope *105*(1):1–7, 1995.

Saitz R, Mayo-Smith MF, Roberts MS, Redmond HA, Bernard DR, Calkins DR: Individualized treatment for alcohol withdrawal: A randomized double-blind controlled trial. JAMA *272*(7):519–523, 1994.

CHLORIDE, SERUM

Norm:

		SI Units
Children and adults	97–107 mEq/L	97–107 mmol/L
Premature infants	95–110 mEq/L	95–110 mmol/L
Full-term infants	96–106 mEq/L	96–106 mmol/L
Panic levels	<80 mEq/L	<80 mmol/L
	>115 mEq/L	>115 mmol/L

Panic Level Symptoms and Treatment:

Symptoms: Impaired mentation, hypotension or hypertension, and cardiac dysrhythmias.

Treatment: Correct the underlying disorder.

Increased: Acidosis (hyperchloremic, nephrotic), alcoholism, alkalosis (respiratory), hyperaldosteronism (primary), anemia, bromism, congestive heart failure, Cushing's disease, dehydration, diabetes insipidus, diarrhea (sodium loss > chloride loss), eclampsia, fever, head trauma, hypercorticoadrenalism, hypernatremia, hyperparathyroidism, hyperventilation, hypoproteinemia, intestinal fistula (sodium loss > chloride loss), nephritis (acute), nephrosis, neurogenic hyperventilation, ostomies, prostatic obstruction, renal failure (acute), salicylate intoxication, seawater aspiration (severe), serum sickness, uremia, ureterosigmoidostomy, and urinary obstruction. Drugs include acetazolamide, ammonium chloride, boracic acid, boric acid, chlorothiazide, cholestyramine, cyclosporin, glucocorticoids, guanethidine sulfate, imipenem-cilastin sodium, oxyphenbutazone, phenylbutazone, sodium bromide, sodium chloride, and spironolactone.

Decreased: Acidosis (diabetic, diarrheal, lactic, metabolic, tubular, respiratory), Addison's disease, anesthesia, burns, CNS disorders, cholera, congestive heart failure, diabetic ketoacidosis, diaphoresis, diarrhea (severe), edema, emphysema, fasting, fever, freshwater aspiration, heat exhaustion, heavymetal poisoning, hypertrophic pyloric stenosis, hypokalemia, hyponatremia, hypoventilation, infections (acute), intestinal obstruction, nephritis, paralytic ileus, pneumonia, pyelonephritis (chronic), pyloric obstruction, renal failure (chronic), rickettsial diseases, suction (gastric), syndrome of inappropriate antidiuretic hormone secretion, typhus fever, ulcerative colitis, uremia, vomiting, Waterhouse-Friderichsen syndrome, and water intoxication. Drugs include aldosterone, amiloride hydrochloride, bumetanide, corticotropin, dextrose infusions (prolonged), ethacrynic acid, furosemide, mercurial diuretics, prednisolone, prednisolone acetate, prednisolone sodium phosphate, prednisolone tebutate, sodium bicarbonate, spironolactone, triamterene, and thiazide diuretics.

Description: Chloride, a hydrochloric acid salt, is the most abundant body anion in the extracellular fluid. It functions in counterbalancing cations such as sodium and also acts as a buffer during oxygen/carbon dioxide exchange in red blood cells. Chloride also aids in digestion, osmotic pressure, and water balance. It is measured in serum, along with other electrolytes to evaluate electrolyte acid-base balance.

Professional Considerations:

1. Consent form NOT required.
2. Preparation:
   A. Tube: Red-top, red/gray-top, or gold-top.
   B. Do NOT draw during hemodialysis.
3. Procedure:
   A. Draw the specimen from an extremity that does not have saline infusing into it. Draw a 3-ml blood sample without a tourniquet, if possible.
   B. The sample may be taken from infants from a capillary heelstick.
   C. Do NOT allow the client to clench/unclench the hand prior to blood drawing.
4. Postprocedure care:
   A. None.
5. Client and family teaching:
   A. Results are normally available in ≤4 hours.
6. Factors that affect results:
   A. Reject hemolyzed specimens.
   B. Any condition accompanied by prolonged vomiting and/or diarrhea will alter levels.
   C. Potassium chloride, ammonium chloride, acetazolamide methyldopa, diazoxide, and bromides may cause falsely elevated results.
   D. Drugs such as ethacrynic acid, furosemide, thiazide diuiretics, and bicarbonate may lead to decreased levels.
7. Other data:
   A. In respiratory acidosis, chloride excretion is a necessary component of renal compensation.
   B. Useful interpretation of the results requires clinical knowledge of the client.

Bibliography:

Chalas J, Francoual J, Lindenbaum A: A reply to: Evaluation of methods for sodium, potassium, and chloride determination in relation to the analytical quality goals. Ann Biol Clin 53(4):239–240, 1995.
Norris MK: Checking chloride levels. Nursing 24(3):76, 1994.

CHLORIDE, SWEAT, SPECIMEN

Norm:

		SI Units
Adults	10–70 mEq/L	10–70 mmol/L
Children	5–45 mEq/L	5–45 mmol/L

Increased: Cystic fibrosis (levels >60 mEq/L are indicative of cystic fibrosis in children <age 20). Also Addison's disease, adrenal insufficiency, diabetes insipidus (hereditary nephrogenic), ectodermal dysplasia, fucosidosis, glucose-6-phosphate-dehydrogenase deficiency, hypothyroidism, malnutrition, mucopolysaccharidosis, and renal failure.

Decreased: Hypoaldosteronism and sodium depletion. Drugs include mineralocorticoids.

Description: Chloride is an electrolyte normally excreted in sweat and urine combined chemically with sodium or other cations. It functions in the maintenance of acid-base balance and electrical neutrality of the body. Sweat chloride levels are found to be especially high in children with cystic fibrosis, a genetic disease that affects exocrine gland functioning, including the sweat glands of the skin, which secrete abnormally high levels of sodium, potassium, and chloride electrolytes. Sweat chloride levels are often high in genetic carriers of the cystic fibrosis genome as well. Genetic carriers have one recessive defective gene and one dominant normal gene and have no other manifestations of the disease. This test involves the stimulation of sweat production by iontophoresis, the painless delivery of a small amount of electric current to the skin.

Professional Considerations:

1. Consent form NOT required.

Risks:
None.

Contraindications:
In clients with dermatitis.

2. Preparation:
   A. Obtain equipment for the iontophoresis and preweighed gauze or filter paper, sterile water, normal saline, forceps, weighing bottle, tape, plastic, and pilocarpine.
3. Procedure: Gibson-Cooke Technique:
   A. Wash and dry the right forearm or right thigh with distilled water.
   B. Place a small amount of the pilocarpine-soaked gauze on the skin of the area to be studied and attach it to

the positive electrode. Place a small amount of the saline-soaked gauze on the skin and attach it to the negative electrode.
   C. Deliver 4 mA of current in 15- to 20-second intervals for 5 minutes.
   D. Remove and discard the electrodes.
   E. Place the preweighed, dry, sterile gauze or filter paper over the pilocarpine gauze site. Cover it with plastic and seal it with waterproof tape.
   F. After 30–40 minutes, droplets visible beneath the plastic indicate an adequate accumulation of sweat.
   G. Remove and discard the tape and plastic.
   H. Remove the gauze or filter paper with forceps and place it directly into a weighing bottle, seal it tightly, and send it to the laboratory.
4. Postprocedure care:
   A. It is normal for the studied area to remain reddened for several hours.
5. Client and family teaching:
   A. The test is not painful but does cause a minor tingling sensation.
   B. Parents are able to stay with the child during the test to help provide distraction.
   C. Skin erythema will fade within 24 hours.
6. Factors that affect results:
   A. Improper cleansing of the test area may cause unreliable results.
   B. The hands have a higher sweat chloride content than arms or legs and thus should be avoided as a study site.
   C. Hot weather could deplete sodium chloride stores and affect the results.
   D. Poor or incomplete sealing of the test site could result in falsely increased chloride levels by allowing evaporation of sweat.
   E. Falsely low values may occur in clients with edema or hypoproteinemia.
   F. Increased levels may be caused by skin rashes or lesions over the testing site.
7. Other data:
   A. A positive sweat test in itself is not diagnostic of cystic fibrosis. The clinical picture and family history are important considerations.
   B. Repetition of both borderline and positive tests is recommended.

Bibliography:

Gibson LE, Cooke RE: A test for concentration of electrolytes in sweat in cystic fibrosis of the pancreas utilizing pilocarpine by iontophoresis. Pediatrics *23*:545–549, 1959.

Hammond KB, Turcios NL, Gibson LE: Clinical evaluation of the macroduct sweat collection system and conductivity analyzer in the diagnosis of cystic fibrosis. J Pediatr *124*(2):255–260, 1994.

Highsmith WE, Burch LH, Zhou Z, Olsen JC, Boat TE, Spock A, Gorvoy JD, Quittel L, Friedman KJ, Silverman LM, et al.: A novel mutation in the cystic fibrosis gene in patients with pulmonary disease but normal sweat chloride concentrations. New Engl J Med *331*(15):974–980, 1994.

CHLORIDE, URINE

Norm:

		SI Units
24-hour Urine		
Adult	110–250 mEq/24 h	110–250 mmol/day
>Age 60	95–195 mEq/24 h	95–195 mmol/day
Spot Urine	15–115 mEq/L	15–115 mmol/L
Child		
Infant	2–10 mEq/L	2–10 mmol/L
12 months–6 years	15–40 mEq/L	15–40 mmol/L
6–10 years		
Male	36–110 mEq/L	36–110 mmol/L
Female	18–74 mEq/L	18–74 mmol/L
10–14 years		
Male	64–176 mEq/L	64–176 mmol/L
Female	36–173 mEq/L	36–173 mmol/L

Increased: Cushing's syndrome, dehydration, hypernatremia, salicylate toxicity, syndrome of inappropriate antidiuretic hormone secretion (SIADHS), and starvation. Drugs include chlorothiazide diuretics and mercurial diuretics.

Decreased: Addison's disease, congestive heart failure (prolonged), diarrhea, diaphoresis, emphysema, low-salt diet, malabsorption syndrome, nasogastric suction (prolonged), pyloric obstruction, and renal damage.

Description: Chloride is the most abundant extracellular anion. It is normally excreted by the kidney to help maintain the normal fluid and electrolyte and acid-base balance of the body. The amount of chloride excreted in the urine is an indication of the state of electrolyte balance.

Professional Considerations:

1. Consent form NOT required.
2. Preparation:
   A. Obtain a clean, 3-L specimen container without preservatives.
   B. Write the beginning time of collection on the laboratory requisition and specimen container.
3. Procedure:
   A. Discard the first morning urine specimen.
   B. Begin to time a 24-hour urine collection.
   C. Save all the urine voided for 24 hours in a clean, 3-L container without preservatives. Refrigeration is unnecessary. Include the urine voided at the end of the 24-hour period.
4. Postprocedure care:

A. Compare the urine quantity in the specimen container with the urinary output record for the test. If the specimen contains less urine than was recorded as output, some of the sample may have been discarded, invalidating the test.
B. Document the quantity of the urine output for the 24-hour collection period on the laboratory requisition.
C. Send the specimen to the laboratory for refrigeration.
5. Client and family teaching:
   A. Save all the urine voided in the 24-hour period and urinate before defecating to avoid loss of urine. If any urine is accidentally discarded, discard the entire specimen and restart the collection the next day.
6. Factors that affect results:
   A. All the urine voided for the 24-hour period must be included to avoid a falsely low result.
   B. Bromides may cause falsely elevated results.
7. Other data:
   A. Dietary intake should be considered when evaluating results. This is a useful test for monitoring the effects of a low-salt diet.

Bibliography:

Meland E, Laerum E, Ulvik RJ: Salt restriction in hypertension—the effect of dietary advice and self monitoring of chloride concentration in urine. Scand J Clin Lab Invest *54*(5):399–404, 1994.

Shankaran S, Liang KC, Ilagan N, Fleischmann L: Mineral excretion following furosemide compared with bumetanide therapy in premature infants. Pediatr Nephrol *9*(2):159–162, 1995.

CHLORPHENTERMINE
(see Amphetamines, Blood)

CHLORPROMAZINE
(see Phenothiazines, Blood

CHOLANGIOGRAM
*(see Endoscopic Retrograde
Cholangiopancreatography,
Diagnostic; Intravenous
Cholangiography, Diagnostic;
Percutaneous Transhepatic
Cholangiography, Diagnostic; or T-
Tube Cholangiography,
Postoperative, Diagnostic)*

CHOLECYSTOGRAPHY RADIOGRAPHY, DIAGNOSTIC

Norm: Good visualization of the gall-bladder; no stones and no filling defects.

Usage: Diagnosis of gallbladder pathology such as stones, polyps, tumors, or duct defects. Usually complaints of right upper quadrant, right epigastric pain, or both, of unknown etiology.

Description: Oral cholecystography is used to study the dye-filled gallbladder by radiographic film. Stones or calculi can be seen as darker shadows, and filling defects indicate polyps or tumors after opacification of the gallbladder by radiopaque contrast medium. The gallbladder and the contour and patency of the cystic duct and hepatic ducts are also studied.

Professional Considerations:

1. Consent form IS required.

Risks:
Respiratory failure, shock, allergic reaction to dye (itching, hives, rash, tight feeling in the throat, shortness of breath, bronchospasm, anaphylaxis, death); renal toxicity.

Contraindications:
Known abdominal infection or inflammation; vomiting; previous allergy to iodine, iopanoic acid, radiographic dye, or shellfish; renal or hepatic failure; and pregnancy, unless the benefits outweigh the risks; jaundice with bilirubin >2 mg/dl; or severe vomiting or diarrhea.

2. Preparation:
    A. *See Client and family teaching.*
    B. Have emergency equipment readily available.
    C. If diarrhea or vomiting occurs before the test, consult the radiologist to see if the test should be rescheduled.
3. Procedure:
    A. A series of radiographic films are taken of the right upper quadrant of the client's abdomen with the client in several positions.
4. Postprocedure care:
    A. The dye is excreted in the urine. Mild dysuria is common.
    B. A fatty meal may enhance dye excretion. The client may resume a normal diet.
    C. Observe for allergic reaction to radiographic dye (listed above) × 24 hours.
5. Client and family teaching:
    A. On the evening prior to the test, eat a low-fat meal, and then fast beginning at midnight before the test or after step B, whichever is earlier.
    B. Take six 0.5-g iopanoic acid tablets by mouth 12 hours prior to the test. The tablets should be taken with a large amount of water at 5-minute intervals. Then fast from food and fluids until the test is completed.
    C. If preparing for the test at home, go to the nearest emergency room if experiencing rash, itching, or hives, or difficulty in breathing after taking iopanoic acid tablets.
    D. The procedure will take approximately 1 hour.
6. Factors that affect results:
    A. Hepatic failure with bilirubin >1.8 mg/dl will interfere with gallbladder visualization. The dye must be processed in the liver before it passes into the gallbladder. The test will be cancelled for a high bilirubin level.
    B. Vomiting or diarrhea will inhibit dye uptake and result in inadequate visualization of the gallbladder. If either occurs, the test should be postponed and the dye readministered. Alternatively, other visualization methods may be used.
    C. A fatty diet will cause the dye to pass through the system too rapidly for gallbladder visualization to be performed 12 hours after the dye tablets are taken.
7. Other data:
    A. Occasionally, after the above procedure, the client is given a fatty meal or Bilevac (fatty synthetic) to test gallbladder contractility. Further radiographs are then taken in 1–2 hours.
    B. Contractility studies may also be accomplished 15 minutes after the first set of radiographs by intravenous injection of fatty sincalide.
    C. Cholecystography is being replaced by

ultrasound, which is now the diagnostic test of choice, or by MRI/CT in selected situations.

Bibliography:

Creasy TS: Assessment of the biliary tract by antegrade cholecystography after percutaneous cholecystostomy in patients with acute cholecystitis. Br J Radiol 66(788):662–666, 1993.

Diehl AK, Schwesinger WH, Holleman DR Jr, Chapman JB, Kurtin WE: Clinical correlates of gallstone composition: distinguishing pigment from cholesterol stones. Am J Gastroenterol 90(6): 967–972, 1995.

CHOLESTEROL, BLOOD

Norm: There is variation in recommended norms in the literature.
(*Note:* Range given applies to a healthy population consuming a typical North American diet.)

Age	Male mg/dl	Male SI Units mmol/L	Female mg/dl	Female SI Units mmol/L
Total Cholesterol				
Adult	(10% higher levels for Afro-Americans)			
20–24	124–218	3.21–5.64	122–216	3.16–5.59
25–29	133–244	3.44–6.32	128–222	3.32–5.75
30–34	138–254	3.57–6.58	130–230	3.37–5.96
35–39	146–270	3.78–6.99	140–242	3.63–6.27
40–44	151–268	3.91–6.94	147–252	3.81–6.53
45–49	158–276	4.09–7.15	152–265	3.94–6.86
50–54	158–277	4.09–7.17	162–285	4.20–7.38
55–59	156–276	4.04–7.15	172–300	4.45–7.77
60–64	159–276	4.12–7.15	172–297	4.45–7.69
65–69	158–274	4.09–7.10	171–303	4.43–7.85
≥70	144–265	3.73–6.86	173–280	4.48–7.25
Child				
Cord blood	44–103	1.14–2.66	50–108	1.29–2.79
≤4	114–203	2.95–5.25	112–200	2.90–5.18
5–9	121–203	3.13–5.25	126–205	3.26–5.30
10–14	119–202	3.08–5.23	124–201	3.21–5.20
15–19	113–197	2.93–5.10	119–200	3.08–5.18

High-Density Lipoprotein Cholesterol (HDL)

Age	Male mg/dl	Male SI Units mmol/L	Female mg/dl	Female SI Units mmol/L
Adult	(Afro-American levels approximately 10 mg/dL higher)			
20–24	30–63	0.78–1.63	33–79	0.85–2.04
25–29	31–63	0.80–1.63	37–83	0.96–2.15
30–34	28–63	0.72–1.63	36–77	0.93–1.99
35–39	29–62	0.75–1.60	34–82	0.88–2.12
40–44	27–67	0.70–1.73	34–88	0.88–2.28
45–49	30–64	0.78–1.66	34–87	0.88–2.25
50–54	28–63	0.72–1.63	37–92	0.96–2.38
55–59	28–71	0.72–1.84	37–91	0.96–2.35
60–64	30–74	0.78–1.91	38–92	0.98–2.38
65–69	30–75	0.78–1.94	35–96	0.91–2.48
≥70	31–75	0.80–1.94	33–92	0.85–2.38
Child				
Cord blood	6–53	0.16–1.37	13–56	0.34–1.45
5–9	38–75	0.98–1.94	36–73	0.93–1.89
10–14	37–74	0.96–1.91	37–70	0.96–1.81
15–19	30–63	0.78–1.63	35–74	0.91–1.91

Age	Male		Female	
	mg/dl	SI Units mmol/L	mg/dl	SI Units mmol/L
Low-Density Lipoprotein Cholesterol (LDL)				
Adult				
20–24	66–147	1.71–3.81	57–159	1.48–4.12
25–29	70–165	1.81–4.27	71–164	1.84–4.25
30–34	78–185	2.02–4.79	70–156	1.81–4.04
35–39	81–189	2.10–4.90	75–172	1.94–4.45
40–44	87–186	2.25–4.82	74–174	1.92–4.51
45–49	97–202	2.51–5.23	79–186	2.05–4.82
50–54	89–197	2.31–5.10	88–201	2.28–5.21
55–59	88–203	2.28–5.26	89–210	2.31–5.44
60–64	83–210	2.15–5.44	100–224	2.59–5.80
65–69	98–210	2.54–5.44	92–221	2.38–5.72
≥70	88–186	2.28–4.82	96–206	2.49–5.34
Child				
Cord blood	20–56	0.52–1.45	21–58	0.54–1.50
5–9	63–129	1.63–3.34	68–140	1.76–3.63
10–14	64–133	1.66–3.44	68–136	1.76–3.52
15–19	62–130	1.61–3.37	59–137	1.53–3.55

		SI Units
Cholesterol Esters	60–75% of total or <210 mg/dl	0.60–0.75 <5.43 mmol/L
Free cholesterol	<50 mg/dl	<1.29 mmol/L
LDL:HDL ratio	<3	<3

Increased Total Cholesterol: Anemia (aplastic), anorexia nervosa, atherosclerosis, bile duct blockage, coronary heart disease, celiac disease, cholestasis, cirrhosis (biliary), congestive heart failure, Cushing's disease, debrancher deficiency, diabetes mellitus (poorly controlled), eclampsia, Forbes' disease, glomerulonephritis, hepatic cholesterol ester storage disease, hepatic phosphorylase deficiency, hypercholesterolemia (idiopathic), hyperlipoproteinemia, hypothyroidism, jaundice (obstructive, cholestatic), leukemia, limit dextrinosis, lipid disorders, lipoidosis, nephrosis, nephrotic syndrome, pancreatectomy, pancreatitis (chronic), pregnancy, starvation (early), stress, type III glycogen deposition disease, type VI glycogen storage disease, and von Gierke's disease. Drugs include amiodarone, anabolic steroids, androgens, catecholamines, chenodeoxycholic acid, cinchophen, chlorpropamide, corticosteroids (glucogenic), cyclosporine, diuretics, epinephrine, epinephrine bitartrate, epinephrine borate, epinephrine hydrochloride, epinephrine racemic, ergocalciferol, isotretinoin, levodopa, miconazole, oral contraceptives, phenytoin, phenytoin sodium, sulfonamides, thiazides.

Decreased Total Cholesterol: Abetalipoproteinemia, acanthocytosis, amylopectinosis, Andersen's disease, anemia (pernicious, hemolytic, hypochromic), Bassen-Kornzweig syndrome, brancher deficiency, cancer, cirrhosis (Laennec's, portal), epilepsy, familial lecithin-cholesterol acyltransferase deficiency (absent cholesterol esters), Gaucher's disease, Hansen's disease, hepatic disease, hepatitis (toxic, viral), hyperthyroidism, hypobetalipoproteinemia, infections (severe), intestinal obstruction, jaundice (hepatocellular), leprosy, liver cellular necrosis, malnutrition, pancreatic carcinoma, porphyria (acute, intermittent), premenstrual time phase, steatorrhea, Tangier disease, tuberculosis, type IV glycogen deposition disease, and uremia. Drugs include allopurinol, aminosalicylic acid, androgens, asparaginase, azathioprine, carbutamide, cholestyramine, chlorpropamide, chlortetracycline, clofibrate, clomiphene, colchicine, colestipol, cyproterone acetate, dextrothyroxine, doxazocin, erythromycin, estrogens, fenfluramine, gemfibrozil, glucagon, haloperidol, heparin sodium, hydralazine, interferon, isoniazid, kanamycin, ketoconazole, levothyroxine sodium, lovastatin, MAO inhibitors, neomycin, niacin, neomycin, phenformin, pravastatin, prazosin, probucol, simvastatin, tetracyclines, thiazides, thyroxine, trimethadione, and vitamin A.

Description: Cholesterol is a sterol compound synthesized exogenously in the liver from dietary fats and endogenously within cells. It is present in all body tissues and is a major component of low-density lipoproteins (LDL), brain and nerve cells, cell membranes, and some gallstones. Hypercholesterolemia, combined with low levels of high-density lipoprotein HDL), increases the risk for developing arteriosclerosis. Levels under 200 mg/dl (5.17 mmol/L, SI units) are desirable. Levels from 200–239 mg/dl (5.17–6.18 mmol/L, SI units) are classified as borderline high, and levels over 239 mg/dl (>6.18 mmol/L, SI units) are classified as high. Cholesterol levels tend to decrease temporarily with major illness or surgery.

Professional Considerations:
1. Consent form NOT required.
2. Preparation:
   A. *See Client and family teaching.*
   B. Tube: Red-top, red/gray-top, or gold-top.
3. Procedure:
   A. Leave the tourniquet on for as short a time as possible and no more than 2 minutes.
   B. *Total cholesterol and cholesterol esters*:
      i. Draw a 1-ml blood sample.
   C. *HDL cholesterol*:
      i. Draw a 1-ml blood sample.
4. Postprocedure care:
   A. Transport the specimen to the laboratory immediately.
5. Client and family teaching:
   A. Consume a diet containing consistent levels of cholesterol for 3 weeks before this test.
   B. If more than total cholesterol will be measured, fast from food and liquids, except for water, for 12–14 hours and from alcohol for 24 hours prior to the test.
   C. The evening meal prior to the test should be free of high-cholesterol foods and have less than 30% total fat content.

D. Drugs affecting the results should be withheld for 24 hours, whenever possible.
E. Desirable cholesterol levels and risk for coronary heart disease are listed in this section in the *Lipid Profile, Blood Test*. These may be used to identify and teach desirable levels to clients.

6. Factors that affect results:
   A. Reject hemolyzed specimens.
   B. Levels may be lower when collected with the client recumbent for 20 minutes or more than in those samples collected when the client is standing erect.
   C. Cholesterol levels should always be drawn at the same time of day after the same type of diet the day before, with the client in the same position.
   D. Drugs which may cause falsely elevated results include ascorbic acid, bromides, chlorpromazine, corticosteroids, iodides, viomycin, and vitamin A.
   E. Drugs that may cause falsely decreased levels include nitrates, nitrites, and propylthiouracil.

7. Other data:
   A. Total cholesterol specimen is stable for 7 days at room temperature when nonhemolyzed.
   B. Cholesterol esters convert to free cholesterol when left at room temperature.
   C. *See also Low-Density Lipoprotein Cholesterol, Blood; and High-Density Lipoprotein Cholesterol, Blood.*

Bibliography:
Jarvik GP, Wijsman EM, Kukull WA, Schellenberg GD, Yu C, Larson EB: Interactions of apolipoprotein E genotype, total cholesterol level, age, sex in prediction of Alzheimer's disease: a case-control study. Neurology *45*(6):1092–1096, 1995.

Lee MJ, Crook T, Noel C, Levinson UM: Detergent extraction and enzymatic analysis for fecal long-chain fatty acids, triglycerides, and cholesterol. Clin Chem *40*(12):2230–2234, 1994.

CHOLINESTERASE II
(see Pseudocholinesterase, Plasma)

CHOLINESTERASE (PSEUDO), PLASMA
(see Pseudocholinesterase, Plasma)

CHORIONIC VILLI SAMPLING, DIAGNOSTIC

Norm: No detection of chromosome/genetic defects.

Usage: Detection of genetic defects, chromosomal abnormalities, and acquired disorders in fetuses in women who are at high risk. Disorders such as hemophilia (factor VIII or IX), cystic fibrosis, mental retardation, Down syndrome, chromosome abnormalities, fragile X syndrome, beta-thalassemia, and Duchenne muscular dystrophy. Infections.

Description: Chorionic villi Sampling (CVS) consists of extracting a small amount of villous tissue directly from the chorion. This procedure can be performed at about 10 weeks' gestation and does not require in vitro culturing of cells because sufficient numbers are directly available in the extracted tissue. The procedure allows prenatal diagnosis at about 2 months' gestation rather than at nearly 5 months' gestation.

Professional Considerations:

1. Consent form IS required.

Risks:

Bleeding, hematoma, infection, intrauterine death, spontaneous abortion. Limb reduction defects may occur, possibly due to vascular accident from decreased perfusion in distal limbs or from thrombosis at the sampling site, or from inadvertent amnion puncture resulting in either amniotic bands or loss of amniotic fluid, with subsequent compression and deformity (Gruber et al. 1994). *See also Amniocentesis and Amniotic Fluid Analysis, Diagnostic.* CVS involves slightly higher fetal loss rate than does amniocentesis, with most estimates ranging from 1 to 2%.

Contraindications:

Morbid obesity, retroverted uterus with intervening bowel.

2. Preparation:
   A. Arrange for a laboratory technician to be present to evaluate the sample on location.
   B. Must have complete family history.
   C. Provide continuous fetal heart tone monitoring.
   D. *See Amniocentesis and Amniotic Fluid Analysis, Diagnostic.*
   E. *See Obstetric Sonogram, Diagnostic.*
3. Procedure:
   A. *Transabdominal CVS:*
      i. The client is positioned supine.
      ii. Under ultrasonic guidance, a long 20-gauge needle is inserted percutaneously through the abdomen into villous tissue.
   B. *Transcervical CVS:*
      i. The client is placed in dorsal lithotomy position.
      ii. Under ultrasonic guidance, a malleable catheter is inserted through the cervix into villous tissue.
      iii. The perineum, vagina, and cervix are prepared with antiseptic solution.
      iv. A sterile speculum is placed in the vagina to allow visualization of the cervix.
      v. The catheter is advanced through the cervix into chorion frondasum under ultrasonic guidance.
4. Postprocedure care:
   A. Suggest maternal serum α-fetoprotein (MSAFP) screening at 15–20 weeks' gestation.
   B. *See Amniocentesis and Amniotic Fluid Analysis, Diagnostic.*
   C. *See Obstetric Sonogram, Diagnostic.*
5. Client and family teaching:
   A. The advantage of CVS, as opposed to amniocentesis, is earlier diagnosis of genetic defects.
   B. Explore the couple's expectations and review the risks and limitations of the test.
   C. Refer the client with abnormal results for genetic counseling.
6. Factors that affect results:
   A. Specimens not large enough invalidate the results.
   B. Specimens not labeled invalidate the results.
7. Other data:
   A. CVS is not indicated if neural tube defect is suspected.
   B. *See also Amniocentesis and Amniotic Fluid Analysis, Diagnostic.*

Bibliography:

Bahado-Singh RO, Morotti R, Pirhonen J, Copel JA, Mahoney MJ: Invasive techniques for prenatal diagnosis: current concepts. J Assoc Acad Minor Phys 6(1):28–33, 1995.

Brambati B: Chorionic villus sampling. Curr Opin Obstet Gynecol. 7(2):109–16, 1995.

Gruber B, Burton BK: Oromandibular-limb hypogenesis syndrome following chorionic villus sampling. Int J Pediatr Otorhinolaryngol 29(1):59–63, 1994.

CHRISTMAS FACTOR, BLOOD

(see Factor IX, Blood)

CHROMIUM, SERUM

Norm: 0.18–0.47 ng/ml (35–90 nmol/L, SI units) or <0.5 mg/L.

Increased: Chromium toxicity.

Decreased: Total parenteral nutrition.

Description: Chromium is a trace element normally found in the body. It may aid amino acid transport, especially to the liver and heart. Chromium may also enhance insulin activity and proper glucose utilization. Industrial exposure to chromium in tanning, electroplating, steel and metal industries, photography, and the paint, dye, and explosives industries may cause toxicity, resulting in liver and kidney impairment, dermatitis, convulsions, and coma. Respiratory tract cancers have been linked to chromium exposure.

Professional Considerations:

1. Consent form NOT required.
2. Preparation:
   A. Tube: Blue-top, metal-free.
3. Procedure:
   A. Draw a 5-ml blood sample.
4. Postprocedure care:
   A. None.
5. Client and family teaching:
   A. Results are normally available within 24–48 hours.
6. Factors that affect results:
   A. Reject hemolyzed specimens.
   B. Results are invalidated if the client has undergone a recent diagnostic test involving the injection of radioactive chromium.
   C. Laboratory equipment used to measure chromium must be free of metal and stainless steel. Measurement must be performed under laminar air flow conditions.
7. Other data:
   A. Occupational exposure causes dermatitis, skin ulcerations, perforations of the nasal septum, asthma, and cancer of the nasal mucosa or lungs.
   B. *See also Cr-51, Blood and Chromium, Urine.*

Bibliography:

Gao M, Levy LS, Faux SP, Aw TC, Braithwaite RA, Brown SS: Use of molecular epidemiological techniques in a pilot study on workers exposed to chromium. Occup Environ Med *51*(10):663–668, 1994.

Granadillo VA, Parra de Machado L, Romero RA: Determination of total chromium in whole blood, blood components, bone, and urine by fast furnace program electrothermal atomization AAS and using neither analyte isoformation nor background correction. Anal Chem *66*(21):3624–3631, 1994.

Losi ME, Amrhein C, Frankenberger WT Jr: Environmental biochemistry of chromium. Rev Environ Contamination and Toxicol *1326*:91–121, 1994.

Raithel HJ, Schaller KH, Kraus T, Lehnert G: Biomonitoring of nickel and chromium in human pulmonary tissue. International Archives of Occupational and Environmental Health *65*(Suppl 1):S197–S200, 1993.

Simpson JR, Gibson RS: Hair, serum, and urine chromium concentrations in former employees of the leather tanning industry. Biol Trace Element Res *32*:155–159, 1992.

CHROMIUM, URINE

Norm:

	SI Units
0.1–2.0 µg/L	1.9–38.4 nmol/L

Increased: Chromium toxicity.

Decreased: Diabetes (children), pregnancy, total parenteral nutrition.

Description: Chromium is a trace element required by the body for its participation in the action of insulin on cell surfaces. Chromium is therefore important in glucose utilization. Deficiencies in chromium are being studied related to glucose intolerance and malnutrition. Chromium is mainly excreted by the kidneys, but it is currently difficult to measure chromium in small amounts in the urine. Chromium toxicity occurs from high exposure in the tanning, electroplating, steel and other metal industries, photography, and the paint, dye, and explosives industries, and may also occur in clients with chronic renal disease. Toxicity may result in liver and kidney impairment, dermatitis, convulsions, and coma. Respiratory tract cancers have been linked to chromium exposure. This test is used to detect chromium toxicity.

Professional Considerations:

1. Consent form NOT required.
2. Preparation:
   A. Prepare a 3-L container for chromium collection by leeching it for 48 hours in 10% nitric acid and then washing it with metal-free, distilled water.
   B. Write the exact starting time of the urine collection on the laboratory requisition.
3. Procedure:
   A. Collect a 24-hour urine specimen in an air-tight, specially prepared 3-L container free of preservatives and metals.
   B. Avoid contamination of the urine with stool.
4. Postprocedure care:
   A. Compare urine quantity in the specimen container with the urinary output record for the test. If the specimen contains less urine than was recorded as output, some of the sample may

have been discarded, invalidating the test.
  B. Document quantity of urine output for the collection period on the laboratory requisition.
5. Client and family teaching:
  A. Save all the urine voided in the 24-hour period and urinate before defecating to avoid loss of urine. If any of the urine is accidentally discarded, discard the entire specimen and restart the collection the next day.
  B. Results are normally available within 24 hours.
6. Factors that affect results:
  A. Falsely elevated values may result from urine exposed to metal (as in collections from a metal urinal or bedpan) or contaminated with stool.
  B. Laboratory equipment used to measure chromium must be free of metal and stainless steel. Measurement must be performed under laminar air flow conditions.
  C. All the urine voided for the 24-hour period must be included to avoid a falsely low result.
7. Other data:
  A. Most laboratories currently use urine as a gross screening for toxicity. Because of the difficulty detecting small amounts of chromium in urine, serum levels are more accurate for determination of the level of toxicity.

Bibliography:

Gao M, Levy LS, Faux SP, Aw TC, Braithwaite RA, Brown SS: Use of molecular epidemiological techniques in a pilot study on workers exposed to chromium. Occup Environ Med 51(10):663–668, 1994.

Gargas ML, Norton RL, Paustenbach DJ, Finley BL: Urinary excretion of chromium by humans following ingestion of chromium Picolinate. Implications for biomonitoring. Drug Metab Dispos 22(4):522–529, 1994.

Granadillo VA, Parra de Machado L, Romero RA: Determination of total chromium in whole blood, blood components, bone, and urine by fast furnace program electrothermal atomization AAS and using neither analyte isoformation nor background correction. Anal Chem 66(21):3624–3631, 1994.

CHROMOSOME ANALYSIS, BLOOD

Norm: A total of 46 chromosomes with 22 matched pairs plus XX for females and XY for males.

Usage: Diagnosis of chromosome abnormalities leading to Down syndrome, other physical or mental retardation, and sex chromosome disorders such as Turner's syndrome or Klinefelter's syndrome; establishes sex in hypogonadism or unclear genitalia; part of the work-up for amenorrhea, infertility, frequent miscarriages, and other chromosomal-related disorders and some leukemias; used in genetic counseling for prospective parents and those with a family history of genetic disease.

Description: Chromosome analysis involves karyotyping human chromosomes from a culture of leukocytes from peripheral blood. Cell replication of the cultured leukocytes is chemically halted in metaphase, and microscopic photographs are taken of the chromosomes within the cell nucleus. The chromosome pictures are enlarged and the chromosomes are paired, sorted, and studied for symmetry of pairs, number of chromosomes, identification of sex chromosomes, and staining patterns.

Professional Considerations:

1. Consent form NOT required.
2. Preparation:
  A. *See Client and family teaching.*
  B. Preschedule this test with the laboratory.
  C. Tube: Green-top.
3. Procedure:
  A. Draw a 7-ml blood sample.
4. Postprocedure care:
  A. Write the date and time of specimen collection on the laboratory requisition.
  B. Send the specimen to the laboratory immediately.
5. Client and family teaching:
  A. Fast for 3 hours and do not eat fatty foods for 12 hours prior to specimen collection.
6. Factors that affect results:
  A. Reject hemolyzed specimens or specimens received more than 24 hours after collection.
7. Other data:
  A. Karyotyping may be completed on other tissues including tumor cells, bone marrow, amniocentesis, or buccal smear.
  B. Some forms of leukemia, especially chronic myelogenous, are noted by chromosome assay of blood.

Bibliography:

Bouffler SD: Whole-chromosome hybridization. Intl Rev Cytol 153:171–232, 1994.

Pathak S, Dave BJ, Gagos S: Chromosome alterations in cancer development and apoptosis. In Vivo 8(5):843–850, 1994.

Royle NJ: The proterminal regions and telomeres of human chromosomes. Adv Genet 32:273–315, 1995.

CHS

(see Pseudocholinesterase, Plasma)

CHYMEX TEST FOR PANCREATIC FUNCTION, DIAGNOSTIC (BENTIROMIDE TEST, CHYMOTRYPSIN)

Norm: Normal exocrine pancreatic function as well as gastric emptying, intestinal absorption, and liver and renal function. Approximately 85 mg *para*-aminobenzoic acid (PABA) in urine within 6 hours after ingestion of Chymex (Bentiromide).

Usage: Noninvasive testing of pancreatic function, and minor role in work-up of malabsorption syndrome.

Description: Chymex is the trade name for bentiromide in glycol solution that is an easy, noninvasive test for pancreatic exocrine function. Normally, pancreatic digestive enzyme chymotrypsin cleaves the bentiromide in the intestine, liberating the PABA, which is then absorbed, processed in the liver to a conjugated arylamine, and excreted by the kidney within 6 hours. The urine test for PABA is the Bretton-Marstial method for analysis of arylamines.

Professional Considerations:

1. Consent form NOT required.

Risks:
Infection.

Contraindications:
The safety of this test is unknown and should therefore be avoided in pregnant women, nursing mothers, and children under age 6. The test is also contraindicated in clients with dysphagia, increased intracranial pressure (due to risk of osmotic shift of free water into brain cells), and congestive heart failure or other states of tenuous fluid balance.

2. Preparation:
   A. *See Client and family teaching.*
   B. Obtain Bentiromide, 500 mg, and a large plastic container for urine collection.
   C. The client should void just prior to the beginning of the study.
3. Procedure:
   A. Administer Bentiromide 500 mg orally, followed by 250 ml of water.

B. Give 250 ml of water orally after 2 hours.
C. Give 500 ml of water orally over the next 4-hour period.
D. Collect all urine during the 6-hour period beginning with ingestion of Bentiromide.
4. Postprocedure care:
   A. Send the urine to the laboratory promptly for an arylamine assay.
   B. A normal diet may be resumed.
5. Client and family teaching:
   A. Avoid other testing for 7 days.
   B. Fast overnight before the test.
   C. Drink plenty of fluids after the test.
6. Factors that affect results:
   A. Poor liver or renal function can interfere with accurate results.
   B. Supplemental pancreatic enzymes may cause false-normal results. They may be discontinued for 5 days prior to the test or 1 day in clients with cystic fibrosis.
   C. Falsely elevated results may be caused by sunscreens.
   D. Drugs that may cause falsely elevated results include acetaminophen, benzocaine, chloramphenicol, lidocaine hydrochloride, multivitamins (some), phenacetin, procainamide hydrochloride, and thiazide diuretics.
7. Other data:
   A. This test is not performed in all laboratories.

Bibliography:

Maringhini A, Nelson DK, Jones JD, Dimagno EP: Is the plasma amino acid consumption test an accurate test of exocrine pancreatic insufficiency? Gastroenterology *106*(2):488–493, 1994.

CHYMOTRYPSIN TEST
(see Chymex Test for Pancreatic Function, Diagnostic)

CIRCULATING ANTICOAGULANT (CAC, LUPUS ANTICOAGULANT), BLOOD

Norm: Negative. No CAC identified.

Positive: Indicates the presence of an inhibitor (CAC). There are two types of CAC: one is a specific factor inhibitor—an immunoglobulin that interferes with the function of any one clotting factor; and a lupus anticoagulant—an immunoglobulin that interferes with phospholipid in coagulation tests.

Description: Circulating anticoagulants (CACs) and lupus anticoagulants develop spontaneously or are acquired in association with diseases or certain medication exposure. Clients with systemic lupus erythematosus, malignancies, or chronic inflammatory diseases such as ulcerative colitis and rheumatoid arthritis are known to develop these antibodies. CACs may also develop during complications postpartum or in clients taking chlorpromazine, or similar drugs. In the laboratory they prolong the PT (prothrombin time), PTT (partial thromboplastin time) or both. CACs are detected by a test called a "mixing study," in which normal plasma is added to client plasma and the PT or PTT repeated. Failure to correct the clotting to normal is a positive test. Additional tests are used to determine whether the CAC is a specific factor inhibitor, or a lupus anticoagulant.

Professional Considerations:

1. Consent form NOT required.
2. Preparation:
   A. Tube: Blue-top.
3. Procedure:
   A. Draw this specimen last or discard 1–2 ml of blood into a syringe or tube, leaving the needle in place.
   B. Attach a second syringe or tube and draw a 5-ml blood sample into a blue-top tube.
   C. Mix the specimen well by gently inverting the tube several times and transport it within 1 hour of collection.
4. Postprocedure care:
   A. Write the collection time on the laboratory requisition.
5. Client and family teaching:
   A. The client must not take IV heparin for 4–8 hours, or SQ heparin for 24 hours. Some other anticoagulant drugs may interfere with the test. Coumadin (Warfarin) does not interfere.
6. Factors that affect results:
   A. Drugs that may cause false-positive results include heparin, hirudin, and argatroban.
   B. Contact of the specimen with the tissue thromboplastin may cause false-negative results. This is the reason for the double-draw procedure.
   C. Reject hemolyzed, diluted, iced, or clotted specimens and specimens received more than 1 hour after collection.
   D. Separate and refrigerate plasma if the test cannot be performed within 2 hours of collection.
7. Other data:
   A. Specific factor inhibitors cause severe bleeding. Severe clinical bleeding is rare with the lupus anticoagulant unless there are other clotting abnormalities such as thrombocytopenia.

Bibliography:

Armitage JB, Hernandez JA, Kaplan HS: Laboratory assessment of circulating anticoagulants. Clin Lab Med *14*(4):795–812, 1994.

Bowie EJ, Thompson JH Jr, Pascuzzi CA, Owen CA Jr. Thrombosis in systemic lupus despite circulating anticoagulants. J Lab Clin Med *62*:416, 1963.

CISTERNOGRAPHY, CSF FLOW SCAN

(see Cisternography, Radionuclide, Diagnostic)

CISTERNOGRAPHY, RADIONUCLIDE (CSF FLOW STUDIES, CSF FLOW SCAN), DIAGNOSTIC

Norm: Normal cerebrospinal fluid (CSF) flow patterns at specific times after intrathecal injection of radiographic material into the lumbar area of the spinal cord.

1 hour:	Basal cisterns.
3–4 hours:	Radioactivity has reached the cerebral area and begun to spread to the ventricles and subarachnoid area.
24 hours:	The flow of radioactivity should be complete to convexities or subarachnoid areas, without leakage or obstruction that would interfere with bilateral symmetry of flow.
48 hours:	Radioactivity is primarily diffuse over the vertex, but not in the brainstem area, as it has been absorbed into the blood circulation. Symmetry is normal.

Usage: Brain atrophy; communicating hydrocephalus; suspected hydrocephalus related to CSF flow blockage (i.e., tumor, cyst, subdural hematoma); CSF leakage (rhinorrhea); cerebrospinal fistulas; CSF leaks after trauma or neurosurgery, identification of dural tear site with basal skull fracture; evaluation of the patency of a CSF shunt; and work-up of central nervous system symptoms such as personality changes, behavioral changes, and other neurologic changes.

Description: A nuclear medicine study of the brain and cerebral blood flow. Injection of a radioisotope into the subarachnoid space through a cisternal or lumbar puncture. The head is scanned at regular intervals to determine the amount of time it takes for the radioisotope to clear from the circulating CSF. Several views are taken at specific times over 24–48 hours.

Professional Considerations:

1. Consent form IS required for the lumbar puncture, the radioactive injection, or the injection by cisternal puncture.

Risks:

Same as for *Lumbar Puncture, Diagnostic.*

Contraindications:

In elevated cerebrospinal fluid pressure; skin infection in lumbar or cisternal area.

2. Preparation:
   A. Inspect the lumbar and cisternal areas for skin infection.
   B. Obtain povidone-iodine, 1–2% Xylocaine, a needle, a syringe, radionuclide, and a sterile lumbar puncture tray including a spinal needle.
   C. Elevated CSF pressure should be ruled out prior to this procedure.
3. Procedure:
   A. *Lumbar injection:*
      i. The client is placed in a lateral position with knees drawn up and chin placed on the chest. A lumbar puncture is performed and CSF pressure is measured. A radionuclide (indium-111, ytterbium-169, iodine-131 bound to RISA) is injected into the lumbar spine space.
      ii. The client is then returned to a hospital room and usually must lie flat between studies, especially for the first series.
      iii. Cisternograms or radiographic scans are completed at 4, 24, and 48 hours.
      iv. The progress and flow pattern of the radiographic material is then studied for diagnostic purposes.
   B. *Cisternal injection:*
      i. Using the lumbar puncture set, a puncture is made directly into the cisterna magna at the base of the skull. A radionuclide (indium-111, ytterbium-169, iodine-131 bound to RISA) is injected into the cisterna magna.

      ii. Cisternograms are obtained in minutes and subsequent studies are performed in 24 and 48 hours.
4. Postprocedure care:
   A. The client should lie flat for 1–4 hours after the injection.
   B. Observe for headache or neurologic changes.
   C. Return the client, when scheduled, to the nuclear medicine department.
5. Client and family teaching:
   A. Notify the nurse or physician of any complaints of headache, dizziness, or nausea.
6. Factors that affect results:
   A. Movement during the scan obscures the views.
   B. Improper injection may cause inadequate visualization.
7. Other data:
   A. Cisternography is an expensive, invasive test.
   B. If improper injection (rather than leak) is suspected, the study should be repeated after at least 1 week. A radiograph of the spine may be used to study a suspected leak in that area.
   C. Health care professionals working in a nuclear medicine area must follow federal standards set by the Nuclear Regulatory Commission. These standards include precautions for handling the radioactive material and monitoring of potential radiation exposure.

Bibliography:

Colquhoun IR: CT cisternography in the investigation of cerebrospinal fluid rhinorrhoea. Clin Radiol 47(6):403–408, 1993.

Eljamel MS, Pidgeon CN, Toland J, Phillips JB, O'Dwyer AA: MRI cisternography, and the localization of CSF fistulae. Neurosurgery 8(4):433–437, 1994.

CK
(see Creatine Kinase, Serum)

CLINISTIX TEST, DIAGNOSTIC
(see Glucose Qualitative, Semiquantitative, Urine)

CLINITEST, DIAGNOSTIC
(see Glucose Qualitative, Semiquantitative, Urine)

CLONAZEPAM, BLOOD

Norm: Negative.

		SI Units
Therapeutic level	10–80 µg/L	32–254 nmol/L
Panic level	≥100 µg/L	≥254 nmol/L

Panic Level Symptoms and Treatment:

Symptoms: Deteriorating level of consciousness, coma.

Treatment:
Stop drug until neurologic status improves, then modify dose.
Provide airway support.
Perform hourly neurologic checks.
Use gastric lavage.
Administer fluids and vasopressors.
Administer CNS antidepressants.
Monitor for seizures and myoclonus while drug is stopped.
Conduct serial monitoring of clonazepam levels.
Forced diuresis and/or hemodialysis will NOT remove benzodiazepines. No information was found on whether peritoneal dialysis will remove these drugs.

Usage: Monitoring for drug abuse; monitoring for therapeutic levels with long-term use and overdose. Treatment of convulsions/myoclonus, sedation, anxiety. Reduce spasticity of cerebral palsy.

Description: Clonazepam is a schedule-IV benzodiazepine used for the treatment of convulsions and myoclonus. Peak levels occur within 2 hours after oral administration. The drug is metabolized in the liver and excreted by the kidneys, with a half-life of 20–40 hours.

Professional Considerations:

1. Consent form NOT required.
2. Preparation:
   A. Tube: Red-top, red/gray-top, or gold-top.
   B. MAY be drawn during hemodialysis.
3. Procedure:
   A. Collect a 5-ml blood sample.
4. Postprocedure care:
   A. If storing, separate and freeze the serum.
5. Client and family teaching:
   A. If an accidental overdose occurs in clients on chronic clonazepam therapy, teach the early signs of overdose (drowsiness, ataxia, slurred speech) for which emergency room treatment must be sought in the future.
   B. For intentional overdose, refer the client for crisis intervention.
6. Factors that affect results:
   A. Concomitant administration of carbamazepine, phenobarbital, or phenytoin may result in subtherapeutic clonazepam values.
7. Other data:
   A. For seizures, dose adjustments are necessary after 90 days due to the development of tolerance.
   B. Physical dependence can occur. Discontinuation must be accomplished by tapering to avoid status epilepticus.
   C. *See also Benzodiazepines, Plasma and Urine.*

Bibliography:

Beauclair L, Fontaine R, Annable L, Holobow N, Chouinard G: Clonazepam in the treatment of panic disorder: a double-blind, placebo-controlled trial investigating the correlation between clonazepam concentrations in plasma and clinical response. J Clin Psychopharmacol *14*(2):111–118, 1994.

Dahlin M, Knutsson E, Nergardh A: Treatment of spasticity in children with low dose benzodiazepine. J Neurol Sci *117*(1–2):54–60, 1993.

Glod CA, Mathieu J: Expanding uses of anticonvulsants in the treatment of bipolar disorder. J Psychosoc Nurs Ment Health Serv *31*(5):37–39, 1993.

Steingard RJ, Goldberg M, Lee D, DeMaso DR: Adjunctive clonazepam treatment of tic symptoms in children with comorbid tic disorders and ADHD. J Am Acad Child Adolesc Psychiatry *33*(3):394–399, 1994.

CLOSTRIDIAL TOXIN, SERUM

Norm: Negative.

Positive: Botulism.

Negative: Absence of microorganism.

Botulism Symptoms and Emergency Treatment:

Symptoms: Diarrhea, dizziness, double-vision, fatigue, gastrointestinal pain, headache, nausea, weakness, vomiting. Cardiac and respiratory paralysis is possible.

Treatment:

1. Establish IV access.
2. Administer trivalent botulism anti-toxin (Connaught Laboratories, LTD). (*Note:* anaphylaxis is possible if the antitoxin is given to clients with asthma, hay fever, horse or horse serum allergies, or past exposure to horse serum.) Follow the package insert instructions for sensitivity testing prior to antitoxin administration.
3. Induce vomiting with syrup of ipecac, if the syrup can be given soon after ingestion of the contaminated food. (Induction of emesis is contraindicated in clients with no gag reflex, or with central nervous system depression or excitation.)
4. Perform gastric lavage, if emesis does not produce the contaminated food.
5. Give activated charcoal slurry.
6. Administer saline cathartic if no ileus is present.
7. Monitor for respiratory decompensation, which may occur suddenly in clients with botulism. Elective intubation is advisable for large ingestions.
8. Notify the state health department and the Centers for Disease Control (404)639–2206. (The medical emergency number is (404)639–2888.)

Description: Clostridia are gram-positive anaerobes of the family *Bacillaceae* characterized by production of exothermic spores, enzymes, and potent endotoxins. *Clostridium* species are found in soil, freshwater, and marine sediments, and some species are part of the human lower gastrointestinal tract. *C. botulinum* causes botulism, a neuroparalytic disease transmitted by the clostridial spores that survive improper cooking of food. Botulism causes acute flaccid paralysis and may lead to death if not treated with antitoxin before the onset of neurologic symptoms. Infant botulism is represented by hypotonia, feeding disruption, and a weak cry. Because of the severity of the disease and the potential for an epidemic among other clients ingesting the affected food, cases of suspected botulism must be immediately reported to the State Department of Health and the Centers for Disease Control. Serum samples are used to confirm the diagnosis via identification of the toxin of *C. botulinum*.

Professional Considerations:

1. Consent form NOT required.
2. Preparation:
   A. Vials: aerobic and anaerobic culture vials.
   B. It may be necessary for this test to be performed by an outside laboratory.
3. Procedure:
   A. Collect a 15- to 20-ml blood sample from each of two sites aseptically in the two culture vials, one for the aerobic and one for the anaerobic culture.
   B. Double the amount of cultures collected for clients on whom antibiotic therapy has been instituted.
4. Postprocedure care:
   A. Note antibiotic therapy on the laboratory requisition.
5. Client and family teaching:
   A. Results may not be available for several days. Empiric therapy is typically started while awaiting results.
6. Factors that affect results:
   A. Antibiotic therapy may interfere with organism identification.
7. Other data:
   A. 20–50 g of stool and the food suspected of causing botulism should also be collected and sent for testing with the serum sample. *See Botulism Diagnostic Procedures, Stool.*

Bibliography:

Brook I: Clostridial infection in children. J Med Microbiol *42*(2):78–82, 1995.

Neu HC: Emerging trends in antimicrobial resistance in surgical infections: A review. Eur J Surg (Suppl A90) (573):7–18, 1994.

CLOSTRIDIUM DIFFICILE TOXIN ASSAY, STOOL

Norm: Negative. No *Clostridium difficile* toxin detected.

Positive: Antibiotic-related pseudomembranous enterocolitis.

Usage: Determine the presence or absence of *Clostridium difficile* toxin A.

Description: *Clostridium difficile* is a large, gram-positive, rod-shaped bacteria that releases two necrotizing toxins (toxin A [enterotoxin] and toxin B [cytotoxin]) causing a potentially fatal pseudomembranous colitis, especially in clients receiving antibiotics. *C. difficile* enterocolitis is the most common cause of diarrheal disease in hospitalized clients. Although it is part of the normal flora of the intestine, antibiotics to which it is resistant may increase the amount of *C. difficile* in the intestine. *C. difficile* enterocolitis is associated most commonly with clindamycin, ampicillin, and cephalosporin therapy, but is possible with any antibiotic therapy. The test includes detection of toxin produced by the organism in the stool of a client.

Professional Considerations:

1. Consent form NOT required.
2. Preparation:
   A. Obtain a sealed plastic feces specimen container, no preservative; a sealed sterile or nonsterile container with lid.
3. Procedure:
   A. Obtain a freshly passed fecal specimen of 25 g solid stool or 25–50 ml of liquid stool in a sterile, tightly sealed plastic container.
4. Postprocedure care:
   A. Send the specimen to the laboratory for processing within 3–4 hours.
   B. The specimen may be refrigerated for up to 24 hours before testing.
   C. Freeze the specimen if the test will not be performed within 24 hours. Transportation to an outside laboratory should be performed with the specimen stored in dry ice.
5. Client and family teaching:
   A. For outpatients, cohabitants should also be tested.
6. Factors that affect results:
   A. Exposure of the specimen to carbon dioxide may deactivate the toxins.
7. Other data:
   A. Results generally take up to 2 days.
   B. Culture is sometimes also prescribed, but often recovers organisms that do not produce toxin.
   C. Many normal infants and up to 21% of adults may have *C. difficile* as a transient or permanent part of their normal flora. Therefore, cultures of *C. difficile* are not diagnostic.
   D. *C. difficile* has been isolated in hospitals from curtains, bookshelves, bedpans, and linens (Marler 1996).

Bibliography:

Bowman RA, Arrow S, Croese L, Riley TV: Evaluation of an enzyme immunoassay kit for the detection of *Clostridium difficile* enterotoxin. Pathology *26*(4):480–481, 1994.

Cartwright CP, Stock F, Beekmann SE, Williams EC, Gill VJ: PCR amplification of rRNA intergenic spacer regions as a method for epidemiologic typing of *Clostridium difficile*. J Clin Microbiol *33*(1):184–187, 1995.

Marler LM: *Clostridium difficile*-associated disease: A complex laboratory-assisted diagnosis. Clin Lab Sci *8*(6):318–320, 1996.

Ratcliff RM, Goodwin AA, Lanser JA: Use of gene amplification to detect *Clostridium difficile* in clinical specimens. Pathology *26*(4):477–479, 1994.

CLOT RETRACTION, SERUM

Norm: 30–60 minutes for beginning of retraction; 1–2 hours for partial clot retraction; 6–24 hours for complete clot retraction.

Increased: Not applicable.

Decreased: Anemia (aplastic), disseminated intravascular coagulation (DIC), factor XIII deficiency, fibrinogen deficiency, fibrinolytic activity (increased), Glanzmann's thrombasthenia, Hodgkin's disease, hyperfibrinogenemia, hypofibrinogenemia, idiopathic thrombocytopenia purpura, leukemia (acute), multiple myeloma, platelet deficiency, platelet dysfunction, polycythemia vera, and thrombocytopenia purpura (secondary).

Description: A test performed on whole blood that determines the length of time required for firm clot formation by platelets and fibrinogen. Clot retraction decreases clot size during formation of the hemostatic plug. Test results indicate platelet and fibrinogen quantity and function. This test is rarely used.

Professional Considerations:

1. Consent form NOT required.
2. Preparation:
   A. Tube: Red-top, red/gray-top, or gold-top.
3. Procedure:
   A. Collect and discard 3 ml of blood, leaving the needle in place in the vein.
   B. Attach a fresh syringe and collect 4–10 ml of blood.
   C. Observe the tube for clotting. When a clot has formed, observe after 2, 6, 12, and 24 hours for retraction from the walls of the test tubes and record findings as no retraction, partial retraction, or complete retraction; time taken for beginning retraction; and complete retraction; clot consistency; amount of serum surrounding clot; and serum cell volume.
4. Postprocedure care:
   A. Observe for bleeding from the venipuncture site for 15 minutes if the client has a known coagulopathy.
5. Client and family teaching:
   A. Results are normally available within 24–48 hours.
6. Factors that affect results:
   A. Hemolysis invalidates results. Reject hemolyzed specimens.
   B. Plastic test tubes prolong the test results.
   C. Low platelet count, aspirin therapy, increased fibrinolysis, and hypofibrino-

genemia will result in abnormal clot retraction.

D. In DIC, afibrinogenemia, and severe hemophilic-state, clot formation may not occur.

7. Other data:

A. This test is only a measure of platelet function and is now considered useful mainly in the diagnosis of Glanzmann's thrombasthenia.

Bibliography:

Carr ME Jr, Carr SL: Fibrin structure and concentration alter clot elastic modulus but do not alter platelet mediated force development. Blood Coagul Fibrinolysis 6(1):79–86, 1995.

Carr ME Jr, Zekert SL: Abnormal clot retraction, altered fibrin structure, and normal platelet function in multiple myeloma. Am J Physiol 266(3, Pt. 2):H1195–H1201, 1994.

Chen YP, O'Toole TE, Leong L, Liu BQ, Diaz-Gonzalez F, Ginsberg MJ: Beta 3 integrin-mediated fibrin clot retraction by nucleated cells: differing behavior of alpha IIb beta 3 and alpha v beta 3. Blood 86(7):2606–2615, 1995.

Pierce JN, Taber KH, Hayman LA: Acute intracranial hemorrhage secondary to thrombocytopenia: CT appearances unaffected by absence of clot retraction. AJNR 15(2):213–215, 1994.

CLOT UREA SOLUBILITY, BLOOD

(see factor XIII)

CO, BLOOD

(see Carbon Monoxide, Blood)

CO₂, BLOOD

(see Carbon Dioxide, Partial Pressure, Blood; and Carbon Dioxide, Total Content, Blood)

COAGULATION FACTOR ASSAY, BLOOD

Norm: Factors VIII, IX, and XII are present and normal.

Usage: Detection of the type of hemophilia or other coagulation abnormalities.

Description: A blood assay completed by special coagulation laboratories to determine the presence of a congenital or acquired blood clotting factor deficiency that may cause hemophilia or other blood coagulation disorders. The client's blood is mixed with normal serum and/or specially prepared plasma or serum with a known specific deficiency. The results are studied for prothrombin time (PT), partial thromboplastin time (PTT), and activated partial thromboplastin time (APTT), as well as clot solubility to urea. The pattern (see table below) of clotting, PT, PTT, and any change when cross-mixed with the special agent plasma gives results that can determine the specific factor deficiency. For example, in hemophilia:

1. Test plasma adsorbed contains only factors XI and XII and so would specifically correct a client's plasma deficiency in these factors and therefore identify the problem.

2. Test plasma aged contains VII, IX, and XI and is known to lack I, V, and VIII.

Professional Considerations:

1. Consent form NOT required.

2. Preparation:

A. Preschedule the study with the special coagulation laboratory.

B. Tube: 2.7-ml blue-top or 4.5-ml blue-top, a control tube, and a waste tube or syringe. Also obtain a container of ice.

3. Procedure:

A. Perform a venipuncture and withdraw 2 ml of blood into a syringe or vacuum tube. Remove the syringe or tube, leaving the needle in place. Attach a second syringe, and draw two blood samples, one in a citrated blue-top tube and the other in a control tube. The sample quantity should be 2.4 ml for a 2.7 ml tube and 4.0 ml for a 4.5-ml tube. Mix the sample gently by inverting the tube several times. Place

COAGULATION FACTOR ASSAY

Hemophilia Type	PT	PTT	Adsorbed Plasma	Aged Normal Serum
Factor VIII	Normal	Increase	Corrects	No change
Factor IX	Normal	Increase	No change	Corrects
Factor XI	Normal	Increase	Partial	Partial
Factor XII	Normal	Increase	Corrects	Corrects

the specimens immediately in the container of ice.
4. Postprocedure care:
   A. Write the collection time on the laboratory requisition.
   B. Refrigerate the specimen during transport, and transport it to the laboratory immediately. The test should be completed within 2 hours.
   C. Observe the venipuncture site closely for any client with known coagulopathy.
5. Client and family teaching:
   A. The client should not have coumadin therapy for 2 weeks or heparin therapy for 2 days.
6. Factors that affect results:
   A. Reject clotted or nonrefrigerated specimens.
   B. The double-draw procedure is required to avoid contact of the blood with tissue thromboplastin, which may cause false-negative results.
   C. Drugs that may cause false-negative

results include bishydroxycoumarin, heparin calcium, heparin sodium, and warfarin sodium.
   D. Oral contraceptives may cause abnormally high levels of factors II, VII, IX, and X.
7. Other data:
   A. It is normal for healthy premature infants to have low (50% of normal) levels of factors II, III, IX, X, XI, and XII, even though a normal premature infant does not bleed spontaneously.

Bibliography:

Hauser I, Schneider B, Lechner K: Post-partum factor VIII inhibitors. A review of the literature with special reference to the value of steroid and immunosuppressive treatment. Thromb Haemost 73(1):1–5, 1995.
Verbruggen B, Novakova I. Wessels H, Boezeman J, van den Berg M, Mauser-Bunschoten E: The Nijmegen modification of the Bethesda assay for factor VIII C inhibitors: improved specificity and reliability. Thromb Haemost 73(2):247–251, 1995.

COCAINE, BLOOD

Norm: None detected.

		SI Units
Therapeutic range	100–500 ng/ml	330–1650 μmol/L
Panic (fatal) level	>1000 ng/ml	> 3300 μmol/L

Panic Level Symptoms and Treatment:

Symptoms: Short-lived CNS and sympathetic stimulation, hypertension, tachypnea, tachycardia, and mydriasis.

Treatment:

Induce emesis if oral ingestion. (*Note:* Induction of emesis is contraindicated in clients with no gag reflex, or with central nervous system depression or excitation.).

Perform gastric lavage if oral ingestion.

Perform whole bowel irrigation for ingested packs of cocaine

Provide airway and cardiac support.

Administer diazepam or phenobarbital for convulsions.

Do NOT use beta blockers.

Provide cool environment or hypothermia if the client is febrile.

Monitor renal function for damage from rhabdomyolysis.

Consider need for continuous ECG monitoring.

Usage: Determination of therapeutic cocaine levels or diagnosis of drug abuse or drug overdose.

Description: Cocaine is a schedule-II, central nervous system stimulant, and local anesthetic used clinically for its bronchodilator and vasoconstrictor effects, which result in increased blood pressure, respiratory rate, and heart rate. It is readily absorbed via mucous membranes, detoxified in the liver, excreted by the kidneys, and acts for 2 hours or less. Cocaine is also a drug of abuse, and street names for it include C, coke, crack, girl, lady, happy dust, gold dust, and stardust. An overdose may lead to cardiopulmonary failure.

Professional Considerations:

1. Consent form NOT required unless the specimen may be used for legal evidence.
2. Preparation:
   A. Tube: Green-top or lavender-top. Also obtain ice.
3. Procedure:
   A. If the specimen will be used as legal evidence, have the specimen collection witnessed.
   B. Draw a 5- to 10-ml blood sample and place the tube immediately on ice.

4. Postprocedure care:
   A. If the specimen will be used as legal evidence, seal the bag and label it as legal evidence. Label the specimen with the exact time drawn, the client's name, and the specimen source. Sign, and have the witness sign, the laboratory requisition. Laboratory personnel in receipt of the specimen must also sign the requisition and record the time of receipt on it.
   B. Transport the specimen to the laboratory immediately.
5. Client and family teaching:
   A. For overdose, refer the client and the family for crisis intervention and psychological support.
   B. Referrals to appropriate rehabilitation centers and therapeutic community programs should be offered to all addicted clients who may be interested.
   C. Cocaine can cause lung and kidney problems, heart attacks, strokes, hallucinations, feelings of suicide, and death. It is an addictive drug. When you stop using cocaine, withdrawal symptoms may include depression, lack of energy, sleep disturbances, chills, muscle aches, fast heartbeat, sweating, and chest pain.
6. Factors that affect results:
   A. Reject specimens not received on ice. Cocaine is rapidly hydrolyzed in blood, and iced specimens must be processed by gas chromatography within 1 hour.
7. Other data:
   A. Because cocaine is so rapidly hydrolyzed, blood specimens would have to be drawn just after use to show positive for abuse. Therefore, levels of urinary cocaine or its metabolite, benzoylecgonine, are more accurate screening methods for drug abuse.
   B. The use of cocaine, even one time, can cause rhabdomyolysis, a disease that causes muscle tissue destruction.

Bibliography:

Baselt RC, Yoshikawa D, Chang J, Li J: Improved long-term stability of blood cocaine in evacuated collection tubes. J Forensic Sci *38*(4):935–937, 1993.

Middleton RM, Kirkpatrick MB: Clinical use of cocaine: a review of the risks and benefits. Drug Safety *9*(3):212–217, 1993.

Ruiz P, Cleary T, Nassiri M, Steele B: Human T lymphocyte subpopulation and NK cell alterations in persons exposed to cocaine. Clin Immunol Immunopathol *70*(3):245–250, 1994.

Sukbuntherng J, Walters A, Chow JJ, Mayersohn M: Quantitative determination of cocaine, cocalthylene (ethylcocaine), and metabolites in plasma and urine by high-performance liquid chromatography. J Pharm Sci *84*(7):799–804, 1995.

COCCIDIOIDOMYCOSIS SKIN TEST, DIAGNOSTIC

Norm: Negative or no skin reaction.

Positive: Skin induration >5 mm diameter indicates exposure to *Coccidioides,* but gives no indication of duration.

Usage: Determine the exposure to fungal infections affecting the pulmonary system.

Description: *Coccidioides immitis* is a fungus found in the soil of dry climates of the southwest United States and Latin America. Spores in the dust are inhaled, causing respiratory infection that is mild, asymptomatic, or may cause acute to chronic pulmonary cavities. A rare 1% of infected individuals develop disseminated disease/infection that is fatal. The course of the disease includes fever, malaise, and respiratory complaints, which are self-limiting, as the client develops antibodies. In the disseminated form, the skin, bones, internal organs, and meninges are infected. This test is performed by injecting a *Coccidioides* antigen sample and observing for signs of an antibody reaction.

Professional Considerations:

1. Consent form NOT required.
2. Preparation:
   A. Obtain an alcohol wipe, a syringe, a subcutaneous needle, and a *Coccidioides* antigen sample.
3. Procedure:
   A. Cleanse the volar aspect of the lower arm with an alcohol wipe and allow it to dry.
   B. Inject 0.1 ml of 1:100 dilution coccidiodin or spherulin (which is more sensitive) subcutaneously.
   C. Circle the injection site with a pen or marker.
4. Postprocedure care:
   A. Read the skin test 24 and 48 hours after the injection.
5. Client and family teaching:
   A. The injection causes a stinging sensation.
   B. Do not wash off the marking until the test is read. Return in 24–48 hours to have the test site read.
6. Factors that affect results:
   A. Low dilution of the antigen preparation (i.e., 1:10) may produce a cross-reaction, indicating other fungal diseases.
   B. The skin test may be negative in the severe, disseminated form of the disease.
7. Other data:
   A. Cross-reactions occur in clients with histoplasmosis.
   B. The advantage of skin testing is that

results are available in approximately 24–48 hours.

C. The main disadvantage is the time period needed to develop antibodies.

Bibliography:

Ravel R (ed): Clinical Laboratory Medicine: Clinical Application of Laboratory Data, 6th ed. St. Louis, MO, Mosby Year Book, 1995.

CODEINE, SERUM AND URINE

Norm: Negative.

		SI Units
Serum		
Therapeutic level	10–100 ng/ml	33–334 nmol/L
Panic level	>200 ng/ml	>668 nmol/L
Urine		
Therapeutic level	5–30 mg/L	
Panic level	31–250 mg/L	

Panic Level Symptoms and Treatment:

Symptoms: CNS depression (including somnolence, convulsions, stupor, coma), ataxia, vomiting, rash and itching of the skin, respiratory depression, miosis, hypotension, and skeletal muscle flaccidity.

Treatment:

Maintain patent airway and support breathing.
Administer vasopressors to support blood pressure.
Perform neurologic checks q 1 hour.
Hemodialysis will NOT remove codeine.

Usage: Codeine therapy and codeine overdose.

Description: Codeine is a schedule-II narcotic analgesic used for relief of mild-to-moderate pain and as an antitussive. It is metabolized by the liver and excreted as norcodeine and conjugated morphine by the kidneys, with a half-life of 2.5–4.0 hours.

Professional Considerations:

1. Consent form NOT required unless the specimen may be used as legal evidence.
2. Preparation:
   A. Obtain a clean urine container.
   B. Tube: Red-top, red/gray-top, or gold-top.
   C. The specimen MAY be drawn during hemodialysis.
3. Procedure:
   A. If the specimen may be used as legal evidence, have the specimen collection witnessed.
   B. *Serum:* Draw a 5-ml blood specimen.
   C. *Urine:* Collect 50 ml of urine in a clean container without preservatives. A fresh specimen may be taken from a urinary drainage bag.
4. Postprocedure care:
   A. If the specimen is being collected for legal purposes, sign, and have the witness sign, the laboratory requisition. Also write the date, time, and specimen source on the requisition. Transport the specimen to the laboratory in a sealed plastic bag labeled as legal evidence. Each person handling the specimen should write the date and time he or she received the specimen on the requisition.
5. Client and family teaching:
   A. In the event of accidental overdose, the early signs of overdose for which to seek emergency treatment include drowsiness, ataxia, and/or slurred speech.
   B. For intentional overdose, refer the client for crisis intervention.
6. Factors that affect results:
   A. Some metabolites may affect urine codeine level; thus, a confirmatory serum codeine measurement must also be drawn.
   B. Lengthened codeine half-life is associated with end-stage renal disease.
7. Other data:
   A. Accidental overdose with codeine-containing cough medications occurs in children.

Bibliography:

Delbeke FT, Debackere M: Influence of hydrolysis procedures on the urinary concentrations of codeine and morphine in relation to doping analysis. J Pharm Biomed Anal *11*(4–5):339–343, 1993.

Lin Z, Lafolie P, Beck O: Evaluation of analytical procedures for urinary codeine and morphine measurements. J Anal Toxicol *18*(3):129–133, 1994.

Tai SS, Christensen RG, Paule RC, Sander LC, Welch MJ: The certification of morphine and codeine in a human urine standard reference material. J Anal Toxicol *18*(1):7–12, 1994.

COGNITIVE TESTS, EVENT-RELATED POTENTIALS, DIAGNOSTIC

Norm: Normal recognition and reaction time.

Usage: Alzheimer's disease, dementia, depression, multiple sclerosis, psychiatric illnesses, and other clinical or experimental situations in which cognitive function disorders are suspected.

Description: A test devised to measure perceptomotor skills, sensory acuity, and ability to discriminate. Attention span is also tested, as the client is asked to indicate it by pressing a button quickly after recognizing certain auditory or visual clues. When combined with evoked potential recordings, the test can give information about possible areas of error (i.e., a psychiatric disorder in which an hysterical loss of hearing shows positive brain response to sound, but the client is unable to respond). Lack of expected response may be found to result from physical hearing loss rather than from psychiatric causes.

Professional Considerations:

1. Consent form NOT required.
2. Preparation:
   A. Obtain earphones, a multichannel recorder with response button, and stimulus equipment.
3. Procedure:
   A. This test is carried out in a specialized psychophysiology laboratory.
   B. The client is seated in a quiet environment in a comfortable chair.
   C. After headphones are placed over the client's ears, a pattern or patterns of auditory cues are given.
   D. The client must respond to the cues by pushing a button as quickly as possible to signify his or her recognition of the proper cue.
   E. Visual cues consisting of patterns of light flashes are also utilized. A multichannel recorder notes the stimulus and response so that the time lapse, as well as correctness of response, can be determined.
   F. In some tests, an evoked potential is also recorded and determined. One electrode (active) is placed between the vertex and the auditory meatus. Neutral electrodes are attached to the ear lobes and an evoked potential recording of the hearing test is obtained along with the above recordings.
4. Postprocedure care:
   A. Remove the headphones.
5. Client and family teaching:
   A. You must cooperate if the results are to be of value. You will be asked to recognize certain demonstrated tones through earphones and respond by pressing the button provided.
6. Factors that affect results:
   A. Hearing loss or visual disorders impair the client's ability to respond to the auditory and visual cues.
   B. The test is not helpful in clients who are unable to cooperate or comprehend the instructions.
   C. Noise or other distractions in the testing environment may interfere with the client's comprehension of the testing cues.
7. Other data:
   A. *See also Brainstem Auditory Evoked Potential, Diagnostic.*

Bibliography:

Flannery J, Korcheck S: Use of the levels of cognitive functioning assessment scale (LOCFAS) by acute care nurses. Appl Nurs Res 6(4):167–169, 1993.

Gottschalk LA: The development, validation, and applications of a computerized measurement of cognitive impairment from the content analysis of verbal behavior. J Clin Psychol 50(3):349–361, 1994.

Marson DC, Cody HA, Ingram KK, Harrell LE: Neuropsychologic predictors of competency in Alzheimer's disease using a rational reasons legal standard. Arch Neurol 52(10):955–959, 1995.

COLD AGGLUTININ SCREEN, BLOOD

Norm: Negative or <1:32. Titers >1:40 are positive.

Usage: This test is indicated when an antibody screen or panel suggests cold autoagglutination because the cold agglutinins are interfering with the examination for irregular antibodies. It also may be performed for hemolytic anemia or as part of the work-up of painful extremities in cold weather (Raynaud's) or other suspected cold reactions as in surgery.

Description: Cold agglutinins are antibodies that are able to agglutinate (clump) type O human blood cells at cold (<20°C) temperatures but not at room or higher temperatures. Cold agglutinins are present in small amounts in the circulation of many people and react at severely cold temperatures (4°C). Increased levels may follow infections. Their presence and reactivity at temperatures of 20°C or below is termed "wide amplitude" cold agglutination. Positive cold agglutinins can cause agglutination or clumping of antigens, which leads to thrombosis, pain in the extremities, and hemolysis.

Professional Considerations:

1. Consent form NOT required.
2. Preparation:
   A. Tube: Red-top, red/gray-top, or gold-top.
3. Procedure:
   A. Draw a 4-ml blood sample.
4. Postprocedure care:
   A. The specimen is separated and then stored at 4°C for 2 hours or overnight.
5. Client and family teaching:
   A. Results are normally available within 48 hours.
6. Factors that affect results:
   A. Reject hemolyzed specimens.
7. Other data:
   A. Autoagglutination can occur in clients with positive results when exposed to cold, and occurs especially in the extremities where body temperatures are normally lowest. It may also occur during surgery, especially during open heart surgery, where the perfusate for bypass is 15–32°C.
   B. Cold agglutinins are not found in normal (room temperature) blood cross-match methods.
   C. This is not to be confused with *Cold Agglutinin Titer*, which is a specific test for *Mycoplasma* pneumonia. The only connection is that among other infections, *Mycoplasma* infection may cause the presence of these cold agglutinins.

Bibliography:

Schwartz RS, Silberstein LE, Berkman EM: Autoimmune hemolytic anemias. *In* Hoffman R, Benz EJ, Shattil SJ, Furie B, Cohen HJ, Silberstein LE (eds): Hematology: Basic Principles and Practice, 2nd ed. New York, Churchill Livingstone, pp 710–729, 1995.

COLD AGGLUTININ TITER, SERUM

Norm: Negative or titer <32 or <1:32.

Positive: Titer >40 or >1:40 in combination with acute respiratory symptoms usually indicates *Mycoplasma pneumoniae* infection, usually *Mycoplasma* pneumonia, viral pneumonia, or primary atypical pneumonia. An agglutination reaction present even at very high titers suggests *M. pneumoniae*, especially if the test is specific for anti-I antigens. Positive titers due to *Mycoplasma pneumoniae* infection rise after about 10 days, peak at 12–25 days, and then diminish by 30 days with an acute infection. Positive titers may also indicate cirrhosis (hypertrophic, syphilitic), hemolytic anemia, Hodgkin's disease, lymphoma, mononucleosis infection, pleuropneumonia-like organism (PPLO), PNH, trypanosomiasis, and tuberculosis (febrile).

Negative: Titer <1:32 is negative for *Mycoplasma pneumoniae* or related infection.

Description: Cold agglutinins are antibodies that cause clumping or agglutination of type O red blood cells at cold temperatures. The cold agglutinin titer tests for cold agglutinins at 2–8°C—those antibodies that result from *Mycoplasma pneumoniae* infection. A titer is the highest dilution of a serum that will demonstrate a specific antigen-antibody reaction. *Mycoplasma pneumoniae* is a nonbacterial infective agent that causes a pneumonia characterized by fever and a nonproductive or nonpurulent cough.

Professional Considerations:

1. Consent form NOT required.
2. Preparation:
   A. Tube: Red-top, red/gray-top, gold-top, or lavender-top.
3. Procedure:
   A. Draw a 4-ml blood sample.
   B. Usually at least two serial samples are taken. The first is taken 1 week after the onset of illness. The second is taken 12–25 days after the onset of illness, and a third may be taken 30 days after the onset.
4. Postprocedure care:
   A. Transport the specimen to the laboratory immediately. The blood is allowed to clot at 37°C and the serum is then separated from the cells and cooled for testing.
5. Client and family teaching:
   A. Results are normally available within 48 hours.
6. Factors that affect results:
   A. Reject hemolyzed specimens or refrigerated specimens. Refrigeration before separation of serum may cause false-negative results.
   B. Antibiotic therapy may decrease antibody production.
   C. False-positive results may occur in clients with malaria, congenital syphilis, peripheral vascular disease, hepatic cirrhosis, anemia, and respiratory diseases. In such cases, the titer pattern is more constant, without peaks.
   D. The sample must not be allowed to clot at room temperature.
7. Other data:
   A. Culture methods for *Mycoplasma*

pneumoniae are available, but the cold agglutinin titer is more reliable for diagnosis. Two serial titers are most helpful, as the *Mycoplasma pneumoniae* titers follow a specific pattern that peaks during the third to fourth week.

B. Serial titers are most helpful, as the *Mycoplasma pneumoniae* titers follow a specific pattern (i.e., peaks during the third to fourth week after infection).

C. Newer cold agglutinin methods that test agglutination reactions specific to major antigen types make this test much more specific. *Mycoplasma pneumoniae* is related to the I-i antigen system. Anti-M or anti-P are associated with other cold agglutinin activity and diseases.

Bibliography:

Schwartz RS, Silberstein LE, Berkman EM: Autoimmune hemolytic anemias. *In* Hoffman R, Benz EJ, Shattil SJ, Furie B, Cohen HJ, Silberstein LE (eds): Hematology: Basic Principles and Practice, 2nd ed. New York, Churchill Livingstone, pp 710–729, 1995.

COLONOSCOPY, DIAGNOSTIC

Norm: The intima of the large intestine is normally orange-pink in color, with folds and smooth indentations covered with mucus. Blood vessels may be visible below the epithelial surface.

Usage: Visualization of the mucosa of the entire colon and terminal ileum. Screening for intestinal abnormalities, including diverticula, polyps, tumors, ulcerative areas, infection, inflammation, irritation, bleeding sites, or strictures. Also used to study and biopsy or remove tumors, polyps, ulcerative colitis, parasitic disease, or other causes of diarrhea.

Description: A fiberoptic endoscopy study in which the lining of the large intestine is visually examined for inflammation or other changes of the mucosal surface and for bleeding sites or strictures.

Professional Considerations:

1. Consent form IS required.

Risks:
Dysrhythmias, hemorrhage, myocardial infarction, perforation of colon, peritonitis, respiratory depression.

Contraindications:
Recent myocardial infarction or pulmonary embolus; retained barium from an earlier study; second or third trimester pregnancy. Sedatives are contraindicated in clients with central nervous system depression.

2. Preparation:
   A. *See Client and family teaching.*
   B. A tap-water enema may be prescribed to be given just prior to the test.
   C. Sedation may be prescribed.
   D. Prepare suction equipment, emergency equipment, naloxone, lubricant, cytology brush, and containers of fixative for cytology specimens.
   E. Record baseline vital signs.
3. Procedure:
   A. The client is positioned lying on the left side with knees flexed and draped for privacy and comfort.
   B. The flexible fiberoptic endoscope is inserted through the anus, and the rectum and colon are visualized.
   C. Specimens may be obtained for cytology.
   D. Photographs are taken of anomalies present.
   E. Polyps may be removed with colonoscopy biopsy forceps or an electrocautery snare.
4. Postprocedure care:
   A. Place the tissue specimens in fixative of 10% formalin. Place the cytology specimens in 95% ethyl alcohol. Label the specimens and send them to the laboratory immediately.
   B. Observe the client and check vital signs every 15–30 minutes until fully recovered. If sedation was used, follow institutional protocol for postsedation monitoring. Typical monitoring includes continuous ECG monitoring and pulse oximetry, with continual assessments (q 5–15 minutes) of airway, vital signs, and neurologic status until the client is lying quietly awake, breathing independently, and responding appropriately to commands spoken in a normal tone.
   C. After the client has fully recovered, he or she may resume a normal diet.
   D. Observe for signs of colon perforation, which include abdominal pain or distension, malaise, fever, purulent rectal drainage, or lower gastrointestinal bleeding.
5. Client and family teaching:
   A. Follow a clear liquid diet for 48 hours prior to the test and resume normal diet after the test.
   B. Bowel preparation is very important. A laxative is usually prescribed the

evening prior to the test, unless contraindicated. Examples are 10 ounces of magnesium citrate or 3 tablespoons of castor oil.

   C. Make arrangements for transportation home after the procedure, because driving is not permitted for 24 hours after receiving sedation.

   D. Take deep, slow breaths during the procedure. The urge to defecate is normal and can be relieved with this type of breathing.

   E. An increase in flatus is normal and minor amounts of blood in the stool are expected after polyp removal.

6. Factors that affect results:

   A. Soap-suds enemas irritate the mucosa, increase mucus production, and hinder visibility.

   B. Barium from any previous gastrointestinal work-up makes colon visualization impossible.

   C. Failure to clean the lower intestine makes colon visualization impossible.

   D. Strictures or other abnormalities from previous surgery, radiation, or severe, chronic inflammatory disease may interfere with passage of the colonoscope.

7. Other data:

   A. The findings from this procedure may be useful to the surgeon during laparotomy to exclude other lesions.

Bibliography:

Bernstein CN, Shanahan F, Weinstein WM: Are we telling patients the truth about surveillance colonoscopy in ulcerative colitis? Lancet *343*(88–89):71–74, 1994.

Church JM: Complete colonoscopy: how often? And if not, why not? Am J Gastroenterol *89*(4):556–560, 1994.

Johnson H Jr: Management of major complications encountered with flexible colonoscopy. J Natl Med Assoc *85*(12):916–920, 1993.

Karasick S, Ehrlich SM, Levin DC, Harford RJ, Rosetti EF, Ricci JA, Beam LM, Gigliotti JV: Trends in use of barium enema examination, colonoscopy, and sigmoidoscopy: is use commensurate with risk of disease? Radiology *195*(3):777–784, 1995.

Lo AY, Beaton H:. Selective management of colonoscopic perforations. J Am Coll Surg *179*(3):333–337, 1994.

COLOR VISION TESTS, DIAGNOSTIC

Norm: The client is able to identify all the colors, symbols, and patterns presented.

Usage: Screening for retinal disease or color vision deficiency.

Description: A test using pseudoisochromatic plates with numbers or letters buried in a matrix of colored dots. Deficits can be genetic and result from one or more of the three-color cone systems, or acquired.

Professional Considerations:

1. Consent form NOT required.
2. Preparation:

   A. Obtain an eye patch or hand-held occluder, test kit, and pointer.

3. Procedure:

   A. One eye is occluded and the test booklet is held approximately 14 inches (35 cm) in front of the unoccluded eye.

   B. Sample plates of different patterns of primary colors with a background of a variety of colors are shown to the client, one at a time.

   C. The client is asked to identify the patterns of the primary colors and to trace the patterns with a pointer.

4. Postprocedure care:

   A. None.

5. Client and family teaching:

   A. Bring corrective glasses or lenses to the test.

   B. There are no food or fluid restrictions.

   C. The test is painless.

6. Factors that affect results:

   A. Conduct the test in a well-lighted area.

   B. Abnormalities of the ocular media, the retina, or the optic nerve can affect results and should be ruled out if color blindness is discovered.

   C. The client may be unable to cooperate and participate in the test.

7. Other data:

   A. Color blindness may include more than one spectrum of color.

Bibliography:

Geier SA, Kronawitter U, Hammel G, Berninger T, Klauss V, Goebel FD: Impairment of colour contrast sensitivity and neuroretinal dysfunction in patients with symptomatic HIV infection or AIDS. Br J Ophthalmol *77*(11):716–720, 1993.

Ing EB, Parker JA, Emerton LA: Computerized colour vision testing. Can J Ophthalmol *29*(3):125–128, 1994.

Tian N, Wu DZ, Liang J: A study of spectral electroretinogram of color vision defects due to macular diseases. Yen Ko Hsueh Pao [Eye Science] *10*(3): 163–167, 1994.

COLORECTAL CANCER ALLELOTYPING FOR CHROMOSOME 17p AND 18q (P53 OR DCC GENE), SPECIMEN AND BLOOD

Norm: Normal gene sequence.

Usage: Detect germline and tumor cell deletions and mutations in the p53 tumor suppressor gene. Absence of normal gene, p53: Bladder, breast, colorectal, esophageal, liver, lung, and ovarian carcinomas, brain tumors, sarcomas, lymphomas, and leukemias. Absence of DCC: colorectal carcinomas.

Description: A tumor suppressor gene is a cellular gene whose loss of function may lead to tumor development. The transformation of a normal colon epithelial cell into a colorectal cancer proceeds through a series of steps. This process is accompanied by a series of genetic changes, which include the inactivation of several tumor suppressor genes. Evidence for involvement of tumor suppressor genes in colorectal tumors comes from the study of chromosomal losses and molecular biologic analysis of tumor DNA. Among those genes known to be lost are p53 and the DCC gene, which are located on chromosomes 17p and 18q, respectively.

Professional Consideration:

1. Consent form IS required for biopsy. *See Biopsy, Site-Specific, Specimen* for risks and contraindications.
2. Preparation:
   A. *See Biopsy, Site-Specific, Specimen.*
   B. Obtain a biopsy bottle for tissue section.
   C. Tube: Yellow-top or lavender-top.
3. Procedure:
   A. Obtain a frozen (solid tumor) specimen.
   B. Draw 2 ml of venous blood.
   C. *See Biopsy, Site-Specific, Specimen.*
4. Postprocedure care:
   A. *See Biopsy, Site-Specific, Specimen.*
   B. The tumor tissue must be sent for genetic analysis. Label and transport the specimen to the pathology department.
5. Client and family teaching:
   A. *See Biopsy, Site-Specific, Specimen.*
6. Factors that affect results:
   A. Small specimens decrease the reliability of the results.
   B. Tissue specimens must not be frozen nor blood specimens clotted.
7. Other data:
   A. The specimen must be >40% tumor.

Bibliography:

Jen J, Kim H, Piantadosi S, Liu ZF, et al.: Allelic loss of chromosome 18Q and prognosis in cancer. N Engl J Med *331*(4):213–221, 1994.

Khine K, Smith DR, Goh HS: High frequency of allelic deletion on chromosome 17p in advanced cancer. Cancer 73:28–35, 1994.

Yaremko ML, Wasylyshyn ML, Westbrook CA, Michelassi F: Oncogenes, suppressor genes, and allele losses in colon cancer. Adv Surg *26*:323–232, 1993.

COLPOSCOPY, DIAGNOSTIC

Norm: Normal appearance of vagina and cervix. Vagina and cervix are free of lesions and no abnormal cells or tissue are present.

Usage: Evaluation of suspicious lesions or suspected cervical or vaginal cancer, evaluation of abnormal cytology of the vagina and cervix, testing for vulvar dystrophy, and screening for cervical abnormalities in women whose mothers were treated with diethylstilbestrol (DES) when pregnant with them.

Description: The visual examination of the vagina and cervix using a lighted colposcope that magnifies the mucosal surfaces. Colposcopy helps diagnose benign and preclinical cancerous lesions of the cervix and vagina.

Professional Considerations:

1. Consent form IS required.

Risks:
Bleeding, infection.

Contraindications:
Biopsy during colposcopy is contraindicated in the presence of anticoagulant therapy, bleeding disorders, thrombocytopenia, or heavy menses.

2. Preparation:
   A. The client should disrobe below the waist.
   B. Obtain a speculum, a 3% acetic acid solution, sterile cotton-tipped swabs, a colposcope, biopsy forceps, a cauterizer, a specimen cup with preservative, and sterile cotton.
3. Procedure:
   A. The client is placed in the lithotomy position and draped for comfort and privacy.
   B. The vagina and cervix are exposed with a speculum.
   C. Cervical mucus is removed with acetic acid.
   D. The colposcope is inserted and the walls of the vagina and cervix are visually examined for color, keratinization, lesions, blood vessel structure, inflammation, atrophy, and erosion. Suspicious areas may be biopsied, and cautery or pressure is used to control bleeding.
4. Postprocedure care:
   A. Vaginal bleeding is not abnormal. Provide a sanitary pad.
5. Client and family teaching:
   A. The procedure lasts about 15 minutes and may cause slight discomfort from the vaginal speculum.

B. A small amount of bleeding may occur due to the sampling of tissue.

C. Results may not be available for several days.

D. Refrain from sexual intercourse until receiving confirmation on a follow-up visit that the biopsy site has healed.

6. Factors that affect results:
   A. Heavy menstrual flow may interfere with adequate visualization of the cervix.

7. Other data:
   A. Colposcopy is helpful in adding information about tumor extension.

Bibliography:

Hartz LE: Quality of care by nurse practitioner delivering colposcopy services. J Am Acad Nurse Practitioners 7(1):23–27, 1995.

Mayeau EJ Jr, Harper MB, Abreo F, Pope JB, Phillips GS: A comparison of the reliability of repeat cervical smears and colposcopy in patients with abnormal cervical cytology. J Fam Pract 40(1):57–62, 1995.

Worthington S, Rubin M: Nurse-midwifery evaluation and management of cervical pathology and the colposcopic examination. J Nurse-midwifery 38(2 Suppl):36S–41S, 1993.

COMPANION, DIAGNOSTIC

(see Glucose Monitoring Machines, Diagnostic)

COMPLEMENT, TOTAL, SERUM (CH$_{50}$)

Norm: 75–160 U/ml (75–160 kU/L, SI units), >33% of plasma CH$_{50}$ (fraction of plasma CH$_{50}$: >0.33, SI units).

Increased: Diabetes mellitus, jaundice (obstructive), mixed connective tissue disease, myocardial infarction (acute), rheumatoid arthritis (adult, severe), thyroiditis, ulcerative colitis, and Wegener's granulomatosis.

Decreased: Allograft rejection, cirrhosis (advanced), glomerulonephritis (poststreptococcal acute, chronic), hemolytic anemia (autoimmune), hepatitis (chronic, active), hypogammaglobulinemia, kwashiorkor, lupus nephritis, malaria, multiple myeloma, rheumatic fever, serum sickness (acute), sinusitis (S. pneumoniae, Neisseria), subacute bacterial endocarditis (SBE), and systemic lupus erythematosus (SLE).

Usage: Evaluate and follow up SLE client's response to therapy; screen for complement component deficiency; evaluate cases of immune complex disease, glomerulonephritis, arthritis, SBE, and cryoglobulinemia. Hypocomplementemia that accompanies some forms of renal disease may indicate immune utilization. Identification and monitoring of immune-related diseases.

Description: The complement system is comprised of a series of proteins that when activated serve to amplify an immune response. Activation of the complement (C) system lends to the elaboration of potent inflammatory mediators, facilitates particle opsonization and clearance, and may result in the direct lysis of altered mammolian cells and certain bacteria. The complement system may be activated by a number of immunologic and non-immunologic stimuli. Complement activation proceeds by either the classical or alternative pathway. (See Complement Components, Serum.) The test for total serum complement evaluates the integrity of the complement cascade. Total complement is depressed during the active phases of immune diseases when various individual components are significantly depressed.

Professional Considerations:

1. Consent form NOT required.
2. Preparation:
   A. Tube: Red-top, red/gray-top, or gold-top.
3. Procedure:
   A. Draw a 3-ml blood sample.
   B. Leave the specimen at room temperature to clot. Then refrigerate it at 4°C for 30 minutes to 1 hour.
4. Postprocedure care:
   A. Send the specimen to the laboratory for immediate testing.
5. Client and family teaching:
   A. Results are normally available within 48 hours.
6. Factors that affect results:
   A. Complement is heat-sensitive and deteriorates rapidly. Send the specimen to the laboratory immediately.
   B. Freeze the specimen at −70°C if it cannot be processed immediately after 1 hour of refrigeration.
7. Other data:
   A. Various individual components (C1–C9) may be depressed only slightly in immune disease and may not have a significant effect on the total complement level.
   B. Low CH$_{50}$ levels tend to correlate with active phases of immune complex diseases such as SLE (especially if associated with nephritis) and cases of glomerulonephritis.
   C. Decreased complement in synovial

fluid may be seen with acute arthritis. Low serum complement levels occur in some clients with severe active rheumatoid factor positive arthritis, and may indicate the development of vasculitis.

D. *See C1q Immune Complex Detection, Serum; C3 Complement, Serum; C3 Proactivator, Serum; C4 Complement, Serum; Complement Components, Serum; and Complement Fixation, Serum.*

Bibliography:

Glovsky MM: Applications of complement determinations in human disease. Ann Allergy 72(6):477-486, 1994.

Norris MK: Checking your patient's complement assay. Nursing 24(1):26, 1994.

Osterland CK: Laboratory diagnosis and monitoring in chronic systemic autoimmune diseases. Clin Chem 40(11):2146–2153, 1994.

Porcel JM, Peakman M, Senaldi G, Vergani D: Methods for assessing complement activation in the clinical immunology laboratory. J Immunol Methods 157(12):1–9, 1993.

COMPLEMENT COMPONENTS, SERUM

Norm:

		SI Units
Classical pathway components		
C1	70,000–200,000U/ml	70–200 MU/L
C1q		
Adult	14.9–22.1 mg/dl	149–221 mg/L
Maternal	9–24.8 mg/dl	90–248 mg/L
Newborn	9–20 mg/dl	90–200 mg/L
C1r		
Adult	0.025–0.10 mg/ml	0.025–0.010 g/L
C1s	0.05–0.10 mg/ml	0.05–0.10 g/L
C2	1.6–3.6 mg/dl	16–36 mg/L
C4		
Adult	10–67.5 mg/dl	100–675 mg/L
Alternative pathway components		
Factor D	1–5 µg/L	1–5 mg/L
C3-proactivator		
Adult	127–278 µg/ml	127–278 mg/L
Properdin		
Adult	10–36.5 µg/ml	10–36.5 mg/L
Cord serum	8.1–23.4 µg/ml	8.1–23.4 mg/L
Regulatory components		
C1-INH	8–24.0 mg/dl	80–240 mg/L
C4-binding protein	18–32 mg/dl	180–320 mg/L
Factor H	40.5–71.7 mg/dl	405–717 mg/L
Factor I	0.025–0.05 mg/ml	25–50 mg/L
Anaphylatoxin inactivator	30–40 µg/ml	30–400 mg/L
S-protein	(mean) 500 µg/ml	(mean) 500 mg/L
C-3 Nephritic factor	Negative	Negative
Split products		
$C3_{desArg}$	<940 ng/ml	<940 µg/L
$C4_{desArg}$	<2.8 µg/ml	<2.8 mg/L
$C5_{desArg}$	<12 ng/ml	<12 µg/L
Bb, Ba	Negative	Negative
C4d	Trace	Trace
SC5b–9	<390 µg/ml	<390 mg/L

		SI Units
Terminal pathway components		
C3		
Adult	83–177 mg/dl	0.83–1.77 g/L
Cord serum	57–116 mg/dl	0.57–1.16 g/L
6 months	74–177 mg/dl	0.74–1.77 g/L
C5		
Adult	4.8–18.5 mg/dl	48–185 mg/L
Cord serum	3.4–6.2 mg/dl	34–62 mg/L
6 months	2.4–6.4 mg/dl	24–64 g/L
C6		
Adult	28–60 µg/ml	28–60 mg/L
Cord serum	6.9–12.7 mg/dl	69–127 mg/L
C7		
Adult	27–80 µg/ml	27–80 mg/L
C8		
Adult	40–106 µg/ml	40–106 mg/L
C9		
Adult	33–250 µg/ml	33–250 mg/L

Usage: Helps diagnose immune-mediated disease and genetic complement deficiency.

Description: The complement system is comprised of a series of proteins that, when activated, serve to amplify an immune response. Complement comprises 10% of serum globulins. Aspiration of the complement (C) system leads to the elaboration of potent inflammatory mediators, facilitates particle opsonization and clearance, and may result in the direct lysis of altered mammolian cells and foreign bacteria. The complement system may be activated by a number of immunologic and nonimmunologic stimuli. Complement activation proceeds by classical and alternative mechanisms. The components C1–C1q, C1r, C1s, C2, and C4 are activated in the classical pathway, which is stimulated when an antigen–antibody reaction occurs. Alternative pathway components, C3 Proactivator, Properdin, and Factor D, are stimulated possibly by mechanisms other than antigen–antibody reactions. C3 and C4 levels are most often used to evaluate the integrity of the classical and alternative pathways. Levels of other individual components may be used to monitor autoimmune activity and identify a genetic deficiency of the individual component(s).

Professional Considerations:

1. Consent form NOT required.

2. Preparation:
   A. Tube: Red-top, red/gray-top, or gold-top.
3. Procedure:
   A. Draw a 7-ml blood sample.
   B. Leave the specimen at room temperature to clot. Then refrigerate at 4°C for 30 minutes to 1 hour.
4. Postprocedure care:
   A. Write the exact specimen collection time on the laboratory requisition.
   B. Send the specimen to the laboratory, where testing should be performed immediately.
5. Client and family teaching:
   A. Results are normally available within 12 hours.
6. Factors that affect results:
   A. Complement is heat-sensitive and deteriorates rapidly.
   B. Reject hemolyzed specimens or specimens received more than 2 hours after collection.
   C. Freeze the specimen at –70°C if it cannot be processed immediately after 1 hour of refrigeration.
7. Other data:
   A. Complement abnormalities in disease are commonly deficiencies rather than increases.
   B. Serial measurements are recommended.
   C. *See C1q Immune Complex Detection, Serum; C3 Complement, Serum; C3 Proactivator, Serum; C4 Complement, Serum; Complement Fixation, Serum; and Complement Total, Serum.*

Bibliography:

Glovsky MM: Applications of complement determinations in human disease. Ann Allergy *72*(6):477–486, 1994.

Norris MK: Checking your patient's complement assay. Nursing *24*(1):26, 1994.

Osterland CK: Laboratory diagnosis and monitoring in chronic systemic autoimmune diseases. Clin Chemistry *40*(11):2146–2153, 1994.

Porcel JM, Peakman M, Senaldi G, Vergani D: Methods for assessing complement activation in the clinical immunology laboratory. J Immunol Methods *157*(1–2):1–9, 1993.

COMPLEMENT FIXATION (CF), SERUM

Norm: Negative test—red cell hemolysis occurs; positive test—absence of red cell hemolysis.

Positive: In the presence of antigen–antibody reactions.

Usage: Detection of antigens, antibodies, or both, during reactions. Clinically, complement fixation is used to detect the presence of anti-DNA, immunoglobulins, and antiplatelet antibodies.

Description: CF is a two-step process based on the principle that one or more of the complement components can be fixed (used) in an antigen–antibody reaction. The test is initiated by adding a known amount of complement to the client's serum. The added complement is then fixed. The second step detects the amount of complement fixed and the proportion of antibody or antigen in the client's serum. The second step is performed by adding antigenic sheep red blood cells to the serum. The remaining unfixed complement will lyse the sheep red blood cells. Therefore, lysis occurs when the complement is unfixed, indicating that the serum is deficient in either antigen or antibody. Lysis does not occur if all the complement is fixed, indicating the presence of antigen and antibody in the serum.

Professional Considerations:

1. Consent form NOT required.
2. Preparation:
   A. Tube: Red-top, red/gray-top, or gold-top.
3. Procedure:
   A. Draw a 3-ml blood sample.
4. Postprocedure care:
   A. None.
5. Client and family teaching:
   A. Two days are required for this test because the second incubation must occur overnight.
6. Factors that affect results:
   A. A contaminated tube may give anti-complementary results.
   B. Gonococcal vaccine may cause a false-positive gonococcal complement fixation test.
   C. Tuberculosis may cause a false-positive leishmaniasis complement fixation test.
   D. Brucellosis and Q fever may cause a false-positive psittacosis complement fixation test.
7. Other data:
   A. *See C1q Immune Complex Detection, Serum; C3 Complement, Serum; C3 Proactivator, Serum; C4 Complement, Serum; Complement Components, Serum; and Complement Total, Serum.*

Bibliography:

Garcia E, Ramirez LE, Monteon V, Sotelo J: Diagnosis of American trypanosomiasis (Chagas' disease) by the new complement fixation test. J Clin Microbiol *33*(4):1034–1035, 1995.

Prager EM, Wilson AC: Information content of immunological distances. Methods Enzymol *224:* 140–152, 1993.

Thacker WL, Talkington DF: Comparison of two rapid commercial tests with complement fixation for serologic diagnosis of *Mycoplasma* pneumonial infections. J Clin Microbiol *33*(5):1212–1214, 1995.

COMPLETE BLOOD COUNT (CBC), BLOOD

Norms:

		SI Units
Hematocrit (HCT)		
Adult females	37–47%	0.37–0.47 L/L
Pregnant		
Trimester 1	35–46%	0.35–0.46 L/L
Trimester 2	30–42%	0.30–0.42 L/L
Trimester 3	34–44%	0.34–0.44 L/L
Postpartum	34–44%	0.34–0.44 L/L
Adult males	40–54%	0.40–0.54 L/L

		SI Units
Children		
Newborn	42–68%	0.42–0.68 L/L
3 months	29–54%	0.29–0.54 L/L
1 year	29–41%	0.29–0.41 L/L
3 years	31–44%	0.31–0.44 L/L
10 years	34–45%	0.34–0.45 L/L

Hemoglobin (HGB)

Adult females	12–16 g/dl	7.4–9.9 mmol/L
Pregnant		
Trimester 1	11.4–15.0 g/dl	7.1–9.3 mmol/L
Trimester 2	10.0–14.3 g/dl	6.2–8.9 mmol/L
Trimester 3	10.2–14.4 g/dl	6.3–8.9 mmol/L
Postpartum	10.4–15.0 g/dl	6.4–9.3 mmol/L
Adult males	14.0–18.0 g/dl	8.7–11.2 mmol/L
Panic low level	<5 g/dl	<3.1 mmol/L
Panic high level	>18 g/dl	>11.2 mmol/L
Children		
Newborn		
Day 1	15.5–24.5 g/dl	9.6–15.2 mmol/L
Days 2–3	19.0 g/dl	11.8 mmol/L
Days 4–8	14.3–22.3 g/dl	8.9–13.8 mmol/L
Days 9–13	16.5 g/dl	10.2 mmol/L
2–8 weeks	10.7–17.3 g/dl	6.6–10.7 mmol/L
3–5 months	9.9–15.5 g/dl	6.1–9.6 mmol/L
6–11 months	11.8 g/dl	7.3 mmol/L
1–2 years	9.0–14.6 g/dl	5.6–9.0 mmol/L
3–9 years	9.4–15.5 g/dl	5.8–9.6 mmol/L
10 years	10.7–15.5 g/dl	6.6–9.6 mmol/L
11–15 years	13.4 g/dl	8.3 mmol/L
Panic levels	<5 g/dl	<3.1 mmol/L
	>18 g/dl	>11.2 mmol/L

Red Blood Cells (RBC)

Adult females	4.0–5.5 million/µl	$4.0–5.5 \times 10^{12}$/L
Pregnant		
Trimester 1	4.0–5.0 million/µl	$4.0–5.0 \times 10^{12}$/L
Trimester 2	3.2–4.5 million/µl	$3.2–4.5 \times 10^{12}$/L
Trimester 3	3.0–4.9 million/µl	$3.0–4.9 \times 10^{12}$/L
Postpartum	3.2–5.0 million/µl	$3.2–5.0 \times 10^{12}$/L
Adult males	4.5–6.2 million/µl	$4.5–6.2 \times 10^{12}$/L
Children		
Newborn		
Day 1	4.1–6.1 million/µl	$4.1–6.1 \times 10^{12}$/L
Days 2–8	5.1 million/µl	5.1×10^{12}/L
Days 9–13	5.0 million/µl	5.0×10^{12}/L
2–8 weeks	3.8–5.6 million/µl	$3.8–5.6 \times 10^{12}$/L
3–5 months	3.8–5.2 million/µl	$3.8–5.2 \times 10^{12}$/L
6–11 months	4.6 million/µl	4.6×10^{12}/L
1–2 years	3.6–5.5 million/µl	$3.6–5.5 \times 10^{12}$/L
3 years	4.5 million/µl	4.5×10^{12}/L
4 years	4.0–5.2 million/µl	$4.0–5.2 \times 10^{12}$/L

		SI Units
Red Blood Cells (RBC) *(continued)*		
Children *(continued)*		
5 years	4.6 million/µl	4.6×10^{12}/L
6–10 years	4.7 million/µl	4.7×10^{12}/L
11–15 years	4.8 million/µl	4.8×10^{12}/L
Mean Cell Volume (MCV)		
Adults	82–93 µ^3	82–98 fl
Children		
Newborn		
Day 1	106 µ^3	106 fl
Days 2–3	105 µ^3	105 fl
Days 4–8	103 µ^3	103 fl
Days 9–13	98 µ^3	98 fl
2–8 weeks	90 µ^3	90 fl
3 months	82 µ^3	82 fl
4–5 months	80 µ^3	80 fl
6–11 months	77 µ^3	77 fl
1 year	78 µ^3	78 fl
2 years	77 µ^3	77 fl
3 years	79 µ^3	79 fl
4–10 years	80 µ^3	80 fl
11–15 years	82 µ^3	82 fl
Mean Cell Hemoglobin (MCH)		
Adults	26–34 pg	1.61–2.11 fmol
Children		
Newborn		
Day 1	38 pg	2.36 fmol
Days 2–3	37 pg	2.30 fmol
Days 4–8	36 pg	2.23 fmol
Days 9–13	33 pg	2.05 fmol
2–8 weeks	30 pg	1.86 fmol
3 months	28 pg	1.73 fmol
4–5 months	27 pg	1.67 fmol
6–11 months	26 pg	1.61 fmol
1–2 years	25 pg	1.55 fmol
3 years	26 pg	1.61 fmol
4–10 years	27 pg	1.67 fmol
11–15 years	28 pg	1.73 fmol
Mean Cell Hemoglobin Concentration (MCHC)		
Adults	31–38%	19.2–23.58 mmol/L
Children		
Newborn		
Day 1	36%	22.34 mmol/L
Days 2–8	35%	21.72 mmol/L
Days 9–13	34%	21.10 mmol/L
2–8 weeks	33%	20.48 mmol/L
3–5 months	34%	21.10 mmol/L
6–11 months	33%	20.48 mmol/L
1–2 years	32%	19.86 mmol/L

		SI Units
3 years	35%	21.72 mmol/L
4–15 years	34%	21.10 mmol/L

White Blood Cells (WBC)

Adult females	4500–11,000/µl	$4.5–11.0 \times 10^9$L
Pregnant		
Trimester 1	6600–14,100/µl	$6.6–14.1 \times 10^9$L
Trimester 2	6900–17,100/µl	$6.9–17.1 \times 10^9$L
Trimester 3	5900–14,700/µl	$5.9–14.7 \times 10^9$L
Postpartum	9700–25,700/µl	$9.7–25.7 \times 10^9$L
Adult males	4500–11,000/µl	$4.5–11.0 \times 10^9$L
Children		
Newborn	9000–30,000/µl	$9.0–30.0 \times 10^9$L
3 months	5700–18,000/µl	$5.7–18.0 \times 10^9$L
1 year	6000–17,500/µl	$6.0–17.5 \times 10^9$L
3 years	5700–16,300/µl	$5.7–16.3 \times 10^9$L
10 years	4500–13,500/µl	$4.5–13.5 \times 10^9$L

Differential White Blood Cells

GRANULOCYTES

Segmented Neutrophil (Segs)	54–62%	0.54–0.62
Adults	3800/µl or mm^3	3800×10^6/L
Children		
Birth	8400/µl or mm^3	8400×10^6/L
12 hours	12,100/µl or mm^3	$12,100 \times 10^6$/L
24 hours	8870/µl or mm^3	8870×10^6/L
1 week	4100/µl or mm^3	4100×10^6/L
2 weeks	3320/µl or mm^3	3320×10^6/L
1–2 months	2750/µl or mm^3	2750×10^6/L
4 months	2730/µl or mm^3	2730×10^6/L
6 months	2710/µl or mm^3	2710×10^6/L
8 months	2680/µl or mm^3	2680×10^6/L
10 months	2600/µl or mm^3	2600×10^6/L
12 months	2680/µl or mm^3	2680×10^6/L
2 years	2660/µl or mm^3	2660×10^6/L
4 years	3040/µl or mm^3	3040×10^6/L
6 years	3600/µl or mm^3	3600×10^6/L
8–14 years	3700/µl or mm^3	3700×10^6/L
16–20 years	3800/µl or mm^3	3800×10^6/L
Band Neutrophils (Bands)	3–5%	0.03–0.05
Adults	620/µl or mm^3	620×10^6/L
Children		
Birth	2540/µl or mm^3	2540×10^6/L
12 hours	3460/µl or mm^3	3460×10^6/L
24 hours	2680/µl or mm^3	2680×10^6/L
1 week	1420/µl or mm^3	1420×10^6/L
2 weeks	1200/µl or mm^3	1200×10^6/L
1 month	1150/µl or mm^3	1150×10^6/L
2 months	1100/µl or mm^3	1100×10^6/L
4–10 months	1000/µl or mm^3	1000×10^6/L
12 months	990/µl or mm^3	990×10^6/L
2 years	850/µl or mm^3	850×10^6/L

		SI Units
Band Neutrophils (Bands) *(continued)*		
Children *(continued)*		
4 years	710/µl or mm^3	710×10^6/L
6 years	670/µl or mm^3	670×10^6/L
8 years	660/µl or mm^3	660×10^6/L
10 years	645/µl or mm^3	645×10^6/L
12–14 years	640/µl or mm^3	640×10^6/L
16–20 years	620/µl or mm^3	620×10^6/L
Eosinophils (Eos)	1–3%	0.01–0.03
Adults	200/µl or mm^3	200×10^6/L
Children		
Birth	400/µl or mm^3	400×10^6/L
12–24 hours	450/µl or mm^3	450×10^6/L
1 week	500/µl or mm^3	500×10^6/L
2 weeks	350/µl or mm^3	350×10^6/L
1 month–1 year	300/µl or mm^3	300×10^6/L
2 years	280/µl or mm^3	280×10^6/L
4 years	250/µl or mm^3	250×10^6/L
6 years	230/µl or mm^3	230×10^6/L
8–20 years	200/µl or mm^3	200×10^6/L
Basophils (Basos)	0–0.75%	0–0.0075
Adults	40/µl or mm^3	40×10^6/L
Children		
Birth–24 hours	100/µl or mm^3	100×10^6/L
1 week–8 years	50/µl or mm^3	50×10^6/L
10–20 years	40/µl or mm^3	40×10^6/L
MONOCYTES (MONOS)	3–7%	0.03–0.07
Adults	300/µl or mm^3	300×10^6/L
Children		
Birth	1050/µl or mm^3	1050×10^6/L
12 hours	1200/µl or mm^3	1200×10^6/L
24 hours–1 week	1100/µl or mm^3	1100×10^6/L
2 weeks	1000/µl or mm^3	1000×10^6/L
1 month	700/µl or mm^3	700×10^6/L
2 months	650/µl or mm^3	650×10^6/L
4 months	600/µl or mm^3	600×10^6/L
6–8 months	580/µl or mm^3	580×10^6/L
10–12 months	550/µl or mm^3	550×10^6/L
2 years	530/µl or mm^3	530×10^6/L
4 years	450/µl or mm^3	450×10^6/L
6 years	400/µl or mm^3	400×10^6/L
8–12 years	350/µl or mm^3	350×10^6/L
14 years	380/µl or mm^3	380×10^6/L
16–18 years	400/µl or mm^3	400×10^6/L
20 years	380/µl or mm^3	380×10^6/L
LYMPHOCYTES (LYMPHS)	25–33%	0.25–0.33
Adults	2500/µl or mm^3	2500×10^6/L
Children		
Birth–12 hours	5500/µl or mm^3	5500×10^6/L
24 hours	5800/µl or mm^3	5800×10^6/L
1 week	5000/µl or mm^3	5000×10^6/L

		SI Units
2 weeks	5500/µl or mm³	5500 × 10⁶/L
1 month	6000/µl or mm³	6000 × 10⁶/L
2 months	6300/µl or mm³	6300 × 10⁶/L
4 months	6800/µl or mm³	6800 × 10⁶/L
6 months	7300/µl or mm³	7300 × 10⁶/L
8 months	7600/µl or mm³	7600 × 10⁶/L
10 months	7500/µl or mm³	7500 × 10⁶/L
12 months	7000/µl or mm³	7000 × 10⁶/L
2 years	6300/µl or mm³	6300 × 10⁶/L
4 years	4500/µl or mm³	4500 × 10⁶/L
6 years	3500/µl or mm³	3500 × 10⁶/L
8 years	3300/µl or mm³	3300 × 10⁶/L
10 years	3100/µl or mm³	3100 × 10⁶/L
12 years	3000/µl or mm³	3000 × 10⁶/L
14 years	2900/µl or mm³	2900 × 10⁶/L
16 years	2800/µl or mm³	2800 × 10⁶/L
18 years	2700/µl or mm³	2700 × 10⁶/L
20 years	2500/µl or mm³	2500 × 10⁶/L

Platelets (Plt)

Adults	150,000–400,000/µl or mm³	150–400 × 10⁹/L
Panic levels	<30,000/µl or mm³	<30 × 10⁹/L
	>1,000,000/µl or mm³	>1000 × 10⁹/L
Children		
Newborn	100,000–300,000/µl or mm³	100–300 × 10⁹/L
3 months	260,000/µl or mm³	260 × 10⁹/L
1–10 years	250,000/µl or mm³	250 × 10⁹/L
Panic levels	<20,000/µl or mm³	<20 × 10⁹/L
	>1,000,000/µl or mm³	>1000 × 10⁹/L

Increased: See individual test listings.

Decreased: See individual test listings.

Description: The complete blood count (CBC) consists of several tests that allow for the evaluation of different cellular components of the blood on a broad spectrum of clients. The items commonly evaluated include hemoglobin, hematocrit, red blood cells, red blood cell indices, white blood cells, white blood cell differential, platelets, and microscopic examination of stained blood smears. Normal levels of the different blood components vary among different age groups, depending on the body's needs and composition (see "Norms," above). The CBC is used for physical examinations, preoperative screening, and evaluation of acute disease or symptoms of anemia or infection. Serial values are often used to track the progress of a variety of diseases and to monitor for side effects resulting from acute or chronic use of drugs that may cause blood dyscrasias. See individual test listings as follows for detailed descriptions of CBC components: *Blood Indices, Blood; Differential Leukocyte Count, Peripheral Blood; Hematocrit, Blood; Hemoglobin, Blood; Platelet Count, Blood; and Red Blood Cell, Blood.*

Professional Considerations:

1. Consent form NOT required.
2. Preparation:
   A. Tube: Lavender-top.
3. Procedure:
   A. To avoid a hemodiluted sample, draw the sample from an extremity that does not have intravenous fluids infusing into it. Leaving the tourniquet in place no longer than 60 seconds, completely fill the tube with a venous blood sample. Invert and gently rotate the tube to thoroughly mix the anticoagulant.
4. Postprocedure care:
   A. Write the specimen collection time on the laboratory requisition.

5. Client and family teaching:
  A. See individual test listings.
  B. Results are normally available within 4 hours.
6. Factors that affect results:
  A. Failure to fill the tube completely with blood causes an improper blood–anticoagulant ratio that yields unreliable values.
  B. The serum sample is stable at room temperature for 10 hours, may be refrigerated for up to 18 hours, and should not be frozen.
  C. *See also individual test listings.*
7. Other data:
  A. *See individual test listings.*

Bibliography:

Dorner K, Schulze S, Reinhardt M, Seeger H, Van Hove L: Improved automated leucocyte counting and differential in newborns achieved by the haematology analyser CELL-DYN 3500. Clin Lab Haematol *17*(1):23–30, 1995.

Higgins C: Full blood count (RBC, Hb, PCV, MCV, MCH, and reticulocytes). Nurs Times *91*(7): 38–40, 1995.

Jones BA, Meier F, Howanitz PJ: Complete blood count specimen acceptability. A College of American Pathologists Q-Probes study of 703 laboratories. Arch Pathol Lab Med *119*(3):203–208, 1995.

Mates M, Heyd J, Souroujon M, Ben Sasson A, Manny N, Hershko C: The haematologist as watchdog of community health by full blood count. QJM *88*(5):333–339, 1995.

COMPUTED TOMOGRAPHIC PERCUTANEOUS TRANSSPLENIC PORTOGRAPHY (CT-PTSP)
(see Splenoportography, Diagnostic)

COMPUTED TOMOGRAPHY, ELECTRON BEAM, DIAGNOSTIC
(see Ultrafast Computed Tomography, Diagnostic)

COMPUTED TOMOGRAPHY OF THE BODY, DIAGNOSTIC

Norm: Negative. No tumor or pathologic activity.

Usage: Determination of the extent of primary and secondary neoplasms of the neck; evaluation of bony and inflammatory abnormalities of the spine and joints, including neoplasms, fractures, dislocations, and congenital anomalies; localization of foreign bodies in the soft tissues, hypopharynx, or larynx, and assessment of airway integrity after trauma; evaluation of retropharyngeal abscesses; investigation of suspected tracheal, thymic, mediastinal, and hilar masses; evaluation of problems identified on chest radiographics; staging of bronchogenic carcinoma and gastrointestinal tumors; detection of aortic aneurysm or aortic dissection; detection, localization, and characterization of lung disease; detection of mediastinal or diaphragmatic herniation; evaluation of musculoskeletal or soft tissue trauma or neoplasms; evaluation of suspected congenital or other abnormalities of specific body organs such as the liver, gallbladder, pancreas, kidneys, adrenal gland, and spleen; identification and localization of sites of hemorrhage; assessment of the organs and structures of the peritoneal cavity and pelvis; and sometimes used to provide imaging identification and guidance for invasive procedures such as abscess drainage or amebic liver abscess, percutaneous biopsy, or aspirate for cytologic or histologic study. For additional uses, see *Bibliography,* below.

Description: Computed tomography (CT) is a radiographic scan that may be performed with or without contrast on virtually any portion of the body. CT is classified as a reconstructive imaging procedure because it produces a picture of the contents of a portion of the body based on the differing densities and composition of body tissues. The picture is obtained by projecting x-rays along all possible lines in the plane of the body. An x-ray detector records the intensity of the x-rays from multiple angles as it is transmitted through the tissue. A computer then reconstructs the differing intensities into pixels that appear in differing shades for differing tissues and represent an anterior-to-posterior "slice" across the plane of the body. CT is used to detect very minor differences in radiographic contrast, providing radiography that portrays boundaries between tissues that are normally indistinguishable to radiographic examination. The tissue contrast differentiation of CT is superior to that of conventional radiography. CT of the body takes longer than CT of the head because of the larger size of the body.

Professional Considerations:

1. Consent form NOT required.

Risks:

Allergic reaction to dye (itching, hives, rash, tight feeling in the throat, shortness of breath, bronchospasm, anaphylaxis, death); renal toxicity; hematoma or infection at the injection site for CT with contrast.

Contraindications:

CT with contrast: Previous allergy to iodine, shellfish, or radiographic dye; renal insufficiency. CT is contraindicated in clients who are unable to lie motionless.

2. Preparation:
   A. For CT with contrast, *see Client and family teaching.*
   B. Remove radiopaque objects such as jewelry, snaps, and electrocardiographic leads with snaps (if possible).
   C. Establish intravenous access for injection of the dye and prepare emergency equipment for a possible hypersensitivity reaction.
3. Procedure:
   A. The client is positioned supine, with his or her head secured and resting on a headrest on a motorized handling table. For spinal studies, the lumbar spine is straightened by flexing the knees and providing a footrest.
   B. The client must lie motionless as the table slowly advances through the circular opening of the scanner. The CT scanner sends a narrow beam of x-rays across the area to be imaged in a linear fashion. While scanning a client, the nonabsorbed x-rays are detected at the same time as the beam is transmitting. This linear scan sequence is repeated at many different angles around the client's body. The data collected consists of a series of profiles that reflect the area visualized at different angles.
   C. If contrast medium is to be used, it is injected intravenously at this time and the scan is repeated. The client is observed for rash or respiratory difficulty, which may indicate reaction to the contrast medium. Reactions usually develop within 30 minutes if the client is allergic to the dye.
4. Postprocedure care:
   A. Replace electrocardiographic (ECG) leads if they were removed.
   B. For CT with contrast, observe for side effects such as headache, nausea, and vomiting. Resume previous diet if no side effects have been noted.
5. Client and family teaching:
   A. The client must lie motionless during the scan. Because this can be a frightening test, it should be described carefully to the client before entering the CT room.
   B. If contrast medium will be used, fast from food and fluids for 4 hours before the CT scan.
6. Factors that affect results:
   A. Unavoidable internal motion of body organs such as the heart and lungs or intentional movement by the client contributes to the appearance of "tuning-fork"-like streaks across the picture.
   B. Radiopaque objects such as jewelry and snaps obscure visualization.
7. Other data:
   A. CT is an expensive, highly technical study.
   B. *See also Chest Tomography, Diagnostic, Ultrafast Computed Tomography, Diagnostic; and Cerebral Computed Tomography, Diagnostic.*

Bibliography:

Cortet B, Flipo RM, Remy-Jardin M, Coquerelle P, Duquesnoy B, Remy J, Delcambre B: Use of high resolution computed tomography of the lungs in patients with rheumatoid arthritis. Ann Rheum Dis 54(10):815–819, 1995.

Frick SL, Sims SH: Is computed tomography useful after simple posterior hip dislocation? J Orthop Trauma 9(5):388–391, 1995.

Goodman LR: Congestive heart failure and adult respiratory distress syndrome. New insights using computed tomography. Radiol Clin North Amer 34(1):33–46, 1996.

Gupta M, Kesarwala H, Gaur S: Amebic liver abscess in a child. Clin Pediatr 35(3):155–156, 1996.

Jeng CM, Wu DY, Shih CC, Lee WY, Kung CH, Lau MK: Computed tomography and magnetic resonance imaging of diffuse pigmented villonodular synovitis: report of a case. J Formos Med Assoc 94(10):638–640, 1995.

COMPUTED TOMOGRAPHY OF THE BRAIN, DIAGNOSTIC
(see Cerebral Computed Tomography, Diagnostic)

CONCENTRATION TEST, URINE

Norm:

		SI Units
Specific gravity	1.025–1.032	1.025–1.032
Osmolality	>800 mOsm/kg water	>800 mmol/kg

Increased: Dehydration.

Decreased: Congestive heart failure, diabetes insipidus, Fanconi's syndrome, hydronephrosis, hypercalcemia, hypokalemia, hypoproteinemia, nephrogenic diabetes insipidus, polycystic kidneys, pyelonephritis (chronic), and sickle cell trait. Drugs include diuretics.

Description: The urine concentration test is an evaluation of renal capacity to concentrate urine in response to fluid deprivation or to dilute the urine in response to fluid overload. Urine specific gravity and osmolality are measured after mild hypernatremia is induced by 12 hours of fluid restriction and deprivation. This test is used to detect renal impairment and evaluate renal tubular function. It is also used to differentiate deficiency of antidiuretic hormone (ADH) from renal insensitivity to ADH. In clients with normal renal function and diabetes insipidus (caused by ADH deficiency), administration of exogenous ADH causes urine osmolality to increase. In clients with renal insensitivity to ADH (nephrogenic diabetes insipidus), the exogenous ADH does not cause an increase in urine osmolality.

Professional Considerations:

1. Consent form NOT required.

Risks:

Hypotension and associated sequelae.

Contraindications:

This test may be contraindicated in clients with subnormal cardiac output, due to the risk of depleting plasma volume.

2. Preparation:
   A. *See Client and family teaching.*
   B. Obtain baseline weight prior to the evening meal before the test and every 4 hours until the test is completed. Terminate the test if weight decreases more than 5% from the baseline weight or for orthostatic hypotension.
   C. Obtain three 500-ml clean containers.
   D. Monitor the client closely throughout the test for symptoms of severe dehydration or for surreptitious intake of fluids.
3. Procedure:
   A. Collect the entire voided urine speci-

mens in separate, refrigerated, clean containers at 0600 (6 A.M.), 0800 (8 A.M.), and 1000 (10 A.M.). Record the exact time and amount of each specimen.
   B. If the test is being performed to differentiate diabetes insipidus from nephrogenic diabetes insipidus, exogenous ADH (vasopressin) is administered intravenously as soon as a plateau in osmolality is reached. A final urine sample is collected, as above, in 1 hour.
4. Postprocedure care:
   A. Resume diet and fluids.
   B. Record the time and amount of each specimen collected on the laboratory requisition.
   C. Refrigerate the specimens until testing.
5. Client and family teaching:
   A. Eat a high-protein dinner the day before the test.
   B. Fluids are restricted to 200 ml the evening before the test, including the evening meal.
   C. Fast from food and fluids from midnight prior to the test until the test is completed.
   D. It is normal to feel very thirsty during the testing period, but you should not drink anything.
6. Factors that affect results:
   A. Failure to follow dietary and fluid restrictions will interfere with results.
   B. Fluid intake over 200 ml caused by intravenous therapy invalidates the results.
   C. Administration of radiographic dyes within 7 days prior to the test may cause increased urine osmolality.
   D. Baseline glucosuria invalidates the results.
7. Other data:
   A. None.

Bibliography:

Dewit L, Anninga JK, Hoefnagel CA, Nooijen WJ: Radiation injury in the human kidney: A prospective analysis using specific scintigraphic and biochemical endpoints. Int J Oncol Biol Physiol 19(4):977–983, 1990.

Sacher RA, McPherson RA: Widmann's Clinical Interpretation of Laboratory Tests. Philadelphia, FA Davis, 1991.

CONDYLOMA LATUM, VULVAR OR ANAL CULTURE FOR CYTOLOGY, SPECIMEN

Norm: Negative findings.

Description: Condyloma latum is a flat, moist, papular growth that appears on the moist skin of the genital and anal areas during the secondary stages of syphilis. It is also called flat condyloma.

Professional Considerations:

1. Consent form NOT required.
2. Preparation:
   A. Verify the collection procedure with the individual laboratory performing the test. Smears may be required to be prepared and fixed at the bedside.
   B. Obtain sterile cotton swabs or Culturette, gloves, and transport medium.
3. Procedure:
   A. *Vulvar sample:* Wipe the vulva with sterile cotton or gauze. Insert a sterile, cotton-tipped swab between the vulva and leave it in place for several seconds for optimum absorption of pathogens.
   B. *Anal sample:* Insert a sterile, cotton-tipped swab into the anus approximately 2 cm. Leave the swab in place several seconds for optimum absorption of pathogens. If feces are obtained, discard the swab and repeat the procedure.
4. Postprocedure care:
   A. Place the swab in the transport medium according to the requirements of the laboratory performing the test.
   B. Send the swab immediately to the laboratory.
5. Client and family teaching:
   A. Refer the client with positive results for follow-up care, which is necessary for prevention and early detection of sequelae.
6. Factors that affect results:
   A. Results are invalidated if the swab dries out before being inoculated onto culture medium or preparing a smear.
7. Other data:
   A. None.

Bibliography:

Pavithran K: Solitary condyloma latum on the umbilicus [letter]. Int J Dermatol *31*(8):597–598, 1992.

Sagerman PM, Kadish AS, Niedt GW: Condyloma acuminatum with superficial spirochetosis simulating condyloma latum. Am J Dermatopathol *15*(2):176–179, 1993.

CONIZATION OF CERVIX (COLD KNIFE CONIZATION), DIAGNOSTIC

Norm: Negative. No abnormal findings.

Usage: Follow-up for abnormal Pap smear; cervical cancer; used when colposcopy, cervical cytology, and colposcopy biopsies yield inconclusive findings.

Description: Conization is a biopsy of the uterine cervix that is performed after cervical smears reveal the presence of intraepithelial neoplasias. It may be performed in conjunction with dilation and curettage. The advantage that conization brings to the diagnostic process is that it provides a sample of the entire lateral margins of the transformation zone of the cervix. Cold knife conization is less expensive than laser conization and produces equally satisfactory specimens for histologic examination. The cold knife method may also be superior to the loop electrosurgical excisional procedure (LEEP) because it does not produce electrocautery artifact that interferes with examination of the cervical margins.

Professional Considerations:

1. Consent form IS required.

Risks:

Hemorrhage, infection, sepsis.

Contraindications:

Anticoagulant therapy, bleeding disorders, thrombocytopenia. Sedatives are contraindicated in clients with central nervous system depression.

2. Preparation:
   A. *See Client and family teaching.*
   B. Preschedule this test with the pathology laboratory. Biopsy specimens must be processed immediately.
   C. Obtain Lugol's solution, a tenaculum, vasopressin, conization knife, suture material, Gelfoam or Surgicel (or electrocautery), and a sterile container.
3. Procedure:
   A. This procedure is usually performed under general anesthesia, although local anesthesia is occasionally used.
   B. The client is placed in a lithotomy position and the cervix is painted with Lugol's solution (Schiller's test) to detect white, pale, or unstained areas, which may indicate lesions.
   C. A suture may be sewn on each side of the cervix to control bleeding. The anterior lip of the cervix is lifted with a tenaculum, and Pitressin (vasopressin) is injected into several areas to control bleeding.
   D. A cone of tissue is removed from the cervical os with a cold knife (Fleming knife). Tissues that did not stain with the Schiller's test are included in the cone. The specimen is transferred immediately to the laboratory in a sterile container, with or without sterile

saline, according to the requirements of the laboratory performing the test.

E. Bleeding may be controlled by packing with Gelfoam or Surgicel, or by cervical sutures or electrocautery.

4. Postprocedure care:
   A. Provide sanitary pads and observe for heavy bleeding, which is abnormal.
   B. Perform standard postanesthesia observations and assessments if general anesthesia or deep sedation was used.

5. Client and family teaching:
   A. If general anesthesia will be used, fast from food and fluids for 8 hours prior to the procedure.
   B. A greenish-grayish discharge from the vagina due to the presence of the Lugol's solution is normal for several days after the test.
   C. Resume previous diet after the procedure.

6. Factors that affect results:
   A. Electrocautery should not be used, as it distorts tissues and impairs diagnosis.

7. Other data:
   A. Conization should be performed in a hospital, rather than in a physician's office.
   B. Conization should be performed before dilation and curettage, which dislodges the cervical epithelium.
   C. Moore et al. (1995) found that residual dysplasia present in cold knife conization specimens was not predictive of residual dysplasia in hysterectomy specimens.

Bibliography:

Mathevet P, Dargent D, Roy M, Beau G: A randomized prospective study comparing three techniques of conization: cold knife, laser, and LEEP. Gynecol Oncol 54(2):175–179, 1994.

Moore BC, Higgins RV, Laurent SL, Marroum MC, Bellitt P: Predictive factors from cold knife conization for residual cervical intraepithelial neoplasia in subsequent hysterectomy. Am J Obstet Gynecol 173(2):361–366, 1995.

CONJUNCTIVAL, FUNGUS, CULTURE

Norm: No growth.

Usage: Conjunctivitis and fungal infections.

Description: Fungi are slow-growing, eukaryotic organisms that can grow on living and nonliving organic materials, and are subdivided into yeasts and molds. Factors that predispose clients to fungal infections by lowering the normal host defense mechanisms include administration of broad-spectrum antibiotics, placement of invasive lines, poor nutritional status, parenteral nutrition, surgery, trauma, and long-term use of steroids. Conjunctival fungal infections appear as spongy, granular growths on the conjunctiva. Although tentative identification of fungi can be made quickly with staining techniques, culture of the organism on special fungal culture media is required to confirm a diagnosis of a fungal infection.

Professional Considerations:

1. Consent form NOT required.
2. Preparation:
   A. Obtain a needle and syringe or sterile scraper, or two sterile swabs and a sterile container.
3. Procedure:
   A. For draining conjunctiva, aspirate or scrape as much exudate as possible with a needle and syringe or sterile scraper.
   B. Send the sample to the laboratory in a sterile container.
   C. Alternatively, with two small, sterile, cotton-tipped, minimally absorbent swabs, obtain a smear of the conjunctiva. Obtain as much specimen as possible.
   D. Place the swabs into sterile tubes.
4. Postprocedure care:
   A. Record any antifungal therapy on the laboratory requisition.
   B. Send the swabs immediately to the laboratory.
5. Client and family teaching:
   A. The culture will not hurt, but a feeling of pressure will be felt along the conjunctivae.
6. Factors that affect results:
   A. Aspiration of pus or exudate yields better results than do swabs.
7. Other data:
   A. The best results are obtained if the culture is taken before antifungal therapy is started.
   B. Because fungi are slow-growing organisms, primary cultures should be held for at least 2 weeks and preferably for 4 weeks or longer before being reported as negative.

Bibliography:

BenEzra D: Current practice: diagnosis and treatment in primary healthcare. Allergy 50(Suppl 21): 30–33, discussion 34–38, 1995.

Vajpayee RB, Gupta SK, Bareja U, Kishore K: Ocular atopy and mycotic keratitis. Ann Ophthalmol 22(10):369–372, 1990.

CONJUNCTIVAL, ROUTINE, CULTURE

Norm: No abnormal growth. Normal flora includes diphtheroids, *Staphylococcus epidermidis*, *Streptococcus* *pneumoniae, Staphylococcus pyogenes,* and *Streptococcus viridans.*

Usage: Used to establish the presence of bacterial or viral pathogens causing blepharitis, chalazion, conjunctivitis, impetigo, and stye.

Description: Conjunctivitis is an inflammation of the eye conjunctiva most commonly caused by *Staphylococci, Chlamydia* (causing inclusion conjunctivitis), *Rickettsiae,* viruses, or parasites. Less commonly, the conjunctiva may be infected by *Gonococcus* and may possibly lead to blindness. Conjunctivitis may also result from allergic processes or injury to the eye. Symptoms of conjunctivitis include redness, swelling, drainage, and itching. This condition is commonly diagnosed via culture and Gram staining or Wright staining of drainage from the lower conjunctiva.

Professional Considerations:

1. Consent form NOT required.
2. Preparation:
   A. Cleanse the skin around the eye.
   B. Obtain an eye swab approved for microbiologic purposes and culture tube (Culturette).
3. Procedure:
   A. Gently but firmly, wipe a sterile, cotton-tipped swab over the inflamed lower conjunctiva or inner canthus, avoiding the eyelashes.
   B. Insert the swab into a Culturette tube and squeeze the ampule of medium.
   C. If the specimen will be tested for *Gonococcus* (most commonly in newborns), place the swab in a Transgrow bottle, not a Culturette tube.
4. Postprocedure care:
   A. Write the antibiotic therapy on the laboratory requisition.
   B. Send the swab to the laboratory immediately.
5. Client and family teaching:
   A. Where inflammation is present, the swab technique may cause transient pain.
   B. Wash hands after touching conjunctival area to avoid spread of infection to others.
6. Factors that affect results:
   A. Results are invalidated if the specimen dries out before being inoculated onto culture medium or preparing a slide for staining.
7. Other data:
   A. The best results are obtained if the culture is taken before antibiotic therapy is started.
   B. Candidal blepharitis is often found in immunosuppressed clients.

Bibliography:

Klapper PE, Cleator GM: Adenovirus cross-infection: a continuing problem. J Hosp Infect *30* (Suppl): 262–267, 1995.

Wasserman D, Asbell PA, Friedman AJ, Bottone EJ: Capnocytophaga ochracea chronic blepharoconjunctivitis. Cornea *14*(5):533–535, 1995.

CONNECTING PEPTIDE, SERUM
(see C-Peptide, Serum)

COOMBS', DIRECT (DIRECT ANTIGLOBULIN TEST), SERUM

Norm: Negative

Positive: Arthritis (rheumatoid), elderly clients, erythroblastosis fetalis, hemolytic anemia (autoimmune, drug-induced), infection, neoplasm, renal disorders, systemic lupus erythematosus, and transfusion reaction. Drugs include (possibly due to IgG erythrocyte sensitization by the drugs) Aminopyrine, cephalosporins, chlorpromazine, dipyrone, ethosuximide, hydralazine hydrochloride, insulin, isoniazid, levodopa, mefenamic acid, melphalan, methyldopa, methyldopate hydrochloride, oxyphenisatin, *para*-aminosalicylic acid, penicillins, phenacetin, phenytoin, phenytoin sodium, procainamide hydrochloride, quinidine gluconate, quinidine polygalacturonate, quinidine sulfate, rifampin, streptomycin sulfate, sulfonamides, and tetracyclines.

Negative: Hemolytic anemia (nonautoimmune, non-drug-induced). Normal finding.

Usage: Used to show antigen-antibody reactions, differentiation of types of hemolytic anemias, testing for suspected erythroblastosis fetalis, and investigation of erythrocyte sensitization by drugs or blood transfusions.

Description: The direct Coombs' test involves adding Coombs' antihuman globulin serum to a client's washed red blood cells and observing for agglutination, which signals the presence of previously undetected IgG antibodies, complement, or immunoglobulins on the surfaces of the client's erythrocytes. The Coombs' antiglobulin contains antibodies to IgG and several complement components. The antibodies detected by the direct Coombs' test are difficult to detect any other way because they are left over from incomplete antigen-antibody reactions and, although present on the erythrocyte surfaces, remain invisible. The Coombs' antiglobulin causes completion of the antigen-antibody reaction, thus making the antibodies identifiable as they begin clumping.

Professional Considerations:

1. Consent form NOT required.
2. Preparation:
   A. Tube: Lavender-top, red-top, red/gray-top, or gold-top.
3. Procedure:
   A. Draw a 7-ml blood sample.
   B. The sample may be obtained from cord blood.
4. Postprocedure care:
   A. Write recent transfusions and drugs on the laboratory requisition.
5. Client and family teaching:
   A. For positive results, the more specific direct Coombs' IgG test is indicated.
6. Factors that affect results:
   A. Reject hemolyzed specimens.
   B. Cord blood contaminated by Wharton's jelly may yield unreliable results.
   C. Cold agglutinins may cause false-positive results.
   D. Drugs that may cause false-negative results in the presence of acquired hemolytic anemia include heparin calcium and heparin sodium.
7. Other data:
   A. This test does not delineate the nature of the antibodies identified.
   B. The test must be completed within 24 hours of specimen collection.
   C. DeAngelis et al. (1994) found a high incidence of positive results in clients with antibodies to HIV and suggest that this test may be helpful as a prognostic indicator for the disease course.
   D. *See also Antibody Identification, Red Cell, Serum.*

Bibliography:

De Angelis V, Biasinutto C, Pradella P, Vaccher E, Spina M, Tirelli U: Clinical significance of positive direct antiglobulin test in patients with HIV infection. Infection 22(2):92–95, 1994.

Fadal RG: IgE-mediated hypersensitivity reactions. Otolaryngol Head Neck Surg. 109(3, Pt 2):565–758, 1993.

Heddle NM, Wentworth P, Anderson DR, Emmerson D, Kelton JG, Blajchman MA: Three examples of Rh haemolytic disease of the newborn with a negative direct antiglobulin test. Transfus Med 5(2):113–116, 1995.

COOMBS', DIRECT IgG, SERUM

Norm: Negative.

Positive: Anemia (hemolytic, drug-induced), erythroblastosis fetalis, leukemia (chronic lymphocytic), and transfusion reaction. Drugs include (possibly due to IgG erythrocyte sensitization by the drugs) aminopyrine, cephalosporins, chlorpromazine, dipyrone, ethosuximide, hydralazine, hydrochloride, insulin, isoniazid, levodopa, mefenamic acid, melphalan, methyldopa, methyldopate hydrochloride, oxyphenisatin, *para*-aminosalicylic acid, penicillins, phenacetin, phenytoin, phenytoin sodium, procainamide hydrochloride, quinidine gluconate, quinidine polygalacturonate, quinidine sulfate, rifampin, streptomycin sulfate, sulfonamides, and tetracyclines.

Description: *See Coombs' Direct, Serum.* This test is more specific than a direct Coombs' test and is performed after a positive direct Coombs' test. The direct Coombs' IgG test mixes Coombs' antiglobulin containing only anti-IgG with the client's washed red blood cells and observing for agglutination, which signals the presence of IgG on the surface of the client's erythrocytes.

Professional Considerations:

1. Consent form NOT required.
2. Preparation:
   A. Tube: Lavender-top
3. Procedure:
   A. Draw a 7-ml blood sample.
4. Postprocedure care:
   A. Write recent transfusions and drugs on the laboratory requisition.
5. Client and family teaching:
   A. Results are normally available within 24 hours.
6. Factors that affect results:
   A. Cold agglutinins may cause false-positive results.
   B. False-negative results may occur in the presence of sensitized erythrocytes with less than 100–300 IgG molecules per cell.
7. Other data:
   A. The test must be completed within 24 hours of specimen collection.

Bibliography:

Girelli G, Perrone MP, Adorno G, Arista MC, Coluzzi S, Damico C, di Giorgio G, Monarca B: A second example of hemolysis due to IgA autoantibody with anti-e specificity. Haematologica 75(2):182–183, 1990.

Ylagen ES, Curtis BR, Wildgen ME, Mass MD, Chaplin H: Invalidation of antiglobulin tests by a high thermal amplitude cryoglobulin. Transfusion 30(2):154–157, 1990.

COOMBS', INDIRECT (INDIRECT ANTIGLOBULIN TEST), SERUM

Norm: Negative.

Positive: Erythroblastosis fetalis, hemolytic anemia (drug-induced), incompatible crossmatch, maternal-fetal Rh incompatibility, and prior transfusion reaction. Drugs include levodopa, mefenamic acid, methyldopa, and methyldopate hydrochloride.

Description: This test detects unexpected circulating antibodies by exposing a client's serum to group O erythrocytes that are not affected by anti-A or anti-B antibodies, but do contain other known antigens. It screens for reactions to RhDu, Kell, and Duffy antigens; pretransfusion blood screening; detection of leukocyte, platelet, or rare antibodies, and screening prenatally for fetomaternal blood incompatibility. In contrast to the direct Coombs' test, which detects antibodies already attached to erythrocytes, the indirect Coombs' test detects the presence of antibodies other than those of the ABO groups that are present in the serum. The test is performed by: (1) mixing erythrocytes containing known antigens to a client's serum and allowing time for unknown antibodies in the client's serum to react with the antigens; and (2) the addition of Coombs' antihuman globulin serum to the mixture and observing for agglutination, indicating the presence of antibodies.

Professional Considerations:

1. Consent form NOT required.
2. Preparation:
   A. Tube: Red-top, red/gray-top, or gold-top.
3. Procedure:
   A. Draw a 10-ml blood sample (adult) or a 2.5-ml blood sample (pediatric).
4. Postprocedure care:
   A. Write recent transfusions and drugs on the laboratory requisition.
5. Client and family teaching:
   A. Results are normally available within 24 hours.
   B. If results are positive, an additional sample may be needed to perform antibody identification.
6. Factors that affect results:
   A. Reject hemolyzed specimens.
   B. Cold agglutinins may cause false-positive results.
7. Other data:
   A. Negative tests on pregnant women during the first 12 weeks' gestation should be repeated at 28 weeks' gestation. A positive test at 28 weeks' gestation indicates the need for antibody identification testing.
   B. This test must be completed within 48 hours of specimen collection.

Bibliography:

Hillyer CD, Schwenn MR, Fulton DR, Meissner HC, Berkman EM: Autoimmune hemolytic anemia in kawasaki disease: A case report. Transfusion 30(8):738–740, 1990.

Zupanska B, Brojer E, McIntosh J, Seyfried H, Howell P: Correlation of monocyte-monolayer assay results, number of erythrocyte-bound IgG molecules, and IgG subclass composition in the study of red cell alloantibodies other than D. Vox Sang 58(4):276–280, 1990.

COPPER (Cu), SERUM

Norm:

		SI Units
Adult females	80–155 µg/dl	12.56–24.34 µmol/L
Pregnant, 40 weeks	118–302 µg/dl	18.53–47.41 µmol/L
Adult males	70–140 µg/dl	10.99–21.98 µmol/L
Children		
≤6 months	20–70 µg/dl	3.14–10.99 µmol/L
Infant	15–65 µg/dl	2.35–10.20 µmol/L
Child	30–150 µg/dl	4.71–23.55 µmol/L

Increased: Alzheimer's disease, anemia (aplastic, pernicious, megaloblastic of pregnancy; iron deficiency), cirrhosis (biliary), elevated C-reactive protein, glomerulonephritis, hemochromatosis, Hodgkin's disease, hyperestrogenemia, hypothyroidism, hyperthyroidism, infection, leukemia, Lofgren syndrome, lymphoma, myocardial infarction, pellagra, pregnancy, rheumatic fever, rheumatoid arthritis, sarcoidosis, and systemic lupus erythematosus. Drugs include carbamazepine, estrogens and oral contraceptives, phenobarbitol, and phenytoin sodium.

Decreased: Burns, hypoproteinemia, kwashiorkor, malabsorption, Menkes' kinky hair syndrome, nephrosis, and Wilson's disease.

Description: Copper is an essential trace element that functions in hemoglobin synthesis and activation of respiratory enzymes. Abnormally low levels cause impaired erythrocyte production and survival time and lowered catabolism by copper-containing enzymes. Copper toxicity causes jaundice, hepatic injury, headache, and vomiting, and may lead to hemolytic shock. This test is most frequently used to aid diagnosis of Wilson's disease, in which serum copper levels are low, urine copper levels are high, and increased amounts of copper are deposited in body tissues.

Professional Considerations:

1. Consent form NOT required.
2. Preparation:
   A. Preschedule this test with the laboratory.
   B. Obtain a stainless steel needle, plastic syringe, and navy-blue-top tube.

C. Do NOT draw during hemodialysis or peritoneal dialysis.
3. Procedure:
   A. Draw a 10-ml blood sample in a plastic syringe, using a stainless steel needle.
   B. Transfer the sample into a navy-blue-top tube without a rubber siliconized stopper.
4. Postprocedure care:
   A. None.
5. Client and family teaching:
   A. Results are normally available within 24 hours.
6. Factors that affect results:
   A. The contact of serum with rubber siliconized stopper yields unreliable results.
7. Other data:
   A. Serum ceruloplasmin and urine copper are usually also evaluated in conjunction with this test.
   B. Serial testing and copper supplementation are recommended for clients with burns.

Bibliography:

Brenner AJ, Harris ED: A quantitative test for copper using bicinchoninic acid. Anal Biochem *226*(1): 80–84, 1995.

Donghi M, Giura R, Antonelli P: Increase of serum copper concentration in Lofgren syndrome. Sarcoidosis *12*(2):147–149, 1995.

Gosling P, Rothe HM, Sheehan TM, Hubbard LD: Serum copper and zinc concentrations in patients with burns in relation to burn surface area. J Burn Care Rehabil *16*(5):481–486, 1995.

COPPER (Cu), URINE

Norm:

		SI Units
All ages	0–60 μg/24 hours	0–0.96 μmol/day
Wilson's disease	>100 μg/24 hours	>1.60 μg/day

Increased: Alzheimer's disease, aminoaciduria, cirrhosis (biliary, Indian childhood), hepatitis (chronic, active), hyperceruloplasminemia, nephrotic syndrome, pellagra, proteinuria, and Wilson's disease (500–1000 mg/dl).

Description: Copper is an essential trace element that functions in hemoglobin synthesis and activation of respiratory enzymes. Abnormally low levels cause impaired erythrocyte production and survival time and lowered catabolism by copper-containing enzymes. Copper toxicity causes jaundice, hepatic injury, headache, and vomiting, and may lead to hemolytic shock. This test is most frequently

used to aid diagnosis of Wilson's disease, in which serum copper levels are low, urine copper levels are high, and increased amounts of copper are deposited in body tissues.

Professional Considerations:

1. Consent form NOT required.
2. Preparation:
   A. Preschedule this test with the laboratory.
   B. Obtain a clean polyethylene, acid-washed container, pH paper, hydrochloric (HCl) or nitric acid, and a 100-ml clean container for the aliquot.
3. Procedure:
   A. Discard the first morning urine specimen.
   B. Begin to time a 24-hour urine collection.

C. Save all the urine voided for 24 hours in a room-temperature, clean, 3-L, polyethylene, acid-washed container. Document the quantity of urine output during the specimen collection period. For catheterized clients, empty the urine drainage bag into the acidified collection container hourly. Include the urine voided at the end of the 24-hour period. Add HCl or nitric acid as needed to maintain pH at 2.

4. Postprocedure care:
   A. Compare the urine quantity in the specimen container with the urinary output record for the test. If the specimen contains less urine than was recorded as output, some of the sample may have been discarded, invalidating the test.
   B. Document the urine quantity on the laboratory requisition.
   C. Send a 100-ml aliquot to the lab.

5. Client and family teaching:
   A. Save all the urine voided in the 24-hour period and urinate before defecating to avoid loss of urine. If any urine is accidentally discarded, discard the entire specimen and restart the collection the next day.

6. Factors that affect results:
   A. All the urine voided for the 24-hour period must be included before taking aliquot, to avoid a falsely low result.
   B. Contact of the specimen with stool or metal invalidates results.

7. Other data:
   A. Serum copper and serum ceruloplasmin are usually also evaluated in conjunction with this test.

Bibliography:

Anderson RA, Bryden NA, Polansky MM, Deuster PA: Acute exercise effects on urinary losses and serum concentrations of copper and zinc of moderately trained and untrained men consuming a controlled diet. Analyst 120(3):867–870, 1995.

COPROPORPHYRIN (UCP), URINE

Norm: Norms vary by laboratory. Some reported ranges are:

		SI Units
24-hour urine		
All	34–234 µg/24 hours	51–351 nmol/day
Adult females	1–57 µg/24 hours	1.5–86 nmol/day
Adult males	0–96 µg/24 hours	0–144 nmol/day
First morning void		
All	0.5–2.3 µg/dl	0.75–3.5 nmol/L

Increased: Acute myocardial infarction, acute poliomyelitis, anemia (hemolytic, pernicious, sideroachrestic), cirrhosis (alcoholic), coproporphyria (erythropoietic), erythroid hyperplasia, exercise, fever, hemochromatosis, Hodgkin's disease, lead poisoning, leukemia, porphyria (congenital erythropoietic), porphyria cutanea tarda, protoporphyria (erythropoietic), thyrotoxicosis, and vitamin deficiencies. Drugs include barbiturates, chloral hydrate, chlordiazepoxide, chlorpropamide, meprobamate, and sulfonamides.

Decreased: Not clinically significant.

Description: Coproporphyrin is a compound formed during the production of the heme portion of hemoglobin. After it is metabolized, small amounts of coproporphyrin can be found in the urine of healthy individuals. Clients with one of the congenital or acquired diseases classified as the "porphyrias" secrete and excrete increased amounts of hemoglobin precursor compounds, including coproporphyrin. This test is most frequently used in conjunction with the measurement of other urine porphyrin levels to differentiate the etiology and type of porphyria occurring.

Professional Considerations:

1. Consent form NOT required.
2. Preparation:
   A. *See Client and family teaching.*
   B. Obtain a 3-L, light-protected, clean specimen container, pH paper, sodium bicarbonate, and a 100-ml light-protected container.
3. Procedure:
   A. *24-Hour urine:*
      i. Discard the first morning urine specimen.
      ii. Begin to time a 24-hour urine collection.
      iii. Collect a 24-hour urine specimen in a refrigerated dark bottle containing 5 g of sodium carbonate. Document the quantity of urine

output and keep the container tightly covered during the specimen collection period. For catheterized clients, maintain the collection bag on ice in a light-protected container and empty the bag into the refrigerated collection container hourly.

   iv. Maintain the pH of the specimen between 6 and 7 by adding sodium bicarbonate as needed. Include the urine voided at the end of the 24-hour period.

   v. At the end of the collection period, mix the specimen gently and transfer a 50-ml aliquot to a light-protected container and cap tightly.

  B. *First morning void:*

   i. Collect the entire first morning voided urine specimen in a light-protected container.

4. Postprocedure care:

  A. Before taking aliquot, compare the urine quantity in a specimen container with a urinary output record for the test. If the specimen contains less urine than was recorded as output, some of the sample may have been discarded, thus invalidating the test.

  B. Send the specimen to the laboratory immediately and refrigerate it until testing.

5. Client and family teaching:

  A. Barbiturates, chloral hydrate, chlorpropamide, sulfonamides, meprobamate, and chlordiazepoxide will induce porphyria and should be stopped 10 days before the test.

  B. Save all the urine voided in the 24-hour period and urinate before defecating to avoid loss of urine. If any urine is accidentally discarded, discard the entire specimen and restart the collection the next day.

6. Factors that affect results:

  A. All the urine voided for the 24-hour period must be included before taking the aliquot, to avoid a falsely low result.

  B. Porphyrins decompose when exposed to light.

  C. Drugs that may cause unreliable results include phenothiazines.

7. Other data:

  A. This test is not specific for lead poisoning.

  B. Uroporphyrin, protoporphyrin, delta-aminolevulinic acid (ALA), and porphobilinogen levels should also be performed.

Bibliography:

Buttery JE, Chamberlain BR, Gee D, Pannall PR: Total porphyrin and coproporphyrin and uroporphyrin fractions in urine measured by second-derivative spectroscopy. Clin Chem 41(1):103–106, 1995.

Jacob K, Doss MO: Composition of urinary coproporphyrin isomers I-IV in human porphyrias. Eur J Clin Chem Clin Biochem 31(10):617–624, 1993.

CORONARY ANGIOGRAPHY, DIAGNOSTIC

(see Cardiac Catheterization, Diagnostic)

CORONARY INTRAVASCULAR ULTRASOUND (CORONARY SONOGRAM, CORONARY ULTRASOUND), DIAGNOSTIC

Norm: Three-dimensional view of the inside of vasculature. Normal coronary vascular anatomy; absence of coronary artery narrowing or occlusion; absence of coronary artery lumenal irregularities.

Usage: Provides information regarding tissue characterization, morphology, and the precise measurement of the dimensions of the coronary arteries; identification of plaque and thrombus, as well as other luminal irregularities; assessment of the coronary arteries before and after coronary angioplasty; identification of the best location for the placement of arterial stents, a coil wire used to keep arteries open in clients with occluded arteries. Helps check for stent expansion after placement of intracoronary stents. Also used for the location of atherosclerotic plaque formation prior to removal during cardiac catheterization.

Description: An invasive ultrasound performed from a transducer within the lumen of the coronary arteries. The intravascular ultrasound uses a tiny transducer, about 1 mm in diameter, which is fed through a catheter leading to the heart from a femoral vessel. Similar to those seen in sonograms and echocardiograms, ultrasound images of the inside of the arteries appear on a monitor, offering a clear picture of the inside of the vessel. The images allow visualization of tears, precise determination of the size and shape of a plaque buildup or blood clot, or evaluation of the effectiveness of an angioplasty. This procedure is extremely useful in the evaluation of left main coronary artery narrowing. It is performed in conjunction with coronary catheterization/angiography. A baseline impression, depicted through tissue differentiation, can provide insight into the progression and degree of coronary artery disease. When used in conjunction with other procedures, the ultrasound requires about 5 minutes.

Professional Considerations:

1. Consent form IS required. Consent for this procedure may be included with the consent for cardiac catheterization/angiography.

Risks:

Prolonged bleeding, hemorrhage, cerebrovascular accident, hypotension, death.

Contraindications:

No different than those for cardiac catheterization.

2. Preparation:
   A. See *Cardiac Catheterization, Diagnostic.* No additional preparation is necessary for this procedure.
3. Procedure:
   A. An 8-french, transducer-tipped catheter is placed over a guidewire into the coronary artery. The sound beam is swept through a series of radial positions within the perimeter of a well-defined cross-sectional plane. The echo information is then converted to a "real time" cross-sectional image of the vessel.
   B. This procedure increases the length of

a cardiac catheterization procedure by approximately 15 minutes and requires a larger dose of heparin.

4. Postprocedure care:
   A. Because additional heparinization is required when this procedure is added to a cardiac catheterization, the immediate postprocedure bedrest requirements may be prolonged.
   B. See *Cardiac Catheterization, Diagnostic.*
5. Client and family teaching:
   A. See *Cardiac Catheterization, Diagnostic.*
6. Factors that affect results:
   A. None found.
7. Other data:
   A. Complications of this procedure include the potential for lifting plaque or thrombus from the vessel lumen because the tip of the transducer actually enters the coronary artery, as well as potential complications listed under *Cardiac Catheterization, Diagnostic.*

Bibliography:

Bolz KD, Fjermeros G, Wideroe TE, Hatlinghus S: Catheter malfunction and thrombus formation on double-lumen hemodialysis catheters: an intravascular ultrasonographic study. Am J Kidney Dis 25(4):597–602, 1995.

Martin BL, Mintz GS: Intravascular Ultrasound. St. Louis, MO, CV Mosby, 1994.

Mehra MR, Ventura HO, Smart FW, Collins TJ, Ramee SR, Stapleton DD: An intravascular ultrasound study of the influence of angiotensin-converting enzyme inhibitors and calcium entry blockers on the development of cardiac allograft vasculopathy. Am J Cardiol 75(12):853–854, 1995.

Tobis JM, Yock PG (eds): Intravascular Ultrasound Imaging. New York, Churchill Livingstone, 1992.

Schlant RC, Alexander RW (eds): The Heart Arteries and Veins. New York, McGraw-Hill, 1994.

CORTISOL, PLASMA OR SERUM

Norm: Peaks occur at about 0800 (8 A.M.) and troughs occur in late afternoon.

		SI Units
Adult		
8–10 A.M..	5–28 µg/dl	138–773 nmol/L
4–6 P.M.	2–14 mg/dl or ½ morning level	55–386 nmol/L
8 P.M.	<50% of morning level	
Child		
8–10 A.M.	15–25 µg/dl	414–690 nmol/L
4–6 P.M.	5–10 µg/dl or ½ morning level	138–276 nmol/L
8 P.M.	<50% of morning level	

Increased: Burns, Cushing's disease, Cushing's syndrome, eclampsia, exercise, hepatic disease (severe), hyperpituitarism, hypertension, hyperthyroidism, infectious disease, obesity, pancreatitis (acute), pregnancy, renal disease (severe), shock, stress (severe, heat, cold, trauma, psychological), surgery, and virilism. Drugs include corticotropin, estrogens, oral contraceptives, and vasopressin.

Decreased: Addison's disease, adrenal insufficiency, adrenogenital syndrome, chromophobe adenoma, craniopharyngioma, hypoglycemia, hypophysectomy, hypopituitarism, hypothyroidism, liver disease, postpartum pituitary necrosis, and Waterhouse-Friderichsen syndrome. Drugs include dexamethasone, dexamethasone acetate, and dexamethasone sodium phosphate.

Description: Cortisol is a steroidal hormone released from the adrenal cortex when stimulated by secretion of adrenocorticotropic hormone (ACTH) from the pituitary gland. Cortisol is normally secreted in a diurnal pattern, with peaks and troughs occurring during specific time periods. This test is most commonly used to aid diagnosis of Cushing's syndrome, in which multiple results compared from A.M. and P.M. reveal no diurnal variation in cortisol levels. However, plasma or serum cortisol levels are less reliable than a 24-hour urine collection for diagnosing or ruling out Cushing's syndrome.

Professional Considerations:

1. Consent form NOT required.
2. Preparation:
   A. *See Client and family teaching.*
   B. Tube: Red-top, red/gray-top, or gold-top tube for serum level; green-top or lavender-top for plasma level.
3. Procedure:
   A. *Plasma level:*
      i. Draw a 1-ml blood sample.
   B. *Serum level:*
      i. Draw a 1-ml blood sample.
4. Postprocedure care:
   A. Write the collection time on the laboratory requisition. Also note the patient status, such as "after ACTH infusion," where applicable.
   B. Send the specimen to the laboratory for immediate spinning.
5. Client and family teaching:
   A. Fast from food and fluids for 4–8 hours before the procedure.
   B. Restrict physical activity for 10–12

hours. The client should be relaxed and recumbent for 30 minutes prior to the test.
6. Factors that affect results:
   A. Reject hemolyzed or lipemic specimens.
   B. Cortisol is secreted in a diurnal pattern. The highest levels occur from 5 to 10 A.M., with peak levels occurring at about 8 A.M.
   C. Specimens collected other than in the morning should be collected before meals.
   D. Collect specimens at the same time each day.
   E. Hypoglycemic states suppress plasma cortisol response.
   F. Falsely increased results may occur from amphetamines, estrogens (within 6 weeks), ethanol, methamphetamines, nicotine, oral contraceptives (within 6 weeks), quinacrine, and spironolactone.
   G. Estrogens during pregnancy and during oral contraceptive use will falsely increase levels by increasing plasma proteins that bind with cortisol.
   H. Falsely decreased results may result when there is a delay in spinning down the sample.
7. Other data:
   A. The specimen is stable at room temperature for 1 week.
   B. Extreme elevation in the morning and no variation in the evening is suggestive of carcinoma.
   C. Newell-Price et al. (1995) found that a single sleeping midnight cortisol level above 50 nmol/L had a 100% accuracy in the diagnosis of Cushing's syndrome, 2% more accurate than the dexamethasone suppression test alone.

Bibliography:

Newell-Price J, Trainer P, Perry L, Wass J, Grossman A, Besser M: A single sleeping midnight cortisol has 100% sensitivity for the diagnosis of Cushing's syndrome. Clin Endocrinol *43*(5):545–550, 1995.

Resnick HS, Yehuda R, Pitman RK, Foy DW: Effect of previous trauma on acute plasma cortisol level following rape. Am J Psychiatry *152*(11):1675–1677, 1995.

CORTISOL, URINE

Norm:

		SI Units
Adult	10–100 µg/day	27–276 nmol/day
Child >age 12	5–55 µg/day	14–152 nmol/day
Child <age 12	2–27 µg/day	5.5–74 nmol/day

Increased: Amenorrhea, Cushing's syndrome, hyperthyroidism, lung cancer (small cell carcinoma), pituitary tumor, pregnancy, and stress. Drugs include corticotropin.

Decreased: Hypothyroidism and renal glomerular dysfunction. Drugs include dexamethasone, dexamethasone acetate, and dexamethasone sodium phosphate.

Description: Cortisol is a steroidal hormone released from the adrenal cortex when stimulated by secretion of adrenocorticotropic hormone (ACTH) from the anterior pituitary gland. Free cortisol is unconjugated cortisol filtered by the renal glomeruli into the urine. Although it comprises under 5% of circulating cortisol, the amount filtered follows the pattern of cortisol secretion from the adrenal cortex. Because it is excreted in a diurnal pattern, a 24-hour urine sample contains the effects of both the peak and trough cortisol levels and is thus a more accurate measurement than serum levels for diagnosing or ruling out Cushing's syndrome in which continuously high levels of cortisol are secreted.

Professional Considerations:
1. Consent form NOT required.
2. Preparation:
   A. *See Client and family teaching.*
   B. Obtain a clean, 3-L urine container to which 10 g of boric acid or 20 ml of 33% acetic acid has been added.
3. Procedure:
   A. Discard the first morning urine specimen.
   B. Save all the urine voided for 24 hours in a refrigerated 3-L container to which 10 g of boric acid has been added. If the specimen is over 1 L, add 10 g of boric acid for each additional liter of urine. Include the urine voided at the end of the 24-hour period. For catheterized clients, keep the drainage bag on ice and empty urine into the collection container hourly.
   C. Alternatively, obtain a room-temperature collection as above in a 3-L container to which 20 ml of 33% acetic acid has been added.
4. Postprocedure care:
   A. Compare the urine quantity in the specimen container with the urinary output record for the test. If the specimen contains less urine than was recorded as output, some of the sample may have been discarded, invalidating the test.
   B. Document the quantity of urine output for the 24-hour period on the laboratory requisition.
   C. The specimen should be frozen until testing occurs.
5. Client and family teaching:
   A. Do not take spironolactone or quinacrine for 7 days before the test.
   B. Because exercise increases cortisol secretion, activity should be restricted 24 hours prior to the test until the collection is complete.
   C. Save all the urine voided in the 24-hour period and urinate before defecating to avoid loss of urine. If any urine is accidentally discarded, discard the entire specimen and restart the collection the next day.
6. Factors that affect results:
   A. Stress during the test increases levels.
   B. All the urine voided for the 24-hour period must be included to avoid a falsely low result.
   C. Falsely increased results may occur from amphetamines, estrogens (within 6 weeks), methamphetamines, nicotine, novosporin, oral contraceptives (within 6 weeks), quinacrine, and spironolactone.
7. Other data:
   A. Also measure creatinine concentration.

Bibliography:
Dolezalova M: Routine high-performance liquid chromatographic determination of urinary unconjugated cortisol using solid-phase extraction and ultraviolet detection. Clin Chim Acta 231(2): 129–137, 1994.
Holder G: External quality assessment of urinary-free cortisol measurement in the UK against a gas chromatography mass spectroscopy reference method. Ann Clin Biochem 32(Pt 1):84–90, 1995.
Kathol RG, Poland RE, Stokes PE, Wade S: Relationship of 24-hour urinary free cortisol to 4-hour salivary morning and afternoon cortisol and cortisone as measured by a time-integrated oral diffusion sink. J Endocrinol Invest 18(5):374–377, 1995.

COXSACKIE A OR B VIRUS TITER, BLOOD

Norm: Negative. Less than a fourfold increase in titer of paired (acute and convalescent) sera.

Positive Coxsackie A: Acute febrile respiratory disease, conjunctivitis (epidemic hemorrhagic), enteroviral carditis, myositis, and viral carditis.

Positive Coxsackie B: Acute febrile respiratory disease, aseptic meningitis (viral), enteroviral carditis, epidemic pleurodynia, meningitis, myocarditis, pericarditis, pleurisy, and viral carditis.

Description: The Coxsackie virus is divided into two antigenically different groups, A and B, and is of the enterovirus family. Enteroviruses are easily transmitted via the fecal-oral route and are associated with epidemics, especially in newborn nurseries. While blood is rarely used for isolation of viruses, serological testing may be performed to detect Coxsackie A virus or Coxsackie B virus antibodies. Twenty-three species of Coxsackie A exist. Types 1, 4, 9, 16, and 23 may infect the heart, causing pericarditis progressing to heart failure. Coxsackie type A is also associated with a severe form of conjunctivitis and with respiratory disease. Six species of Coxsackie B exist. Types 1–5 may infect the heart, causing pericarditis progressing to heart failure. These same types may cause pleurodynia, a disease of limited duration (1 week) in which the client experiences the acute onset of chest or abdominal pain along with fever and headache. Types 2–5 cause most cases of viral meningitis. This test involves measuring the antibody levels in both an acute and convalescent sample of blood to detect an increase in the titer. It is a neutralization test in which diluted samples (1:2, 1:8, 1:32, 1:128, 1:512) are mixed with Coxsackie A virus or Coxsackie B virus, inoculated onto a cell culture system, and observed for antigen-antibody reactions for up to 7 days. Enterovirus antibodies respond very quickly to infection; thus, the earlier the acute sample is collected, the better the chance of detecting a positive test.

Professional Considerations:

1. Consent form NOT required.
2. Preparation:
   A. Preschedule the test with the laboratory.
   B. Tube: Red-top, red/gray-top, or gold-top.
3. Procedure:
   A. Draw a 3- to 4-ml blood sample.
   B. Collect an acute-phase sample promptly after symptoms appear and no more than 1 week after onset.
   C. Collect the convalescent sample 2–3 days after the onset of symptoms or 2–3 weeks after the acute-phase sample.
4. Postprocedure care:
   A. Label the specimen as either the acute sample or the convalescent sample.

B. The test should be specified as either *Coxsackie A Virus Titer* or *Coxsackie B Virus Titer.*
C. Transport the specimen immediately to the laboratory. The sample should be clotted at room temperature, with serum and clot then separated and saved for simultaneous testing with the convalescent sample.
5. Client and family teaching:
   A. Results may not be available for several days.
6. Factors that affect results:
   A. Transportation of the serum to an outside laboratory may result in clot disintegration and hemolysis, thus invalidating the test.
   B. After separation, samples are stable up to 6 weeks when refrigerated. Longer storage requires freezing at $\leq -20°C$.
   C. Paired sera should be tested at the same time in the same laboratory.
   D. False-negative Coxsackie A virus results may occur when the acute-phase titer is elevated due to past Coxsackie A virus infection.
   E. False-negative Coxsackie B virus results may occur when the acute-phase titer is elevated due to past Coxsackie B virus infection.
7. Other data:
   A. Other tests performed to detect Coxsackie A virus or Coxsackie B virus infection include swabs of feces and the throat.

Bibliography:

Druyts-Voets E, Van Renterghem L, Gerniers S: Coxsackie B virus epidemiology and neonatal infection in Belgium. J Infect 27(3):311–316, 1993.

Lennette DA: Collection and preparation of specimens for virological examination. *In* Lennette EH, Balows A, Hausler WJ, Shadomy HJ (eds): Manual of Clinical Microbiology. Washington, DC, American Society for Microbiology, 1985, pp 687–693.

Zaher SR, Kassem AS, Hughes JJ: Coxsackie virus infections in rheumatic fever. Indian J Pediatr 60(2):289–298, 1993.

CPA

(see Carotid Phonoangiography, Diagnostic)

C-PEPTIDE (CONNECTING PEPTIDE), SERUM

Norm:

		SI Units
C-peptide		
Adult ≤age 60	≤4.0 ng/ml	≤4.0 µg/L
Female >age 60	1.4–5.5 ng/ml	1.4–5.5 µg/L
Male >age 60	1.5–5.0 ng/ml	1.5–5.0 µg/L
Insulin/glucose ratio <0.3		

Usage: Factitious (self-medication) hypoglycemia due to exogenous insulin overdose or insulin abuse; detection of fasting hypoglycemia and/or insulinoma by failure to suppress C-peptide production with exogenous insulin administration; evaluation following pancreatectomy for residual islet tissue; and evaluation of insulin reserve in insulin-dependent diabetics.

Increased: Islet cell tumor. Drugs include oral hypoglycemic agents and sulfonylureas.

Decreased: Diabetes mellitus.

Description: C-peptide is an inactive, amino acid residue degradation product of proinsulin. It is formed as a byproduct during the endogenous conversion of proinsulin to insulin in the pancreatic beta-cells and its release is unaffected by exogenous insulin administration. C-peptide levels normally correlate with insulin levels because it is released by the beta-cells in amounts similar to endogenous insulin release. This test is helpful in estimating endogenous insulin levels when insulin assay is falsely elevated by insulin antibodies.

Professional Considerations:

1. Consent form NOT required.
2. Preparation:
   A. Tube: Red-top, red/gray-top or gold-top, and gray-top, and a container of ice.
3. Procedure:
   A. Draw a 7-ml blood sample for insulin and C-peptide in a chilled, red-top tube.
   B. Pack the sample for insulin in ice.

C. Draw a 5-ml blood sample for glucose in a gray-top tube.
4. Postprocedure care:
   A. Write the collection time on the laboratory requisition.
   B. Transport the specimen to the laboratory immediately.
   C. The serum should be immediately separated in a chilled centrifuge and frozen in a plastic tube.
5. Client and family teaching:
   A. A fast from food and fluids for 8 hours may be required before sampling.
6. Factors that affect results:
   A. Reject hemolyzed specimens.
   B. Recent radioactive scans invalidate the results.
   C. C-peptide levels do not always correlate with intrinsic insulin levels in obese clients and clients with islet cell tumors.
   D. Hepatic dysfunction causes elevated levels.
7. Other data:
   A. Perform the C-peptide measurement and insulin measurement on the same sample.

Bibliography:

Chiodera P, Volpi R, Capretti L, Speroni G, Caffarri G, Colla R, Caiazza A, Coiro V: Influence of residual C-peptide secretion on the arginine vasopressin response to hypoglycaemia and metoclopramide in insulin-dependent diabetes. Eur J Clin Invest 25(8):568–573, 1995.

Kullmer T, Gabriel H, Jungmann E, Haak T, Morbitzer D, Usadel KH, Kindermann W: Increase of serum insulin and stable c-peptide concentrations with exhaustive incremental graded exercise during acute hypoxia in sedentary subjects. Exp Clin Endocrinol Diabetes 103(3):156–161. 1995.

CPK

(see Creatine Kinase, Serum)

Cr-51 (CHROMIUM) RED CELL SURVIVAL, BLOOD

Norm:

Plasma radioactivity half-life	≤2 hours
Tagged Cr-51 red cell half-life	25–35 days
Gamma scan	Only slight spleen, liver, and bone marrow radioactivity

Increased: Thalassemia minor.

Decreased: Anemia (congenital nonspherocytic, idiopathic acquired hemolytic, megaloblastic of pregnancy, pernicious, sickle cell), elliptocytosis (with hemolysis), hemoglobin C disease, hemoglobinuria (paroxysmal nocturnal), leukemia (chronic lymphatic), spherocytosis (hereditary), and uremia.

Description: Red cell survival time is measured by tagging a sample of the client's red blood cells (RBCs) with radioactive Cr-51. Over a 4-week period, blood samples are periodically measured for radioactivity levels to determine the amount of time taken for the tagged RBCs to disappear from the circulation. Major body organs may also be scanned with a gamma camera to locate concentrations of radioactivity. The test aids in identifying the cause of anemia and sites of RBC destruction.

Professional Considerations:

1. Consent form NOT required.

Risks:

Bleeding, infection, hematoma.

Contraindications:

Active bleeding extended clotting times, breast-feeding, and pregnancy.

2. Preparation:
   A. For procedures 3A–C below, collect a sterile glass beaker containing sodium chromate.
   B. For procedures 3D–F, tubes: green-top and lavender-top.
3. Procedure:
   A. Draw a 30-ml blood sample and mix it with 100 mCi of Cr-51 (sodium chromate).
   B. Incubate overnight.
   C. Inject the mixture intravenously into the client.
   D. 30 minutes later, draw a 6-ml blood sample in a lavender-top tube for measurement of baseline volumes of blood and red cells.
   E. 24 hours later, draw a 6-ml blood sample in a green-top tube. Send the specimen to the laboratory for a same-day measurement of hematocrit and of Cr-51 with a scintillation well counter.
   F. Repeat procedure 3E every 1–3 days for 4 weeks.
   G. After the last sample is drawn, draw a 6-ml blood sample in a lavender-top tube for comparison measurement of blood and red cell volumes.
4. Postprocedure care:
   A. None.
5. Client and family teaching:
   A. No isolation is necessary.
6. Factors that affect results:
   A. Conditions that decrease red cell volume or the proportion of tagged red cells to nontagged red cells, including blood draws, blood transfusions, chronic occult extravascular blood loss, and hemorrhage, will simulate decreased survival time.
7. Other data:
   A. Normal tests are seen in hemoglobin C *trait* and sickle cell *trait* and elliptocytosis without hemolysis.
   B. Normal red cell half-life is 60 days.
   C. This test may also be used to predict the viability of donated red blood cells.

Bibliography:

Anderson G, Gray LS, Mintz PD: Red cell survival studies in a patient with anti-Tca. Am J Clin Pathol 95(1):87–90, 1995.

Myhre BA, Marcus CS, Wheeler NC: The prediction of autologous red cell survival. Ann Clin Lab Sci 20(4):258–262, 1990.

C-REACTIVE PROTEIN, SERUM

Norm:

		SI Units
Qualitative	Negative	
Quantitative		
Adult	68–8200 ng/ml	68–8200 µg/L
	or 20 mg/dl	
	or <8 µg/ml	
Cord blood	10–350 ng/ml	10–350 µg/L

Positive (>1:2 titer): Crohn's disease, empyema, gout, inflammation, Hodgkin's disease, lymphoma, malignant tumor, meningitis, myocardial infarction, myxoma (of heart left atrium), necrosis, nephritis, peritonitis, pharyngitis (streptococcal), pneumonia (pneumococcal), postcommissurotomy syndrome, postoperatively (first week), pregnancy (after month 3), renal infarction, rheumatic fever (acute), rheumatoid arthritis (acute), sepsis, systemic lupus erythematosus, trauma (surgical), and tuberculosis.

Usage: Monitoring of rheumatoid arthritis and rheumatic fever inflammatory processes, differentiation of Crohn's disease from ulcerative colitis, and detection of the presence or exacerbation of inflammatory processes.

Description: C-reactive protein is an abnormal serum glycoprotein produced by the liver during acute inflammation. Because it disappears rapidly when inflammation subsides, its detection signifies the presence of a current inflammatory process. C-reactive protein interacts with the complement cascade and is detected by antiserum via immunoassays.

Professional Considerations:

1. Consent form NOT required.
2. Preparation:
   A. Tube: Red-top.
3. Procedure:
   A. Draw a 2-ml blood sample.
4. Postprocedure care:
   A. Transport the specimen to the laboratory for immediate testing.
   B. Do not refrigerate the specimen.
5. Client and family teaching:
   A. Fast from food and fluids for 4 hours before sampling.
6. Factors that affect results:
   A. Drugs that may cause false-positive results include oral contraceptives.
   B. Drugs that may cause false-negative results due to suppression of inflammation include NSAIDS, steroids, and salicylates.
   C. Presence of an intrauterine device may cause inflammation, which produces a positive test.

D. Overnight refrigeration of the sample may produce a false-positive result.
7. Other data:
   A. Useful in monitoring postoperative inflammatory complications.
   B. Yentis, Soni, and Sheldon (1995) found daily measurements of C-reactive protein to correlate with resolution of sepsis. Specifically, "A decrease in CRP by 25% or more from the previous day's level was a good indicator of resolution of sepsis, with a sensitivity of 97%, specificity 95% and predictive value of 97%.

Bibliography:

Kasperska-Czyzyk T, Heding LG, Tronier B: The serum concentration of insulin, C-peptide, and proinsulin in patients with acute pancreatitis. Int J Pancreatol 17(2):167–171, 1995.

Smith RP, Lipworth BJ: C-Reactive protein in simple community-acquired pneumonia. Chest (4): 1028–1031, 1995.

Yamazaki H, Oi H, Matsushita M, Inoue T, Tang JT, Inoue T: C-reactive protein as an indicator of effect and of adverse reaction to transcatheter arterial embolization. Radiat Med 13(4):163–165, 1995.

Yentis SM, Soni N, Sheldon J: C-reactive protein as an indicator of resolution of sepsis in the intensive care unit. Intensive Care Med 21(7):602–605, 1995.

CREATINE KINASE (CK), SERUM

Norm: Results are method-dependent and should be compared with the reference values of the laboratory performing the test.

	SI Units
Creatine Kinase—Total	
Adult females 5–25 µg/ml	
10–135 IU/L	
5–35 mU/ml	
Ambulatory 10–70 U/L	0.17–1.16 µKat/L
≤Age 60 10–55 U/L	0.17–0.92 µKat/L
>Age 60 16–80 U/L	0.27–1.33 µKat/L
Adult males 5–35 µg/ml	
20–170 IU/L	
5–55 mU/ml	
Ambulatory 25–90 U/L	0.42–1.50 µKat/L
<Age 61 12–80 U/L	0.20–1.33 µKat/L
Age 61–70 20–110 U/L	0.33–1.83 µKat/L
>Age 70 22–90 U/L	0.37–1.50 µKat/L
Children	
Newborn 65–580 IU/L at 30°C	
10–200 U/L	0.17–3.33 µKat/L
Male 0–70 IU/L at 30°C	
Female 0–50 IU/L at 30°C	

Total levels may be normal in acute myocardial infarction, even when the CK-MB isoenzyme is elevated. In general, total CK trends in acute myocardial infarction are:

Initial rise:	2–6 hours after onset of damage.
Peak levels:	18–36 hours after onset of damage.
Return to baseline:	3–6 days.

		SI Units
Creatine Kinase Isoenzymes	**% of Total CK**	**Fraction of Total CK**
CK_1-BB (brain)	0–3	0–0.03
CK_2-MB (heart)	0–6	0–0.06
CK_3-MM (muscle)	90–97	0.90–0.97

CK_2-MB trends in acute myocardial infarction:

Initial rise:	4–8 hours after onset of damage.
Peak levels:	18–24 hours after onset of damage.
Return to baseline:	3 days after onset of damage.

Increased Total CK: Amyotrophic lateral sclerosis, anoxia, atresia (biliary), bowel injury, brain tumor, burns (thermal, electrical), cancer (breast, lung, oat cell, gastrointestinal, prostatic), carbon monoxide poisoning, cardiomyopathy (cobalt-beer), carbon monoxide poisoning, carrier state (for Duchenne's muscular dystrophy), cerebrovascular accident, CNS trauma, coma (hepatic), convulsions, coughing (severe), delirium tremens, dermatomyositis, eosinophilia-myalgia syndrome, exercise, head injury, hemodialysis, hypokalemia (severe), hypothermia, hypothyroidism, infarction (bowel, cerebral, myocardial, prostate), intoxication (alcohol, salicylate), intramuscular injection (recent), labor, leptospirosis, malignant hyperthermia, meningoencephalitis, muscle spasms, muscular dystrophy (Duchenne's, limb-girdle, fascioscapulohumeral), myocarditis, myoglobinuria, myopathy (from alcoholism), myotonic dystrophy, myxedema, necrosis of striated muscle, organ rejection (heart transplant), parturition, polymyositis, postictal state, pregnancy, prostate injury, psychosis (acute with agitation), pulmonary edema, pulmonary embolism, renal failure, renal insufficiency (chronic), Reye's syndrome, rhabdomyolysis, Rocky Mountain spotted fever, shock, skeletal muscle disorders, status epilepticus, striated muscle atrophy (acute), subarachnoid hemorrhage, surgery (bowel, cardiac, CNS, prostate), tachycardia, thyrotoxicosis, toxic shock syndrome (day 7), trauma (muscular), typhoid fever, and very muscular people.

Increased CK_1-BB (Brain): Anoxia, atresia (biliary), cancer (breast, gastrointestinal, oat cell, prostatic, widespread malignancies), cerebrovascular accident (hemorrhage, infarction), hemodialysis, hypothermia, intestinal necrosis, labor, malignant hyperthermia, renal failure, shock, surgery (CNS), and uremia.

Increased CK_2-MB (Heart): Anoxia, burns (electrical, thermal), cancer (lung), carbon monoxide poisoning, cardiomyopathy (cobalt-beer), collagen vascular diseases, congestive heart failure (rare), coronary angiography (rare), coronary insufficiency (rare), hypothermia, hypothyroidism, malignant hyperthermia, muscular dystrophy (Duchenne's), myocardial infarction, myocarditis, myoglobinuria (severe), polymyositis, pulmonary embolism, renal insufficiency (chronic), Reye's syndrome, rhabdomyolysis, Rocky Mountain spotted fever, surgery (cardiac, valve replacement), systemic lupus erythematosus, and trauma (cardiac).

Increased CK_3-MM (Muscle): Cardiac catheterization (with myocardial damage), cardioversion, coronary arteriography (with myocardial damage), hypothyroidism, intramuscular injections, muscle trauma, myocardial infarction, psychosis (acute with agitation), Reye's syndrome, shock, surgery, and trauma (skeletal muscle).

Decreased Total CK: Addison's disease, anterior pituitary hyposecretion, connective tissue disease, hepatic disease (alcoholic), low muscle mass, metastatic neoplasia, and pregnancy (first half). Drugs include steroids.

Decreased CK_1-BB, CK_2-MB, CK_3-MM): Not applicable.

Description: Creatine kinase is an enzyme found in muscle and brain tissue and reflects tissue catabolism due to cell trauma. It catalyzes creatine-creatinine metabolism. The test is performed to detect myocardial or skeletal muscle damage or central nervous system damage resulting in increased tissue catabolism from those areas. Determination of the type of tissue damage (tissue undergoing increased catabolism) occurring can be performed by performing the CK isoenzymes test that measures the three types of isoenzymes that make up total CPK: CK_1-BB, CK_2-MB, and CK_3-MM. CK_1-BB is found mainly in brain tissue, but also in the smooth muscle, thyroid gland, lungs, and prostate gland. CK_2-MB is found mainly in cardiac muscle, but also in the tongue, diaphragm, and skeletal muscle (scant amount). CK_3-MM is found mainly in skeletal muscle. The isoenzyme test is usually repeated at 8- to 12-hour intervals to track trends characteristic of specific types of cell damage. Most recently, test kits have been developed that allow detection of CK_3-MM and CK_2-MB isoforms earlier than the traditional methods for CK isoenzyme detection.

Professional Considerations:

1. Consent form NOT required.
2. Preparation:
   A See *Client and family teaching.*
   B. Tube: Red-top, red/gray-top, or gold-top.
3. Procedure:
   A. Collect a 5-ml blood sample.
4. Postprocedure care:
   A. Send the specimen to the laboratory immediately.
   B. Refrigerate the specimen if measurement will be delayed more than 2 hours. Separate the serum and freeze it if the test will not be performed within 24 hours of collection.
   C. If isoenzyme measurement is desired, specify this on the laboratory requisition.

5. Client and family teaching:
   A. If the test is for skeletal muscle disorder evaluation, the client should avoid strenuous physical activity for 24 hours before the test.
   B. Avoid ingestion of alcohol for 24 hours before the test.
   C. Withhold drugs that would affect the test results (see below) for 24 hours before the test, when possible.
6. Factors that affect results:
   A. Necessary intramuscular (IM) injections should be given after or at least 1 hour before this test.
   B. Hemolysis invalidates the results.
   C. Invasive procedures and other factors that elevate CK include cardiac catheterization (with myocardial injury), cardioversion, coronary arteriography (with myocardial injury), electric shock, electrocautery, electromyography, intramuscular injections, and muscle massage (recent).
   D. Drugs that may cause falsely increased CK values include aminocaproic acid, clofibrate, codeine, dexamethasone, dexamethasone acetate, dexamethasone sodium phosphate, digoxin, epsilon-aminocaproic acid, ethanol, furosemide, glutethimide, guanethidine, halothane, heroin, imipramine, lithium carbonate, meperidine hydrochloride, morphine sulfate, phenobarbital, and succinylcholine chloride.
7. Other data:
   A. CK is considered to be a marker for Duchenne's muscular dystrophy.
   B. Evaluation of myocardial infarction should also include LDH isoenzyme measurements every 24 hours.
   C. In clients suspected of acute myocardial infarction, CK-MB testing alone may reveal more information than total CK level, which may not show an elevation initially.

Bibliography:

Canalias F, Saco Y, Gella FJ: Comparison of kits for the determination of creatine kinase activity in serum. Eur J Clin Chem Clin Biochem *33*(8): 535–539, 1995.

Delanghe JR, De Buyzere ML, De Scheerder IK, Cluyse LP, Thierens HM: Characteristics of creatine release during acute myocardial infarction, unstable angina, and cardiac surgery. Clin Chem *41*(6, Pt 1):928–933, 1995.

Mair J, Morandell D, Genser N, Lechleitner P, Dienstl F, Puschendorf B: Equivalent early sensitivities of myoglobin, creatine kinase MB mass, creatine kinase isoform ratios, and cardiac troponins I and T for acute myocardial infarction. Clin Chem *41*(9):1266–1272, 1995.

Ravkilde J, Nissen H, Horder M, Thygesen K: Independent prognostic value of serum creatine kinase isoenzyme MB mass, cardiac troponin T and myosin light chain levels in suspected acute myocardial infarction. Analysis of 28 months of follow-up in 196 patients. J Am Coll Cardiol *25*(3): 574–581, 1995.

CREATINE KINASE ISOENZYMES (CK ISOENZYMES), SERUM
(see Creatine Kinase, Serum)

CREATINE PHOSPHOKINASE (CK, CPK), SERUM
(see Creatine Kinase, Serum)

CREATINE, URINE

Norm:

		SI Units
Adults	<6% of urine creatinine	
Adult females	≤80 mg/24 hours	0–615 μmol/day
Pregnant	≤12% of urine creatinine	
Adult males	≤40 mg/24 hours	0–307 μmol/day
Infants	Equal to urine creatinine	
Children	≤30% of urine creatinine	

Increased: Acromegaly, Addison's disease, amyotonia congenita, burns, children (growth state), Cushing's syndrome, diabetes mellitus, disseminated lupus erythematosus, fractures, hyperthyroidism, hypothyroidism, infections, injuries (crushing), leukemia, male eunuchoidism, muscular dystrophy, myasthenia gravis, myoglobinuria (acute paroxysmal), myopathy (alcoholic), myotonia (congenital Thompsen's disease), myotonic dystrophy, neurogenic atrophy, poliomyelitis, polymyositis, pregnancy, puerperium, starvation, and raw meat diet.

Decreased: Hypothyroidism.

Description: Creatine is a compound that functions in anaerobic muscle metabolism by combining with phosphate to yield energy used in intense muscle activity for short periods of time. Normally, phosphocreatine breaks down into creatinine, which is then excreted in the urine. In some conditions, particularly muscle diseases, creatine is released in increased amounts into the bloodstream and can be measured in the urine.

Professional Considerations:

1. Consent form NOT required.
2. Preparation:
   A. Obtain a clean, 3-L, 24-hour urine container with toluene preservative.
3. Procedure:
   A. Discard the first morning urine specimen.
   B. Save all the urine voided for 24 hours in a refrigerated, clean, 3-L container to which toluene preservative has been added. Include the urine voided at the end of the 24-hour period. For catheterized clients, keep the drainage bag on ice and empty urine into the refrigerated collection container hourly.
4. Postprocedure care:
   A. Compare the urine quantity in the specimen container with the urinary output record for the test. If the specimen contains less urine than was recorded as output, some of the sample may have been discarded, invalidating the test.
   B. Document urine quantity on the laboratory requisition.
   C. Send the entire specimen to the lab.
5. Client and family teaching:
   A. Save all the urine voided in the 24-hour period and urinate before defecating to avoid loss of urine. If any urine is accidentally discarded, discard the entire specimen and restart the collection the next day.
6. Factors that affect results:
   A. All the urine voided for the 24-hour period must be included to avoid a falsely low result.
   B. Drugs that may cause falsely elevated results include caffeine, corticosteroids, corticotropin, cortisone acetate, desoxycorticosterone acetate, desoxycorticosterone pivalate, methyltestosterone, nitrofurantoin, nitrofurantoin sodium, phenolsulfonphthalein, and sodium benzoate.
   C. Drugs that may cause falsely decreased results include anabolic steroids, androgens, and thiazide diuretics.
   D. The results may be increased after 3 weeks of pregnancy.
7. Other data:
   A. Nahas et al. (1993) suggest this test may be useful as a marker for testicular damage.

Bibliography:

Beyer C: Creatine measurement in serum and urine with an automated enzymatic method. Clin Chem *39*(8):1613–1619, 1993.

Beyer C, Alting IH, Backer ET: Measurement of creatine in urine by creatinase, sarcosine oxidase, and peroxidase reevaluated. Clin Chem *39*(8):1743–1744,1993

Nahas K, le Net JL, Provost JP, Tomaszewski KE: An investigation of urinary creatine excretion as a potential marker for testicular damage. Hum Exp Toxicol *12*(2):173–176, 1993.

CREATININE, SERUM

Norms:

		SI Units
Jaffe, manual method	0.8–1.5 mg/dl	70–133 µmol/day
Jaffe, kinetic or enzymatic method		
Adults		
Females	0.5–1.1 mg/dl	44–97 µmol/L
Males	0.6–1.2 mg/dl	53–106 µmol/L
Elderly	May be lower	May be lower
Children		
Cord blood	0.6–1.2 mg/dl	53–106 µmol/L
Newborn	0.8–1.4 mg/dl	71–124 µmol/L
Infant	0.7–1.7 mg/dl	62–150 µmol/L
Age 1 female	≤0.5 mg/dl	≤44 µmol/L
Age 1 male	≤0.6 mg/dl	≤53 µmol/L
Age 2–3 female	≤0.6 mg/dl	≤53 µmol/L
Age 2–3 male	≤0.7 mg/dl	≤62 µmol/L
Age 4–7 female	≤0.7 mg/dl	≤62 µmol/L
Age 4–7 male	≤0.8 mg/dl	≤71 µmol/L
Age 8–10 female	≤0.8 mg/dl	≤71 µmol/L
Age 8–10 male	≤0.9 mg/dl	≤80 µmol/L
Age 11–12 female	≤0.9 mg/dl	≤80 µmol/L
Age 11–12 male	≤1.0 mg/dl	≤88 µmol/L
Age 13–17 female	≤1.1 mg/dl	≤97 µmol/L
Age 13–17 male	≤1.2 mg/dl	≤106 µmol/L
Age 18–20 female	≤1.2 mg/dl	≤106 µmol/L
Age 18–20 male	≤1.3 mg/dl	≤115 µmol/L

Increased: Values are 20–40% higher in the late afternoon than in the morning. Acromegaly, allergic purpura, amyloidosis, analgesic abuse, azotemia (prerenal, postrenal), congenital hypoplastic kidneys, congestive heart failure, diabetes mellitus, diet (high meat content), gigantism, glomerulonephritis (chronic), Goodpasture's syndrome, gout, hemoglobinuria, high dietary intake, hypovolemic shock, hyperthyroidism, intestinal obstruction, Kimmelstiel-Wilson syndrome, metal poisoning, multiple myeloma, muscle destruction, nephritis, nephropathy (hypercalcemic, hypokalemic), nephrosclerosis, polyarteritis nodosa, polycystic disease, pyelonephritis, renal artery stenosis or thrombosis, renal cortical necrosis, renal failure, renal vein thrombosis, renal tuberculosis, rheumatoid arthritis (active), scleroderma, sickle cell anemia, subacute bacterial endocarditis, systemic lupus erythematosus, testosterone therapy, toxic shock syndrome, uremia, and urinary obstruction. Drugs include acetohexamide, androgens, arginine, bromsulphalein, captopril, cephalosporins, cimetidine, cincophen, clofibrate, corticosteroids, diacetic acid, diuretics, disopyramide phosphate, fosinopril, fructose, gentamicin sulfate, glucose, hydralazine hydrochloride, hydroxyurea, lipomul, lithium carbonate, mannitol, meclofeamate sodium, methicillin sodium, metoprolol tartrate, minoxidil, mithramycin, nitrofurantoin, propranolol, protein, pyruvate, sulfonamides, streptokinase, testosterone, testosterone cypionate, testosterone enanthate, testosterone propionate, triamterine, and viomycin.

Decreased: Diabetic ketoacidosis (artifactual decrease) and muscular dystrophy. Drugs include cefoxitin sodium, cimetidine, chlorpromazine, chlorprothixene, marijuana, thiazide diuretics, and vancomycin.

Description: Creatinine is produced continuously as a nonprotein end product of anaerobic energy-producing creatine-phosphate metabolism in skeletal muscle. Because it is continually and easily excreted by the renal system, increased levels indicate a slowing of the glomerular filtration rate. Creatinine is thus a very specific indicator of renal function, revealing the balance between creatinine formation and excretion. A diurnal variation in creatinine may be related to meals, with troughs occurring around 0700 (7 A.M.) and peaks occurring around 1900 (7 P.M.).

Professional Considerations:

1. Consent form NOT required.
2. Preparation:
   A. Tube: Red-top, red/gray-top, or gold-top.
   B. Do NOT draw during hemodialysis.
3. Procedure:
   A. Draw a 1-ml blood sample.
4. Postprocedure care:
   A. Send the specimen to the laboratory promptly and refrigerate it until tested.

5. Client and family teaching:
   A. Avoid excessive exercise for 8 hours and avoid excessive red meat intake for 24 hours before the test.
6. Factors that affect results:
   A. Some clients with longstanding chronic renal failure may have normal levels.
   B. Drugs that may cause falsely elevated levels include amphotericin B, ascorbic acid, barbiturates, capreomycin sulfate, carbutamide, cefoxitin sodium, cephalothin sodium, chlorthalidone, clonidine, colistin sulfate, dextran, doxycycline hyclate, kanamycin, levodopa, methyldopa, methyldopate hydrochloride, para-aminohippurate, phenolsulfonphthalein, and sulfobromophthalein.
7. Other data:
   A. The specimen will remain stable for 1 week when refrigerated and for 1 month when frozen.

Bibliography:

Gennaro MC, Abrigo C, Marengo E, Baldin C, Martelletti MT: Determination of creatinine in human serum. Statistical intercalibration of methods. Analyst *120*(1):47–51, 1995.

Salive ME, Jones CA, Guralnik JM, Agodoa LY, Pahor M, Wallace RB: Serum creatinine levels in older adults: relationship with health status and medications. Age Ageing *24*(2):142–150, 1995.

Thienpont LM, Van Landuyt KG, Stockl D, De Leenheer AP: Candidate reference method for determining serum creatinine by isocratic HPLC: validation with isotope dilution gas v chromatography-mass spectrometry and application for accuracy assessment of routine test kits. Clin Chem *41*(7):995–1003, 1995.

van den Anker JN, de Groot R, Broerse HM, Sauer PJ, van der Heijden BJ, Hop WC, Lindemans J: Assessment of glomerular filtration rate in preterm infants by serum creatinine: comparison with inulin clearance. Pediatrics *96*(6):1156–1158, 1995.

CREATININE, URINE

Norms:

		SI Units
Adult	14–26 mg/kg/24 hours	124–230 µmol/kg/day
Female	600–1800 mg/24 hours	5.3–16 µmol/day
Male	800–2000 mg/24 hours	7–18 µmol/day
Child	8–22 mg/kg/24 hours	71–195 µmol/kg/day

Increased: Fever and tissue catabolism. Values are 20–40% higher in the late afternoon than in the morning.

Decreased: Decreased renal perfusion, glomerulonephritis, cystic kidney disease, polymyositis, pyelonephritis (chronic bilateral), and shock (hypovolemic).

Description: Creatinine is produced continuously as a nonprotein end product of anaerobic energy-producing creatine-phosphate metabolism in skeletal muscle. It is continually and easily excreted by the renal system via glomerulofiltration. Decreased levels of urine creatinine indicate a slowing of the glomerular filtration rate. Creatinine is thus a very specific indicator of renal function. A diurnal variation in creatinine may be related to meals, with troughs occurring around 0700 and peaks occurring around 1900. Because this test involves the collection of a 24-hour urine sample, it captures the effects of both peaks and troughs of creatinine levels.

Professional Considerations:

1. Consent form NOT required.
2. Preparation:
   A. Obtain a clean, 3-L, 24-hour urine container.
3. Procedure:
   A. Discard the first morning urine specimen.
   B. Save all the urine voided for 24 hours in a refrigerated, clean, 3-L container with or without a preservative. Include the urine voided at the end of the 24-hour period. For catheterized clients, keep the drainage bag on ice and empty it into the refrigerated collection container hourly.
4. Postprocedure care:
   A. Compare the urine quantity in the specimen container with the urinary output record for the test. If the specimen contains less urine than was recorded as output, some of the sample may have been discarded, invalidating the test.
   B. Document the quantity of urine output and the beginning and ending times of collection on the laboratory requisition.
   C. Send the specimen to the laboratory immediately and refrigerate it until tested.

5. Client and family teaching:
   A. Save all the urine voided in the 24-hour period and urinate before defecating to avoid loss of urine. If any urine is accidentally discarded, discard the entire specimen and restart the collection the next day.
6. Factors that affect results:
   A. Failure to include all the urine voided for the 24-hour period yields a falsely low result.
   B. Failure to refrigerate the specimen throughout the collection period yields a falsely low result.
   C. Drugs that may cause falsely elevated results include amphotericin B, ascorbic acid, barbiturates, capreomycin sulfate, carbutamide, cefoxitin sodium, cephalothin sodium, chlorthalidone, clonidine, colistin sulfate, dextran, doxycycline hyclate, kanamycin, levodopa, methyldopa, methyldopate hydrochloride, para-aminohippurate, phenolsulfonphthalein, sulfobromophthalein.
   D. Drugs that may cause falsely decreased results include anabolic steroids, androgens, and thiazides.
7. Other data:
   A. Urine creatinine is stable when refrigerated for 1 week, and when frozen for 1 month.

Bibliography:

Fujita T, Takata S, Sunahara Y: Enzymatic rate assay of creatinine in serum and urine. Clin Chem *39*(10):2130–2136, 1993.

CREATININE CLEARANCE, 12- OR 24-HOUR, URINE

(see Creatinine Clearance, Serum, Urine)

CREATININE CLEARANCE, SERUM, URINE

Norm: Corrected to 1.73 m of body surface area.

| | Adult Female | | Adult Male | |
| | | SI Units | | SI Units |
Age	ml/min	ml/sec	ml/min	ml/sec
≤20	84	1.4	90	1.5
21–30	90	1.5	96	1.6
31–40	96	1.6	102	1.7
41–50	102	1.7	108	1.8
51–60	108	1.8	114	1.9
61–70	114	1.9	120	2.0
71–80	120	2.0	126	2.1
81–90	126	2.1	132	2.2
91–100	132	2.2	138	2.3

	Child	
Age	ml/min	SI Units ml/sec
<1	72	1.2
1	45	0.8
2	55	0.9
3	60	1.0
4–5	71–73	1.2
6–7	64–67	1.1
8	72	1.2
9	83	1.4
10–11	89–92	1.5
12	109	1.8
13–14	86	1.4

Increased: Not applicable.

Decreased: Acute tubular necrosis, atherosclerosis (of renal artery), congestive heart failure, dehydration, elderly clients, glomerulonephritis, malignancy (bilateral renal), nephrosclerosis, obstruction (renal artery), phenacetin, polycystic kidney disease, pyelonephritis (advanced bilateral chronic), shock (cardiogenic, hypovolemic), thrombosis (renal vein), and tuberculosis (renal). Drugs include aminoglycosides, amphotericin B, and penicillins.

Description: Creatinine is produced continuously as a nonprotein end product of anaerobic energy-producing creatine metabolism in skeletal muscle. It is continually and easily excreted by the renal system via glomerular filtration. The creatinine clearance test measures both a blood sample and a urine sample to determine the rate at which creatinine is being cleared from the blood by the kidneys. Specifically, "clearance" means the amount of blood cleared of creatinine in 1 minute and is independent of urine flow rate. Decreased results occur when over 50% of renal nephrons are damaged, thus indicating impaired glomerular filtration. Creatinine clearance is thus a very specific indicator of renal function, revealing the balance between creatinine formation and excretion.

Professional Considerations:

1. Consent form NOT required.
2. Preparation:
   A. *Urine collection:* Obtain a clean, 3-L, 24-hour urine bag or bottle.
   B. *Serum collection:* Tube: Red-top, red/gray-top, or gold-top.
   C. Do NOT draw the specimen during hemodialysis.
3. Procedure:
   A. *Urine collection:*
      i. Discard the first morning urine specimen.
      ii. Begin to time a 24-hour urine collection. (2-, 6-, or 12-hour urine collections can also be performed, but a 24-hour specimen is preferable.)
      iii. Save all the urine voided for 24 hours in a refrigerated, clean, 3-L container with or without a preservative. Include the urine voided at the end of the 24-hour period. For catheterized clients, keep the drainage bag on ice and empty into the refrigerated collection container hourly.
   B. *Serum collection:*
      i. Because the glomerular filtration rate remains stable, the serum specimen can be drawn at any time during the urine collection period. Draw a 7-ml blood sample in a red-top tube for serum creatinine.
4. Postprocedure care:
   A. Compare the urine quantity in the specimen container with the urinary output record for the test. If the specimen contains less urine than was recorded as output, some of the sample may have been discarded, invalidating the test.
   B. Document the quantity of the urine output as well as the beginning and ending times for the 24-hour period on the laboratory requisition.
   C. Send the 24-hour urine specimen to the laboratory immediately and refrigerate it until tested.
   D. Urine creatinine is stable for 1 week when refrigerated and for 1 month when frozen.

5. Client and family teaching:
   A. Avoid strenuous exercise for 8 hours before the test.
   B. For the urine test, save all the urine voided in the 24-hour period and urinate before defecating to avoid loss of urine. If any urine is accidentally discarded, discard the entire specimen and restart the collection the next day.
6. Factors that affect results:
   A. Failure to refrigerate the specimen throughout the collection period allows the creatinine to decompose, causing falsely low results.
   B. Drugs that may cause falsely elevated results include amphotericin B, ascorbic acid, barbiturates, capreomycin sulfate, carbutamide, cefoxitin sodium, cephalothin sodium, chlorthalidone, clonidine, colistin sulfate, dextran, doxycycline hyclate, kanamycin, levodopa, methyldopa, methyldopate hydrochloride, *para*-aminohippurate, phenolsulfonphthalein, and sulfobromophthalein.
   C. Drugs that may cause falsely decreased results include anabolic steroids, androgens, and thiazides.
7. Other data:
   A. None.

Bibliography:

Bertino JS Jr: Measured versus estimated creatinine clearance in patients with low serum creatinine values [published erratum appears in Ann Pharmacother 1994 Jun 28(6):811]. Ann Pharmacother 27(12):1439–1442, 1993.

Bhatla B, Moore HL, Nolph KD: Modification of creatinine clearance by estimation of residual urinary creatinine and urea clearance in CAPD patients. Adv Perit Dial 11:101–105, 1995.

Flynn FV: Assessment of renal function: Selected developments. Clin Biochem 23(1):49–54, 1990.

Paap CM, Nahata MC: Prospective evaluation of ten methods for estimating creatinine clearance in children with varying degrees of renal function. J Clin Pharm Ther 20(2):67–73, 1995.

Sokoll LJ, Russell RM, Sadowski JA, Morrow FD: Establishment of creatinine clearance reference values for older women. Clin Chem 40(12):2276–2281, 1994.

Van Lente F, Suit P: Assessment of renal function by serum creatinine and creatinine clearance: Glomerular filtration rate estimated by four procedures. Clin Chem 35(12):2326–2330, 1989.

CRYOFIBRINOGEN, PLASMA

Norm: Negative. No cryofibrinogen noted.

Positive: : Familial Mediterranean fever (acute), hemophilia, infections (neonatal), hepatitis C viral infection, multiple myeloma, neoplasms, thromboembolic conditions, toxemia of pregnancy, and scleroderma. Also associated with conditions exhibiting cryoglobulins. Drugs include oral contraceptives.

Description: Cryofibrinogen is a complex of fibrinogen and protein fragments that precipitates at 0–4°C and redissolves when warmed. Cryofibrinogenemia refers to the presence of these precipitated complexes in plasma, but not in serum. It is associated with elevations in alpha$_1$-antitrypsin, haptoglobin, alpha$_2$-macroglobulin, and hyperfibrinogenemia. Symptoms include sensitivity to cold, including urticaria, bleeding, and blood vessel damage. Cryofibrinogenemia has been associated with thromboembolic conditions, inflammatory processes, and malignancies. Cryofibrinogens have also been detected secondary to purpura and gangrene from peripheral occlusion. Positive tests require a study of cold precipitable proteins in order to differentiate cryofibrinogen from cryoglobulins.

Professional Considerations:

1. Consent form NOT required.
2. Preparation:
   A. Tube: Blue-top, black-top, or lavender-top, depending on the individual laboratory requirements. Also obtain a container of warm water.
   B. The client should not receive heparin therapy for 2 days.
3. Procedure:
   A. Draw a 7-ml blood sample. Place the tube in the container of warm water.
4. Postprocedure care:
   A. Write the collection time on the laboratory requisition.
   B. Transport the specimen to the laboratory immediately. The specimen should be allowed to clot at 37°C. A portion of plasma is kept at room temperature and another portion is refrigerated overnight. The samples are then compared for gel or white particle formation. If present, the sample is incubated ½ hour at 37°C. Absence of the gel or white particles after incubation indicates a positive test.
5. Client and family teaching:
   A. Heparin therapy within 2 days prior to the test may cause false-negative results.
6. Factors that affect results:
   A. Reject specimens received more than 2 hours after collection.
7. Other data:
   A. Cryofibrinogen is not to be confused with cryoglobulins, which precipitate from *serum*, rather than plasma, during cold conditions.
   B. At least 24 hours is required for results.

Bibliography:

Ishimura E, Nishizawa Y, Shoji S, Okumura M, Nishitani H, Kim CW, Watanabe Y, Wakasa K, Morii H,

Kashgarian M: Heat-insoluble cryoglobulin in a patient with essential type I cryoglobulinemia and massive cryoglobulin-occlusive glomerulonephritis. Am J Kidney Dis *26*(4):654–657, 1995.

Jantunen E, Soppi E, Neittaanmaki H, Lahtinen R: Essential cryofibrinogenaemia, leukocytoclastic vasculitis and chronic purpura. J Intern Med *234*(3): 331–333, 1993.

Tanaka K, Aiyama T, Imai J, Morishita Y, Fukatsu T, Kakumu S: Serum cryoglobulin and chronic hepatitis C virus disease. Am J Gastroenterol *90*(10):1847–1852, 1995.

CRYOGLOBULIN, SERUM
(see Cryoglobulin, Qualitative, Serum)

CRYOGLOBULIN, QUALITATIVE, SERUM

Norm: Negative.

Positive Type I Cryoglobulin: Leukemia (chronic lymphocytic), lymphoma, multiple myeloma, and Waldenström's macroglobulinemia.

Positive Type II Cryoglobulin: Lymphoma, mixed essential cryoglobulinemia, multiple myeloma, rheumatoid arthritis, and Sjögren's syndrome.

Positive Type III Cryoglobulin: Chronic infection, cytomegalovirus infection, endocarditis (infective), glomerulonephritis (poststreptococcal), hepatitis (acute viral, chronic active), infectious mononucleosis, kalaazar, leprosy, polymyalgia rheumatica, primary biliary cirrhosis, rheumatoid arthritis, scleroderma, Sjögren's syndrome, systemic lupus erythematosus, and tropical splenomegaly syndrome.

Positive Type I, II, or III: Hodgkin's disease, infection (viral), and Raynaud's disease.

Description: Cryoglobulins are abnormal serum proteins that precipitate at low laboratory temperatures and redissolve after being warmed. They cannot be identified by serum protein electrophoresis. Cryoglobulin presence in the serum causes vascular problems most commonly of the extremities and is usually associated with immunological disease. Three types may be delineated to help differentiate the type of disease occurring. This test involves obtaining a "cryocrit" by observing for cold precipitation of cryoglobulin after at least 72 hours of storage at 4°C and confirm-

ing the reversibility of the reaction by rewarming the serum sample.

Professional Considerations:

1. Consent form NOT required.
2. Preparation:
   A. *See Client and family teaching.*
   B. Tube: Red-top, red/gray-top, or gold-top.
   C. The syringe and red-top tube should be warmed to 37°C to prevent loss of cryoglobulins.
3. Procedure:
   A. Draw a 10-ml blood sample in a tube that has been prewarmed to body temperature.
4. Postprocedure care:
   A. Keep the specimen warm and send it to the laboratory immediately for warmed clotting at 37°C.
5. Client and family teaching:
   A. Fast from food and fluids for 8 hours before the test.
   B. Clients with positive tests should avoid exposure to cold temperatures.
   C. Results may not be available for several days.
6. Factors that affect results:
   A. After separation of serum from the clot and subsequent serum centrifugation, refrigerate the sample for 3–7 days. Testing the sample before the end of the precipitation period may yield incorrect results. .
7. Other data:
   A. The serum should be kept under observation for 1 week to detect late-forming cryoglobulins.
   B. Cryoglobulins are not to be confused with cryofibrinogen, which precipitates from *plasma,* rather than serum, in cold conditions.

Bibliography:

Ferri C, Mannini L, Bartoli V, Gremignai G, Genovesi-Evert F, Oristofani R, Albanese B, Pasero G, Bombardieri S: Blood viscosity and filtration abnormalities in mixed cryoglobulinemia patients. Clin Exp Rheumatol *8*(3):271–281, 1990.

Hambley H, Vetters JM: Artifacts associated with a cryoglobulin. Postgrad Med J *65*(762):241–243, 1989.

Sikander F, Salgaonkar DS, Joshi VR: Cryoglobulin studies in systemic lupus erythematosus. J Postgrad Med *35*(3):139–143, 1989.

CRYPTOCOCCAL ANTIGEN TITER, CEREBROSPINAL FLUID (CSF), SPECIMEN

Norm: Negative.

Positive: Titers of 1:8 or more indicate active meningitic *Cryptococcus neoformans* infection, Titers of 1:4 are highly suggestive of meningitic *Cryptococcus neoformans* infection.

Description: *Cryptococcus* is a yeast member of the Fungi Imperfecti group found in the soil and in contaminated bird droppings. It is thought to be transmitted to humans by inhalation from the environment. Normal host defense mechanisms prevent *Cryptococcus* from causing disease. Clients with Hodgkin's disease, sarcoidosis, acquired immune deficiency syndrome, diabetes, and those on corticosteroid therapy are more susceptible to cryptococcal infection. *Cryptococcus neoformans* is the genus most commonly causing pathology in humans, with chronic meningitis being the most common manifestation. Antigen detection enables earlier diagnosis than does culture. This test uses latex agglutination to detect the presence of the cryptococcal antigen in a sample of cerebrospinal fluid. The results are reported in titers, with the level of titer corresponding to the extent of infection. Serial titers may be used to monitor response to therapy.

Professional Considerations:

1. Consent form IS required for the spinal tap. See *Lumbar Puncture, Diagnostic*, for risks and contraindications.
2. Preparation:
   A. *See Lumbar Puncture, Diagnostic.*
3. Procedure:
   A. 5–10 ml of cerebrospinal fluid is collected through a needle inserted into the spinal canal between L3-4 or L4-5 or directly from the ventricles of the brain during special procedures. *See Lumbar Puncture, Diagnostic.*
4. Postprocedure care:
   A. *See Lumbar Puncture, Diagnostic.*
   B. Transport the specimen to the laboratory immediately.
5. Client and family teaching:
   A. *Cryptococcus* is not thought to be transmitted directly from person to person. Isolation of the clients with positive results is unnecessary.
6. Factors that affect results:
   A. False-positive results may occur in clients with rheumatoid arthritis. This cross-reaction may be eliminated by treating the sample with pronase or boiling the sample with disodium EDTA.
   B. Tanner et al. (1994) recently demonstrated sensitivities of 93–100% and specificity of 93–98% in five commercially available kits for testing for cryptococcal antigen titer in cerebrospinal fluid.
7. Other data:
   A. Amphotericin B and 5-fluocytosine are used to treat cryptococcal infections.

B. A positive culture is required to confirm diagnosis of cryptococcal infections.
C. *See Lumbar Puncture, Diagnostic* for procedural contraindications.
D. *See also Cryptococcal Antigen Titer, Serum* for further information about the disease.

Bibliography:

Hay RJ: Cryptococcosis, AIDS, and clinical trials. [commentary]. Lancet *34*: 530, 1995.
Robinson GR: Images in clinical medicine: Severe cryptococcal pneumonia. N Engl J Med *332*(26): 1752, 1995.
Tanner DC, Weinstein MP, Fedorciw B, Joho KL, Thorpe JJ, Reller L: Comparison of commercial kits for detection of cryptococcal antigen. J Clin Microbiol *32*(7):1680–1684, 1994.

CRYPTOCOCCAL ANTIGEN TITER, SERUM

Norm: Negative.

Positive: Titers of 1:8 or more are indicative of active disseminated *Cryptococcus neoformans* infection; titers of 1:4 are highly suggestive of disseminated *C. neoformans* infection.

Description: *Cryptococcus* is a yeast member of the Fungi Imperfecti group found in the soil and in contaminated bird droppings. It is thought to be transmitted to humans by inhalation from the environment. Normal host defense mechanisms prevent *Cryptococcus* from causing disease. Clients with Hodgkin's disease, sarcoidosis, acquired immune deficiency syndrome, and those on corticosteroid therapy are more susceptible to cryptococcal infection. *C. neoformans* is the genus most commonly causing pathology in humans, with chronic meningitis being the most common manifestation. Other types of cryptococcal disease involve the lungs, the cutaneous tissue, the skeletal system, and a disseminated infection. Serologic antigen detection allows earlier diagnosis than does culture. This test involves using latex agglutination to detect the presence of the cryptococcal antigen in a sample of serum. Detection of the cryptococcal antigen in serum usually indicates systemic cryptococcosis. Results are reported in titers, with the level of titer corresponding to the extent of infection. Serial titers may be used to monitor response to therapy.

Professional Considerations:

1. Consent form NOT required.
2. Preparation:
   A. Tube: Red-top, red/gray-top, or gold-top.
3. Procedure:
   A. Draw a 10-ml blood sample.
4. Postprocedure care:
   A. Transport the specimen to the laboratory immediately.
5. Client and family teaching:
   A. *Cryptococcus* is not thought to be transmitted directly from person to person. Isolation of the client is unnecessary.
   B. Results may not be available for several days.
6. Factors that affect results:
   A. False-positive results may occur in clients with rheumatoid arthritis. This cross-reaction may be eliminated by treating the sample with pronase or boiling the sample with disodium EDTA.
   B. Tanner et al. (1994) found significant differences in sensitivity among five commercially available kits that test for cryptococcal antigen in serum. Kits that pretreat the specimen with pronase had greater specificity (97%) than kits that do not pretreat with pronase (83%).
7. Other data:
   A. Amphotericin B and 5-fluorocytosine are used to treat cryptococcal infections.
   B. A positive culture is required to confirm diagnosis of cryptococcal infections.

Bibliography:

Eberhardt TH: False-positive reactions in cryptococcal antigen determination. Am J Clin Pathol *100*(3): 364, 1993.

Powderly WG, Cloud GA, Dismukes WE, Saag MS: Measurement of cryptococcal antigen in serum and cerebrospinal fluid: value in the management of AIDS-associated cryptococcal meningitis. Clin Infect Dis *18*(5):789–792, 1994.

Tanner DC, Weinstein MP, Fedorciw B, Joho KL, Thorpe JJ, Reller L: Comparison of commercial kits for detection of cryptococcal antigen. J Clin Microbiol *32*(7):1680–1684, 1994.

CRYPTOCOCCUS ANTIBODY TITER, SERUM

Norm: Negative.

Positive: Titers ≥1:2 are highly suggestive of cryptococcal infection. Positive IFA at titers of ≥1:16 are diagnostic for cryptococcosis.

Description: *Cryptococcus* is a yeast member of the Fungi Imperfecti group found in the soil and in contaminated bird droppings. It is thought to be transmitted to humans by inhalation from the environment. Normal host defense mechanisms prevent *Cryptococcus* from causing disease. Clients with Hodgkin's disease, sarcoidosis, acquired immune deficiency syndrome, diabetes mellitus, and those on corticosteroid therapy, are more susceptible to cryptococcal infection. *C. neoformans* is the genus most commonly causing pathology in humans, with chronic meningitis being the most common manifestation. Other types of cryptococcal disease involve the lungs, the cutaneous tissue, the skeletal system, and a disseminated infection. Serologic antibody detection allows earlier diagnosis than does culture. This test involves using two tests (indirect fluorescent-antibody and tube agglutination) to detect the presence of the cryptococcal antibody in a sample of serum. The results are reported as the highest dilution demonstrating agglutination when serum is combined with yeast cells.

Professional Considerations:

1. Consent form NOT required.
2. Preparation:
   A. Tube: Red-top, red/gray-top, or gold-top.
3. Procedure:
   A. Obtain a 5-ml blood sample.
4. Postprocedure care:
   A. None.
5. Client and family teaching:
   A. *Cryptococcus* is not thought to be transmitted directly from person to person. Isolation of the client is unnecessary.
6. Factors that affect results:
   A. False-negative results may occur in the presence of increased circulating antigens as the disease progresses. Results may then become positive as drug therapy lowers antigen levels.
   B. False-positive results may occur in the presence of antibodies from past cryptococcal infections.
7. Other data:
   A. Amphotericin B and 5-fluocytosine are used to treat cryptococcal infections.
   B. A positive culture is required to confirm diagnosis of cryptococcal infections.

Bibliography:

Mukherjee J, Cleare W, Casadevall A: Monoclonal antibody mediated capsular reactions (Quellung) in Cryptococcus neoformans. J Immunol Methods *184*(1):139–143, 1995.

CRYPTOSPORIDIUM DIAGNOSTIC PROCEDURES, STOOL

Norm: Negative.

Usage: AIDS.

Description: To detect the presence of *Cryptosporidium,* a coccidian obligate parasite that inhabits the intestinal mucosa and respiratory tracts of many animals and can cause diarrhea in humans. In clients with intact immune systems, cryptosporidiosis is self-limited to 2 weeks or less. In immuno-compromised clients, the disease causes a severe diarrhea lasting weeks to years. In this test, *Cryptosporidium* oocysts must be distinguished from yeast cells. Iodine stains are used to differentiate yeast cells, which do stain, from *Cryptosporidium* oocysts, which do not stain. An acid-fast stain is then performed on a smear of fixed or unfixed stool to confirm the presence of *Cryptosporidium.* In a positive test, *Cryptosporidium* oocysts stain bright red, but yeast cells do not stain.

Professional Considerations:

1. Consent form NOT required.
2. Preparation:
   A. Clarify the collection procedure with the individual laboratory that will be performing the test. Preschedule this test with the laboratory because testing must be done on a freshly collected specimen.
   B. Obtain a clear container.
3. Procedure:
   A. Collect a 20-g sample of stool directly into a wide-mouth, water-tight, clean container.
   B. Some laboratories require that the stool specimen be preserved immediately with a 10% formalin solution or sodium acetate–acetic acid formalin.
   C. If the client is unable to defecate into the container, substitute a sheet of waxed paper and transfer the specimen into the container.
   D. Repeat the collection every other day for a total of three specimens.
4. Postprocedure care:
   A. If a fixative is used, document the consistency of the fresh sample on the laboratory requisition or include a sample of unfixed specimen in a separate container.
   B. Transport the specimen to the laboratory immediately.
5. Client and family teaching:
   A. Contamination of the stool specimen with urine or toilet water invalidates the results.
6. Factors that affect results:
   A. Antimicrobial therapy causes false-negative results. The test should be repeated 5–10 days after discontinuation of antibiotic therapy.
   B. Do not use polyvinyl alcohol (PVA) fixative.
7. Other data:
   A. Handle the specimen cautiously to prevent self-contamination. *Cryptosporidium* is highly contagious.

Bibliography:

Chappell CL, Okhuysen PC, Sterling CR, DuPont HL: Cryptosporidium parvum: intensity of infection and oocyst excretion patterns in healthy volunteers. J Infect Dis 173(1):232–236, 1996

Cryptosporidium in water supplies: the second Badenoch report. Commun Dis Rep 5(46):245–248, 1995.

CSF ANALYSIS, CSF EXAMINATION

(see Cerebrospinal Fluid, Glucose, Specimen; Cerebrospinal Fluid, Immunoglobulin G, Immunoglobulin G Ratios and Immunoglobulin G Index; Immunoglobulin G Synthesis Rate, Specimen; Cerebrospinal Fluid, Routine Analysis, Specimen; and Cerebrospinal Fluid, Routine, Culture and Cytology)

CSF FLOW STUDIES, DIAGNOSTIC

(see Cisternography, Radionuclide, Diagnostic)

CT-PTSP

(see Splenoportography, Diagnostic)

CT SCAN

(see Cerebral Computed Tomography, Diagnostic; Chest Tomography, Diagnostic; Computed Tomography of the Body, Diagnostic; and Tomography, Paranasal Sinuses, Diagnostic)

CULDOSCOPY, DIAGNOSTIC

Norm: Normal structure and arrangement of the pelvic organs; absence of inflammatory processes, lesions, adhesions, or ectopic pregnancy; and patent fallopian tubes.

Usage: Aids in the diagnosis of endometriosis, pelvic adhesions, and pelvic abnormalities not diagnosable by palpation. Exploratory procedure for adhesions or tubal blockage causing sterility or for suspected salpingitis, ectopic pregnancy, pelvic pain, or pelvic inflammatory disease.

Description: The direct visualization of the pelvic organs through a culdoscope inserted through the cul-de-sac (rectovaginal septum) of the vagina into the pelvis. The culdoscope, or pelvic endoscope, is a surgical instrument with a fiberoptic light source, lens, and light hood. Although visualization of the pelvic organs is more difficult with culdoscopy than with laparoscopy, the procedure poses less risk to the woman.

Professional Considerations:

1. Consent form IS required.

Risks:

Inadvertent amniocentesis, pain.

Contraindications:

In instances of cul-de-sac mass, fixed uterine retrodisplacement, acute gynecologic infections, thickened nodular uterosacral ligaments, and in clients who are unable to maintain a knee-chest position.

2. Preparation:
    A. Pain medication may be prescribed.
    B. The client should void just prior to the procedure and disrobe below the waist or wear a gown.
    C. Obtain an antiseptic solution; a culdoscope; a cannula and a trocar; sterile water in a warmer; perineal retractor; a speculum; a tenaculum; a local anesthetic; two needles; two syringes; indigo carmine dye; a pillow; and an absorbable suture material.
    D. The culdoscope is prewarmed in a sterile solution.
    E. Insert an indwelling urinary catheter to prevent bladder distention from urine.
3. Procedure:
    A. The client is placed face-down in the knee-chest position with her thighs perpendicular to the examination table and her shoulders supported with shoulder rests.
    B. A perineal retractor is inserted to expose the vaginal vault and the area is cleansed with an antiseptic solution.

C. A speculum is inserted through the vagina to elevate the perineum, and a tenaculum is used to pull the cervix toward the symphysis pubis, thus exposing the cul-de-sac.
D. The rectovaginal septum is injected with local anesthetic in several places.
E. The trocar is inserted through a cannula and pushed through the vaginal wall at the cul-de-sac and then removed. Upon removal, pneumoperitoneum occurs, aided by the knee-chest position, as air rushes into the peritoneal cavity.
F. The culdoscope is connected to the fiberoptic light cord and inserted through the cannula into the peritoneal cavity, and the angled lens system is manipulated to methodically inspect the pelvic organs. Organs and structures inspected include the posterior uterine surface, fallopian tubes and ovaries, uterosacral ligaments, pelvic peritoneum, appendix, rectum, and sigmoid colon.
G. Dye may be injected into the uterus through the cervix, and the fallopian tubes inspected for patency.
H. The culdoscope is removed and the woman is assisted into a prone position with a pillow under the abdomen to force air out of the abdominal cavity. The cannula is removed and the cul-de-sac sutured with absorbable sutures.
4. Postprocedure care:
    A. Notify the physician for more than a small amount of bleeding or for fever, chills, or an increase in abdominal pain.
5. Client and family teaching:
    A. You may experience abdominal cramping for several days after the procedure, until the air dissipates.
6. Factors that affect results:
    A. The value of this procedure depends on the skill of the operator.
7. Other data:
    A. Microsurgical repair of adnexal structures is sometimes performed with culdoscopy.

Bibliography:

Corson SL, Sedlacek TV, Hoffman JJ: Greenhill's Surgical Gynecology, 5th ed. Chicago, Year Book Medical Publishers, 1986.

Sherer DM, Abramowicz JS: Inadvertent amniocenteses occurring during unrelated invasive diagnostic procedures in the third trimester. Am J Perinatol 10(6):412–413, 1993.

CULTURE, BLOOD

(see Blood Culture, Blood; and Blood Culture with Antimicrobial Removal Device, Culture)

CULTURE, CEREBROSPINAL FLUID, SPECIMEN
(see Cerebrospinal Fluid, Routine, Culture and Cytology, Specimen)

CULTURE, ROUTINE, SPECIMEN

Norm: No growth, normal flora.

Usage: Abscess, auditory infestations, bites (animal, human), blepharitis, body cavity drainage or fluids, inflammation, otitis externa, otitis media, respiratory secretions, ulcerations, and wounds (draining, surgical, traumatic).

Description: Laboratory cultures of specimens taken from various body substances are performed to isolate and identify pathogenic microorganisms causing disease. This test involves the direct microscopic inspection of a Gram-stained smear of an organism after it is grown in selected media.

Professional Considerations:

1. Consent form NOT required.
2. Preparation:
   A. Obtain the proper specimen container for the site (see the table at the bottom of the page).
   B. Label multiple collections of the same test sequentially.
   C. Wear a mask to prevent inhalation of airborne microorganisms expelled with coughing while collecting tracheal or nasopharyngeal specimens.
3. Procedure:
   A. A separate specimen should be obtained for each test.
   B. *Ear culture:* Insert a cotton-tipped Culturette ⅛ to ¼ inch into the external auditory canal and rotate the swab. Remove the swab without touching

any other parts of the ear. Insert the swab into the Culturette tube and squeeze the end of the tube to release the media contents.
   C. *Eye culture:* Swab the inner canthus of the eye with a sterile cotton-tipped Culturette swab. Insert the swab into the Culturette tube and squeeze the end of the tube to release the medium contents.
   D. *Nasal culture:* Have the client clear the nose of excess secretions and tilt back the head. Insert the cotton-tipped Culturette into the nostril until it reaches the posterior nares and swab it in a circular motion two times. Leave the swab in place for 15 seconds. Slowly remove the swab and place it in the Culturette tube. Squeeze the swab end of the tube to release the medium contents. Repeat this procedure using the other nostril for nares culture.
   E. *Nasopharyngeal culture:* Have the client tilt back the head and open the mouth. While depressing the tongue with a tongue blade, gently swab the tonsillar area from left to right. Also swab any reddened or purulent areas. Remove the swab without touching any other parts of the mouth. Insert the swab into the Culturette tube and squeeze the end of the tube to release the media contents.
   F. *Sputum culture:* A first morning sputum specimen is recommended. Chest clapping, postural drainage, and/or aerosol therapy may be helpful in mobilizing tenacious secretions just prior to sputum collection. Have the client cough deeply several times and expel the mucus contents mobilized into a wide-mouthed, sterile specimen cup. Instruct the client to avoid otherwise contaminating the cup's inside or edges. Tightly cap the cup.
   G. *Sputum, tracheal, culture:* Ventilated clients should be hyperoxygenated before starting the procedure. Place the sputum trap in-line between the suc-

CULTURE, ROUTINE, SPECIMEN

Site	Type of Sterile Container
Ear	Cotton swab Culturette
Eye	Cotton swab Culturette
Nasal	2 Cotton swab Culturettes
Nasopharyngeal	Cotton swab Culturette
Site drainage	Cotton swab Culturette
Sputum	Sterile cup with lid
Sputum, tracheal	Sputum trap
Wound, superficial	Cotton swab Culturette
Wound, deep	Sterile syringe

tion tubing and suction catheter. Maintain the trap in an upright position. Using a sterile technique, insert the suction catheter tip into the tracheostomy, endotracheal tube, or nares and advance it into the trachea without applying suction. In 10 seconds or less, apply suction and obtain 3–5 ml of mucus for culture in the trap and remove the suction catheter. Cap the sputum trap.

H. *Wound, superficial site drainage:* Swab the site with the cotton-tipped end of a Culturette. Avoid touching the surrounding skin with the tip. Place the swab into the Culturette tube and squeeze the swab end to release the media contents. Large wounds should have several separate cultures performed from different areas of the wound.

I. *Wound, deep:* Aspirate drainage with a syringe and needle from deep inside the wound. Remove the syringe, expel the air into sterile gauze, and either cap the needle with a rubber stopper or cork, or inject the contents into anaerobic culture medium. Transport the specimen to the laboratory immediately.

4. Postprocedure care:
   A. Label the container with the specimen collection date and time.
   B. Place the specimen in a sealed plastic bag.
   C. Write any recent antibiotic or antifungal therapy on the laboratory requisition.
   D. Send the specimen to the laboratory immediately. Do not refrigerate it.

5. Client and family teaching:
   A. The specimen collection procedure is typically painless, unless pressure is placed on an area of inflammation.
   B. *Sputum collection:* Deep coughs are necessary to produce sputum, rather than saliva. To produce the proper specimen, take several breaths in, without fully exhaling each, then expel sputum with a "cascade cough."
   C. Clients started on empiric therapy should continue taking drugs unless and until test results are found to be negative.

6. Factors that affect results:
   A. Antibiotic or antifungal therapy initiated before the specimen is taken may produce false-negative results. Obtain the culture before starting this therapy for the most accurate identification of the causative bacteria and the best clinical results.

7. Other data:
   A. Results for most microorganisms will not be available for 48–72 hours. Fungi and mycobacteria may take several weeks. Gram stains requested should be available within 1 hour.

B. Normal mouth flora include *Actinomyces,* anaerobic and aerobic (nongroup A) streptococci, anaerobic spirochetes, *Enterobacteriaceae, Haemophilus influenzae, Lactobacillus, Pneumococcus, Bramhamella catarrhalis, Bacteroides* species, *Candida* fungi, nonpathogenic *Neisseria, N. meningitidis, Staphylococcus aureus, S. epidermidis, S. pyogenes,* and *Veillonella* species.

C. Normal throat flora include alpha and nonhemolytic streptococci, *Bacteroides, Candida* fungi, *Corynebacteria* species, *Enterobacteriacea, H. influenzae, N. meningitidis, nonpathogenic Neisseria, Pneumococcus, S. aureus,* and *S. pyogenes.*

D. Normal nasal flora in small amounts include *B. catarrhalis, C. albicans,* diphtheroids, *H. influenza, Neisseria* species (except *N. gonorrhoeae* and *N. meningitidis), S. aureus, S. epidermidis, S. pneumoniae,* and *S. pyogenes.*

E. Normal ear flora include *S. epidermidis, Corynebacterium,* and *S. aureus.*

F. Normal eye flora include diphtheroids, *Enterobacteriacea, Haemophilus* species, *Moraxella* species, *Neisseria* species, *Pneumococcus, Sarcina, S. epidermidis,* and *S. pyogenes.*

G. Nasal cultures should generally be limited to situations where throat specimens are not easily obtained, as throat cultures are usually more advantageous for diagnosing upper respiratory tract infections.

Bibliography:

Hill WM: Routine detection of Trichomonas vaginalis in genital specimens using culture in microtitre trays. Br J Biomed Sci *52*(2):93–96, 1995.

Roddey OF Jr, Clegg HW, Martin ES, Swetenburg RL, Koonce EW: Comparison of throat culture methods for the recovery of group A streptococci in a pediatric office setting. JAMA *274*(23):1863–1865, 1995.

Wilson ML, Weinstein MP, Mirrett S, Reimer LG, Feldman RJ, Chuard CR, Reller LB: Controlled evaluation of BacT/alert standard anaerobic and FAN anaerobic blood culture bottles for the detection of bacteremia and fungemia. J Clin Microbiol *33*(9):2265–2270, 1995.

CULTURE, ROUTINE, STOOL
(see Stool Culture, Routine)

CULTURE, SKIN, SPECIMEN

Norm: Negative.

Usage: Abscesses, acne, anthrax, athlete's foot, burn infections, candidiasis, carbuncles, erysipelas, folliculitis, herpes simplex, *Microsporum au-*

douinii for ringworm of the scalp, ova or mites scrapings for scabies, pruritus, psoriasis, pyoderma, *Staphylococcus aureus* or group A beta-hemolytic streptococci for impetigo, *Streptococcus pyogenes*, tinea cruris, warts, yaws, and other skin infections.

Description: A sample of infected lesions of the skin is incubated and the growth patterns, bacterial cell staining, and microscopic appearance are studied for determination of the organism causing the disease process. The most common skin pathogens are *Aspergillus, Blastomyces, Candida, Coccidioides immitis, Cryptococcus, Enterococci, Histoplasma capsulatum, Microsporum, Penicillium, Proteus, Rhizopus, Rhodotorula, Sporothrix schenckii, Staphylococci, Streptococci,* and *Trichophyton* species.

Professional Considerations:

1. Consent form NOT required.
2. Preparation:
   A. Obtain 70% alcohol, sterile water, a sterile scalpel or spatula, and a sterile Petri dish or anaerobic swab culture tubes as indicated.
3. Procedure:
   A. Cleanse the lesion site with 70% alcohol and then rinse with sterile water to eliminate the effect of alcohol on any bacteria. Allow the site to dry.
   B. Scrape the edge of the lesion to obtain tissue samples and/or purulent drainage with a sterile scalpel or spatula. Place the sample in a sterile petri dish.
   C. For an anaerobic culture, obtain purulent drainage samples from deep in the wound on a swab and carefully place them in an anaerobic culture medium.
4. Postprocedure care:
   A. Apply a dry, sterile dressing as needed.
5. Client and family teaching:
   A. If started on empiric therapy, you should continue taking the prescribed drug(s) unless and until the test results are found to be negative.
6. Factors that affect results:
   A. Obtain specimens before starting antibiotics for the most accurate bacterial identification and best clinical outcome.
   B. For burned clients, viable skin rather than eschar yields the best results.
   C. Chances of inadequate sampling of the lesion can be reduced by taking several separate samplings of the lesion and/or exudate.
7. Other data:
   A. Minor normal flora of the skin include *Staphylococcus aureus*, fungi of the pityriasis types, and *S. epidermidis*, which may proliferate in clients with poor immune systems and invasive wounds.

Bibliography:

Dimri GP, Lee X, Basile G, Acosta M, Scott G, Roskelley C, Medrano EE, Linskens M, Rubelj I, Pereira-Smith O, et al.: A biomarker that identifies senescent human cells in culture and in aging skin in vivo. Proc Natl Acad Sci USA *92*(20): 9363–9367, 1995.

Le Poole IC, Van den Wijngaard RM, Westerhof W, Dormans JA, Van den Berg FM, Verkruisen RP, Dingemans KP, Das PK: Organotypic culture of human skin to study melanocyte migration. Pigment Cell Res *7*(1):33–43, 1994.

Varani J, Perone P, Inman DR, Burmeister W, Schollenberger SB, Fligiel SE, Sitrin RG, Johnson KJ: Human skin in organ culture. Elaboration of proteolytic enzymes in the presence and absence of exogenous growth factors. Am J Pathol *146*(1): 210–217, 1995.

CULTURE, THROAT, FOR *CORYNEBACTERIUM*, SPECIMEN

Norm: Negative.

Positive: Diphtheria.

Description: *Corynebacterium* is an anaerobic, gram-positive, non-acid-fast, motile bacteria that does not produce endospores. *C. diphtheriae* liberates a cytotoxin that causes diphtheria, an acute infection of the oropharynx, larynx, nose, and other mucous membranes marked by a characteristic patchy gray pseudomembrane over a lesion surrounded by reddened, inflamed tissue. The mode of transmission is usually direct contact with the discharges from lesions of an infected client. Culture of the throat is taken for incubation and study of the appearance and growth patterns of bacteria, as well as the microscopic appearance and staining properties to identify the presence or absence of *Corynebacterium*.

Professional Considerations:

1. Consent form NOT required.
2. Preparation:
   A. *See Client and family teaching.*
   B. Obtain a tongue blade, sterile swab, and Culturette.
   C. Call the laboratory so it can have on hand the special culture medium for *C. diphtheriae*.
3. Procedure:
   A. With the client's head tilted back and mouth opened, depress the tongue with the tongue blade. Have the client

say "Ah" to elevate the uvula and expose the infective lesions.

B. Shine a light into the oropharynx to locate the characteristic gray lesions. Remove the patchy gray pseudomembrane by rubbing it firmly with a sterile swab.

C. Press a sterile Culturette swab firmly against the lesion for a few seconds. For asymptomatic clients, culture the tonsillar fossae, the posterior pharynx, and the retrouvular areas.

D. Remove the swab, taking care to avoid touching any area except the infected site.

4. Postprocedure care:

A. Return the swab to the Culturette tube and crush the ampule of the medium.

B. Transport the specimen to the laboratory immediately. The specimen should be refrigerated if it is not tested immediately.

5. Client and family teaching:

A. Antiseptic gargles or mouthwashes prior to the procedure may prevent bacterial growth. Avoid using these products for 8 hours before the test.

B. Erythromycin is used to treat this disease.

C. If started on empiric therapy, you should continue taking the prescribed drug(s) unless and until the test results are found to be negative.

D. Results are normally available within 4 days.

6. Factors that affect results:

A. Obtain cultures before starting antibiotics.

7. Other data:

A. Diphtheria is communicable for up to 4 weeks from the appearance of the bacilli in the lesions.

B. A positive throat culture may also indicate a carrier state.

C. Cultures of the nose and the pseudomembrane are also helpful in making a positive diagnosis.

D. Toxic strains of this disease have recently been found in Russia, and nontoxogenic strains have been isolated with increasing frequency in the United Kingdom via prospective screening at sexually-transmitted-disease clinics.

Bibliography:

Wilson AP: The return of Corynebacterium diphtheriae: the rise of non-toxigenic strains. J Hosp Infect *30* (Suppl): 306–312, 1995.

Wilson AP: Treatment of infection caused by toxigenic and non-toxigenic strains of Corynebacterium diphtheriae. J Antimicrobiol Chemother *35*(6): 717–720, 1995.

CULTURE, URINE
(see Culture, Routine, Specimen)

CUTANEOUS IMMUNOFLUORESCENSE BIOPSY, DIAGNOSTIC

Norm: A descriptive, interpretive report of histologic study findings is made.

Usage: Bulbous pemphigoid, dermatitis herpetiformis, herpes gestationis, and pemphigus; indicated in the investigation of cutaneous forms of lupus erythematosus, blistering disease, and vasculitis; also used to confirm the histopathology of skin lesions and to follow the results of treatment.

Description: A biopsy of the skin is taken for direct epidermal immunofluorescent study. Direct immunofluorescence is a histologic technique whereby the skin sample is treated with fluorescein-conjugated human immunoglobulin antisera, then incubated and examined under ultraviolet light. Deposition of human immunoglobulins and complement components in skin tissue and lesions (indicating pathology) is identified and differentiated by the immunofluorescent patterns demonstrated.

Professional Considerations:

1. Consent form IS required.

Risks:
Bleeding, infection.

Contraindications:
May be contraindicated in bleeding disorders, anticoagulated states, and immunocompromised states.

2. Preparation:

A. Obtain punch forceps, an antiseptic solution, gauze, and a sterile specimen container.

3. Procedure:

A. A 4-mm punch biopsy or surgically excised specimen of involved or uninvolved skin is obtained.

B. The specimen is quick-frozen in liquid nitrogen and stored at −70°C. If the specimen is to be shipped to an outside lab, it is preserved in Michel holding solution with the pH maintained between 7.0 and 7.4.

4. Postprocedure care:

A. Apply a dry, sterile dressing to the biopsy site.

5. Client and family teaching:

A. The test typically is transiently painful.

B. Place pressure over the site for 5 minutes if bleeding occurs.
C. Results may not be available for several days.
6. Factors that affect results:
   A. Amount of biopsy <4 mm is insufficient.
   B. The reliability of immunofluorescence technique is affected by factors such as age and site of the lesion, type of immunofluorescence, and type of immunoglobulin. For this reason, histopathology should also be used to confirm the results.
7. Other data:
   A. The final report may take up to 3 days.

Bibliography:

al-Suwaid AR, Venkataram MN, Bhushnurmath SR: Cutaneous lupus erythematosus: comparison of direct immunofluorescence findings with histopathology. Int J Dermatol 34(7):480–482, 1995.

Burrows NP, Bhogal BS, Russell Jones R, Black MM: Clinicopathological significance of cutaneous epidermal nuclear staining by direct immunofluorescence. J Cutan Pathol 20(2):159–162, 1993.

CXR, DIAGNOSTIC
(see Chest X-Ray, Diagnostic)

CYANIDE, BLOOD

Norm:

		SI Units
Serum		
Nonsmoker	0.004 mg/L	0.15 µmol/L
Smoker	0.006 mg/L	0.22 µmol/L
Panic (lethal) level	>0.1 mg/L	>3.7 µmol/L
Nitroprusside therapy	0.01–0.06 mg/L	0.37–2.21 µmol/L
Whole Blood		
Nonsmoker	0.016 mg/L	0.59 µmol/L
Smoker	0.041 mg/L	1.52 µmol/L
Panic (lethal) level	>1 mg/L	>37 µmol/L
Nitroprusside therapy	0.05–0.5 mg/L	1.9–19 µmol/L

Panic Level Symptoms and Treatment::

Symptoms: Headache, dizziness, abdominal pain and nausea, confusion, labored breathing, syncope, convulsions, and coma prior to respiratory failure. Loss of consciousness, metabolic acidosis, and cardiopulmonary failure are the three most common signs of cyanide poisoning in clients who die from this problem.

Treatment: Amyl nitrite, sodium nitrite, sodium thiosulfate.

Usage: Cyanide poisoning and monitoring of cyanide levels during nitroprusside therapy.

Description: A determination of the presence of cyanide in the blood. Cyanide is a very toxic chemical that inactivates cellular respiration enzymes (cytochrome oxidase), poisoning their functional activity and causing death from asphyxia. The major cause of death from cyanide poisoning is suicide.

Professional Considerations:
1. Consent form NOT required.
2. Preparation:
   A. Tube: Lavender-top, black-top, or green-top.
3. Procedure:
   A. Completely fill the tube with blood.
4. Postprocedure care:
   A. If cyanide poisoning is suspected, monitor neurologic and respiratory status closely and have emergency intubation equipment and oral airway available.
5. Client and family teaching:
   A. None.
6. Factors that affect results:
   A. An insufficient blood sample may cause falsely low results.
7. Other data:
   A. None.

Bibliography:

Borgohain R, Singh AK, Radhakrishna H, Rao VC, Mohandas S: Delayed onset generalised dystonia after cyanide poisoning. Clin Neurol Neurosurg *97*(3):213–215, 1995.

Demedts P, Wauters A, Franck F, Neels H: Monitoring of cyanocobalamin and hydroxocobalamin during treatment of cyanide intoxication [letter]. Lancet *346*(8891–8892):1706–1707, 1995.

Rosenow F, Herholz K, Lanfermann H, Weuthen G, Ebner R, Kessler J, Ghaemi M, Heiss WD: Neuro-

logical sequelae of cyanide intoxication—the patterns of clinical, magnetic resonance imaging, and positron emission tomography findings. Ann Neurol *38*(5):825–828, 1995.

Yen D, Tsai J, Wang LM, Kao WF, Hu SC, Lee CH, Deng J: The clinical experience of acute cyanide poisoning. Am J Emerg Med *13*(5):524–528, 1995.

CYCLIC ADENOSINE MONOPHOSPHATE (cAMP, CYCLIC AMP), SERUM AND URINE

Norm:

		SI Units
Serum	5.6–10.9 ng/ml	17–33 nmol/L
Urine		
Total cAMP	112–188 mg/L	340–570 nmol/L
cAMP portion of creatinine	3–5 mmol/g of creatinine	
cAMP portion of glomerular filtrate	6.6–15.5 mg/L	20–47 mmol/L
cAMP nephrogenous portion of glomerular filtrate	<9.9 mg/L	<30 nmol/L

Increased: Hyperparathyroidism, malignant processes combined with hypercalcemia, and pseudohyperparathyroidism.

Decreased: Hypoparathyroidism and pseudohypoparathyroidism.

Description: Nephrogenous cyclic adenosine monophosphate (cAMP) is an enzyme that increases in production in the renal tubules in response to parathyroid hormone. cAMP influences the rate of cell protein synthesis and indirectly affects renal reabsorption of phosphate, gastrointestinal calcium absorption, and skeletal calcium mobilization. cAMP in urine is the result of renal tubular cAMP secretion, and glomerular-filtered cAMP. Thus, by comparing the serum and urine levels of cAMP with the glomerular filtration rate, the portion of cAMP secreted by the tubules can be estimated. There is some evidence that it may be secreted in a diurnal pattern. In clients with hyperparathyroidism, increased levels of nephrogenous cAMP are usually found as a result of excess parathyroid hormone production. A 24-hour urine collection may reveal increased levels of cAMP as a result of excess parathyroid hormone in the system.

Professional Considerations:

1. Consent form NOT required.
2. Preparation:
   A. *See Client and family teaching.*
   B. Preschedule this test with the laboratory.
   C. Tube: Red-top, red/gray-top, or gold-top for the serum sample.
   D. Obtain a 3-L container with hydrochloric acid (HCl) preservative for the urine sample.
   E. The client should lie recumbent throughout the urine collection.
   F. For 24-hour collections, discard the first morning urine specimen and write the beginning time on the laboratory requisition.
3. Procedure:
   A. *Serum collection:* Draw a 5-ml blood sample.
   B. *Urine collection:* Collect a 2- or 24-hour urine sample for cAMP and creatinine in a refrigerated, 3-L container. For 24-hour collections, include the urine voided at the end of the 24-hour period. For catheterized clients, keep the drainage bag on ice and empty urine into the acidified collection container hourly.
4. Postprocedure care:
   A. *Serum sample:*
      i. Write the specimen collection time on the laboratory requisition.
      ii. Transport the specimen to the laboratory immediately for serum separation.
      iii. Freeze the specimen if the test

cannot be performed immediately.

B. *Urine sample:*
   i. Compare the urine quantity in the specimen container with the urinary output record for the test. If the specimen contains less urine than was recorded as output, some of the sample may have been discarded, invalidating the test.
   ii. Write the ending time of collection and the total urine volume on the laboratory requisition.
   iii. Send the specimen to the laboratory immediately and refrigerate it until testing.

5. Client and family teaching:
   A. Limit physical exertion for 4 hours before the urine test.
   B. Urinate before defecating to avoid loss of urine for the urine test. If any urine is accidentally discarded, discard the entire specimen and restart the collection the next day.
   C. Results may not be available for more than 24 hours.

6. Factors that affect results:
   A. Reject serum specimens received more than 1 hour after collection.
   B. Radioactive scans within 7 days prior to the test invalidate the serum and urine results.
   C. Impaired renal function precludes the value of this urine test, as results cannot be relied upon for diagnosis.
   D. All the urine voided for the 24-hour period must be included to avoid a falsely low result.

7. Other data:
   A. For differentiation of hypoparathyroidism from pseudohypoparathyroidism, *see Cyclic Adenosine Monophosphate Provocation Test, Urine.*

Bibliography:

Rossi AG, Cousin JM, Dransfield I, Lawson MF, Chilvers ER, Haslett C: Agents that elevate cAMP inhibit human neutrophil apoptosis. Biochem Biophys Res Commun *217*(3):892–899, 1995.

Vilaboa NE, Calle C, Perez C, de Blas E, Garcia-Bermejo L, Aller P: cAMP increasing agents prevent the stimulation of heat-shock Protein 70 (HSP70) gene expression by cadmium chloride in Human myeloid cell lines. J Cell Sci *108* (Pt 8):2877–2883, 1995.

CYCLIC ADENOSINE MONOPHOSPHATE PROVOCATION TEST, URINE

Norm: Positive: A 10- to 20-fold increase, or 3.6–4 mmol.

Negative: Type I Pseudohypoparathyroidism.

Description: A test that measures cyclic adenosine monophosphate (cAMP) response to parathyroid hormone administration. cAMP is an enzyme that influences the rate of cell protein synthesis, and indirectly affects renal reabsorption of phosphate, gastrointestinal calcium absorption, and skeletal calcium mobilization. In normal clients and those with idiopathic or postoperative hypoparathyroidism, parathyroid hormone administration causes increased renal tubular production of cAMP. In clients with pseudohypoparathyroidism, a genetically transmitted, autosomal dominant disease resulting in tissue resistance to the effects of parathyroid hormone, the infusion fails to increase production of cAMP in the renal tubules, resulting in a negative test.

Professional Considerations:
1. Consent form NOT required.

Risks:
Allergic reaction to parathyroid hormone (itching, hives, rash, tight feeling in the throat, shortness of breath, bronchospasm, anaphylaxis, death).

Contraindications:
Positive parathyroid hormone skin test. This test is contraindicated in hypercalcemia.
Precaution:
Use cautiously when digitalis has been administered and in renal impairment, cardiac disease, or sarcoidosis.

2. Preparation:
   A. Preschedule this test with the laboratory.
   B. Obtain 300 U of parathyroid hormone and reconstitute it with sterile water for injection, as directed on the container.
   C. Obtain a needle, a syringe, and a 1-L urine collection container with hydrochloric acid (HCl) preservative.
   D. Establish intravenous access with 5% dextrose in water.
   E. Have emergency equipment readily available.

3. Procedure:
   A. Have the client empty the bladder.
   B. Attach a new collection bag on ice for catheterized clients.

C. Administer the prescribed dose of parathyroid hormone over 15 minutes.

D. Save all the urine collected in a refrigerated, 1-L container with HCl preservative. For catheterized clients, empty the drainage bag into the collection container hourly.

E. Three hours after the completion of the infusion, mix the container gently and collect a 50- to 100-ml aliquot for cAMP measurement.

4. Postprocedure care:

A. Send the specimen to the laboratory immediately. Refrigerate the specimen until testing.

B. Observe the client for lethargy, anorexia, nausea, vomiting, vertigo, or abdominal cramps that could result from the mobilization of calcium stores by parathyroid hormone administration.

5. Client and family teaching:

A. You will not be permitted to drive for 24 hours after the test and should make arrangements for someone else to drive you home.

6. Factors that affect results:

A. Radioactive scans within 7 days prior to the test invalidate the results.

7. Other data:

A. None.

Bibliography:

Dooper MW, Timmermans A, Weersink EJ, De Monchy JG, Kauffman HF: Defect in potentiation of adenyl cyclase correlates with bronchial hyperreactivity. J Allergy Clin Immunol 96(5, Pt 1):628–634, 1995.

Montminy MR, Gonzalez GA, Yamamoto KK: Characteristics of the cAMP response unit. Metabolism 39(9, Suppl 2):6–12, 1990.

CYCLIC AMP

(see Cyclic Adenosine Monophosphate, Serum and Urine)

CYSTINE, QUALITATIVE, URINE

Norm: Negative.

Positive: Congenital cystinuria, Fanconi's syndrome, Lowe's syndrome, nephrolithiasis, nephrotoxicity (due to heavy metals), pyelonephritis (acute), renal tubular acidosis, and Wilson's disease.

Description: Cystine is an amino acid normally absent or present in only low amounts in the urine. In conditions causing cystinuria over 300 mg/day, smooth, waxy cystine stones form in the kidneys and may be passed into the urine. Positive qualitative results should be followed by a 24-hour collection for cystine measurement, because random samples may demonstrate peaks of cystine excretion in the urine.

Professional Considerations:

1. Consent form NOT required.

2. Preparation:

A. Obtain a clean container.

3. Procedure:

A. Obtain a random urine specimen of 20 ml. A fresh specimen may be taken from a urinary drainage bag.

4. Postprocedure care:

A. Send the specimen to the laboratory immediately.

5. Client and family teaching:

A. Results are normally available within 24 hours.

6. Factors that affect results:

A. Drugs that may cause false negative results include penicillamine.

7. Other data:

A. This test should be scheduled before an intravenous pyelogram.

B. This is not a test for cystinosis, in which the urine cystine may be normal or only slightly elevated.

Bibliography:

Lindell A, Denneberg T, Hellgren E, Jeppsson JO, Tiselius HG: Clinical course and cystine stone formation during tiopronin treatment. Urol Res 23(2):111–117, 1995.

Lindell A, Denneberg T, Jeppsson JO, Tiselius HG: Measurement of diurnal variations in urinary cystine saturation. Urol Res 23(4):215–220, 1995.

CYSTOGRAPHY, RETROGRADE, DIAGNOSTIC

Norm: Normal and intact structure of the urethra, bladder, and ureter orifices; normal location of bladder; and absence of rupture, fistula, or tumor.

Usage: Detection of neurogenic bladder, calculi, fistulas, bladder tumors, bladder diverticuli, and hematoma or rupture in the bladder.

Description: Retrograde cystography is the injection of contrast dye and sometimes air through a catheter into the bladder followed by radiographs of the pelvis and bladder with the client in several positions.

Professional Considerations:

1. Consent form IS required.

Risks:

Bleeding, infection, urinary tract obstruction, allergic reaction to dye (itching, hives, rash, tight feeling in the throat, shortness of breath, bronchospasm, anaphylaxis, death), renal toxicity.

Contraindications:

History of allergy to radiographic dye, iodine, or shellfish; in urethral obstruction or during the acute phase of a urinary tract infection.

2. Preparation:
   A. Obtain a straight urinary catheter and a catheter insertion tray, 50–300 ml of radiographic dye, and a syringe.
   B. The client should disrobe below the waist or wear a gown.
   C. Obtain baseline vital signs.
   D. Have emergency equipment readily available.
3. Procedure:
   A. The client is positioned supine on the radiographic table.
   B. A baseline kidney-ureter-bladder (KUB) radiograph is taken.
   C. 200–300 ml (50–100 ml for infants) of radiographic dye is instilled into the bladder by a catheter inserted through the urethra.
   D. After the catheter is clamped, the client is assisted to several different positions by a tilt table; the physical position changes for radiographic examination of the bladder and surrounding areas.
   E. The catheter is unclamped, the bladder fluid allowed to drain, and final radiographs are taken.
4. Postprocedure care:
   A. Monitor vital signs every 15 minutes × 4, then every 30 minutes × 2, then hourly × 4, then every 2 hours until 24 hours after the test.
   B. Encourage the oral intake of fluids where not contraindicated.
   C. Observe for signs of allergic reaction to the dye (listed above) × 24 hours.
   D. Observe for urinary retention, or symptoms of urinary tract infection (fever; chills; tachycardia; tachypnea; abdominal, flank or suprapubic pain; hesitancy and frequency; dysuria; and hematuria. Notify the physician for any of these signs.
   E. *See Client and family teaching.*
5. Client and family teaching:
   A. A clear liquid diet and a cathartic the day before the test may improve the clarity of the results by minimizing intestinal gas and the amount of stool.
   B. After the procedure, save all the urine voided for the next day and report chills or painful urination. Blood in the urine that lasts more than 4–6 hours is abnormal.

6. Factors that affect results:
   A. This test should not be performed within 1 week of a previous intestinal barium examination.
   B. The clarity of the radiographic images may be diminished by the presence of excess gas or stool in the lower gastrointestinal tract.
7. Other data:
   A. None.

Bibliography:

Brown FL: Retrograde cystography. In Hamilton HK, Cahill M (eds): Diagnostics, 2nd ed. Springhouse, PA, Springhouse Corporation, 1986, pp 965–966.

Leibovitch I, Rowland RG, Little JS Jr, Foster RS, Bihrle R, Donohue JP: Cystography after radical retropubic prostatectomy: Clinical implications of abnormal findings. Urology *46*(1):78–80, 1995.

Miller KT, Moshyedi AC: Systemic reaction to contrast media during cystography [letter]. Am J Roentgenol *164*(6):1551, 1995.

Mouratidis B, Lomas F, Hurley B: Anastomotic leak of pancreatic transplant demonstrated by radionuclide cystography. Clin Nucl Med *20*(8):742–743, 1995.

Treves ST, Zurakowski D, Bauer SB, Mitchell KD, Nichols DP: Functional bladder capacity measured during radionuclide cystography in children. Radiology *198*(1):269–272, 1996.

CYSTOMETRY, DIAGNOSTIC

Norm: Normal filling pattern. Absence of residual urine; sensation of fullness at 300–500 ml, urge to void at 150–450 ml; filling bladder pressure constant until capacity reached with contraction of capacity. Normal thermal sensation when hot and cold sterile fluids are introduced into the bladder.

Usage: Evaluation of detrusor muscle function and tonicity, determination of etiology of bladder dysfunction, and differentiation of the type of neurogenic bladder dysfunction.

Description: Cystometry involves assessment of bladder neuromuscular function after instillation of measured quantities of fluid and/or air and evaluating the client's neurologic sensations and muscular responses. It also includes assessment of the voiding flow pattern for abnormalities. Neuromuscular dysfunction of the bladder can occur when lesions interfere with the neural pathways that transmit bladder reflexes to the brain or with progressive diseases, congenital malformations, strokes, or postoperatively. Cystometry is most often performed in a physician's office or clinic.

Professional Considerations:

1. Consent form IS required.

Risks:

Clients with cervical spinal cord lesions may exhibit autonomic dysreflexia (bradycardia, hypertension, flushing, diaphoresis, and headache) during instillation of fluid or carbon dioxide. Intravenous propantheline bromide may help to counteract this response.

Contraindications:

This procedure is contraindicated in the acute phase of urinary tract infection and in urethral obstruction.

2. Preparation:
   A. Obtain a gas cystometer, a cystometric set, a 16F catheter (smaller for children), and an irrigation solution of sterile 0.9% saline or sterile, distilled water.
   B. The client should disrobe below the waist or wear a gown.
3. Procedure:
   A. The client urinates into a funnel attached to a machine that plots the amount, flow, and time of voiding on a graph.
   B. Residual urine volume, if any, is then measured via the insertion of an indwelling catheter.
   C. As the client lies in a supine position, thermal sensation is evaluated by the client's reported sensations in response to the instillation of 30–60 ml of room-temperature 0.9% sterile saline solution, followed by 30–60 ml of 29–32°C, 0.9% sterile saline solution through the catheter into the bladder.
   D. The fluid is then drained from the bladder.
   E. The client's sensations to bladder filling are measured next by connecting the catheter to a cystometer and instilling measured amounts of sterile fluid or carbon dioxide into the bladder.
   F. The cystometer measures and graphically records bladder pressure and volume, along with the client's reported descriptions of sensations, such as when he or she first feels the urge to void or feels unable to go any longer without voiding, and any reported discomfort.
   G. The instillation is stopped when the client feels uncomfortably full or if it is determined that there is an absence of filling sensation.
   H. The air or fluid and catheter are re-

moved or the client may be asked to void the fluid.
   I. The test may be repeated in standing or sitting positions or after the administration of bladder tone stimulants such as bethanechol chloride.
4. Postprocedure care:
   A. Encourage the oral intake of fluids when not contraindicated; 125 ml/hour for 24 hours is desirable.
   B. Monitor fluid intake and urine output for 24 hours.
   C. Observe for urinary retention, symptoms of urinary tract infection (fever; chills; tachycardia; tachypnea; abdominal, suprapubic, or flank pain; hesitancy and frequency; dysuria; and hematuria).
   D. Hematuria for more than 4–6 hours is abnormal. More postprocedure discomfort may be experienced after carbon dioxide instillation than after irrigant instillation.
   E. Analgesics may be prescribed for bladder spasms.
5. Client and family teaching:
   A. You must lie very still during the test.
   B. You may experience bladder spasms and see blood in your urine after the procedure. Spasms occurring for longer than 24 hours or bloody urine for more than 4–6 hours is abnormal. Call the physician if either of these occurs.
6. Factors that affect results:
   A. Antihistamines may interfere with bladder function by causing relaxation.
   B. Movement during the test may interfere with bladder reflexes.
7. Other data:
   A. None.

Bibliography:

Palmer MA, Desmond AD: Simultaneous measurement of urethral opening pressure and urethral cross-sectional area during voiding cystometry. Br J Urol 73(3):275–278, 1994.

Wall LL, Wiskind AK, Taylor PA: Simple bladder filling with a cough stress test compared with subtracted cystometry for the diagnosis of urinary incontinence. Am J Obstet Gynecol 171(6): 1472–1477, discussion 1477–1479, 1994

Yeung CK, Godley ML, Duffy PG, Ransley PG: Natural filling cystometry in infants and children. Br J Urol 75(4):531–537, 1995.

CYSTOSCOPY, DIAGNOSTIC

Norm: Normal structure and function of the bladder; absence of strictures, tumors, or bladder calculi; and absence of inflammation or purulent secretions.

Usage: Evaluation and differentiation of urinary tract disorders, method for obtaining bladder and ureteral biopsies, sometimes used for excision of small tumors, and evaluation of suspected urinary tract malformation in children.

Description: Cystoscopy is the direct, transurethral visualization of the bladder and urethra with the use of a lighted, magnifying cystoscope with a variety of lenses. The cystoscope is a metal instrument with a solid obturator that is placed inside a sheath within the urethra. Flexible cystoscopy is becoming more widely used as an alternative to rigid cystoscopy. Cystoscopy is indicated after other tests such as cystography show abnormalities, or for symptoms such as dysuria, frequency, or incontinence. The procedure may be performed in a hospital or in a physician's office.

Professional Considerations:

1. Consent form IS required.

Risks:

Bleeding, infection, urinary tract obstruction.

Contraindications:

Acute inflammations of the urethral passage. Sedatives are contraindicated in clients with central nervous system depression.

2. Preparation:
   A. *See Client and family teaching.*
   B. Obtain a cystoscopy tray, disinfectant or surgical scrub solution, a genitourinary irrigant, drapes, sterile gloves, a cystoscope and light source, urethral dilators (sounds), filiforms and followers, and two or three sterile specimen containers (for possible biopsy, urine for culture and sensitivity, and a urine sample for cytology).
   C. A sedative may be prescribed.
   D. The client should disrobe below the waist or wear a gown.
   E. Obtain baseline vital signs.
   F. Pad the lithotomy stirrups.
   G. Have emergency equipment readily available.
3. Procedure:
   A. The client is positioned in the supine position on the cystoscopic table for possible administration of general or regional anesthesia.
   B. The client is then placed in the lithotomy position for external genitalia cleansing and draping and cystoscopic examination.
   C. After local anesthesia (if used) is instilled into the bladder and retained for a few minutes, the urethra is progressively dilated, and a cystoscope is inserted through the urethra.
   D. Urine specimens for culture or cytology may be removed through the cystoscope.
   E. The bladder is filled with genitourinary irrigant solution and the lighted cystoscope is used with magnification to directly examine the interior walls, structures, and contents of the bladder.
   F. The bladder is inspected for tumors, calculi, diverticula, obstructions, and strictures.
   G. A biopsy of the bladder or ureters may be taken, and tiny tumors may also be excised through the cystoscope, with bleeding controlled via electrocautery.
4. Postprocedure care:
   A. For general anesthesia, monitor vital signs every 15 minutes × 4, then every 30 minutes × 2, then every 2 hours × 2. Typical postanesthesia monitoring also includes continuous ECG monitoring and pulse oximetry, with continual assessments (q 5–15 minutes) of airway and neurologic status, until the client is lying quietly awake, is breathing independently, and responds appropriately to commands spoken in a normal tone.
   B. For local anesthesia, assist the client to a chair until strength has returned to baseline or for at least 30 minutes.
   C. Encourage oral intake of fluids: 125 ml/h × 24–48 hours when not contraindicated.
   D. Monitor fluid intake and urine output × 24 hours.
   E. Observe for urinary retention, or symptoms of urinary tract infection (fever, chills, pain [abdominal, suprapubic, or flank], tachypnea, tachycardia, hesitancy and frequency, dysuria, and hematuria). Notify the physician if any of these signs occur.
   F. Observe for hematuria. Pink urine is normal initially, but should clear. Frank hematuria or clotting is abnormal. Dysuria lasting more than 4–6 hours is abnormal.
   G. Analgesics may be prescribed for bladder spasms, and sitz or tub baths may help decrease generalized genital area discomfort.
   H. Resume diet.
5. Client and family teaching:
   A. Do not exercise vigorously for 14 days before the procedure.
   B. Arrange for someone to drive you home, as you will not be permitted to drive for 24 hours after the procedure.
   C. For general anesthesia, fast from food and fluids for 8 hours. For local anesthesia, consume only clear liquids for 8 hours. You may be required to take

in a large amount of fluids to promote urine flow during the procedure.

D. Clients receiving local anesthesia may feel the urge to void while the cysto-scope is in place.

E. After the procedure, drink 6–8 glasses of water or other fluids per day for 2 days (unless contraindicated). Watch for warning symptoms of complica-tions (see above). Report chills, fever, dysuria, or frank blood in the urine.

F. Do not have sexual relations until healing is confirmed by the physician.

6. Factors that affect results:
   A. None.
7. Other data:
   A. Urethroscopy or retrograde pyelogram may also be combined with cystoscopy.
   B. Cystoscopy may also be used as a ther-apeutic procedure to crush and re-move calculi, perform bladder irriga-tion, resect tumors, or perform a transurethral resection of the prostate gland.
   C. The use of intraurethral lidocaine gel has not been shown to decrease client pain during rigid cystoscopy. Anxiety has been shown to positively correlate with pain perception.

Bibliography:

Knoblauch NO, Rinning H, Knudsen P, Lund L, Nielsen KT: Routine use of ultrasound and flexi-ble cystoscopy in the control of benign bladder tumours. Int Urol Nephrol 26(4):431–436, 1994.

Madsen FA, Bruskewitz RC: Cystoscopy in the evalua-tion of benign prostatic hyperplasia. World J Urol 13(1):14–16, 1995.

O'Sullivan DC, Chilton CP: Flexible cystoscopy. Br J Hosp Med 51(7):340–345, 1994.

Rana A, Rashwan HM, West OF, Stow J, Ng PE, Chisholm GD: Air insufflation versus water irri-gation during flexible cystoscopy: a prospective randomized study. Br J Urol 74(3):311–314, 1994.

Stein M, Lubetkin D, Taub HC, Skinner WK, Haber-man J, Kreutzer ER: The effects of intraurethral lidocaine anesthetic and patient anxiety on pain perception during cystoscopy. J Urol 151(6): 1518–1521, 1994.

CYSTOURETHROGRAPHY, VOIDING, DIAGNOSTIC

Norm: Normal formation of bladder and urethra, normal excretion of con-trast medium through the urethra, and absence of retrograde movement of contrast medium into the ureters.

Usage: Detection of urinary tract con-genital anomalies, vesicoureteral re-flux, neurogenic abnormalities, enlarged prostate gland, urethral stric-tures, and bladder diverticula or polyps.

Description: Using fluoroscopy or radiography, voiding cystourethrogra-phy demonstrates the bladder filling via contrast medium instillation through a catheter into the bladder and then shows exiting of the contrast medium during voiding.

Professional Considerations:

1. Consent form IS required.

Risks:

Bleeding, hematuria, infection, urinary tract obstruction, allergic reaction to dye (itching, hives, rash, tight feeling in the throat, shortness of breath, bronchospasm, anaphylaxis, death), renal toxicity.

Contraindications:

Previous allergy to radiographic dye, iodine or shellfish; in the acute phase of a urinary tract infection; urinary tract obstruction; during pregnancy or breast-feeding; recent bladder surgery; and urethral obstruction, evulsion, or transection. Sedatives are contraindicated in clients with central nervous system depression.

2. Preparation:
   A. *See Client and family teaching.*
   B. Obtain a balloon catheter, a contrast medium, and a syringe or tubing for instillation of the contrast medium.
   C. The client should disrobe below the waist.
   D. A sedative may be prescribed. Elder & Longenecker (1995) demonstrated safety of Midazolam use for excessively frightened children undergoing void-ing cystourethrography.
   E. Have emergency equipment readily available.

3. Procedure:
   A. After the client is positioned supine, a balloon catheter is inserted through the urethra into the bladder and the balloon is inflated.
   B. The bladder is filled with contrast medium via gravity or syringe instilla-tion and the catheter is clamped.
   C. Radiographic or fluoroscopic films of the lower urinary tract are taken with the client in several positions.
   D. The catheter is then removed and the client must void in a right-sided or left-sided position with the lower leg flexed at the hip. Male testes should be shielded by lead before voiding begins.
   E. Several more radiographic or fluoro-scopic films of the lower urinary tract are taken during voiding.
   F. If the client is unable to void, the blad-

der area is gently pressed to stimulate voiding.

4. Postprocedure care:
   A. Encourage oral intake of fluids, 125 ml/hour × 24 hours when this is not contraindicated.
   B. Monitor fluid intake and urine output for quantity and hematuria × 24 hours. Hematuria or dysuria that lasts more than 4–6 hours is abnormal.
   C. Observe for signs of allergic reaction to the dye (listed above) × 24 hours.
   D. Observe for urinary retention, or symptoms of urinary tract infection (fever, chills, pain [abdominal, suprapubic, or flank], tachypnea, tachycardia, hesitancy and frequency, dysuria, and hematuria). Notify physician for anuria × 8 hours, or for any of the above signs.
   E. Analgesics may be prescribed for bladder spasms, and sitz or tub baths may help decrease generalized genital area discomfort.

5. Client and family teaching:
   A. You should arrange for someone to drive you home.
   B. A clear liquid diet and a cathartic may be prescribed the day before the exam.
   C. The urge to void during the procedure is normal.
   D. Drink 6–8 glasses of water or other fluids per day for 2 days (unless contraindicated). Watch for warning symptoms of complications (see above). Report chills, fever, dysuria, or frank blood in the urine.

6. Factors that affect results:
   A. Although the clearest films result from the recumbent position, standing films are sometimes used for clients unable to void while lying down.
   B. Intestinal barium studies within 1 week prior to the test or the presence of a large amount of gas in the lower bowel may inhibit the clarity of the films.

7. Other data:
   A. None.

Bibliography:

Brown FL: Voiding cystourethrography. In Hamilton HK, Cahill M (eds): Diagnostics, 2nd ed. Springhouse, PA, Springhouse Corporation, 1986, pp 988–990.

Dardenne AN: Anaphylactoid reactions during voiding cystourethrography [letter]. Am J Roentgenol 164(6):1551–1552, 1995.

Elder JS, Longenecker R: Premedication with oral midazolam for voiding cystourethrography in children: safety and efficacy. Am J Roentgenol 164(5):1229–1232, 1995.

Kleniman PK, Diamond DA, Karellas A, Spevak MR, Nimkin K, Belanger P: Tailored low-dose fluoroscopic voiding cystourethrography for the reevaluation of vesicourethral reflux in girls. Am J Roentgenol 162(5):1151–1154, 1994.

Mussurakis S, Sprigg A, Steiner M: Patterns of integration and clinical value of voiding cystourethrography in the work-up of urinary tract infection in children. Eur Urol 28(2):165–170, 1995.

CYSTS AND NIPPLE DISCHARGE, DIAGNOSTIC

(see Cytologic Study of Breast Cyst, Diagnostic; or Cytologic Study of Nipple Discharge, Diagnostic)

CYTOCHEMICAL STAIN

(see Leukocyte Cytochemistry, Specimen)

CYTOLOGIC STUDY, SPECIMEN

(see Bronchial Washing, Specimen, Diagnostic; Brushing Cytology, Specimen, Diagnostic; Cerebrospinal Fluid, Routine, Culture and Cytology, Specimen; Cytologic Study of Breast Cyst, Effusions, Gastrointestinal Tract, Nipple Discharge, Respiratory Tract, or Urine, Diagnostics; Needle Aspiration Cytology, Specimen; Ocular Cytology, Specimen; Oral Cavity Cytology, Specimen)

CYTOLOGIC STUDY OF BREAST CYST, DIAGNOSTIC

Norm: Absence of cells indicating malignancy or infection.

Usage: Determine if the breast lesion is a mass or a cyst, and determine if malignant cells are present.

Description: Breast cyst cytology is the microscopic study of the fluid or cells obtained by fine-needle aspiration. The lesion may have been detected by breast examination and/or mammogram. The fluid is fixed and examined by the cytologist on a microscopic slide. Any cells in the cyst fluid are studied for diagnosis of neoplasm, infective process, and, rarely, tuberculosis of the breast.

Professional Considerations:

1. Consent form NOT required. *See Needle Aspiration, Diagnostic* for procedure-specific risks and contraindications.
2. Preparation:
   A. Obtain a 21- or 23-gauge long needle, a 10-ml syringe, sterile 0.9% saline, a red- or marble-top glass tube or gold-seal plastic tube, and a clean jar.
   B. The client should disrobe above the waist.
   C. Position the client for comfort and accessibility to the cyst and drape him or her for privacy.

3. Procedure:
   A. The aspiration site is identified. The skin is cleansed with an alcohol wipe and allowed to dry.
   B. The suspect mass is immobilized by one hand, while the needle is inserted with the other hand.
   C. Fluid is aspirated by drawing back on the syringe.
   D. A fluid drop is placed on a clean slide and the thin edge of a second slide is used to produce a smear.
   E. The slide is then fixed immediately in 95% ethyl alcohol in a clean jar.
   F. If more than a minute amount of fluid has been aspirated, place the remaining fluid in a red- or marble-top tube.
   G. If the specimen is minute, rinse the needle with 10 ml of sterile 0.9% saline and place the rinsed material into the tube.
   H. Label the slide and the aspirate or wash with the client's name, and indicate the specimen source, noting which breast.
4. Postprocedure care:
   A. Apply pressure to the aspiration site for a short time.
   B. Write the pertinent clinical information on the laboratory requisition.
   C. Send the specimens to the laboratory for immediate evaluation.
5. Client and family teaching:
   A. This is the diagnostic procedure of choice for breast cysts in pregnant women because there are no x-rays or anesthesia required.
   B. This is a sterile procedure that takes approximately 10 minutes, with minimal discomfort.
   C. Watch the area for the next 72 hours for redness, drainage, and swelling, and check for fever over 101°F (38.3°C); report any of these signs to the physician or nurse.
   D. Results are normally available within 48 hours.
6. Factors that affect results:
   A. Immediate fixation of the smear prevents drying of the sample and distortion of the findings due to contamination.
   B. Some cytologists prefer specimens that were allowed to dry before being placed in the fixative. These should be specifically labeled, as they are stained differently for study.
   C. An insufficient sample may result when the breast lesion is not penetrated or it contains no fluid.
7. Other data:
   A. Aspiration is an inexpensive screening procedure for evaluating breast lesions. It decreases the necessity of open surgical biopsy for a definitive diagnosis.
   B. This test is more reliable than nipple discharge cytology for ruling out neoplasms.

C. Culture of the aspirate is usually obtained for a complete work-up.

Bibliography:

Chalas E, Valea F: The gynecologist and surgical procedures for breast disease [review]. Clin Obstet Gynecol *37*(4):948–953, 1994.

de la Torre M, Lindholm K, Lindgran A: Fine needle aspiration cytology of tubular breast carcinoma and radial scar. Acta Cytol *38*(6):884–890, 1994.

Hindle WH, Payne PA, Pan EY: The use of fine-needle aspiration in the evaluation of persistent palpable dominant breast masses [see comments]. Am J Obstet Gynecol *168*(6, Pt 1):1818–1819, 1993.

Sagin HB, Kiroglu Y, Aksoy F: Hydatid cyst of the breast diagnosed by fine needle aspiration biopsy. A case report. Acta Cytologica *38*(6):965–967, 1994.

CYTOLOGIC STUDY OF EFFUSIONS, DIAGNOSTIC

Norm: No tumor cells or infection.

Usage: Gout, lymphoproliferative disease, infections of and/or fistulas into serous cavities, metabolic arthritis, metastatic neoplasms, myeloproliferative disease, rheumatoid arthritis, rheumatoid pleuritis, systemic lupus erythematosus, and pulmonary TB.

Description: An effusion is an abnormal collection of fluid occurring most commonly in the pericardial sac, abdomen, pleural space, and synovial cavities. Effusions may be transudate due to hydrostatic pressure differences or exudate due to tumors or infective processes. Effusion cytology is the microscopic study of the fluid aspirate of the particular effusion used to differentiate the cause and type of effusion and to characterize and identify the source of infection or the tumor type.

Professional Considerations:

1. Consent form IS required for the procedure used to obtain the specimen. See individual procedures for procedure-specific risks and contraindications.
2. Preparation:
   A. Check PT and PTT. This procedure may be contraindicated in clients with coagulation defects.
   B. Obtain the appropriate procedure tray, sterile gloves and drapes, povidone-iodine solution, and 1–2% Xylocaine. If a large effusion is to be drained, obtain a heparinized vacuum bottle, and tubing with a clamp or stopcock.
   C. Obtain baseline vital signs.
   D. For a pericardiocentesis, monitor ECG continuously throughout the procedure.
   E. For small or loculated effusions, an ultrasound or CT guided tap will in-

crease the chance of obtaining a specimen.

3. Procedure:
   A. Position the client appropriately for the procedure to be performed.
   B. Cleanse the aspiration site and surrounding skin with povidone-iodine solution and allow it to dry.
   C. Overlay the aspiration site with sterile drapes.
   D. Obtain two 3- to 10-ml samples of fluid using a sterile technique via arthrocentesis, pericardiocentesis, paracentesis, or thoracentesis. Place one specimen in a heparinized tube and one in a nonheparinized tube for evaluation and cytology.

4. Postprocedure care:
   A. For a thoracentesis, a postprocedure chest x-ray MUST be performed to check for a possible pneumothorax.
   B. Monitor vital signs for indications of bleeding or hemodynamic changes.
   C. Write the name, date, source of fluid, and symptoms on the laboratory requisition.
   D. Send the specimen to the laboratory immediately. Refrigerate specimens not examined immediately.

5. Client and family teaching:
   A. This is a sterile procedure that takes up to 1 hour and may include moderate discomfort.
   B. It is very important to stay as still as possible during the procedure to avoid injury and complications.
   C. Results are normally available within 72 hours.

6. Factors that affect results:
   A. Results are most accurate when the specimen is examined within 1 hour of collection.

7. Other data:
   A. This method is usually more sensitive than blind biopsy for diagnosis of pleural malignancies.

Bibliography:

Chiyoda S, Kinoshita T, Miwa M: Monoclonal integration of HTLV-1 in pleural effusion cells in a seropositive patient with tuberculosis pleuritis. Int J Hematol 61(1):35–38, 1995.

Garcia LW, Ducatman BS, Wang HH: The value of multiple fluid specimens in the cytological diagnosis of malignancy. Mod Pathol 7(6):665–668, 1994.

McCalmont TH, McLeod DL, Kerr RM, Hopkins MB, Geisinger KR: Fatal disseminated herpesvirus infection with hepatitis. A peritoneal fluid cytologic warning. Arch Pathol Lab Med 118(5):566–567, 1994.

Ruitenbeek T, Gouw AG, Poppema S: Immunocytology of body cavity fluids. MOC-31, a monoclonal antibody discriminating between mesothelial and epithelial cells. Arch Pathol Lab Med 118(3):265–269, 1994.

Stewart RJ, Perry K, Bowie RD, O'Dea DJ: Peritoneal cytology for suspected acute appendicitis: an economic evaluation. Health Econ 3(5):321–332, 1994.

CYTOLOGIC STUDY OF GASTROINTESTINAL TRACT, DIAGNOSTIC

Norm: Normal cells of the gastrointestinal tract. No tumor cells or infection.

Usage: Cytologic examination of exfoliation of the mucosa of the gastrointestinal tract to diagnose benign, precancerous, or malignant lesions of the esophagus, stomach, and duodenum. Also for amyloidosis, microscopic colitis, Crohn's disease, granulomatous inflammation, gastritis, *Helicobacter pylori*, leiomyosarcoma, lymphoma, intestinal spirochetosis, melanosis coli, Mélétrier's disease, pernicious anemia, schistosomiasis, toxic drug effect on gastric mucosa, and Whipple's disease.

Description: Brushings or fine-needle aspirations of the mucosa of the upper gastrointestinal tract are performed during endoscopic examination. Washings of the mucosa for a specimen via a nasogastric tube may be performed when endoscopy is not available or is contraindicated and neoplasm is clinically suspected. Brushings of the colon or rectum can be made via proctosigmoidoscopy.

Professional Considerations:

1. Consent form NOT required for nasogastric tube method. Consent form IS required for endoscopy and sigmoidoscopy.

Risks:

See individual procedures for risks and contraindications.

Contraindications:

Severe gastrointestinal bleeding, varices (gastric or esophageal), and clients who are unable to cooperate.

2. Preparation:
   A. Preschedule this test with the laboratory.
   B. If colon washing is to be performed, administer oral cathartic as prescribed and collect the last bowel movement prior to the test to send to the laboratory with the washing specimen.
   C. For collection of gastric washings for cytology, obtain a nasogastric (NG) tube, a lubricant, 0.9% saline, a syringe, a 500-ml clean container, a 50% ethyl alcohol fixative, and dry ice.

D. For collection of endoscopic brushings for cytology, obtain endoscopic equipment, a brush, glass slides labeled with the client's name, a clean container of 95% alcohol or other fixative required by the specific laboratory, and dry ice or 50% ethyl alcohol.

E. For colon washing, obtain enema tube, 0.9% saline, a large airtight plastic container, and dry ice or 50% ethyl alcohol.

F. *See Upper Gastro-Duodeno-Jejunoscopy, Diagnostic; Barium Enema, Diagnostic; Proctoscopy, Diagnostic; or Sigmoidoscopy, Diagnostic* for other preparations, as would be appropriate for the procedure being performed.

3. Procedure:

   A. *Gastric washing:*

      i. Insert a nasogastric tube.

      ii. Withdraw gastric contents with a Toomey syringe and discard.

      iii. Instill 300–500 ml of 0.9% saline solution into the stomach through the NG tube.

      iv. Have the client roll 360° four or five times.

      v. Aspirate all the gastric contents into a clean, sealed container.

   B. *Endoscopic brushings for cytology:*

      i. During endoscopy, a brushing is taken from specific lesions of the esophagus, the stomach, or the duodenal area.

      ii. The brush should be rolled onto a slide to cover at least a 1.5-cm diameter area.

      iii. The slide should be immediately placed into a container of 95% ethyl alcohol or other required fixative.

   C. *Colon washing:* Colon washing is performed just prior to barium enema washing.

      i. Insert the enema tubing into the colon through the rectum.

      ii. Instill 100 ml of 0.9% saline solution through the tubing.

      iii. Have the client roll 360° several times.

      iv. Drain the fluid out of the enema tubing and instill it into an airtight container.

   D. *Colon or rectal brushing:*

      i. Insert the proctoscope or sigmoidoscope.

      ii. Take a brushing from the lesion sites.

      iii. The brush should be rolled onto a slide to cover at least a 1.5-cm diameter area.

4. Postprocedure care:

   A. Either pack the specimen in dry ice or preserve it with 50% ethyl alcohol.

   B. Write the time and source of the specimen collection on the laboratory requisition. Each separate brushing sample

should be labeled with the anatomic site of collection.

C. Transport the specimen to the cytotechnologist in the pathology laboratory immediately for fixing and microscopic examination.

D. Remove the nasogastric or enema tube.

E. Resume normal diet.

F. *See Upper Gastro-Duodeno-Jejunoscopy, Diagnostic; Barium Enema, Diagnostic; Proctoscopy, Diagnostic; or Sigmoidoscopy, Diagnostic* for other postprocedure care, as appropriate for the procedure being performed.

5. Client and family teaching:

   A. Eat a soft diet for the evening meal prior to the test.

   B. Fast from food for 8–12 hours and from water for 1 hour before the procedure.

6. Factors that affect results:

   A. Washings may be performed twice. Discarding the first aspirate and sending the second aspirate for study may be more reliable, especially for gastric neoplasms.

   B. Contamination of the specimen with food or barium invalidates the results.

   C. Reject specimens not packed in dry ice or not received promptly after collection.

   D. Reject slides that were allowed to dry before fixing, or those received without fixative.

   E. Reject unlabeled slides.

7. Other data:

   A. This is not as effective a diagnostic tool as radiography or endoscopy with biopsy.

   B. A negative report does not rule out malignancy.

   C. Gastroscopy-guided brushings are preferable to gastric washings for cytologic study.

   D. Proctosigmoidoscopic smears to investigate diarrhea should be performed with no preparation of the bowel as the exudate may be washed away, the mucosa distorted, trauma of the mucosa induced, or the evidence of disease obscured or altered.

Bibliography:

Das DK, Pant CS: Fine needle aspiration cytologic diagnosis of gastrointestinal tract lesions. A study of 78 cases. Acta Cytol 38(5):723–729, 1994.

Debongnie JC, Mairesse J, Donnay M, Dekoninck X: Touch cytology. A quick, simple, sensitive screening test in the diagnosis of infections of the gastrointestinal mucosa. Arch Pathol Lab Med 118(11):1115–1118, 1994.

O'Donoghue JM, Horgan PG, O'Donohoe MK, Byrne J, O'Hanlon DM, McGuire M, Given HF: Adjunctive endoscopic brush cytology in the detection of upper gastrointestinal malignancy. Acta Cytol 39(1):28–34, 1995.

CYTOLOGIC STUDY OF NIPPLE DISCHARGE, DIAGNOSTIC

Norm: Absence of tumor cells or infection.

Usage: Diagnosis of inflammatory disease, intraductal papilloma, mammary dysplasia with ectasia of the ducts, metastasis or suspected malignancy of the breast, and papillomatosis.

Description: Nipple discharge is considered abnormal except in lactating or pregnant women, although some discharge is caused by medication. Several nipple discharge smears are fixed on glass slides and microscopically studied for the presence of abnormal cells indicating neoplasm or infection, and rarely, tuberculosis of the breast.

Professional Considerations:

1. Consent form NOT required.
2. Preparation:
   A. Explain the procedure. The client who assists should hold the fixative bottle under the breast so that the slide can be immediately placed in the fixative.
   B. Obtain warmed sterile saline, 6–12 clean glass slides, 6–12 clean glass bottles of 95% ethyl alcohol, labels, and cotton or gauze.
   C. The client should disrobe above the waist.
   D. Position the client so it is convenient to obtain the specimen, and drape him or her for privacy.
3. Procedure:
   A. Vigorously cleanse the nipple, then soak it in warm saline on a cotton or gauze pad for 10–15 minutes and pat it dry.
   B. Gently strip the subareolar area with a thumb and forefinger, moving toward the nipple tip. Continue until a pea-sized droplet of fluid is expressed.
   C. Place the frosted side of a clean glass microscope slide on the nipple and quickly slide it across the nipple tip to obtain a smear of fluid.
   D. Immediately place the slide into a small jar of 95% ethyl alcohol fixative.
   E. Label the jar with the number of the smear and whether it was taken from the right or left breast. This is especially important when both breasts are studied.
   F. Repeat steps 3A–E until four to six slides from each breast are obtained, if possible.
4. Postprocedure care:
   A. Write a description of the discharge and the client's name, age, clinical symptoms, and which breast is being studied on the laboratory requisition.
   B. Send the specimens to the laboratory immediately.
   C. Cleanse the breast and nipple as needed.
5. Client and family teaching:
   A. The procedure takes about 10 minutes.
   B. Results are normally available within 48 hours.
   C. About 3% of breast cancers and 10% of benign lesions of the breast are associated with nipple discharge. Negative cytology does not rule out a malignancy.
6. Factors that affect results:
   A. Immediate fixation of the smear prevents drying of the sample and distortion of the findings due to contamination.
   B. Several (rather than 1 or 2) slides improve results because later smears include more abnormal cells, if present.
   C. Medications that affect hormonal balance and that may cause nipple discharge include chlorpromazines, digitalis, diuretics, oral contraceptives, phenothiazines, and steroids.
7. Other data:
   A. Mammography and biopsy or aspiration are more reliable diagnostic procedures for breast malignancy.

Bibliography:

Carty NJ, Mudan SS, Ravichandran D, Royle GT, Taylor I: Prospective study of outcome in women presenting with nipple discharge. Ann Coll Surg Engl 76(6):387–389, 1994.

Hou MF, Huang TJ, Huang YS, Hsieh JS: A simple method of duct cannulation and localization for galactography before excision in patients with nipple discharge. Radiology 195(2):568–569, 1995.

Motomura K, Koyama H, Noguchi S, Inaji H, Azuma C: Detection of c-erbB-2 gene amplification in nipple discharge by means of polymerase chain reaction. Breast Cancer Res Treat 33(1):89–92, 1995.

Ohuchi N, Furuta A, Mori S: Management of ductal carcinoma in situ with nipple discharge. Intraductal spreading of carcinoma is an unfavorable pathologic factor for breast-conserving surgery. Cancer 74(4):1294–1302, 1994.

CYTOLOGIC STUDY OF RESPIRATORY TRACT, DIAGNOSTIC

Norm: Negative.

Usage: Diagnosis of respiratory neoplasms or premalignant cell changes related to chronic inflammation, inhaled toxins, tuberculosis, or asthma; and diagnosis of respiratory bacterial, viral, or parasitic infections.

Description: Respiratory tract cytology is the microscopic study of the number and type of cells of the respiratory tract and/or sputum to detect the presence of cells abnormal for that specimen, including tumor or pretumor cells or evidence of an infective process. Any anomalies of cells are correlated to clinical data for diagnosis.

Professional Considerations:

1. Consent form NOT required unless the sample for study is obtained via bronchoscopy.
2. Preparation:
   A. An aerosol treatment just prior to specimen collection may help to mobilize respiratory secretions.
3. Procedure:
   A. Three early-morning specimens are obtained.
   B. Have the client rinse the mouth with water.
   C. Instruct the client to inhale deeply and then exhale with a deep, expulsive cough, and expectorate sputum directly into a sterile, wide-mouthed container.
   D. Alternatively, bronchial secretions may be removed directly during bronchoscopy or via nasotracheal suctioning using a specimen trap.
4. Postprocedure care:
   A. Write the client's name, the date, the specimen source, the specimen number, the diagnosis, and the clinical symptoms on the laboratory requisition.
   B. Send the specimen to the laboratory immediately.
5. Client and family teaching:
   A. Results are normally available within 72 hours.
   B. To produce a deep sputum specimen, rather than saliva, take several deep breaths, without fully exhaling between them. When you feel as though you cannot take any more breaths, cough out forcefully and catch the sputum in the sterile cup.
   C. The results may have to be confirmed via culture or biopsy.
6. Factors that affect results:
   A. The results are most accurate when examined within 1 hour of collection.
   B. The results are invalid if the sample is saliva, rather than respiratory secretions.
7. Other data:
   A. About 15% of results are false-negatives.
   B. Sputum cytology is more likely to be negative in a client with small cell carcinoma than in one with non-small cell carcinoma of the lung.
   C. Culture and/or biopsy are usually more reliable than cytology for diagnosis of respiratory tract neoplasm or infection.

Bibliography:

Konstan MW, Hilliard KA, Norvell TM, Berger M: Bronchoalveolar lavage findings in cystic fibrosis patients with stable, clinically mild lung disease suggest ongoing infection and inflammation. [Published erratum appears in Am J Respir Crit Care Med 151(1):260.] Am J Respir Crit Care Med 150(2):448–454, 1994.

Maesaki S, Kohno S, Mashimoto H, Araki J, Asai S, Hara K: Detection of *Cryptococcus neoformans* in bronchial lavage cytology: report of four cases. Intern Med 34(1):54–57, 1995.

Piaton E, Grillet-Ravigneaux MH, Saugier B, Pellet H: Prospective study of combined use of bronchial aspirates and biopsy specimens in diagnosis and typing of centrally located lung tumors. Br Med J 310(6980):624–627, 1995.

Redington AE, Springall DR, Ghatei MA, Lau LC, Bloom SR, Holgate ST, Polak JM, Howarth PH: Endothelia in bronchoalveolar lavage fluid and its relation to airflow obstruction in asthma. Am J Respir Crit Care Med 151(4):1034–1039, 1995.

Sutinen S, Riska H, Backman R, Sutinen SH, Froseth B: Alveolar lavage fluid (ALF) of normal volunteer subjects: cytologic, immunocytochemical, and biochemical reference values. Respir Med 89(2):85–92, 1995.

CYTOLOGIC STUDY OF URINE, DIAGNOSTIC

Norm: Normal type and amount of squamous and epithelial cells of the urinary tract and little or no cellular debris; red blood cell count (RBC) ≤ 3; white blood cell count (WBC) ≤ 4; no abnormal cells such as cytomegalic inclusion bodies, malignant cells, parasites, or yeasts.

Usage: Anemia (hemolytic), cerebral metachromatic leukodystrophy, cytomegalovirus infection (cytomegalic inclusion bodies), measles (cytomegalic inclusion bodies), renal hemosiderosis, screening for premalignant cell changes, transplant rejection, urinary tract infections (herpes virus, fungal, schistosoma, others), urinary tract inflammation (epithelial cells, RBC, WBC), and urinary tract primary or metastatic cancer (malignant cells).

Description: Urine cytology is the microscopic study of cells in urine to detect the presence of abnormal cells, including tumor or pretumor cells or evidence of an infective process. Any abnormalities found are correlated to clinical data for a diagnosis of urinary tract neoplasm, infection, or other diseases that may affect the urine.

Professional Considerations:

1. Consent form NOT required.
2. Preparation:
   A. Obtain a sterile container.

B. Hydrate the client ½ to 1 hour prior to specimen collection.

3. Procedure:
   A. Urine cytology involves centrifuging and filtering the urine, or cytocentrifuging, staining, and examining the filtered sediment.
   B. For a voided specimen, have the client urinate directly into a sterile container. Tightly cover the container.
   C. Catheterization may be used if it is otherwise difficult to obtain the specimen or if a high urinary tract lesion is suspected.

4. Postprocedure care:
   A. Send the specimen to the laboratory immediately.

5. Client and family teaching:
   A. Discard the first morning void if collecting the sample in the morning. With the next void, urinate directly into the container, then cap it tightly.
   B. Results are normally available within 48 hours.

6. Factors that affect results:
   A. An early-morning specimen is unsuitable, as cell death occurs in the bladder overnight.
   B. Recent instrumentation may cause cell injury or changes that give false-positive results.
   C. Hypotonic solutions used as washing during cystourethroscopy procedures may alter the results by directly affecting cell structure and appearance.
   D. Chemotherapeutic agents such as cyclophosphamide may alter the results.

7. Other data:
   A. A voided specimen is preferred except when specific study of high urinary tract areas is needed. Urine from each ureter may be studied and compared.
   B. Cytomegalovirus (CMV) can be diagnosed via urine cytology. Several specimens are recommended because cytomegalovirus is not shed continuously. The presence of CMV in the urine may indicate CMV disease or an asymptomatic reactivation of CMV disease.

Bibliography:

Burrows L, Knight R, Kupfer S, Panico M, Palearas A, Solomon M: The diagnostic accuracy of urine cytological analysis in the rapid assessment of acute renal allograft dysfunction. Transplant Proc 27(1):1044–1045, 1995.

Meloni AM, Peier AM, Haddad FS, Powell IJ, Block AW, Huben RP, Todd I, Potter W, Sandberg AA: A new approach in the diagnosis and follow-up of bladder cancer. FISH analysis of urine, bladder washings, and tumors. Cancer Genet Cytogenet 71(2):105–118, 1993.

Radio SJ, Stratta RJ, Linder J, Wisecarver JL, Taylor RJ, Markin RS: Histological confirmation of acute rejection detected by urine cytology in pancreas transplant recipients. Transplant Proc 26(2):529–530, 1994.

Roberti I, Reisman L, Burrows L, Lieberman KV: Urine cytology and urine flow cytometry in renal trans-

plantation—a prospective double blind study. Transplantation 59(4):495–500, 1995.

Rupp M, O'Hara B, McCullough L, Saxena S, Olchiewski J: Prostatic carcinoma cells in urine specimens. Cytopathology 5(3):164–170, 1994.

CYTOLOGY, SPECIMEN
(see Cytologic Study, Specimen)

CYTOLOGY, URINE
(see Cytologic Study of Urine, Diagnostic)

CYTOMEGALIC INCLUSION DISEASE, CYTOLOGY, URINE

Norm: Negative for inclusion body cells.

Positive: Cytomegalovirus infections of a disseminated type.

Description: Cytomegalovirus is a member of the herpesvirus family and causes cytomegalic inclusion disease, a generalized infection of infants and small children caused by intrauterine, natal, or postnatal exposure to infected secretions (blood, cervical secretions, urine, saliva, breast milk, or semen). The mode of transmission to immunocompromised clients is unknown. Cytomegalic inclusion disease symptoms may range from none in healthy-appearing children to generalized symptoms of a severe infection, and is characterized by the presence of intranuclear or intracellular inclusion bodies in the kidney that are excreted in the urine. The disease may also affect the salivary glands, lung, liver, pancreas, and brain, where inclusion bodies may also be found. Severe symptoms may be fatal.

Professional Considerations:
1. Consent form NOT required.
2. Preparation:
   A. Obtain a clean-catch urine kit.
   B. Hydrate the client for ½ to 1 hour.
   C. The specimen should be obtained at least 3 hours after the last void, but should not be the first morning void.
3. Procedure:
   A. Urine cytology involves centrifuging and filtering the urine, or cytocentrifuging, staining, and examining the filtered sediment.
   B. The clean-catch urine technique must be used to decrease the risk of specimen contamination. *See clean-catch collection instructions in the test Body Fluid, Routine, Culture.*

C. A fresh specimen may be taken from a clean urinary drainage bag.

4. Postprocedure care:
   A. Send the specimen to the laboratory immediately.

5. Client and family teaching:
   A. Provide collection instructions (above) if the client will be obtaining the specimen independently.
   B. This test is one of the most reliable and rapid methods for diagnosing cytomegalovirus infection. Several specimens are recommended because cytomegalovirus is not shed continuously.

6. Factors that affect results:
   A. Specimens should be tested within 6 hours.

7. Other data:
   A. Cytomegalic inclusion bodies are often found in clients with cancer undergoing chemotherapy and in transplant clients receiving immunosuppressive drugs.
   B. Inclusion bodies may also be found in smears and brushings from other sources, such as bronchoalveolar lavage fluid and biopsies of cytomegalovirus infected tissues.

Bibliography:

Abulafia D, DuBeshter B, Dawson AE, Sherer DM: Presence of cytomegalovirus inclusion bodies in a recurrent ulcerative vaginal lesion. Am J Obstet Gynecol *169*(5):1179–1180, 1993.

Bajanowski T, Wiegand P, Brinkmann B: Comparison of different methods for CMV detection. Int J Legal Med *106*(4):219–222, 1994.

Grefte A, van der Guessen M, van Son W, The TH: Circulating cytomegalovirus (CMV)-infected endothelial cells in patients with a active CMV infection. J Infect Dis *167*(2):270–277, 1993.

Teot LA, Ducatman BS, Giesinger KR: Cytologic diagnosis of cytomegaloviral esophagitis. A report of three acquired immunodeficiency syndrome-related cases. Acta Cytol *37*(1)93–96, 1993.

CYTOMEGALOVIRUS ANTIBODY, SERUM

Norm: Negative.

IgM   <1:8
IgH   <1:8 for those exposed
IgG   <1:16 for those exposed

Positive: A fourfold increase in the antibody titer between the acute and convalescent specimens or IgM >1:8 in a single specimen indicates a primary cytomegalovirus infective process. Cytomegalovirus (CMV) infections include congenital CMV, spontaneous CMV mononucleosis (heterophil-negative mononucleosis), post-transfusion CMV mononucleosis, and CMV in immunosuppressed clients. Disseminated infections may cause CMV retinitis, esophagitis, hepatitis, and ileocolitis.

Description: Cytomegalovirus is a herpes virus. The virus is present in a large segment of the population early in life without causing apparent disease. Serologic prevalence studies show that 60–90% of U.S. adults, depending on socioeconomic level, are positive for antibodies to CMV. Since the presence of disease is unusual, host factors predisposing to the disease should be investigated when the disease is manifested. CMV mononucleosis usually occurs in older adults compared to Epstein-Barr mononucleosis, and presents with a lower incidence of pharyngitis and lymphadenopathy. Congenital CMV may cause a variety of developmental abnormalities and neurologic deficits in the infant or young child. In the immunosuppressed client, pulmonary or systemic infections may occur. Clients receiving tissue transplants (liver, heart, lung, kidney, and bone) are also at high risk for manifested infections. CMV immune status should be performed on all organ transplant candidates before surgery. Blood for transfusion to seronegative transplant clients and all premature neonates should be from donors without CMV antibodies.

Professional Considerations:

1. Consent form NOT required.
2. Preparation:
   A. Tube: Red-top, red/gray-top, or gold-top.
3. Procedure:
   A. Draw a 3-ml blood sample. Label the tube as the acute sample.
   B. 10–14 days later, repeat the test and label the tube as the convalescent sample.
4. Postprocedure care:
   A. Results are normally available within 72 hours.
5. Client and family teaching:
   A. It is important to return in 10 days to 2 weeks for follow-up sampling to see if the infection is clearing up.
   B. Acyclovir, gancyclovir, and foscarnet are used for treatment of cytomegalovirus infections.
6. Factors that affect results:
   A. False-positive low titer results may occur in clients exposed to the Epstein-Barr virus, but a high titer confirms CMV. May also be falsely positive in those with rheumatoid factor in their serum.
7. Other data:
   A. The titer is not valid for the study of infants <6 months of age, because they may have maternal antibodies present in their serum.
   B. In a CMV-positive client, CMV may be

cultured from urine. The presence of the virus in the urine may indicate CMV disease or an asymptomatic reactivation of CMV. The finding of a positive CMV blood culture has a much higher correlation with the presence of CMV disease.

C. CMV antibody titers are of little value in determining the presence of CMV infection in immunocompromised clients because of the high incidence of CMV seropositive clients in the general public. Viral isolation is necessary for diagnosis.

Bibliography:

Gerna G, Sarasini A, Percivalle E, Zavattoni M, Baldanti F, Revello MG: Rapid screening for resistance to ganciclovir and foscarnet of primary isolates of human cytomegalovirus from culture-positive blood samples. J Clin Microbiol *33*(3): 738–741, 1995.

Hillyer CD, Emmens RK, Zago-Novaretti M, Berkman EM: Methods for the reduction of transfusion-transmitted cytomegalo-virus infection: filtration versus the use of seronegative donor units [review]. Transfusion *34*(10):929–934, 1994.

Newkirk MM, Watanabe Duffy KN, Leclerc J, Lambert N, Shiroky JB: Detection of cytomegalovirus, Epstein-Barr virus and herpes virus-6 in clients with rheumatoid arthritis with or without Sjögren's syndrome. Br J Rheumatol *33*(4):317–322, 1994.

St. George K, Rinaldo CR Jr.: Effects of enhancing agents on detection of cytomegalovirus in clinical specimens. J Clin Microbiol *32*(8):2024–2027, 1994.

D & C
(see Dilation and Curettage)

D-DIMER TEST (FIBRIN DEGRADATION FRAGMENT), BLOOD

Norm: 0–0.5 µg/mL

Positive: Indicates in vivo fibrinolytic activity.

Usage: Acute thrombosis, including arterial, coronary, pulmonary, and deep vein, defibrination therapy, disseminated intravascular coagulation, fibrinolysis (primary and secondary), fibrinolytic therapy post-operative, malignancy, pregnancy, (especially postpartum period), pre-eclampsia, sickle cell anemia vaso-occlusive crisis, surgery, and unstable angina.

Description: An assay to measure the amount of clot breakdown products specific for cross-linked fragments (D-dimer) derived from fibrin. The test can be performed on whole blood without the removal or interference of fibrinogen. It does not distinguish lysis of physiologic and pathologic thrombi, but distinguishes between fibrinogenolysis and fibrinolysis.

Professional Considerations:

1. Consent form NOT required.
2. Preparation:
   A. Tube: Blue-top if other coagulation tests are being drawn at the same time. Otherwise obtain a red-top, red/gray-top, or gold-top tube.
3. Procedure:
   A. Completely fill a blue-top tube or draw a 5-ml sample in a red-top, red/gray-top, or gold-top tube.

B. The specimen is stable for 8 hours at room temperature or for 6 months at –20° C.
4. Postprocedure care:
   A. Assess the client for other signs of thrombosis, emboli, or veno-occlusive disease.
5. Client and family teaching:
   A. Results are normally available within 48 hours.
6. Factors that affect results.
   A. D-dimer levels increase with increasing levels of tumor marker CA 125 in ovarian cancer, and with increasing titers of rheumatoid factors.
7. Other data:
   A. May be of use in veno-occlusive disease associated with sequelae of bone marrow transplant in oncology.

Bibliography:

Bouman CS, Ypma ST, Sybesma JP: Comparison of the efficacy of D-dimer, fibrin degradation products and prothrombin fragment 1+2 in clinically suspected deep venous thrombosis. Thromb Res *77*(3):225–234, 1995.

Ginsberg JS, Wells PS, Brill-Edwards P, Donovan D, Panju A, van Beek EJ, Patel A: Application of a novel and rapid whole blood assay for D-dimer in patients with clinically suspected pulmonary embolism. Thromb Haemost *73*(1):35–38, 1995.

Hager K, Platt D: Fibrin degeneration product concentrations (D-dimers) in the course of ageing. Gerontology *41*(3):159–165, 1995.

Panchenko E, Dobrovolsky A, Davletov K, Titaeva E, Kravets A, Podinovskaya J, Karpov Y: D-dimer and fibrinolysis in patients with various degrees of atherosclerosis. Eur Heart J *16*(1):38–42, 1995.

DEEP VEIN THROMBOSIS SCAN, DIAGNOSTIC
(see I-125-Labeled Fibrinogen Leg Scan, Diagnostic)

DEHYDROEPIANDROSTERONE SULFATE (DHEA-S), SERUM AND URINE, 24-HOUR

Norm:

		SI Units
Serum		
Adult female	0.5–2.8 µg/ml	
	or 200–800 ng/dl	
Premenopausal	60–340 µg/dl	1.6–8.9 µmol/L
	or 820–3380 ng/ml	
Postmenopausal	<130 µg/dl	
	or 100–610 ng/ml	
Pregnant (term)	230–1170 ng/ml	
Adult male	130–550 µg/dl	3.4–14.4 µmol/L
	or 270–1400 ng/dl	
Prepubertal male	2000–3350 ng/ml	
Newborn	1670–3640 ng/ml	
Child	100–600 ng/dl	
Urine		
Female	0.2–1.8 mg/day	0.7–6.2 µmol/day
Male	0.2–2 mg/day	0.7–6.9 µmol/day

Increased: Adrenal cortex adenoma and carcinoma, Cushing's disease, ectopic ACTH-producing tumors, female acne and hirsutism, oligomenorrhea in female athletes, polycystic ovarian syndrome, Stein-Leventhal syndrome, and virilizing congenital adrenal hyperplasia.

Decreased: Primary and secondary adrenal insufficiency. Low levels in amniotic fluid indicate anencephaly in the fetus.

Description: Dehydroepiandrosterone (DHEA-S) is the most abundant steroid in the circulation. It arises primarily from the adrenal cortex and is converted to testosterone. Although not androgenic itself, it is a specific and stable marker of adrenal androgen production. Levels are normally elevated in neonates and then decrease markedly until the age of 7. At puberty, increased levels of DHEA-S from the adrenals result in the axillary and pubic hair growth, preceding gonadal androgen secretion.

Professional Considerations:

1. Consent form NOT required.
2. Preparation:
   A. *Blood test:* Tube: Red-top, red/gray-top, gold-top, or green-top.
   B. *Urine test:* Obtain a 3-L, 24-hour urine jug without preservative.
3. Procedure:
   A. *Blood test:* Obtain a 1-ml blood sample.
   B. *Urine test:*
      i. Discard the first morning urine specimen.
      ii. Save all the urine voided for 24 hours. Include the urine voided at the end of the 24-hour period. For catheterized clients, keep the drainage bag on ice and empty urine into the collection container hourly.
4. Postprocedure care:
   A. Freeze the serum specimen if it is not tested within 1 hour.
   B. *Urine:*
      i. Compare the urine quantity in the specimen container with the urinary output record for the test. If the specimen contains less urine than was recorded as output, some urine may have been discarded, thus invalidating the test.
      ii. Document the quantity of urine output for the collection period on the laboratory requisition.
      iii. It is best to send the entire specimen to the laboratory so that it can be measured and mixed well before being tested.
5. Client and family teaching:
   A. Avoid radionuclide scans for 24 hours before this test.
   B. *Urine:* Save all the urine voided in the 24-hour period and urinate before defecating to avoid loss of urine. If any urine is accidentally discarded, discard the entire specimen and restart the collection the next day.

C. Results are normally available within 24 hours.

6. Factors that affect results:
   A. Radionuclides administered in the last 24 hours may increase results.
   B. Phenytoin and carbamazepine cause DHEA-S levels to decrease.

7. Other data:
   A. For those who exercise strenuously, such as marathon runners, DHEA-S levels will be elevated at the completion of the exercise period and for up to 36 hours after.
   B. Levels decline with age in men and women. Individuals differ in the amount of DHEA-S secreted and, for unknown reasons, DHEA-S levels positively correlate with longevity.

Bibliography:

Carmina E, Lobo RA: Evidence for increased androsterone metabolism in some normoandrogenic women with acne. J Clin Endocrinol Metab 76(5): 1111–1114, 1993.

Gilad S, Chayen R, Tordjman K, Kish E, Stern N: Assessment of 5 alpha-reductase activity in hirsute women: comparison of serum androstanediol glucuronide with urinary androsterone and aetiocholanolone excretion. Clin Endocrinol 40(4): 459–464, 1994.

Zwicker H, Rittmaster RS: Androsterone sulfate: physiology and clinical significance in hirsute women. J Clin Endocrinol Metab 76(1):112–116, 1993.

DENVER II DEVELOPMENTAL SCREENING TEST, DIAGNOSTIC

Norm: Infant or child is able to pass the age-related items.

Usage: Developmental screening and monitoring test for infants and children that can be used during pediatric health care visits and by public health nurses in well child clinics.

Description: The infant or child being test is observed for age-related items that measure gross motor, fine motor/adaptive, language, and cliental-social development. The test was first developed and used in 1967. It was revised in 1990 to make it more reliable and valid, to include infants under 30 months of age, and to include adjustments for cultural and ethnic differences. A parent questionnaire is part of the test, allowing parents to participate and give their input. It is recommended that these reported items also be observed during the testing.

Professional Considerations:

1. Consent form NOT required.
2. Preparation:
   A. Provide a quiet environment.
3. Procedure:
   A. Each child is observed/tested on items that are selected on the basis of chronological age.
   B. The full test takes about 30 minutes. A shorter version can be accomplished with a high rate of reliability for identifying abnormalities by selecting the three items in each sector that are closest to but not to the left of the age line.
4. Postprocedure care:
   A. Children who do not pass items all other children of their age are able to do should be considered for further evaluation.
   B. Mild development delays are noted by items in a "caution" category. These are items the child does not pass that are passed by 75–90% of children the same age.
   C. The test needs to be interpreted within the context of the overall progress and situation of the child.
5. Client and family teaching:
   A. The test usually takes less than 1 hour and helps identify potential developmental problems in the child.
   B. A parent or person familiar to the child will be asked to stay with the child during the screening.
   C. Results are completely available within 48 hours.
6. Factors that affect results:
   A. Environmental distractions interfere with validity of the results.
   B. Testing by untrained clients. Screening should be performed only by clients who have successfully completed a written and an observational proficiency test.
7. Other data:
   A. Accuracy can be improved by frequent rescreening.
   B. Rescreening at intervals may reinforce suspicions of developmental delay.
   C. Parents' opinions and concerns about their children's developmental skills and interests should be sought and addressed.

Bibliography:

Faller HS, Graham-Wilson P, Howlett MS: The McDenver at McDonald's. J Nurs Educ 32(1):40–41, 1993.

Frankenburg WK, Dodds J, Archer P, Bresnick B, Maschka P, Edelman N, Shapiro H: Denver II Technical Manual. Denver: Denver Developmental Materials, Inc., 1990a.

Frankenburg WK, Dodds J, Archer P, Bresnick B, Maschka P, Edelman N, Shapiro H: Denver II Screening Manual. Denver: Denver Developmental Materials, Inc., 1990b.

Wade G: Update on the Denver II. Pediatric Nurs 18(2):140–141, 1992.

11-DEOXYCORTISOL (COMPOUND S) TEST, DIAGNOSTIC

Norm: 0–2 mg/dl (0–57.72 nmol/L, SI units).

Usage: Basal levels aid in diagnosis of adrenal carcinoma and congenital adrenal hyperplasia; used to measure response when Metyrapone is given to diagnosing adrenal insufficiency and Cushing's disease.

Description: Blood test used to determine a specific metabolic block in the synthesis of cortisol. Cortisol is synthesized by two successive hydroxylations of 17 alpha-hydroxyprogesterone. The first results in 11-deoxycortisol, which is then catalyzed by 11 beta-hydroxylase to yield cortisol. This test is used in conjunction with the Metyrapone test to diagnose primary and secondary adrenal insufficiency. Metyrapone blocks the conversion of 11-deoxycortisol to cortisol, which then stimulates the adrenals to produce more 11-deoxycortisol. A blood level of 11-deoxycortisol that is not elevated after Metyrapone administration indicates the presence of adrenal insufficiency.

Professional Considerations:

1. Consent form NOT required.
2. Preparation:
   A. Tube: Green-top.
3. Procedure:
   A. Obtain a 7-ml blood sample.
4. Postprocedure care:
   A. Deliver the specimen to the laboratory immediately. Separate and freeze the plasma.
5. Client and family teaching:
   A. Results are normally available within 48 hours.
6. Factors that affect results:
   A. Results are increased if the client is taking any glucocorticoids, such as hydrocortisone, dexamethasone, or prednisone.
7. Other data:
   A. 11-deoxycortisol has no glucocorticoid activity.
   B. *See also Metyrapone Test.*

Bibliography:

Kraan GP, Hartstra J, Wolthers BG, van der Molen JC, Nagel GT, Drayer NM, Zijlstra RW, Kruizinga WH: Synthesis and identification of twelve A-ring reduced 6 alpha-and 6 beta-hydroxylated compounds derived from 11-deoxycortisol, corticosterone, and 11-dehydrocorticosterone. J Steroid Biochem Mol Biol 49(2–3):233–244, 1994.

Kraan GP, van Wee CJ, Wolthers BG, Rouwe CW, Drayer NM, de Bruin R: Kinetics and metabolism of 11-deoxycortisol in a patient with congenital adrenal hyperplasia due to 11 beta-hydroxylase deficiency. J Steroid Biochem Mol Biol 44(1):29–37, 1993.

Kraan GP, van Wee KT, Wolthers BG, van der Molen JC, Nagel GT, Drayer NM, van Leusen D: Synthesis and characterization of the 6 alpha- and 6 beta-hydroxylated derivatives of corticosterone, 11-dehydrocorticosterone, and 11-deoxycortisol. Steroids 58(10):495–503, 1993.

DESIPRAMINE
(see Tricyclic Antidepressants, Plasma or Serum)

DEXAMETHASONE SUPPRESSION TEST, DIAGNOSTIC

Norm: 24-hour urines should be <50% baseline.

Plasma cortisol	<5 µg/dl
Urine-free cortisol	<25 µg/24 hours
Urine for 17-OHCS	4 µg/24 hours

Positive: High levels of serum cortisol and 17-OHCS are present after dexamethasone is administered. Occurs in adrenal hyperplasia, adrenal tumors, Cushing's disease, depression, and oat cell cancer of the lung.

Description: Screening test for Cushing's disease and for depression. The test can be performed following a low or high dose of dexamethasone, or as an overnight test with a morning blood draw. Dexamethasone is a potent synthetic glucocorticoid that is used to test the integrity of the hypothalamic-pituitary-adrenal axis. When given to normal clients, it decreases the production of cortisol and other adrenal steroids through the usual feedback systems. In clients with Cushing's disease or depression there is no suppression of ACTH. The low test dose is for screening. If positive, a high-dose test is given to determine the cause of Cushing's disease. If there is suppression with the high-dose test, it indicates a pituitary origin of the excess cortisol. If there is no suppression, it indicates an adrenal or ectopic tumor.

Professional Considerations:

1. Consent form NOT required.
2. Preparation:
   A. Obtain a 3-L plastic container.
   B. Tube: Green-top, red-top, red/gray-top, or gold-top.

C. Baseline values for plasma cortisol, urine-free cortisol, and urine 17-OHCS should be known.

3. Procedure:

A. Obtain a 5-ml blood sample for plasma cortisol level.

B. Overnight test consists of administering 1 mg of dexamethasone orally at 1100 (11:00 A.M.) followed by venipuncture for cortisol level the next day at 0800 (8:00 A.M.).

C. The low-dose test includes a baseline measure of urine-free cortisol or 17-OHCS followed by oral dexamethasone 0.5 mg every 6 hours for 2 days followed by a 24-hour urine for free cortisol or 17-OHCS collected on day 2.

D. The high-dose test includes a baseline measure of urine-free cortisol or 17-OHCS followed by oral dexamethasone 2 mg every 6 hours for 2 days followed by a 24-hour urine for urine-free cortisol or 17-OHCS collected on day 2.

4. Postprocedure care:

A. Send the blood sample to the laboratory within 30 minutes for serum separation and freezing.

5. Client and family teaching:

A. Oral dexamethasone will be given at a specific time the evening before the blood sampling. The blood and urine samples will be collected at specific times the next day.

B. *Urine:* Save all the urine voided in the 24-hour period and urinate before defecating to avoid loss of urine. If any urine is accidentally discarded, notify the physician immediately, as the test results will be invalid.

6. Factors that affect results:

A. Failure to ingest oral dexamethasone, and radioactive scan performed within the last 24 hours, will elevate the results. For depressed clients, methylene blue is added to the dexamethasone tablets and urinary excretion of the dye is monitored to indicate that the drug was ingested.

B. False-positives occur with acute illnesses, alcoholism, anorexia nervosa, dehydration, severe depression, diabetes (unstable), electroconvulsive therapy post-treatment day 1, fever, malnutrition, nausea, obesity, pregnancy, high stress, and temporal lobe disease. Drugs include barbiturates, carbamazepine, estrogens, glutethimide, meprobamate methaqualone, methyprylon, oral contraceptives, phenytoin, reserpine, rifampin, spironolactone, stilbestrol, and tetracycline.

C. False-negatives occur with Addison's disease, hypopituitarism, and in clients who metabolize dexamethasone at an abnormally slow rate. Drugs include benzodiazepines (high-dose), corticosteroids, and cyproheptadine.

7. Other data:

A. Levels in some clients with Cushing's disease may be suppressed by 50%, but these clients can be identified by the metyrapone test.

B. As a screening test for depression it is 90% specific and 45% sensitive.

C. *See also Metyrapone Test, Serum.*

Bibliography:

Avgerinos PC, Yanovski JA, Oldfield EH, Nieman LK, Cutler GB Jr.: The metyrapone and dexamethasone suppression tests for the differential diagnosis of the adrenocorticotropin-dependent Cushing syndrome: a comparison [see comments]. Ann Intern Med *121*(5):318–327, 1994.

Bernini GP, Argenio GF, Cerri F, Franchi F: Comparison between the suppressive effects of dexamethasone and loperamide on cortisol and ACTH secretion in some pathological conditions. J Endocrinol Invest *17*(10):799–804, 1994.

Montwill J, Igoe D, McKenna TJ: The overnight dexamethasone test is the procedure of choice in screening for Cushing's syndrome. Steroids *59*(5):296–298, 1994.

Yanovski JA, Cutler GB Jr., Chrousos GP, Nieman LK: Corticotropin-releasing hormone stimulation following low-dose dexamethasone administration. A new test to distinguish Cushing's syndrome from pseudo-Cushing's states [see comments]. JAMA *269*(17):2232–2238, 1993.

DHEA, SERUM
(see Dehydroepiandrosterone Sulfate, Serum)

DIALYZABLE CALCIUM, SERUM
(see Calcium, Ionized, Blood)

DIASCAN, DIAGNOSTIC
(see Glucose Monitoring Machines, Diagnostic)

DIAZEPAM, SERUM

Norm: Negative.

		SI Units
Therapeutic range	100–1000 ng/ml	0.35–3.51 µmol/L
Panic level	>5000 ng/ml	>17.55 µmol/L
Lethal level		720 µg/ml

Panic Level Symptoms and Treatment:

Symptoms: Ataxia, cyanosis, coma, convulsions, diminished reflexes, mental confusion, respiratory depression, somnolence, and slurred speech, vertigo.

Treatment:

Perform gastric lavage with warm tap water or 0.9% saline if within 2 hours of ingestion.

Administer activated charcoal.

Monitor for central nervous system depression.

Protect airway. Support breathing with oxygen and mechanical ventilation, if necessary.

Do NOT induce emesis.

Implement seizure precautions.

Flumazenil has been used as a competitive antagonist to reverse the profound effects of benzodiazepine overdose. Use of Flumazenil is contraindicated if concomitant tricyclic antidepressants were taken.

Do NOT use barbiturates.

Forced diuresis and/or hemodialysis will NOT remove benzodiazepines to any significant extent. No information was found on whether peritoneal dialysis will remove these drugs.

Increased: Drug abuse, overdose, and suicide.

Description: Benzodiazepine derivative that acts on the limbic and subcortical levels of the central nervous system, producing sedation, skeletal muscle relaxation, and anticonvulsant effects. Absorbed from gastrointestinal tract, metabolized by the liver, excreted in the urine and stool, peak plasma concentration is 1–2 hours, half-life is 21–46 hours, and steady-state levels occur in 5–10 days.

Professional Considerations:

1. Consent form NOT required unless sample is being collected as legal evidence.
2. Preparation:
   A. Tube: Red-top, red/gray-top, or gold-top.
   B. MAY be drawn during hemodialysis.

3. Procedure:
   A. Have the specimen collection witnessed if being collected for legal evidence.
   B. Obtain a 5-ml blood sample.
   C. For a therapeutic dose evaluation, draw the sample 2 hours after oral ingestion of diazepam.
4. Postprocedure care:
   A. For specimens collected for legal evidence, write the client's name, date, exact time of collection, and specimen source on the lab requisition. Sign, and have the witness sign, the lab requisition.
   B. Transport the specimen to the laboratory immediately in a sealed plastic bag marked as legal evidence. All persons handling the specimen should sign and mark the time of receipt on the laboratory requisition.
   C. Observe for side effects of ataxia, drowsiness, lethargy, nystagmus, nausea, tinnitus, and vertigo, which often subside after continued therapy.
5. Client and family teaching:
   A. Discuss the need for psychological intervention with the family and the client if panic or lethal doses have been determined. Refer for crisis intervention for intentional overdose.
   B. Expect intensive care unit placement for severe overdose.
   C. Death is rare in overdose when diazepam is taken alone.
6. Factors that affect results:
   A. None.
7. Other data:
   A. *See also Benzodiazepines, Plasma and Urine.*

Bibliography:

Gaudreault P, Guay J, Thivierge RL, Verdy I: Benzodiazepine poisoning. Clinical and pharmacological considerations and treatment [review]. Drug Safety 66(4):247–265, 1991.

Spivey WH, Roberts JR, Derlet RW: A clinical trial of escalating doses of flumazenil for reversal of suspected benzodiazepine overdose in the emergency department. Ann Emerg Med 22(12):1813–1821, 1993.

Takatori T, Tomii S, Terazawa K, Negao M, Kanamori M, Tomaru Y: A comparative study of diazepam levels in bone marrow versus serum, saliva, and brain tissue. Int J Legal Med 104(4):185–188, 1991.

Viani A, Rizzo G, Carrai M, Pacifici GM: The effect of ageing on plasma albumin and plasma protein binding of diazepam, salicylic acid and digitoxin in healthy subjects and patients with renal impairment. Br J Clin Pharmacol 33(3): 299–304, 1992.

DIETHYLPROPION

(see Amphetamines, Blood)

DIFFERENTIAL LEUKOCYTE COUNT (DIFF), PERIPHERAL BLOOD

Norm:

		SI Units
White Blood Cells (WBC)		
Adult females	4500–11,000/µl	$4.5–11.0 \times 10^9$/L
Pregnant		
Trimester 1	6600–14,000/µl	$6.6–14.1 \times 10^9$/L
Trimester 2	6900–17,100/µl	$6.9–17.1 \times 10^9$/L
Trimester 3	5900–14,700/µl	$5.9–14.7 \times 10^9$/L
Postpartum	9700–25,700/µl	$9.7–25.7 \times 10^9$/L
Adult males	4500–11,000/µl	$4.5–11.0 \times 10^9$/L
Children		
Newborn	9000–30,000/µl	$9.0–30.0 \times 10^9$/L
3 months	5700–18,000/µl	$5.7–18.0 \times 10^9$/L
1 year	6000–17,500/µl	$6.0–17.5 \times 10^9$/L
3 years	5700–16,300/µl	$5.7–16.3 \times 10^9$/L
10 years	4500–13,500/ul	$4.5–13.5 \times 10^9$/L
Differential White Blood Cells		
GRANULOCYTES		
Segmented Neutrophils (Segs)	54–62%	0.54–0.62
Adult	3800/µl	3800×10^6/L
Children		
Birth	8400/µl	8400×10^6/L
12 hours	12,100/µl	$12,100 \times 10^6$/L
24 hours	8870/µl	8870×10^6/L
1 week	4100/µl	4100×10^6/L
2 weeks	3320/µl	3320×10^6/L
1–2 months	2750/µl	2750×10^6/L
4 months	2730/µl	2730×10^6/L
6 months	2710/µl	2710×10^6/L
8 months	2680/µl	2680×10^6/L
10 months	2600/µl	2600×10^6/L
12 months	2680/µl	2680×10^6/L
2 years	2660/µl	2660×10^6/L
4 years	3040/µl	3040×10^6/L
6 years	3600/µl	3600×10^6/L
8–14 years	3700/µl	3700×10^6/L
16–20 years	3800/µl	3800×10^6/L
Band Neutrophils (Bands)		
Proportion	3–5%	0.03–0.05
Adults	620/µl	620×10^6/L
Children		
Birth	2540/µl	2540×10^6/L
12 hours	3460/µl	3460×10^6/L
24 hours	2680/µl	2680×10^6/L
1 week	1420/µl	1420×10^6/L
2 weeks	1200/µl	1200×10^6/L
1 month	1150/µl	1150×10^6/L
2 months	1100/µl	1100×10^6/L
4–10 months	1000/µl	1000×10^6/L

		SI Units
Band Neutrophils (Bands) *(continued)*		
Children *(continued)*		
12 months	990/μl	990×10^6/L
2 years	850/μl	850×10^6/L
4 years	710/μl	710×10^6/L
6 years	670/μl	670×10^6/L
8 years	660/μl	660×10^6/L
10 years	645/μl	645×10^6/L
12–14 years	640/μl	640×10^6/L
16–20 years	620/μl	620×10^6/L
Eosinophils (Eos)		
Proportion	1–3%	0.01–0.03
Adults	200/μl	200×10^6/L
Children		
Birth	400/μl	400×10^6/L
12–24 hours	450/μl	450×10^6/L
1 week	500/μl	500×10^6/L
2 weeks	350/μl	350×10^6/L
1 month–1 year	300/μl	300×10^6/L
2 years	280/μl	280×10^6/L
4 years	250/μl	250×10^6/L
6 years	230/μl	230×10^6/L
8–20 years	200/μl	200×10^6/L
Basophils (Basos)		
Proportion	0–0.75%	0–0.0075
Adult	40/μl	40×10^6/L
Children		
Birth–24 hours	100/μl	100×10^6/L
1 week–8 years	50/μl	50×10^6/L
10–20 years	40/μl	40×10^6/L
MONOCYTES (MONOS)		
Proportion	3–7%	0.03–0.07%
Adults	300/μl	300×10^6/L
Children		
Birth	1050/μl	1050×10^6/L
12 hours	1200/μl	1200×10^6/L
24 hours–1 week	1100/μl	1100×10^6/L
2 weeks	1000/μl	1000×10^6/L
1 month	700/μl	700×10^6/L
2 months	650/μl	650×10^6/L
4 months	600/μl	600×10^6/L
6–8 months	580/μl	580×10^6/L
10–12 months	550/μl	550×10^6/L
2 years	530/μl	530×10^6/L
4 years	450/μl	450×10^6/L
6 years	400/μl	400×10^6/L
8–12 years	350/μl	350×10^6/L
14 years	380/μl	380×10^6/L
16–18 years	400/μl	400×10^6/L
20 years	380/μl	380×10^6/L

		SI Units
LYMPHOCYTES (LYMPHS)		
Proportion	25–33%	0.25–0.33
Adults	2500/µl	2500×10^6/L
Children		
Birth–12 hours	5500/µl	5500×10^6/L
24 hours	5800/µl	5800×10^6/L
1 week	5000/µl	5000×10^6/L
2 weeks	5500/µl	5500×10^6/L
1 month	6000/µl	6000×10^6/L
2 months	6300/µl	6300×10^6/L
4 months	6800/µl	6800×10^6/L.
6 months	7300/µl	7300×10^6/L
8 months	7600/µl	7600×10^6/L
10 months	7500/µl	7500×10^6/L
12 months	7000/µl	7000×10^6/L
2 years	6300/µl	6300×10^6/L
4 years	4500/µl	4500×10^6/L
6 years	3500/µl	3500×10^6/L
8 years	3300/µl	3300×10^6/L
10 years	3100/µl	3100×10^6/L
12 years	3000/µl	3000×10^6/L
14 years	2900/µl	2900×10^6/L
16 years	2800/µl	2800×10^6/L
18 years	2700/µl	2700×10^6/L
20 years	2500/µl	2500×10^6/L

Increased White Blood Cell Count: Abscess, actinomycosis, amebiasis, Andersen's disease, anemia (acquired hemolytic), anorexia, anoxia, anthrax, appendicitis, bacterial infections, blastomycosis, bronchitis, burns, chickenpox, cholecystitis (acute), choledocholithiasis, cholera, cirrhosis (with necrosis), colon cancer, convulsive seizures, Crohn's disease, croup, Cushing's syndrome, cytomegalovirus, dengue fever, diphtheria, dissecting aortic aneurysm, diverticulitis, diverticulosis, dysproteinemia, eclampsia, electrical injury, emotional stress, empyema (acute subdural), endocarditis, Epstein-Barr virus, erythroblastosis fetalis, exercise, exposure to ultraviolet light, fascioliasis, fatty liver, fever of undetermined origin, G-6-PD deficiency, gangrene, glomerulonephritis (poststreptococcal), gout (acute), halothane toxicity, heart transplant rejection, hemorrhage, hepatitis (alcoholic), hepatoma, hookworm, Hodgkin's disease, idiopathic myelofibrosis, infection (bacterial, parasitic), infectious mononucleosis, intestinal obstruction, ketoacidosis, lactic acidosis, legionnaires' disease, leukemia, leukocytosis, lymphoma, meningitis, menstruation, myocardial infarction, myocarditis, pancreatitis, peritonitis, pneumonia, pneumomediastinum, poisoning (arthropods, chemicals, metals, venom), polycythemia vera, postoperative surgical stress, pregnancy, paroxysmal tachycardia, preleukemia, pylephlebitis, rat-bite fever, red blood cell hemolysis, retroperitoneal fibrosis, rheumatic fever, rubeola, sepsis, shock, smallpox, stress, strongyloidiasis, suppurative cholangitis, systemic lupus erythematosus, tonsillitis, toxic shock syndrome, transfusion reaction, trauma, trichuriasis, tuberculosis, tularemia, tumor necrosis, ulcers, ultraviolet irradiation, uremia, yellow fever, visceral larva migrans, Wegener's granulomatosis, and Weil's disease. Drugs include allopurinol, anesthetics, atropine sulfate, barbiturates, diethylcarbamazine, epinephrine bitartrate, epinephrine borate, epinephrine hydrochloride, erythromycin, steroids, streptomycin sulfate, and sulfonamides.

Increased Neutrophils: Acute infections, allergies, anemia, anoxia, anxiety, appendicitis, asthma, burns, cancer, chickenpox, cholecystitis, cholera, colitis, Cushing's syndrome dermatitis, diabetic acidosis, Di Guglielmo disease, diphtheria, diverticulitis, diverticulosis, eclampsia, electroconvulsive therapy treatment, empyema, emphysema, endocarditis, fear, G-6-PD deficiency, gangrene, gout, hemorrhage, inflammation, ketoacidosis, labor and delivery, leukemia, leukocytosis, lymphoma, meningitis (purulent), myocardial infarction, osteomyelitis, otitis media, pancreatitis, panic, peritonitis, pernicious anemia, pneumonia, poisoning (carbon monoxide, lead, mercury, arsenic, turpentine), polycythemia vera, postoperative surgical stress, pulmonary infarction, pyelonephritis, pyemia, rheumatic fever, rheumatoid arthritis, salpingitis, scarlet fever, septicemia, smallpox, smoking, thyroiditis, tonsillitis, transfusion reaction, typhus, and uremia. Drugs include acetylcholine, benzene, carbon monoxide, casein, chlorpropamide, corticosteroids, corticotropin, digitalis, epinephrine, ethylene glycol, histamine, heparin, insect venoms, lead, lithium, mercury, potassium chloride, and turpentine.

Increased Bands: Pharyngitis.

Increased Segmented: Pernicious anemia.

Increased Eosinophils: Addison's disease, allergies, atheroembolic renal disease, asthma, brucellosis, cancer (bone, brain, ovary, testes), chorea, coccidioidomycosis, dermatitis, diverticulitis, diverticulosis, eczema, gangrene, hay fever, Hodgkin's disease, leprosy, leukemia (chronic granulocytic), leukocytosis, Löffler's syndrome, malaria, metastatic carcinoma, parasitic infections, pemphigus, pernicious anemia, phlebitis, polycythemia vera, psoriasis, pruritus due to jaundice, radiation therapy, rheumatoid arthritis, rhinitis, sarcoidosis, scarlet fever, sickle cell anemia, splenectomy, Sjögren's syndrome, thrombophlebitis, tuberculosis, and ulcerative colitis. Drugs include antibiotics (associated with allergic reactions), allopurinol, aminosalicylic acid, anticonvulsants, cephalosporins, chlorpropamide, digitalis, heparin, imipramine, methotrexate, nitrofurantoin, penicillin, phenothiazine, procainamide, procarbazine, propranolol, quinidine, streptomycin, sulfonamides, and tetracycline.

Increased Basophils: Allergic reaction to food/drugs/inhalants, chickenpox, chronic myelogenous leukemia, erythroderma, Heinz-body anemia, Hodgkin's disease, hypothyroidism, irradiation, leukocytosis, myelofibrosis, myxedema, nephrosis, periarteritis nodosa, polycythemia vera, serum sickness, sinusitis, smallpox, splenectomy, ulcerative colitis, and urticaria. Drugs include antithyroids, desipramine, and estrogens.

Increased Lymphocytes: Brucellosis, cytomegalovirus, diverticulitis, diverticulosis, endocarditis, hepatitis, Hurler's syndrome, infectious mononucleosis, leukocytosis, lymphocytic leukemia, pertussis, syphilis, toxoplasmosis, and xerostomia. Drugs include aspirin, carbon disulfate poisoning, haloperidol, lead intoxication, levodopa, phenytoin, and tetrahydrochloride poisoning.

Increased Monocytes: Brucellosis, carbon disulfide poisoning, Epstein-Barr virus, Hodgkin's disease, leukemia (AML, CML), leukocytosis, multiple myeloma, phosphorus poisoning, rheumatoid arthritis, salmonellosis, sarcoidosis, syphilis, systemic lupus erythematosus, tetrahydrochloride poisoning, tuberculosis, and ulcerative colitis. Drugs include haloperidol and methsuximide.

Decreased White Blood Cell Count: Agranulocytosis, AIDS, alcoholism, anaphylactic shock, anemia (aplastic, pernicious), amyloidosis, anorexia nervosa, anthrax, arsenic poisoning, brucellosis, cachexia, chemical toxicity, chemotherapy, cirrhosis, Colorado tick fever, dengue fever, disseminated lupus erythematosus, Felty's syndrome, Gaucher's disease, heavy chain disease, hepatitis (infectious, viral), Hodgkin's disease, hypersplenism, hypothermia, idiopathic myelofibrosis, infection (severe bacterial, viral), influenza, legionnaires' disease, leishmaniasis, leukemia (some forms), leukopenia, lymphoma, measles, mononucleosis, myxedema, paratyphoid fever, pharyngitis, pneumocystis pneumonia, preleukemia, protein therapy, psittacosis, Q fever, radiation therapy, renal trauma, rheumatic fever, rubella, sepsis neonatorum, shock, Sjögren's syndrome, stiff-man syndrome, stomatitis, strongyloidiasis, toxoplasmosis, tuberculosis, tularemia, and typhoid fever. Drugs include acetaminophen, aminoglutethimide, aminopyrine, antibiotics, antineoplastics, antithyroids, arsenicals, aurothioglucose, bismuth, chloramphenicol, chloroquine phosphate, diazepam, diethylcarbamazine, ethotoin, furosemide, immunosuppressives, meprobamate, methyldopa, methyldopate hydrochloride, methsuximide, phenothiazines, phenylbutazone, phenytoin, phenytoin sodium, primidone, procainamide hydrochloride, quinacrine hydrochloride, quinine sulfate, sulfonamides, and vitamin A.

Decreased Neutrophils: Acromegaly, Addison's disease agranulocytosis, anaphylactic shock, anorexia nervosa, aplastic anemia, brucellosis, cachexia, carcinoma, Chediak-Higashi syndrome, chemotherapy, cirrhosis, Colorado tick fever, dengue fever, Felty's syndrome, folic acid deficiency, Gaucher's disease, hypersplenism, hypopituitarism, hypothyroidism, infections, infectious hepatitis, infectious mononucleosis, influenza, iron deficiency anemia, kala-azar, malaria, measles, mumps, myelofibrosis, myeloma, paratyphoid fever, paroxysmal nocturnal hemoglobinuria, pernicious anemia, pneumonia, psittacosis, radiation therapy, Rocky Mountain spotted fever, rubella, rubeola, sarcoma, septicemia, thyrotoxicosis, tularemia, typhoid fever, vitamin B_{12} deficiency, and yellow fever. Drugs include alcohol, aminophylline, antipyrine, aminopyrine, ampicillin, arsenic, aspirin, barbiturates, carbimazole, cephalothin, chemotherapeutic agents, chloramphenicol, chlorpromazine, chlorpropamide, cinchophen, DDT, diazepam, dinitrophenol, diuretics, electroconvulsive therapy treatment, gold salts, imipramine, indomethacin, isoniazid, mephenytoin, 6-mercaptopurine, methaphenolene hydrochloride, methicillin, *p*-aminobenzoic acid, penicillin, phenacetin, phenylbutazone, phenylhydrazine, phenytoin, procainamide, quinine, rauwolfia, streptomycin, sulfonamides, tolbutamide, tripelennamine hydrochloride, and urethan.

Decreased Eosinophils: Acromegaly, anemia (aplastic), coccidioidomycosis, congestive heart failure, Cushing's syndrome, disseminated lupus erythematosus, eclampsia, fascioliasis, Goodpasture's syndrome, hypersplenism, infections, infectious mononucleosis, schistosomiasis, and stress. Drugs include adrenocorticotropic hormone, corticotropin, epinephrine glucocorticoids, methysergide, niacin, niacinamide, procainamide, and thyroxine.

Decreased Basophils: Acute infection, anaphylaxis, Cushing's syndrome, hyperthyroidism, ovulation, pregnancy, radiation therapy, thyrotoxicosis, and stress. Drugs include chemotherapy, corticosteroids, corticotropin, procainamide, and thiotepa.

Decreased Lymphocytes: Aplastic anemia, Cushing's syndrome, Hodgkin's disease, immunoglobulin deficiencies, leukemia (chronic granulocytic, monocytic), lymphosarcoma, renal failure, systemic lupus erythematosus, thymic hypoplasia in children, and uremia. Drugs include asparaginase, chlorambucil, cortisone, epinephrine, glucocorticoids, lithium, mechlorethamine, niacin, nitrogen mustard, and radiation therapy to the lymphatics.

Decreased Monocytes: Aplastic anemia and hairy-cell leukemia.

Description: The differential white blood cell count (Diff) assesses each leukocyte distribution on two stained glass slides of peripheral blood. One hundred white blood cells are identified and then classified (differentiated) according to their morphology. A relative percentage of each type of cell is then determined and reported. White blood cells (leukocytes) function in the body's immune defense system. Three main types of white blood cells exist: granulocytes, monocytes, and lymphocytes, and are identified and counted via microscopic examination of stained blood films. *Granulocytes,* manufactured by bone marrow, are subdivided into neutrophils, eosinophils, and basophils, and function in bacterial phagocytosis. Neutrophils are further subclassified as either segmented or band neutrophils. Segmented neutrophils (Segs) are more mature and comprised of two to five lobes, which increase (shift to the right) during pathologic conditions. Band neutrophils (Bands) are less mature and increase in number (shift to the left) during conditions causing increased white blood cell (WBC) production. Eosinophils are leukocytes that contain course round granules. Eosinophils become active in the later stages of inflammation. These cells act as phagocytes and are active in allergic reactions and parasitic infections. Eosinophils are under the influence of the adrenal cortex. *Monocytes* manufactured by bone marrow function both in antigen recognition and phagocytosis of cellular debris. *Lymphocytes* formed by the lymphatic system function in humoral and cell-mediated immune responses to foreign antigens.

Professional Considerations:

1. Consent form NOT required.
2. Preparation:
   A. Tube: Lavender-top glass or lavender-sealed plastic.
3. Procedure:
   A. Draw a 3.5-ml blood sample.
   B. Do not leave tourniquet in place longer than 60 seconds.
4. Postprocedure care:
   A. Apply pressure at the site of the venipuncture because bleeding may occur due to disease entity.
   B. Record the collection time because counts vary according to time of day.
5. Client and family teaching:
   A. Results are normally available within 24 hours.
6. Factors that affects results:
   A. In leukemia, cryofibrinogenemia, and cryoglobulinemia, WBC results performed on an electronic cell counter are unreliable. The counts must be performed manually.
   B. The most accurate leukocyte counts are obtained from capillary punctures. For EDTA-anticoagulated blood (lavender-top tube), the most accurate counts are obtained within 4 hours of the specimen collection.
   C. The serum sample is stable at room temperature for 10 hours and refrigerated for 18 hours and should not be frozen.
   D. Leukocyte differential relative values reported as percentages should be converted to absolute values by multiplying the percent by the total WBC count prior to interpretation.
7. Other data:
   A. "Shift to the left" means there is an increased number of immature neutrophils in the peripheral blood. Neutrophils are usually illustrated from left (young cells) to right (mature cells) in

the differential. A low total WBC count with a left shift indicates a recovery from bone marrow depression or an infection of such intensity that the demand for neutrophils in the tissue is greater than the capacity of the bone marrow to release them in the circulation. A high total WBC count with a left shift indicates an increased release of neutrophils by the bone marrow in response to an overwhelming infection or inflammation.

B. "Shift to the right" means cells have more than the usual number of nuclear segments. This is found in liver disease, Down syndrome, or megaloblastic and pernicious anemia.

C. The eosinophil count may be used in conjunction with the Thorn test to evaluate adrenocortical stimulation.

D. An automated WBC may not reveal the "shifts."

Bibliography:

Bjornestad E, Lie RT, Janssen CW Jr.: The diagnostic potential of some routine laboratory tests. Br J Clin Pract *47*(5):243–245, 1993.

Eriksson S, Granstrom L, Carlstrom A: The diagnostic value of repetitive preoperative analyses of C-reactive protein and total leucocyte count in patients with suspected acute appendicitis. Scand J Gastroenterol *29*(12):1145–1149, 1994.

Gallagher EJ, Brooks F, Gennis P: Identification of serious illness in febrile adults. Am J Emerg Med *12*(2):129–133, 1994.

Korppi M, Kroger L, Laitinen M: White blood cell and differential counts in acute respiratory viral and bacterial infections in children. Scand J Infect Dis *25*(4):435–440, 1993.

DIGITAL SUBTRACTION ANGIOGRAPHY (DSA) AND TRANSVENOUS-DIGITAL SUBTRACTION, DIAGNOSTIC

Norm: Normal carotid arteries, vertebral arteries, abdominal aorta and branches, renal arteries, and peripheral vessels.

Usage: Aneurysms, aortic valvular stenosis, arterial occlusion, bypass surgery (postoperative), carotid stenosis, hepatocellular carcinoma, jugular tumors, nutcracker renal phenomenon, pheochromocytoma, pulmonary emboli, thoracic outlet syndrome, and ulcerative plaques.

Description: A noninvasive computer imaging procedure that allows examination of the arteries in the body following an IV injection of contrast medium. Images of the cardiac region are subtracted from images obtained after contrast medium injection as the dense images of soft tissue and bone are removed by the computer. There is less discomfort and risk of complications than with an arteriogram, but visualization of the arteries is less precise, and visualization of stenotic lesions in sequential branches may not occur.

Professional Considerations:

1. Consent form IS required.

Risks:

Allergic reaction to dye (itching, hives, rash, tight feeling in the throat, shortness of breath, bronchospasm, anaphylaxis, death), aphasia, hemiplegia, hemorrhage, paresthesia, thromboemboli, infection, renal toxicity from contrast medium.

Contraindications:

Recent myocardial infarction, severe renal failure, previous allergy to dye, iodine, or shellfish; during pregnancy or breast-feeding.

2. Preparation:
   A. Assess for normal renal function.
   B. Have emergency equipment readily available.
   C. Glycogen may be administered intravenously to reduce motion artifacts by stopping peristalsis.
   D. Record baseline vital signs.
3. Procedure:
   A. A local anesthetic is given over the basilic or cephalic veins in the antecubital area.
   B. Venous catheterization is performed and iodine contrast medium is injected at a rate of 14 ml/second.
   C. Radiographic images are taken of arteries made visible by the contrast medium.
4. Postprocedure care:
   A. Monitor vital signs every 15 minutes until stable.
   B. Observe the puncture site of catheterization for infection, hemorrhage, and hematoma.
   C. Force fluids after the procedure to help

flush the contrast medium through the kidneys. A liter of IV fluid may be given as a precautionary measure to clients having an increased risk of developing renal toxicity from the contrast medium, such as the elderly, and clients with dehydration, diabetes, or multiple myeloma.
   D. Monitor renal function (BUN and creatinine) for 2 days after the procedure in all clients to be sure the levels remain normal. If the levels become abnormally elevated, indicating nephrotoxicity, continuous IV fluids should be given until the levels return to normal limits. An adverse reaction to IV contrast medium should be noted in a prominent place on the chart and the client informed that he or she should not receive a contrast medium in the future.
   E. If the study is necessary in a client with renal insufficiency, a newer, less nephrotoxic agent should be used, even though it is more expensive, and the client should be well hydrated.
5. Client and family teaching:
   A. You must remain still during the procedure.
   B. The procedure takes approximately 45 minutes.
6. Factors that affect results:
   A. Small amounts of motion by the individual including swallowing and respirations obscure results.
   B. Intracardiac or intra-arterial injection of contrast medium can also obscure results.
7. Other data:
   A. The femoral vein may also be used for catheterization.

Bibliography:

Derdeyn CP, Moran CJ, Cross DT, Grubb RL Jr, Dacey RG Jr: Intraoperative digital subtraction angiography: a review of 112 consecutive examinations. Am J Neuroradiol 16(2):307–318, 1995.

Garbagnati F, Spreafico C, Marchiano A, Frigerio LF, Patelli G, Gervasoni A, Giovannardi G, Damascelli B: Carbon dioxide digital subtraction angiography in oncological-interventional radiology. Tumori 81(1):52–55, 1995.

van Rooij WJ, den Heeten GJ, Sluzewski M: Pulmonary embolism: diagnosis in 211 patients with use of selective pulmonary digital subtraction angiography with a flow-directed catheter. Radiology 195(3):793–797, 1995.

Yamagiwa I, Obata K, Saito H, Washio M: Intravenous digital subtraction angiography for the evaluation of renal artery blood flow following the removal of a neuroblastoma. Surg Today 24(11):973–977, 1994.

DIGITOXIN, SERUM

Norm: Negative.

		SI Units
Therapeutic values	10–32 ng/ml	13.1–41.9 nmol/L
Panic level	>35 ng/ml	45.8 nmol/L

Panic Level Symptoms and Treatment:

Symptoms: Anorexia, hyperkalemia, mental status changes, nausea, vomiting, diarrhea, and visual distortion in which objects appear yellow or green or have a halo around them. Serious toxic symptoms are bradycardia and atrioventricular (AV) nodal block.

Treatment:

1. Continuous ECG monitoring is necessary. Watch for prolonged PR-interval, widening QRS-interval, lengthening QTc, and AV block.
2. Transcutaneous pacing for rhythms progressing to AV block.
3. Discontinue medication.
4. For acute overdose, empty the stomach by inducing emesis (with extreme caution) with syrup of ipecac or by gastric lavage or warm 0.9% saline or tap water. Do NOT induce emesis if signs of central nervous system depression are evident or if the client has no gag reflex.
5. Give activated charcoal.
6. Treat hypokalemia with a potassium supplement.
7. Treat hyperkalemia with IV glucose and insulin.
8. For potentially life-threatening toxicity, administer digoxin-specific antibody fragments (Fab). The dose depends on the amount of digitoxin to be neutralized, usually 240 mg (six 40-mg vials reconstituted with sterile water to provide a solution of 10 mg/mL) given via IV push or as an infusion over 15–30 minutes.
9. Hemodialysis will NOT remove digitoxin, but will be helpful in treating serious hyperkalemia.

Usage: Prophylactic management and treatment of heart failure and to control the ventricular rate in atrial fibrillation or atrial flutter. May also be used to treat and prevent recurrent paroxysmal atrial tachycardia. Monitoring of serum levels is performed during initial digitoxin therapy, if toxicity is suspected from symptoms, and for assessment of medication compliance. After a stable dose is established, routine monitoring is not usually necessary.

Description: Long-acting cardiac glycoside with a half-life is 5–7 days, and with peak concentrations occurring in 1–3 hours; 90% is metabolized in the liver and excreted in the urine. The main property of a cardiac glycoside is its positive inotropic effect on the myocardium. It also decreases the conduction velocity through the AV node and prolongs the effective refractory period of the AV node.

Professional Considerations:

1. Consent form NOT required.
2. Preparation:
   A. Tube: Red-top, red/gray-top, or gold-top.
   B. Specimens should be drawn 6–8 hours after the last dose of digitoxin.
   C. The specimen MAY be drawn during hemodialysis.
3. Procedure:
   A. Draw a 3-ml blood sample.
4. Postprocedure care:
   A. If toxic levels are found, withhold the drug and notify the physician.
   B. Be sure to request the right drug level. There will be an error in results if digoxin is requested instead of digitoxin.
5. Client and family teaching:
   A. Results are normally available within 24 hours.
   B. If activated charcoal was given for elevated levels, the client should drink 4–6 glasses of water each day for 2 days to prevent constipation. The activated charcoal will also cause stools to be black for a few days.
   C. A rebound of the digitoxin level may occur 2–3 days after Fab administration.
6. Factors that affect results:
   A. Radioactive tracer within 24 hours falsely elevates results.
   B. Recent administration of digoxin may increase results.
   C. Serum potassium, calcium, or magnesium imbalances may falsely elevate results.
   D. Drug interactions include cholestyramine, heparin, kaolin-pectin, neomycin, phenobarbital, phenytoin, quinidine, rifampin, and verapamil, which may elevate results.
   E. Results may be elevated in hepatic or renal dysfunction.
7. Other data:
   A. Treatment of supraventricular tachycardia and atrial fibrillation may need to have drug levels in the high therapeutic range.
   B. Digoxin is a metabolite of digitoxin, so digoxin-specific antibody fragments are effective in the treatment of toxicity.
   C. Use with caution in the elderly.
   D. Toxicity usually results from hepatic or renal dysfunction, hypokalemia, hypothyroidism, severe hypoxic heart or respiratory disease, or variations in the client response to the dose.

Bibliography:

Doucet J, Fresel J, Hue G, Moore N: Protein binding of digitoxin, valproate and phenytoin in sera from diabetics. Eur J Clin Pharmacol *45*(6):577–579, 1993.

Duncker GI, Kisters G, Grille W: Prospective, randomized, placebo-controlled, double-blind testing of colour vision and electroretinogram at therapeutic and subtherapeutic digitoxin serum levels. Opthalmologica *208*(5):259–261, 1994.

Nokhodian A, Santos SR, Kirch W: Digitoxin and its metabolites in patients with liver cirrhosis. Eur J Drug Metab Pharmacokinet *18*(2):207–213, 1993.

Schmitt K, Tulzer G, Hackel F, Sommer R, Tulzer W: Massive digitoxin intoxication treated with digoxin-specific antibodies in a child. Pediatr Cardiol *15*(1):48–49, 1994.

DIGOXIN, SERUM

Norm: Negative.

		SI Units
Therapeutic level	0.5–2.0 ng/ml	0.6–2.6 nmol/L
Dysrhythmias	1.5–2.0 ng/ml	1.9–2.6 nmol/L
Congestive heart failure	0.8–1.5 ng/ml	1.0–1.9 nmol/L
Panic level (adult)	>2.4 ng/ml	>3.2 nmol/L
Panic level (children)	>3.0 ng/ml	>3.8 nmol/L

Panic Level Symptoms and Treatment:

Symptoms: Anorexia, hyperkalemia, mental status changes, nausea, vomiting, diarrhea, and visual distortion in which objects appear yellow or green or have a halo around them. Serious toxic symptoms are bradycardia and AV nodal block.

Treatment:

1. Continuous ECG monitoring is necessary. Watch for prolonged PR-interval, widening QRS-interval, lengthening QTc, and AV block.
2. Transcutaneous pacing for rhythms progressing to AV block.
3. Discontinue medication.
4. For acute overdose soon after ingestion, empty stomach by inducing emesis with syrup of ipecac or by gastric lavage or warm 0.9% saline or tap water. Do NOT induce emesis if signs of central nervous system depression are evident or if the client has no gag reflex.
5. Give activated charcoal.
6. Treat hypokalemia with potassium supplement.
7. Treat hyperkalemia with IV glucose and insulin.
8. For potentially life-threatening toxicity, administer digoxin-specific antibody fragments (Fab). The dose depends on the amount of digoxin to be neutralized, usually 240 mg (six 40-mg vials reconstituted with sterile water to provide a solution of 10 mg/mL) given via IV push or as an infusion over 15–30 minutes. Hemodialysis and peritoneal dialysis will NOT remove digoxin, but will be helpful in treating serious hyperkalemia. Hemoperfusion WILL remove digoxin.

Usage: Prophylactic management and treatment of heart failure, and to control the ventricular rate in atrial fibrillation or atrial flutter. May also be used to treat and prevent recurrent paroxysmal atrial tachycardia. Monitoring of serum levels is performed during initial digoxin therapy, if toxicity is suspected from symptoms, and for assessment of medication compliance. After a stable dose is established, routine monitoring is not usually necessary.

Description: Cardiac glycoside with prompt action, and less prolonged effect than digitoxin, that is rapidly excreted in the urine. Half-life is 32–51 hours in adults and 11–50 hours in children, with peak concentrations reached in 1–5 hours. Steady-state levels are reached after 7–11 days in adults and after 2–10 days in children. The main property of a cardiac glycoside is its positive inotropic effect on the myocardium. It also decreases the conduction velocity through the AV node and prolongs the effective refractory period of the AV node.

Professional Considerations:

1. Consent form NOT required.
2. Preparation:
   A. Tube: Red-top, red/gray-top, or gold-top.

B. Specimens should be drawn 6–8 hours after last dose of digoxin.

C. MAY be drawn during hemodialysis.

3. Procedure:

A. Draw a 1-ml blood sample.

4. Postprocedure care:

A. Be sure to request the right drug level to be drawn. There will be an error in results if digitoxin is requested instead of digoxin.

B. If toxic levels are found, withhold the drug and notify the physician.

5. Client and family teaching:

A. Results are normally available within 24 hours.

B. A rebound of the digitoxin level may occur 2–3 days after Fab administration.

6. Factors that affect results:

A. Radioactive tracer within 24 hours may falsely elevate results.

B. Serum potassium, calcium, or magnesium imbalances may increase results.

C. Drug interactions include amiodarone, antacids, cholestyramine, erythromycin, flecainide, heparin, ibuprofen, kaolin-pectin, neomycin, phenobarbital, phenytoin, quinidine, rifampin, and verapamil, which may increase results.

D. Results may be elevated in hepatic or renal dysfunction.

7. Other data:

A. Treatment of supraventricular tachycardia and atrial fibrillation may need to have drug levels in the high therapeutic range.

B. Use with caution in the elderly.

C. Toxicity usually results from hepatic or renal dysfunction, hypokalemia, hypothyroidism, severe hypoxic heart or respiratory disease, or variations in the client response to the dosage.

D. Anticonvulsants have been reported to increase hepatic clearance of digoxin.

E. Common names include Lanoxicaps, Lanoxin, Digoxin Elixir, and Lanoxin Elixir.

Bibliography:

Chan T, Vilke GM, Williams S: Bidirectional tachycardia associated with digoxin toxicity. J Emerg Med 13(1):89, 1995.

Gardner TW, Klein R, Moss SE, Ferris FL 3rd, Remaley NA: Digoxin does not accelerate progression of diabetic retinopathy. Diabetes Care 18(2):237–240, 1995.

Guinta A, Maione S, Arnese MR, Giacummo A, Liucci GA, Palma M, de Campora P, Cangianiello S, Condorelli M: Effects of intravenous digoxin on pulmonary venous and transmitral flows in patients with chronic heart failure of different degrees. Clin Cardiol 18(1):2733, 1995.

Ibanez C, Carcas AJ, Frias J, Abad F: Activated charcoal increases digoxin elimination in patients. Int J Cardiol 48(1):27–30, 1995.

Jones KW, Howell RR: Digoxin dosing: an alternate approach. J S C Med Assoc 91(3):112–113, 1995.

DILATION AND CURETTAGE (D & C), DIAGNOSTIC

Norm: No abnormal cells.

Usage: Acquired and congenital cervical stenosis, cancer, diagnosis and treatment of abnormal uterine bleeding, dysmenorrhea, insertion of an IUD, insertion of a radium device for treatment of cancer, pedunculated leiomyomas, preceding a hysterography or hysteroscopy, and uterine polyps.

Description: A widening of the cervical canal with a dilator and then a scraping of the uterine canal with a curette. The test is performed for diagnostic purposes less frequently than in the past, as other modalities, such as endometrial biopsy and pelvic ultrasound have become available for use. D & C is usually performed therapeutically after an incomplete abortion or miscarriage.

Professional Considerations:

1. Consent form IS required.

Risks:

The primary complication is perforation of the uterus. If a perforation occurs and the client is stable, a laparoscopy can be performed to evaluate the perforation. If a perforation is suspected during a suction curettage, a laparoscopy must be performed to continue the procedure to be sure that bowel is not aspirated into the uterus. If the client becomes unstable, emergency surgery is necessary.

Contraindications:

Clients with coagulopathies or active vaginal infections.

2. Preparation:

A. Ascertain any drug allergies.

B. Perineal shave may be preferred.

C. The client should void prior to procedure.

D. An enema may be prescribed prior to the procedure.

E. An intravenous line may be initiated.

F. Obtain containers of 10% formalin solution for tissue specimens.

G. Measure and document baseline vital signs.

3. Procedure:
   A. Regional or general anesthesia is initiated.
   B. The cervical canal is dilated with a dilator and the uterine canal is scraped with a curette.
   C. Tissue specimens are placed in containers of 10% formalin and sent to the laboratory for analysis. If an infection is suspected, part of the specimen should be placed in a sterile container without fixative and sent to the laboratory for culture and sensitivity.

4. Postprocedure care:
   A. Assess vital signs every 15 minutes until stable and then every hour × 4 following general anesthesia. Additional monitoring after general anesthesia typically includes continuous ECG monitoring and pulse oximetry, with continual assessments (q 5–15 minutes) of airway, vital signs, and neurologic status until the client is lying quietly awake, is breathing independently, and responds appropriately to commands spoken in a normal tone.
   B. Following regional anesthesia, assess vital signs when the procedure is completed and continue to monitor if unstable.
   C. Assess the perineal pad for color and amount of drainage.
   D. Assess for postanesthesia sensation.
   E. Assess and medicate for cramping.

5. Client and family teaching:
   A. The procedure takes approximately 45 minutes.
   B. The procedure is accompanied by cramping similar to menstrual cramps. Medications will be given to keep this tolerable.
   C. Call the physician for signs of infection: fever >101°F (38.3°C), pelvic or vaginal pain, purulent vaginal drainage, or for excessive bleeding.

6. Factors that affect results:
   A. None found.

7. Other data:
   A. None.

Bibliography:

Feldman S, Cook EF, Harlow BL, Berkowitz RS: Predicting endometrial cancer among older women who present with abnormal vaginal bleeding. Gynecol Oncol 56(3):376–381, 1995.

Feldman S, Shapter A, Welch WR, Berkowitz RS: Two-year follow-up of 263 patients with post/perimenopausal vaginal bleeding and negative initial biopsy. Gynecol Oncol 55(1):56–59, 1994.

Holmes LB: Possible fetal effects of cervical dilation and uterine curettage during the first trimester of pregnancy. J Pediatr 126(1):131–134, 1995.

Lajinian S, Margono F, Mroueh J: Sonographic appearance of suspected iatrogenic uterine perforation. A case report. J Reprod Med 39(11):911–912, 1994.

DINITROPHENYLHYDRAZINE (DNPH) TEST, DIAGNOSTIC

Norm: Normal amino acid screen.

Usage: Cystinuria, Hartnup's homocystinuria disease, maple syrup urine disease, oasthouse urine disease, PKU, tyrosinemia, tyrosinosis, lactic acidosis, fructose-1,6-diphosphatase deficiency, ketosis, seizures, and unexplained mental retardation.

Description: Metabolic screening test to detect inherited disorders in the metabolism of branched-chain amino acids.

Professional Considerations:

1. Consent form NOT required.
2. Preparation:
   A. Obtain a clean specimen container.
3. Procedure:
   A. Obtain a 15-ml random urine specimen.
4. Postprocedure care:
   A. Keep the urine sample refrigerated or frozen.
5. Client and family teaching:
   A. Results are normally available within 72 hours.
6. Factors that affect results:
   A. Radiopaque contrast dye may increase the results.
   B. Falsely elevated results occur if valproic acid, penicillin derivatives, and/or benzoic acid preservatives have been ingested within three days of the urine collection.
7. Other data:
   A. A 24-hour urine sample may also be obtained.
   B. Peritoneal dialysis may be used to clear amino acids from the body.
   C. One of the branched-chain amino acids produces a metabolite that causes the urine to smell like maple syrup.
   D. The test can also be performed on a newborn heel stick blood spot as part of the neonatal screening for metabolic disorders.

Bibliography:

Cabello ML, Garcia AM, Dalmau J, Dominguez C, Conde C: An asymptomatic variant of maple syrup urine disease without organic aciduria. J Inherit Metab Dis 17(1):115–116, 1994.

Chace DH, Hillman SL, Millington DS, Kahler SG, Roe CR, Naylor EW: Rapid diagnosis of maple syrup urine disease in blood spots from newborns by tandem mass spectrometry. Clin Chem 41(1): 62–68, 1995.

Gouyon JB, Desgres J, Mousson C: Removal of branched-chain amino acids by peritoneal dialysis, continuous arteriovenous hemofiltration, and continuous arteriovenous hemodialysis in rabbits: implication for maple syrup urine disease treatment. Pediatr Res 35(3):357–361, 1994.

Kahler SG, Sherwood WG, Woolf D, Lawless ST, Zaritsky A, Bonham J, Taylor CJ, Clarke JT, Durie P, Leonard JV: Pancreatitis in patients with organic acidemias. J Pediatr 124(2):239–243, 1994.

DIPYRIDAMOLE-THALLIUM SCAN
(see Heart Scan, Diagnostic)

DIRECT ANTIGLOBULIN TEST
(see Coombs', Direct, Serum)

DISOPYRAMIDE PHOSPHATE, SERUM

Norm:

Therapeutic	2–5 µg/ml
Panic level	>7 µg/ml

Panic Level Symptoms and Treatment:

Symptoms: Prolonged QT interval and ventricular tachycardia, heart failure, hypotension.

Treatment:

Stop medication.
Monitor ECG for R-on-T phenomenon.
Support airway, breathing, and blood pressure.
Hemodialysis WILL remove disopyramide. No information was found on peritoneal dialysis' effect on disopyramide levels.

Usage: Monitoring for therapeutic dosage during disopyramide phosphate.

Description: A quinidinelike type 1a antidysrhythmic agent used to treat atrial and ventricular dysrhythmias. It depresses myocardial responsiveness, slows automaticity and raises cardiac tissue threshold, prolonging the effective refractory period. It also prolongs cardiac conduction. Disopyramide is metabolized by the liver, with a half-life of 4–10 hours. Up to 80% is excreted in the urine. Steady-state levels are reached after 25–30 hours.

Professional Considerations:

1. Consent form NOT required.
2. Preparation:
   A. Note the time the last dose was taken.
   B. Note on the laboratory requisition if the client is taking phenytoin, as this may cause decreased levels of disopyramide phosphate.
   C. Obtain a siliconized red-top or gold-sealed tube.
   D. Do NOT draw this specimen during hemodialysis.
3. Procedure:
   A. Draw a 1-ml blood sample.
   B. Draw a peak sample 2–3 hours after the oral dose.
   C. Draw a trough sample just before the next dose.
4. Postprocedure care:
   A. Assess the results prior to administration of the next dose.
5. Client and family teaching:
   A. The next dose of medication is dependent on these test results.
   B. Explain the need and timing of the peak and trough blood samples.
6. Factors that affect results:
   A. Results are elevated in renal and hepatic dysfunction.
   B. Blood levels are difficult to monitor, as the levels of free (unbound) disopyramide change considerably over a dosing interval.
   C. Metabolism increases with concomitant treatment with phenobarbital, phenytoin, and rifampin.
7. Other data:
   A. Other trade names include DSP, Napamide, Norpace, and Rythmodan.
   B. Metabolite has an anticholinergic effect, causing dry mouth, urinary retention, constipation, blurred vision, exacerbation of glaucoma, and dryness of bronchial secretions.
   C. Use with caution with myasthenia gravis as it may precipitate a crisis.
   D. Do not use with clients in heart failure or shock.
   E. More than 6 µg/mL may be needed to suppress ventricular dysrhythmias.
   F. Enhances the effect of warfarin and oral antihyperglycemics. Does not affect digoxin and digitoxin levels.

Bibliography:

Bursill JA, Wyse KR, Campbell TJ: Quinidine but not disopyramide prolongs cardiac Purkinje fiber action potentials after a pause. J Cardiovasc Pharmacol 23(5):833–837, l994.

Kumagai K, Gondo N, Matsuo K, Annoura M, Moroe K, Nakashima Y, Hiroki T, Arkawa K: Wavelength index: a predictor of the response to disopyramide in paroxysmal lone atrial fibrillation. Cardiology 85(3–4):184–192, 1994.

Pollick C: Effects of disopyramide on diastolic function in hypertrophic cardiomyopathy [letter; comment]. Am J Cardiol 75(8):652, 1995.

Shimizu A, Fukatani M, Tanigawa M, Kaibara M, Konoe A, Isomoto S, Centurion DA, Yano K, Hashiba K: Mechanism of the suppression of repetitive atrial firing by isoproterenol-comparison with disopyramide. Int J Cardiol 43(2):175–183, 1994.

DNA PLOIDY (STEMLINE DNA ANALYSIS), SPECIMEN

Positive: Aneuploid, polyploid.

Negative: Diploid.

Usage: Breast cancer prognosis.

Description: Malignant cells demonstrate greater proliferation than do normal cells and tend to have disordered cellular division whereby aneuploid DNA is present in individual cells. This abnormality increases with the degree of malignancy. Clinical studies indicate that the proportion of proliferating cells in a breast tumor biopsy and the degree of aneuploidy have prognostic significance for breast cancer. Longer disease-free periods after treatment tend to occur in individuals whose tumor has lower degrees of proliferation and fewer aneuploid cells.

Professional Considerations:

1. A consent form IS required for the biopsy itself but not for the test performed.
2. Preparation:
   A. Obtain a sterile formalin specimen container.
   B. The specimen may be obtained by needle or surgical biopsy.
3. Procedure:
   A. Place the tissue specimen in a sterile formalin specimen container.
4. Postprocedure care:
   A. Send the specimen to pathology as soon as possible.
5. Client and family teaching:
   A. DNA ploidy is only one means of measuring the degree of malignancy and prognosis of breast cancer. Other prognostic factors include status of axillary nodes, presence of estrogen and progesterone receptors, tumor size and extension into chest wall or skin, and distant metastasis.
   B. Use a mild analgesic for biopsy site pain.
6. Factors that affect results:
   A. An inadequate sample size may yield false-negative results.
7. Other data:
   A. DNA ploidy analysis may offer additional prognostic information in individuals with prostatic adenocarcinoma, lymphoma, bladder carcinoma, renal cell carcinoma, malignant melanoma, and head and neck cancers.
   B. Relatively few cells are needed to perform DNA ploidy flow cytometry. Therefore, tumors and response to treatment can be monitored for changes in the DNA content of the cells by serial needle biopsy.

Bibliography:

Carmichael MJ, Veltri RW, Partin AW et al.: Deoxyribonucleic acid ploidy analysis as a predictor of recurrence following radical prostatectomy for stage T2 disease. J Urol *153*:1015–1019, 1995.

Hupperts PS, Schutte B, van Assche C, et al.: Ploidy and S-phase fractions (SPF) of primary breast cancers and their nodal metastases. Breast Cancer Res Treat *32*:197–202, 1994.

Koester SK, Maenpaa JU, Wiebe VJ, et al.: Flow cytometry: Potential utility in monitoring drug effects in breast cancer. Breast Cancer Res Treat *32*:57–65, 1994.

DNPH, DIAGNOSTIC
(see Dinitrophenylhydrazine Test, Diagnostic)

DOPPLER ULTRASOUND FLOW STUDIES, DUPLEX DOPPLER ULTRASOUND FLOW STUDIES, DIAGNOSTIC

Norm: Normal blood flow velocity.

Usage: Evaluate blood flow through carotid arteries or peripheral blood vessels. Diagnose carotid artery disease, deep vein thrombosis (DVT), or peripheral vascular disease.

Description: A noninvasive, hand-held, mechanical ultrasound velocity detector that, through acoustical gel, records sound waves reflected from moving RBCs along veins and arteries. A duplex Doppler study adds real-time imaging to the pulsed, gated Doppler technique, giving a video display, which allows for better differentiation between arterial and venous flow. Low-frequency waves indicate low-velocity blood flow.

Professional Considerations:

1. Consent form NOT required.
2. Preparation:
   A. See *Client and Family Teaching.*
3. Procedure:
   A. For peripheral blood studies, pressure cuffs are placed on the extremities; the Doppler probe is used like a stethoscope. Takes 30 minutes.
   B. For carotid blood flow, the brachial pressure is taken and the Doppler flow meter is pressed against the neck region, temporarily compressing the temporal and carotid arteries to obtain blood flow signals. A disparity of 30 mmHg indicates arterial obstruction.
4. Postprocedure care:
   A. Maintain bedrest until otherwise instructed.

5. Client and family teaching:
   A. Do not smoke within 30 minutes before the test.
   B. The test takes less than 60 minutes, can be performed at the bedside, and is painless.
   C. Results are normally available within 24 hours.
6. Factors that affect results:
   A. Anxiety, diabetes, or nicotine constricts blood flow.
7. Other data:
   A. Intramural calcification may inhibit sound penetration, leading to false-positive results.
   B. Most accurate for diagnosis of proximal DVT, but less reliable in isolated calf vein thrombi.
   C. See also Ankle/Brachial Index, Diagnostic.

Bibliography:

Grady-Benson JC, Oishi CS, Hanson PB, Colwell CW Jr, Otis SM, Walker RH: Routine postoperative duplex ultrasonography screening and monitoring for the detection of deep vein thrombosis. A survey of 110 total hip arthroplasties. Clin Orthop (307):130–141, 1994.

Lin, HJ, Yip PK, Liu HM, Hwang BS, Chen RC: Noninvasive hemodynamic classification of carotid-cavernous sinus fistulas by duplex carotid sonography. J Ultrasound Med 13(2):105–113, 1994.

Maiuri F, Gallicchio B, Iaconetta G, Serra LL, Bernardo A: Intraplaque hemorrhage of the carotid arteries: diagnosis by duplex scanning. J Neurosurg Sci 38(2):87–92, 1994.

Meyer CS, Blebea J, Davis K Jr., Fowl RJ, Kempczinski RF: Surveillance venous scans for deep venous thrombosis in multiple trauma patients. Ann Vasc Surg 9(1):109–114, 1995.

DOXEPIN, BLOOD
(see Tricyclic Antidepressants, Plasma or Serum)

DRUG SCREEN, BLOOD
(see Toxicology, Drug Screen, Blood)

DRUG SCREEN, URINE
(see Toxicology, Drug Screen, Urine)

DVT SCAN
(see I-125 Labeled Fibrinogen Leg Scan, Diagnostic)

D-XYLOSE ABSORPTION TEST (XYLOSE TOLERANCE TEST), DIAGNOSTIC, SERUM OR URINE

Norm:

		SI Units
Serum		
Adults	25–40 mg/dl between 1 and 2 hours after ingestion of d-Xylose	1.67–2.66 mmol/L
Children	10–33% of dose ingested, or >30 mg/dl	2.01 mmol/L
>10 years old	>16% of 25-g dose	
Urine		
Adults	4 g of xylose excreted in 5 hours	
Children	16–33% excreted in 5 hours	

Increased: Disaccharidase deficiencies, Hodgkin's disease, malabsorption, and scleroderma.

Decreased: Amyloidosis, celiac disease, cystic fibrosis, diarrhea, massive bacterial overgrowth in small bowel, Whipple's disease, and any other jejunal mucosal disease.

Description: d-Xylose is a pentose (sugar) that is not metabolized by the body and is normally absorbed by the proximal small bowel and excreted unchanged by the kidney into the urine. The test is used to distinguish malabsorption from maldigestion.

Professional Considerations:
1. Consent form NOT required.
2. Preparation:
   A. See Client and family teaching.
   B. Obtain a large brown urine container and three red-top, marble-top, or gold-top tubes.

C. Assess renal function laboratory data (BUN, creatinine).

3. Procedure:
   A. At 0800 (8 A.M.), instruct the client to void and discard the sample.
   B. Draw a fasting blood sample.
   C. Give 25 g of d-Xylose dissolved in 250 ml water by mouth. Give a smaller weight-based amount to children.
   D. Follow with 500 ml of water orally.
   E. No further fluids or food should be given until the test is completed.
   F. Collect all the urine voided for 5 hours following ingestion of d-Xylose in a refrigerated container.
   G. Draw 7-ml blood specimens for d-Xylose levels 60 and 120 minutes following ingestion of d-Xylose.

4. Postprocedure care:
   A. Resume fluids and diet as prescribed.

5. Client and family teaching:
   A. Adults must fast for 8 hours and children for 4 hours prior to drinking prescribed d-Xylose.
   B. Do not eat foods containing pentose: fruits, jams, jellies, and pastries.
   C. The test involves specifically timed specimens.
   D. The test takes several hours. Bring reading material or other diversions to the test.

6. Factors that affect results:
   A. Drugs that will increase absorption in the intestines include aspirin, atropine, and indomethacin.

B. Poor renal function will decrease urinary output, and vomiting will decrease the amount of d-Xylose consumed and/or absorbed.

C. The urine output of d-Xylose may be decreased by dehydration, renal insufficiency, third spacing of fluid, and hypothyroidism, but these will not affect the serum levels.

D. Massive bacterial overgrowth in the small bowel may decrease the amount of d-Xylose available for absorption by the small bowel and therefore decrease the serum and urine levels.

7. Other data:
   A. Since an abnormal d-Xylose test suggests small bowel mucosal disease, a biopsy should be performed as the next step.

Bibliography:

Ehrenpyeis ED, Ganger DR, Kochvar GT, Patterson BK, Craig RM: D-xylose malabsorption: characteristic findings in patients with the AIDS wasting syndrome and chronic diarrhea. J Acquir Immune Defic Syndr 5(10):1047–1050, 1992.

Kadry Z, Furukawa H, Abu-Elmagd K, Manez R, Venkataramanan R, Tzakis A, Reyes J, Nour B, Fung J, Todo S, et al.: Use of the D-xylose absorption test in monitoring intestinal allografts. Transplant Proc 26(3):1645, 1994.

Peled Y, Doron D, Laufer H, Bujanover Y, Gilat T: D-xylose absorption test. Urine or blood? Dig Dis Sci 36(2):188–192, 1991.

EAR, ROUTINE, CULTURE
(see Culture, Routine, Specimen)

EASTERN EQUINE ENCEPHALITIS VIRUS TITER, SPECIMEN

Norm: Titer <1:10.

Positive: A fourfold increase in titer between acute and convalescent specimens supports the diagnosis of eastern equine encephalitis.

Negative: Normal finding or bacterial infection.

Description: Eastern equine encephalitis is an inflammation of the brain caused by an arbovirus that attacks the central nervous system. The mode of transmission to humans is through the bite of a mosquito of the genus *Culex*.

Professional Considerations:

1. Consent form NOT required.
2. Preparation:
   A. Tube: Red-top, red/gray-top, or gold-top.

B. Assess for fever and symptoms of meningitis and meningioencephalitis, including convulsions, abnormal reflexes, extremity rigidity, and bulging of the fontanelle in infants. In children, assess for headache, drowsiness of 2–3 days, nausea, and vomiting. In adults, assess for frontal headache, photophobia, nausea, and vomiting.

3. Procedure:
   A. Draw a 7-ml blood sample.

4. Postprocedure care:
   A. Send the specimen to the laboratory immediately.
   B. Draw a convalescent sample 14 days later.

5. Client and family teaching:
   A. The convalescent sample will be drawn in 2 weeks to see if the treatment is working.
   B. The mortality rate in the United States is 65–75%. Survivors often have significant neurologic disabilities.

6. Factors that affect results:
   A. Failure to collect a convalescent sample will result in the inability to show a ris-

ing of antibody titer between the acute and convalescent phases of the disease.

7. Other data:
   A. Common hosts include mosquitos, birds, ducks, fowl, and horses.

Bibliography:

Roehrig JT, Hunt AR, Chang GJ, et al.: Identification of monoclonal antibodies capable of differentiating antigenic varieties of eastern equine encephalitis viruses. Am J Trop Med Hyg 42(4):394–398, 1990.

Weaver SC, Scott TW, Rico-Hesse R: Molecular evolution of eastern equine encephalomyelitis virus in North America. Virology 182(2):774–784, 1991.

EBCT

(see Ultrafast Computed Tomography, Diagnostic)

ECG

(see Electrocardiogram, Diagnostic)

ECHINOCOCCOSIS SEROLOGICAL TEST, BLOOD

Norm: IHA 1:2–1:64.

Usage: Echinococcosis.

Description: Echinococcosis is a tapeworm infection common among clients in contact with sheep or cattle. Any member of the dog family may serve as a definitive host for the adult tapeworm. Dogs are infected by feeding on the offal of domestic animals, or on animal parts at butchering time. Children are at a high risk of ingesting eggs excreted by dogs because of their close contact with their pet dogs. Humans are the intermediate host. The eggs become bloodborne and form cysts in the liver and other parts of the body. It may take 5–20 years for a cyst to grow large enough to cause symptoms.

Professional Considerations:

1. Consent form NOT required.
2. Preparation:
   A. Tube: Red-top, red/gray-top, or gold-top.
   B. Obtain recent history for possible animal contact.
3. Procedure:
   A. Draw a 7-ml blood sample.
4. Postprocedure care:
   A. Surgical resection of the cyst is the treatment of choice.
   B. Aspiration of the cyst contents should not be attempted for a diagnosis because of the danger of rupture and leakage of the contents. This could cause an acute allergic reaction, anaphylactic shock, or dissemination of the infection.

5. Client and family teaching:
   A. Results are normally available within 72 hours.
6. Factors that affect results:
   A. False-positive results may occur in clients with a history of cirrhosis, collagen disease, systemic lupus erythematosus, or schistosomiasis.
7. Other data:
   A. Positive titers occur in 35–50% of cases with hydatid lung cysts, and in 85% with hydatid liver cysts.
   B. Removal of the cyst does not dramatically lower the antibody titer. It may persist for years.

Bibliography:

Afsar H, Yagci F, Meto S, Aybasti N: Hydatid disease of the kidney: evaluation and features of diagnostic procedures. J Urol 151(3):567–570, 1994.

Awad Mohammad Ael-N, Ray CJ, Karcioglu ZA: Echinococcus cysts of the orbit and substernum [letter]. Am J Opthalmol 118(5):676–678, 1994.

Babba H, Messedi A, Masmoudi S, Zribi M, Grillot R, Ambriose-Thomas P, Beyrouti I, Sahnoun Y: Diagnosis of human hydatidosis: comparison between imagery and six serologic techniques. Am J Trop Med Hyg 50(1):64–68, 1994.

Baijal SS, Basarge N, Srinadh ES, Mittal BR, Kumar A: Percutaneous management of renal hydatidosis: a minimally invasive therapeutic option. J Urol 153(4):1199–1201, 1995.

Vaizey CJ, Sanne I, Gilbert JM: Periappendiceal hydatidosis: an unusual cause of right iliac fossa pain. Br J Surg 81(9):1371–1372, 1994.

ECHOCARDIOGRAM (ECHO, HEART SONOGRAM, HEART ULTRASOUND), DIAGNOSTIC

Norm: No abnormalities.

Usage: Atrial septal defect, aortic stenosis or regurgitation, atrial tumors, bradycardia, cardiomyopathy, congenital heart disease, effusion (pericardial), embolization of artery, endocarditis, idiopathic hypertrophic subaortic stenosis, lymphoma metastasis, Marfan's syndrome, mitral regurgitation or stenosis, mitral valve prolapse, myocardial infarction postevaluation for wall motion abnormalities, myocarditis, panic disorder, patent ductus arteriosus, pericarditis, subacute bacterial endocarditis (SBE), transposition of the great arteries, tricuspid atresia, ventricular septal defect, and other cardiac defects.

Description: An echocardiogram is a noninvasive, acoustic imaging procedure that determines the size, shape, position, thickness, and movements of the heart valves, walls, and chambers during each cardiac cycle. It records the echoes created by the deflection of short pulses of an ultrasonic beam off of the cardiac structures onto an oscilloscope. The time required for the ultrasonic beam to be reflected back to the transducer from differing densities of tissue is converted by a computer to an electrical impulse displayed on an oscilloscopic screen to create a two-dimensional picture of the heart in different projections. The resolution of the oscilloscope recording obtained is determined by the frequency of the beam. Lower frequencies penetrate further, but provide less resolution than higher frequencies. An echocardiogram can also be performed transesophageal (TEE) with the transmitter inserted into the esophagus similar to an endoscope. This gives a clearer view of the valves and endocardium especially in the presence of obesity or severe chronic obstructive pulmonary disease (COPD).

Professional Considerations:

1. Consent form NOT required.
2. Preparation:
   A. The client should disrobe above the waist or wear a gown.
3. Procedure:
   A. With the client in a supine or recumbent position, conductive gel is placed over the third and fourth intercostal spaces to the left of the sternum.
   B. A transducer is angled directly over the intercostal spaces or beneath the xiphoid process to direct ultrasonic waves that are displayed on the oscilloscopic machine and printed in the M (motion) mode on a recorder.
   C. The client may also be placed on the left side to obtain a different view of the heart and may occasionally be asked to perform certain maneuvers or to inhale amyl nitrite (a gas with a slightly sweet odor) to record changes in heart function.
   D. For a transesophageal echocardiogram, the throat is anesthetized with spray and the transducer is passed orally into the esophagus. (*See Transesophageal Sonogram, Diagnostic* for more information).
4. Postprocedure care:
   A. Remove the conductive gel from the skin.
   B. For a transesophageal echocardiogram, oral fluids must be held until the local anesthesia is no longer in effect and the gag reflex has returned.
5. Client and family teaching:
   A. The procedure takes 30–60 minutes,

can be performed at the bedside, and is painless.
   B. Remain as still as possible.
   C. Results are normally available within 24 hours.
6. Factors that affect results:
   A. Thick chests, COPD, obesity, or chest wall abnormalities/scar tissue or dressings may alter the display of ultrasonic waves on the recorder.
   B. Better resolution can be obtained for children than for adults because their thinner, less dense chest wall enables use of a higher frequency, shorter wavelength sound.
   C. Improper placement of the transducer.
7. Other data:
   A. Very sensitive test in detecting pericardial effusion.
   B. Side effects of amyl nitrite, which has a short duration of action, are dizziness, flushing, and tachycardia.
   C. *See also Stress Test, Pharmacologic, Diagnostic.*

Bibliography:

Dans AL, Bossone EF, Guyatt GH, Fallen EL: Evaluation of the reproducibility and accuracy of apex beat measurement in the detection of echocardiographic left ventricular dilation. Can J Cardiol *11*(6):493–497, 1995.

Lopes LM, Cha SC, de Moraes EA, Zugaib M: Echocardiographic diagnosis of fetal Marfan syndrome at 34 weeks' gestation. Prenat Diagn *15*(2):183–185, 1995.

McPherson DD, Sirna S, Collins SM, Ross AF, Moyers JR, Kane BJ, Hiratzka LF, Marcus ML, Kerber RE: Can atherosclerotic coronary arteries vasodilate? An intraoperative high-frequency epicardial echocardiographic study. Am J Cardiol *76*(1):21–25, 1995.

Nakagawa T, Tanouchi J, Nishino M, Ito T, Ohnishi S, Tanahashi H, Yamada Y, Abe H: Transesophageal echocardiography combined with magnetic resonance imaging for detecting venous anomalies in dextrocardia. A case report [review]. Angiology *46*(6):531–535, 1995.

Spes CH, Mudra H, Schnaack SD, Klauss V, Rieber J, Reichle F, Kruger TM, Uberfuhr P, Angermann CE, Theisen K: Dobutamine stress echocardiography for detection of transplant coronary vasculopathy: comparison with angiography and intracoronary ultrasound. Transplant Proc *27*(3): 1973–1974, 1995.

ECHOENCEPHALOGRAM
(see Brain Sonogram, Diagnostic)

ECHOGRAM/ECHOGRAPHY
(see Abdominal Aorta Sonogram, Diagnostic; Brain Sonogram, Diagnostic; Breast Sonogram, Diagnostic; Echocardiogram, Diagnostic; Eye and Orbit Sonograms, Diagnostic; Gallbladder and Biliary System Sonogram, Diagnostic; Gynecologic Sonogram, Diagnostic; Kidney Sonogram, Diagnostic; Liver Sonogram, Diagnostic; Lymph Node

and Retroperitoneal Sonogram, Diagnostic; Obstetric Sonogram, Diagnostic; Pancreas Sonogram, Diagnostic; Prostate Sonogram Diagnostic; Spleen Sonogram, Diagnostic; Thyroid Sonogram, Diagnostic; Transesophageal Sonogram, Diagnostic; or Urinary Bladder Sonogram, Diagnostic)

EEG
(see Electroencephalogram, Diagnostic)

EGD
(see Esophagogastroduodenoscopy, Diagnostic)

EKG
(see Electrocardiogram, Diagnostic)

EKG, SIGNAL-AVERAGED, DIAGNOSTIC
(see Signal-Averaged Electrocardiography, Diagnostic)

ELECTROCARDIOGRAM (ECG, EKG), DIAGNOSTIC

Norm: Normal sinus rhythm, no dysrhythmias.

Usage: Anesthesia, angina pectoris, anxiety, dysrhythmias, atrial septal defect, beriberi, bradycardia, carbon monoxide poisoning, chest pain, coarctation of the aorta, congestive heart failure, effusion (pericardial), emergency monitoring, endocarditis, heart murmur, ischemia, myocardial infarction (MI), pacemaker function, palpitations, panic disorder, patent ductus arteriosus, pericarditis, preoperative evaluation, pulmonic stenosis, respiratory distress, surgery, syncope, tetralogy of Fallot, transposition of the great arteries, tricuspid atresia, ventricular hypertrophy, ventricular septal defect, and yellow fever.

Description: Recording of the heart's electrical current using electrodes from 12 different leads: bipolar limb leads I, II, III; augmented limb leads AVR, AVL, AVF; and precordial chest leads V_1–V_6. The heart's electrical activity takes three forms on the ECG: the P-wave, which signifies atrial depolarization; the QRS complex, which signi-

fies ventricular depolarization; and the T-wave, which signifies ventricular repolarization. This test identifies conduction abnormalities, dysrhythmias, monitors recovery from MI, and helps evaluate the effectiveness of cardiac medications. Single lead tracings monitor the presence and type of electrical conduction during cardiac emergencies and during insertion of a temporary transvenous pacemaker.

Professional Considerations:
1. Consent form NOT required.
2. Preparation:
   A. The client should disrobe above the waist.
   B. Cleanse the skin where the electrodes will be placed by rubbing it lightly with an alcohol wipe, then scraping gently with the edge of an electrode.
   C. Check the paper supply.
3. Procedure:
   A. *Single-channel recording:*
      i. The client is positioned supine.
      ii. Five electrodes are placed over clean fleshy skin with the conductor ends pointing upward. Electrodes are positioned on the right arm, the left arm, the right leg, and the left leg; the lead is sequentially repositioned for 6-second recording at locations V_1-V_6 on the chest.
      iii. The machine is turned on, and the recording is begun.
      iv. In nonautomatic machines, turn the lead selector to lead I and run it for 6 seconds for each lead from I through AVF. Then, turn the lead selector to neutral and determine the proper placement for leads V_1–V_6 before recording. The position of V_1 is at the fourth intercostal space, right sternal border. V_2 is at the fourth intercostal space, left sternal border. V_3 is midway between V_2 and V_4. V_4 is at the left midclavicular line at the fifth intercostal space. V_5 follows V_4 in a straight line over the fifth intercostal space to the anterior axillary line, and V_6 follows V_5 in a straight line over the fifth intercostal space to the left midaxillary line.
      v. The procedure takes 15 minutes.
      vi. During emergencies, three electrodes can be placed for monitoring: the white lead on the right upper chest, the black lead on the left upper chest, and the red lead on the lower left lateral chest.
   B. *Simultaneous 12-channel recording:*
      i. The client is positioned supine.
      ii. The limb leads are connected to electrodes and each is attached to a limb.

iii. Leads V_1–V_6 are connected to electrodes and attached to the chest wall in the locations described under procedure A.iv.

iv. The machine is activated and a simultaneous recording of all 12 channels is printed automatically by the electrocardiograph machine.

v. The procedure takes 5–10 minutes.

4. Postprocedure care:
   A. Label the ECG with name, room number, date, time, and episodes of chest pain during the procedure.
   B. Remove the electrodes and cleanse the skin of any residual conductive gel.

5. Client and family teaching:
   A. You should not move or talk during the procedure.

6. Factors that affect results:
   A. Body movement, poor skin cleansing, or improper electrode placement procedure produces artifact, which may necessitate repeating the test.
   B. The results should be interpreted in comparison with prior electrocardiograms, if available.

7. Other data:
   A. MI produces three changes on the ECG: elevated ST indicates formation of ischemia, and then the T wave flattens and inverts with an enlarged Q-wave appearing, which indicates necrosis.
   B. See also Holter Monitor, Diagnostic; and Signal-Averaged Electrocardiography, Diagnostic.
   C. The abbreviation "EKG" is often spoken and written instead of the more proper "ECG" to decrease confusion with "EEG" (electroencephalogram).

Bibliography:

Daoud EG, Pitt A, Armstrong WF: Electrocardiographic response during dobutamine stress echocardiography. Am Heart J 129(4):672–677, 1995.

Fesmire FM: ECG diagnosis of acute myocardial infarction in the presence of left bundle-branch block in patients undergoing continuous ECG monitoring. Ann Emerg Med 26(1):69–82, 1995.

Garland JL, Wolfson Ab: Routine admission electrocardiography in emergency department patients. Ann Emerg Med 23(2):275–280, 1994.

Horton LA, Mosee S, Brenner J: Uses of the electrocardiogram in a pediatric emergency department. Arch Pediatr Adolesc Med 148(2):184–188, 1994.

Velanovich V: Preoperative screening electrocardiography: predictive value for postoperative cardiac complications. South Med J 87(4):431–434, 1994.

ELECTROENCEPHALOGRAM (EEG), DIAGNOSTIC

Norm: No abnormal patterns.

Usage: Alzheimer's disease, brain cancer, brain death, central nervous system pain, dementia, epilepsy, focal brain lesions, insomnia, Jacob-Creutzfeldt disease, migraine headaches, myoclonus, narcolepsy, seizure disorders, sleep disorders, status epilepticus, vertigo, and tremor. Helps differentiate acute delirium from psychiatric illness, and the pseudodementia of depression from organic dementia.

Description: Recording of electric potentials based on the distribution of waveforms with different frequencies and amplitudes that are generated by the cerebral cortex of the brain.

Professional Considerations:

1. Consent form NOT required.

2. Preparation:
   A. See Client and family teaching.
   B. Check to see if certain medications must be withheld, such as anticonvulsants.
   C. Shampoo hair the night before and avoid any hair additives or cosmetics.

3. Procedure:
   A. The client is positioned in a supine position. Up to 25 electrodes, attached to a cap, are placed on the scalp. The scalp is cleaned and pricked at each site of the electrode and a small amount of conduction paste is applied. When all electrodes are correctly positioned with good skin contact, the cap is secured under the chin and recording begins.
   B. The client may be asked to follow several commands so that a baseline may be recorded. These commands may include opening/closing the eyes, blinking, swallowing, and hyperventilating. The client may also be stimulated with a repetitively flashing light.

4. Postprocedure care:
   A. Remove the cap with the electrodes.
   B. Reinstate medications that were withheld.

5. Client and family teaching:
   A. Do NOT drink cola, tea, coffee, or alcohol or eat chocolate up to 8 hours before the test.
   B. It is important to remain still during the test.
   C. The procedure takes up to 2 hours.

6. Factors that affect results:
   A. Fasting that results in hypoglycemia may decrease response time, leading to an abnormal pattern.
   B. Oily hair or hair spray interferes with the accuracy of the recording.
   C. Movement, sweating, and muscle tension may interfere with the tracing.

7. Other data:
   A. Petit mal shows spikes and waves of three cycles per second.
   B. Grand mal shows many high-voltage spikes and waves.
   C. Intracranial lesions show slow delta waves or unilateral beta waves.

D. A normal EEG may support diagnoses of retardation, depression, or schizophrenia.
E. Brain death is indicated by a flat line except for artifacts.
F. Encephalopathies show diffuse slowing of background activity.
G. Rapid activity is present in drug withdrawal states.
H. A single negative EEG should not rule out a seizure disorder. Serial or repeated EEG tracings are necessary.

Bibliography:

Nowack WJ, Jordan R: Propofol, seizures and generalized paroxysmal fast activity in the EEG. Clin Electroencephalogr 25(3):110–114, 1994.

Serafetinides EA: EEG in psychiatry. J Clin Psychiatry 54(10):397, 1993.

Shinner S, Kang H, Berg AT, Goldensohn ES, Hauser WA, Moshe SL: EEG abnormalities in children with a first unprovoked seizure. Epilepsia 35(3) 471–476, 1994.

Wical BS: Neonatal seizures and electrographic analysis: evaluation and outcomes [review]. Pediatr Neurol 10(4):271–275, 1994.

ELECTROLYTES, PLASMA OR SERUM

(see also Anion Gap, Blood; Carbon Dioxide, Blood; Chloride, Serum; Potassium, Serum; and Sodium, Plasma or Serum)

Norm:

		SI Units
Anion gap	7–17 mEq/L	7–17 mmol/L
Carbon dioxide, total content		
Adults	22–30 mEq/L or 38–50 mmHg	22–30 mmol/L
Panic levels	<15 mEq/L or >50 mEq/L	<15 mmol/L >50 mmol/L
Neonates–2 years	32–44 mmHg	
Children >2 years	22–26 mEq/L	22–26 mmol/L
Chloride		
Children and adults	97–107 mEq/L	97–107 mmol/L
Premature infants	95–110 mEq/L	95–110 mmol/L
Full-term infants	96–106 mEq/L	96–106 mmol/L
Panic levels	<80 mEq/L or >115 mEq/L	<80 mmol/L >115 mmol/L
Potassium		
Adults	3.5–5.3 mEq/L	3.5–5.3 mmol/L
Premature infants		
Cord blood	5.0–10.2 mEq/L	5.0–10.2 mmol/L
2 Days	3.0–6.0 mEq/L	3.0–6.0 mmol/L
Full-term newborn		
Cord blood	5.6–12.0 mEq/L	5.6–12.0 mmol/L
Newborn	3.7–5.0 mEq/L	3.7–5.0 mmol/L
Infants	4.1–5.3 mEq/L	4.1–5.3 mmol/L
Children	3.4–4.7 mEq/L	3.4–4.7 mmol/L
Panic levels		
Adults	<2.5 mEq/L or >6.6 mEq/L	<2.5 mmol/L or >6.6 mmol/L
Newborn	<2.5 mEq/L or >8.1 mEq/L	<2.5 mmol/L or >8.1 mmol/L
Sodium		
Adults	136–145 mEq/L	136–145 mmol/L
Umbilical cord	116–166 mEq/L	116–166 mmol/L
Infants	139–146 mEq/L	139–146 mmol/L
Children	138–145 mEq/L	138–145 mmol/L

Usage: Evaluate the four electrolytes at once and compare their relative values. Evaluate acid-base balance and determine the anion gap [$Na^+ - (Cl^- + HCO_3^-)$].

Description: The electrolyte panel is a series of tests performed on one tube of blood. The tests commonly included are *Anion Gap, Blood; Carbon Dioxide, Blood; Chloride, Serum; Potassium, Serum; and Sodium, Plasma or Serum.* See individual test listings for further description.

Professional Considerations:

1. Consent form NOT required.
2. Preparation:
   A. Tube: Red-top, red/gray-top, or gold-top.
   B. Do not allow the client to clench/unclench the hand prior to blood drawing.
   C. Do NOT draw specimens during hemodialysis.
3. Procedure:
   A. Collect the specimen without a tourniquet or quickly after tourniquet application, to prevent stasis.
   B. Using a 20-gauge or larger needle, draw a 5-ml blood sample.
   C. Do not aspirate strongly or push plunger into the vacuum tube too forcefully.
4. Postprocedure care:
   A. Write the collection time on the laboratory requisition.
   B. Transport the specimen to the laboratory within 15 minutes.
5. Client and family teaching:
   A. Do NOT clench/unclench the fist prior to blood drawing.
   B. Results are normally available within 24 hours.
6. Factors that affect results:
   A. Hemolysis of the specimen abnormally elevates the potassium level and invalidates results.
7. Other data:
   A. See individual test listings.

Bibliography:

Elias F M, Merkouropoulos M, Tsianos EV, Siamopoulos KC: Acid-base and electrolyte abnormalities in alcoholic patients. Miner Electrolyte Metab *20*(5):274–281, 1994.

Moon PF, Kramer GC: Hypertonic saline-dextran resuscitation from hemorrhagic shock induces transient mixed acidosis. Crit Care Med *23*(2): 323–331, 1995.

Omvik P, Myking OL: Unchanged central hemodynamics after six months of moderate sodium restriction with or without potassium supplement in essential hypertension. Blood Press *4*(1):32–41, 1995.

Vasuyattakul S, Lertpattanasuwan N, Vareesangthip K, Nimmannit S, Nilwarangkur S: A negative anion gap as a clue to diagnose bromide intoxication. Nephron *69*(3):311–313, 1995.

ELECTROLYTES, URINE
(see also Chloride, Urine; Potassium, Urine; Sodium, Urine)

Norm:

		SI Units
Chloride		
Adults	110–250 mEq/24 hours or 9 g/L	110–250 mmol/day
Children	15–115 mEq/L	15–115 mmol/L
Potassium		
Adults (intake-dependent)	25–123 mEq/24 hours	25–123 mmol/day
Children	17–57 mEq/24 hours	17–57 mmol/day
Sodium		
Adults	75–200 mEq/24 hours	75–200 mmol/day
Children		
Newborn	14–40 mEq/24 hours	14–40 mmol/day
6–10 years		
Females	20–69 mEq/24 hours	20–69 mmol/day
Males	41–115 mEq/24 hours	41–115 mmol/day
10–14 years		
Female	48–168 mEq/24 hours	48–168 mmol/day
Male	63–177 mEq/24 hours	63–177 mmol/day

Usage: Evaluate renal function and fluid volume status by noting the amount of each electrolyte excreted and determine the anion gap $[(Na^+ + K^+) - Cl^-]$.

Description: Urine electrolyte testing involves a series of tests performed on a sample of urine. The urine specimen may be random or a timed 12-hour or 24-hour urine. Tests commonly included are *Chloride, Urine; Potassium, Urine; and Sodium, Urine.* See individual test listings for further description.

Professional Considerations:

1. Consent form NOT required.
2. Preparation:
   A. Obtain a specimen container or 3-L container without preservatives or a pediatric urine collection device/bag and tape, depending on whether the sample is to be a random sample or a 24-hour urine collection.
   B. Write the beginning time of the collection on the laboratory requisition and the specimen container.
   C. Note the diuretic or glucocorticoid therapy on the laboratory requisition.
3. Procedure:
   A. Obtain a random fresh urine specimen from a void or a urinary catheter drainage bag.
   B. For a 24-hour specimen, discard the first morning urine specimen.
   C. Save all the urine voided for 24 hours in a refrigerated, clean, 3-L container without preservatives. Document the quantity of the urine output during the specimen-collection period. Include urine voided at the end of the 24-hour period. For catheterized clients, keep the drainage bag on ice and empty the urine into the collection container hourly.
   D. Pediatric/infant specimen collection:
      i. Place the child in a supine position with the knees flexed and the hips externally rotated and abducted.
      ii. Cleanse, rinse, and thoroughly dry the perineal area.
      iii. To prevent the child from removing the collection device/bag, a diaper may be placed over the genital area.
      iv. *Females:* Tape the pediatric collection device/bag to the perineum. Starting at the area between the anus and vagina, apply the device/bag in an anterior direction.
      v. *Males:* Place the pediatric collection device/bag over the penis and scrotum and tape it to the perineal area.
      vi. Empty the collection device/bag into the refrigerated collection container hourly.

4. Postprocedure care:
   A. For a 24-hour specimen, compare the urine quantity in the specimen container with the urinary output record for the test. If the specimen contains less urine than was recorded as output, some of the sample may have been discarded, invalidating the test.
   B. Document the quantity of urine and the collection ending time on the laboratory requisition.
   C. Send the specimen to the laboratory and refrigerate it.
   D. *See also individual test listings.*
5. Client and family teaching:
   A. Save all the urine voided in the 24-hour period and urinate before defecating to avoid loss of urine. Avoid contaminating the urine with toilet tissue or stool. If any urine is accidentally discarded, discard the entire specimen and restart the collection the next day.
6. Factors that affect results:
   A. All the urine voided for the 24-hour period must be included in the 24-hour specimen to avoid a falsely low result.
   B. For spot urine testing, potassium levels are higher at night than in the morning, and sodium levels are higher in the morning than at night.
   C. *See also individual test listings.*
7. Other data:
   A. Urine osmolality is often requested at the same time as urine electrolytes.
   B. *See also individual test listings.*

Bibliography:

Dyer AR, Shipley M, Elliott P: Urinary electrolyte excretion in 24 hours and blood pressure in the INTERSALT Study. I. Estimates of reliability. The INTERSALT Cooperative Research Group. Am J Epidemiol *139*(9):927–939, 1994.

Ruilope LM, Lahera V, Araque A, Suarez C, Rodicio JL, Romero JC: Electrolyte excretion and sodium intake [review]. Am J Med Sci 307 (Suppl 1): S107–S111, 1994.

Van Savage JG, McSherry SA, Lepor H, Mohler JL: Effects of alpha-adrenergic agonist on neobladder water and electrolyte transport. Urology *43*(3): 324–327, 1994.

ELECTROMYELOGRAM

(see Electromyogram and Nerve Conduction Studies, Diagnostic)

ELECTROMYOGRAM (EMG) AND NERVE CONDUCTION STUDIES (ELECTROMYELOGRAM), DIAGNOSTIC

Norm: For nerve conduction studies, the normal physiologic state is minimal activity at rest and a normal conduction velocity of 40 to 80 m/s (meters per second) after a nerve is stimulated. For an EMG, there should be no electrical activity from a muscle when it is at rest, and an orderly recruitment of voluntary motor unit potentials with gradually increasing voluntary motor muscle effort.

Usage: Amyotrophic lateral sclerosis, Bell's palsy, beriberi, botulism, carpal tunnel syndrome, cervical disc disease with nerve root compression, dermatomyositis, diabetic peripheral neuropathy, Eaton-Lambert syndrome, lesions affecting anterior horn cells, motor neuron disease, muscular dystrophy, myasthenia gravis, myopathy, myositis, nerve entrapment, neuropathy, poliomyelitis, polymyositis, polyneuropathy, and radiculopathy.

Description: For a nerve conduction test, electrodes are applied over the nerves and muscles being studied. Nerve conduction measurements are performed by electrically stimulating a nerve at one point and recording the velocity of the response either at the muscle for a motor nerve, or at some distance along the sensory nerve. Nerve conduction studies only directly test the portion of the nerve between the two sites. They do not detect damage more proximal or more distal to the nerve segments tested. The studies also only measure the speed of conduction in the largest and fastest conducting fibers of peripheral nerves, and so are most sensitive to changes in these fibers. For an EMG, needle electrodes are inserted into the muscles being studied to measure electrical activity during voluntary muscle contraction. When used in combination, the two tests can help differentiate the type of problem. A client may have a normal nerve conduction study with an abnormal EMG, or slowing of the nerve conduction with a normal EMG response.

Professional Considerations:

1. Consent form IS required.

Risks:
Dizziness, headache, hematoma.

Contraindications:
Anticoagulant therapy, bleeding disorders, cardiac pacemaker.

2. Preparation:
   A. *See Client and family teaching.*
   B. Muscle relaxants, anticholinergics, and cholinergics should be withheld with consent of the physician.
   C. If enzyme levels are to be drawn (AST, CK, LD), they should be drawn before the electrodiagnostic studies, or not until 5 days after the studies.
3. Procedure:
   A. Use a quiet room and a comfortable position for the client.
   B. For a nerve conduction study, place electrodes over the muscles and sensory nerves to be studied. Use a conduction gel for contact, and tape the electrodes in place. An electric shock is given proximal to the electrodes and the velocity of conduction is recorded.
   C. For an EMG, needle electrodes are inserted into selected muscles and electrical activity is recorded at rest and with muscle contraction.
   D. The results are recorded on tape or viewed on an oscilloscope.
4. Postprocedure care:
   A. Remove all the electrodes and clean off the conduction gel.
   B. Assess for bleeding or hematoma at needle insertion sites.
5. Client and family teaching:
   A. Do not eat or drink food or beverages containing caffeine such as coffee, tea, and cola; do not smoke for 3 hours prior to the procedure.
   B. The procedure takes 1 to 2 hours.
   C. The needle electrodes are uncomfortable when inserted and when the muscle into which they are inserted is moved. They also mildly damage and inflame the muscle. If a muscle biopsy may be required, the muscle to be biopsied should not be tested.
   D. For the nerve conduction test, the electrical shocks are uncomfortable.
6. Factors that affect results:
   A. Pain.
   B. Muscle relaxants, cholinergics, and anticholinergic medications.
7. Other data:
   A. These procedures are performed to extend clinical findings, not to replace clinical findings.
   B. Useful in differentiating between myopathy and neuropathy.
   C. An EMG can recognize denervation in muscles that is difficult to assess by physical exam. It can also differentiate muscle wasting due to neuropathic or myopathic disorders from disuse atrophy.

Bibliography:

Carter GT, McDonald CM, Chan TT, Margherita AJ: Isolated femoral mononeuropathy to the vastus lateralis: EMG and MRI findings. Muscle Nerve *18*(3):341–344, 1995.

Cheong DM, Vaccaro CA, Salanga VD, Waxner SD,

Phillips RC, Hanson MR: Electrodiagnostic evaluation of fecal incontinence. Muscle Nerve *18*(6): 612–619, 1995.

Haig AJ, Talley C, Grobler LJ, LeBreck DB: Paraspinal mapping: quantified needle electromyography in lumbar radiculopathy. Muscle Nerve *16*(5):477–484, 1993.

Morgenlander JC, Sanders DB: Spontaneous EMG activity in the extensor digitorum brevis and abductor hallucis muscles in normal subjects. Muscle Nerve *17*(11):1346–1347, 1994.

Rondinelli RD, Robinson LR, Hassanein KM, Stolov WC, Fujimoto WY, Rubner DE: Further studies on the electrodiagnosis of diabetic peripheral polyneuropathy using discriminant function analysis. Am J Phy Med Rehabil *73*(2):116–123, 1994.

ELECTROMYOGRAPHY (EMG), DIAGNOSTIC

(see Electromyogram and Nerve Conduction Studies, Diagnostic)

ELECTRON BEAM CT

(see Ultrafast Computed Tomography, Diagnostic)

ELECTRON MICROSCOPY (CARDIOMYOPATHY, NERVE TISSUE, SMALL BOWEL MUCOSA), DIAGNOSTIC

Norm: No abnormality or disease noted.

Usage: Adriamycin cardiotoxicity, cardiomyopathy, Hand-Schuller-Christian disease, liver disease, neuropathy, renal disease, tumors, and Whipple's disease.

Description: An examination of a thin section of tissue for microscopic evaluation. Used to define tumor classification when light microscopy is insufficient.

Professional Considerations:

1. Consent form NOT required for this test.
2. Preparation:
   A. Prepare for the surgical excision.
   B. Obtain a sterile container filled with 0.9% saline.
3. Procedure:
   A. Obtain a fresh unfixed tissue specimen and place it in a container of 0.9% saline.
4. Postprocedure care:
   A. Deliver the specimen to the laboratory immediately so the proper fixative can be applied.
5. Client and family teaching:
   A. Results are normally available within 72 hours.
6. Factors that affect results:
   A. Specimens should NOT be placed in formalin.

7. Other data:
   A. Useful in diagnosing or differentiating leukemia/lymphoma, sarcoma, endocrine, and brain tumors.
   B. This is an expensive and time-consuming procedure.

Bibliography:

Aharinejad S, MacDonald IC, MacKay CE, Mason-Savas A: New aspects of microvascular corrosion casting: a scanning transmission electron and high-resolution intravital video microscopic study. Microsc Res Tech *26*(6):473–488, 1993.

Faisant N, Gallant DJ, Bouchet B, Champ M: Banana starch breakdown in the human small intestine studied by electron microscopy. Eur J Clin Nutr *49*(2):98–104, 1995.

Gelb AB, Van Meter SH, Billingham ME, Berry GJ, Rouse RV: Infantile histiocytoid cardiomyopathy—myocardial or conduction system hamartoma: what is the cell type involved? Hum Pathol *24*(11):1226–1231, 1993.

ELECTRONYSTAGMOGRAPHY (EYE MOVEMENT) TEST, DIAGNOSTIC

Norm: Normal eye movement free of nystagmus.

Usage: Brain lesion, dizziness, unilateral hearing loss, nystagmus, tinnitus, and vertigo.

Description: Technique for recording eye movements allowing exact quantification of physiologic and pathologic nystagmus. The test picks up subtle spontaneous nystagmus and also helps differentiate peripheral from central nystagmus. The battery of tests includes visual ocular control, the search for pathological nystagmus with fixation and with eyes open in darkness, and measurement of induced physiologic nystagmus (caloric and rotational). The test can be helpful in identifying a vestibular lesion and localizing it within the peripheral and central pathways. It also provides serial tracings to compare a client's pattern over time.

Professional Considerations:

1. Consent form NOT required.

Risks:

Water caloric test: perforation of the ear drum.

Contraindications:

In clients with pacemakers. Do NOT use water caloric test on clients with a perforated ear drum.

2. Preparation:
   A. None.
3. Procedure:
   A. Small electrodes are taped to the skin on either side of each eye.
   B. Tests include calibration, gaze nystagmus, pendulum tracking, optokinetics, positional tests, and water caloric test.
      i. *Calibration test:* The client holds head straight and fixed and follows with the eyes, a stylus, from the right side to the middle and then to the left side.
      ii. *Gaze nystagmus test:* The client must close his or her eyes and perform an arithmetic task for 30 seconds while eye motion is recorded. Then, eye motion is recorded with the eyes open and fixed looking straight ahead.
      iii. *Pendulum tracking:* A 20-second eye motion recording is made as the client looks straight ahead and follows a pendulum with the eyes. This is followed by a 30-second recording of eye motion as the client stares straight ahead with the eyes closed.
      iv. *Optokinetics test:* Two 30-second recordings of eye motion are made as the client stares straight ahead and then follows a target across the visual field from right to left and then from left to right.
      v. *Positional tests:* A 5-second baseline recording of eye motion is obtained, followed by a recording of eye motion as the client follows the following nine commands:
         a. "With head erect and eyes forward, turn your head quickly to the right."
         b. "With head erect and eyes forward, turn your head quickly to the left."
         c. "Sit erect with eyes closed and quickly lie flat on your back with your eyes still closed."
         d. "Sit up quickly from the lying position with your eyes closed."
         e. "Lie on your back with your eyes closed and quickly turn your body and head to the right."
         f. "Lie on your back with your eyes closed and turn your body and head to the left."
         g. "Sit erect with your eyes forward and closed and lay your head back quickly so it hangs over the back of the chair."
         h. "Quickly pick up your head from over the back of the chair to the erect position."
         i. "Quickly put your head back to the right so that it hangs over the back right side of the headrest on the chair and then re-

peat this by putting your head to the left so it hangs over the back left side of the headrest on the chair."
      vi. *Water caloric test:* The client is positioned at a 30-degree head-of-bed elevation with the eyes closed. Water is instilled directly into the ear canal so that it hits the tympanic membrane, while eye motion is simultaneously recorded. This is followed by a 60-second recording with the eyes open, and a final recording with the eyes closed until nystagmus disappears, or for 3 minutes.
4. Postprocedure care:
   A. Remove electrodes.
   B. Assess for dizziness, nausea, and/or weakness.
5. Client and family teaching:
   A. The test takes less than 1 hour.
   B. The client must be cooperative and able to follow commands to ensure the accuracy of the test results.
6. Factors that affect results:
   A. CNS stimulants will increase eye movement and depressants will decrease eye movement.
   B. Poor eyesight.
   C. Loose electrodes.
   D. Requires considerable cooperation on the part of the client, and skill on the part of the operator in conducting and interpreting the test.
7. Other data:
   A. Results are reported as normal, borderline, or abnormal.

Bibliography:

Alvord LS, Herr RD: ENG in the emergency room: subtest results in acutely dizzy patients. J Am Acad Audiol 5(6):384–389, 1994.

Houston HG, Watson DR: A review of computerized electronystagmography technology [review]. Br J Audiol 28(1):41–46, 1994.

Larijani GE, Gratz I, Afshar M: Postoperative nystagmus and nausea. Ann Pharmacother 28(2): 179–181, 1994.

Nakamura T, Kanayama R, Aoyagi M, Kato I, Koike Y: Computer analysis for routine electronystagmography tests. Acta Otolaryngol 511(Suppl):109–113, 1994.

Panosian MG, Paige GD: Nystagmus and postural instability after headshake in patients with vestibular dysfunction. Otolaryngol Head Neck Surg 112(3):399–404, 1995.

ELECTROPHYSIOLOGIC STUDY (EPS), DIAGNOSTIC

Norm: Negative for ability to induce dysrhythmias. Normal cardiac conduction system mapping. No reentrant pathways identified.

Usage: To document the anatomy and physiologic substrates of episodic dysrhythmias by reproducing them so the mechanism can be identified. Helps diagnose cardiac conduction defects, circous reentry, ectopic foci, syncope of unexplained cause, tachydysrhythmias, and ventricular preexcitation syndromes; evaluates the effectiveness of antidysrhythmic medications or ablation; helps determine proper choice of a pacemaker; maps the cardiac conduction system prior to ablation; determines the need for an implanted defibrillator to prevent sudden cardiac death; and recording of intracardiac electrocardiograms.

Description: Electrophysiologic study involves the introduction of an electrode catheter under fluoroscopy through a peripheral vein or artery and into the cardiac chambers/sinuses and performing programmed electrical stimulation of the heart. Clients who may require EPS include survivors of sudden cardiac death, those with syncope with other than cardiac causes ruled out, and clients with dysrhythmias. Clients who usually require repeat EPS are those who have undergone antidysrhythmic therapy or catheter ablation since the last study. EPS is usually performed in a special laboratory or operating room by a cardiologist, with a specially trained registered nurse and a technician in attendance, certified in ACLS (Advanced Cardiac Life Support).

Professional Considerations:

1. Consent form IS required.

Risks:

Arterial injury (rare), cardiac perforation/rupture, cerebrovascular accident, fatal dysrhythmias, death, hemorrhage (rare), infection, insertion site hematoma, major venous thrombosis, myocardial infarction, pericardial effusion, pulmonary embolus.

Contraindications:

Bleeding disorders, thrombocytopenia. Sedatives are contraindicated in clients with central nervous system depression.

2. Preparation:
   A. Antidysrhythmic drugs are usually dis-

continued for several days prior to the test, when tolerated, for initial EPS. For evaluation of effectiveness of antidysrhythmic therapy, drug levels should reach a steady state prior to EPS. This may take several days or even a few weeks for drugs such as amiodarone.
   B. The client should fast from food overnight and from fluids for 4 hours prior to the test.
   C. Establish intravenous access.
   D. If left ventricular stimulation is planned that requires an arterial EPS route, preheparinization may be prescribed.
   E. Have emergency cart and defibrillator/cardioverter readily available.
   F. A sedative may be prescribed.
   G. Obtain baseline vital signs. Monitor vital signs and level of consciousness continuously throughout the procedure. Observe respiratory status closely throughout the procedure, especially if a sedative is administered.

3. Procedure:
   A. The client is positioned on the procedure table and the peripheral pulses distal to the insertion site are marked. The location and baseline quality of the pulses are documented.
   B. A baseline electrocardiogram is obtained. The leads are left in place for continuous cardiac monitoring.
   C. The insertion site is cleansed with povidone-iodine, allowed to dry, and draped.
   D. A cordis is introduced, using the Seldinger technique, through a femoral, brachial, subclavian, or jugular vein. An arterial approach is used for stimulation of the left ventricle. A size 5F, 6F, or 7F electrode catheter is advanced under fluoroscopy to the heart.
   E. Intracardiac electrocardiograms are recorded.
   F. After verifying proper catheter position, the following or any combination may be performed, depending on the purpose of the study (an amnestic such as midazolam may be administered prior to induction of dysrhythmias):
      i. Mapping of the electrical system and pathways, with characterization of the electrical properties of the cardiac conduction system.
      ii. Measurement of conduction times, refractory periods, and recovery times of different portions of the heart.
      iii. Pacing of the atria may be performed, and extrastimuli may be added at specific intervals, to evaluate whether they can stimulate dysrhythmias.
      iv. Attempts to induce dysrhythmias by delivery of a small electrical

charge to specific locations of the chamber walls.

v. Overdrive pacing.

vi. Antidysrhythmic drug effectiveness may be evaluated by administering the drug to terminate stimulated dysrhythmias.

G. Induced dysrhythmias that are poorly tolerated (i.e., cause hypotension, loss of consciousness) may be terminated by overdrive pacing, cardioversion, or defibrillation.

H. The catheter is removed, and pressure is applied to the site for 10 minutes, or at least until 10 minutes after bleeding stops. A pressure dressing is placed over the site.

4. Postprocedure care:

A. Assess and document the following every 15 minutes × 4, then every 30 minutes × 4, then hourly × 4, then every 4 hours until 24 hours after the procedure.

i. Vital signs.

ii. Insertion site for bleeding or hematoma.

iii. Color, motion, temperature, sensation, and the presence and quality of pulses in the extremity distal to the insertion site as compared to baseline, and the opposite extremity. Notify the physician for any changes from baseline assessment.

B. If deep sedation was used, follow institutional protocol for postsedation monitoring. Typical monitoring includes continuous ECG monitoring and pulse oximetry, with continual assessments (q 5–15 minutes) of airway, vital signs, and neurologic status until the client is lying quietly awake, is breathing independently, and responds appropriately to commands spoken in a normal tone.

C. For bleeding at insertion site, apply firm pressure for 10 minutes. If bleeding continues after 10 minutes, continue holding pressure, and notify physician.

D. A sandbag may be placed over the insertion site for several hours.

E. Maintain continuous electrocardiographic monitoring and observe for dysrhythmias for at least 24 hours.

F. Resume diet.

G. If antidysrhythmic drugs were administered during EPS or begun after EPS, observe cardiac monitor pattern for their effect.

5. Client and family teaching:

A. Fast from food from midnight the night before the procedure. Fluids may be taken up to 4 hours prior to the test but no caffeine is permitted.

B. The procedure takes up to 8 hours.

C. Because this procedure can be frightening, good explanations are necessary. Inform the client of the following information: you will have to lie as motionless as possible on your back, and feelings of flushing, anxiousness, dizziness, and palpitations are common during EPS. EPS will cause abnormal heart rhythms, and the doctors, nurses, and technicians are skilled at quickly treating these rhythms. The procedure may take 1–8 hours. After EPS, you must lie with the extremity distal to the insertion site motionless for several (usually 8) hours, and a sandbag may be in place over the site. Vital signs, the insertion site, and affected extremity circulation will be checked frequently after EPS.

6. Factors that affect results:

A. Antidysrhythmic drugs that are not completely cleared from the body prior to initial EPS may result in a falsely normal study.

7. Other data:

A. Subsequent treatment based on EPS findings may include antidysrhythmic drugs, ablation, implantation of an implantable cardioverter defibrillator (ICD), implantation of a rapid atrial pacemaker (overdrive pacing), combinations of the above, or other techniques.

B. *See also HIS Bundle Electrophysiology, Diagnostic.*

Bibliography:

Fisher JD, Kim SG, Ferrick KJ, Roth JA: Serial electrophysiologic-pharmacologic studies for the control of ventricular arrhythmias [review]. Coronary Artery Dis 5(8):653–664, 1994.

Reiter MJ, Mann DE, Reiffel JE, Hahn D, Hartz V: Significance and incidence of concordance of drug efficacy predictions by Holter monitoring and electrophysiological study in the ESVEM Trial. Electrophysiologic Study Versus Electrocardiographic Monitoring [see comments]. Circulation 91(7):1988–1995, 1995.

Riggio DW, Peters RW, Feliciano Z, Gottlieb SS, Shorofsky SR, Gold MR: Acute electrophysiologic effects of amiodarone in patients with congestive heart failure. Am J Cardiol 75(16):1158–1161, 1995.

Tung RT, Bajaj AK: Safety of implantation of a cardioverter-defibrillator without general anesthesia in an electrophysiology laboratory. Am J Cardiol 75(14):908–912, 1995.

EMG

(see Electromyogram and Nerve Conduction Studies, Diagnostic)

ENDOMETRIUM, ANAEROBIC, CULTURE

Norm: No growth of anaerobic bacteria.

Positive: Actinomycosis, endometriosis, and pelvic inflammatory disease.

Description: The endometrium is the interior uterine mucosal layer formed of epithelium. This is the uterine layer that proliferates and sheds in response to hormonal effects throughout the menstrual cycle. Because the uterus is an anaerobic environment, anaerobic endometrial infections may cause symptoms of severe abdominal pain and bloating, menstrual irregularities, and infertility problems. Endometrial culture is performed when any of the above are suspected.

Professional Considerations:

1. Consent form NOT required.
2. Preparation:
   A. Obtain disinfectant, a sterile syringe, a vaginal speculum, and an anaerobic transport tube.
3. Procedure:
   A. Place the client in the dorsal lithotomy position with feet in the stirrups and drape her for comfort and privacy.
   B. Insert the vaginal speculum, disinfect the cervix; then, using a sterile syringe, aspirate material through the cervical os.
   C. Expel air bubbles from the syringe and place the collected material into the anaerobic tube.
4. Postprocedure care:
   A. Provide a sanitary pad for the client for minor bleeding.
   B. Transport the specimen to the laboratory within 30 minutes.
   C. Include the site of the specimen and list any recent antibiotic therapy on the laboratory requisition.
5. Client and family teaching:
   A. A feeling of pelvic cramping similar to a strong menstrual cramp is normally felt during insertion of the aspiration tube through the cervix. Prostaglandin inhibitors, such as ibuprofen or naproxen sodium, will lessen the discomfort and may be taken before and/or after the procedure.
   B. Minor spotting on a sanitary pad is normal during the 24 hours after the procedure.
   C. Notify the physician for excessive bleeding, or for purulent drainage, increasing pelvic pain, or fever >101°F (38.3°C).
   D. Take showers, rather than tub baths, for 3–4 days.
   E. Do not have sexual relations for 7 days after the procedure.
   F. Results are normally available within 72 hours.
6. Factors that affect results:
   A. Do not refrigerate the sample(s).
7. Other data:
   A. This test is not optimal for fungus culture.

B. Actinomycosis may be associated with endometritis and pelvic inflammatory disease from use of IUD contraception.

Bibliography:

Chatwani A, Amin-Hanjani S: Incidence of actinomycosis associated with intrauterine devices. J Reprod Med *39*(8):585–587, 1994.

Faro S, Martens M, Maccato M, Hammill H, Pearlman M: Vaginal flora and pelvic inflammatory disease. Am J Obstet Gynecol *169*(2, Pt 2):470–474, 1993.

ENDOSCOPIC RETROGRADE CHOLANGIOPANCREATOGRAPHY (ERCP), DIAGNOSTIC

Norm: Patent bile ducts, duodenal papilla, pancreatic ducts, and gallbladder.

Usage: Determine the cause of cirrhosis, evaluate jaundice, diagnose cholangitis, pancreatic cancer, pancreatitis, pancreatic cysts, pancreatic ductal lesions, pancreas divisum, and papillary stenosis. After the ERCP, via endoscopy, cysts can be drained, stones can be removed from the common bile duct, and stents can be placed across biliary or pancreatic strictures.

Description: Endoscopic retrograde cholangiopancreatography (ERCP) is the radiographic viewing of the hepatobiliary tree and pancreatic ducts through an endoscope using contrast medium injected through the ampulla of Vater.

Professional Considerations:

1. Consent form IS required.

Risks:

Cholangitis, dysrhythmias, pancreatitis, perforation of intestine, peritonitis.

Contraindications:

Anticoagulant therapy, bleeding disorders, thrombocytopenia, renal insufficiency. Sedatives are contraindicated in clients with central nervous system depression.

2. Preparation:
   A. A kidney, ureter, and bladder (KUB) flat plate radiograph of the abdomen is taken to determine an absence of barium.
   B. *See Client and family teaching.*

C. Obtain a topical anesthetic, sedative, and endoscope.

D. Establish intravenous access.

3. Procedure:

A. A topical anesthetic is applied to the oropharyngeal area.

B. Sedatives are given intravenously.

C. The client is placed in the left lateral position.

D. The endoscope is inserted through the esophagus to the stomach and then into the duodenum.

E. The client is then placed in the prone position, the papilla is cannulated with a catheter, and contrast dye is injected into the pancreatic and/or bile ductal system.

F. Several radiographs are taken and then biopsies may be taken if desired.

4. Postprocedure care:

A. The client should have nothing by mouth until the gag reflex returns.

B. If deep sedation was used, follow institutional protocol for postsedation monitoring. Typical monitoring includes continuous ECG monitoring and pulse oximetry, with continual assessments (q 5–15 minutes) of airway, vital signs, and neurologic status until the client is lying quietly awake, is breathing independently, and responds appropriately to commands spoken in a normal tone.

C. Assess for the complication of urinary retention.

5. Client and family teaching:

A. Fast from food and fluids for 12 hours before and after the procedure until the gag reflex returns.

B. The procedure takes approximately 1 hour.

6. Factors that affect results:

A. Retained barium can obstruct viewing.

7. Other data:

A. Up to 95% of the pancreatic duct and 85% of the biliary duct can be visualized by an experienced physician.

B. Useful in differentiating surgical from medical jaundice.

Bibliography:

Kent AL, Cox MR, Wilson TG, Padbury RT, Toouli J: Endoscopic retrograde cholangiopancreatography following laparoscopic cholecystectomy. Aust NZ J Surg 64(6):407–412, 1994.

Neuhaus H, Feussner H, Ungeheuer A, Hoffman W, Siewert JR, Classen M: Prospective evaluation of the use of endoscopic retrograde cholangiography prior to laparoscopic cholecystectomy. Endoscopy 24(9):745–749, 1992.

Wyllie R, Kay MR: Application of gastrointestinal endoscopy in infants and children. Curr Opin Pediatr 6(5):568–573, 1994.

ENTAMOEBA HISTOLYTICA, SEROLOGIC TEST, BLOOD

Norm: Negative, IHA titer <1:128, CF titer <1:8.

Positive: Diarrhea, dysentery, and liver abscess. A fourfold rise in titer supports the diagnosis of *Entamoeba* infection.

Negative: Bacterial infection of the intestines.

Description: *Entamoeba histolytica* is a protozoa that causes intestinal disease, transmitted in infected food and water by flies and by direct contact. Abscesses may form on the liver, lungs, and brain, causing fatalities.

Professional Considerations:

1. Consent form NOT required.

2. Preparation:

A. *See Client and family teaching.*

B. Tube: Red-top, red/gray-top, or gold-top.

3. Procedure:

A. Draw a 7-ml blood sample.

4. Postprocedure care:

A. Resume previous diet.

B. Draw convalescent sample 14–21 days after acute sample.

5. Client and family teaching:

A. Fast from food and fluids from midnight until after the test has been completed.

B. *Entamoeba histolytica* amebiasis is treated with metronidazole, except during pregnancy.

C. Return in 2–3 weeks to have a follow-up sample drawn. This will help determine whether the infection is responding to treatment.

6. Factors that affect results:

A. Ulcerative colitis may cause false-positive results.

7. Other data:

A. Serology may remain positive for as long as 2 years after curative therapy.

B. *Entamoeba histolytica* amebiasis is a reportable disease in most areas.

Bibliography:

Proctor EM: Laboratory diagnosis of amebiasis [review]. Clin Lab Med 11(4):829–859, 1991.

Salta RA, Martinez-Palomo A, Canales L, et al.: Suppression of T-lymphocyte response to *Entamoeba histolytica* antigen by immune sera. Infect Immunol 58(12):3941–3946, 1990.

Shandil RK, Vinayak VK: Cytopathogenicity of *Entamoeba histolytica* to human intestinal epithelial cells: inhibition by monoclonal antibodies and sera from amoebic patients. Jpn J Med Sci Biol 44(4):159–169, 1991.

EOS, BLOOD
(see Differential Leukocyte Count, Peripheral Blood)

EOSINOPHIL COUNT, BLOOD
(see Differential Leukocyte Count, Peripheral Blood)

EOSINOPHIL SMEAR, SPECIMEN

Norm: No eosinophils.

Usage: Evaluate allergic airway inflammation in clients with asthma.

Description: Eosinophils are found in increased numbers in the sputum of clients with allergic airway inflammation. An induced sputum is a useful noninvasive method for studying the inflammation.

Professional Considerations:

1. Consent form NOT required.
2. Preparation:
   A. Obtain two glass slides, a sterile applicator, and a sterile container.
3. Procedure:
   A. Obtain a sputum specimen in a sterile container, or induce a sputum specimen by giving the client an aerosol inhalation treatment with 0.9% saline and then encouraging him or her to cough.
4. Postprocedure care:
   A. The requisition must state the site of the specimen.
5. Client and family teaching:
   A. Deep coughs are necessary to produce sputum, rather than saliva. To produce the proper specimen, take several breaths in, without fully exhaling each, then expel sputum with a "cascade cough" and catch the sputum in the container.
   B. Results are normally available in 24 hours.
6. Factors that affect results:
   A. Reject slides received in cytology fixative.
7. Other data:
   A. Over 80% eosinophils in relation to total neutrophils suggests asthma.

Bibliography:

Eller J, Lapa E, Silva JR, Poulter LW, Lode H, Cole PJ: Cells and cytokines in chronic bronchial infection. Ann N Y Acad Sci 725:331–345, 1994.

Fahy JV, Liu J, Wong H, Boushey HA: Analysis of cellular and biochemical constituents of induced sputum after allergen challenges: a method for studying allergic airway inflammation. J Allergy Clin Immunol 93(6):1031–1039, 1994.

EP

(see Protoporphyrin, Free Erythrocyte, Blood)

EPHEDRINE

(see Amphetamines, Blood)

EPINEPHRINE, BLOOD

(see Catecholamines, Plasma)

EPS, DIAGNOSTIC

(see Electrophysiologic Study, Diagnostic)

EPSTEIN-BARR VIRUS (EBV), SEROLOGY, BLOOD

Norm: Negative, no virus found.

Increased: Burkitt's lymphoma, Epstein-Barr virus, head and neck tumors, Hodgkin's, infectious hepatitis, infectious mononucleosis, lymphocytic leukemia, nasopharyngeal carcinoma, sarcoidosis, and systemic lupus erythematosus.

Description: Epstein-Barr virus is a B-lymphocyte human herpesvirus that is the causative agent of infectious mononucleosis. The mode of transmission is through direct contact with the saliva of an infected client. Signs and symptoms, after a 4- to 8-week incubation period, include malaise, anorexia, chills, fever, cervical lymphadenopathy, pharyngitis splenomegaly, hepatitis, and peripheral atypical lymphocytosis. An Epstein-Barr virus panel is drawn, which includes four antibody levels: IgM VCA (viral capsid antigen), IgG VCA, EA (early antigen), and EBNA (Epstein-Barr nuclear antigen). The pattern of reactivity is helpful in distinguishing recent primary infection, reactivated infection, or remote inactive infection. Individual labs will give their reference range.

Professional Considerations:

1. Consent form NOT required.
2. Preparation:
   A. Tube: Red-top, red/gray-top, or gold-top.
   B. Write the date of the onset of illness on the laboratory requisition.
3. Procedure:
   A. Draw a 3-ml blood sample.
4. Postprocedure care:
   A. Refrigerate the serum after separation.
5. Client and family teaching:
   A. Results are normally available within 72 hours.
6. Factors that affect results:
   A. Cytomegalovirus in clients who have had organ transplants will cause a positive result for EBV serology.
   B. Post-transfusion reactions of blood and blood products will cause a temporary increase in EBV serology.
   C. False-positive results occur in clients with collagen vascular disease such as rheumatoid arthritis, leukemia, lymphoma, or HIV.

7. Other data:
  A. Up to 20% of people are negative for heterophil antibodies (*Monospot Screen, Blood*) with infectious mononucleosis.
  B. In the presence of clinical findings of infectious mononucleosis with negative heterophile and specific viral antibody tests, primary cytomegalovirus infection should be considered.
  C. Antibody titers for EBV are needed only if there is a question of a false-positive on the Monostat rapid slide test for EBV.
  D. Many people with chronic fatigue syndrome present with high antibody titers for EBV, but these are probably unrelated to the disease process.
  E. *See also Monospot Screen, Blood.*

Bibliography:

Benedetto A, Camporiondo MP, Di Caro A, Gallone D, Garbuglia AR, Sette P, Zaniratti MS: Predominance of Epstein-Barr virus DNA in immature CD21-deficient B-lymphocytes from HIV-infected patients [letter]. AIDS 7(2):292–293, 1993.

Cirone M, De Maria R, D'Alessandro A, Frati L, Faggioni A, Ragona G: Epstein-Barr virus DNA is present both in CD10/ cd77 positive and negative subsets of human tonsillar lymphocytes. Cancer Letters 89(1):125–128, 1995.

Lam KM, Whittle H, Grzywacz M, Crawford DH: Epstein-Barr virus-carrying B cells are large, surface IgM, IgD-bearing cells in normal individuals and acute malaria patients. Immunology 82(3):383–388, 1994.

Miyashita E, Thorley-Lawson DA: A new form of Epstein-Barr virus latency in vivo. Curr Top Microbiol Immunol 194:135–144, 1995.

ERCP

(see Endoscopic Retrograde Cholangiopancreatography, Diagnostic)

ERGONOVINE MALEATE TEST, DIAGNOSTIC

Usage: Aids in the diagnosis of coronary spasm during coronary arteriography, echocardiography, and electrophysiologic studies in clients with variant angina and no major occlusions of the coronary arteries.

Description: Erognovine stimulates contractions of vascular smooth muscle. It is administered during the cardiac procedure to produce and evaluate the effects of the resulting coronary artery spasm. The IV initial phase half-life is 1–5 minutes. The terminal phase half-life is 0.5–2.0 hours.

Professional Considerations:

1. Consent form IS required.

Risks:

Adverse drug effects may occur with Ergonovine: nausea and vomiting; dizziness; headache; tinnitus; diaphoresis; palpitations; transient chest pain; dyspnea; thrombophlebitis; hematuria; water intoxication; nasal congestion; diarrhea; and allergic phenomena, including shock. Ergonovine-induced hypertension has been accompanied by headaches, severe dysrhythmias, seizures, and cerebrovascular accidents. Hypotension has also been reported. *See also individual procedures for procedure-specific risks.*

Contraindications/Precautions:

Previous allergy to ergot, hypertension, pregnancy, toxemia, untreated hypocalcemia. Use Ergonovine with extreme caution in the presence of renal or hepatic dysfunction, coronary artery disease, peripheral vascular disease, or sepsis. *See also individual procedures for procedure-specific contraindications.*

2. Preparation:
  A. *See the listing for the procedure that is being performed.*
3. Procedure:
  A. 0.1–0.4 mg of ergonovine maleate is given slowly intravenously with dilution.
4. Postprocedure care:
  A. *See the specific procedure for postprocedure care.*
  B. Observe for adverse drug effects (listed under *Risks.*
5. Client and family teaching:
  A. Inform the client about the approximate time length of the procedure that will be used in conjunction with ergonovine administration.
6. Factors that affect results:
  A. None found.
7. Other data:
  A. Hypertension may occur if the client is given the IV dose too rapidly or without dilution, or if ergonovine is used along with a regional anesthetic or vasoconstrictor.
  B. This drug is also used to stimulate contractions of the uterus to prevent and treat postpartum and postabortion hemorrhage caused by uterine atony.

Bibliography:

Attenhofer C, Speich R, Salomon F, Burkhard R, Amann FW: Ventricular fibrillation in a patient with exercise-induced anaphylaxis, normal coronary arteries, and a positive ergonovine test. Chest 105(2):620–622, 1994.

Chimienti M, Negroni MS, Pusineri E, Regazzi MB, Inglese L, Klersy C, De Ambroggi L: Once daily felodipine in preventing ergonovine-induced myocardial ischemia in Prinzmetal's variant angina. Eur Heart J 15(3):389–393, 1994.

Fournier JA, Sanchez A, Cortacero JA: Selective ergonovine-induced coronary artery spasm and ST-segment alternans after blunt thoracic trauma. Int Cardiol 47(3):290–292, 1995.

Song JK, Park SW, Kim JJ, Doo YC, Kim WH, Park SJ, Lee SJ: Values of intravenous ergonovine test with two-dimensional echocardiography for diagnosis of coronary artery spasm. J Soc Echocardiogr 7(6):607–615, 1994.

Watanabe K, Inomata T, Miyakita Y, Takahashi M, Suzuki T, Koyama S, et al.: Electrophysiologic study and ergonovine provocation of coronary spasm in unexplained syncope. Jpn Heart J 34(2): 171–182, 1993.

ERYTHROCYTE, BLOOD
(see Red Blood Cells, Blood)

ERYTHROCYTE PROTOPORPHYRIN (EP), BLOOD
(see Protoporphyrin, Free Erythrocyte, Blood)

ERYTHROCYTE SEDIMENTATION RATE, BLOOD
(see Sedimentation Rate, Erythrocyte, Blood)

ERYTHROPOIETIN, SERUM

Norm: 7–36 milli-immunochemical units/ml.

Increased: Aplastic anemia, acute lymphocytic leukemia, cerebellar hemangioblastomas, chronic obstructive pulmonary disease, hepatoma, high altitudes, hypoxia, nephrectomy, nephroblastoma, pheochromocytoma, pregnancy, kidney transplant rejection, renal cancer, and renal cysts.

Decreased: Autoimmune diseases, Hodgkin's disease, polycythemia rubra vera, and renal failure (chronic).

Description: Erythropoietin is a glycoprotein produced in the peritubular cells in the renal cortex of the kidney. It is released in response to renal hypoxia and stimulates the formation and development of erythrocytes in the bone marrow.

Professional Considerations:
1. Consent form NOT required.
2. Preparation:
   A. Tube: Red-top, red/gray-top, or gold-top.
3. Procedure:
   A. Draw a 5-ml blood sample.
4. Postprocedure care:
   A. Note on the laboratory requisition the amount of oxygen delivery, as oxygen influences erythrocyte function.
5. Client and family teaching:
   A. The results are normally available within 24 hours.
6. Factors that affect results:
   A. Morning values are higher than afternoon values due to the diurnal rhythm of secretion.
   B. Blood donation increases serum values.
7. Other data:
   A. Useful in differentiating primary from secondary polycythemia.
   B. May not reliably detect ectopic erythropoietin-like substances, so neoplasia cannot be excluded.

Bibliography:

Kendall RG, Jeffries R, Cavill I, Norfolk DR: Relationship between endogenous erythropoietin levels, reticulocyte count, and reticulocyte RNA distribution. A study of anemic patients with and without renal failure. Ann NY Acad Sci 718:353–355, 1994.

Lee HY, Kim HS, Kang SW, Kang DH, Yoo HM, Choi KH, Han DS, Kim YS, Park KI: Serum erythropoietin levels after living-donor renal allografts. Transplant Proc 26(4):2151–2153, 1994.

Nowicki M: Erythropoietin and hypertension. J Hum Hyperten 9(2):81–88, 1995.

Sanders HN, Rabb HA, Bittle P, Ramirez G: Nutritional implications of recombinant human erythropoietin therapy in renal disease. J Am Diet Assoc 94(9):1023–1029, 1994.

Wood PA, Hrushesky WJ: Cisplatin-associated anemia: an erythropoietin deficiency syndrome. J Clin Invest 95(4):1650–1659, 1995.

ESOPHAGEAL ACIDITY TEST (TUTTLE TEST), DIAGNOSTIC

Norm:

Esophageal pH >5.0.
Esophageal reflux: pH ≤5.0

Usage: Helps diagnose gastroesophageal reflux.

Description: A test that evaluates the integrity of the esophageal sphincter by measuring the pH of gastric and esophageal contents using a pH electrode attached to an esophageal catheter introduced through the mouth and esophagus. This test may be performed in conjunction with esophageal manometry.

Professional Considerations:

1. Consent form IS required.

Risks:

Aspiration and chemical bronchitis, vasovagal response.

Contraindications:

Clients at high risk for poor tolerance of a vasovagal reaction (i.e., clients with known cardiac instability).

2. Preparation:
   A. *See Client and family teaching.*
   B. Verify that the client has fasted.
   C. Obtain a gastric catheter with a pH electrode, and 300 ml of 0.1%N hydrochloric acid (HCl).
   D. Establish intravenous access. Have a 0.9% saline and atropine on hand for use in the event a vasovagal response occurs.
   E. The client should void just prior to the test.
3. Procedure:
   A. Place the client in a high Fowler's position.
   B. Assess for vasovagal reaction, dysrhythmia, cyanosis, or coughing during the procedure.
   C. Introduce the catheter with a pH electrode through the mouth to the back of the throat. Instruct the client to swallow, perform the Valsalva maneuver, or lift the legs to stimulate reflux to catheter level; then determine the pH.
   D. If the pH is normal, pass the catheter into the stomach, instill 300 ml of 0.1%N HCl over 3 minutes, and repeat item 3B.
4. Postprocedure care:
   A. Assess vital signs every 30 minutes × 2. Extend assessments as needed if the client was treated for a vasovagal reaction during the procedure.
5. Client and family teaching:
   A. Fast from midnight before the test and avoid smoking for 24 hours prior to the test.
   B. Do not drink alcohol for 24 hours before the test.
   C. The physician may want you to stop taking adrenergic blockers, antacids, anticholinergics, cimetidine, cholinergics, corticosteroids, and reserpine for 24 hours before the test. Check with your doctor before stopping any of your medicine.

   D. You must swallow a catheter with a small electrode attached, which will measure the amount of acid in your esophagus and stomach. After the measurements are taken, the electrode will be slowly pulled out of your stomach.
   E. The test takes 30 minutes or less.
   F. The results are immediately available.
6. Factors that affect results:
   A. Antacids, anticholinergics, and cimetidine may decrease pH. Adrenergic blockers, cholinergics, corticosteroids, ethanol, and reserpine may increase pH.
7. Other data:
   A. None.

Bibliography:

Farkkila MA, Ertama L, Katila H, Kuusi K, Paavolainen M, Varis K: Globus pharyngis, commonly associated with esophageal motility disorders. Am J Gastroenterol *89*(4):503–508, 1994.

Thorne SM: Mother's internal working models with infants with gastroesophageal reflux. Maternal-Child Nurs J *22*(2):39–48, 1994.

ESOPHAGEAL MANOMETRY, DIAGNOSTIC

Norm:

"Congruent esophageal pressures bilaterally; smooth progression of motility and peristalsis in a proximal-to-distal pattern, absence of spasm.

Diurnal variations in distal and proximal pressure amplitudes, distal duration, and propulsive contractions.

Median proportion of propulsive waves: 56%.

Median proportion of simultaneous waves: 10%.

No significant difference in the elderly population." (Adamek, 1994)

Usage: Assessment and diagnosis of dysphagia, esophageal reflux, spasm, and motility abnormalities, hiatal hernia.

Description: In esophageal manometry, a multilumen esophageal catheter is introduced through the mouth and oropharynx into the esophagus, and pressures along the esophagus are measured as the client performs a series of swallowing maneuvers. The test helps identify locations of abnormal contractions and peristalsis in the esophagus, as well as areas of increased pressure that would indicate esophageal spasm. The test may be performed in conjunction with the esophageal acidity (Tuttle) test and the acid perfusion (Bernstein) test. It has been used extensively in the research setting in the study of esophageal motility disorders and is less commonly used in the clinical setting.

Professional Considerations:

1. Consent form IS required.

Risks:

Vasovagal reaction, dysrhythmia, cyanosis, or coughing.

Contraindications:

Clients at high risk for poor tolerance of a vasovagal reaction (i.e., clients with known cardiac instability).

2. Preparation:
   A. Verify that the client has fasted.
   B. The client should void just prior to the test.
   C. Obtain a gastric catheter, a swallowing sensor, water, and a syringe.
3. Procedure:
   A. Place the client in a high Fowler's position.
   B. Introduce the catheter through the mouth to the back of the throat. Instruct the client to swallow the catheter several times, until it has passed into the esophagus to the proper level.
   C. Reposition the client in a supine position.
   D. Attach the swallowing sensor to the client's neck.
   E. The client is then asked to swallow small amounts of water injected into the mouth with a syringe and the esophageal pressures are measured. This is followed by several dry swallows with corresponding pressure measurements.
4. Postprocedure care:
   A. Assess vital signs every 30 minutes × 2. Extend assessments as needed if the client was treated for a vasovagal reaction during the procedure.
   B. Observe for cholinergic side effects: bradycardia, dizziness, diaphoresis, flushing, muscle cramping, nausea, urinary urgency, and vomiting.
5. Client and family teaching:
   A. Fast from midnight before the test and avoid smoking for 24 hours prior to the test.
   B. Do not drink alcohol, or take adrenergic blockers, antacids, anticholinergics, cimetidine, cholinergics, corticosteroids, and reserpine for 24 hours before the test.

C. Arrange for transportation home, as you will not be allowed to drive for 12–24 hours after receiving edrophonium chloride.
D. You must swallow a catheter with a small electrode attached. You will then be asked to swallow several times, first with small amounts of water injected into the mouth, then without water. The catheter and neck sensor will measure the pressures in the esophagus as you swallow. After the measurements are taken, the catheter will be slowly pulled out of the stomach.
E. The test takes 30 minutes or less.
6. Factors that affect results:
   A. None.
7. Other data:
   A. *See also Acid Perfusion Test, Diagnostic* and *Esophageal Acidity Test, Diagnostic.*

Bibliography:

Adamek RJ, Wegener M, Wienbeck M, Gielen B: Long-term esophageal manometry in healthy subjects. Evaluation of normal values and influence of age. Dig Dis Sci *39*(10):2069–2073, 1994.

American Gastroenterological Association: An American Gastroenterological Association medical position statement on the clinical use of esophageal manometry. Gastroenterology *107*(6):1865, 1994.

Chang FY, Lee CT, Yeh CL, Lee SD, Chu LS: Correlation of esophageal manometry and radionuclide esophageal transit in normal subjects. Chin J Physiol *38*(1):43–46, 1995.

Kahrilas PJ, Clouse RE, Hogan WJ: American Gastroenterological Association technical review on the clinical use of esophageal manometry. Gastroenterology *107*(6):1865–1884, 1994.

Leite LP, Castell DO: Ambulatory esophageal manometry in the evaluation of unexplained chest pain. Dig Dis *13*(3):145–152, 1995.

ESOPHAGEAL RADIOGRAPHY, DIAGNOSTIC

Norm: Normal size and normal peristalsis.

Usage: Achalasia; esophageal varices; esophagitis; locating a foreign body; gastrointestinal bleeding; guidance for balloon dilatation of stricture; head and neck cancer; impaction; hiatus hernia; polyps.

Description: A radiographic and fluoroscopic examination of the esophagus for patency, structure, and motility. When examined in conjunction with the stomach, duodenum, and upper jejunum, this test is known as an upper GI series.

Professional Considerations:

1. Consent form IS required.

Risks:
This procedure carries minimal risks.

Contraindications:
Dysphagia, ileus.

2. Preparation:
   A. Verify that the client has fasted.
3. Procedure:
   A. A plain radiograph of the esophagus is taken in the supine position.
   B. Barium sulfate, approximately 400 ml, is then swallowed with the client in a standing position in front of the fluoroscope, and radiographs are again taken.
   C. Follow-up radiographs at 24 hours may be performed.
   D. The procedure takes 45 minutes.
4. Postprocedure care:
   A. Resume diet.
   B. Observe for passage of barium in the stool for 2–3 days.
   C. A laxative may be needed to evacuate barium.
   D. Encourage the oral intake of fluids to help prevent barium impaction.
5. Client and family teaching:
   A. Fast from food and fluids from midnight on, before the test.
   B. Drink 4–6 glasses of water per day (unless contraindicated) for 2–3 days after the test to promote barium excretion. Barium stools will look grayish-white. Notify health care provider if unable to pass barium in stool within 3 days.
   C. Results are normally available within 24 hours.
6. Factors that affect results:
   A. Retained barium from a previous examination interferes with the quality of the radiographic images.
7. Other data:
   A. Esophageal varices are difficult to identify and are usually a sign of liver cirrhosis.
   B. Barium comes in flavors, but is still described as unpleasant to swallow.

Bibliography:

Cole TJ, Turner MA: Manifestations of gastrointestinal disease on chest radiographs. Radiographics *13*(5):1013–1034, 1993.

DeVault KR, Castell DO: Current diagnosis and treatment of gastroesophageal reflux disease. Mayo Clin Proc *69*(9):867–876, 1994.

Halama AR: Clinical approach to the dysphagic patient. Acta Otorhinolaryngol Belg *48*(2):119–126, 1994.

McNicholas MM, Gibney RG, MacErlaine DP: Radiologically guided balloon dilatation of obstructing gastrointestinal strictures. Abdom Imaging *19*(2):102–107, 1994.

Shaffer HA Jr, de Lange EE: Gastrointestinal foreign bodies and strictures: radiologic interventions. Curr Probl Diagn Radiol *23*(6):205–249, 1994.

ESOPHAGOGASTRO-DUODENOSCOPY (EGD), DIAGNOSTIC

Norm: Normal upper gastrointestinal tract (i.e., esophageal mucosa is smooth and pink, with visible submucosal blood vessels; stomach mucosa is comprised of continuous, deeper red rugal folds; duodenal lining is covered with villi. All surfaces are free of ulcers, varices, bleeding, and lesions.

Usage: Biopsy, cancer, dysphagia, esophagitis, gastric ulcers, hiatal hernia, Mallory-Weiss tear, odynophagia (painful swallowing), postoperative examination of the gastrointestinal (GI) tract and upper GI bleeding.

Description: Visualization of the esophagus, stomach, and upper duodenum with a fiberoptic scope that has a lighted mirror lens on the end.

Professional Considerations:
1. Consent form IS required.

Risks:
Gastrointestinal perforation and hemorrhage, aspiration, infection, respiratory arrest, death.

Contraindications:
Zenker's diverticulum or large aortic aneurysm. Sedatives are contraindicated in clients with central nervous system depression.

2. Preparation:
   A. Verify that the client has fasted.
   B. The client should urinate and attempt to defecate prior to the procedure to increase comfort.
   C. The client should remove dentures, partial plates, and jewelry.
   D. Assess for allergies to anesthetics.
   E. Establish intravenous access.
   F. Obtain specimen containers, one with 95% ethyl alcohol, the other with 10% formaldehyde; an endoscope, and an intravenous sedative.
   G. Measure and record heart rate, blood pressure, and respiratory rate.
   H. Attach electrodes for continuous ECG monitoring and initiate continuous pulse oximetry measurement.
   I. Atropine may be prescribed to dry secretions prior to the test.
3. Procedure:
   A. A topical, bitter-tasting anesthetic is

applied to the throat and a mouth guard inserted if the client has teeth.
B. Intravenous sedation is given.
C. The endoscope is inserted into the esophagus and slowly advanced to the duodenum.
D. Air is instilled to distend any area to aid in visualization.
E. Biopsies and/or photos may be taken.

4. Postprocedure care:
A. If deep sedation was used for the procedure, follow institutional protocol for postsedation monitoring. Typical monitoring includes continuous ECG monitoring and pulse oximetry, with continual assessments (q 5–15 minutes) of airway, vital signs, and neurologic status until the client is lying quietly awake, is breathing independently, and responds appropriately to commands spoken in a normal tone.
B. Resume previous diet after the gag reflex returns and sedation has worn off, usually 2 hours following the procedure.
C. Observe for signs of perforation: pain, fever, dyspnea, tachycardia, cyanosis, and pleural effusion.

5. Client and family teaching:
A. Ambulatory clients should arrange for transportation home, because they will not be allowed to drive for 12 hours after the procedure.
B. Fast from food and fluids for 8 hours before the test.
C. You may receive medication to dry secretions during the test and this will cause a dry mouth. Sedation may also be used to cause a relaxed state that may or may not result in sleeping through the test. After a local anesthetic is sprayed in the back of the throat, you will be positioned lying on the side, and the flexible scope will be inserted through the mouth. Suction will remove any draining saliva. Pressure may be felt as the scope advances through the esophagus into the stomach. Feelings of bloating but not pain are common.
D. The procedure lasts about 40 minutes.
E. Results are normally available within 24 hours.

6. Factors that affect results:
A. If the client moves excessively during the procedure, the risk of perforation is increased.

7. Other data:
A. Emergency EGD diagnostic accuracy is 80–85%.

Bibliography:

Ibach MB, Grier JF, Goldman DE, LaFontaine S, Gholson CF: Diagnostic considerations in evaluation of patients presenting with melena and nondiagnostic esophagogastroduodenoscopy. Dig Dis Sci 40(7):1459–1462, 1995.

Pope JB, Mayeaux EJ Jr, Harper MB: Effectiveness and safety of esophagogastroduodenoscopy in family practice: experience at a university medical center. Fam Med 27(8):506–511, 1995.

ESR

(see Sedimentation Rate, Erythrocyte, Blood)

ESTERASE STAIN, DIAGNOSTIC

Norm: Descriptive interpretation by hematologist.

Usage: Leukemia.

Description: Stain of bone marrow to distinguish normal and leukemic cells of neutrophils, monocytes, and their precursors.

Professional Considerations:

1. Consent form NOT required.
2. Preparation:
   A. Obtain glass slides, a lancet, a capillary tube, and a bone marrow tray.
3. Procedure:
   A. Obtain a bone marrow specimen and a fingerstick collection for peripheral blood smear.
4. Postprocedure care:
   A. Assess the bone marrow aspiration site for bleeding and/or hematoma.
   B. The client must lie flat for 1–2 hours after the procedure.
   C. Send the specimen slides to the laboratory immediately.
5. Client and family teaching:
   A. Bone marrow aspiration is very painful, but only for a brief moment.
   B. Results are normally available within 24 hours.
6. Factors that affect results:
   A. Poor bone marrow sample will decrease the amount and/or quality of the cells, leading to inaccurate interpretation.
7. Other data:
   A. Staining of fresh specimens enhances assessment.
   B. *See also Bone Marrow Aspiration Analysis, Specimen* for professional considerations related to the bone marrow aspiration procedure.

Bibliography:

Drexler HG, Minowada J: Morphological, immunophenotypical and isoenzymatic profiles of human leukemia cells and derived T-cell lines. Hematol Oncol 7(2):115–125, 1989.

Ross DW: Monocyte esterase deficiency: Familial or environmental? [letter]. J Clin Pathol 43(11):963–964, 1990.

ESTRADIOL, SERUM

Norm:

		SI Units
Menstruating females		
Early cycle	20–170 pg/ml	73–626 pmol/L
Midcycle	70–500 pg/ml	258–1840 pmol/L
Late cycle	45–340 pg/ml	166–1251 pmol/L
Postmenopausal	15–18 pg/ml	18.4–66 pmol/L
Females taking oral contraceptives	12–50 pg/ml	44–184 pmol/L
Adult males	10–50 pg/ml	37–184 pmol/L
Prepubertal males	2–8 pg/ml	11–29 pmol/L

Increased: Adrenal tumors, cirrhosis, gynecomastia in males, hyperthyroidism, Klinefelter's syndrome, liver tumors, ovarian neoplasm, polycystic ovary syndrome.

Decreased: Amenorrhea, anorexia nervosa, hypopituitarism, infertility, menopause, osteoporosis, ovarian hypofunction, pituitary disease, and polycystic ovary syndrome.

Description: Estradiol is an estrogenic hormone secreted by the ovary and by the placenta that acts on the mucosa of the uterus to stimulate endometrial growth in preparation for the progestational stage. Other actions include follicle-stimulating hormone (FSH) suppression and luteinizing hormone (LH) stimulation. Estradiol levels help evaluate ovarian function, menstrual abnormalities, feminization disorders, and estrogen-producing tumors. Estradiol production diminishes or stops during menopause. Witt et al. (1995) found that basal estradiol levels helped predict success with artificial insemination by donor sperm. Goldin et al. (1994) found that a high-fiber diet reduced serum estradiol.

Professional Considerations:

1. Consent form NOT required.
2. Preparation:
   A. Tube: Red-top, red/gray-top, or gold-top.
3. Procedure:
   A. Draw a 3-ml blood sample.
4. Postprocedure care:
   A. Write the collection time, and the client's sex and present menstrual cycle phase on the laboratory requisition.
   B. Transport the specimen to the laboratory immediately for spinning and freezing within 1 hour.
5. Client and family teaching:
   A. Results are normally available within 24 hours.
6. Factors that affect results:
   A. Reject the specimen if the client has had a radioactive scan within 7 days.
   B. Highest levels occur 1 day before the LH surge, and again after corpus luteum formation.
   C. Drugs that may falsely elevate results include ampicillin, cascara, cortisone (large doses), diethylstilbestrol, hydrochlorothiazide, meprobamates, phenazopyridine, prochlorperazine, and tetracyclines.
7. Other data:
   A. The specimen is stable at room temperature for 1 week, in a frost-free refrigerator for 1 year, and in a nondefrosting freezer for 3 years.
   B. This test should not be used to evaluate fetal well-being, because it does not measure estriol.

Bibliography:

Elias AN, Stone SC, Tayyanipour R, Pandian MR, Rojas FJ, Gwinup G: Relationship between serum estradiol concentration and IGF-I, IGF-II, and IGF-binding proteins in patients with premature ovarian failure on short-term estradiol therapy. Int J Fertil Menopausal Stud *40*(4):196–201, 1995.

Goldin BR, Woods MN, Spiegelman DL, Longcope C, Morrill-LaBrode A, Dwyer JT, Gualtieri LJ, Hertzmark E, Gorbach SL: The effect of dietary fat and fiber on serum estrogen concentrations in premenopausal women under controlled dietary conditions. Cancer *74*(3, Suppl):1125–1131, 1994.

Witt BR, Barad DH, Barg P, Cohen BL, Lindheim SR, Testaiuti L, Amin HK: Basal serum follicle stimulating hormone (FSH) and estradiol levels as predictors of pregnancy in unstimulated donor insemination cycles. J Assist Reprod Genet *12*(3):157–160, 1995.

Yamamoto M, Hibi H, Katsuno S, Miyake K: Serum estradiol levels in normal men and men with idiopathic infertility. Int J Urol *2*(1):44–46, 1995.

ESTRADIOL RECEPTOR AND PROGESTERONE RECEPTOR IN BREAST CANCER, DIAGNOSTIC

Norm:

		SI Units
Negative	<6 fmol/mg cytosol protein	<6 nmol/kg cytosol protein
Borderline	6–10 fmol/mg cytosol protein	6–10 nmol/kg cytosol protein
Positive	>10 fmol/mg cytosol protein	>10 nmol/kg cytosol protein

Usage: Breast cancer.

Description: Estradiol, an estrogen hormone that is secreted almost entirely by the ovary, is most abundant in premenopausal women. Progesterone is a hormone excreted by the corpus luteum of the ovary that reaches its peak during the middle of the luteal phase of menstruation. Both of these hormones may create an environment where certain breast cancers can grow more prolifically. Therefore, knowing if a type of cancer grows in the presence of a certain hormone makes treatment modalities for decreasing levels of that hormone realistic. In this test, a sample of breast tissue is tested for the presence of estradiol and progesterone receptors. Hence, breast tissue, at least 1 g, is removed by excision or needle biopsy for identification as positive or negative for estradiol and progesterone receptors.

Professional Considerations:

1. Consent form IS required for biopsy. See *Biopsy, Site-Specific, Specimen* for procedure-specific risks and contraindications.
2. Preparation:
   A. Obtain a specimen jar; a waxed cardboard container or a plastic tube without fixative; and a needle biopsy tray.
3. Procedure:
   A. Local anesthetic is not used, because it can destroy estradiol receptors.
   B. 0.2–1.0 g of breast cancer tissue is removed by excision or needle biopsy, separated from fat and normal tissue, and placed in a dry jar, waxed cardboard container, or plastic tube that

does NOT contain formalin or saline. Label the specimen.
   C. Transport the fresh specimen to the laboratory immediately, prior to surgical wound closure.
   D. The specimen must be frozen quickly with liquid nitrogen, dry ice acetone, or cryostat within 20 minutes of collection.
4. Postprocedure care:
   A. Apply a dry, sterile dressing to the site.
5. Client and family teaching:
   A. A small sample of breast tissue will be removed with a hollow needle. The breast will not be numbed with an anesthetic, because this can cause false-negative results, so there will be discomfort for a short time. The procedure takes a few minutes and leaves no scar.
   B. Use mild analgesia for postprocedure pain, if needed.
   C. Results may not be available for several days.
6. Factors that affect results:
   A. Specimens not frozen within 20 minutes will falsely decrease results.
   B. Antiestrogen preparations taken within the last 2 months may cause a negative estradiol receptor response.
7. Other data:
   A. 50–70% of breast cancers are positive.

Bibliography:

Graham JD, Roman SD, McGowan E, Sutherland RL, Clarke CL: Preferential stimulation of human progesterone receptor B expression by estrogen in T-47D human breast cancer cells. J Biol Chem *270*(51):30693–30700, 1995.

Schodin DJ, Zhuang Y, Shapiro DJ, Katzenellenbogen BS: Analysis of mechanisms that determine dominant negative estrogen receptor effectiveness. J Biol Chem *270*(52):31163–71, 1995.

Tellez C, Jordan VC: Hormonal treatment of advanced breast cancer. Surg Oncol Clin North Amer *4*(4):751–777, 1995.

ESTRIOL, SERUM, 24-HOUR URINE
Norm:

	Total Estriol	SI Units

Serum

A diurnal pattern is present, with the highest levels occurring in the mid- to late afternoon.

Weeks of pregnancy		
30–32	31–330 ng/ml	108–1145 nmol/L
34–36	45–350 ng/ml	156–902 nmol/L
36–38	48–570 ng/ml	167–1978 nmol/L
40	95–460 ng/ml	330–1596 nmol/L

Urine

Week 30 of pregnancy	≥9 mg/24 hours
Females, nonpregnant	0–54 mg/24 hours
Males	0.3–2.4 mg/24 hours
Children	0.3–2.4 mg/24 hours
Panic level	4 ng/ml or 40% below the average of two prior values

Increased: Feminizing tumors, true precocious puberty, liver cirrhosis, and multiple pregnancy. Drugs include oxytocin.

Decreased: Anencephaly, abortion, anemia, choriocarcinoma, diabetes mellitus, erythroblastosis fetalis, fetal adrenal aplasia, fetal Down syndrome, fetal growth retardation, fetal encephalopathy, gynecomastia, hepatic disease, hemoglobinopathy, hydatidiform mole, intrauterine death, menopause, postmaturity, preeclampsia, and Rh immunization. Drugs include betamethasone, cascara, corticosteroids (large doses), dexamethasone, diuretics, glutethimide, estrogens, mandelamine, meprobamate, penicillins, phenazopyridine, phenolphthalein, probenecid, and Senna.

Description: Estriol is an estrogen synthesized in the placenta by a fetal hormone. Serum estriol levels are used to evaluate fetal and placental function for abnormalities such as growth retardation and fetal death. Low serum estriol has been associated with increased risk for X-linked ichthyosis. Estriol levels must be evaluated in consideration of the number of weeks gestation, because levels vary during pregnancy. Because serum levels fluctuate throughout the day, serial levels over time are used to evaluate the status of the fetus and the placenta.

Professional considerations:

1. Consent form NOT required.
2. Preparation:
   A. Tube: Red-top, red/gray-top, or gold-top.
   B. Obtain a clean, 3-L container without preservative.
3. Procedure:
   A. *Serum test:* Draw a 5-ml blood sample.
   B. *Urine test:*
      i. Discard the first morning urine specimen.
      ii. Begin to time a 24-hour urine collection.
      iii. Save all the urine voided for 24 hours in a clean, 3-L container. Document the quantity of urine output during the specimen collection period. Include the urine voided at the end of the 24-hour period.
4. Postprocedure care:
   A. Mix the 24-hour urine specimen gently, and obtain a 100-ml aliquot to send to the laboratory.
5. Client and family teaching:
   A. Discard the first specimen of the morning, then save all the urine voided in a 24-hour period and urinate prior to defecation to avoid loss of urine. If any urine is accidentally discarded, discard the entire specimen and restart the collection the next day.
   B. Results are normally available within 24 hours after completion of the urine collection.
   C. Refer pregnant clients with low serum estriol levels for genetic counseling.
6. Factors that affect results:
   A. Draw serum levels at the same time of the day for each sample.

B. Reject the specimen if the client has had a radioactive scan within 48 hours.

7. Other data:

A. Single values are not as meaningful as a trend in a series of measurements.

Bibliography:

David M, Israel N, Merksamer R, Bar-Nizan N, Borochowitz Z, Bar-el H, Yehudai I, Dar H: Very low maternal serum unconjugated estriol and prenatal diagnosis of steroid sulfatase deficiency. Fetal Diagn Ther 10(2):76–79, 1995.

Keren DF, Canick JA, Johnson MZ, Schaldenbrand JD, Haning RV Jr, Hackett R: Low maternal serum unconjugated estriol during prenatal screening as an indication of placental steroid sulfatase deficiency and X-linked ichthyosis. Am J Clin Pathol 103(4):400–403, 1995.

Saller DN Jr, Canick JA, Palomaki GE, Knight GJ, Haddow JE: Second-trimester maternal serum alpha-fetoprotein, unconjugated estriol, and hCG levels in pregnancies with ventral wall defects. Obstet Gynecol 84(5):852–855, 1994.

ESTROGEN RECEPTOR ASSAY, TISSUE SPECIMEN

(see Estradiol Receptor and Progesterone Receptor in Breast Cancer, Diagnostic)

ESTROGENS, NONPREGNANT, 24-HOUR, URINE

(see Estrogens, Serum and 24-Hour Urine)

ESTROGENS, SERUM AND 24-HOUR URINE

Norm:

	Total Estrogens	SI Units
Serum	pg/ml	ng/L
Premenopausal females	60–400	60–400
Postmenopausal females	<130	<130
Males	20–80	10–130
Children	<25	<25
24-Hour Urine	g/g Creatinine	mg/mol Creatinine
Adult females		
Follicular phase	7–65	0.79–7.35
Midcycle peak	32–104	3.62–11.75
Luteal phase	8–135	0.90–15.26
Adult males	4–23	0.45–2.60

Increased in Serum: Amenorrhea, fibrocystic disease, feminizing tumors, corpus luteum cyst, hypogonadism in males, and Stein-Leventhal syndrome. Drugs include cascara, chlortetracycline, estrogens, levodopa, oral contraceptives, phenothiazines, tetracyclines, and vitamins.

Increased in Urine: Adrenocortical tumor, ovarian or testicular tumors, and virilization. Drugs include acetazolamide (in pregnant women), cascara, clomiphene, chlortetracycline, corticotropin, hydrochlorothiazide (in pregnant women), levodopa, phenothiazines, testosterone, tetracyclines, and vitamins.

Decreased in Serum: Amenorrhea, anorexia nervosa, dysmenorrhea, infertility, menopause, menorrhagia, menstruation, metrorrhagia, osteoporosis, psychogenic stress, and Turner's syndrome. Drugs include acetazolamide, cascara, glucose, hydrochlorothiazide, phenothiazines, tetracyclines, and vitamins.

Decreased in Urine: Amenorrhea, menopause, ovarian dysfunction, and Simmonds' disease. Drugs include acetazolamide, cascara, glucose, hydrochlorothiazide, phenothiazines, senna, tetracyclines, and vitamins.

Description: Estrogen is a hormone produced in the ovaries, testes, placenta, and adrenals that influences the development and maintenance of the female sex organs. Estrogen levels in females fluctuate in predictable amounts throughout the menstrual cycle, with the highest amounts produced during ovulation and the levels greatly decreasing during the latter phase of the cycle. Decreasing estrogen and rising progesterone levels signal the body that pregnancy has not occurred and leads to sloughing of the uterine lining. Serum and urine tests may be performed independently.

Professional Considerations:

1. Consent form NOT required.
2. Preparation:
   A. Tube: Red top, red/gray-top, or gold-top. Also obtain ice.
   B. Obtain urine collection bottle containing 10-ml glacial acetic acid or boric acid.
3. Procedure:
   A. *Serum:* Draw a 1.5-ml blood sample. Place the specimen on ice.
   B. Discard the first morning void, then collect all the urine voided in a refrigerated, 24-hour urine bottle containing glacial acetic acid. For catheterized clients, keep the drainage bag on ice and empty the bag into a refrigerated collection container hourly.
4. Postprocedure care:
   A. Write the client's age, sex, and current menstrual cycle phase on the laboratory requisition. For urine samples, document the quantity of urine output and the ending time for the 24-hour collection on the laboratory requisition.
   B. Place the blood or urine specimen on ice. Deliver to the laboratory within 30 minutes after the collection has been completed.
5. Client and family teaching:
   A. Discard the first specimen of the morning, then save all the urine voided in a 24-hour period and urinate prior to defecation to avoid loss of urine. If any urine is accidentally discarded, discard the entire specimen and restart the collection the next day.
   B. Results are normally available within 48 hours.
6. Factors that affect results:
   A. Reject the specimen if the client has received a radioactive scan within the last 48 hours.
   B. An incomplete urine specimen may cause falsely decreased results.
7. Other data:
   A. Do NOT use this test in pregnant females or to assess fetal well-being, as it does not measure estriol.

Bibliography:

Ji AJ, Nunez MF, Machacek D, Ferguson JE, Iossi MF, Kao PC, Landers JP: Separation of urinary estrogens by micellar electrokinetic chromatography. J Chromatogr B Biomed Appl 669(1):15–26, 1995.

Sepkovic DW, Bradlow HL, Ho G, Hankinson SE, Gong L, Osborne MP, Fishman J: Estrogen metabolite ratios and risk assessment of hormone-related cancers. Assay validation and prediction of cervical cancer risk. Ann NY Acad Sci 768:312–316, 1995.

Spratt DI, Longcope C, Cox PM, Bigos ST, Wilbur-Welling C: Differential changes in serum concentrations of androgens and estrogens in post menopausal women with acute illness. J Clin Endocrinol Metab 76(6):1542–1547, 1993.

ETHANOL, BLOOD

(see Alcohol, Blood or Toxicology, Volatiles Group by GLC, Blood or Urine)

ETHCHLORVYNOL, BLOOD

Norm: Negative.

		SI Units
Therapeutic level	5–10 µg/ml	35–70 µmol/L
Toxic level	>20 µg/ml	>138 µmol/L
Panic level	>25 µg/ml	>150 µmol/L

Panic Level Symptoms and Treatment:

Symptoms: Nausea, vomiting, hypotension, bradycardia, respiratory depression, hypothermia, coma.

Treatment:

Monitor for noncardiogenic pulmonary edema.
Protect airway and support breathing.
Perform gastric lavage with warm tap water or normal saline if the client is treated soon after ingestion.
Give activated charcoal.
Seizure precautions: use phenobarbital or diazepam or restart ethychlorvynol, then taper drug if convulsions occur.
Administer resin or charcoal hemoperfusion if comatose
(*Note:* Hemodialysis and peritoneal dialysis will NOT remove ethychlorvynol from the bloodstream);
Provide cardiovascular and respiratory support of symptoms.

Usage: Drug abuse and overdose.

Description: A nonbarbiturate sedative-hypnotic drug that is absorbed through the gastrointestinal tract and metabolized in the liver, with a half-life of up to 20 hours. Duration of action is 5 hours.

Professional Considerations:

1. Consent form NOT required.
2. Preparation:
   A. Tube: Red-top or red/gray top.
   B. Do NOT use alcohol wipe at venipuncture site.
   C. The specimen MAY be drawn during hemodialysis.
3. Procedure:
   A. Cleanse the site with povidone-iodine, then draw a 5-ml blood sample.
4. Postprocedure care:
   A. Monitor cardiovascular, respiratory, and neurologic status for symptoms of overdose and provide support as needed.
5. Client and family teaching:
   A. For accidental overdose, teach client and family about proper dosing and side effects, as well as interactions of the drug with alcohol and the signs for which medical attention must be sought.
   B. For intentional overdose, refer the client and family for psychiatric counseling and crisis intervention.
   C. Referrals to appropriate rehabilitation centers and therapeutic community programs should be offered to all addicted clients who may be interested.
   D. If activated charcoal was given for elevated levels, the client should drink 4–6 glasses of water each day for 2 days to prevent constipation. The activated charcoal will cause stools to be black for a few days.
6. Factors that affect results:
   A. Peak blood levels occur 1.0–1.5 hours after ingestion.
   B. The refrigerated specimen remains stable at 0–6°C for several days.
7. Other data:
   A. Sedative effects are potentiated by alcohol.
   B. Ethchlorvynol interacts with monoamine oxidase (MAO) inhibitors, tricyclic antidepressants, alcohol, barbiturates, central nervous system depressants, and oral anticoagulants. Transient delirium reported when used concurrently with amitriptyline.
   C. Intravenous use may precipitate pleural effusion.

Bibliography:

Blanch L, Roussos C, Brotherton S, Michel RP, Angle MR: Effect of tidal volume and PEEP in ethchlorvynol-induced asymmetric lung injury. J Appl Physiol 73(1):108–116, 1992.
Yagi K, Baudendistel LJ, Dahms TE: Ibuprofen reduces ethchlorvynol lung injury: possible role of blood flow distribution. J Appl Physiol 72(3):1156–1165, 1992.

ETHOSUXIMIDE, BLOOD

Norm: Negative.

		SI Units
Therapeutic level	40–100 µg/ml	280–710 µmol/L
Panic level	>200 µg/ml	>1420 µmol/L

Overdose Symptoms and Treatment:

Symptoms: Nausea, vomiting, lethargy.

Treatment:
Give activated charcoal slurry.
Administer saline cathartic unless client has an ileus.
Give sorbitol cathartic.
Do gastric lavage if soon after ingestion.
Protect airway and support breathing.
Administer neurologic checks q 1 hour.
Forced diuresis is not helpful.
Hemodialysis WILL remove ethosuximide.

Increased: Drug abuse and overdose.

Decreased: Absence of Ethosuximide use and convulsions during ethosuximide use.

Description: Anticonvulsant used in the treatment of petit mal seizures. Depresses motor cortex and elevates central nervous system (CNS) threshold to stimuli. Absorbed from the gastrointestinal (GI) tract. Half-life of 40–60 hours in adults and 30–50 hours in children. Metabolized by the liver and excreted slowly in the urine. Steady-state levels are reached after 8–12 days in adults and 6–10 days in children.

Professional Considerations:

1. Consent form NOT required.
2. Preparation:
   A. Tube: Green-top, red/gray-top, or gold-top.
   B. Do NOT draw during hemodialysis.
3. Procedure:
   A. Draw a 1-ml blood sample.
4. Postprocedure care:
   A. Monitor for overdose symptoms and provide support as needed.
5. Client and family teaching:
   A. Results are normally available within 24 hours.
   B. Seek medical attention if early warning signs of drug overdose are noted: fatigue, drowsiness, confusion, difficulty waking up, slurred speech, unsteady gait.
   C. If activated charcoal was given for elevated levels, the client should drink 4–6 glasses of water each day for two days to prevent constipation. The activated charcoal will cause stools to be black for a few days.
   D. Referrals to appropriate rehabilitation centers and therapeutic community programs should be offered to all addicted clients who may be interested.
6. Factors that affect results:
   A. Peak levels occur 2–4 hours after dose.
7. Other data:
   A. Side effects include a lupuslike syndrome.
   B. Neurotoxic interaction with valproate is possible.
   C. Hypersensitivity to succinimides may cause adverse reactions, including pancytopenia, dizziness, myopia, vaginal bleeding, urticaria, swelling of tongue, and hirsutism.

Bibliography:

Villen T, Bertilsson L, Sjoqvist F: Nonstereoselective disposition of ethosuximide in humans. Ther Drug Monit 12(5):514–516, 1990.

ETHYL ALCOHOL
(see Alcohol, Blood or Toxicology, Volatiles Group by GLC, Blood or Urine)

ETHYLENE GLYCOL, SERUM AND URINE

Norm: Serum and urine: Negative.

Serum panic level	>2 mmol/L
Serum lethal level	>20 mmol/L

Poisoning Symptoms and Treatment:

Symptoms:

1. Within the first hour, the client appears drunk, followed by coma with convulsions.
2. In the first 12 hours, hypertension and leukocytes occur.
3. Within 12–24 hours, cardiopulmonary failure, acute renal failure, and metabolic acidosis occur. Other symptoms include abdominal pain and tetany.

Treatment:

Both hemodialysis and peritoneal dialysis WILL remove ethylene glycol.
Administer ethanol to saturate the compound.

Usage: Poisoning, either accidental or intentional, by alcoholics.

Description: Ethylene glycol is a compound contained in antifreeze that, when ingested and metabolized, causes toxicity to the body. After ingestion, oxalic acid is excreted by the kidneys, causing oxalate crystals in the urine, acidosis, tetany, and renal failure. The minimum lethal dose is approximately 100 ml, but any amount ingested may produce toxic symptoms. Half-life is 3 hours without treatment, 2.5 hours with dialysis, and 17 hours with concomitant oral ethanol.

Professional Considerations:

1. Consent form NOT required.
2. Preparation:
   A. *Serum:* Tube: Gray-top, red/gray-top, or gold-top.
   B. Do NOT draw during hemodialysis.
   C. *Urine:* Obtain a clean specimen container.
3. Procedure:
   A. *Serum:* Draw a 1-ml blood sample.
   B. *Urine:* Obtain a random urine sample in a clean container.
4. Postprocedure care:
   A. Store the blood or urine sample at 4°C.
   B. Observe for seizures or coma, and assess for renal failure.
5. Client and family teaching:
   A. Explain the possible side effects of ethylene glycol ingestion (described above) and that the client will require

intensive care monitoring for up to 48 hours or longer.
6. Factors that affect results:
    A. An uncooperative client may require catheterization to obtain a urine specimen.
7. Other data:
    A. Ethyl glycol can also be detected in gastric secretions.

Bibliography:

Bjellerup P, Kallner A, Kollind M: GLC determination of serum-ethylene glycol, interferences in ketotic patients. J Toxicol Clin Toxicol *32*(1):85–87, 1994.

Blanchard DE, Desjardins PR: A rapid measurement of ethylene glycol. Clin Biochem *27*(1):25–30, 1994.

Malmlund HO, Berg A, Karlman G, et al.: Considerations for the treatment of ethylene glycol poisoning based on analysis of two cases. J Toxicol Clin Toxicol *29*(2):231–240, 1991.

ETOH, BLOOD

(see Alcohol, Blood or Toxicology, Volatiles Group by GLC, Blood or Urine)

EUGLOBULIN CLOT LYSIS, BLOOD

Norm: Lysis in 1.5–4 hours.
Panic level: 100% lysis in 1 hour.

Panic Level Symptoms and Treatment:

Symptoms: Bleeding from wounds, phlebotomy sites, intracerebrally.

Treatment:
Discontinue any drugs (listed below) contributing to shortened lysis time.
Place the client on bleeding precautions.
Monitor neurologic status for signs of intracerebral bleeding.

Usage: Urokinase and streptokinase monitoring.

Decreased or Shortened Lysis Time: Disseminated intravascular coagulation (DIC), fibrinolysis, hemorrhage, pancreatic or pulmonary surgery, and pyrogen reactions. Drugs include asparaginase, clofibrate, dextran, epinephrine, streptokinase, and urokinase.

Description: Euglobulin clot lysis gives a measure of fibrinogen activity

by measuring plasminogen and plasminogen activator, which are proteins important in preventing fibrin clot formations.

Professional Considerations:

1. Consent form NOT required.
2. Preparation:
    A. Tube: 2.7-ml blue-top or a 4.5-ml blue-top and a control tube and a waste tube or syringe. Also obtain a container of ice.
    B. Schedule the test with the laboratory before drawing blood, as the sample must be centrifuged within 30 minutes of obtaining it.
3. Procedure:
    A. Avoid taking the sample from an extremity into which intravenous fluids are infusing.
    B. Withdraw 2 ml of blood into a syringe or vacuum tube. Remove the syringe or tube, leaving the needle in place. Attach a second syringe, and draw two blood samples, one in a citrated blue-top tube and the other in a control tube. The sample quantity should be 2.4 ml for a 2.7-ml tube and 4.0 ml for a 4.5-ml tube. Place the specimens immediately in a container of ice.
4. Postprocedure care:
    A. Deliver specimens to the laboratory for processing within 30 minutes.
5. Client and family teaching:
    A. Avoid strenuous physical activity for 1 hour prior to sampling.
6. Factors that affect results:
    A. Aminocaproic acid (Amicar) neutralizes urokinase and streptokinase.
    B. Lysis time may be shortened in clients who have exercised within the last hour.
    C. Venipuncture that is rough, including pumping the fist or massaging the vein, may shorten lysis time.
7. Other data:
    A. Heparin does not affect results.
    B. *See also Diluted Whole Blood Clot Lysis, Blood.*

Bibliography:

Asakura H, Jokaji H, Saito M, et al.: Changes in plasma levels of tissue-plasminogen activator/inhibitor complex and active plasminogen activator inhibitor in patients with disseminated intravascular coagulation. Am J Hematol *36*(3):176–183, 1991.

Marsh N: Does heparin stimulate fibrinolysis? Br J Haemotol *72*(2):163–167, 1990.

Sirridge MS, Reaner S: Laboratory Evaluation of Hemostasis and Thrombosis, 3rd ed. Philadelphia, Lea and Febiger, 1983, pp 173–174.

EXACTECH, DIAGNOSTIC

(see Glucose Monitoring Machines, Diagnostic)

EXCRETION FRACTION OF FILTERED SODIUM, BLOOD AND URINE

Norm: 1–2 excretion fraction (F).

Increased: Acute tubular necrosis, renal failure, uremia, and urinary obstruction. Drugs include diuretics.

Decreased: Azotemia, glomerulonephritis, and hepatorenal syndrome.

Description: A sensitive and specific test for acute tubular necrosis that requires assays of both urine and serum sodium and creatinine. The excretion fraction is calculated by the equation:

$$\frac{\text{Urine Sodium}}{\text{Plasma Sodium}} \times \frac{\text{Plasma Creatinine}}{\text{Urine Creatinine}} \times 100$$

Professional Considerations:
1. Consent form NOT required.
2. Preparation:
   A. Tube: Red-top, red/gray-top, or gold-top. Also obtain a urine cup.
   B. List diuretics on the laboratory requisition.
3. Procedure:
   A. Obtain a 10-ml random urine specimen.
   B. Draw a 7-ml blood sample.
4. Postprocedure care:
   A. Send specimens to the laboratory within 2 hours.
5. Client and family teaching:
   A. Results are normally available within 12 hours.
6. Factors that affect results:
   A. See individual tests (*Sodium, Plasma, Urine, Creatinine Plasma, Urine*).
7. Other data:
   A. Timed specimens are not required.

Bibliography:

Espinel CH, Gregory AW: Differential diagnosis of acute renal failure. Clin Nephrol *13*:73–77, 1980.
Lieberthal W, Levinsky NG: Treatment of acute tubular necrosis. Semin Nephrol *10*(6):571–583, 1990.
Rasmussen HH, Ibels LS: Acute renal failure. Multivariate analysis of causes and risk factors. Am J Med *73*:211, 1982.

EXOPHTHALMOMETRY TEST, DIAGNOSTIC

Norm: 12–20 mm. Eyes differ by <3 mm.

Usage: Cellulitis, endophthalmos, exophthalmos, periostitis, retinoblastoma, thyroid disease, tumors of the eye, and xanthomatosis.

Description: Measures the amount of forward protrusion of the eye by using an exophthalmometer. The exophthalmometer is a horizontal, calibrated bar with movable 45-degree mirrors on both sides.

Professional Considerations:
1. Consent form NOT required.
2. Preparation:
   A. If previous exam results are available, calibrate the bar to the baseline reading.
3. Procedure:
   A. Position client upright, facing the examiner, with eyes on the same level.
   B. Hold the horizontal bar of the exophthalmometer in front of the client's eyes and parallel to the floor.
   C. Move the two concave carriers against the lateral orbital margins and record the reading.
   D. Measure each eye separately.
   E. Have the client fixate his or her right eye on your left eye. Using the locked inclined mirrors, superimpose the apex of the right cornea on the scale, and record the reading.
   F. Repeat the procedure with the client's left eye fixated on the examiner's right eye and record the reading.
4. Postprocedure care:
   A. For abnormal results, refer to a specialist.
5. Client and family teaching:
   A. The test is painless.
6. Factors that affect results:
   A. Failure to set calibrated bar at baseline.
7. Other data:
   A. Use of steroids may contribute to exophthalmos.

Bibliography:

Hunter PD, Baker SS: The treatment of enophthalmos by orbital injection of fat autograft. *120*(8):835–839, 1994.
Kratky V, Hurwitz JJ: Hertel exophthalmometry without rim contact. *101*(5):931–937, 1994.

EXTRACORPOREAL SHOCK WAVE LITHOTRIPSY
(see Lithotripsy, Diagnostic)

EXTRACTABLE NUCLEAR ANTIGEN (ENA COMPLEX), SERUM
(see Anti-SM Test, Diagnostic; and Anti-RNP Test, Diagnostic)

EYE AND ORBIT SONOGRAMS (EYE AND ORBIT ECHOGRAMS, EYE AND ORBIT SONOGRAMS), DIAGNOSTIC

Norm: Negative for foreign body, cyst, inflammation, tumor, retinal detachment, or optic nerve atrophy. Orbit is of proper size, shape, and concavity.

Usage: Alternative to direct ophthalmoscopic visualization of the interior of the eye when cataract, fundal opacity, or vitreous hemorrhage is present; detection of intraocular foreign body or tumor; detection of retrobulbar optic nerve, optic nerve atrophy, or optic nerve tumor; differentiation of intraocular melanoma; eye measurement prior to lens implant; and evaluation of fundal abnormalities, intactness of retina, and the vitreous humor.

Description: Evaluation of the eye and orbit via the creation of an oscilloscopic picture from the echoes of high-frequency sound waves passing over the eye and eyelid (acoustic imaging). The time required for the ultrasonic beam to be reflected back to the transducer from differing densities of tissue is converted by a computer to an electrical impulse displayed on an oscilloscopic screen to create both a linear waveform and a two-dimensional dot-pattern picture of the structures. The B-scan mode is used to evaluate the optic disc, and the A-scan mode is used to evaluate optic nerve disease. Water immersion of the eye may also be used in conjunction with the eye sonogram to enhance images of the anterior part of the globe. The immersion of the transducer in water lifts it away from the eye, while still preventing air from obscuring the image. The transducer provides the best picture when it is at least 5–8 mm away from the structures being imaged. A newer method, ultrasound biomicroscopy, is able to provide even better images of the relationship of the structures of the anterior globe of the eye than is conventional immersion ultrasonography.

Professional Considerations:

1. Consent form NOT required.
2. Preparation:
   A. A sedative or general anesthetic may be used for children being evaluated for retinoblastoma or other purposes. The child should fast from food and fluids for 4 hours if general anesthesia will be used.
   B. Remove metal objects such as eyeglasses or jewelry from the client's head and neck.
   C. Obtain anesthetic eyedrops and conductive gel. If water immersion is to be performed, obtain an ocular drape and 0.9% sterile saline.
3. Procedure:
   A. The client is positioned supine in bed or on a procedure table.
   B. After anesthetic eye drops are administered, a transducer coated with conductive gel is slowly passed over a clear, methylcellulose eyeform applied to the eye to form an airtight seal. The resulting waveform provides eye measurements and helps delineate the presence of abnormal tissue or structure.
   C. The eye cup is removed and the eyelid closed. The gel-coated transducer is then slowly passed over the eyelid. A two-dimensional image of the eye and orbit are displayed on the oscilloscope.
   D. *Water immersion* (sometimes performed):
      i. A waterproof drape is fastened around the orbit.
      ii. After anesthetic drops are instilled, the eyelid is retracted and the eye is flooded with warm, sterile 0.9% saline.
      iii. The transducer is immersed into the water and moved slowly across the eye.
      iv. The client may be asked to move the eye in specific directions.
      v. The water is then drained and the drape removed.
   E. The procedure takes less than 30 minutes. Permanent photographs of the oscilloscopic recordings are made.
4. Postprocedure care:
   A. Remove conductive gel from the eyelid(s) after the anesthetic effects have worn off (to prevent corneal damage).
   B. If general anesthesia was administered, monitor vital signs every 15 minutes × 4, then every 30 minutes × 2, then hourly × 4. Additional monitoring typically includes continuous ECG monitoring and pulse oximetry, with continual assessments (q 5–15 minutes) of airway, vital signs, and neurologic status until the client is lying quietly awake, is breathing independently, and responds appropriately to commands spoken in a normal tone.
5. Client and family teaching:
   A. The procedure is noninvasive, painless, and poses no risk; it is important for you to relax the eyelid during the procedure.

B. You may hear an echo that sounds like repetitious humming or a musical note as the eye structures reflect the ultrasonic beam.

C. Avoid rubbing your eyes until the anesthetic effects have worn off (about ½ hour). Infants or small children may need to be restrained during this time.

6. Factors that affect results:
    A. None found.
7. Other data:
    A. None found.

Bibliography:

Doro D: Optic neuropathies: Diagnostic role of standardized echography. Metab Ophthalmol 13(2–4): 67–71, 1990.

Mrochuk J: Introduction to diagnostic ophthalmic ultrasound for nurses in ophthalmology. J Ophthalmol Nurs Technol 9(6):234–239, 1990.

Pavlin CJ, Harasiewicz K, Sherar MD, et al.: Clinical use of ultrasound biomicroscopy. Ophthalmology 98(3):287–295, 1991.

Romijn RL, Thijssen JM, Oosterveld BJ, et al.: Ultrasonic differentiation of intraocular melanomas: parameters and estimation methods. Ultrason Imaging 12(1):27–55, 1991.

Verbeek AM, Mitropoulos P: Diagnostic ultrasound: an aid in the differentiation of anterior segment lesions of the eye. Int Ophthalmol 15(3):205–212, 1991.

EYE CULTURE AND SENSITIVITY, DIAGNOSTIC

(see Conjunctival, Routine, Culture; and Conjunctival, Fungus, Culture)

EYE RADIOGRAPHY (X-RAY OF THE EYE), DIAGNOSTIC

Norm: Normal, no foreign bodies or masses.

Usage: Foreign bodies, fractures, and tumors.

Description: An invasive radiographic examination of the eye performed to determine the location of foreign body, tumor mass, or fracture of the orbit.

Professional Considerations:

1. Consent form IS required.

Risks:
Allergic reaction to contrast media (itching, hives, rash, tight feeling in the throat, shortness of breath, bronchospasm, anaphylaxis, death); renal toxicity from contrast medium.

Contraindications:
Previous allergy to iodine, shellfish, or contrast media; renal insufficiency.

2. Preparation:
    A. Have emergency equipment readily available.
3. Procedure:
    A. After the client's head is immobilized, he or she is asked to stare at a fixed point.
    B. Oxygen is injected between the capsule and sclera to detect a foreign body or into the muscle cone to detect masses.
    C. Iodine contrast may also be injected and radiography taken within 15 minutes due to the quick absorption rate.
    D. The total exam takes 40 minutes.
    E. For more precise localization, magnetic resonance imaging (MRI) is used.
4. Postprocedure care:
    A. Medicate for pain if required.
5. Client and family teaching:
    A. A head immobilizer will be used because any movement will blur the radiographic images. If needed, numbing medicine will be used to minimize discomfort during the procedure.
6. Factors that affect results:
    A. Motion of the client during radiography obscures the results.
    B. Artifacts in the film holder may cast shadows.
7. Other data:
    A. Meningiomas and papillomas are tumors that usually displace the eye.

Bibliography:

Griffiths HS, Sarno C: Contemporary Radiology: An Introduction to Imaging. Philadelphia, WB Saunders, 1979.

Hiatt RL: Eye trauma in children. South Med J 84(6):747–750, 1991.

Provenzale JM, Weber AL, Klintworth CK, McLendon RE: Radiologic–pathologic correlation. Bilateral retinoblastoma with coexistent pinealoblastoma (trilateral retinoblastoma). Am J Neuroradiol 16(1):157–165, 1995.

FACTOR, FITZGERALD (HIGH MOLECULAR WEIGHT KININOGEN), PLASMA

Norm: Activated partial thromboplastin time (APTT) normal or 25–35 seconds (ellagic acid activation products) or 30–45 seconds (diatomaceous earth activation products) after mixing the sample with plasma known to be deficient for the Fitzgerald factor.

Increased: Congenital deficiency of the Fitzgerald factor, factor XI (sometimes), factor XII deficiency (sometimes), and high molecular weight kininogen deficiency. Drugs include bishydroxycoumarin, heparin calcium, heparin sodium, and warfarin sodium.

Decreased: Not applicable.

Description: Fitzgerald factor deficiency is a rare, autosomal recessive trait affecting the intrinsic pathway of coagulation that results in an abnormal APTT and coagulation time without other factor deficiencies. Fitzgerald factor interferes with plasminogen activation, immune pathway activation, and generation of the vasoactive polypeptide bradykinin. The client is asymptomatic for bleeding.

Professional Considerations:

1. Consent form NOT required:
2. Preparation:
   A. Preschedule this test with the laboratory.
   B. Tube: 2.7- or 4.5-ml blue-top. Also obtain ice.
3. Procedure:
   A. Withdraw 2 ml of blood into a syringe or vacuum tube. Remove the syringe or tube, leaving the needle in place. Attach a second syringe, and draw a 2.4-ml sample in a 2.7-ml tube or a 4.0-ml sample in a 4.5-ml tube. Place the specimens immediately in a container of ice.
   B. Gently tilt the tube five or six times to mix.
4. Postprocedure care:
   A. Place the specimen on ice immediately.
   B. Write the collection time on the laboratory requisition.
   C. Transport the specimen to the laboratory immediately, discard the ice, and refrigerate the specimen. The sample should be centrifuged and refrigerated within 1 hour of collection. Freeze the plasma if the test will not be performed within 24 hours of specimen collection.
5. Client and family teaching:
   A. The client should not have warfarin therapy for 2 weeks or heparin therapy for 2 days before the test.
   B. Results are normally available within 24 hours.
6. Factors that affect results:
   A. Failure to discard the first 1–2 ml of blood may result in specimen contamination with tissue thromboplastin.
   B. Reject hemolyzed or clotted specimens, specimens not completely mixed, tubes partially filled with blood, specimens diluted or contaminated with heparin, specimens not placed on ice, or specimens received more than 1 hour after collection.
7. Other data:
   A. Compare results to prior PTT and APTT.
   B. *See Partial Thromboplastin Time; and Activated Partial Thromboplastin Substitution Test.*

Bibliography:

Matsueda R, Umeyama H, Puri RN, Bradford HN, Coleman RW: Design and synthesis of a kinogen-based selective inhibitor of thrombin-induced platelet aggregation. 7(1):32–35, 1994.

Vaziri ND, Gonzales EC, Wang J, Said S: Blood coagulation, fibrinolytic, and inhibitory proteins in end stage renal disease: Effect of hemodialysis. 23(6):828–835, 1994.

FACTOR, FLETCHER (PREKALLIKREIN), PLASMA

Norm: Activated partial thromboplastin time (APTT) normal or 30–45 seconds (diatomaceous earths activator) after mixing the sample with plasma known to be deficient for the Fletcher factor.

Increased: Fletcher factor deficiency, hepatic disease, prekallikrein deficiency, and uremia. Drugs include bishydroxycoumarin, heparin sodium, heparin calcium, and warfarin sodium.

Decreased: Not applicable.

Description: Rare condition of prolonged APTT and prekallikrein deficiency. The APTT shortens only after prolonged contact activation. The deficiency is thought to be inherited as an autosomal recessive trait in which the client is asymptomatic for bleeding. Fletcher factor is thought to function as a necessary component in the activation of factor XI and XII. To detect a deficient Fletcher factor, an APTT test is conducted on the sample and then repeated with a diatomaceous earth activator and lengthened incubation time from 3 to 10 minutes. The deficiency is suggested if the second APTT test is corrected.

Professional Considerations:

1. Consent form NOT required:
2. Preparation:
   A. Preschedule this test with the laboratory.
   B. Tube: 2.7-ml or 4.5-ml blue-top. Also obtain ice.
3. Procedure:
   A. Withdraw 2 ml of blood into a syringe or vacuum tube. Remove the syringe or

tube, leaving the needle in place. Attach a second syringe, and draw a 2.4-ml sample in a 2.7-ml tube or a 4.0-ml sample in a 4.5-ml tube. Place the specimens immediately in a container of ice.

   B. Gently tilt the tube five or six times to mix.

4. Postprocedure care:

   A. Place the specimen on ice immediately.

   B. Write the collection time on the laboratory requisition.

   C. Transport the specimen to the laboratory immediately, discard the ice, and refrigerate the specimen. The sample should be centrifuged and refrigerated within 1 hour of collection. Freeze the plasma if the test will not be performed within 24 hours of collection.

5. Client and family teaching:

   A. The client should not have warfarin therapy for 2 weeks or heparin therapy for 2 days before the test.

   B. Results are normally available within 24 hours.

6. Factors that affect results:

   A. Failure to discard the first 1–2 ml of blood may result in specimen contamination with tissue thromboplastin.

   B. Reject hemolyzed or clotted specimens, specimens not completely mixed, tubes partially filled with blood, specimens not received on ice, specimens diluted or contaminated with heparin, or specimens received more than 1 hour after collection.

   C. Ellagic acid activation products should not be used for this test.

7. Other data:

   A. Compare results to prior PT and APTT.

   B. *See Partial Thromboplastin Time; and Activated Partial Thromboplastin Substitution Test.*

Bibliography:

Fossum S, Hoem NO, Johannesen S, Korpberget M, Nylund E, Sandum S, Briseid K: Contact factors in plasma from women on oral contraception: significance of factor XI for the measured activity of factor XII. Throm Res *74*(5):477–485, 1994.

Tayeh MA, Olson ST, Shore JD: Surface induced alterations in the kinetic pathway for cleavage of human high molecular weight kinogen by plasma kallikrein. J Biol Chem *269*(23):16318–16325, 1994.

Weide I, Romisch J Simmet T: Contact activation triggers stimulation of the monocyte 5-lipooxygenase pathway via plasmin. Blood *83*(7):1941–1951, 1994.

FACTOR I, PLASMA

(see Fibrinogen, Plasma)

FACTOR II (PROTHROMBIN), BLOOD

(see Prothrombin Time, Blood)

FACTOR V (LABILE FACTOR, PROACCELERIN, AC-GLOBULIN), BLOOD

Norm: 50–150% of normal (control sample) activity. Half-life is 12–36 hours.

Increased: Not applicable.

Decreased: Alpha-globulin deficiency, disseminated intravascular coagulation, factor V deficiency, factor V inhibitors (circulating), fibrinogenolysis, hepatic disease, labile factor deficiency, leukemia (acute), parahemophilia, postoperatively, proaccelerin deficiency, and radioactive phosphorus therapy. Drugs include ansindione, bishydroxycoumarin, dicumarol, phenprocoumon, and warfarin sodium.

Description: Factor V is a vitamin K-dependent glycoprotein synthesized in the liver. It is part of the prothrombin-converting complex that functions in the extrinsic pathway of blood clotting. Specifically, it is a cofactor that accelerates the conversion of prothrombin to thrombin. Factor V deficiency is an inherited, autosomal recessive condition that occurs with equal frequency in men and women. The symptoms can be mild to severe and include bruising easily, frequent nosebleeds, menorrhagia, and prolonged bleeding after traumatic episodes, including operative and dental procedures. The test is performed by first performing a prothrombin time (PT) on the client's plasma. A factor V-deficient plasma substrate is then mixed with the client's plasma and the degree of correction in the PT is determined and compared to the degree of correction obtained by normal plasma.

Professional Considerations:

1. Consent form NOT required:
2. Preparation:

   A. Preschedule this test with the laboratory.

   B. Tube: 2.7- or 4.5-ml blue-top. Also obtain ice.

3. Procedure:

   A. Withdraw 2 ml of blood into a syringe or vacuum tube. Remove the syringe or tube, leaving the needle in place. Attach a second syringe, and draw a 2.4-ml sample in a 2.7-ml tube or a 4.0-ml sample in a 4.5-ml tube. Place the specimens immediately in a container of ice.

B. Gently tilt the tube five or six times to mix.

4. Postprocedure care:
   A. Place the specimen on ice immediately.
   B. For clients with coagulopathy, hold pressure over the sampling site for at least 5 minutes and observe the site closely for development of a hematoma.
   C. Write the collection time on the laboratory requisition.
   D. Take the iced specimen to the laboratory immediately, as factor V is labile in drawn blood samples.

5. Client and family teaching:
   A. The client should not have warfarin therapy for 2 weeks or heparin therapy for 2 days before the test.
   B. Results are normally available within 24 hours.
   C. Seek medical attention for signs of bleeding (i.e., hematoma, bleeding of gums, wounds, petechiae, confusion, changing level of consciousness).

6. Factors that affect results:
   A. Failure to discard the first 1–2 ml of blood may result in specimen contamination with tissue thromboplastin.
   B. Reject hemolyzed or clotted specimens, specimens not completely mixed, tubes partially filled with blood, specimens not on ice, specimens diluted or contaminated with heparin, or specimens received more than 2 hours after collection.
   C. Some drugs that may cause shortened prothrombin time include meprobamate, barbiturates, ethchlorvynol, glutethimide, oral contraceptives, and vitamin K.
   D. Some drugs that may cause prolonged prothrombin time include antibiotics, chloral hydrate, hydroxyzine hydrochloride, hydroxyzine pamoate, iothiouracil, methylthiouracil, phenylbutazone, phenyramidol, phosphorus (toxicity), propylthiouracil, salicylates, sulfonamides, tolbutamide, and vitamin A.

7. Other data:
   A. Coagulation factor roman numerals identify order of discovery rather than their order in the stages of clot formation.
   B. Platelet transfusion is a common treatment.
   C. *See Partial Thromboplastin Time; and Activated Partial Thromboplastin Substitution Test.*

Bibliography:

Beauchamp NJ, Daly ME, Cooper PC, Preston FE, Peake IR: Rapid two-stage PCR for detecting factor VG1691A mutation. Lancet *344*(8923):694–695, 1994.

Smid WM, DeWolf JT, Nijland JH, Bom VJ, Van der Meer J: Severe bleeding caused by an inhibitor to coagulation factor V: a case report. Blood Coagul Fibrinolysis *5*(1):133–137, 1994.

FACTOR VII (STABLE FACTOR, PROCONVERTIN, AUTOPROTHROMBIN I), BLOOD

Norm: 50–150% of normal (control sample) activity. Half-life is 6 hours.

Increased: Pregnancy (late) and thromboembolism, uremia. Drugs include oral contraceptives.

Decreased: Factor VII deficiency, hemorrhagic disease of the newborn, hepatic carcinoma, hepatitis, jaundice (obstructive), kwashiorkor, proconvertin autoprothrombin I deficiency, stable factor deficiency, and vitamin K deficiency. Drugs include ansindione, bishydroxycoumarin, dicoumarol, dicumarol, phenprocoumon, and warfarin sodium.

Description: Factor VII is a vitamin K-dependent beta globulin synthesized in the liver. It is activated in the extrinsic pathway during blood clotting, and in turn activates tissue thromboplastins, with excess amounts of factor VII present in serum and plasma when clotting is completed. Both forms of the rare factor VII deficiency are autosomal recessive and affect both males and females. Bleeding symptoms may be severe, including cerebral hemorrhage. The test is performed by first performing a prothrombin time (PT) on the client's plasma. A factor VII-deficient plasma substrate is then mixed with the client's plasma and the degree of correction in the PT is determined and compared to the degree of correction obtained by normal plasma.

Professional Considerations:

1. Consent form NOT required:
2. Preparation:
   A. Preschedule this test with the laboratory.
   B. Tube: 2.7-ml or 4.5-ml blue-top.
3. Procedure:
   A. Withdraw 2 ml of blood into a syringe or vacuum tube. Remove the syringe or tube, leaving the needle in place. Attach a second syringe, and draw a 2.4-ml sample in a 2.7-ml tube or a 4.0-ml sample in a 4.5-ml tube. Place the specimen immediately in a container of ice.
   B. Gently tilt the tube five or six times to mix.

4. Postprocedure care:
   A. For clients with coagulopathy, hold pressure over the sampling site for at least 5 minutes and observe the site closely for development of a hematoma.
   B. Write the collection time on the laboratory requisition.
   C. Transport the specimen to the laboratory immediately. Centrifuge and leave the specimens at room temperature.
5. Client and family teaching:
   A. The client should not have coumarin therapy for 2 weeks before the test.
   B. Results are normally available within 24 hours.
   C. Seek medical attention for signs of bleeding (i.e., hematoma, bleeding of gums, wounds, petechiae, confusion, changing level of consciousness).
6. Factors that affect results:
   A. Failure to discard the first 1–2-ml of blood may result in specimen contamination with tissue thromboplastin.
   B. Reject hemolyzed or clotted specimens, specimens not completely mixed, tubes partially filled with blood, specimens not refrigerated, or specimens received more than 2 hours after collection.
   C. Cold temperatures activate factor VII. Do not refrigerate or freeze the plasma.
   D. Drugs that may cause shortened PT include barbiturates, dorimide, ethchlorvynol, glutethimide, meprobamate, oral contraceptives, and vitamin K.
   E. Some drugs that may cause prolonged prothrombin time include antibiotics, chloral hydrate, hydroxyzine hydrochloride, hydroxyzine pamoate, iothiouracil, methylthiouracil, phenylbutazone, phosphorus (toxicity), propylthiouracil, salicylates, tolbutamide, and vitamin A.
7. Other data:
   A. After separation of plasma, factor VII is stable for 4 days at 25–37°C.
   B. *See Prothrombin Time.*
   C. Coagulation factor roman numerals identify order of discovery rather than their order in the stages of clot formation.

Bibliography:

Bremme K, Wramsby H, Andersson O, Wallin M, Blomback M: Do lowered factor VII levels at extremely high endogenous estradiol levels protect against thrombin formation? Blood Coagul Fibrinolysis 5(2):205–210, 1994.

Kario K, Matsuo T, Matsuo M, Koide M, Yamada T, Nakamura S, Sakata T, Kato H, Miyata T: Marked increase of activated factor VII in uremic patients. Thromb Haemost 73(5):763–767, 1995.

Miller GJ, Stirling Y, Howarth DJ, Cooper JC, Green FR, Lane A, Humphries S: Dietary fat intake and plasma factor VII antigen concentration [letter]. Thromb Haemost 73(5):893, 1995.

FACTOR VIII (ANTIHEMOPHILIA FACTOR, AHF), BLOOD

Norm: 50–150% of normal (control sample) activity.

Mild deficiency	5–25%
Moderately severe deficiency	1–5%
Severe deficiency	<1%
von Willebrand's disease	1–50%
Plasma level	≈100 µg/L

Increased: Coronary artery disease, exercise, hyperthyroidism, hypoglycemia, macroglobulinemia, pregnancy, and surgery. Drugs include oral contraceptives and sudden discontinuance of bishydroxycoumarin and warfarin sodium.

Decreased: Disseminated intravascular coagulation, factor VIII inhibitor (from childbirth, multiple myeloma, neoplasms, penicillin allergy, rheumatoid arthritis, or systemic lupus erythematosus), fibrinolysis, hemophilia A and von Willebrand's disease.

Description: Factor VIII is a glycoprotein thought to be made up of two components that are easily dissociated. One component contains von Willebrand Factor (vWf). The second component contains factor VIII Ag, a protein antigen, and factor VIII (measured by this test), which refers to the coagulant activity. Factor VIII is the antihemophilia (A) factor essential for thromboplastin generation in stage I of the intrinsic coagulation pathway. Factor VIII deficiency is usually transmitted as a sex-linked, recessive condition. This test is performed by first performing a partial thromboplastin Time (PTT) on the client's plasma. A Factor VIII-deficient plasma substrate is then mixed with the client's plasma and the degree of correction in the PTT is determined and compared to the degree of correction obtained by normal plasma.

Professional Considerations:

1. Consent form NOT required.
2. Preparation:
   A. Preschedule this test with the laboratory.
   B. Tube: 2.7- or 4.5-ml blue-top. Also obtain ice.
3. Procedure:
   A. Withdraw 2 ml of blood into a syringe

or vacuum tube. Remove the syringe or tube, leaving the needle in place. Attach a second syringe, and draw a 2.4-ml sample in a 2.7-ml tube or a 4.0-ml sample in a 4.5-ml tube. Place the specimen immediately in a container of ice.

B. Gently tilt the tube five or six times to mix.

4. Postprocedure care:
   A. For clients with coagulopathy, hold pressure over sampling site for at least 5 minutes and observe site closely for development of a hematoma.
   B. Transport the specimen to the laboratory immediately, discard the ice, and refrigerate the specimen. The sample should be centrifuged and refrigerated within 1 hour. Freeze the plasma if the test will not be performed within 24 hours of collection.

5. Client and family teaching:
   A. The client should not have warfarin therapy for 2 weeks or heparin therapy for 2 days before the test.
   B. Results are normally available within 24 hours.

6. Factors that affect results:
   A. Failure to discard the first 1–2 ml of blood may result in specimen contamination with tissue thromboplastin.
   B. Reject hemolyzed or clotted specimens, specimens not completely mixed, tubes partially filled with blood, specimens not on ice, or specimens received more than 1 hour after collection.

7. Other data:
   A. Coagulation factor roman numerals identify order of discovery rather than their order in the stages of clot formation.
   B. There is currently less than optimal standardization of this test.
   C. Previous terminology used for factor VIII includes factor VIIIC, AHG, and AHF.
   D. *See also Partial Thromboplastin Time, Plasma and Activated Partial Thromboplastin Substitution Test, Diagnostic.*

Bibliography:

Amano K, Arai M, Koshihara K, et al.: Autoantibody to factor VIII that has less reactivity to factor VII/von Willebrand factor complex. Am J Hematol 49(4):310–317, 1995.

Antonarakis SE, Rossiter JP, Young M, et al.: Factor VIII gene inversions in severe hemophilia A: results of an international consortium study. Blood 86(6):2206–2212, 1995.

Windsor S, Lyng A, Taylor SA, et al.: Severe haemophilia A in a female resulting from two de novo factor VIII mutations. Br J Haematol 90(4):906–909, 1995.

FACTOR VIII R:Ag, BLOOD

(see von Willebrand Factor Antigen, Blood)

FACTOR IX (CHRISTMAS FACTOR, HEMOPHILIC FACTOR B, PLASMA THROMBOPLASTIN COMPONENT, PTC), BLOOD

Norm: 50–150% of normal (control sample) activity. Plasma level about 4 mg/L. Half-life is 20 hours.

Increased: Not applicable.

Decreased: Hemophilia B (Christmas disease), hepatic disease, nephrotic syndrome, and vitamin K deficiency. Drugs include ansindione, bishydroxycoumarin, dicoumarol, dicumarol, heparin calcium, heparin sodium, phenprocoumon, and warfarin sodium.

Description: Factor IX is a vitamin K-dependent beta globulin essential in stage I of the intrinsic coagulation system as an influence on the amount of thromboplastin available. It is deficient in the inherited, sex-linked disease of hemophilia B, with bleeding symptoms similar to hemophilia A, but usually milder. Factor IX deficiency may also be acquired in severe hepatic dysfunction. The test is performed by first performing a partial thromboplastin time (PTT) on the client's plasma. A factor IX-deficient plasma substrate is then mixed with the client's plasma and the degree of correction in the PTT is determined and compared to the degree of correction obtained by normal plasma.

Professional Considerations:

1. Consent form NOT required.
2. Preparation:
   A. Preschedule this test with the laboratory.
   B. Tube: 2.7- or 4.5-ml blue-top. Also obtain ice.
3. Procedure:
   A. Withdraw 2 ml of blood into a syringe or vacuum tube. Remove the syringe or tube, leaving the needle in place. Attach a second syringe, and draw a 2.4-ml sample in a 2.7-ml tube or a 4.0-ml sample in a 4.5-ml tube.
   B. Gently tilt the tube five or six times to mix.
4. Postprocedure care:
   A. Place the specimen on ice immediately.
   B. For clients with coagulopathy, hold pressure over the sampling site for at least 5 minutes and observe the site closely for development of a hematoma.

C. Write the collection time on the laboratory requisition.

D. Transport the specimen to the laboratory immediately. The specimen should be centrifuged and refrigerated within 2 hours, where it will remain stable for several weeks.

5. Client and family teaching:
   A. The client should not have coumarin therapy for 2 weeks or heparin therapy for 2 days before the test.
   B. Results are normally available within 24 hours.
   C. Seek medical attention for signs of bleeding (i.e., hematoma, bleeding of gums, wounds, petechiae, confusion, changing level of consciousness).

6. Factors that affect results:
   A. Reject hemolyzed or clotted specimens, specimens not completely mixed, tubes partially filled with blood, specimens not refrigerated, specimens diluted or contaminated with heparin, or specimens received more than 2 hours after collection.
   B. Failure to discard the first 1–2 ml of blood may result in specimen contamination with tissue thromboplastin.

7. Other data:
   A. Coagulation factor roman numerals identify order of discovery rather than their order in the stages of clot formation.
   B. *See also Partial Thromboplastin Time, Plasma and Activated Partial Thromboplastin Substitution Test, Diagnostic.*

Bibliography:

Givens TB, Fischer TJ, Callahan JB: Improvements in accuracy and reproducibility of quantitative clotting factor assays by use of a novel approach for modeling reference curves. Comput Biol Med *24*(6):463–471, 1994.

Gordon EM, Tang H, Salazar RL, Kohn DB: Expression of coagulation factor IX (Christmas factor) in human hepatoma (HepG2) cell cultures after retroviral vector-mediated transfer. Am J Pediatr Hematol Oncol *15*(2):196–203, 1993.

Nielsen LR, Scheibel E, Ingerslev J, Schwartz M: Detection of ten new mutations by screening the gene encoding factor IX of Danish hemophilia B patients. Thromb Haemost *73*(5):774–778, 1995.

FACTOR X (STUART-PROWER FACTOR), BLOOD

Norm: 50–150% of normal (control sample) activity. Plasma level about 12 mg/L. Half-life is 30–50 hours.

Increased: Normal pregnancy. Drugs include oral contraceptives.

Decreased: Factor X deficiency, hepatic disease, and vitamin K deficiency. Drugs include ansindione, bishydroxycoumarin, dicoumarol, dicumarol, phenprocoumon, and warfarin sodium.

Description: A vitamin K-dependent proenzyme alphaglobulin active in both the intrinsic and extrinsic coagulation pathways. Factor X deficiency can be inherited, and also acquired in severe hepatic dysfunction and causes usually mild bleeding and prolonged prothrombin time (PT) and activated partial thromboplastin time (APTT). The test is performed by first performing a PT on the client's plasma. A Factor X-deficient plasma substrate is then mixed with the client's plasma and the degree of correction in the PT is determined and compared to the degree of correction obtained by normal plasma.

Professional Considerations:

1. Consent form NOT required.
2. Preparation:
   A. Preschedule this test with the laboratory.
   B. Tube: 2.7- or 4.5-ml blue-top.
3. Procedure:
   A. Withdraw 2 ml of blood into a syringe or vacuum tube. Remove the syringe or tube, leaving the needle in place. Attach a second syringe, and draw a 2.4-ml sample in a 2.7-ml tube or a 4.0-ml sample in a 4.5-ml tube.
   B. Gently tilt the tube five or six times to mix. Place the specimen immediately in a container of ice.
4. Postprocedure care:
   A. For clients with coagulopathy, hold pressure over the sampling site for at least 5 minutes and observe the site closely for development of a hematoma.
   B. Transport the specimen to the laboratory immediately. The specimens should be left at room temperature, with the stopper in place until tested within 24 hours.
5. Client and family teaching:
   A. The client should not have coumarin therapy for 2 weeks or heparin therapy for 2 days before the test.
   B. Results are normally available within 24 hours.
   C. Seek medical attention for signs of bleeding (i.e., hematoma, bleeding of gums, wounds, petechiae, confusion, changing level of consciousness).
6. Factors that affect results:
   A. Failure to discard the first 1–2 ml of blood may result in specimen contamination with tissue thromboplastin.
   B. Reject hemolyzed or clotted specimens, specimens not completely mixed, tubes partially filled with blood, specimens

diluted or contaminated with heparin, or specimens received more than 2 hours after collection.

C. Some drugs that may cause shortened prothrombin time include barbiturates, dorimide, dormtabs, ethchlorvynol, glutethimide, meprobamate, oral contraceptives, and vitamin K.

D. Some drugs that may cause prolonged prothrombin time include antibiotics, chloral hydrate, hydroxyzine hydrochloride, hydroxyzine pamoate, iothiouracil, methylthiouracil, phenylbutazone, phosphorus (toxicity), propylthiouracil, salicylates, tolbutamide, and vitamin A.

7. Other data:
A. Coagulation factor roman numerals identify order of discovery rather than their order in the stages of clot formation.
B. *See Partial Thromboplastin Time, Plasma.*

Bibliography:

Gentry R, Ye L, Nemerson Y: Surface-mediated enzymatic reactions: simulations of tissue factor activation of factor X on a lipid surface. Biophys J *69*(2):362–371, 1995.

Phillippou H, Adami A, Boisclair MD, Lane DA: An ELISA for factor X activation peptide: application to the investigation of thrombogenesis in cardiopulmonary bypass. Br J Haematol *90*(2):432–437, 1995.

FACTOR XI (PLASMA THROMBOPLASTIN ANTECEDENT, PTA), BLOOD

Norm: 65–135% of normal (control sample) activity. Plasma level about 7 mg/dl. Half-life is 40–80 hours.

Increased: Not applicable.

Decreased: Congenital heart disease, factor XI deficiency, hepatic disease, newborns (transient), pregnancy, and vitamin K deficiency. Drugs include ansindione, bishydroxycoumarin, dicoumarol, dicumarol, heparin calcium, heparin sodium, phenprocoumon, and warfarin sodium.

Description: Factor XI is a beta globulin active in stage I of the intrinsic coagulation pathway and missing, defective, or deficient in hemophilia C, an inherited, autosomal recessive deficiency that occurs in both sexes and causes prolonged coagulation evidenced by mild bleeding after surgical procedures. The test is

performed by first performing a partial thromboplastin time (PTT) on the client's plasma. A factor XI-deficient plasma substrate is then mixed with the client's plasma and the degree of correction in the PTT is determined and compared to the degree of correction obtained by normal plasma.

Professional Considerations:

1. Consent form NOT required.
2. Preparation:
A. Preschedule this test with the laboratory.
B. Tube: 2.7- or 4.5-ml blue-top. Also obtain ice.
3. Procedure:
A. Withdraw 2 ml of blood into a syringe or vacuum tube. Remove the syringe or tube, leaving the needle in place. Attach a second syringe, and draw a 2.4-ml sample in a 2.7-ml tube or a 4.0-ml sample in a 4.5-ml tube.
B. Gently tilt the tube five or six times to mix.
4. Postprocedure care:
A. Place the specimen on ice immediately.
B. For clients with coagulopathy, hold pressure over the sampling site for at least 5 minutes and observe the site closely for development of a hematoma.
C. Write the collection time on the laboratory requisition.
D. Transport the specimen to the laboratory immediately, discard the ice, and refrigerate ther specimens. The sample should be centrifuged and refrigerated within 2 hours.
5. Client and family teaching:
A. The client should not have warfarin therapy for 2 weeks or heparin therapy for 2 days before the test.
B. Results are normally available within 24 hours.
C. Seek medical attention for signs of bleeding (i.e., hematoma, bleeding of gums, wounds, petechiae, confusion, changing level of consciousness).
6. Factors that affect results:
A. Failure to discard the first 1–2 ml of blood may result in specimen contamination with tissue thromboplastin.
B. Reject hemolyzed or clotted specimens, specimens not completely mixed, tubes partially filled with blood, specimens not refrigerated, specimens diluted or contaminated with heparin, or specimens received more than 2 hours after collection.
C. The test for factor XI deficiency must be performed on a freshly collected specimen.

D. Freezing the specimen may falsely elevate results.
7. Other data:
A. Coagulation factor roman numerals identify order of discovery rather than their order in the stages of clot formation.
B. *See also Partial Thromboplastin Time, Plasma and Activated Partial Thromboplastin Substitution Test, Diagnostic.*

Bibliography:

Bolton-Maggs PH, Patterson DA, Wensley RT, Tuddenham EG: Definition of the bleeding tendency in factor XI deficient kindreds: a clinical and laboratory study. Thromb Haemost 73(2):194–202, 1995.

Briseid K, Hoem NO, Johannesen S, Haug K: Amidolytic assay of factor XI in human plasma: significance of kallikrein for the activity measured. Thromb Res 78(3):239–250, 1995.

FACTOR XII (HAGEMAN FACTOR), BLOOD

Norm: 50–150% of normal (control sample) activity. Plasma level: 23–47 mg/ml. Half-life is 52–60 hours.

Increased: After exercise.

Decreased: Factor XII deficiency, nephrotic syndrome, and pregnancy.

Description: Factor XII is a beta globulin or gamma globulin enzyme, the active form of which initiates the intrinsic coagulation pathway. Its deficiency is inherited as an autosomal recessive defect with bleeding symptoms usually absent and causes a prolonged partial thromboplastin time (PTT). The test is performed by first performing a PTT on the client's plasma. A factor XI-deficient plasma substrate is then mixed with the client's plasma, and the degree of correction in the PTT is determined and compared to the degree of correction obtained by normal plasma.

Professional Considerations:

1. Consent form NOT required.
2. Preparation:
A. Preschedule this test with the laboratory.
B. Tube: 2.7- or 4.5-ml blue-top. Also obtain ice.

3. Procedure:
A. Withdraw 2 ml of blood into a syringe or vacuum tube. Remove the syringe or tube, leaving the needle in place. Attach a second syringe, and draw a 2.4-ml sample in a 2.7-ml tube or a 4.0-ml sample in a 4.5-ml tube.
B. Gently tilt the tube five or six times to mix.
4. Postprocedure care:
A. Place the specimen on ice immediately.
B. For clients with coagulopathy, hold pressure over the sampling site for at least 5 minutes and observe the site closely for development of a hematoma.
C. Write the collection time on the laboratory requisition.
D. Transport the specimen to the laboratory immediately, discard the ice, and refrigerate the specimen. The sample should be centrifuged and refrigerated within 2 hours. Freeze the plasma if the test will not be performed within 24 hours of collection.
5. Client and family teaching:
A. The client should not have warfarin therapy for 2 weeks or heparin therapy for 2 days before the test.
B. Results are normally available within 24 hours.
C. Seek medical attention for signs of bleeding (i.e., hematoma, bleeding of gums, wounds, petechiae, confusion, changing level of consciousness).
6. Factors that affect results:
A. Failure to discard the first 1–2 ml of blood may result in specimen contamination with tissue thromboplastin.
B. Reject hemolyzed or clotted specimens, specimens not completely mixed, tubes partially filled with blood, specimens not refrigerated, specimens diluted or contaminated with heparin, or specimens received more than 2 hours after collection.
7. Other data:
A. Coagulation factor roman numerals identify order of discovery rather than their order in the stages of clot formation.
B. *See also Partial Thromboplastin Time, Plasma and Activated Partial Thromboplastin Substitution Test, Diagnostic.*

Bibliography:

Shibayama Y, Brunnee T, Kaplan AP, Reddigari S: Activation of human Hageman factor (factor XII) in the presence of zinc and phosphate ions. Braz J Med Biol Res 27(8):1817–1828, 1994.

Wallock M, Arentzen C, Perkins J: Factor XII deficiency and cardiopulmonary bypass. Perfusion 10(1):13–16, 1995.

Winter M, Gallimore M, Jones DW: Should factor XII assays be included in thrombophilia screening? Lancet 346(8966):52, 1995.

FACTOR XIII (FIBRIN STABILIZING FACTOR, CLOT UREA SOLUBILITY), BLOOD

Norm: Clot is insoluble in 5 M urea for at least 24 hours. Half-life of factor XIII is 100 hours.

Increased: Factor XIII is more often increased than decreased in most clients.

Decreased: Agammaglobulinemia, factor XIII deficiency, hepatic disease, hyperfibrinogenemia, lead poisoning, multiple myeloma, and postoperatively.

Description: Factor XIII is an alpha globulin which, in its active form, stabilizes fibrin clots. Its deficiency is a rare, inherited, autosomal recessive condition that may result in symptoms ranging from abnormal bleeding from cuts and in joints, to cerebral hemorrhage and infant death from umbilical cord hemorrhage. The test is performed by adding calcium chloride to the sample and clotting the mixture at 37°C for ½ hour, then placing the clot in 5 M urea and observing hourly for clot dissolution. Clots from clients with factor XIII deficiency will dissolve within 1–3 hours.

Professional Considerations:

1. Consent form NOT required.
2. Preparation:
   A. Tube: 2.7- or 4.5-ml blue-top. Also obtain ice.
3. Procedure:
   A. Withdraw 2 ml of blood into a syringe or vacuum tube. Remove the syringe or tube, leaving the needle in place. Attach a second syringe, and draw a 2.4-ml sample in a 2.7-ml tube or a 4.0-ml sample in a 4.5-ml tube. Place the specimens immediately in a container of ice.
   B. Gently tilt the tube five or six times to mix.
4. Postprocedure care:
   A. Place the specimens on ice immediately.
   B. For clients with coagulopathy, hold pressure over the sampling site for at least 5 minutes and observe the site closely for development of a hematoma.
   C. Write the collection time on the laboratory requisition.
   D. Transport the specimens to the laboratory immediately, discard the ice, and refrigerate the specimens.
5. Client and family teaching:
   A. The client should not have warfarin therapy for 2 weeks or heparin therapy for 2 days before the test.
   B. Results are normally available within 24 hours.
   C. Seek medical attention for signs of bleeding (i.e., hematoma, bleeding of gums, wounds, petechiae, confusion, changing level of consciousness).
6. Factors that affect results:
   A. Reject hemolyzed or clotted specimens, specimens not completely mixed, tubes partially filled with blood, specimens not refrigerated, specimens diluted or contaminated with heparin, or specimens received more than 2 hours after collection.
   B. The presence of only 1% of normal levels of factor XIII is enough to provoke a normal test result.
7. Other data:
   A. Coagulation factor roman numerals identify order of discovery rather than their order in the stages of clot formation.

Bibliography:

Ballerini G, Gemmati D, Moratelli S, Morelli P, Serino: A photometric method for the dosage of factor XIII applied to the study of chronic hepatopathies. Throm Res *78*(5):451–456, 1995.

Song YC, Sheng D, Taubenfeld SM, Matsueda GR: A microtiter assay for factor XIII using fibrinogen and biotinylcadaverine as substrates. Anal Biochem *223*(1):88–92, 1994.

FAT, SEMIQUANTITATIVE, STOOL

Norm:

Neutral fat	<50 globules/HPF
Fatty acids	<100 globules/HPF

Increased: Amyloidosis, beta-lipoprotein deficiency, bile salt deficiency, blind loop syndrome, celiac disease, cystic fibrosis, diarrhea, diverticulosis, enteritis, hepatobiliary disease, hypogammaglobulinemia, increased peristalsis, ingestion of castor oil or mineral oil, intestinal fistula, lymphangiectasis, lymphoma, pancreatic disease (cancer, chronic pancreatitis, enzyme deficiency, mucoviscoidosis), postoperatively (bowel resection), sprue, Whipple's disease, and Zollinger-Ellison syndrome.

Description: Fecal fat is measured to aid diagnosis of conditions causing poor absorption of dietary fat, resulting in steatorrhea.

Professional Considerations:

1. Consent form NOT required.
2. Preparation:
   A. Obtain a clean plastic specimen container and a clean toilet seat hat catcher.

B. The client is to ingest a 60 g fat/day diet for 3–6 days.

C. Avoid use of suppositories, oily lubricants, or mineral oil in the perianal or genital areas for 3 days prior to and during specimen collection.

3. Procedure:

A. Collect 20 ml of stool in a clean glass or plastic container.

4. Postprocedure care:

A. Cleanse the anal area.

5. Client and family teaching:

A. Explain the need to avoid use of rectal, vaginal, or genital-area oils, lubricants, or suppositories for 3 days prior to the test. The client should urinate before defecating, then defecate sample into the hat catcher and transfer the stool sample to the specimen container with a wooden spatula.

B. Results may take several days.

6. Factors that affect results:

A. Send fresh random stool samples to the laboratory within 2 hours.

7. Other data:

A. Bedtime laxatives may be needed for constipated clients.

B. Some malabsorption syndromes such as tropical sprue may not show increased fecal fat.

Bibliography:

DeCurtis M, Kempson C, Ventura V, et al.: The relationship between fecal fat and water in very-low-birth-weight infants. J Pediatr Gastroenterol Nutr 11(1):63–65, 1990.

Hussain Y, Guzelhan C, Odink J, et al.: Comparison of the inhibition of dietary fat absorption by full versus divided doses of orlistat. J Clin Pharmacol 34(11):1121–1125, 1994.

FAT, URINE

Norm: Negative.

Positive: Acute tubular nephrosis, azotemia (prerenal), fat embolism, nephritis (acute interstitial, chronic interstitial), nephrotic syndrome, polycystic kidney disease, and renal failure (chronic).

Negative: Normal finding in up to 50% of clients with fat embolism.

Description: Urine fat occurs most commonly in nephrotic syndrome and fat or cholesterol embolism. When nephrotic syndrome is suspected, fat is found in renal epithelial cells and casts; thus the urine sediment is examined microscopically for fat. When fat embolism occurs, fat is found freely floating in the urine. Therefore, the urine is agitated gently to allow free fat to float, and the surface contents are skimmed and stained with a fat stain.

Professional Considerations:

1. Consent form NOT required.

2. Preparation:

A. Obtain a 10-ml clean plastic vial.

B. Write the suspected diagnosis on the laboratory requisition to ensure that the proper test method is used.

3. Procedure:

A. Collect a clean void of 8 ml of urine. A fresh specimen may be taken from a urinary drainage bag.

4. Postprocedure care:

A. Cleanse the area around the urethral meatus.

5. Client and family teaching:

A. Explain the procedure for cleansing the urethral area.

B. Results are normally available within 24 hours.

6. Factors that affect results:

A. Reject specimens contaminated with oil.

B. The presence of corn starch in the genital area may cause false-positive results.

7. Other data:

A. The gross appearance of urine being cloudy may indicate fat in the urine.

Bibliography:

Galeano NF, Darling P, Lepage G, et al.: Taurine supplementation of a premature formula improves fat absorption in preterm infants. Pediatr Res 22(1):67–71, 1987.

Rosman HS, Davis TP, Reddy D, et al.: Cholesterol embolization: Clinical findings and implications. J Am Coll Cardiol 15(6):1296–1299, 1990.

FDP, BLOOD

(see Fibrin Breakdown Products, Blood)

FEBRILE AGGLUTININS, SERUM

Norm: Negative, or less than a fourfold rise in titer between acute and convalescent samples.

Normal Dilutions:

Salmonella antibody	<1:80
Brucellosis antibody	<1:80
Tularemia antibody	<1:40
Rickettsial antibody	<1:40

Usage: Suspected infection with *Brucella,* paratyphoid, *Proteus, Rickettsia,* Rocky Mountain spotted fever, salmonellosis, tularemia, typhoid, or typhus.

Description: Febrile agglutination tests are performed to identify the cause of febrile illnesses. Bacterial antibodies to the above organisms will agglutinate in vitro if present in the serum.

Professional Considerations:

1. Consent form NOT required.
2. Preparation:
   A. Tube: Red-top, red/gray-top, or gold-top.
3. Procedure:
   A. Draw a 10-ml blood sample and label it as the acute sample. Repeat the test every 3–5 days. Draw the final sample in 10–14 days and label it as the convalescent sample.
4. Postprocedure care:
   A. Send the specimens to the laboratory immediately.
5. Client and family teaching:
   A. Two samples must be taken about 2 weeks apart to identify a trend in levels that can pinpoint the cause of the fever. The client may be treated empirically before the second sample is taken.

6. Factors that affect results:
   A. Reject hemolyzed specimens.
   B. Chronic exposure to or vaccination against the above organisms may cause high titers.
   C. Immunosuppressed clients may be infected but have low or negative titers.
   D. Antibiotic therapy causes low initial titers.
   E. Brucella antigen skin tests may elevate titers.
   F. Many cross-reactions are possible.
7. Other data:
   A. Results are given in the highest dilution in which a positive reaction with the antigen occurs.
   B. A blood culture for the above organisms should be performed concurrently.

Bibliography:

Gale DA, Everard CO, Carrington DG, et al.: Leptospiral antibodies in patients from a barbadian general practice. Eur J Epidemiol 6(2):150–155, 1990.
Van Savage J, Decker MD, Edwards KM, et al.: Natural history of pertussis antibody in the infant and effect on vaccine response. J Infect Dis *161*(3):487–492, 1990.

FECAL FAT, QUANTITATIVE, 72-HOUR, STOOL

Norm:

Adult, 60 g fat/day diet	2–6 g/24 hours or <20% of total solids
Adult, fat-free diet	<4 g/day
Breast-fed infant	<1 g/day
Child up to 6 years old	<2 g/day

Increased: Amyloidosis, beta-lipoprotein deficiency, bile salt deficiency, blind loop syndrome, celiac disease, Crohn's disease, cystic fibrosis, diarrhea, diverticulosis, enteritis, hepatobiliary disease, hypogammaglobulinemia, increased peristalsis, ingestion of castor oil or mineral oil, intestinal fistula, lymphangiectasis, lymphoma, pancreatic disease (cancer, chronic pancreatitis, enzyme deficiency, mucoviscoidosis), postoperatively (bowel resection), sprue (celiac), Whipple's disease, and Zollinger-Ellison syndrome.

Description: Fecal fat is measured to aid diagnosis of conditions causing poor absorption of dietary fat resulting in steatorrhea. The value of this test is that the amount of dietary fat intake is known and used in evaluation of the results.

Professional Considerations:

1. Consent form NOT required.
2. Preparation:
   A. Obtain 500-ml clean plastic containers, dry ice, and a clean toilet seat hat catcher.
3. Procedure:
   A. Collect all stools, using a hat catcher in the toilet, on the fourth, fifth, and sixth days of the specified diet and place the stools in the clean plastic containers.
   B. Keep the specimen containers refrigerated during the collection period.
4. Postprocedure care:
   A. Freeze the specimens on dry ice if the testing will not be performed within 24 hours.
   B. Record the date and time of each specimen collected.
5. Client and family teaching:
   A. The client is to ingest a 50- to 150-g fat/day diet for 3–6 days.
   B. Avoid suppositories, oily lubricants, or mineral oil in the perianal or genital areas for 3 days prior to and during collection.
   C. Avoid contaminating the stool with urine or toilet paper.
   D. Results may take several days.
6. Factors that affect results:
   A. Reject specimens submitted in improper containers such as cartons, coffee cans, or plastic bags.

B. False-negative results are most commonly caused by failure to collect all stools.

7. Other data:

A. Bedtime laxatives may be needed for constipated clients.

B. Some clients with malabsorption syndromes such as tropical sprue may not show increased fecal fat excretion.

Bibliography:

Welburg JW, Monkelbaan JF, De Vries EG, et al.: Effects of supplemental dietary calcium on quantitative and qualitative fecal fat excretion in man. Ann Nutr Metab *38*(4):185–191, 1994.

FECAL LEUKOCYTE, STOOL, DIAGNOSTIC

Norm: No leukocytes present.

Usage: Determine the type of diarrhea, invasive or noninvasive, to the mucosa of the colon. If no fecal leukocytes are present in the stool specimen, an antidiarrheal medication can be given. If fecal leukocytes are present, an antidiarrheal medication should not be given. The results of this test will be readily available, whereas a culture will take several days.

Description: The presence of fecal leukocytes in the stool indicates that the cause of the diarrhea is an organism or process that is breaking the mucosal barrier of the colon, such as *Salmonella, Shigella, Amoeba, Campylobacter, Helicobacter, or Yersinia* infections, Crohn's disease, and chronic inflammatory bowel disease. Fecal leukocytes are usually not present in infectious processes that do not invade the mucosa, such as "viral enteritis," toxin-mediated diarrhea, or infections with noninvasive *E. coli*. The absence of blood and fecal leukocytes usually means the diarrhea process is transient and can by treated symptomatically. *Clostridium difficile* may or may not be associated with leukocytes in the stool, so if it is sus-

pected, a stool culture should be sent and no anti-diarrheal agent given until the results are back and negative.

Professional Considerations:

1. Consent form is NOT required.
2. Preparation:
   A. Obtain a stool specimen container.
3. Procedure:
   A. Instruct the client to collect a stool sample, or use a bedpan so that the sample can be obtained.
   B. Send the specimen to the laboratory.
4. Postprocedure care:
   A. Keep the rectal area as clean and as dry as possible to prevent skin breakdown.
   B. If diarrhea is frequent, encourage fluids and check serum electrolytes for abnormalities.
5. Client and family teaching:
   A. Avoid contaminating the stool with toilet tissue or urine.
   B. Results are normally available within 48 hours.
6. Factors that affect results:
   A. None.
7. Other data:
   A. Stool cultures should be obtained from all clients with fecal leukocytes to differentiate acute infection from inflammatory bowel syndrome. In the absence of fecal leukocytes, stool cultures are usually negative.

Bibliography:

Huicho L, Sanchez D, Contreras M, Paredes M, Murga H, Chinchay L, Guevara G: Occult blood and fecal leukocytes as screening tests in childhood infectious diarrhea: an old problem revisited. Pediatr Infect Dis J *12*(6):474–477, 1993.

Marx CE, Morris A, Wilson ML, Reller LB: Fecal leukocytes in stool specimens submitted for *Clostridium difficile* toxin assay. Diagn Microbiol Infect Dis *16*(4):313–315, 1993.

Yong WH, Mattia AR, Ferraro MJ: Comparison of fecal lactoferrinlates agglutination assay and methylene blue microscopy for detection of fecal leukocytes in *Clostridium difficile*-associated disease. J Clin Microbiol *32*(5):1360–1361, 1994.

Zins BJ, Tremaine WJ, Carpenter HA: Collagenous colitis: mucosal biopsies and association with fecal leukocytes. Mayo Clin Proc *70*(5):430–433, 1995.

FENFLURAMINE, BLOOD
(see Amphetamines, Blood)

FERRIC CHLORIDE TEST, DIAGNOSTIC

Norm: Negative, no color change.

Usage: Amino acid disorders, drug ingestion, and metabolic disorders.

Description: A nonspecific random urine test that produces color reactions with certain conditions.

Condition	Color change
Alcoholism	Red or red-brown
Alkaptonuria	Blue or green, fades quickly
Diabetes	Red or red-brown
Drug ingestion	
Acetophenetidines	Red
Aminosalicylic acid	Red-brown
Antipyrines	Red
Cyanates	Red
Phenol derivative	Violet
Phenothiazines	Purple-pink
Salicylates	Stable purple
Histidinemia	Green or blue-green
Maple syrup urine disease	Blue
Phenylketonuria	Blue or blue-green, fades to yellow
Starvation	Red or red-brown
Tyrosinosis	Green, fades in seconds
Other products	
Alpha-ketobuturic acid	Purple, fades to red-brown
Bilirubin	Blue-green
Orthohydroxyphenyl acetic acid	Mauve
Orthohydroxyphenyl pyruvic acid	Red
Pyruvic acid	Deep gold-yellow or green
Xanthurenic acid	Deep green, later brown

Professional Considerations:

1. Consent form NOT required.
2. Preparation:
   A. Obtain a clean container.
   B. Cleanse the area around the urethral meatus.
3. Procedure:
   A. Collect an early morning random specimen of 4 ml of urine in a clean container. A fresh specimen may be taken from a urinary drainage bag.
   B. Add 10% FeCl by drops to 1–2 ml of urine.
4. Postprocedure care:
   A. If the specimen will not be analyzed immediately, acidify the urine to a pH of <4; or else freeze the sample immediately at –20°C for no longer than 1 week.

5. Client and family teaching:
   A. If the client will collect the sample, teach the proper method for cleansing the urethral meatus.
   B. Results are normally available within 12 hours.
6. Factors that affect results:
   A. Dietary intake high in phenylalanine.
   B. Levodopa medication.
7. Other data:
   A. The contents of a wet diaper may be used.

Bibliography:

Scott RE, Ward VL, Grinstead GF, et al.: Melanogenuria: Laboratory evaluation of the qualitative Thormahlen and ferric chloride tests and their clinical utility. Clin Chem *34*(3):582–585, 1988.

FERRITIN, SERUM

Norm:

		SI Units
Adult females		
≤40 years	11–122 ng/ml	11–122 µg/L
>40 years	12–263 ng/ml	12–263 µg/L
Adult males	15–200 ng/ml	15–200 µg/L
Children		
Newborn	25–200 ng/ml	25–200 µg/L
1 month	200–600 ng/ml	200–600 µg/L

		SI Units
Children *(continued)*		
2–5 months	50–200 ng/ml	50–200 µg/L
6 months	7–140 ng/ml	7–140 µg/L
1–15 years	7–140 ng/ml	7–140 µg/L

Increased: Anemia (chronic, hemolytic, megaloblastic, pernicious, sideroblastic), carcinoma (generalized, hepatic), cirrhosis, hemochromatosis (idiopathic), hepatic disease (acute, chronic), hepatic necrosis, hepatitis, hepatoma, Hodgkin's disease, hyperthyroidism, inflammation (chronic), iron intake (excessive dietary or by blood transfusion), leukemia, jaundice (obstructive), multiple myeloma, polycythemia, renal disease (chronic), rheumatoid arthritis, siderosis, thalassemia (major, minor), and tissue trauma. Drugs include iron.

Decreased: Anemia (iron-deficiency), hemodialysis, inflammatory bowel disease, pregnancy, and surgery (gastrointestinal).

Description: An iron-storing protein manufactured in the liver, spleen, bone marrow, tumor cells, and sites of inflammation. Evaluation of ferritin levels is most often performed in the differential diagnosis of several types of anemia.

Professional Considerations:

1. Consent form NOT required.
2. Preparation:
   A. Tube: Red-top, red/gray-top, or gold-top.
3. Procedure:
   A. Draw a 1-ml blood sample.
4. Postprocedure care:
   A. Centrifuge and freeze samples.
5. Client and family teaching:
   A. Results may not be available for several days.
6. Factors that affect results:
   A. Reject specimens if the client had a radioactive scan within 48 hours prior to specimen collection.
7. Other data:
   A. Hemolyzed samples are acceptable.

Bibliography:

Bell H, Skinningsrud A, Raknerud N, Try K: Serum ferritin and transferrin saturation in patients with chronic alcoholic and non-alcoholic liver disease. J Intern Med *236*(3):315–322, 1994.

Castro O, Poillon WN, Finke H, Massac E: Improvement of sickle cell anemia by iron limited erythropoiesis. Am J Hematol *47*(2):74–81, 1994.

Tikhibault PK, Wlodarczyk J: Correlation of serum ferritin levels and postsclerotherapy pigmentation. A prospective study. J Dermatol Surg Oncol *20*(10):684–686, 1994.

FETAL HEMOGLOBIN (HbF), BLOOD

Norm:

Adults	0–2% of total hemoglobin
Children	
Newborn	60–90% of total hemoglobin
1–5 months	<75% of total hemoglobin
6–12 months	<5% of total hemoglobin
1–20 years	<2% of total hemoglobin

Increased: Anemia (aplastic, megaloblastic, nonhereditary refractory normoblastic, pernicious, refractory, sickle cell, spherocytic), bone marrow metastasis, diabetes, Down syndrome, erythroleukemia, hereditary persistence of fetal hemoglobin, hyperthyroidism, hypothyroidism, infants (small-for-gestational-age, chronic intrauterine anoxia, developmental abnormalities), leukemia, lymphoma, macroglobulinemia, multiple myeloma, myelofibrosis, paroxysmal nocturnal hemoglobinuria, pregnancy (fetal blood leakage into mother's blood), spherocytosis, thalassemia (major, minor), thyrotoxicosis, trisomy 13–15, D trisomy, and trisomy 21. Drugs include anticonvulsants.

Decreased: Multiple chromosome abnormality (C/D translocation).

Description: Fetal hemoglobin, HbF, the hemoglobin present during fetal development, contains a polypeptide globin chain that is different from adult hemoglobin. It comprises most of the hemoglobin of a newborn's red blood cells. Over the first 6 months of life, most of the fetal hemoglobin is replaced by adult hemoglobin, although a small portion of HbF may persist throughout the lifespan. This test is most often used to differentiate thalassemia and other hemoglobinopathies in which abnormalities may be found in the polypeptide globin chains.

Professional Considerations:
1. Consent form NOT required.
2. Preparation:
   A. Tube: Lavender-top or green-top.
3. Procedure:
   A. Draw a 2-ml blood sample.
4. Postprocedure care:
   A. None.
5. Client and family teaching:
   A. Results may take several days.
6. Factors that affect results:
   A. Reject specimens older than 4 days at room temperature.
7. Other data:
   A. Sample is stable at room temperature for 4 days.

Bibliography:

Franco RS, Barker R, Miller MA, et al.: Fetal hemoglobin and potassium in isolated transferrin receptor positive dense sickle reticulocytes. Blood *84*(6): 2013–2020, 1994.

Park VM, Bravo RR, Price JO, et al.: A model system using fetal hemoglobin to distinguish fetal cells enriched from maternal blood. Ann NY Acad Sci *731*:133–135, 1994.

FETAL HEMOGLOBIN STAIN
(see Betke-Kleihauer Stain, Diagnostic)

FETAL MONITORING, EXTERNAL, DIAGNOSTIC

Norm: Fetal heart rate (FHR) and variability normal.

Fetal heart rate (FHR)   120–160 bpm.
FHR variability   5–25 bpm.

Usage: Monitoring FHR and uterine contractions, evaluation of fetal effects of stressed and nonstressed situations, assessment of the need for internal fetal monitoring, and monitoring of fetal well-being during the oxytocin challenge test.

Description: A noninvasive test in which an electronic transducer is placed on the pregnant abdomen to amplify the FHR while a cardiotachometer records FHR, and pressure sensors record uterine contractions. External fetal monitors record fluctuations in the baseline FHR and detect variability between beats. This test is able to detect FHR accelerations and decelerations in response to uterine contractions.

Professional Considerations:
1. Consent form NOT required.
2. Preparation:
   A. Obtain a fetal heart monitor and an electroconductive gel.
   B. Cleanse the transducer and transducer connections.
3. Procedure:
   A. The client is placed in a semi-Fowler's or left lateral position with the abdomen exposed.
   B. The transducer is coated with electroconductive gel and strapped over the abdominal area with the most distinct fetal heart tones. For active labor, this is the fundus.
   C. The alarm limits for FHR are set, and test recordings are started to ensure that the system is functioning properly.
   D. For active labor, baseline FHR is recorded and calculated over a 10-minute period and then monitored continuously as labor progresses. The recording is evaluated for abnormalities in FHR and FHR response to contractions, drugs, or maternal position.
   E. Transducer location may need adjustment in response to fetal movement in utero.
4. Postprocedure care:
   A. Weekly external fetal monitoring is indicated for diabetes, hypertension, fetal growth retardation, and pregnancy over 42 weeks' gestation.
5. Client and family teaching:
   A. For antepartal testing, the client should eat a full meal just prior to the test.
   B. The test poses no risk of harm to the client or the fetus.
6. Factors that affect results:
   A. Maternal position may cause fetal distress. The left-side lying position best promotes oxygen delivery to the fetus.
   B. Maternal obesity may interfere with the adequacy of recordings.
   C. Artifact may result from poor transducer connections, or dried electroconductive gel on the transducer.
7. Other data:
   A. Events that cause changes in the FHR recordings during active labor are handwritten on the graphic recording. These include maternal movement, administration of drugs, and procedures.

Bibliography:

Wapner RJ, Weisberg M: External fetal monitoring. *In* Hamilton HK, Cahill M (eds): Diagnostics, 2nd ed. Springhouse, PA, Springhouse Corporation, 1986, pp 723–726.

Ware DJ, Devoe LD: The nonstress test. Reassessment of the "gold standard." Clin Perinatol, *21*(4):779–796, 1994.

FETAL MONITORING, INTERNAL, DIAGNOSTIC

Norm:

Fetal heart rate (FHR)	120–160 bpm
FHR variability	5–25 bpm

Maternal Contractions and Intrauterine Pressure During Labor:

Prelabor	<3 contractions over 10 minutes
	25–40 mmHg contraction pressure
First stage	<6 contractions over 10 minutes
	8–12 mmHg baseline pressure
	30–40 mmHg contraction pressure
Second stage	1 contraction about every 2 minutes
	10–20 mmHg baseline pressure
	50–80 mmHg contraction pressure

Usage: Monitoring of beat-to-beat variability of FHR. Rate and pressure monitoring of uterine contractions. Often used as an adjunct to external fetal monitoring. More accurate than external fetal monitoring in cases of maternal obesity.

Description: During this invasive monitoring procedure, a sterile fetal scalp electrode and a uterine catheter are inserted through the vaginal canal for the purpose of FHR and uterine contraction measurements during labor after 3-cm cervical dilation. Internal monitoring enables a better assessment of the effect of labor on the fetus than does external fetal monitoring.

Professional Considerations:

1. Consent form IS required.

Risks:

Maternal uterine perforation; intrauterine infection; and fetal scalp infection, abscess, or hematoma.

Contraindications:

Active genital herpes.

Precaution:

Test should be performed only when the fetal presenting part is the head.

2. Preparation:
   A. Obtain an antiseptic solution, a fetal scalp electrode and guide, a pressure catheter for intrauterine contraction monitoring, a catheter guide, a transducer, a fetal heart monitor, and a topical antibiotic.
3. Procedure:
   A. The client is placed in a dorsal lithotomy position.

B. The perineal area is cleansed with antiseptic solution.
C. A vaginal examination is performed to measure cervical dilation and identify a fetal scalp location over bone for electrode placement.
D. The electrode is guided through the vaginal canal and cervical os and gently screwed into place on the fetal scalp.
E. The electrode wires are connected to the fetal monitor via a maternal thigh plate coated with electroconductive gel. Correct placement and functioning of the system are verified when an FHR signal is demonstrated by the fetal monitor.
F. The fluid-filled catheter for monitoring uterine contractions is then guided into place through the cervix a shallow distance into the uterus. The distal end is connected to a pressure transducer for continuous monitoring of intrauterine pressure.

4. Postprocedure care:
   A. Cleanse the fetal scalp electrode site with antiseptic and apply the antibiotic after delivery.
5. Client and family teaching:
   A. Internal fetal monitoring poses risks (listed above) but provides much better assessment of how well the fetus is tolerating the labor process than does external fetal monitoring.
6. Factors that affect results:
   A. Drugs that affect the sympathetic and parasympathetic nervous systems may influence FHR.
   B. The maternal position may cause fetal distress. The left-side lying position best promotes oxygen delivery to the fetus.
7. Other data:
   A. None.

Bibliography:

Schifrin BS: Polemics in perinatology: The electronic fetal monitoring guidelines. J Perinatol *10*(2): 188–192, 1990.

Spence MR, Harwell T: Invasive fetal monitoring and human immunodeficiency virus transmission [letter; comment]. Am J Obstet Gynecol *172*(1, Pt 1):243–244, 1995.

Wapner RJ, Weisberg M: External fetal monitoring. *In* Hamilton HK, Cahill M (eds): Diagnostics, 2nd ed. Springhouse, PA, Springhouse Corporation, 1986, pp 727–730.

FETOSCOPY, DIAGNOSTIC

Norm: Normal fetal development. Absence of neural tube defects.

Usage: Diagnosis of malformation of the fetus. Detection of neural tube defect. Blood samples may be obtained to test for sickle cell anemia and hemophilia.

Description: Fetoscopy is an endoscopic procedure that allows direct examination of the fetus via the fetoscope.

Professional Considerations:

1. Consent form IS required.

Risks:

Abortion or premature labor; amnionitis (antibiotics may be given prophylactically to prevent this complication).

Contraindications:

Anteriorly placed placenta, bleeding disorder, hypertensive crisis, incompetent cervix, history of spontaneous abortion or premature labor.

2. Preparation:
   A. To prevent excessive fetal activity during the procedure, the mother may be given meperidine (Demerol), which crosses the placenta and quiets the fetus.
   B. Obtain a local anesthetic and a fetoscopy tray.
3. Procedure:
   A. The abdominal wall of the mother is anesthetized with a local anesthetic.
   B. An ultrasound examination is then used to locate the fetus and placenta.
   C. A small incision is made in the abdominal wall, and the fetoscope is inserted through the abdominal wall into the amniotic cavity. The fetus is visualized for obvious malformations, such as neural tube defects.
4. Postprocedure care:
   A. Apply a dry, sterile dressing to the fetoscopy site.

5. Client and family teaching:
   A. This procedure poses risks (listed above).
   B. A local anesthetic will be used to prevent pain. The client will feel pressure as the fetoscope is inserted.
   C. The test takes about 40 minutes.
6. Factors that affect results:
   A. Excessive movement of the mother may obscure results.
7. Other data:
   A. None.

Bibliography:

Lawrence L: Fetal heart monitoring with a fetoscope. Midwifery Today Childbirth Education *24*:30–34, 1993.

FETUS EXAMINATION AFTER DEATH

(see Autopsy, Diagnostic)

FIBRIN BREAKDOWN PRODUCTS (FIBRIN DEGRADATION PRODUCTS, FDP), BLOOD

Norm: 2–10 µg/ml. Panic range: >40 µg/ml.

Increased: Abruptio placentae, aneurysm, blood transfusion reaction, brain damage, burns, carcinomatosis, cirrhosis (alcoholic), congenital heart disease, deep vein thrombosis, disseminated intravascular coagulation, internal bleeding (newborns), intrauterine death, myocardial infarction, organ rejection (renal transplant), parturition, postcesarean birth, preeclampsia, pregnancy (third trimester), pulmonary embolism, pulmonary infarction, renal disease, respiratory distress (newborns), sepsis, shock, sunstroke, surgical complications, and tissue damage (extensive). Drugs include barbiturates (large doses causing coma), streptokinase, and urokinase.

Decreased: Not clinically significant.

Description: Seven split products result from splitting fibrin or fibrinogen as a result of attack by plasmin during dissolution of fibrin clots. These split products, labeled A, B, C, D, E, X, and Y, indicate recent clotting activity. Greatly increased amounts interfere with hemostatic plug formation and indicate abnormal amounts of fibrinolysis. Levels over 40 mg/ml are highly suggestive of disseminated intravascular coagulation.

Professional Considerations:

1. Consent form NOT required.
2. Preparation:
   A. Tube: 2.7- or 4.5-ml blue-top. Also obtain ice.
3. Procedure:
   A. Withdraw 2 ml of blood into a syringe or vacuum tube. Remove the syringe or tube, leaving the needle in place. Attach a second syringe, and draw a 2.4-ml sample in a 2.7-ml tube or a 4.0-ml sample in a 4.5-ml tube. Place the specimens immediately in a container of ice.
   B. Gently tilt the tube until a clot forms.
4. Postprocedure care:
   A. For clients with coagulopathy, hold pressure over the sampling site for at least 5 minutes and observe the site closely for development of a hematoma.
   B. Place the specimens on ice.
5. Client and family teaching:
   A. Results are normally available within 4 hours.
   B. Seek medical attention for signs of bleeding (i.e., hematoma, bleeding of gums, wounds, petechiae, confusion, changing level of consciousness).
6. Factors that affect results:
   A. Reject specimens of nonclotted blood.
   B. Reject specimens if the tube is mixed vigorously.
   C. If heparin is to be administered, do so after this specimen is drawn.
7. Other data:
   A. This test does not distinguish between conditions producing primary fibrinolysin activity and those producing secondary fibrinolysin activity.

Bibliography:

de Maat MP, Nieuwenhuizen W, Knot EA, van Buuren HR, Swart GR: Measuring plasma fibrinogen levels in patients with liver cirrhosis. The occurrence of proteolytic fibrin(ogen) degradation products and their influence on several fibrinogen assays. Thromb Res 78(4):353–362, 1995.

Gaffney PJ, Edgell T, Creighton-Kempsford LJ, Wheeler S, Tarelli E: Fibrin degradation product (FnDP) assays: analysis of standardization issues and target antigens in plasma. Br J Haematol 90(1):187–194, 1995.

Gravlee GP, Arora S, Lavender SW, et al.: Predictive value of blood clotting test in cardiac surgical patients. Ann Thorac Surg 58(1):216–221, 1994.

Leavell KJ, Peterson MW, Gross TJ: The role of fibrin degradation products in neutrophil recruitment to the lung. Am J Respir Cell Mol Biol 14(1):53–60, 1996.

FIBRIN DEGRADATION FRAGMENT

(see D-dimer, Blood)

FIBRIN DEGRADATION PRODUCTS, BLOOD

(see Fibrin Breakdown Products, Blood)

FIBRIN SPLIT PRODUCTS, PROTAMINE SULFATE TEST, BLOOD

Norm: Negative test.

Positive Test: Deep vein thrombosis, disseminated intravascular coagulation (DIC), infarcts, postoperative blood vessel clots, and pulmonary embolism.

Description: Protamine sulfate added to the blood sample helps differentiate between conditions producing secondary fibrinolysin (positive test) and conditions producing primary fibrinolysin (negative test). It is primarily used as a screening test for DIC, which produces secondary fibrinolysin.

Professional Considerations:

1. Consent form NOT required.
2. Preparation:
   A. Tube: Blue-top.
   B. Perform this test prior to implementing heparin therapy.
3. Procedure:
   A. Draw a 3-ml blood sample.
4. Postprocedure care:
   A. For clients with coagulopathy, hold pressure over the sampling site for at least 5 minutes and observe the site closely for development of a hematoma.
   B. Write the collection time on the laboratory requisition.
   C. Do NOT shake the tube or place it on ice.
   D. Transport the specimen to the laboratory immediately for incubation.
5. Client and family teaching:
   A. Results are normally available within 2 hours.
   B. Seek medical attention for signs of bleeding (i.e., hematoma, bleeding of gums, wounds, petechiae, confusion, changing level of consciousness).
6. Factors that affect results:
   A. Reject hemolyzed specimens or specimens received more than 2 hours after collection.
   B. Drugs that may produce a false-positive result include heparin calcium and heparin sodium.
7. Other data:
   A. Assess for signs of shock from bleeding: tachycardia, hypotension, and clammy cold skin.

Bibliography:

von Eckardstein A, Heinrich J, Funke H, Schulte H, Schonfeld R, Kohler E, Steinmetz A, Assmann G: Glutadine polymorphism in apo A-IV affects plasma concentrations of lipoprotein(a) and fibrin split products in coronary heart disease patients. Arterioscler Thromb 13(2):240–246, 1993.

FIBRIN STABILIZING FACTOR, BLOOD

(see Factor XIII, Blood)

FIBRINOGEN (FACTOR I), PLASMA

Norm: Quantitative is 150–400 mg/dl (1.5–4.5 g/L, SI units).

Increased: Arthritis (rheumatoid), familial paroxysmal peritonitis (familial Mediterranean fever, periodic disease), hepatitis, infection (acute), and menstruation.

Decreased: Abortion (septic, missed), anemia (acquired hemolytic), burns (severe), carcinoma (prostate, lung, metastasis), circulating fibrinogen inhibitors, cirrhosis, coagulation factor deficiency, congenital fibrinogen disorders (afibrinogenemia, hypofibrinogenemia, dysfibrinogenemia), cryoglobulinemia, disseminated intravascular coagulation (DIC), eclampsia, embolism (amniotic fluid, fat, meconium), leukemia, lymphoma, macroglobulinemia, multiple myeloma, newborns, septicemia, shock, snakebite, thrombotic thrombocytopenic purpura, transfusion reaction, and trauma. Drugs include asparaginase, phenobarbital drug poisoning, urokinase, and streptokinase.

Description: Fibrinogen (factor I) is a heat-stable, complex polypeptide that converts to the insoluble polymer of fibrin after thrombin enzymatic action and combines with platelets to clot the blood. Synthesized in the liver, fibrinogen increases in diseases associated with tissue damage or inflammation. There is some evidence that it may be useful as a predictor of arteriosclerotic disease. This test is performed by adding thrombin to the client's plasma and measuring the amount of time taken for clotting to occur at standard dilutions. The amount of fibrin is then calculated based on the thrombin clotting time.

Professional Considerations:

1. Consent form NOT required.
2. Preparation:
   A. Tube: 2.7- or 4.5-ml blue-top.
3. Procedure:
   A. Withdraw 2 ml of blood into a syringe or vacuum tube. Remove the syringe or tube, leaving the needle in place. Attach a second syringe, and draw two blood samples, one in a citrated blue-top tube and the other in a control tube. The sample quantity should be 2.4-ml for a 2.7-ml tube and 4.0 ml for a 4.5 ml tube. Draw a 5-ml blood sample in a sodium citrate-anticoagulated blue-top tube.
4. Postprocedure care:
   A. For clients with coagulopathy, hold pressure over sampling site for at least 5 minutes and observe site closely for development of a hematoma.
   B. Transport the specimens to the laboratory immediately for spinning. The specimens are then stable for 3 days when refrigerated.
5. Client and family teaching:
   A. Seek medical attention for signs of bleeding (i.e., hematoma, bleeding of gums, wounds, petechiae, confusion, changing level of consciousness).
6. Factors that affect results:
   A. Reject hemolyzed specimens or tubes partially filled with blood.
7. Other data:
   A. Active bleeding or administration of a blood transfusion within 1 month prior to the test invalidates results.
   B. Normally, a prothrombin time and an activated partial thromboplastin time can also be performed on this specimen.
   C. *See also Partial Thromboplastin Time, Plasma.*

Bibliography:

DeMatt MP, Nieuwenhuizen W, Knot EA, et al.: Measuring fibrinogen levels in patients with lever cirrhosis. The occurrence of proteolytic fibrin degradation products and their influence on several fibrinogen assays. Throm Res 78(4):353–362, 1995.

Lip GY, Lowe GD, Metcalfe MJ, et al.: Effects of warfarin therapy on plasma fibrinogen, Von Willebrand factor, and fibrin D Dimer in left ventricular dysfunction secondary to coronary artery disease with and without aneurysms. Am J Cardiol 76(7):453–458, 1995.

FIBRINOGEN UPTAKE, DIAGNOSTIC

(see I-125-Labeled Fibrinogen Leg Scan, Diagnostic)

FIBRINOLIGASE, BLOOD

(see Factor XIII, Blood)

FIBROBLAST SKIN CULTURE

Norm: Requires interpretation.

Usage: Gardner's syndrome, hereditary tyrosinemia (type 1), Hurler's syndrome, Marfan's syndrome, and mucopolysaccharidosis.

Description: Fibroblasts, large stellate spindle-shaped connective tissue cells, are common in developing or repairing tissues, where they are associated with protein and collagen synthesis. The test is used to help identify gene coding for genetic diseases through cytogenetic study.

Professional Considerations:

1. Consent form IS required.

Risks:
Bleeding, infection.

Contraindications:
None.

---

2. Preparation:
   A. Obtain povidone-iodine solution, a sterile needle, a knife, and a sterile container.
3. Procedure:
   A. Cleanse the site to be biopsied with povidone-iodine solution and allow it to dry.
   B. Raise the skin with a sterile needle.
   C. Excise a 2-mm skin snip just below the needle with the knife.
   D. Place the skin snip in a sterile container.
4. Postprocedure care:
   A. Send the skin biopsy without fixative to the laboratory.
5. Client and family teaching:
   A. The test involves taking a tiny sample of skin for testing. Pain is minimal enough that a local anesthetic is often not needed.
6. Factors that affect results:
   A. None.
7. Other data:
   A. A scleral punch may also be used for the biopsy.

Bibliography:

Freedland M, Karmiol S, Rodriguez J, Normolle D, Smith D Jr, Garner W: Fibroblast responses to cytokines are maintained during aging. Ann Plast Surg 35(3):290–296, 1995.

Ulrich-Merzenich G, Bhonde RR: Donor site, age, and health affect fibroblast growth in culture [letter]. In Vitro Cell Dev Biol Anim 31(7):494–496, 1995.

Zhang LQ, Laato M, Muona P, Penttinen R, Oikarinen A, Peltonen J: A fibroblast cell line cultured from a hypertrophic scar displays selective downregu- lation of collagen gene expression: barely detectable messenger RNA levels of the pro alpha 1(III) chain of type III collagen. Arch Dermatol Res 287(6):534–538, 1995.

FLAT PLATE X-RAY OF ABDOMEN (KIDNEY-URETER-BLADDER, KUB, SCOUT FILM), DIAGNOSTIC

Norm: Kidneys equal in size, with the left slightly higher than the right. Ureters are not seen. The bladder appears as a shadow.

Usage: Gross evaluation of the abdominal structures and contents for size, position, and structure. Screening for urinary tract abnormalities or for paralytic ileus or other gastrointestinal abnormalities.

Description: A plain film (noncontrast) anteroposterior radiograph of the abdominal area taken with the client supine. This test is commonly called a kidneys, ureters, and bladder (KUB) because the positioning and x-ray angle emphasizes visualization of these structures. However, other abdominal structures such as the liver, gallbladder, or aorta are also visualized with this radiograph. The test is usually performed as a screening for abnormalities following nonspecific urinary or gastrointestinal symptoms. Films are examined for organ and vessel location and size, symmetry, gas patterns, location of fluid, and calcification of structures. This radiograph may be performed at the bedside with a portable x-ray camera.

Professional Considerations:

1. Consent form NOT required.
2. Preparation:
   A. Practitioners should stand behind the x-ray camera at a safe distance (≥11 feet) during x-ray exposure. A film badge should be worn by any professional working in an area with frequent x-rays being taken. A lead apron should be worn by the professional if remaining with the client during the radiograph.
3. Procedure:
   A. Position the client supine on an x-ray table (or in bed for a portable x-ray), with arms held over the head.
   B. Shield the male penis and testicles during x-ray exposure.
4. Postprocedure care:
   A. None.

5. Client and family teaching:
   A. Breathe out and hold breath as an anterior to posterior view radiograph is taken.
   B. Results are normally available within 1–2 hours.
6. Factors that affect results:
   A. Poor visualization may be due to the presence of air, stool, or barium in the gastrointestinal tract; or to obesity or ascites.

7. Other data:
   A. Confirmation of abnormalities diagnosed by this procedure requires further testing.

Bibliography:

Dalla-Palma L, Stacul F, Bazzocchi M, et al.: Ultrasonography and plain film versus intravenous urography in ureteric colic. Clin Radiol *1*(5):333–336, 1993.

FLECAINIDE, PLASMA OR SERUM

Norm: Negative.

		SI Units
Therapeutic trough	0.2–1.0 µg/ml	0.5–2.4 µmol/L
Panic level	>1.0 mg/µl	>2.4 mmol/L

Overdose Symptoms and Treatment:

Symptoms: Overdose will produce effects that are extensions of pharmacologic effects. AV nodal escape rhythms and prolongation of QRS and QT intervals. ECG abnormalities associated with overdose have included regular ventricular tachycardia with a right bundle branch that progressed to polymorphous tachycardia; substantial prolongation of the PR and JT intervals, widened p waves. Sudden death may occur.

Treatment: Symptomatic and supportive care with ECG, blood pressure, and respiratory monitoring. There is no specific antidote. Hemodialysis will NOT remove flecainide.

Increased: Hepatic or renal dysfunction. Drugs include amiodarone, cimetidine, and propranolol.

Decreased: Drugs include phenobarbital and rifampin.

Description: Flecainide is a class 1 C antidysrhythmic used for ventricular dysrhythmias. It is metabolized and excreted by the liver and kidneys, with a half-life of 20 hours and steady-state levels reached by 3–5 days after starting therapy.

Professional Considerations:

1. Consent form NOT required.
2. Preparation:
   A. If the client is also taking propranolol or quinidine, indicate this on the laboratory requisition.
   B. Tube: Red-top, red/gray-top, gold-top, or green-top.
   C. MAY be drawn during hemodialysis.
3. Procedure:
   A. Draw the blood sample just prior to the next scheduled dose.
   B. Draw a 2-ml blood sample.
4. Postprocedure care:
   A. Send the specimen to the laboratory promptly. Serum or plasma must be separated within 2 hours.
5. Client and family teaching:
   A. Results are normally available within 24 hours.
6. Factors that affect results:
   A. Propranolol and quinidine cause unreliable results when the spectrofluorometric method is used.
7. Other data:
   A. Plasma levels >1.2 µg/ml in clients with renal dysfunction are associated with serious side effects and sudden death.

Bibliography:

Epstein AE, Hallstrom D, et al.: Mortality following ventricular arrhythmia suppression by encainide, flecainide and moricizine after MI: the original design concept of Cardiac Arrhythmia Suppression Trail. JAMA *270*(20):2451–2456, 1993.

Ever J, Eichelbaum m, Kroemer HK: Unpredictability of Flecainide plasma concentrations in patients with renal failure: relationship to side effects and sudden death? Ther Drug Monit *4*:349–351, 1994.

FLUCYTOSINE, SERUM

Norm:

		SI Units
Therapeutic level	25–100 µg/ml	195–775 µmol/L
Panic level	>125 µg/ml	>970 µmol/L

Panic Level Symptoms and Treatment:

Symptoms: Panic levels correlate poorly with clinical symptoms. May have adverse effects on renal, hepatic, and hematopoietic systems.

Treatment: Flucytosine can be eliminated by hemodialysis (50%); peritoneal dialysis; and in part, by hemofiltration.

Usage: Monitoring for therapeutic and toxic levels of the drug.

Description: An orally effective, systemic antifungal drug that is a secondary agent often used in conjunction with amphotericin B for treating serious, deep-seated mycotic infections due to *Candida* and *Cryptococcus* species. Is less effective but less toxic than amphotericin B. Ancobon is well absorbed, well distributed throughout the body, and the majority is excreted unchanged by the kidneys. Half-life is 3–6 hours.

Professional Considerations:

1. Consent form NOT required.
2. Preparation:
   A. Tube: Red-top, red/gray-top, or gold-top or green-top.
   B. Do NOT draw during hemodialysis.
3. Procedure:
   A. Draw a 5-ml blood sample 2 hours after oral administration for peak levels and immediately prior to oral administration for trough levels.
4. Postprocedure care:
   A. None.
5. Client and family teaching:
   A. Inform the client or the family of the rationale for the test.
   B. Results are normally available in 24 hours.
6. Factors that affect results:
   A. Ancobon half-life may increase up to 200 hours in clients with renal failure.
7. Other data:
   A. None.

Bibliography:

Krcmery S, Masar O, Krcmery V: Nosocomial Torulopsis glabrate fungemia with shock in a pregnant woman successfully treated with high doses of fluconazole and delivery of healthy child [letter]. J Chemother 7(3):253, 1995.

Lau AH, Kronfol NO: Elimination of flucytosine by continuous hemofiltration. Am J Nephrol 15(4): 327–331.

Terrell CL, Hughes CE: Antifungal agents used for deep-seated mycotic infections. Mayo Clin Proc 67(1):69–91, 1993.

FLUORESCEIN ANGIOGRAPHY (EYE FUNDUS), DIAGNOSTIC

Norm: No leakage of dye from blood vessels of the retina during any of the following phases.

Filling Stage: Begins 12–15 seconds after dye injection; noted when retinal vessels begin filling with dye.

Choroidal Flush: The retina fluoresces and appears evenly mottled throughout the capillaries.

Arterial Stage: Noted when arteries begin to fill with dye.

Arteriovenous Stage: Noted when arteries have filled with dye and veins begin to fill with dye.

Venous Stage: The arteries have emptied and the veins have filled and emptied.

Late Stage: ½–1 hour after injection, the dye has circulated throughout the body and recirculation of the retinal vessels can be seen.

Usage: Evaluation of retinopathy, tumors, retinal circulation abnormalities (occlusion, stenosis, dilation, aneurysm, arteriovenous shunt), or papilledema. Identification of leakage and retinal thickening for subsequent laser treatment.

Description: A radiographic examination of the retinal vasculature after rapid injection of fluorescein dye. Fluorescein angiography provides rapid and direct acquisition of sequential images of the vasculature and the ability to manipulate the fluorescein images with the computer. For example, the processor can adjust for fluorescein leakage into the vitreous, cataracts, or cloudy corneas. It also provides the ability to display fluorescein images and color fundus images for comparison during laser treatment. The rapidly available images are also used to help explain the disease process to the client being examined.

Professional Considerations:

1. Consent form IS required.

Risks:

Allergic reaction (itching, hives, rash, tight feeling in the throat, shortness of breath, bronchospasm, anaphylaxis, death), or seizure reaction to sodium fluorescein.

Contraindications:

Previous allergy to sodium fluorescein; clients who are unable to keep their eyes open for the test.

2. Preparation:
   A. Obtain mydriatic eye drops and 5% or 10% sodium fluorescein.
   B. Administer mydriatic eye drops as prescribed 15–30 minutes prior to the test.
   C. Insert a heparin lock intravenously.
   D. Have emergency equipment, including diazepam or phenytoin, available in case of allergic or seizure reaction.
3. Procedure:
   A. Dilating eye drops are administered.
   B. The client's chin and forehead rest against the fundus camera, and one arm is extended to the side.
   C. The client is instructed to open the eyes very wide, close the mouth, and look forward. The client can blink normally.
   D. Baseline fundus photographs are taken.
   E. Fluorescein dye is injected quickly and may cause facial flushing or nausea.
   F. Photographs of the fundus of the eye are taken every second for 25–45 seconds. Late-phase photographs are taken 30 minutes later, if needed.
4. Postprocedure care:
   A. Discontinue the heparin lock.
5. Client and family teaching:
   A. Clients with glaucoma should omit mydriatic eye drops the day of the test.

B. Do not drive for at least 2 hours after the test.
C. Protective eyewear may be necessary for at least 2 hours after the test if the environment is bright or sunny.
D. Yellow discoloration of the skin and urine is normally present for up to 2 days.
6. Factors that affect results:
   A. Cataracts may interfere with fundal view.
7. Other data:
   A. None.

Bibliography:

Anand R: Fluorescein angiography. Part 1: Technique and normal study. J Opthal Nurs Technol 8(2): 48–52, 1989.

Anand R: Fluorescein angiography. Part 2: Clinical applications. J Opthal Nurs Technol 8(3):102–107, 1989.

Dyer D, Brant A, et al.: Angiographic features and outcome of questionable recurrent choroidal neovascularization. Am J Ophthalmol 120(4):497–505, 1995.

Sapira JD, Olofinboba, Scheiderman L: The funduscopic examination: the more you know what to look for, the more you see. Consultant 35(10): 1443–1449, 1995.

Weinhaus R, Burke J, Delori F, Snodderly D: Comparison of flourescein angiography with microvascular anatomy of macaque retinas. Exp Eye Res 61(1):1–16, 1995.

FLUORESCENT RABIES ANTIBODY (FRA), SPECIMEN

Norm: Negative. Requires interpretation.

Positive: Rabies.

Description: The rabies rhabdovirus causes an acute viral infection of the central nervous system of a variety of animals characterized by neurotropic ribonucleic acid (RNA) viral presence in the saliva, urine, feces, brain, and spinal cord. This virus is occasionally transmitted to humans by an infected skunk, squirrel, cat, bat, dog, or other animal, and is 99% fatal if symptoms appear before treatment is instituted. The serum of a human bitten by a rabid animal is examined via immunofluorescence to detect a significant serum antibody rise. This test can be used for antemortem diagnosis in clients who have never received rabies vaccine or passive antibody.

Professional Considerations:

1. Consent form NOT required.
2. Preparation:
   A. Tube: Red-top, red/gray-top, or gold-top.
3. Procedure:
   A. Draw a 7-ml human blood sample and send it to the laboratory along with an-

imal brain. *(See Animals and Rabies, Negri Bodies.)*

4. Postprocedure care:
   A. None.
5. Client and family teaching:
   A. Results are normally available in 24 hours.
   B. Both preexposure and postexposure prophylaxis is available against rabies.
6. Factors that affect results:
   A. None.
7. Other data:
   A. Animal survival for 10 days makes rabies unlikely.
   B. Rabies is a reportable disease in most areas, as are animal bites.

Bibliography:

Fishbein DB, Robinson LE: Rabies. New Engl J Med *329*(22):1632, 1993.

Weisberg D: Rabies: a growing threat. Curr Health *22*(2):13–16, 1995.

FLUORESCENT TREPONEMAL ANTIBODY-ABSORBED DOUBLE-STAIN (FTA-ABS DS) TEST, SERUM

Norm: Nonreactive.

Usage: Serologic confirmation of syphilis when nontreponemal tests are positive.

Description: Syphilis is a complex, sexually transmitted disease characterized by a wide range of symptoms that imitate other diseases and is caused by the organism *Treponema pallidum*. This test provides the most sensitive detection of treponemal antibodies for syphilis in all stages. It differentiates biologic false-positives from true syphilis positives and can help diagnose syphilis when definite clinical signs are present but other tests are negative. This test is positive in the treponemal diseases of bejel, pinta, syphilis, and yaws. Before testing, the serum is treated to remove antibodies that could cause false-positive results. The technique involves using fluorescence microscopy with special filters that decrease the amount of natural fluorescence from the background of the specimen. Fluorescein-conjugated antibodies to IgG are added as a counterstain to the stained specimen and the treponemes are identified as they fluoresce in combination with the antibodies.

Professional Considerations:

1. Consent form NOT required.
2. Preparation:
   A. Tube: Red-top, red/gray-top, or gold-top.
3. Procedure:
   A. Draw a 3-ml blood sample.
4. Postprocedure care:
   A. None.
5. Client and family teaching:
   A. Results are normally available in 24 hours.
   B. If testing positive:
      i. Notify all sexual contacts from the last 90 days (if early stage) to be tested for syphilis.
      ii. Syphilis can be cured with antibiotics. These may worsen the symptoms for the first 24 hours.
      iii. Do not have sex for 2 months and until after repeat testing has confirmed that the syphilis is cured. Use condoms after that for 2 years. Return for repeat testing every 3–4 months for the next 2 years to make sure the disease is cured.
      iv. Do not become pregnant for 2 years, because syphilis can be transmitted to the fetus.
      v. If left untreated, syphilis can damage many body organs, including the brain, over several years' time.
6. Factors that affect results:
   A. Reject hemolyzed specimens or chylous serum samples.
   B. False-positive results may be due to antinuclear antibodies, drug abuse, elevated or abnormal globulins, pregnancy, or systemic lupus erythematosus (beaded pattern).
7. Other data:
   A. This test may remain positive indefinitely for clients previously infected with syphilis. Thus, it is not useful for monitoring clinical response to treatment for syphilis.
   B. Borderline results necessitate repeating the test.

Bibliography:

Woods GL: Update on laboratory diagnosis of sexually transmitted diseases. Clin Lab Med *15*(3):665–684, 1995.

FLUOROSCOPY, DIAGNOSTIC

Norm: Requires interpretation. Usually: symmetric, synchronous pulmonary and diaphragmatic motion. Diaphragmatic excursion = 2–4 cm. Absence of calcification in the coronary arteries.

Usage: Assessment of diaphragmatic function; localization of lung mass for percutaneous biopsy, mediastinal mass, pleural effusion, pleural lesion, and pulmonary disease; screening tool for detection of coronary artery disease; infrequent applications of fluoroscopy other than of the chest include gastrointestinal imaging, venography, myelography, and genitourinary fluoroscopy.

Description: A radiographic examination of pulmonary motion using a fluoroscopic screen containing calcium tungstate crystals, which fluoresce when struck by x-rays. When the x-ray passes through the body, dense areas allow less radiation to pass through onto the fluoroscopic screen than do less dense areas. The resulting pattern of light and dark areas aids in the diagnosis of pathophysiologic conditions. Fluoroscopy can reveal subtle nodular or parenchymal calcifications and coronary artery calcifications better than regular radiographs. The test takes about 5 minutes and includes less than 1 minute of x-ray exposure.

Professional Considerations:

1. Consent form IS required.

Risks:
Radiation exposure, infection.

Contraindications:
Pregnancy and during breastfeeding.

2. Preparation:
   A. The client should remove all upper-body clothing, jewelry, and metal items.
3. Procedure:
   A. The client stands with the chest between the x-ray tube and the fluoroscopic screen.
   B. Remove electrocardiographic monitoring leads and patches containing metal snaps, and safety pins. Move invasive lines out of the fluoroscopic field, if possible.
   C. Wear a lead apron if remaining in the room.
   D. Proceed with fluoroscopy. The client turns in different projections for the procedure.
4. Postprocedure care:
   A. None.
5. Client and family teaching:
   A. Inform the client or family of the rationale for the test.
   B. The client must remove all jewelry or

metal objects from the trunk of the body.
   C. The client must not be pregnant.
   D. Results will be available following the examination of the procedure results by a radiologist.
6. Factors that affect results:
   A. Metallic objects may interfere with the quality of films obtained via fluoroscopy.
7. Other data:
   A. A videotape of the film may be made for later examination.
   B. Fluoroscopy delivers more radiation than does a chest x-ray.

Bibliography:

Ricciardello M, McLean D: Assesment of fluoroscopic systems with a simple test. Australas Phys Eng Sci Med *18*(2):104–113, 1995.

Shao W, Chung T, Berdon W, et al.: Fluoroscopic diagnosis of laryngeal asthma (paradoxical vocal cord motion). Am J Roentgenol *165*(5):1229–1231, 1995.

FLUOROSCOPY OF THE SMALL INTESTINE, DIAGNOSTIC

Norm: Requires interpretation by a radiologist.

Usage: Detection of biliary tract obstruction or strictures. Detection of gastrointestinal inflammation, tumors, lesions, or other structural changes. Diagnosis of hiatal hernia.

Description: A radiographic examination of intestinal motion using a fluoroscopic screen containing calcium tungstate crystals, which fluoresce when struck by x-rays. When the x-ray passes through the body, dense areas allow less radiation to pass through onto the fluoroscopic screen than do less dense areas. The resulting pattern of light and dark areas aids in the diagnosis of pathophysiologic conditions. This procedure can be used with the addition of barium. A nasogastric tube is placed in the duodenum for the purpose of administering dilute barium directly into the small bowel. Fluoroscopy takes about 5 minutes.

Professional Considerations:

1. Consent form IS required.

Risks:
Hemorrhage, infection, perforation, peritonitis. Complications of nasogastric tube insertion include

bleeding, dysrhythmias, esophageal perforation, laryngospasm and decreased mean PO_2.

Contraindications:
Pregnancy and during breast-feeding. Nasogastric tube insertion is contraindicated in esophageal varices.

2. Preparation:
   A. The client should fast for 12 hours.
   B. The client should remove jewelry and metal items.
3. Procedure:
   A. Position the client with abdomen between the x-ray tube and the fluoroscopic screen.
   B. Insert a nasogastric tube if needed.
   C. Wear a lead apron if remaining in the room.
   D. Proceed with fluoroscopy. The client turns in different projections for the procedure.
4. Postprocedure care:
   A. None.
5. Client and family teaching:
   A. Inform the client or the family of the rationale for the test.

B. If barium is used in conjunction with this test, the client should increase fluid intake, if condition permits, until barium has passed through. If necessary, a mild cathartic can be used to aid in this process.
C. Fluoroscopy delivers more radiation than does a chest x-ray.
6. Factors that affect results:
   A. Metallic objects may interfere with the quality of films obtained by fluoroscopy.
7. Other data:
   A. A videotape of the film may be made for later examination.

Bibliography:

Laufer I: Define the appropriate use of enteroclysis in managing patients. Am J Roentgenol 165(5): 1297–1299, 1995.

Olsson R, Castell J, Castell D, Ekberg O: Solid state computerized manometry improves diagnostic yield in pharyngeal dysphagia: simultaneous videoradiography and manometry in dysphagia patients with normal barium swallows. Abdom Imaging 20(3):230–235, 1995.

FLUPHENAZINE
(see Phenothiazines, Blood)

FLURAZEPAM, SERUM

Norm: Negative.

	Therapeutic Ranges	SI Units
Hydroxyethylflurazepam metabolite	0–4 ng/ml	0–9 nmol/L
n-Desalkylflurazepam metabolite	10–140 ng/ml	21–300 nmol/L
Flurazepam panic level	>2000 ng/ml	>4300 nmol/L

Panic Level Symptoms and Treatment:

Symptoms: Dizziness, somnolence, impaired coordination, slurred speech, confusion, coma, and diminished reflexes. Hypotension, respiratory depression, and apnea may occur if the dose has been large.

Treatment:

1. Do gastric lavage within warm tapwater or 0.9% saline if within 2 hours of ingestion.
2. Give activated charcoal.
3. Monitor for central nervous system depression.
4. Protect airway. Support breathing with oxygen and mechanical ventilation, if necessary.
5. Do NOT induce emesis.
6. Implement seizure precautions.
7. Flumazenil has been used as a competitive antagonist to reverse the profound effects of benzodiazepine overdose. Use of Flumazenil is contraindicated if concomitant tricyclic antidepressants were taken.
8. Do NOT use barbiturates.
9. Forced diuresis and/or hemodialysis will NOT remove benzodiazepines. No information is available on whether peritoneal dialysis will remove these drugs.

Positive: Drug abuse, overdose, and seizures.

Negative: Absence of drug in serum.

Description: Flurazepam is a schedule-IV, long-acting benzodiazepine anxiolytic and hypnotic used for the treatment of insomnia and irregular sleeping habits. Flurazepam depresses the central nervous system and relaxes the skeletal muscles. It is absorbed from the gastrointestinal tract within 1 hour, metabolized by the liver, and excreted via the kidneys, with a half-life of up to 100 hours.

Professional Considerations:

1. Consent form NOT required.
2. Preparation:
   A. Tube: Red-top, red/gray-top, or gold-top.
   B. MAY be drawn during hemodialysis.
3. Procedure:
   A. Draw a 5-ml blood sample.
4. Postprocedure care:
   A. None.
5. Client and family teaching:
   A. Inform the client/family of the rationale for the test.
   B. Results are normally available within 24 hours.
   C. If activated charcoal was given for elevated levels, the client should drink 4–6 glasses of water each day for 2 days to prevent constipation. The activated charcoal will also cause stools to be black for a few days.
6. Factors that affect results:
   A. None.
7. Other data:
   A. *See also Benzodiazepines, Plasma and Urine.*

Bibliography:

Krska J, MacLeod TN: Sleep quality and the use of benzodiazepine hypnotics in general practice. J Clin Pharm Ther *20*(2):91–96, 1995.

Mendelson WB: Effects of flurazepam and zolpidem on the perception of sleep in normal volunteers. Sleep *18*(2):88–91, 1995.

FLURAZEPAM HYDROCHLORIDE

(see Benzodiazepines, Plasma and Urine)

FOLEY CATHETER TIP, CULTURE

(see Foreign Body, Routine, Culture)

FOLIC ACID, RED BLOOD CELLS, BLOOD

Norm: Folate present in packed cells (ng/ml).

		SI Units
Adults		
<Age 61	95–500 ng/ml	215–1132 nmol/L
>Age 60	150–450 ng/ml	340–1020 nmol/L

Increased: Folic acid supplements.

Decreased: Alcoholism, anemia (pure vitamin B_{12} deficiency, hemolytic megaloblastic, pernicious, sickle cell), blind loop syndrome, celiac disease, Crohn's disease, dermatitis herpetiformis, diet (inadequate intake), folate coenzyme dysfunction, hepatic disease, lactation (without increased dietary folate), leukopenia, hemodialysis, hyperthyroidism, infants, iron and folate deficiency, leukemia (acute myelomonocytic), malabsorption syndromes, malignancy, malnutrition, myeloproliferative disease, myelosclerosis, neoplastic diseases, pregnancy (without increased dietary folate), renal failure, sprue (tropical, nontropical), thrombocytopenia, and vitamin B_{12} deficiency. Drugs include aminopterin, anticoagulants (chronic), anticonvulsants, chloroquine hydrochloride, chloroquine phosphate, ethanol, glutethimide, hydroxychloroquine sulfate, isoniazid, methotrexate, oral contraceptives (long-term), phenytoin, phenytoin sodium, primaquine phosphate, pyrimethamine, quinacrine hydrochloride, quinine sulfate, and sulfonamides.

Description: Folic acid (folate) is a vitamin/amino acid needed for normal functioning of red and white blood cells. It is formed by bacteria in the intestines, stored in the liver, and found in foods such as eggs, milk, leafy vegetables, yeast, liver, and fruits. Folate is absorbed in the jejunum and functions in the metabolism of amino acids and nucleotides, affecting all tissues that undergo a large amount of cell multiplication. Folate deficiency causes megaloblastic anemia, and eventually leukopenia and thrombocytopenia. Folic acid is thought to play a role in birth defects such as spina bifida, anencephaly, and orofacial clefts.

Symptoms of deficiency take about 3 months to appear and can be caused by inadequate intake, increased body demand, or folate antagonism by drugs. Red blood cells contain more folate than does the serum, and this measurement of folic acid is less sensitive to recent dietary intake of folic acid than is the serum folic acid test.

Professional Considerations:

1. Consent form NOT required.
2. Preparation:
   A. Tube: Red-top, red/gray-top, or gold-top, and lavender-top; and ascorbic acid.
3. Procedure:
   A. Draw a 5-ml blood sample in a red-top tube.
   B. Draw a 5-ml blood sample in a lavender-top tube.
   C. Prepare a hemolysate by adding 0.5 ml of EDTA blood to 4.5 ml of ascorbic acid and freeze immediately.
4. Postprocedure care:
   A. Protect the specimen from light by inserting it in a paper bag.
5. Client and family teaching:
   A. Results are normally available within 24 hours.
6. Factors that affect results:
   A. Reject specimens if the client had a radioactive scan within 48 hours prior to specimen collection.
   B. Bacterial contamination of the specimen may invalidate the results.
7. Other data:
   A. The same specimen from step 3A may be used for serum folic acid level.
   B. The recommended dietary intake of folate is 400 mg/day.

Bibliography:

Tomson T, Lindbom U, et al.: Red cell folate levels in pregnant epileptic women. Euro J Clin Pharmacol 48(39):305–308, 1995.

Ubbink JB: Is an elevated circulating maternal homocysteine concentration a risk factor for neural tube defects? Nutr Rev 53(6):173–175, 1995.

FOLIC ACID, SERUM

Norm:

		SI Units
Adults		
<Age 61	1.8–9 ng/ml	4.1–20.4 nmol/L
>Age 60	1.2–12 ng/ml	4.1–27.2 nmol/L

Increased: Folic acid supplements.

Decreased: Alcoholism, anemia (pure vitamin B_{12} deficiency, hemolytic, megaloblastic, pernicious, sickle cell), blind loop syndrome, celiac disease, Crohn's disease, dermatitis herpetiformis, diet (inadequate intake), folate coenzyme dysfunction, hepatic disease, lactation (without increased dietary folate), leukopenia, hemodialysis, hyperthyroidism, infants, iron and folate deficiency, leukemia (acute myelomonocytic), malabsorption syndromes, malignancy, malnutrition, myeloproliferative disease, myelosclerosis, neoplastic diseases, pregnancy (without increased dietary folate), renal failure, sprue (tropical, nontropical), thrombocytopenia, and vitamin B_{12} deficiency. Drugs include aminopterin, anticoagulants (chronic), anticonvulsants, chloroquine hydrochloride, chloroquine phosphate, ethanol glutethimide, hydroxychloroquine sulfate, isoniazid, methotrexate, oral contraceptives (long-term), phenytoin, phenytoin sodium, primaquine phosphate, pyrimethamine, quinacrine hydrochloride, quinine sulfate, and sulfonamides.

Description: Folic acid (folate) is a vitamin/amino acid needed for normal functioning of red and white blood cells. It is formed by bacteria in the intestines, stored in the liver, and found in foods such as eggs, milk, leafy vegetables, yeast, liver, and fruits. Folate is absorbed in the jejunum and functions in the metabolism of amino acids and nucleotides, affecting all the tissues that undergo a large amount of cell multiplication. Folate deficiency causes megaloblastic anemia, and eventually leukopenia and thrombocytopenia. Folic acid is thought to play a role in birth defects such as spina bifida, anencephaly, and orofacial clefts. Symptoms of deficiency take about 3 months to appear and can be caused by inadequate intake, increased body demand, or folate antagonism by drugs. Serum contains less folate than do the red blood cells. This measurement of folic acid is more sensitive to recent dietary intake of folic acid than is the red blood cell folic acid test.

Professional Considerations:

1. Consent form NOT required.
2. Preparation:
   A. Tube: Red-top, red/gray-top, or gold-top.
   B. *See Client and family teaching.*
3. Procedure:
   A. Draw a 1-ml blood sample prior to any injections of vitamin B_{12}.
4. Postprocedure care:
   A. Protect the specimen from light by inserting it in a paper bag.
   B. Transport the specimen to the laboratory and refrigerate the serum until tested.
   C. If the specimen will not be tested within 24 hours, the serum should be frozen at $-10°C$ and protected from light.
5. Client and family teaching:
   A. Do not eat food 8 hours before sampling. Water is permitted.
   B. Results are normally available within 24 hours.
6. Factors that affect results:
   A. Reject hemolyzed specimens and samples not frozen or not protected from light.
   B. Hemolysis falsely elevates results.
   C. Drugs that are folate antagonists, such as methotrexate and pentamidine, may induce a deficiency state.
   D. Levels may decrease in clients on oral contraceptives.
7. Other data:
   A. The same specimen may be used for one portion of the red blood cell folic acid level test.
   B. Levels fall below normal 21–28 days after deficiency begins.

Bibliography:

Adams MJ, Khoury MJ, et al.: Elevated midtrimester serum methylmalonic acid levels as a risk factor for neural tube defects. Teretology *51*(5):311–317, 1995.

Leeb BF, Witzmann G, et al.: Folic acid and cyanocobalamin levels in serum and erythrocytes during low-dose methotrexate therapy of rheumatoid arthritis and psoriatic arthritis patients. Clin Exp Rheumatol *13*(4):459–463, 1995.

Stolzenberg R: Possible folate deficiency with postsurgical infections. Nutr Clin Pract *9*(6):247–250, 1994.

FOLLICLE-STIMULATING HORMONE (FSH, FOLLITROPIN), SERUM

Norm:

Normal ranges will vary among laboratories and are dependent upon which international system of measurement is used.

		SI Units
Adult females		
Premenopausal	4–30 mIU/ml	4–30 IU/L
Follicular phase	2–25 mIU/ml	2–25 IU/L
Midcycle peak	10–90 mIU/ml	10–90 IU/L
Luteal phase	2–25 mIU/ml	2–25 IU/L
Pregnant	Low to undetectable	
Menopausal	40–250 mIU/ml	40–250 IU/L
Postmenopausal	40–250 mIU/ml	40–250 IU/L
Adult males	4–25 mIU/ml	4–25 IU/L
Children, prepubertal	5–13 mIU/ml	5–13 IU/L

Increased: Acromegaly (early), amenorrhea (primary), anorchism, castration, gonadal failure, hyperpituitarism, hypogonadism, hypothalamic tumor, hysterectomy, Klinefelter's syndrome, male climacteric, menopause, menstruation, orchiectomy, ovarian failure, pituitary tumors, precocious puberty, premature menopause, seminiferous tubule failure, seminoma, Stein-Leventhal syndrome (polycystic ovary syndrome), testicular agenesis, testicular destruction (due to radiation or mumps orchitis), testicular failure, testicular feminization syndrome (complete), and Turner's syndrome (primary hypogonadism).

Decreased: Adrenal hyperplasia, amenorrhea (secondary), anorexia nervosa, anovulatory menstrual cycle, delayed puberty, hypogonadotropinism, hypophysectomy, hypothalamic dysfunction, neoplasm (adrenal, ovarian, testicular), panhypopituitarism, and prepubertal child. Drugs include chlorpromazine, estrogens, oral contraceptives, progesterone, and testosterone.

Description: When released from the anterior pituitary gland, follicle-stimulating hormone (FSH) in women promotes maturation of the ovarian follicle, which produces estrogen. As levels of estrogen rise, luteinizing hormones are produced. Together, FSH and luteinizing hormone induce ovulation. In men, FSH produces spermatogenesis, and the luteinizing hormone stimulates the secretion of androgens. This test aids in the differential diagnosis of hypogonadism, infertility, menstrual disorders, and precocious puberty.

Professional Considerations:

1. Consent form NOT required.
2. Preparation:
   A. Tube: Red-top, red/gray-top, or gold-top or lavender-top.
3. Procedure:
   A. Draw a 1-ml blood sample between 6 and 7 A.M.
4. Postprocedure care:
   A. Write the beginning date of the female's last menstruation on the laboratory requisition.
   B. Send the specimen to the laboratory immediately for separation and freezing of serum.

5. Client and family teaching:
   A. Results are normally available within 24 hours.
   B. Repeating of the test is often required to ensure an accurate diagnosis.
6. Factors that affect results:
   A. Reject hemolyzed specimens or if the client had a radioactive scan within 48 hours.
   B. Radionuclides cause a falsely decreased FSH level.
   C. Values should be compared with the norms for the laboratory performing the test.
7. Other data:
   A. Several daily specimens are recommended, due to episodic release of FSH from the pituitary gland.

Bibliography:

Daya S, Gunby J, et al.: Randomized controlled trial of follicle stimulating hormone versus human menopausal gonadotropin in in-vitro fertilization. Hum Reprod *10*(6):1392–1396, 1995.

Latronico, Anasti J, et al.: Brief report: testicular and ovarian resistance to luteinizing hormone caused by inactivating mutations of the luteinizing hormone-receptor gene. New Engl J Med *334*(8): 507–513, 1996.

Unzer SR, dos-Santos JE, et al.: Alternatives in plasma gonadotropins and sex steroid levels in obese ovulatory and chronically anovulatory women. J Reprod Med *40*(7):516–520, 1995.

FOLLICLE-STIMULATING HORMONE (FSH, FOLLITROPIN), URINE

Norm:

		SI Units
Adult females	3–12 IU/24 hours	3–12 IU/day
Follicular phase	2–15 IU/24 hours	2–15 IU/day
Midcycle peak	8–60 IU/24 hours	8–60 IU/day
Luteal phase	2–10 IU/24 hours	2–10 IU/day
Menopausal	35–100 IU/24 hours	35–100 IU/day
Adult males	2–18 IU/24 hours	2–18 IU/day
>Age 61	Higher	
Female children		
Neonate–12 months	<1.4 IU/24 hours	<1.4 IU/day
12 months–8 years	<4.0 IU/24 hours	<4.0 IU/day
9–10 years	1–4 IU/24 hours	1–4 IU/day
11–12 years	1–8 IU/24 hours	1–8 IU/day
13–14 years	1–10 IU/24 hours	1–10 IU/day
Male children		
Neonate–12 months	<1.4 IU/24 hours	<1.4 IU/day
12 months–8 years	<4.5 IU/24 hours	<4.5 IU/day
9–10 years	1–5 IU/24 hours	1–5 IU/day
11–12 years	1.5–5 IU/24 hours	1.5–5 IU/day
13–14 years	2–12 IU/24 hours	2–12 IU/day

Increased: Acromegaly (early), amenorrhea (primary), anorchism, castration, gonadal failure, hyperpituitarism, hypogonadism, hypothalamic tumor, hysterectomy, Klinefelter's syndrome, male climacteric, menopause, menstruation, orchiectomy, ovarian failure, pituitary tumors, precocious puberty, premature menopause, seminiferous tubule failure, seminoma, Stein-Leventhal syndrome (polycystic ovary syndrome), testicular agenesis, testicular destruction (due to radiation or mumps orchitis), testicular failure, testicular feminization syndrome (complete), and Turner's syndrome (primary hypogonadism).

Decreased: Adrenal hyperplasia, amenorrhea (secondary), anorexia nervosa, anovulatory menstrual cycle, delayed puberty, hypogonadotropinism, hypophysectomy, hypothalamic dysfunction, neoplasm (adrenal, ovarian, testicular), panhypopituitarism, and prepubertal child. Drugs include chlorpromazine, estrogens, oral contraceptives, progesterone, and testosterone.

Description: When released from the anterior pituitary gland, follicle-stimulating hormone (FSH) in women promotes maturation of the ovarian follicle, which produces estrogen. As levels of estrogen rise, luteinizing hormones are produced. Together, FSH and luteinizing hormone induce ovulation. In men, FSH produces spermatogenesis, and luteinizing hormone stimulates the secretion of androgens. Urine FSH levels are more useful than serum levels because a 24-hour collection will reflect both the peaks and lows of the episodic FSH secretion. This urine test aids in the differential diagnosis of hypogonadism, infertility, menstrual disorders, and precocious puberty.

Professional Considerations:
1. Consent form NOT required.
2. Preparation:
   A. Obtain a 3-L container with boric acid additive.
   B. Write the beginning time of the collection on the laboratory requisition.
3. Procedure:
   A. Discard the first morning urine specimen.
   B. Collect all the urine voided in a 24-hour period in a refrigerated, 3-L container to which 10 g of boric acid has been added. Document the quantity of urine output during the collection pe-

riod. Include the urine voided at the end of the 24-hour period. For catheterized clients, keep the drainage bag on ice and empty urine into the collection container hourly.
4. Postprocedure care:
   A. Write the total amount of urine in the 24-hour sample on the laboratory requisition.
   B. Gently mix the container and send a 50-ml aliquot to the lab.
5. Client and family teaching:
   A. Save all the urine voided in the 24-hour period and urinate before defecating to avoid loss of urine. If any urine is accidentally discarded, discard the entire specimen and restart the collection the next day.
   B. Results are normally available within 24 hours.
   C. A repeat of the test is required to ensure an appropriate diagnosis.
6. Factors that affect results:
   A. Radionuclides cause a falsely decreased FSH level.
7. Other data:
   A. Several 24-hour urine specimens are recommended, due to episodic release of FSH from the pituitary gland.

Bibliography:
Balasch J, Fabregules F, et al.: Further characterization of the luteal phase inadequacy after gonadotropin-releasing hormone agonist-induced ovulation in gonadotropin-stimulated cycles. Hum Reprod 10(6):1377–1381, 1995.
Nielsen AH, Hagemann A, et al.: Regulation of angiotensin II receptor expression in ovarian follicles. A review. Adv Exp Med Biol 377:407–410, 1995.

FOLLITROPIN, SERUM
(see Follicle-Stimulating Hormone, Serum)

FOLLITROPIN, URINE
(see Follicle-Stimulating Hormone, Urine)

FOREIGN BODY, ROUTINE, CULTURE

Norm: No growth.

Usage: Aids diagnosis of infection due to invasive lines, catheters, and other foreign bodies. Part of the workup for suspected septic processes in clients on hyperalimentation or with other invasive lines. Determination of sensitivity of line sepsis microorganisms to antibacterial therapy.

Description: Includes the culturing of heart valves, dialysis catheters, Swan-Ganz or other central line tip, and intrauterine devices. Test also includes culture of indwelling urinary catheters. Nosocomial urinary tract infections associated with the presence of indwelling urinary catheters account for up to 40% of urinary tract infections.

Professional Considerations:

1. Consent form NOT required.
2. Preparation:
   A. Obtain povidone-iodine, a sterile container or a red-top tube, and sterile gloves.
   B. For urinary catheter tip culture, obtain sterile scissors, a 20-ml syringe, and a sterile specimen cup or red-top tube.
3. Procedure:
   A. *Invasive lines:*
      i. Remove the line site dressing.
      ii. Cleanse the line insertion site and surrounding skin with povidone-iodine and allow to dry.
      iii. Remove the invasive line, taking care not to contaminate the distal portion with skin or other objects.
      iv. Insert the tip (distal end) into a sterile, red-top tube or sterile container. Cut the distal 1.5-inch tip with sterile scissors, allowing the tip to drop into the container.
   B. *Indwelling urinary catheter:*
      i. Remove the water filling the balloon of the catheter using a syringe.
      ii. Remove the catheter, using sterile gloves and being careful not to contaminate the tip.
      iii. While holding the tip over or inside a sterile container, cut off at least 1 inch with sterile scissors and allow the tip to fall into the container.
      iv. Close the container.
4. Postprocedure care:
   A. Write the type of catheter and the removal site on the requisition.
   B. Write the collection time on the laboratory requisition.
   C. Transport the specimen to the laboratory within 1 hour.
   D. Do not refrigerate or incubate the specimen.
5. Client and family teaching:
   A. Specimen collection is usually painless.
   B. Incubation of the culture may take 24–48 hours.
6. Factors that affect results:
   A. Reject specimens if received more than 2 hours after collection.
   B. Contamination of the urinary catheter specimen with the external genital area may obscure the validity of the results. This is a frequent occurrence in the collection of the tip.
7. Other data:
   A. Irritation of the urethra is minimized

by totally deflating the balloon, which holds from 5 to 30 ml of sterile water.

Bibliography:

Ascher D, Shoupe B, et al.: Comparison of standards and quantitative blood cultures in the evaluation of children with suspected central venous line sepsis. Diagn Microbiol Infect Dis 15(6):499–503, 1992.

Rush K, Haller L: Patient Factors and central line infection. Clin Nurs Res 4(4):397–410, 1995.

FRA, SPECIMEN

(see Fluorescent Rabies Antibody, Specimen)

FRACTIONAL URINE, SPECIMEN

(see Urinalysis, Fractional, Urine)

FREE CALCIUM, SERUM

(See Calcium, Ionized, Blood)

FREI SKIN TEST FOR LYMPHOGRANULOMA VENEREUM, DIAGNOSTIC

Norm: Negative.

Usage: Aids in the diagnosis of lymphogranuloma venereum (LGV).

Description: Lymphogranuloma venereum is a sexually transmitted disease caused by *Chlamydia trachomatis* of immunotypes L1–L3, resulting in suppurative inguinal adenitis several days to several weeks after exposure. The most common mode of transmission is through sexual contact. The Frei test is not diagnostically specific. Clients with the disease become positive at about 3 weeks after the initial infection.

Professional Considerations:

1. Consent form NOT required.

Risks:

Allergic reaction to LGV injection; infection.

Contraindications:

Previous allergy to chicken eggs.

2. Preparation:
   A. Obtain a 1-ml syringe with a needle and LGV antigen for intradermal injection.
3. Procedure:
   A. Inject intradermally 0.1 ml of heat-inactivated, egg-grown LGV.

B. Inject a control substance made from a normal yolk sac at another intradermal site.

C. Read the skin test in 48–72 hours. The test is positive if the test site has a raised papular area ≥ 6 × 6 mm and the control site reaction is ≤ 5 × 5 mm.

4. Postprocedure care:
   A. List the injection site location on the client's record.

5. Client and family teaching:
   A. Results will be available in 48–72 hours.

6. Factors that affect results:
   A. Chlamydial infections that share the same group antigen will produce a positive Frei test.

7. Other data:
   A. Licensed Frei test antigens are not available commercially in the United States.
   B. Clients testing positive will always test positive on any future Frei tests.
   C. Delayed positive reactions are possible for several days.

Bibliography:

Blanchard TJ, Mabey DC: Chlamydial infections. Br J Clin Pract *48*(4):201–205, 1994.

Buntin DM: The 1993 sexually transmitted disease treatment guidelines. Semin Dermatol *13*(4): 269–274, 1994.

Martin DH, Mroczkowski TF: Dermatologic manifestations of sexually transmitted disease other than HIV. Infect Dis Clin North Am *8*(3):533–582, 1994.

FROZEN TISSUE SECTION, DIAGNOSTIC

Norm: Interpreted by pathologist.

Usage: Rapid diagnosis on biopsied tissue while surgery is in progress.

Description: The rapid freezing and slicing of tissue for pathologic examination and interpretation. Using frozen tissue section samples as a basis for diagnosis, while NOT 100% accurate, has consistently proven to be a highly accurate method for *rapid* diagnosis. This method may also be used for fluorescent microscopy and for identification of fats and enzymes undetectable by other methods.

Professional Considerations:

1. Consent form IS required for the procedure used to obtain the specimen. See *Biopsy, Site-Specific, Specimen* for procedure-specific risks and contraindications.

2. Preparation:
   A. Preoperative teaching involving the type of procedure required for the sampling to proceed; for example, anesthesia-induced procedure requires . . .

B. *See Client and family teaching.*

3. Procedure:
   A. Place the moistened, fixed or unfixed tissue on a freezing microtome table.
   B. Allow carbon dioxide to enter the table through the side perforations.
   C. Freeze the tissue and slice it into thin sections via the cryostat.
   D. Attach the frozen section to a glass slide.
   E. Stain the nucleus of the cells with a hematoxylin dye.
   F. Stain the cytoplasm of the cells with eosin dye.
   G. Examine the slide microscopically and interpret.

4. Postprocedure care:
   A. *See individual procedure listings.*

5. Client and family teaching:
   A. Preparation for the procedure is necessary.
   B. Fast from food and fluids for 12 hours before the procedure.
   C. Call the physician for signs of infection at the procedure site: increasing pain, redness, swelling, purulent drainage, or for fever >101°F.
   D. Supply information on possible support groups available for the diagnosis.

6. Factors that affect results:
   A. Poor tissue sample.

7. Other data:
   A. Microscopic examination is often able to confirm a diagnosis of a specific lesion.
   B. Frozen sections have been reported as false-positives and false-negatives. A fresh section is best for accuracy.

Bibliography:

Biesemer KW, Dent GA, Pryzwansky KB, Folds JD: A comparison study of frozen-section immunoperoxides and flow cytometry for immunophenotypic analysis of lymph node biopsies. Clin Diagn Lab Immunol *1*(3):299–303, 1994.

Ferreiro JA, Myers JL, Bostwick DG: Accuracy of frozen section diagnosis in surgical pathology; review of a 1 year experience with 24,880 cases at Mayo Clinic Rochester. Mayo Clin Proc *70*(12): 1137–1141, 1995.

Fujita M, Suzuki Y, et al.: The validity of intraoperative frozen section diagnosis based on video-microscopy (telepathology). Gen Diagn Pathol *141*(2): 105–110, 1995.

FRUCTOSAMINE, SERUM

Norm:

Normal ranges vary according to method.

Adult

Nondiabetic	1.5–2.7 mmol/L
Diabetic	>2.0–5.0 mmol/L
Child	5% below adult levels

Usage: Evaluate diabetic control, reflecting glucose concentrations over a shorter time period (2–3 weeks) than that represented by glycated hemoglobin (hemoglobin A_{1c}) (4–8 weeks). Can be used as an index of longer-term control than glucose levels especially in diabetic clients with abnormal hemoglobin, in clients with gestational diabetes, and in children with type I diabetes.

Professional Considerations:

1. Consent form is NOT required.
2. Preparation:
   A. Tube: Red-top, red/gray-top, or gold-top.
   B. *See Client and family teaching.*
3. Procedure:
   A. Draw a 5-ml blood sample.
4. Postprocedure care:
   A. None.
5. Client and family teaching:
   A. Abstain from food and drink 12 hours prior to the test.
   B. Results are normally available within 24 hours.
6. Factors that affect results:
   A. Albumin levels <3.0g/dL may falsely lower fructosamine concentrations.
7. Other data:
   A. Hemoglobin, ascorbic acid, and ceruloplasmin inhibit fructosamine generation.

Bibliography:

Hughes PF, Agarwal M, Newman P, Morrison J: An evaluation of fructosamine estimation in screening gestational diabetes mellitus. Diabet Med *12*(8):708–712, 1995.

Hutchesson AC, Smith JM: Contribution of serum globulins to total fructosamine in patients treated by haemodialysis. Ann Clin Biochem *32*(Pt 4):419–421, 1995.

Tahara Y, Shima K: Kinetics of HbA1c, glycated albumin, and fructosamine and analysis of their weight functions against preceding plasma glucose level. Diabetes Care *18*(4):440–447, 1995.

FRUCTOSE CHALLENGE TEST, DIAGNOSTIC

Norm: Clients with hereditary fructose intolerance show a decrease in serum glucose, carbon dioxide, and phosphate, and an increase in serum lactate, potassium, uric acid, and magnesium, while levels for normal clients remain fairly stable. They also show a decrease in urine phosphorus excretion and a greater increase in urine urate, lactate, alanine, and magnesium than do normal clients. Serum and urine fructose levels rise and fall at about the same rate for both groups.

Usage: Diagnosis of hereditary fructose intolerance.

Description: Fructose is a carbohydrate found in fruit and honey and is also a product of sucrose hydrolysis. Hereditary fructose intolerance is an autosomal-recessive condition involving an abnormality in fructose-1-phosphate aldolase in the liver, small intestine, and kidneys. Clients with this condition may exhibit hematologic abnormalities (hypoglycemia, hypophosphatemia, hyperuricemia, hypokalemia) and renal abnormalities (malfunctioning tubules, bicarbonaturia, aminoaciduria, phosphaturia). Infants with hereditary fructose intolerance who receive repeated dietary fructose fail to thrive, and exhibit vomiting, jaundice, hypotonia, impaired liver function, bleeding disorders, and possibly death. Clients with the condition develop an aversion to fruit and sweets and are able to live a normal life with a diet free of these foods. The fructose tolerance test involves administering a body-weight-adjusted dose of intravenous fructose and measuring the change in serum and urine value of the components it is known to affect.

Professional Considerations:

1. Consent form IS required.

Risks:

Profound hypoglycemia.

Contraindications:

Alcohol consumption, dizziness.

2. Preparation:
   A. Preschedule this test with the laboratory.
   B. *See Client and family teaching.*
   C. Insert an intravenous line of 0.9% sterile saline at a keep-open rate in one arm.
   D. Insert an indwelling urinary catheter 2 hours prior to the test.
   E. Obtain ten red-top, red/gray-top, or gold-top tubes and reagent strips for testing blood glucose.
3. Procedure:
   A. Due to the risk of profound hypoglycemia in susceptible clients, blood glucose should be measured frequently throughout the test with reagent strips.
   B. A 2-hour baseline urine sample is collected and measured for urate, phosphorus, lactate, alanine, magnesium, and fructose.
   C. A 10-ml blood sample in a red-top tube

is drawn for baseline measurement of fructose, glucose, phosphate, potassium, magnesium, lactate, carbon dioxide, and uric acid.

D. The client lies recumbent while a bolus of 20% solution of fructose at a dose of 200 mg/kg of body weight is injected over 1 minute for children and over 2 minutes for adults.

E. Venous blood samples are drawn immediately after injection and after 5, 10, 15, 20, 30, 45, 60, 90, and 120 minutes in a red-top tube from the arm opposite the injection for the components measured in step 3B.

F. A 2-hour postinjection urine sample is collected and measured for urate, phosphorus, lactate, alanine, magnesium, and fructose.

4. Postprocedure care:
   A. Write beginning and ending times of each collection on the laboratory requisition.
   B. Transport the urine specimen to the laboratory immediately for testing.
   C. Continue to observe for signs of hypoglycemia 4–6 hours after testing.

5. Client and family teaching:
   A. The diet should be free of fructose and sucrose for 3 weeks.
   B. Fast from food for 8 hours before the test.
   C. Take instant glucose, followed by protein such as cheese, if feeling shaky, agitated, or cool and clammy after the test.

6. Factors that affect results:
   A. Abnormally low fructose levels may result if the urine specimen is not tested when it is still fresh.

7. Other data:
   A. Infants fed with a sucrose-containing formula that is hydrolyzed to fructose will exhibit more severe symptoms than breast-fed infants, who are usually asymptomatic, because lactose is not catabolized by the fructose enzyme.
   B. Liver biopsies examined for metabolites of fructose may also be used for diagnosis of hereditary fructose intolerance.
   C. Treatment for hereditary fructose intolerance is a fructose-free and sucrose-free diet.

Bibliography:

Kerner JA: Formula allergy and intolerance. Gastroenterol Clin North Am 24(1):1–25, 1995.

Wilson JD, Robertson T, Whiley M: Hereditary fructose intolerance in an adult [letter]. Aust NZ J Med 24(3):259–260, 1995.

FSH, SERUM
(see Follicle-Stimulating Hormone, Serum)

FSH, URINE
(see Follicle-Stimulating Hormone, Urine)

FTA-ABS, SERUM
(see Fluorescent Treponemal Antibody Absorption, Serum)

FUNGAL ANTIBODY SCREEN, BLOOD

Norm: Negative.

Usage: Rapid detection of antifungal antibodies. Monitoring effectiveness of therapy for fungal infections.

Description: Fungi are slow-growing, eukaryotic organisms that can grow on living and nonliving organic materials, and are subdivided into yeasts and molds. Only a few fungi species infect humans. Normal host defense mechanisms limit the damage they cause superficially. Viral serology for fungal antibodies aids in the diagnosis of aspergillosis, blastomycosis, coccidioidomycosis, cryptococcosis antigen, fungal infections, histoplasmosis, and sporotrichosis antibodies. Antibodies to fungi may be found soon after infection and rise as the infection progresses. Diagnosis of a fungal infection is confirmed when the convalescent sample demonstrates a rise in titer from the acute sample.

Professional Considerations:

1. Consent form NOT required.
2. Preparation:
   A. Tube: Red-top, red/gray-top, or gold-top.
   B. *See Client and family teaching.*
3. Procedure:
   A. Draw a 10-ml blood sample.
   B. Acute and convalescent samples are required. Obtain the acute sample as soon as possible after onset. Draw the convalescent sample in 1–2 weeks.
4. Postprocedure care:
   A. Send the specimen to the laboratory for immediate separation and freezing of the serum.
5. Client and family teaching:
   A. Fast for 12 hours before the test.
   B. A repeat specimen is required in 1–2 weeks.
   C. The treatment will usually be started prophylactically.
6. Factors that affect results:
   A. Reject hemolyzed specimens, tubes partially filled with blood, or speci-

mens received more than 2 hours after collection.

B. Recent fungal antigen skin tests may cause falsely high results.

C. Blastomycosis and histoplasmosis antigens may cross-react to cause falsely high results.

D. False-negative results may be due to immunosuppression from mycoses.

7. Other data:

A. Factors that predispose clients to fungal infections by lowering the normal host defense mechanisms include administration of broad-spectrum antibiotics, invasive lines, poor nutritional status, parenteral nutrition, surgery, trauma, long-term use of steroids, and chemotherapy for cancer treatment.

Bibliography:

Csasdevall A: Antibody immunity and invasive fungal infection. Infect Immun 63(11):421–428, 1995.

Klinger L: Candida antigen and antibody essays [letter]. Acta Paediator 84(8):964, 1995.

Pfaller MA: Epidemiology of fungal infections: the promise of molecular typing. Clin Infest Dis 20(6):1535–1539, 1995.

FUNGIZONE, BLOOD
(see Amphotericin B, Blood)

FUNGUS, CEREBROSPINAL FLUID, CULTURE
(see Cerebrospinal Fluid, Routine, Culture and Cytology, Specimen)

G-6-PD, BLOOD
(see Glucose-6-Phosphate Dehydrogenase, Quantitative and Screen, Blood)

GALACTOKINASE, BLOOD

Norm:

Adults	12.1–39.7 mμ/g Hgb
Children	
2–18 years	11.0–53.6 mμ/g Hgb
<2 years	11.0–150.0 mμ/g Hgb
Infants	3–4 times adult values

Increased: Not clinically significant.

Decreased: Galactokinase deficiency galactosemia and juvenile cataracts.

Description: Galactokinase is an enzyme that functions in the metabolism of galactose to glucose in the liver, a deficiency of which may result in galactosemia. Galactokinase deficiency is one of three forms of galactosemia, an autosomal recessively transmitted inborn error of metabolism characterized by the inability to convert galactose into glucose. This form of galactosemia results in the appearance of infantile/childhood cataracts.

Professional Considerations:

1. Consent form NOT required.

2. Preparation:

A. Preschedule this test with the laboratory.

B. Tube: Green-top, and a container of ice.

3. Procedure:

A. Draw a 7-ml blood sample.

4. Postprocedure care:

A. Place the specimen on ice immediately.

B. Write the collection time on the laboratory requisition.

C. Send the specimen to the laboratory within 2 hours. Keep the specimen on ice until tested.

5. Client and family teaching:

A. Results are normally available within 24 hours.

B. Diet counseling is strongly recommended if the test is positive.

C. Stress the importance of follow-up.

D. Refer clients with positive results for genetic counseling.

6. Factors that affect results:

A. Reject specimens that were not placed on ice or were not received in the laboratory within 2 hours after collection.

7. Other data:

A. Homozygotes have a form of galactosemia with cataracts but without mental retardation or liver disease.

Bibliography:

Berry GT, Nissim I, Lin Z, et al.: Endogenous synthesis of galactose in normal men and patients with hereditary galactosaemia. Lancet 346(8982):1073–1074, 1995.

Jakob C, Kleijer WJ, Allen J, Holton JB: Prenatal diagnosis of galactosemia. Eur J Pediatr 154(7, Suppl 2):S33–S36, 1995.

GALACTOSE CLEARANCE TEST, DIAGNOSTIC
(see Galactose Loading Test, Diagnostic)

GALACTOSE LOADING TEST (GALACTOSE TOLERANCE TEST, GALACTOSE CLEARANCE TEST), DIAGNOSTIC

Norm: Values are for adults. Infants and children clear galactose more rapidly.

		SI Units
Oral Test (Galactose Tolerance Test)		
Whole blood		
1-hour specimen	40–60 mg/dl	2.22–3.33 mmol/L
Total of 30-, 60-, 90-, and 120-minute specimens	<110 mg/dl	<6.11 mmol/L
Urine		
Normal	<2 g/5 hours	<11.1 mmol/5 hours
Borderline	2–3 g/5 hours	11.1–16.7 mmol/5 hours
Abnormal	>3 g/5 hours	>16.7 mmol/5 hours
Intravenous Test (Galactose Clearance Test)		
Whole blood		
45-minute specimen	<99 mg/dl	<5.45 mmol/L
1-hour specimen	<43 mg/dl	<2.34 mmol/L
75-minute specimen	Almost none	Almost none
2-hour specimen	<0 mg/dl	0 mmol/L

Usage: Evaluation of liver functioning, differentiation of obstructive jaundice from hepatocellular jaundice, and evaluation of the amount of functioning liver mass.

Increased: Cirrhosis, hepatitis (acute), hepatocellular jaundice, hyperthyroidism, and metastasis to the liver.

Decreased: Not clinically significant.

Description: Galactose is a monosaccharide obtained from lactose after metabolism by the lactase enzyme. The liver functions in maintenance of the blood sugar level by several mechanisms, including conversion of carbohydrates to glucose. One mechanism by which this is accomplished is by the conversion of galactose to glucose, which is subsequently stored as glycogen. In liver disease, the conversion of galactose to glucose is delayed, resulting in elevated blood and urine galactose levels in timed specimens. The galactose loading test involves the administration of oral or intravenous galactose, followed by timed measurements of blood and urine galactose. In hepatocellular jaundice or diminished functioning liver mass, results are abnormally elevated, but in short-term obstructive jaundice of less than 21 days' duration, results are normal.

This test is seldom used because of its nonspecificity, due to the liver's proportionately large reserve functional capacity.

Professional Considerations:

1. Consent form NOT required.
2. Preparation:
   A. *See Client and family teaching.*
   B. For the oral test, 4 of each: needles, syringes, and green-top tubes; a clean 2-L urine collection container; and 40 g of galactose dissolved in 250 ml of water.
   C. For the intravenous test, 5 of each: needles, syringes, and green-top tubes; and galactose aqueous solution for injection.
   D. Establish intravenous access.
   E. For the oral test, the client should be well hydrated throughout the collection period to promote urine formation.
3. Procedure:
   A. Draw a 5-ml blood sample.
   B. Label the tube as the baseline sample.
   C. *Oral test (galactose tolerance test):*
      i. Administer 40 g of galactose in 250 ml of water orally and record the time.
      ii. Exactly 30 minutes after ingestion of the mixture, draw a 5-ml blood sample.
      iii. Repeat the blood sample collection at 60, 90, and 120 minutes after ingestion.
      iv. Record the collection time and time elapsed since solution ingestion on the label of each tube.
      v. 5 hours after ingestion of the galac-

tose solution, collect all the urine voided in a clean, refrigerated container. The client should empty his or her bladder completely at the end of 5 hours. For a continuous drainage catheter collection, keep the drainage bag on ice.

D. *Intravenous test (galactose clearance test):*

   i. Administer intravenously: galactose 50 g/100-ml aqueous solution in a dose of 0.5 g/kg of body weight.

   ii. Record the time of administration.

   iii. Exactly 45 minutes after galactose injection, draw a 5-ml blood sample.

   iv. Repeat the blood sample collection at 60, 75, and 120 minutes after injection.

   v. Record the collection time and the time elapsed since the solution injection on the label of each tube.

4. Postprocedure care:

  A. Send all the specimens to the laboratory immediately after collection.

  B. Urine specimens should be refrigerated if not tested immediately.

  C. Remove the intravenous line.

5. Client and family teaching:

  A. Fast for 8 hours before the test.

  B. The test requires drinking a galactose solution and having blood samples drawn at specific intervals for 2 hours afterward.

  C. Bring reading material or some other diversionary activity.

  D. Results are normally available within 24 hours.

6. Factors that affect results:

  A. Renal failure may cause elevated blood values and delayed renal excretion of galactose.

  B. Delayed absorption due to gastrointestinal tract abnormalities may falsely elevate the results of the oral test (galactose tolerance test).

  C. Drugs that may increase results include ascorbic acid.

7. Other data:

  A. Glucose and fructose tolerance tests may also be used to evaluate hepatic metabolism of carbohydrates.

  B. This test should not be used to diagnose galactosemia due to the danger of hypoglycemia and hypokalemia. It has been replaced by the following tests: *Galactokinase, Blood; Galactose-1-Phosphate, Blood; Galactose-1-Phosphate Uridyl Transferase, Erythrocyte, Blood; Galactose-1-Phosphate Uridyl Transferase, Qualitative, Blood;* and *Galactose, Screening Test for Galactosemia, Urine.*

Bibliography:

Gibson JB, Berry GT, Mazur AT, et al.: Effect of glucose and galactose loading in normal subjects on red and white blood cell uridine diphosphate sugars. Biochem Mol Med 55(1):8–14, 1995.

Hu OY, Tang HS, Chang CL: The influence of chronic lobular hepatitis on pharmacokinetics of cefoperazone—a novel galactose single-point method as a measure of residual liver function. Biopharm Drug Dispos 15(7):563–576, 1994.

GALACTOSE-1-PHOSPHATE, BLOOD

Norm: <1 mg% galactose-1-phosphate per 100 ml of lysed packed red blood cells. 18.5–28.5 U/g hemoglobin.

Increased: Transferase deficiency (classical) galactosemia.

Description: Galactose-1-phosphate is a metabolite that results after the action of galactokinase on galactose. It is found in red blood cells, subsequently converted to glucose-1-phosphate by galactose-1-phosphate uridyl transferase, and used for energy by the body. In clients with galactosemia who are ingesting milk and milk products, the level of galactose-1-phosphate rises and may become toxic. This test is used to monitor the dietary compliance of clients with galactosemia.

Professional Considerations:

1. Consent form NOT required.

2. Preparation:

  A. Preschedule this test with the laboratory.

  B. Tube: Green-top.

3. Procedure:

  A. Draw a 2-ml blood sample and gently invert the tube three times.

4. Postprocedure care:

  A. Write the collection time on the laboratory requisition.

  B. Refrigerate specimens until tested.

5. Client and family teaching:

  A. Results are normally available within 24 hours.

  B. If results are positive, the client and family will require diet counseling regarding a galactose-free diet.

  C. Galactose toxicity may cause failure to thrive, liver dysfunction, mental retardation, and vomiting/diarrhea.

6. Factors that affect results:

  A. Reject specimens received in the laboratory more than 3 hours after collection.

7. Other data:

  A. None.

Bibliography:

Gitzelmann R: Galactose-1-phosphate in the pathophysiology of galactosemia. Eur J Pediatr 154(7, Suppl 2):S45–S49, 1995.

Kaufman FR, McBride-Chang C, et al.: Cognitive functioning, neurologic status and brain imaging in classical galactosemia. Eur J Pediatr 154(7, Suppl 2):S2–S5, 1995.

GALACTOSE-1-PHOSPHATE URIDYL TRANSFERASE, ERYTHROCYTE, BLOOD

Norm:

		SI Units
Adult	5.9–9.5 µmol/h/ml	98–158 U/L
Heterozygote	2.0–4.8 µmol/h/ml	33–80 U/L
Homozygote	0.0 mmol/h/ml	0.0 U/L
Other norms		
Normal	18–28 U/g Hgb	
Possible carrier state	5–18.5 U/g Hgb	

Increased: Not applicable.

Decreased: Galactose-1-phosphate uridyl transferase deficiency and transferase deficiency (classical) galactosemia.

Description: Galactose-1-phosphate uridyl transferase is an enzyme active in the metabolism of galactose to glucose in the liver. It catalyzes the conversion of galactose-1-phosphate into glucose-1-phosphate. Deficiency of galactose-1-phosphate uridyl transferase is the most common cause of galactosemia. In this test, measurements of this enzyme are performed on the hemolysate of washed erythrocytes.

Professional Considerations:

1. Consent form NOT required.
2. Preparation:
   A. Tube: Green-top, and a container of ice.
3. Procedure:
   A. Draw a 2-ml blood sample and then gently invert the tube three times.
4. Postprocedure care:
   A. Place the specimen immediately on ice.
5. Client and family teaching:
   A. If the results are positive, the client and family will require diet counseling regarding a galactose-free diet.
6. Factors that affect results:
   A. Reject the specimen if it contains recently transfused blood to avoid a possible false-negative result.
   B. Reject hemolyzed specimens or specimens not received on ice.
7. Other data:
   A. Treat galactosemia with a lactose-free diet.
   B. *See also Galactose-1-Phosphate Uridyl Transferase, Qualitative, Blood.*

Bibliography:

Gitzelmann R: Partial deficiency of galactose-1-phosphate uridyl transferase. Eur J Pediatr *154*(7, Suppl 2):S40–S44, 1995.

Segal S: Galactosemia unsolved. Eur J Pediatr *154*(7, Suppl 2):S97–S102, 1995.

GALACTOSE-1-PHOSPHATE URIDYL TRANSFERASE, QUALITATIVE, BLOOD

Norm: Negative.

Positive: Transferase-deficiency (classical) galactosemia.

Description: A qualitative screen for galactosemia and differential diagnosis of milk intolerance in the newborn. This enzyme catalyzes the conversion of galactose-1-phosphate into glucose-1-phosphate in the liver. Galactosemia is an autosomal recessively transmitted inborn error of metabolism characterized by the inability to convert galactose into glucose. This causes deposits of galactose-1-phosphate in body tissues, resulting in vomiting, diarrhea, failure-to-thrive, liver dysfunction, splenomegaly, and cataracts in the infant. Symptoms appear a few days after a milk diet is started. Deficiency of galactose-1-phosphate uridyl transferase is the most common form of galactosemia. Early detection of galactosemia enables institution of a lactose-free diet and avoidance of complications of galactose toxicity. The test involves examining specially treated filter paper with a drop of dried blood under fluorescent lights after timed exposure to ultraviolet light. In a negative test (enzyme present), the blood fluoresces. In a positive test (enzyme absent), the blood will not fluoresce.

Professional Considerations:

1. Consent form NOT required.
2. Preparation:
   A. Preschedule this test with the laboratory.
   B. Write the client's birth date on the laboratory requisition.
   C. Obtain a galactosemia screening filter paper.

3. Procedure:
   A. Obtain three drops of blood from an infant heelstick on the lateral curvature of the heel.
   B. Place each drop in a circle on galactosemia screening filter paper and allow to dry.
   C. Heparinized blood may also be used (green-top tube).
4. Postprocedure care:
   A. Apply a dressing to the heelstick site.
   B. Label the filter paper with the client's name and identification.
   C. Store the specimen at room temperature. Protect it from heat if it is transferred to an outside laboratory.
5. Client and family teaching:
   A. Results are normally available within 24 hours.
   B. If results are positive, the family will require diet counseling regarding a galactose-free diet.
6. Factors that affect results:
   A. This test should be performed during the first 3 days after the infant is born.
   B. False-negative results may occur up to 3 months after blood transfusion, if the Beutler-Baluda screening method is used.
7. Other data:
   A. Treat galactosemia with a lactose-free diet.
   B. Blood testing is considered more reliable than urine testing in screening for galactosemia.
   C. Positive results should be confirmed with a quantitative galactose-1-phosphate uridyl transferase measurement.

Bibliography:
Lai K, Langley SD, Singh RH, et al.: A prevalent mutation for galactose among black Americans. J Pediatr *128*(1):89–95, 1996.
Schweitzer S: Newborn mass screening for galactosemia. Eur J Pediatr *154*(7, Suppl 2):S37–S39, 1995.

GALACTOSE, SCREENING TEST FOR GALACTOSEMIA, URINE

Norm: <10 mg/dl. Galactostix has a lower limit of sensitivity of 100 mg/dl.

Increased: Galactokinase deficiency, galactose-1-phosphate uridyl transferase deficiency, and galactosemia.

Description: A urine screen for galactosemia and differential diagnosis of milk intolerance in the newborn after a positive Benedict's or Clinitest result and a negative glucose oxidase test for glucose. Urine galactose measurements are performed by chromatography.

Professional Considerations:
1. Consent form NOT required.
2. Preparation:
   A. Obtain a clean container with a lid, pediatric urine collection device, and tape.
3. Procedure:
   A. Obtain at least a 10-ml random urine specimen in a clean container.
   B. Place the infant supine, with the knees flexed and the hips externally rotated and abducted.
   C. Cleanse, rinse, and thoroughly dry the perineal area.
   D. To prevent the child from removing the collection device, a diaper may be placed over the genital area.
   E. *Females:* Tape the pediatric collection device to the perineum. Starting at the area between the anus and vagina, apply the device in an anterior direction.
   F. *Males:* Place the pediatric collection device over the penis and scrotum and tape it to the perineal area.
4. Postprocedure care:
   A. Send the specimens to the laboratory and refrigerate them if not tested immediately.
5. Client and family teaching:
   A. If the results are positive, the family will require diet counseling regarding a galactose-free diet.
   B. Results are normally available within 24 hours.
6. Factors that affect results:
   A. None found.
7. Other data:
   A. Blood testing is more reliable than urine testing in screening for galactosemia.
   B. Positive results should be confirmed with a quantitative galactose-1-phosphate uridyl transferase measurement.
   C. *See also Galactose-1-Phosphate Uridyl Transferase, Qualitative, Blood.*

Bibliography:
Elsas LJ, Langley S, et al.: A molecular approach to galactosemia. Eur J Pediatr *154*(7, Suppl 2):S21–S27, 1995.
Schweitzer S: Newborn mass screening for galactosemia. Eur J Pediatr *154*(7, Suppl 2):17–19, 1995.

GALACTOSE TOLERANCE TEST, DIAGNOSTIC
(see Galactose Loading Test, Diagnostic)

GALLBLADDER SERIES
(see Cholecystography Radiography, Diagnostic)

GALLBLADDER AND BILIARY SYSTEM SONOGRAM, DIAGNOSTIC

Norm:

Gallbladder

Appearance	Sonolucent; free of sludge or stones
Location	Anterior to the right kidney, lateral to the pancreas and duodenum
Shape	Circular on transverse scans
	Pear-shaped on longitudinal scans
	7–10 cm long and 2–3 cm wide with a capacity of 30–50 ml
Walls	Sharply defined and smooth, 1–2 mm thick

Cystic duct

Appearance	Not sonolucent due to luminal; Heister's valves visible
Shape	Serpentine

Common bile duct

Shape	Linear; internal diameter <6 mm

Hepatic duct

Lumen	Internal diameter <4 mm

Usage: Diagnosis of cholelithiasis and cholecystitis; and differential diagnosis of the cause of jaundice (obstructive versus nonobstructive).

Description: Evaluation of the gallbladder, cystic duct, and common bile duct via the creation of an oscilloscopic picture from the echoes of high-frequency sound waves passing over these areas. The time required for the ultrasonic beam to be reflected back to the transducer from differing densities of tissue is converted by a computer to an electrical impulse displayed on an oscilloscopic screen to create a three-dimensional picture of the gallbladder and biliary duct system. This test is used when cholecystography cannot confirm a suspected diagnosis. The presence of sludge causes low-level echoes in the interior of the gallbladder. Acute cholecystitis causes the walls to appear thickened and sonolucent, due to edema. Cholelithiasis is demonstrated by a dilated interior, with shadows present. Biliary tree gas causes shadows. Polyps appear as sharply defined masses, while carcinoma appears as a poorly defined mass. In obstructive jaundice, dilation of the gallbladder and biliary duct system is detected.

Professional Considerations:

1. Consent form NOT required.

Risks:

If sincalide is given: infection.

Contraindications:

Administration of sincalide is contraindicated in pregnancy and in children.

2. Preparation:
   A. *See Client and family teaching.*
   B. Some scans may require intravenous access.
3. Procedure:
   A. The client is positioned supine and instructed to hold his or her breath during the scans.
   B. A lubricated transducer is passed slowly over the right upper quadrant of the abdomen with transverse scans (moving from the midline to the right side) taken every 1 cm from the xiphoid process to the right subcostal area.
   C. As the gallbladder borders are identified, they are marked on the client's skin.
   D. Longitudinal and oblique scans are then taken every 5 mm between the marked borders of the gallbladder.
   E. The client is then turned to a steep, left lateral decubitus position, and the scan is repeated from the right costal margin.
   F. The client may then be positioned upright to observe for a movement of suspected stones away from the walls of the gallbladder or cystic duct.
   G. If contractility of the gallbladder is to be evaluated, intravenous sincalide may be injected, or a fatty meal may be ingested and the scan repeated in 30 minutes.
   H. Photographs are taken of the oscilloscopic display.

4. Postprocedure care:
   A. Remove the lubricant from the skin.
   B. Resume previous diet.
5. Client and family teaching:
   A. Consume a diet free of fat the day before the test.
   B. Fast for 8–12 hours before the sonogram, but drink plenty of fluids.
   C. It is important to lie as motionless as possible during the sonogram.
6. Factors that affect results:
   A. Gallstones appear as shadows when well mixed with bile, but if the gallbladder is full of stones, shadows are difficult to detect.
   B. Sinaclide may cause nausea. Movement during nausea may interfere with results.
   C. Dehydration interferes with adequate contrast between organs and body fluids.
   D. Very small stones (<1–2 mm) in the gallbladder must be differentiated from polyps by repositioning the client. The stones will move downward with gravity, while polyps will remain stable.
   E. The more abdominal fat present, the greater the attenuation (reduction in sound wave amplitude and intensity), which interferes with the clarity of the picture.
7. Other data:
   A. Gallbladder cancer cannot usually be diagnosed by sonography.

Bibliography:

Kapoor BS, Agarwal AK, Khanna NN: Prediction of gall stone composition by ultrasound: implications for non-surgical therapy. Br J Radiol 68(809):459–462, 1995.

Kirsner JB: The scientific growth of gastroenterology during the 20th century. The 1994 G. Brohee Lecture. Dig Dis Sci 40(9):1851–1858, 1995.

GALLBLADDER SCAN
(see Hepatobiliary Scan, Diagnostic)

GALLIUM SCAN
(see Gallium Scan of Bone, Brain, Breast, or Liver, Diagnostic)

GALLIUM SCAN OF BONE, DIAGNOSTIC

Norm: Normal patterns of bone gallium uptake as interpreted by a nuclear medicine physician.

Usage: Detection of osteomyelitis, joint infections, and metastatic bone neoplasms (Wilm's tumor).

Description: Nuclear medicine scan using gallium-67 citrate to localize inflammatory lesions of the bone, bone marrow, and cartilage. While the bones normally take up the gallium-67 citrate, abnormal areas of inflammation or tumors appear as areas of increased uptake of the radiopharmaceutical.

Professional Considerations:

1. Consent form IS required.

Risks:
Allergic reaction to the radiopharmaceutical (itching, hives, rash, tight feeling in the throat, shortness of breath, bronchospasm, anaphylaxis, death), infection.

Contraindications:
Previous allergic reaction to the same radiopharmaceutical. This test is usually contraindicated during pregnancy and breast-feeding.

2. Preparation:
   A. Inject the client with a Gallium-67 citrate radiopharmaceutical intravenously 48–72 hours prior to the test. Exception: for the detection of acute inflammatory lesions, scan at 6–24 hours and then again at 48–72 hours.
   B. If the pelvis will be scanned, the bladder should be emptied completely just prior to the procedure.
   C. *See Client and family teaching.*
3. Procedure:
   A. The client is positioned under the gamma camera or a scintillation camera.
   B. Serial images are obtained anteriorly and posteriorly while an uptake probe and detector head measure the radiation emissions.
   C. The client must lie motionless throughout the scan.
4. Postprocedure care:
   A. *See Client and family teaching.*
5. Client and family teaching:
   A. Increase oral intake of fluids, where not contraindicated, beginning 24 hours prior to the scan.
   B. The scan takes 30–60 minutes and is painless.
   C. The camera will make clicking noises during the scan.
   D. It is important to lie motionless during the scan.
   E. Drink 6–8 glasses of water and other fluids each day for 2 days after the test (unless contraindicated).
   F. Results are normally available 24 hours following the completion of the scan.

6. Factors that affect results:
   A. Lesions that are <1–2 cm in size will not be detectable with a gallium scan.
   B. False-positive results may be obtained in the presence of leukopenia.
7. Other data:
   A. Gallium is excreted by the kidney and colon in 24–48 hours.
   B. This test does not distinguish between benign and malignant lesions.
   C. Health care professionals working in a nuclear medicine area must follow federal standards set by the Nuclear Regulatory Commission. These standards include precautions for handling the radioactive material and monitoring of potential radiation exposure.

Bibliography:

Cogswell A, Howman-Giles R, Bergin M: Bone and gallium scintigraphy in children with rhabdomyosarcoma: a 10-year review. Med Pediatr Oncol 22(1):15–21, 1994.

Gashen E, Zwas ST, Sadan M, Kronenberg J: The combined use of classified bone and gallium scans in the management of frontal sinusitis. Nucl Med Commun 15(5):361–366, 1994.

Martin RD, Rieckenbrauck N: The role of the bone-gallium scan in sternal osteomyelitis. Ann Plast Surg 30(4):320–322, 1995.

GALLIUM SCAN OF BRAIN, DIAGNOSTIC

Norm: Normal pattern of brain tissue gallium uptake as interpreted by a nuclear medicine physician.

Usage: Screening and localizing intracranial neoplasms, identification of cerebrovascular accident or tumor recurrence following surgical excision, and differentiation of localized inflammations of central nervous system (abscesses).

Description: A nuclear medicine scan in which radiopharmaceutical Ga-67 or Ga-68 is injected intravenously and a scintillation camera is used to obtain photographs of the meninges and brain soft tissue 24–48 hours later. The gallium is transported to the brain tissue via cerebrospinal fluid and plasma, where it binds to the transferrin receptor sites of soft tissue cells of neutrophilic lactoferrin. Tumors and inflammatory lesions frequently contain large concentrations of these two proteins. A positive scan will have distinct patterns of gallium uptake that differ from normal tissue uptake. For example, neoplasms will appear as dense areas with increased gallium uptake, while inflammatory lesions (most frequently abscesses) appear on the scan as well-localized areas of increased gallium uptake that are encapsulated. Finally, cerebral hemorrhages will differ from normal gallium uptake, appearing as irregular, diffuse areas of uptake. This is due to the vascular occlusion and tissue damage associated with cerebrovascular accidents.

Professional Considerations:
1. Consent form IS required.

Risks:
Allergic reaction to the radiopharmaceutical (itching, hives, rash, tight feeling in the throat, shortness of breath, bronchospasm, anaphylaxis, death), infection.

Contraindications:
Previous allergic reaction to the same radiopharmaceutical. This procedure is usually contraindicated during pregnancy and breast-feeding.

2. Preparation:
   A. The client is injected intravenously with radiopharmaceutical Ga-67 or Ga-68 from 6 to 48 hours prior to the scan.
   B. See Client and family teaching.
3. Procedure:
   A. The client is positioned under the scintillation camera and serial images are obtained from anterior; posterior; lateral; and, occasionally, vertex views.
   B. The client must lie motionless throughout the scan.
4. Postprocedure care:
   A. See Client and family teaching.
5. Client and family teaching:
   A. Increase oral intake of fluids, where not contraindicated, beginning 24 hours prior to the scan.
   B. The scan takes 30–60 minutes and is painless.
   C. The camera may touch the body and will make a clicking noise during the scan.
   D. It is important to lie motionless during the scan.
   E. Drink 6–8 glasses of water and other fluids each day for 2 days after the test (unless contraindicated).
   F. Results are normally available 24 hours following the completion of the scan.
6. Factors that affect results:
   A. Lesions <1–2 cm in size may not be detectable with a gallium scan.
   B. Lesions located at the base of the

brain, such as pituitary adenomas, may be difficult to detect due to the increased vascularity of the area and the difficulty in positioning the camera for clear images.

C. False-positive results may be obtained in the presence of leukopenia.

D. Pediatric neoplasms will most frequently appear intrafrontally, while adult neoplasms will most often be located supratentorially.

7. Other data:

A. Gallium is excreted by the kidney and colon in 24–48 hours.

B. Gallium scanning does not differentiate malignant from benign tumors.

C. Health care professionals working in a nuclear medicine area must follow federal standards set by the Nuclear Regulatory Commission. These standards include precautions for handling the radioactive material and monitoring of potential radiation exposure.

Bibliography:

Becker W: The contribution of nuclear medicine to patients with infection. Eur J Nucl Med *22*(10): 1195–1211. 1995.

Hagemeister FB, Purugganan R, Podoloff Da, et al.: The gallium scan predicts relapse in patients with Hodgkin's disease treated with combination modality therapy. Ann Oncol *5*(Suppl 2):59–63, 1994.

GALLIUM SCAN OF BREAST, DIAGNOSTIC

Norm: Normal pattern of breast gallium uptake as interpreted by a nuclear medicine physician.

Usage: Detection and location of tumor or inflammatory lesions of the breast, evaluation of lymphomas, and identification of recurrent tumors following chemotherapy or radiation therapy.

Description: Nuclear medicine scan using Gallium-67 citrate to localize neoplasms and inflammatory lesions of the breast tissues and lymph nodes. It is believed that the gallium binds to the transferrin and lactoferrin circulating in plasma and soft tissue. Tumors and lesions containing neutrophils also have a large concentrations of these two betaglobulins, causing the gallium clearance to be slower than in normal tissue. Therefore, these abnormalities appear on the scan as abnormally large concentrations of gallium uptake.

Professional Considerations:

1. Consent form IS required.

Risks:

Allergic reaction to the radiopharmaceutical (itching, hives, rash, tight feeling in the throat, shortness of breath, bronchospasm, anaphylaxis, death), infection.

Contraindications:

Previous allergic reaction to a radiopharmaceutical. This procedure is usually contraindicated during pregnancy and breast-feeding.

2. Preparation:

A. The client is injected with a Gallium-67 citrate radiopharmaceutical intravenously 48–72 hours prior to the scan.

B. *See Client and family teaching.*

3. Procedure:

A. The client is positioned either erect or recumbent under a gamma camera or rectilinear scanner in the nuclear medicine department.

B. Serial images are obtained anteriorly and posteriorly, and occasional lateral views may be required.

C. The client must lie motionless during the scan.

4. Postprocedure care:

A. *See Client and family teaching.*

5. Client and family teaching:

A. Increase intake of fluids, where not contraindicated, beginning 24 hours prior to the scan.

B. The camera will make clicking noises during the scan.

C. It is important to lie motionless during the scan.

D. Drink 6–8 glasses of water and other fluids per day × 2 days after the scan.

6. Factors that affect results:

A. Breast tissue has an increased affinity for gallium uptake during pregnancy, lactation, and menarche. These conditions may produce a false-positive result.

B. Drugs that may cause false-positive results include oral contraceptives.

C. Lesions <1–2 cm in size may not be detectable with a gallium scan.

7. Other data:

A. Gallium is excreted by the kidney and colon in 24–48 hours.

B. Gallium scanning does not differentiate malignant from benign tumors.

C. The scan takes 30–60 minutes to perform.

D. Health care professionals working in a nuclear medicine area must follow federal standards set by the Nuclear Regulatory Commission. These standards include precautions for handling the radioactive material and monitoring of potential radiation exposure.

Bibliography:

Berbari N, Johnson DH, Cunha BA: Respiratory syncytial virus pneumonia in a heart transplant recipient presenting as fever of unknown origin by
gallium scan. Heart Lung 24(3):257–259, 1995.

Elahi N, Bayar N, Caner B, et al.: Imaging of an undifferentiated epidermoid carcinoma with Tc-99m
MIB. Clin Nucl Med 20(5):467–468, 1995.

GALLIUM SCAN OF LIVER, DIAGNOSTIC

Norm: Symmetrical patterns of liver gallium uptake. Requires interpretation by nuclear medicine physician.

Usage: Detection of hepatomas, abscesses, biopsy sites, alcoholic cirrhoses; and evaluation of recurrent lymphomas or tumors following chemotherapy and radiation therapy.

Description: Nuclear medicine scan of the liver using gallium-67 citrate radiopharmaceutical. Normal liver tissue will absorb gallium in a symmetrical fashion. Abscesses appear as a "rim sign," heavily concentrated areas of gallium uptake surrounding a cold center. The cold center is an area where no inflammation exists. Abscesses are rich with lactoferrin in the neutrophils, and gallium appears to bind to the lactoferrin, making the abscess visible. Tumors appear as heavily concentrated areas of gallium with normal symmetrical gallium uptake in the surrounding liver tissue.

Professional Considerations:

1. Consent form IS required.

Risks:

Allergic reaction to radiopharmaceutical (itching, hives, rash, tight feeling in the throat, shortness of breath, bronchospasm, anaphylaxis, death), infection.

Contraindications:

Previous allergic reaction to a radiopharmaceutical. This procedure is usually contraindicated during pregnancy and breast-feeding.

2. Preparation:
   A. The client is injected with a gallium-67 citrate radiopharmaceutical intravenously 48–72 hours prior to the scan.
   B. *See Client and family teaching.*
3. Procedure:
   A. The client is positioned either erect or recumbent under a gamma camera or rectilinear scanner in the nuclear medicine department.
   B. Serial images are obtained anteriorly and posteriorly, and occasionally, lateral views may be required.
   C. The client must lie motionless during the scan.
4. Postprocedure care:
   A. *See Client and family teaching.*
5. Client and family teaching:
   A. Increase oral intake of fluids, where not contraindicated, 24 hours prior to the scan.
   B. A clear-liquid diet may be prescribed for the day before the test.
   C. Cleansing enemas may be prescribed the morning before the test.
   D. The camera will make clicking noises during the scan.
   E. The scan takes 30–60 minutes to perform.
   F. Drink 6–8 glasses of water and other fluids per day × 2 days (where not contraindicated) after the scan.
6. Factors that affect results:
   A. Normal hepatic gallium uptake may obscure the detection of abnormal para-aortic nodes in Hodgkin's disease, resulting in a false-negative scan.
   B. Localization of neutrophils labeled with gallium into fresh operative sites and inflamed peritoneum limit their usefulness in clients who have recently undergone surgery.
7. Other data:
   A. Gallium is excreted by the kidney and colon in 24–48 hours.
   B. Gallium scanning does not differentiate malignant from benign tumors.
   C. Health care professionals working in a nuclear medicine area must follow federal standards set by the Nuclear Regulatory Commission. These standards include precautions for handling the radioactive material and monitoring of potential radiation exposure.

Bibliography:

Lantz MM, Bourque MD, Slavin JD, et al.: Splenic-
perisplenic infected hematoma detected on radi-
ogallium-radiocolloid subtraction study. Clin
Nucl Med 20(7):649–650, 1995.

Noguchi M, Muto M, Yanagidaira H, et al.: A case of an
intra-atrial tumor thrombus from hepatocellular
carcinoma first indicated by 67 Ga-citrate scintigraphy. Ann Nucl Med 9(1):39–42, 1995.

GAMMA GLOBULIN (IgG, QUANTITATIVE IgG), PLASMA

Norm:

		SI Units
Adults	550–1750 mg/dl	5.5–17.5 g/L
Children		
Pediatric cord blood	660–1800 mg/dl	6.6–18 g/L
Newborn	831–1231 mg/dl	8.3–12.3 g/L
1–3 months	311–549 mg/dl	3.1–5.5 g/L
4–6 months	241–613 mg/dl	2.4–6.1 g/L
7–12 months	442–880 mg/dl	4.4–8.8 g/L
13–24 months	553–971 mg/dl	5.5–9.7 g/L
2–3 years	709–1075 mg/dl	7.1–10.8 g/L
3–5 years	701–1257 mg/dl	7.0–12.6 g/L
6–8 years	667–1179 mg/dl	6.7–11.8 g/L
9–11 years	889–1359 mg/dl	8.9–13.6 g/L
12–16 years	822–1170 mg/dl	8.2–11.7 g/L

Increased: AIDS, chronic granulomatous infections, cystic fibrosis of the pancreas, hepatitis (chronic), hyperimmunization, infection, juvenile rheumatoid arthritis, Laënnec's cirrhosis, multiple myeloma (IgG myeloma), myxoma of left atrium of heart, pulmonary tuberculosis, serum protein monoclonal gammopathy, Sjögren's syndrome, and systemic lupus erythematosus. Drugs include aminophenazone, anticonvulsants, asparaginase, ethotoin, hydralazine hydrochloride, mephenytoin, methadone, oral contraceptives, phenylbutazone, phenytoin, and phenytoin sodium prompt.

Decreased: Agammaglobulinemia, heavy chain disease, IgA myeloma, leukemia (chronic lymphocytic), lymphoid aplasia, macroglobulinemia, nephrotic syndrome, and type I dysgammaglobulinemia. Drugs include cancer chemotherapeutic agents, dextrans, methylprednisolone, methylprednisolone acetate, methylprednisolone sodium succinate, and phenytoin.

Description: Protein IgG is the major immunoglobulin of blood that possesses antibody activity against viruses, some bacteria, and toxins. It is the only immunoglobulin that crosses the placenta. Used to evaluate humoral immunity, monitor therapy in IgA G myeloma, and evaluate clients, especially those with a propensity to infections.

Professional Considerations:

1. Consent form NOT required.
2. Preparation:
   A. *See Client and family teaching.*
   B. Tube: Red-top, red/gray-top, or gold-top.
3. Procedure:
   A. Draw a 5-ml blood sample.
4. Postprocedure care:
   A. Note vaccinations, immunizations, or toxoid administration within the previous 6 months on the laboratory requisition.
   B. Note administration of blood products within the prior 6 weeks on the laboratory requisition.
   C. Send the specimen to the laboratory immediately.
5. Client and family teaching:
   A. Do not eat or drink, except for water, for 12 hours before sampling.
   B. Results are normally available within 24 hours.
6. Factors that affect results:
   A. Vaccination, immunization, and toxoid administration within 6 months prior to the test may affect results.
   B. Receipt of blood products within 6 weeks prior to the test may affect results.
   C. Drug or radiation treatment for cancer may cause decreased results.
7. Other data:
   A. Electrophoresis is a more precise measurement for gamma globulins.

Bibliography:

Czaja AJ, Carpenter HA, Santrach PJ, Moore SB: Significance of human leukocyte antigens DR3 and DR4 in chronic viral hepatitis. Dig Dis Sci 40(10):2098–2106, 1995.

Nash MC, Shah V, Reader JA, Dillion MJ: Anit-neutrophil cytoplasmic anti-bodies and anti-endothelial cell antibodies are not increased in Kawasaki disease. Br J Rheumatol 34(9):882–887, 1995.

GAMMA-GLUTAMYL TRANSFERASE, BLOOD

(see Gamma-Glutamyl Transpeptidase, Blood)

GAMMA-GLUTAMYL TRANSPEPTIDASE (GGTP, GAMMA-GLUTAMYLTRANSFERASE), BLOOD

Norm:

Adult females	4–25 U
	9–31 mU/ml
	3.5–13 IU/L
	3–33 U/L at 37°C
Adult males	7–40 U
	12–38 mU/ml
	4–23 IU/L
	9–69 U/L at 37°C
Children	
Cord blood	190–270 U/L at 37°C
Premature infants	<140 U/L at 37°C
1–3 days	56–233 U/L at 37°C
4–21 days	0–130 U/L at 37°C
3–12 weeks	4–120 U/L at 37°C
3–6 months, female	5–35 U/L at 37°C
3–6 months, male	5–65 U/L at 37°C
>6 months, female	15–85 IU/L
>6 months, male	5–55 IU/L
1–15 years	0–23 U/L at 37°C

Usage: Evaluation of progression of liver disease and hepatic metastasis, screening for alcoholism, and as legal evidence in rape.

Increased: Acetaminophen toxicity, alcoholism, alpha1-antitrypsin deficiency, biliary atresia, cholecystitis (due to biliary obstruction), cholestasis (intrahepatic), cirrhosis (biliary, Laënnec's), congestive heart failure, fatty liver, hepatic carcinoma (metastatic), hepatitis (acute, chronic), jaundice (obstructive), lipoid nephrosis, liver disease, myocardial infarction, obesity (extreme), pancreatic carcinoma, pancreatitis (acute), primary biliary cirrhosis, renal carcinoma, and systemic lupus erythematosus. Drugs include glutethimide, methaqualone, phenobarbital, phenytoin, and phenytoin sodium.

Decreased: Not clinically significant.

Description: GGTP is a biliary excretory enzyme that assists in the transfer of amino acids and peptides across cellular membranes. It is found in the liver, kidneys, pancreas, brain, heart, salivary glands, and prostate gland. Progression of carcinoma is associated with increasing levels, and regression of carcinoma is associated with decreasing GGTP levels.

Professional Considerations:

1. Consent form NOT required.
2. Preparation:
   A. *See Client and family teaching.*
   B. Tube: Red-top, red/gray-top, or green-top.
3. Procedure:
   A. Draw a 1-ml blood sample.
4. Postprocedure care:
   A. The specimen may be frozen.
5. Client and family teaching:
   A. Fast, except for drinking water, for 8 hours and refrain from drinking alcohol for 24 hours before the test.
6. Factors that affect results:
   A. Reject hemolyzed specimens.
   B. Elevation may occur with phenytoin or phenobarbital therapy; one of the alternate tests, leucine aminopeptidase (LAP), or 5' nucleotides, is preferable in such clients.
7. Other data:
   A. The stability of specimens is as follows: room temperature, 5 days; refrigerated, 7 days; frozen (–20°C), 90 days.
   B. GGTP is more accurate than alkaline

phosphatase for hepatic disease because it is unaffected by abnormalities of skeletal muscles.

Bibliography:

Blumber D, Hochwald S, Pinto J, Burt M: Altered glutathione metabolism in the tumor-bearing state. Ann Surg Oncol 2(4):332–335, 1995.

Mican JM, DiBisceglie AM, et al.: Hepatic involvement in mastocytosis: clinicopathologic correlation in 41 cases. Hepatology 22(4, Pt 1):1163–1170, 1995.

GAS VENTILATION LUNG SCAN, DIAGNOSTIC

Norm: Radioactive gas is distributed equally in both lungs with normal "wash-in" and "wash-out" phases.

Usage: Used in conjunction with a lung perfusion scan to diagnose, identify, and evaluate regions of lung tissue that are not ventilated during respirations. Some conditions in which this may occur include pulmonary embolism, chronic obstructive pulmonary disease, and parenchymal disease (bronchogenic carcinoma).

Description: A nuclear medicine scan in which the client inhales air mixed with radiolabeled gas (xenon-133) via a mask. A gamma camera images the gas distribution of the posterior lung fields through three phases: phase 1 is the "wash-in" phase in which the buildup of radioactive gas occurs. In phase 2, equilibrium occurs. Phase 3 is the "wash-out" phase, in which the gas is removed from the lungs. Decreased areas of ventilation will appear lighter with longer than normal wash-out phases.

Professional Considerations:

1. Consent form NOT required.

Risks:
Dizziness, fetal damage.

Contraindications:
In clients who are unable to follow directions.

2. Preparation:
   A. Obtain baseline vital signs and continue to monitor vital signs every 10–15 minutes.
   B. Remove jewelry and metal objects.
3. Procedure:
   A. The client is positioned erect or supine throughout the scan.
   B. The client inhales a mixture of air and radioactive xenon-133 gas through a mask and holds his or her breath for 20 seconds. For mechanically ventilated clients, krypton-85 gas should be substituted for xenon-133.
   C. The client's chest is scanned with a gamma camera as he or she exhales.
4. Postprocedure care:
   A. None.
5. Client and family teaching:
   A. The test is painless and takes about 15–30 minutes.
   B. Results are normally available following interpretation by a radiologist.
6. Factors that affect results:
   A. An improperly fitting or loose seal on the ventilation mask interferes with the proper mixing of air and gas and allows radioactive gas to contaminate the surrounding air.
7. Other data:
   A. None.

Bibliography:

Huygen PE, Gultuna I, Ince C, et al.: A new ventilation inhomogeneity index from multiple breath indicator gas wash out tests in mechanically ventilated patients. Crit Care Med 21(8):1149–1158, 1995.

McConnell TR, Laubach CA, Clark BA: Value of gas exchange analysis in heart disease. J Cardiopulm Rehabil 15(4):257–261, 1995.

GASTRIC ACID ANALYSIS TEST (PEPTAVLON STIMULATION TEST), DIAGNOSTIC

Norm: Within normal limits.

	SI Units

Basal (Prestimulation) Acid Output (BAO)
is the gastric acid secreted without stimulation:

Adult female		
Normal	1–4 mEq/h	1–4 mmol/h
Duodenal ulcer	3–8 mEq/h	3–8 mmol/h
Gastric carcinoma	0–3 mEq/h	0–3 mmol/h
Gastric ulcer	1–3 mEq/h	1–3 mmol/h

		SI Units
Adult female *(continued)*		
Atrophic gastritis	0 mEq/h	0 mmol/h
Pernicious anemia	0 mEq/h	0 mmol/h
Zollinger-Ellison syndrome	>20 mEq/h	>20 mmol/h
Adult male		
Normal	2–5 mEq/h	2–5 mmol/h
Duodenal ulcer	5–10 mEq/h	5–10 mmol/h
Gastric carcinoma	0–3 mEq/h	0–3 mmol/h
Gastric ulcer	1–5 mEq/h	1–5 mmol/h
Atrophic gastritis	0 mEq/h	0 mmol/h
Pernicious anemia	0 mEq/h	0 mmol/h
Zollinger-Ellison syndrome	>20 mEq/h	>20 mmol/h

Maximum (Stimulated) Acid Output (MAO)
is the gastric acid output following stimulation
(sum of four 15-minute specimens):

Adult female		
Normal	7–15 mEq/h	7–15 mmol/h
Duodenal ulcer	10–20 mEq/h	10–20 mmol/h
Gastric carcinoma	0–5 mEq/h	0–5 mmol/h
Gastric ulcer	5–15 mEq/h	5–15 mmol/h
Atrophic gastritis	0 mEq/h	0 mmol/h
Pernicious anemia	0 mEq/h	0 mmol/h
Zollinger-Ellison syndrome	35–60 mEq/h	35–60 mmol/h
Adult male		
Normal	5–26 mEq/h	5–26 mmol/h
Duodenal ulcer	15–35 mEq/h	15–35 mmol/h
Gastric carcinoma	0–20 mEq/h	0–20 mmol/h
Gastric ulcer	10–20 mEq/h	10–20 mmol/h
Atrophic gastritis	0 mEq/h	0 mmol/h
Pernicious anemia	0 mEq/h	0 mmol/h
Zollinger-Ellison syndrome	35–60 mEq/h	35–60 mmol/h

BAO:MAO Ratio		
Normal	1:2.5–1:5.0	0.3–0.6
Gastric ulcer/gastric carcinoma		20%
Gastric ulcer/duodenal ulcer		20–40%
Duodenal ulcer/Zollinger-Ellison syndrome		40–60%
Zollinger-Ellison syndrome		>60%

Peak Acid Output (PAO) is 2 × (total values of the
two highest 15-minute MAO samples).

Basal to PAO Ratio	
Adult female	0.23
Adult male	0.29

Usage: Diagnosing and evaluating atrophic gastritis, duodenal ulcer, gastric carcinoma, gastric ulcer, menetrier's disease, pernicious anemia, postoperative stomal ulcer, and Zollinger-Ellison syndrome.

Increased: Duodenal ulcer, gastric ulcers in some cases, peptic ulcer disease, pyloric ulcer, and Zollinger-Ellison syndrome. Drugs include adrenergic blockers, alseroxylon, caffeine, calcium salts, cholinergics, corticosteroids, deserpidine, ethanol, rescinnamine, and reserpine.

Decreased: Achlorhydria, anemia (pernicious), gastric atrophy, gastric neoplasm, gastric ulcer, and gastritis. Drugs include antacids, anticholinergics, beta-blocking agents, cimetidine, famotidine, nizatidine, ranitidine hydrochloride, and tricyclic antidepressants.

Description: Gastric acid consists of hydrochloric acid (HCl), electrolytes, and mucus, and is colorless and very acidic, with a pH of <2.5. It is normally secreted by the parietal cells of the stomach in response to the presence of gastrin during the gastric phase of digestion. In the presence of tumors, ulcerative disease, or pernicious anemia, the rate of gastric acid secretion can be accelerated or diminished. The Peptavlon (pentagastrin) stimulation test involves a 1-hour aspiration of stomach secretions. A basal and four 15-minute collections are made after subcutaneous injection of Peptavlon. Peptavlon normally stimulates gastric acid secretion within 10 minutes, with peaks occurring at approximately 30 minutes. By measuring the rate and volume of gastric acid secretion in response to Peptavlon, gastric function can be evaluated. Pernicious anemia and atrophic gastritis result in hyposecretion of gastric acid. Hypersecretion and the rate of secretion can indicate location and type of ulcerative disease, Zollinger-Ellison syndrome, and the need for surgical intervention.

Professional Considerations:

1. Consent form NOT required.
2. Preparation:
   A. *See Client and family teaching.*
   B. Obtain a Levin tube, lubricant, 8 clean plastic containers without preservative, a Toomey syringe, suction equipment, a marker or grease pencil, and Peptavlon (pentagastrin).
   C. Prepare the suction apparatus and tubing.
3. Procedure:
   A. Position the client sitting or lying on the left side.
   B. Insert a Levin tube with a radiopaque tip through the client's nose or mouth into the stomach. Position the Levin tube tip in the lumen below the stomach fundus and confirm the placement via radiography or fluoroscopy.
   C. Reposition the client to a sitting position and wait at least 10 minutes before proceeding further.
   D. Apply low continuous suction to the Levin tube. At 15 and 30 minutes, withdraw two specimens with a Toomey syringe and discard the aspirate.
   E. Begin continuous aspiration of gastric contents, using the syringe, for a total of 60 minutes. Collect the aspirate into the collection containers (labeled 1, 2, 3, 4), using a new collection container every 15 minutes until the basal acid output collection is complete.
   F. Administer Peptavlon 6 mg/kg body weight subcutaneously and begin poststimulation collections, as in step 3E, immediately. The poststimulation collection should continue for 1 hour. Observe for hypersensitivity reaction.
4. Postprocedure care:
   A. Send all 8 containers identified as basal or poststimulation to the laboratory for analysis.
   B. Remove the Levin tube.
   C. Refrigerate the specimens if testing will be delayed more than 4 hours.
   D. Resume previous diet.
   E. Observe for nausea and vomiting.
5. Client and family teaching:
   A. Fast from food after the evening meal the day before testing and from water for 1 hour prior to the test.
   B. Do not smoke or chew gum, and avoid stressful situations for 4 hours before the test.
   C. The test involves the insertion of a tube through the nose into the stomach and periodic removal of the stomach contents with a syringe through the tube. The test may cause symptoms of indigestion because a drug that stimulates gastric acid secretion is given. Mild, temporary discomfort may be experienced during the tube insertion.
   D. The test takes more than 3 hours. Bring reading material or other diversional activity.
6. Factors that affect results:
   A. Histamine antagonists or anticholinergics and antacids should be discontinued 72 and 12 hours before the test. If, however, the objective is to test the effectiveness of a histamine antagonist on acid secretions, the drugs should be continued and the basal output of gastric acid should be performed 1 hour after administration of a morning dose.
   B. Stimuli that may increase gastric acid production include smoking, the sight or odor of food, or stimuli that cause the client to become angry, fearful, or depressed.
7. Other data:
   A. Peptavlon use in children is not indicated.

B. The test must be used with caution in conditions of esophageal varices, esophageal diverticula, esophageal stenosis, malignant neoplasm of the esophagus, aortic aneurysm, gastric hemorrhage, and congestive heart failure.

Bibliography:

Feldman M: Suppression of acid secretion in peptic ulcer disease. J Clin Gastroenterol *20*(Suppl 1): S1–S6, 1995.
Meko JB, Norton JA: Management of patients with Zollinger-Ellison syndrome. Ann Rev Med *46* (6DR):395–411, 1995.

GASTRIC ACID SECRETION, GASTRIC ACID STIMULATION, DIAGNOSTIC

Norm: Within normal limits.

		SI Units

Basal (Prestimulation) Acid Output (BAO)
is the gastric acid secreted without stimulation:

Adult female		
Normal	1–4 mEq/h	1–4 mmol/h
Duodenal ulcer	3–8 mEq/h	3–8 mmol/h
Gastric carcinoma	0–3 mEq/h	0–3 mmol/h
Gastric ulcer	1–3 mEq/h	1–3 mmol/h
Atrophic gastritis	0 mEq/h	0 mmol/h
Pernicious anemia	0 mEq/h	0 mmol/h
Zollinger-Ellison syndrome	>20 mEq/h	>20 mmol/h
Adult male		
Normal	2–5 mEq/h	2–5 mmol/h
Duodenal ulcer	5–10 mEq/h	5–10 mmol/h
Gastric carcinoma	0–3 mEq/h	0–3 mmol/h
Gastric ulcer	1–5 mEq/h	1–5 mmol/h
Atrophic gastritis	0 mEq/h	0 mmol/h
Pernicious anemia	0 mEq/h	0 mmol/h
Zollinger-Ellison syndrome	>20 mEq/h	>20 mmol/h

Maximum (Stimulated) Acid Output (MAO)
is the gastric acid output following stimulation
(sum of four to eight 15-minute specimens):

Adult female		
Normal	7–15 mEq/h	7–15 mmol/h
Duodenal ulcer	10–20 mEq/h	10–20 mmol/h
Gastric carcinoma	0–5 mEq/h	0–5 mmol/h
Gastric ulcer	5–15 mEq/h	5–15 mmol/h
Atrophic gastritis	0 mEq/h	0 mmol/h
Pernicious anemia	0 mEq/h	0 mmol/h
Zollinger-Ellison syndrome	35–60 mEq/h	35–60 mmol/h
Adult male		
Normal	5–26 mEq/h	5–26 mmol/h
Duodenal ulcer	15–35 mEq/h	15–35 mmol/h
Gastric carcinoma	0–20 mEq/h	0–20 mmol/h
Gastric ulcer	10–20 mEq/h	10–20 mmol/h
Atrophic gastritis	0 mEq/h	0 mmol/h
Pernicious anemia	0 mEq/h	0 mmol/h
Zollinger-Ellison syndrome	35–60 mEq/h	35–60 mmol/h

		SI Units
BAO:MAO Ratio		
Normal	1:2.5–1:5	0.3–0.6
Gastric ulcer/gastric carcinoma		20%
Gastric ulcer/duodenal ulcer		20–40%
Duodenal ulcer/Zollinger-Ellison syndrome		40–60%
Zollinger-Ellison syndrome		>60%

Peak Acid Output (PAO) is 2 × (total values of the two highest 15-minute MAO samples).

Basal to PAO Ratio	
Adult female	0.23
Adult male	0.29

Usage: Diagnosis and evaluation of duodenal ulcer, gastric carcinoma, gastric ulcer, pernicious anemia, postoperative stomal ulcer, and Zollinger-Ellison syndrome.

Increased: Duodenal ulcer, gastric ulcers in some cases, peptic ulcer disease, pyloric ulcer, and Zollinger-Ellison syndrome. Drugs include adrenergic blockers, alseroxylon, caffeine, calcium salts, cholinergics, corticosteroids, deserpidine, ethanol, rescinnamine, and reserpine.

Decreased: Achlorhydria, anemia (pernicious), gastric atrophy, gastric neoplasm, gastric ulcer, and gastritis. Drugs include antacids, anticholinergics, beta-blocking agents, cimetidine, famotidine, nizatidine, ranitidine hydrochloride, and tricyclic antidepressants.

Description: Gastric acid is secreted by the parietal cells of the stomach in response to neurologic and hormonal stimulation. Gastric acid is secreted during the gastric phase of digestion and aids in the breakdown of proteins and in the absorption of vitamin B_{12}, folic acid, and iron. It consists of hydrochloric acid (HCl), electrolytes, enzymes, and mucus. It is colorless and very acidic, with a pH of <2.5. In the presence of tumors, ulcerative disease, or pernicious anemia, the rate of gastric acid secretion by the parietal cells can be altered. A diagnostic gastric acid stimulation test involves aspirating and collecting basal and maximal acid outputs. Histalog (betazole, a histamine analog) or histamine diphosphate is injected intramuscularly to stimulate

gastric acid secretion. By measuring the rate and volume of gastric acid, gastric function can be evaluated.

Professional Considerations:
1. Consent form NOT required.

Risks:
Allergic reaction to injection (itching, hives, rash, tight feeling in the throat, shortness of breath, bronchospasm, anaphylaxis, death).

Contraindications:
Positive skin test. Use of histamine diphosphate is contraindicated for clients who have a history of asthma, paroxysmal hypertension, urticaria, or other allergic conditions. Histalog (betazole hydrochloride) has a lower incidence of side effects.

2. Preparation:
   A. Perform a skin test to determine hypersensitivity by injecting 0.1 ml of Histalog or histamine diphosphate subcutaneously. Wait 30 minutes for a reaction to occur. If the wheal exceeds 10 mm in diameter, do not perform the stimulation portion of this test.
   B. Obtain a Levin tube, lubricant, 8–12 clean plastic containers without preservative, a Toomey syringe, suction equipment, a marker or grease pencil, and histamine diphosphate or Histalog.
   C. Prepare suction apparatus and tubing.
   D. *See Client and family teaching.*
3. Procedure:
   A. Position the client sitting or lying on the left side.
   B. Insert a Levin tube with a radiopaque tip through the client's nose or mouth

into the stomach. Position the tube tip in the lumen below the stomach fundus and confirm the placement via radiography or fluoroscopy.

C. Reposition the client to a sitting position and wait at least 10 minutes before proceeding further.

D. Apply low continuous suction to the Levin tube. At 15 and 30 minutes, withdraw two specimens with a Toomey syringe and discard the aspirate.

E. Begin continuous aspiration of the gastric contents, using the syringe, for a total of 60 minutes. Collect the aspirate into the collection containers (labeled 1, 2, 3, 4), using a new collection container every 15 minutes until basal acid output collection is complete.

F. Administer Histalog (betazole hydrochloride) 0.5 mg/kg body weight, or histamine diphosphate 0.1 mg/kg body weight, intramuscularly, and begin poststimulation collections, as in step 3E, immediately. Observe for hypersensitivity reaction.

G. Poststimulation collection should continue for 1 hour (4 specimens) if histamine diphosphate was used, or for 2 hours (8 specimens) if Histalog was used.

4. Postprocedure care:
   A. Send all 8–12 containers, identified as basal or poststimulation, to the laboratory.
   B. Remove the Levin tube.
   C. Resume previous diet.
   D. Observe for nausea and vomiting.

5. Client and family teaching:
   A. Fast from food for 12 hours and from water for 1 hour prior to the procedure.
   B. Do not smoke or chew gum, and avoid stressful situations for 4 hours before the test.
   C. The test involves the insertion of a tube through the nose into the stomach and periodic removal of the stomach contents with a syringe through the tube. The test may cause symptoms of indigestion because a drug that stimulates gastric acid secretion is given. Mild, temporary discomfort may be experienced during tube insertion.
   D. The test takes more than 2 hours.
   E. Results are normally available within 24 hours.

6. Factors that affect results:
   A. Histamine antagonists or anticholinergics and antacids should be discontinued 72 and 12 hours before the test. If, however, the objective is to test the effectiveness of a histamine antagonist on acid secretions, the drugs should be continued and the basal output of gastric acid should be performed 1 hour after administration of a morning dose.
   B. Stimuli that may increase gastric acid production include smoking, the sight or odor of food, or stimuli that cause

the client to become angry, fearful, or depressed.

C. Peak acid output after Histalog may not occur until the second hour after administration.

7. Other data:
   A. None.

Bibliography:

Bergann C, Sarem-Aslani A, Ratge D, et al.: Inadequate response to H2-receptor antagonist. Absence of parietal cell camp-stimulating autoantibodies. Dig Dis Sci 40(12):2678–2683, 1995.

Tunio AM, Hobsley M: Epidermal growth factor in saliva and gastric juice response to histamine. Gut 37(3):335–339, 1995.

GASTRIC ANALYSIS, SPECIMEN

Norm:

Bile	Absent or minimal
Mucus	Appears evenly mixed
Blood	Absent or scant
Fasting acidity	2.5 mEq/L
Quantity produced	62 ml/hour
pH	1.0–2.5

Usage: Anemia (pernicious), stomach pain and burning, ulcers, and Zollinger-Ellison syndrome. Can also determine the presence of *Helicobacter pylori*.

Description: This test analyzes the contents of the stomach for acidity, appearance, and volume.

Professional Considerations:

1. Consent form NOT required.

Risks:

Complications of nasogastric tube insertion include bleeding, dysrhythmias, esophageal perforation, laryngospasm, and decreased mean PO_2.

Contraindications:

Esophageal varices.

2. Preparation:
   A. The client should fast for 12 hours.
   B. The client should not smoke tobacco or chew gum for 6 hours.
   C. Obtain a nasogastric tube, a lubricant, a Toomey syringe, and a clean container.

3. Procedure:
   A. Pass a nasogastric tube into the stomach.
   B. Aspirate all gastric contents into a clean container.

C. Remove the nasogastric tube.
4. Postprocedure care:
   A. Refrigerate the sample if not tested within 4 hours.
5. Client and family teaching:
   A. Fast for 12 hours, and do not chew gum or smoke cigarettes for 6 hours prior to the test.
   B. The test involves the insertion of a tube through the nose into the stomach and removal, with a syringe, of the gastric contents through the tube. The insertion may be uncomfortable and may cause a pressurelike feeling or may cause you to gag and cough. You will be asked to take sips of water and swallow to make the tube insertion easier. Removal of the stomach contents causes no pain.
   C. Further tests may be indicated, based on the results of this analysis.
6. Factors that affect results:
   A. Stimuli that may increase gastric acid production include chewing gum, smoking, the sight or odor of food, or stimuli that cause the client to become angry, fearful, or depressed.
   B. Drugs that may increase gastric acid production include adrenergic block-

ers, caffeine, calcium salts, cholinergics, corticosteroids, ethanol, and reserpine.
   C. Drugs that may decrease gastric acid production include antacids, anticholinergics, beta-blocking agents, cimetidine, famotidine, nizatidine, ranitidine hydrochloride, and tricyclic antidepressants.
   D. Use of Hemoccult slides, as opposed to Gastroccult slides, may lead to a false-negative result if the pH of the gastric secretion is <4.
7. Other data:
   A. Small amounts of bile may be present due to gagging during insertion of the nasogastric tube.
   B. Scant amounts of blood may be present due to trauma during insertion of the nasogastric tube.

Bibliography:

Meko JB, Norton JA: Management of patients with Zollinger-Ellison syndrome. Ann Rev Med 46(6DR): 395–411, 1995.

Namavar F, Roosendaal R, Kuipers EJ, et al.: Presence of *Helicobacter pylori* in the oral cavity, oesophagus, stomach and faeces patients with gastritis. Eur J Clin Microbiol Infect Dis 14(3):234–237.

GASTRIC ANALYSIS, BASAL NOCTURNAL ACID OUTPUT, DIAGNOSTIC

Norm:

		SI Units
Basal Acid Output (BAO)		
Adult female		
Normal	1–4 mEq/h	1–4 mmol/h
Duodenal ulcer	3–8 mEq/h	3–8 mmol/h
Gastric carcinoma	0–3 mEq/h	0–3 mmol/h
Gastric ulcer	1–3 mEq/h	1–3 mmol/h
Atrophic gastritis	0 mEq/h	0 mmol/h
Pernicious anemia	0 mEq/h	0 mmol/h
Zollinger-Ellison syndrome	>20 mEq/h	>20 mmol/h
Adult male		
Normal	2–5 mEq/h	2–5 mmol/h
Duodenal ulcer	5–10 mEq/h	5–10 mmol/h
Gastric carcinoma	0–3 mEq/h	0–3 mmol/h
Gastric ulcer	1–5 mEq/h	1–5 mmol/h
Atrophic gastritis	0 mEq/h	0 mmol/h
Pernicious anemia	0 mEq/h	0 mmol/h
Zollinger-Ellison syndrome	>20 mEq/h	>20 mmol/h

Usage: Aids diagnosis of pernicious anemia, duodenal or stomal ulcer, Menetrier disease, and Zollinger-Ellison syndrome.

Increased: Duodenal ulcer, gastric ulcers in some cases, peptic ulcer disease, pyloric ulcer, and Zollinger-Ellison syndrome. Drugs include adrenergic blockers, alseroxylon, caffeine, calcium salts, cholinergics, corticosteroids, deserpidine, ethanol, rauwolfia, rescinnamine, and reserpine.

Decreased: Achlorhydria, anemia (pernicious), gastric atrophy, gastric neoplasm, gastric ulcer, and gastritis. Drugs include antacids, anticholinergics, beta-blocking agents, cimetidine, famotidine, nizatidine, ranitidine hydrochloride, and tricyclic antidepressants.

Description: Basal nocturnal acid output is the rate of secretion of acid by the stomach when the client is calm and resting, after a 12-hour fast, and at least 24 hours after the last dose of medications that increase or decrease gastric acid. It is measured in millimoles of titratable acidity per hour.

Professional Considerations:

1.   Consent form NOT required.

Risks:

Complications of nasogastric tube insertion include bleeding, dysrhythmias, esophageal perforation, laryngospasm, and decreased mean PO_2.

Contraindications:
Esophageal varices.

2.   Preparation:
     A.   *See Client and family teaching.*
     B.   Obtain a Levin tube, a lubricant, four clean plastic containers without preservative, a Toomey syringe, suction equipment, and a marker or grease pencil.
     C.   Prepare the suction apparatus and tubing.
3.   Procedure:
     A.   Position the client sitting or lying on the left side.
     B.   Insert a Levin tube with a radiopaque tip through the client's nose or mouth into the stomach. Position the tube tip in the lumen below the stomach fundus and confirm the placement via radiography or fluoroscopy.
     C.   Reposition to a sitting position. Wait at least 10 minutes before proceeding further.
     D.   Apply low, continuous suction to the Levin tube. At 15 and 30 minutes, withdraw two specimens with a Toomey syringe and discard the aspirate.
     E.   Begin continuous aspiration of gastric contents using the syringe, for a total of 60 minutes. Collect the aspirate into the collection containers (labeled 1, 2, 3, 4), using a new collection container every 15 minutes until basal acid output collection is complete.

4.   Postprocedure care:
     A.   Send all four sequentially labeled containers to the laboratory.
     B.   The specimens should be refrigerated if not tested within 4 hours.
     C.   Remove the nasogastric tube.
     D.   Resume previous diet.
5.   Client and family teaching:
     A.   Fast for 12 hours, and do not chew gum or smoke cigarettes during the 6 hours prior to the test.
     B.   The test takes about 2 hours. Bring reading material or other diversions.
     C.   The test involves the insertion of a tube through the nose into the stomach and removal, with a syringe, of the gastric contents through the tube. The insertion may be uncomfortable and may cause a pressurelike feeling or cause you to gag and cough. You will be asked to take sips of water and swallow to make the tube insertion easier. Removal of the stomach contents causes no pain.
6.   Factors that affect results:
     A.   Reject specimens if contaminated with bile.
     B.   Stimuli that may increase gastric acid production include smoking, the sight or odor of food, or stimuli that cause anger, fear, or depression.
     C.   The amount of gastric acid increases as body weight increases.
7.   Other data:
     A.   This test is sometimes followed by stimulation of gastric acid production with pentagastrin or histamine. *See also Gastric Acid Analysis Test, Diagnostic; and Gastric Acid Stimulation Test, Diagnostic.*

Bibliography:

Graziani G, Como G, et al.: Effect of gastric acid secretions on intestinal phosphate and calcium absorption in normal subjects. Nephrol Dial Transplant *19*(3):1376–1380, 1995.

Jensen RT: Zollinger-Ellison syndrome: past present and future. Yale J Biol Med *67*(3–4):195–214, 1994.

GASTRIC ASPIRATE, ROUTINE, CULTURE

Norm: Negative. No growth.

Usage: Aids in the diagnosis pulmonary as well as gastrointestinal infections.

Positive: Growth of microorganisms may be secondary to carcinoma or to puncture of the stomach with concomitant peritonitis or intra-abdominal abscess.

Description: This test is performed

by withdrawing a small sample of gastric aspirate through a nasogastric tube and culturing the sample for the growth of microorganisms.

Professional Considerations:

1. Consent form NOT required.

Risks:

Complications of nasogastric tube insertion include bleeding, dysrhythmias, esophageal perforation, laryngospasm and decreased mean PO_2.

Contraindications:

Esophageal varices.

2. Preparation:
   A. Obtain a nasogastric tube, a lubricant, a sterile syringe, and a sterile specimen tube.
3. Procedure:
   A. Pass a nasogastric tube into the stomach.
   B. Using a sterile syringe, aspirate a minimum of 2 ml of gastric contents into the sterile tube.
   C. Remove the nasogastric tube.
4. Postprocedure care:
   A. Write the collection time on the laboratory requisition.
   B. Send the sample to the laboratory within 30 minutes.
5. Client and family teaching:
   A. The test involves the insertion of a tube through the nose into the stomach and removal, with a syringe, of the gastric contents through the tube. The insertion may be uncomfortable and may cause a pressurelike feeling or cause you to gag and cough. You will be asked to take sips of water and swallow to make the tube insertion easier. Removal of the stomach contents causes no pain.
   B. Do not swallow sputum just prior to or during the procedure. Suction will be provided to help remove sputum from the back of the mouth.
   C. Results are normally available within 48 hours.
6. Factors that affect results:
   A. Reject specimens received more than 30 minutes after collection.
7. Other data:
   A. The esophagus and stomach are the two usually sterile areas of the gastrointestinal tract.
   B. Clients who are unable to expectorate sputum may swallow it, thus contaminating their gastric aspirate.

Bibliography:

Riordan SM, McIver CJ, Dumcombe UB, Bolin TD: Bacteriologic analysis of mucosal biopsy specimens for detecting small intestinal bacterial growth. Scand J Gastroenterol *30*(7):681–685, 1995.

Schaaf HS, Beyer N, Gie RP, et al.: Respiratory tuberculosis in childhood: the diagnostic value of clinical features and special investigations. Pediatr Infect Dis J *14*(3):189–194, 1995.

GASTRIC CYTOLOGY, SPECIMEN

(see Cytologic Study of Gastrointestinal Tract, Diagnostic)

GASTRIC pH, SPECIMEN

Norm: 1.0–2.5.

Increased: Duodenal ulcer, evaluation following vagotomy, marginal ulcer, peptic ulcer disease, and Zollinger-Ellison syndrome.

Decreased: Achlorhydria, hypochlorhydria, and pernicious anemia.

Description: Gastric pH expresses hydrogen ion concentration of the gastric contents. It is a reflection of the amount of hydrochloric acid (HCl) produced by the parietal cells of the stomach in response to gastrin stimulation.

Professional Considerations:

1. Consent form NOT required.

Risks:

Complications of nasogastric tube insertion include bleeding, dysrhythmias, esophageal perforation, laryngospasm, and decreased mean PO_2.

Contraindications:

Esophageal varices.

2. Preparation:
   A. Obtain a nasogastric tube, a lubricant, a syringe, a clean container, and a pH Test-Tape.
   B. *See Client and family teaching.*
3. Procedure:
   A. Pass a nasogastric tube into the stomach.
   B. Aspirate a minimum of 2 ml of gastric contents into the clean container.
   C. Dip the pH Test-Tape into the specimen and compare the color change with that on the Test-Tape container.
   D. Remove the nasogastric tube.

4. Postprocedure care:
   A. None.
5. Client and family teaching:
   A. Do not eat for 8 hours prior to the test. Do not smoke cigarettes or chew gum for 4 hours prior to the test. Avoid stressful situations during the 4 hours immediately prior to the test.
   B. The test involves the insertion of a tube through the nose into the stomach and removal, with a syringe, of the gastric contents through the tube. The insertion may be uncomfortable and may cause a pressurelike feeling or cause you to gag and cough. You will be asked to take sips of water and swallow to make the tube insertion easier.

6. Factors that affect results:
   A. Stimuli that may increase gastric acid production include smoking, the sight or odor of food, or stimuli that cause anger, fear, or depression.
7. Other data:
   A. Gastric carcinoma is associated with decreased acidity.

Bibliography:

Feldman M: Suppression of acid secretion in peptic ulcer disease. J Clin Gastroenterol 20(Suppl 1): S1–S6, 1995.

Neumann MJ, Meyer CT, Dutton JC, Smith R: Hold that x-ray: aspirate pH and auscultation prove enteral tube placement. J Clin Gastroenterol 20(4): 293–295, 1995.

Niv Y, Abu-Aivd S, Neumann G: Further applications of blood gas analysis to gastric acidity determination Clin Chim Acta 215(1):9–19, 1993.

GASTRIN, SERUM

Norm:

		SI Units
Fasting		
≤Age 60	<100 pg/ml	<47.7 pmol/L
	or <200 pg/ml	<95.4 pmol/L
>Age 60		
Upper 15% of population	100–800 pg/ml	47.7–381.6 pmol/L
Postprandial	95–250 pg/ml	45.3–119.2 pmol/L
Zollinger-Ellison syndrome	≤60,000 pg/ml	≤28,620 pmol/L
	Often 100–500 pg/ml	Often 47.7–238.3 pmol/L

Increased: Achlorhydria, anemia (pernicious), atrophic gastritis, carcinoma (of the body of the stomach), duodenal ulcer, elderly clients, gastric ulcer, G-cell hyperplasia (antrum of the stomach), hypercalcemia (chronic), hyperparathyroidism, hypochlorhydria, peptic ulcer disease (with Zollinger-Ellison syndrome), postvagotomy, pyloric obstruction with gastric distension, renal disease (chronic, end-stage), short-bowel syndrome, uremia, and Zollinger-Ellison syndrome. Drugs include acetylcholine chloride, calcium carbonate, calcium chloride, cholinergics, and insulin.

Decreased: Drugs include anticholinergics and tricyclic antidepressants.

Description: Gastrin is a hormone secreted by the G-cells of the antrum of the stomach and by the pancreatic islets of Langerhans. Its secretion is stimulated by alkalinity; by distension of the stomach antrum; by vagal stimulation (such as chewing, tasting, or smelling); and by the presence of peptides, amino acids, alcohol, or calcium in the stomach. Its secretion is inhibited by gastric acidity via a negative feedback system. Gastrin is absorbed into the blood and returned to the stomach, where it stimulates the secretion of gastric acid under the mediation of histamine. Other effects of gastrin include increased gastrointestinal motility, and stimulation of insulin, pepsin, and intrinsic factor secretion. Catabolism of gastrin occurs in the kidneys. Serum gastrin measurement is accomplished via radioimmunoassay.

Professional Considerations:

1. Consent form NOT required.
2. Preparation:
   A. *See Client and family teaching.*
   B. Tube: Red-top, red/gray-top, or gold-top.
3. Procedure:
   A. Draw a 2-ml blood sample.
4. Postprocedure care:
   A. Write the collection time on the laboratory requisition.
5. Client and family teaching:
   A. Fast from food for 12 hours and from alcohol for 24 hours prior to the test.

B. Do not chew gum or smoke cigarettes for 4 hours prior to the test.

C. Results are normally available within 24 hours.

6. Factors that affect results:

A. Reject hemolyzed specimens, specimens drawn in anticoagulated tubes, or specimens not received in the laboratory within 30 minutes after collection.

B. Reject grossly lipemic samples, which may yield falsely elevated serum gastrin values as determined by radioimmunoassay.

C. Food, especially high-protein food, causes an increase in gastrin secretion.

D. Hypoglycemia caused by insulin increases gastrin secretion.

E. Drugs that may indirectly cause increased gastrin secretion in response to drug suppression of gastric acidity include antacids, beta-blocking agents, cimetidine, famotidine, nizatidine, and ranitidine hydrochloride.

F. Drugs that may indirectly cause depressed gastrin secretion in response to drug-stimulated increased gastric acidity include adrenergic blockers, alseroxylon, caffeine, calcium salts, corticosteroids, deserpidine, ethanol, rauwolfia, rescinnamine, and reserpine.

7. Other data:

A. 15–26% of clients with Zollinger-Ellison syndrome have Wermer's syndrome: hyperparathyroidism, islet cell tumors, pituitary tumors, Cushing's syndrome, and hyperthyroidism.

Bibliography:

Moreira V, Martin-de-Argila C, Erdozain JC: Serum gastrin and secretin test in Zollinger-Ellison syndrome [letter]. Lancet *347*(8996):270.

Notat-Francesco V, Samual S, Kanakamedala S, Straus EW: Accuracy and precision of serum gastrin measurement in commercial laboratories. J Assoc Acad Minor Phys *6*(4):130–133, 1995.

GASTROINTESTINAL CANCER ANTIGEN
(see CA 19–9, Blood)

GASTROSCOPY OR GASTRO-DUODENAL-JEJUNOSCOPY (GJD), DIAGNOSTIC

Norm: Cardiac and pyloric sphincters are intact. Rugal folds of the stomach are continuous. No blood or lesions are detected. Blood vessels are not visible.

Usage: Detection of gastric cancer, gastric ulcer, gastritis, hiatal hernia, and Mallory-Weiss tears; investigation of unexplained weight loss or dysphagia; and to obtain brushings of gastric mucosa to help determine infectious states such as *H. pylori infection*.

Description: Gastroscopy involves the insertion through the esophagus of a lighted flexible fiberoptic endoscope into the stomach and upper portion of the small intestine, with concurrent visual examination of the mucosal lining for active bleeding sites, varices, ulcers or perforations, lesions, or tears. The procedure takes approximately 30 minutes. Gastro-duodenal-jejunoscopy involves advancing the instrument further into the small intestine to evaluate the integrity of the jejunum, as well as any structural or obstructive abnormalities.

Professional Considerations:

1. Consent form IS required.

Risks:

Gastrointestinal perforation and hemorrhage, peritonitis, aspiration, respiratory arrest, death.

Contraindications:

Thrombocytopenia. Sedatives are contraindicated in clients with central nervous system depression.

2. Preparation:

A. *See Client and family teaching.*

B. Dentures should be removed.

C. A sedative may be prescribed.

D. Obtain baseline vital signs.

E. Obtain a blood pressure cuff, Xylocaine spray, a suction machine and tubing, an endoscope, pulse oximetry, and a gastroscopy cart. A cardiac monitor may be required with some clients.

3. Procedure:

A. A blood pressure cuff is left in place on the client's arm, and vital signs along with pulse oximetry are monitored on an individual basis throughout the procedure.

B. The mouth and oropharynx are anesthetized locally.

C. Oral secretions are suctioned or allowed to drain out as they accumulate.

D. The client is placed in a left lateral position with the head tilted forward.

E. As the endoscope is advanced into the esophagus, the head is slowly tilted back.

F. The esophagus and cardiac sphincter are examined as the endoscope is advanced. The endoscope is rotated clockwise as it is advanced into the stomach and the stomach lining, and the cardiac and pyloric sphincters are examined. The scope is advanced through the pylorus into the duodenal bulb and beyond the bulb apex into the second portion of the pH duodenum. Advancement can continue into the jejunum as well. Photographs of suspicious areas and biopsies or brushings may also be taken. Sclerotherapy is commonly performed during this procedure if active bleeding is noted. Polypectomies are also common. The endoscope is slowly withdrawn.

4. Postprocedure care:
    A. Fasting is required until the gag reflex returns.
    B. Continue assessment of respiratory status. If deep sedation was used, follow institutional protocol for postsedation monitoring. Typical monitoring includes continuous ECG monitoring and pulse oximetry, with continual assessments (q 5–15 minutes) of airway, vital signs, and neurologic status until the client is lying quietly awake, is breathing independently, and responds to commands spoken in a normal tone.
    C. Observe for symptoms of complications, which may include hypotension, pallor, tachycardia (from bleeding), shoulder, neck, back, or abdominal pain (from perforation), or tachypnea and rales due to pulmonary edema after thoracic perforation.
5. Client and family teaching:
    A. Fast from food and fluids for 8–12 hours before the procedure.
    B. Arrange for someone else to drive you home, as clients receiving sedation should not drive until 24 hours later.
    C. It is important to swallow when asked, as the endoscope is inserted through the mouth and advanced into the stomach.
6. Factors that affect results:
    A. The client must be able to swallow.
7. Other data:
    A. This test is to be performed with caution in clients with perforated ulcer, aortic aneurysm, recent bleeding esophageal varices, or Zenker's diverticulum.
    B. Complications of this procedure include esophageal, thoracic, gastric, or diaphragmatic perforation.

Bibliography:

Ibach MB, Grier JF, et al.: Diagnostic considerations in evaluation of patients presenting with melena and nondiagnostic esophagogastro-duodenoscopy. Dig Dis Sci *40*(7):1459–1462, 1995.

Melleney EM, Lambertini L, Willoughby CP: Pulse oximetry monitoring during non-sedated upper gastrointestinal endoscopy. Postgrad Med J *71*(837):433–434, 1995.

Narvaez-Rodriguez I, Saez-de-Santamaria J, et al.: Cytologic brushing as a simple and rapid method in the diagnosis of *Helicobacter pylori* infection. Acta Cytol *39*(5):916–919, 1995.

GENITAL, BACILLUS HAEMOPHILUS DUCREYI, CULTURE

Norm: No growth.

Usage: Distinguishes genital chancroid from other genital ulcerations such as syphilis, herpes genitalis, lymphogranuloma venereum, granuloma inguinale, and traumatic ulcer.

Description: The causative agent of the chancroid genital ulcer *Haemophilus ducreyi* is a nonmotile, gram-negative bacillus transmitted by direct sexual contact. It is more common in warm climates than in cold climates and is contagious until completely healed.

Professional Considerations:

1. Consent form NOT required.
2. Preparation:
    A. Obtain one or more of the following culture media: agar supplemented with IsoVitale X, agar with CVA enrichment, agar with vancomycin (3 mg/L).
3. Procedure:
    A. Cleanse the ulcer and the area surrounding it with three culture kit towelettes. Cleanse the ulcer from front to back and discard each towelette after one pass from front to back.
    B. Swab the base of the ulcer with a sterile cotton swab and transfer the culture directly onto one or more culture media.
4. Postprocedure care:
    A. Transport the culture to the laboratory immediately.
5. Client and family teaching:
    A. Describe the procedure above if the client is to collect the specimen independently.
    B. Results are normally available in 48 hours.
6. Factors that affect results:
    A. For successful growth, inoculation of the culture medium must be performed immediately.
    B. The isolation rate is improved when more than one type of medium is used.
7. Other data:
    A. If the results are negative, the test should be repeated due to common difficulty in growing *H. ducreyi*.

Bibliography:

Trees DL, Morse SA: Chancroid and *Haemophilus ducreyi*: an update. Clin Microbiol Rev *8*(3): 357–375, 1995.

Woods GL: Update on laboratory diagnosis of sexually transmitted diseases. Clin Lab Med *15*(3):665–684, 1995.

GENITAL, *CANDIDA ALBICANS,* CULTURE

Norm: No growth of *Candida*. Normal flora present.

Usage: Candidiasis, moniliasis, urethritis, and vulvovaginitis.

Description: *Candida albicans* is a fungus that is often part of the normal human skin flora but that may also be transmitted sexually. It may cause infections of the skin, nails, and mucous membranes, and may also cause a disseminated infection in debilitated individuals. Predisposing factors for *C. albicans* infections include diabetes mellitus, general debilitation, and broad-spectrum antibiotic therapy. *C. albicans* is a common cause of vaginitis in females.

Professional Considerations:

1. Consent form NOT required.
2. Preparation:
   A. Obtain three or four towelettes, a Culturette or sterile cotton swab, and a red-top tube.
3. Procedure:
   A. Collect the specimen as described for *Genital, Routine, Culture*. Alternatively, swab the urethral orifice, vulva, or vagina with a sterile cotton swab and place it in a sterile tube.
4. Postprocedure care:
   A. Document the specimen source and site, the symptoms, recent antibiotic therapy, and the collection time on the laboratory requisition.
   B. Send the specimen to the laboratory within 2 hours.
5. Client and family teaching:
   A. Results are normally available within 24–48 hours.
   B. *C. albicans* infection is curable with topical medication. The medication must be continued for the full course of treatment to cure the infection.
   C. Future prevention for *C. albicans* infection should include avoidance of nylon pantyhose and underwear and, if the client is diabetic, include maintenance of normal blood glucose levels.
   D. Do not have sexual relations until your physician confirms that the infection is gone.
   E. Do not use feminine hygiene sprays or douche during the treatment.
6. Factors that affect results:
   A. Results may be negative if antibiotic therapy was started prior to specimen collection.
   B. Results are invalidated if the specimen is refrigerated.
7. Other data:
   A. At least 48 hours are required for results.

Bibliography:

Fricker-Hidalgo H, Lebeau B, Kervroedan P, et al.: Auxacolor, a new commercial system for feast identification: evaluation of 182 strains comparatively with ID 32C. Ann Biol Clin Paris *53*(4): 221–225, 1995.

Nyirjesy P, Seeney SM, Grody MH, et al.: Chronic fungal vaginitis: the value of cultures. Am J Ostet Gynecol *173*(3, Pt 1):820–823, 1995.

GENITAL, *NEISSERIA GONORRHOEAE,* CULTURE

Norm: All sites: negative for *Neisseria gonorrhoeae*.

Vaginal culture	Normal flora
Vulval culture	Normal flora
Urethral culture	Normal flora
Prostatic fluid culture	No growth
Endocervical culture	No growth

Usage: Cervicitis, dysuria, endometritis, epididymitis, gonorrhea, menstrual irregularities, pelvic inflammatory disease, pelvic peritonitis, perihepatitis, proctitis, prostatitis, salpingitis, urethral stricture, urethritis, vaginitis, and vulvovaginitis.

Description: *Neisseria gonorrhoeae* is a pyogenic, gram-negative, oxidase-positive cocci that is an obligate parasite of humans. It is the causative organism of the sexually transmitted infection gonorrhea. *N. gonorrhoeae* inhabits the mucous membranes of the genital tract, and may also be found in the oral mucosa of clients who engage in oral sex. Symptoms include dysuria, purulent urethral discharge, proctitis, and pharyngitis. Females are often asymptomatic. Left untreated, gonorrhea leads to skin lesions, arthritis, meningitis, and reproductive problems. *N. gonorrhoeae* is most often found in the urethra of males and the cervix and perineum of females.

Professional Considerations:

1. Consent form NOT required.
2. Preparation:
   A. Wait 1 hour after urination to collect urethral specimens.
   B. Obtain three or four towelettes, a Culturette or cotton swab, and culture media (Transgrow, Jembec, or Thayer-Martin).
3. Procedure:
   A. Collect the specimen as described for *Genital, Routine, Culture*, with the exception that the specimen may also be inoculated directly onto culture media.
   B. A rectal culture may also be collected

for suspected gonorrheal proctitis by inserting a sterile Culturette swab into the rectum. The swab should be held in place for 15 seconds, then removed and placed in the Culturette tube.

4. Postprocedure care:
   A. Write the specimen source and site, time of collection, sex, age, symptoms, and recent antibiotic therapy on the laboratory requisition.
   B. Transport the specimen to the laboratory within 1 hour. If it was inoculated directly onto Thayer-Martin medium, transport the specimen to the laboratory immediately and insert it into a carbon dioxide incubator.
5. Client and family teaching:
   A. Review the specimen collection procedure with the client.
   B. Results are normally available within 48 hours.
   C. Gonorrhea infection is treatable with antibiotics.
   D. If the results are positive, provide the client with the appropriate information on sexually transmitted diseases.
      i. Notify all sexual partners from the last 90 days to be tested for gonorrhea infection.
      ii. Do not have sexual relations until your physician confirms that the infection is gone.
   E. Do not use feminine hygiene sprays or douche during the treatment.
   F. Wear underpants and pantyhose that have a cotton lining in the crotch.
   G. Take showers instead of tub baths until the infection is gone.
6. Factors that affect results:
   A. Reject specimens received more than 30 minutes after collection.
   B. Do not refrigerate samples. *N. gonorrhoeae* is easily destroyed by cold.
7. Other data:
   A. None.

Bibliography:

Seigel WM, Golden NH, Weinberg S, Sacker IM: Hyperendemic penicillinase-producing Neisseria gonorrhoeae genital infection in an inner city population. J Adolesc Health *16*(1):41–44, 1995.

Turner A, Gough KR, Jephcott AE: Comparison of 3 methods for culture confirmation of Neisseria Gonorrhea strains currently circulating in UK. J Clin Pathol *48*(10):919–923, 1995.

GENITAL, ROUTINE, CULTURE

Norm:

Vaginal culture	Normal flora.
Vulval culture	Normal flora.
Urethral culture	Normal flora.
Prostatic fluid culture	No growth.
Endocervical culture	No growth.

Usage: Cervicitis, endometriosis, fungal infections, gonorrhea, pelvic inflammatory disease, peritonitis, and toxic shock syndrome with positive *Staphylococcus aureus*.

Description: Used to identify pathogenic organisms causing genital tract or abdominal pain, inflammation, discharge, or other symptoms.

Professional Considerations:

1. Consent form NOT required.
2. Preparation:
   A. Obtain three or four towelettes and a Culturette.
3. Procedure:
   A. *Female:*
      i. Cleanse the vulva and/or perineal area with three or four culture kit or microbiological towelettes. Cleanse the area from front to back and discard each towelette after one pass from front to back.
      ii. Swab the urethral orifice, vulva or vagina, or genital lesions or discharge with a Culturette swab, and insert the swab into the Culturette tube. Squeeze the tube tip to release the ampule of medium.
      iii. For cervical specimens, place the client in a dorsal lithotomy position and drape her for comfort. Insert a vaginal retractor, lubricated with water only, into the vaginal vault. Using a speculum, gently compress the cervix, to express exudate. Insert a sterile, cotton-tipped swab into the center of the cervical os. Wait 10–15 seconds for absorption to occur, then gently turn the swab 360 degrees. Remove the swab and place it in a Culturette tube.
   B. *Male:*
      i. Retract the foreskin of the penis. Cleanse the tip of the penis with three or four microbiological or culture kit towelettes. Cleanse in an outward circular motion and discard each towelette after one use.
      ii. Forming a ring around the base of the penis with the fingers, strip fingers toward the distal tip, causing urethral discharge to accumulate at the urethral orifice. Place a sterile cotton-tipped swab into the urethral orifice and hold it there for 10–15 seconds to allow the swab to absorb the discharge. Remove the swab and place the sample into a Culturette tube.
4. Postprocedure care:
   A. Transport the specimen to the laboratory within 2 hours.
   B. Do NOT refrigerate the sample.

5. Client and family teaching:
   A. Review the specimen collection procedure (above) with client.
   B. Results are normally available within 24–48 hours.
6. Factors that affect results:
   A. Write the specimen source and site, time of collection, sex, age, symptoms, and recent antibiotic therapy on the laboratory requisition.
   B. Refrigeration destroys many pathogenic organisms.
7. Other data:
   A. Cultures may also be taken of the vaginal walls or of prostatic discharge.
   B. Normal vaginal flora may include aerobic streptococci (groups B and D), anaerobic streptococci, *Candida* fungi, *C. vaginalis*, diphtheroids (*Corynebacteria* species), gram-negative anaerobes such as *Bacteroides* or *Lactobacilli*, *Staphylococcus aureus*, *S. epidermidis*, or *Veillonella*.

Bibliography:

Henderson CE, Egre H, Turk R, et al.: Aminorrhexis lowers the incidence of positive cultures for group B streptococci. Am J Obstet Gynecol *168*(2):624–625, 1993.

Read JS, Klebanoff MA: Sexual intercourse during pregnancy and preterm delivery: effects of vaginal microorganism. The Vaginal Infection and Prematurity Study Group. Am J Obstet Gynecol *168*(2):514–519, 1993.

GENTAMICIN, BLOOD

Norm:

		SI Units
Peak therapeutic level	4–8 μg/ml	8–12 μmol/L
Peak panic level	>12 μg/ml	>24 μmol/L
Trough therapeutic level	<2 μg/ml	<4 μmol/L
Trough panic level	>2 μg/ml	>4 μmol/L

Overdose Symptoms and Treatment:

Symptoms: Loss of hearing, acute tubular necrosis.

Treatment: Both hemodialysis and peritoneal dialysis WILL remove Gentamicin.

Usage: Evaluation of appropriateness of dosing during gentamicin therapy.

Description: Gentamicin is an aminoglycoside antibiotic effective against gram-positive and gram-negative bacteria, including *Pseudomonas aeruginosa, Klebsiella, Proteus, Escherichia,* and *Serratia.* It is excreted by the kidney, with accumulation in renal tubular cells. The half-life is 2–3 hours, with steady-state levels reached in 10–15 hours in clients with normal renal function. Gentamicin has a narrow range of therapeutic value. Thus, it is important to monitor gentamicin levels throughout therapy, beginning from the time it reaches a steady state. In clients with baseline renal impairment, monitoring should be initiated sooner than recommended in this procedure.

Professional Considerations:

1. Consent form NOT required.
2. Preparation:
   A. Tube: Red-top, red/gray-top, or gold-top.
   B. Write any recent antibiotic therapy on the laboratory requisition.
   C. Do NOT draw during hemodialysis.
3. Procedure:
   A. For every 8-hour gentamicin administration, levels should be measured after dose number 5. For every 12-hour dosing, levels should be measured after dose number 3.
   B. Draw a 1-ml blood sample. Draw a trough specimen just prior to the gentamicin dose. Draw a peak specimen 30 minutes to 3 hours after completion of the intravenous dose or 15–60 minutes after completion of the intramuscular dose.
4. Postprocedure care:
   A. Label the tube and laboratory requisition with the specimen collection time and indicate whether it is a peak or trough specimen.
   B. Send the specimen promptly to the laboratory. The sample should be spun within 1 hour, with the serum then frozen or refrigerated until testing.
5. Client and family teaching:
   A. The test helps determine whether the antibiotic is being given at the safe and effective dose.
   B. The trough level is drawn before the antibiotic dose and the peak level is drawn after the dose.

C. Results are normally available within 24 hours.
6. Factors that affect results:
   A. Increased results may be due to gentamicin nephrotoxicity.
7. Other data:
   A. Daily creatinine and Beta$_2$-microglobulin levels should be monitored during gentamicin therapy.
   B. Gentamicin nephrotoxicity is more likely to occur when other nephrotoxic drugs are administered during gentamicin therapy.
   C. Clients receiving gentamicin should have their hearing assessed before starting therapy, and then every day until therapy is completed. Intake and output should be monitored closely throughout gentamicin therapy.
   D. Controlled mechanical ventilation has been shown to decrease levels of gentamicin.

Bibliography:

Adhikari M, Coovadia YM, Singh D: A 4-year study of neonatal meningitis: clinical and microbiological findings. J Trop Pediatr *41*(2):81–85, 1995.
Van Goor H, de Graaf JS, Kooi K, Bleichrodt RP: Gentamycin reduces bacteremia and mortality rates associated with the treatment of experimental peritonitis with recombinant tissue plasminogen activator. J Am Coll Surg *181*(1):38–42, 1995.

GGTP, BLOOD
(see Gamma-Glutamyltranspeptidase, Blood)

GICA
(see CA 19–9, Blood)

GILCHRIST'S SKIN TEST
(see Blastomycosis Skin Test, Diagnostic)

GLOBULIN, PLASMA

Norm:

Total		2.5 g% of protein
Alpha$_1$	0.1–0.4 g/dl	1–5% of total
Alpha$_2$	0.4–1.0 g/dl	4.6–14% of total
Beta	0.5–1.5 g/dl	7.3–15% of total
Gamma	0.5–1.7 g/dl	8–21% of total

Increased Alpha$_1$ Globulin: Burns, carcinomatosis, focal episodes due to tumors, chemical injury, dehydration, diabetes mellitus, glomerulonephritis, Hodgkin's disease, inflammation (acute), lymphoma, necrosis, pregnancy, trauma, and ulcerative colitis. Drugs include estrogens.

Increased Alpha$_2$ Globulin: Acute infection, adrenal insufficiency, allergies, asthma, burns (haptoglobin, ceruloplasmin), carcinomatosis, chemical injury (haptoglobin, ceruloplasmin), Cushing's syndrome, dehydration, diabetes mellitus (advanced), focal episodes due to tumors (haptoglobin, ceruloplasmin), Hodgkin's disease, hypernephroma, hyperparathyroidism, hyperthyroidism, hypoalbuminemia, infarction (haptoglobin, ceruloplasmin), inflammation (haptoglobin, ceruloplasmin), leukemia (myelogenous), lymphoma, myxedema, necrosis (haptoglobin, ceruloplasmin), nephrotic syndrome, nephrosis, peritonitis (familial paroxysmal), pregnancy, rheumatic fever, rheumatoid arthritis, sarcoidosis, systemic lupus erythematosus, trauma (haptoglobin, ceruloplasmin), and ulcerative colitis. Drugs include adrenocorticosteroids (haptoglobin) and estrogens (ceruloplasmin).

Increased Beta Globulin: Biliary cirrhosis, chickenpox, chronic iron deficiency anemia (transferrin), carcinoma (complement), cirrhosis, Cushing's disease (complement), dehydration, diabetes mellitus, dysproteinemia (familial, idiopathic), hepatitis (viral), hypercholesterolemia, hyperparathyroidism, hypothyroidism, macroglobulinemia, malignant hypertension (complement), nephrosis, nephrotic syndrome, nonfasting specimen, pregnancy (transferrin), obstructive jaundice, polyarteritis nodosa (complement), and sarcoidosis.

Increased Gamma Globulin: Amyloidosis, aortic arch syndrome, bacterial endocarditis, carcinoma, chickenpox, Crohn's disease, chronic inflammations, chronic lymphocytic leukemia, cirrhosis, congestive heart failure, cryoglobulinemia, cystic fibrosis, dehydration, Hashimoto's disease, hepatitis (viral), Hodgkin's disease, hypergammaglobulinemia, infection, leukemia (myelocytic, monocytic, myelogenous), liver disease, lymphogranuloma venereum, macroglobulinemia, malignant lymphoma, myasthenia gravis, multiple myeloma, myxedema, myxoma of left heart atrium, obstructive jaundice, polymyositis, retroperitoneal fibrosis, rheumatic fever, rheumatoid arthritis, sarcoidosis, systemic lupus erythematosus, temporal arteritis, tertiary syphilis, toxoplasmosis, trichinosis, tuberculosis, visceral larva migrans, and Waldenström's macroglobulinemia.

Decreased Alpha$_1$ Globulin: Alpha1-antitrypsin deficiency, hepatitis (viral), malabsorption, nephrotic syndrome, scleroderma, and starvation.

Decreased Alpha$_2$ Globulin: Hepatitis (viral), liver disease (haptoglobin), malabsorption, malnutrition (ceruloplasmin), megaloblastic anemia (haptoglobin) nephrotic syndrome (ceruloplasmin), protein-losing enteropathy (ceruloplasmin), red blood cell hemolysis (haptoglobin), scleroderma, starvation, and Wilson's disease (Ceruloplasmin). Drugs include estrogens (haptoglobin).

Decreased Beta Globulin: Atransferrinemia (transferrin), autoimmune disease, malabsorption, protein malnutrition (transferrin), scleroderma, starvation, steatorrhea, systemic lupus erythematosus, and ulcerative colitis.

Decreased Gamma Globulin: Asthma, allergies, amyloidosis, Bruton's disease, Cushing's syndrome, heavy chain disease, hyperglycinemia, hypogammaglobulinemia, leukemia (lymphocytic), lymphoma, malabsorption, nephrosis, nephrotic syndrome, malabsorption, protein-losing enteropathy, scleroderma, starvation, steatorrhea, thymic tumor, and ulcerative colitis.

Description: Globulins are plasma proteins formed mainly in the liver, but also in the lymphatic and reticuloendothelial systems. There are three types of proteins in the family of globulins: alpha, beta, and gamma. Alpha$_1$ globulin consists of alpha$_1$-antitrypsin, alpha$_1$-acid glycoprotein, alpha-fetoprotein, cortisol-binding protein, and thyroxine-binding globulin. Alpha$_2$ globulin consists of haptoglobin, alpha$_2$-macroglobulin, and ceruloplasmin. Beta globulin consists of transferrin, beta-lipoprotein, and complement components. Gamma globulin consists of IgG, IgA, IgM, IgD, and IgE antibodies. Functions served by the globulins include buffers in acid-base balance; transporters of constituents of blood such as lipids, vitamins, hormones, iron, copper, and enzymes; and antibody activity.

Professional Considerations:

1. Consent form NOT required.
2. Preparation:
   A. *See Client and family teaching.*
   B. Tube: Red-top, red/gray-top, or gold-top.
3. Procedure:
   A. Draw a 7-ml blood sample.
4. Postprocedure care:
   A. Vaccinations and immunizations within the prior 6 months should be noted on the laboratory requisition.
   B. Blood product administration or antitoxin administration within the prior 6 weeks should be noted on the laboratory requisition.
5. Client and family teaching:
   A. Fast for 8 hours before the test.
6. Factors that affect results:
   A. Reject hemolyzed specimens.
7. Other data:
   A. The globulin level may be estimated by subtracting albumin from total protein.

Bibliography:

Chimps E, Skinner C: Intravenous immunoglobulin: Implications for use in the neurological patient. J Neurosci Nurs 26(1):8–17, 1994.

Timmerman PR: Intravenous immunoglobulin in oncology nursing practice. Oncol Nurs Forum 20(1):69–75, 1993.

GLOMERULAR BASEMENT MEMBRANE ANTIBODY, SERUM

Norm: Negative.

Positive: Antiglomerular basement membrane disease, including glomerulonephritis (crescentic), and Goodpasture's syndrome.

Description: Antibodies specific for the glomerular basement membrane (GBM) bind to specific antigens, causing an immune response leading to various anti-GBM diseases. This test identifies the presence of circulating GBM antibodies and is positive in 87% of clients with anti-GBM associated

Goodpasture's syndrome and 60% of clients with anti-GBM associated glomerulonephritis. Goodpasture's syndrome is a rare disease characterized by necrotizing glomerulonephritis and hemorrhagic pneumonitis, which may result in renal failure and death.

Professional Considerations:

1. Consent form NOT required.
2. Preparation:
   A. *See Client and family teaching.*
   B. Tube: Red-top, red/gray-top, or gold-top.
3. Procedure:
   A. Draw a 4-ml blood sample.
4. Postprocedure care:
   A. Transport the specimen to the laboratory immediately.
   B. Freeze the serum if the test is not run immediately.
5. Client and family teaching:
   A. Fast (except for water) for 8 hours before the test.
6. Factors that affect results:
   A. Antibiotic administration may produce a false-negative result.
   B. Up to 20% of results may be false-negatives.
7. Other data:
   A. In addition to a specimen of blood, a kidney or lung biopsy may also be evaluated for the presence of the antibody.

Bibliography:

Burns AP, Fisher M, Li P, et al.: Molecular analysis of HLA class II genes in Goodpasture's disease. QJM 88(2):93–100, 1995.

Ito Y, Fukatsu A, Baba M, et al.: Pathogenic significance of interleukin-6 in a patient with antiglomerular basement membrane antibody-induced glomerulonephritis with multinucleated giant cells. Am J Kidney Dis 26(1):72–79, 1995.

GLUCAGON, PLASMA

Norm: Norms vary by laboratory.

		SI Units
Big glucagon	34–192 pg/ml	34–192 ng/L
Proglucagon	<28 pg/ml	<28 ng/L
Glucagon	2–60 pg/ml	2–60 ng/L
Small glucagon	8–54 pg/ml	8–54 ng/L
Adult	20–100 pg/ml	20–100 ng/L
Cord blood	0–215 pg/ml	0–215 ng/L
Newborn–3 days	0–1750 pg/ml	0–1750 ng/L
4 days–14 years	0–148 pg/ml	0–148 ng/L

Increased: Acromegaly, burns, cirrhosis, Cushing's syndrome, diabetes mellitus (average 1525 ± 578 pg/ml [1525 ± 578 ng/L]), diabetic ketoacidosis, familial hyperglucagonemia, glucagonoma (levels >900 pg/ml [900 ng/L, SI units]), hyperosmolality, hypoglycemia, pancreatic islet cell lesion, pancreatitis (acute, severe), pheochromocytoma, postoperatively, renal failure (average 500–580 pg/ml, 500–580 ng/L), stress, trauma, and uremia. Drugs include amino acids, cholecystokinin-pancreozymin, danazol, gastrin, glucocorticoids, insulin, nifedipine, and sympathomimetic amines.

Decreased: Cystic fibrosis, hypoglycemia (related to chronic pancreatitis), idiopathic glucagon deficiency, insulinoma, neoplastic replacement of pancreas, status post pancreatectomy, and pancreatitis (chronic). Drugs include atenolol, pindolol, propranolol, and secretin.

Description: Glucagon is a peptide hormone manufactured in and secreted by the alpha cells of the pancreatic islets of Langerhans. Hypoglycemia, beta-adrenergics, and amino acids stimulate the secretion of glucagon, while increasing insulin levels inhibit its secretion. Glucagon increases blood glucose by increasing the breakdown of glycogen to glucose and stimulates activity of phosphorylase, the enzyme that initiates the first step in gluconeogenesis. This test is most often used as an aid in the diagnosis of glucagonoma, an alpha islet cell neoplasm occurring most often in females after menopause, and hypoglycemia caused by chronic pancreatitis or idiopathic glucagon deficiency.

Professional Considerations:

1. Consent form NOT required.
2. Preparation:
   A. *See Client and family teaching.*
   B. Tube: Lavender-top, and ice.

3. Procedure:
   A. Draw a 10-ml blood specimen into a chilled tube.
   B. Place the specimen immediately on ice.
4. Postprocedure care:
   A. Send the specimen to the laboratory immediately.
   B. Current administration of insulin and/or catecholamines should be noted on the laboratory requisition.
5. Client and family teaching:
   A. Fast for 10–12 hours before test.
   B. Because exercise and stress elevate plasma glucagon levels, the client should be relaxed and recumbent for 30 minutes before the test.
6. Factors that affect results:
   A. Results are invalidated if the client had a radioactive scan within 48 hours.
   B. Reject hemolyzed specimens.
   C. Prolonged fasting, stress, or current use of insulin or catecholamines may elevate glucagon levels.
7. Other data:
   A. Due to influence on glucagon secretion, serum insulin and glucose should also be measured.
   B. This test should not be performed for poorly controlled diabetics.
   C. Stimulation or suppression tests may be needed to confirm a diagnosis of idiopathic glucagon deficiency or hypoglycemia caused by chronic pancreatitis.

Bibliography:

Buggy J, Livingston JN, Rabin DU: Glucagon: Glucagon-like peptide I receptor chimeras reveal domains that determine specificity of glucagon binding. J Biol Chem *270*(13):7474–7478, 1995.

Stroop SD, Kuestner RE, Serwold TF, et al.: Chimeric human calcitonin and glucagon receptors reveal two dissociable calcitonin interaction sites. Biochem *34*(3):1050–1057, 1995.

GLUCOCHEK, DIAGNOSTIC
(see Glucose Monitoring Machines, Diagnostic)

GLUCOMETER, DIAGNOSTIC
(see Glucose Monitoring Machines, Diagnostic)

GLUCOSCAN, DIAGNOSTIC
(see Glucose Monitoring Machines, Diagnostic)

GLUCOSE ALERT, DIAGNOSTIC
(see Glucose Monitoring Machines, Diagnostic)

GLUCOSE-6-PHOSPHATE DEHYDROGENASE (G-6-PD), QUANTITATIVE, BLOOD

Norm: Norms vary according to the test method used:
140–280 U/billion cells.
125–280 U/dl packed red blood cells.
8.6–18.6 U/g hemoglobin.
4.5–10.8 U/g hemoglobin.

Zinkham Method (30°C):		SI Units
Newborn	7.8–14.4 U/g Hb	0.50–0.93 MU/mol Hb
	226–418 U/10^{12} Ercs	0.23–0.42 nU/L Erc
	2.65–4.90 U/ml Ercs	2.65–4.90 kU/L Ercs
Adult	5.5–9.3 U/g Hb	0.35–0.60 MU/mol Hb
	160–270 U/10^{12} Ercs	0.16–0.27 nU/L Erc
	1.87–3.16 U/mL Ercs	1.87–3.16 kU/L Ercs

Increased: Anemia (pernicious, megaloblastic), hepatic coma, hyperthyroidism, myocardial infarction, and Werlhof's disease (idiopathic thrombocytopenic purpura).

Decreased: Anemia (congenital nonspherocytic hemolytic), favism, congenital G-6-PD deficiency, and nonimmunologic hemolytic disease of the newborn.

Description: Glucose-6-phosphate dehydrogenase (G-6-PD) is an enzyme normally present in the erythrocytes. This enzyme is part of the pentose phosphate pathway that metabolizes glucose and functions to protect cells from damage by oxidizing agents. This test measures G-6-PD levels in red blood cells, thereby detecting deficiencies of this enzyme. G-6-PD deficiency is a sex-linked genetic disorder found mostly in males that results in hemolysis of erythrocytes, producing anemia after the receipt of certain drugs. Drugs that may precipitate hemolytic episodes in affected individuals include acetanilid, acetylphenylhydrazine, antipyrine, ascorbic acid, aspirin, chloramphenicol, nalidixic acid, naphthalene, nitrofurantoin, nitrofuran, pentaquine phenacetin, phenylhydrazine, primaquine, probenecid, quinacrine, quinidine, quinine, sulfonamides, and vitamin K. Other precipitants include diabetic acidosis, fava bean ingestion, infections (viral, bacterial), and septicemia.

Professional Considerations:

1. Consent form NOT required.
2. Preparation:
   A. Tube: Lavender-top, blue-top, or green-top.
3. Procedure:
   A. Draw a 3-ml blood sample.
   B. Invert the tube gently several times to mix the sample.
   C. Handle the sample gently to prevent hemolysis.
4. Postprocedure care:
   A. Recent blood transfusion or current/recent ingestion of antimalarials, aspirin, fava beans, nitrofurantoin, phenacetin, sulfonamides, or vitamin K should be noted on the laboratory requisition.
5. Client and family teaching:
   A. Refer the client with elevated levels for long-term medical follow-up care.
   B. Clients testing positive should receive thorough disease teaching, including which drugs place the client at risk for a hemolytic episode.
   C. Refer positive clients for genetic counseling.
6. Factors that affect results:
   A. Reject hemolyzed specimens to avoid false-negative results.
   B. False-negative results may occur after a blood transfusion or a hemolytic episode.
7. Other data:
   A. Several methods are available to test for G-6-PD deficiency. The method utilized by the particular laboratory determines the type of blood tube used.
   B. G-6-PD deficiency is demonstrated most frequently in African Americans, Greeks, Sardinians, and Sephardic Jews.

Bibliography:

Luzzatto L: About hemoglobins, G6PD and parasites in red cells. Exper *51*(3):206–208, 1995.

Yuregir GT, Aksoy K, Arpaci A, et al.: Studies on red cell glucose-6-phosphate dehydrogenase: evaluation of reference values. Ann Clin Biochem *31*(Pt 1):50–55, 1994.

GLUCOSE-6-PHOSPHATE DEHYDROGENASE (G-6-PD) SCREEN, BLOOD

Norm: Enzyme activity detected.

Increased: Not applicable.

Decreased: Anemia (congenital nonspherocytic hemolytic), favism, congenital G-6-PD deficiency, and nonimmunologic hemolytic disease of the newborn.

Description: G-6-PD is an enzyme normally present in erythrocytes. This enzyme is part of the pentose phosphate pathway that metabolizes glucose and functions to protect cells from damage by oxidizing agents. This test measures G-6-PD levels in red blood cells, thereby detecting deficiencies of this enzyme. G-6-PD deficiency is a sex-linked genetic disorder found mostly in males that results in hemolysis of erythrocytes, producing anemia after the receipt of certain drugs. Drugs that may precipitate hemolytic episodes in affected individuals include acetanilid, acetylphenylhydrazine, antipyrine, ascorbic acid, aspirin, chloramphenicol, nalidixic acid, naphthalene, nitrofurantoin, nitrofuran, pentaquine, phenacetin, phenylhydrazine, primaquine, probenecid, quinacrine, quinidine, quinine, sulfonamides, and vitamin K. Other precipitants include diabetic acidosis, fava bean ingestion, infections (viral, bacterial), and septicemia.

Professional Considerations:

1. Consent form NOT required.
2. Preparation:
   A. Tube: Lavender-top.
3. Procedure:
   A. Draw a 2-ml blood sample.
   B. Invert the tube gently several times to mix the sample.
   C. Handle the sample gently to prevent hemolysis.
4. Postprocedure care:
   A. Recent blood transfusion or current/recent ingestion of antimalarials, aspirin, fava beans, nitrofurantoin, phenacetin, sulfonamides, or vitamin K should be noted on the laboratory requisition.
5. Client and family teaching:
   A. Results are normally available within 24 hours.
   B. Clients testing positive should receive thorough disease teaching, including which drugs place the client at risk for a hemolytic episode.
   C. Refer positive clients for genetic counseling.

6. Factors that affect results:
   A. Reject hemolyzed specimens to avoid false-negative results.
   B. False-negative results may occur after a blood transfusion or a hemolytic episode.
7. Other data:
   A. G-6-PD deficiency is demonstrated most frequently in African Americans, Greeks, Sardinians, and Sephardic Jews.

Bibliography:

Boo NY, Ainoon BO, Ooi LH, et al.: Glucose-6-phosphate dehydrogenase enzyme activity of normal term Malaysian neonates of different ethnic origins. J Paediatr Health *30*(3):273–274, 1994.

Muggeo M, Moghetti P, Querena M, et al.: Mononuclear leukocytes from obese patients with type II diabetes have reduced activity of hexokinase, 9-phosphofructokinase and glucose-6-phosphate dehydrogenase. Horm Metab Res *25*(3):160–164, 1993.

GLUCOSE, BLOOD

Norm: Dependent on time and content of last meal. In normal clients, glucose levels return to the fasting level (given in these norms) within 2 hours after the last meal.

		SI Units
Whole Blood		
Adults	60–89 mg/dl	3.3–4.9 mmol/L
>Age 60	68–98 mg/dl	3.8–5.4 mmol/L
Children		
Cord blood	38–82 mg/dl	2.1–4.6 mmol/L
Premature infant	17–51 mg/dl	0.9–2.8 mmol/L
Neonate	25–51 mg/dl	1.4–2.8 mmol/L
Newborn–24 hours	34–51 mg/dl	1.9–2.8 mmol/L
Newborn >24 hours	42–68 mg/dl	2.3–3.8 mmol/L
Children	51–85 mg/dl	2.8–4.7 mmol/L
Serum		
Adults	70–105 mg/dl	3.9–5.8 mmol/L
>Age 60	80–115 mg/dl	4.4–6.4 mmol/L
Children		
Cord blood	45–96 mg/dl	2.5–5.3 mmol/L
Premature infants	20–60 mg/dl	1.1–3.3 mmol/L
Neonates	30–60 mg/dl	1.7–3.3 mmol/L
Newborn–24 hours	40–60 mg/dl	2.2–3.3 mmol/L
Newborn >24 hours	50–80 mg/dl	2.8–4.4 mmol/L
Child	60–100 mg/dl	3.3–5.5 mmol/L

Note: Whole-blood glucose values are about 15% less than serum glucose values, due to greater dilution.

Panic Levels		SI Units
Adults	<40 mg/dl	<2.2 mmol/L
	or >700 mg/dl	or >38.6 mmol/L
Neonates	<30 mg/dl	<1.6 mmol/L
	or >300 mg/dl	>1.6 mmol/L

Panic Level Symptoms and Treatment—Increased:

Symptoms: Abdominal pain, fatigue, muscle cramps, nausea, polyuria, thirst, and vomiting.

Treatment: Subcutaneous and/or intravenous injection of insulin per sliding scale. Intravenous insulin is typically administered via continuous infusion for panic levels accompanied by reduced level of consciousness. Hourly adjustments are based on subsequent blood glucose measurements.

Hourly neurologic checks.
Hourly intake and output.
Monitor for hypokalemia as side-effect of treatment.

Panic Level Symptoms and Treatment—Decreased:

Symptoms: Confusion, headache, hunger, irritability, nervousness, restlessness, sweating, and weakness.

Treatment: Administer oral form of glucose followed by oral ingestion of carbohydrates. For neonates or unconscious clients, give IV glucose or IV/IM glucagon.

Increased: Acromegaly, anesthesia, burns, carbon monoxide poisoning, cerebrovascular accident, convulsions, Cushing's disease, Cushing's syndrome, cystic fibrosis, diabetes mellitus, eclampsia, encephalitis, gigantism, hemochromatosis, hemorrhage, hyperthyroidism, hyperpituitarism, hyperadrenalism, hypertension, hypervitaminosis A (chronic), infections, injury, malnutrition (chronic), meningitis, myocardial infarction, obesity, pancreatic carcinoma, pancreatic insufficiency, pancreatitis (chronic) pheochromocytoma, pituitary adenoma, pregnancy, shock, subarachnoid hemorrhage, stress, trauma, and Wernicke's encephalopathy. Drugs include anabolic steroids, androgens, arginine, ascorbic acid, asparaginase, aspirin, baclofen, benzodiazepines, bisacodyl (prolonged use), chlorpromazine, chlorthalidone, cimetidine, clonidine, corticosteroids, corticotropin, dextran, dextrothyroxine, diazoxide, disopyramide phosphate, epinephrine, epinephrine bitartrate, epinephrine borate, epinephrine hydrochloride, estrogens, ethacrynic acid, furosemide, glucose infusions, haloperidol, imipramine, isoproterenol hydrochloride, heparin calcium, heparin sodium, hydralazine hydrochloride, indomethacin, isoniazid, levodopa, levothyroxine sodium/T4, lithium carbonate, magnesium hydroxide, (prolonged high doses), mercaptopurine, methimazole, methyldopa, methyldopate (hydrochloride), nalidixic acid, nicotine, nicotinic acid, oral contraceptives, oxazepam, para-aminosalicylic acid, phenolphthalein, phenytoin, phenytoin sodium, progestins, promethazine hydrochloride, propranolol (in diabetics), propylthiouracil, reserpine, ritodrine hydrochloride, terbutaline sulfate, tetracyclines, thiazides, thyroglobulin, thyroid, tolbutamide (SMA methodology), and triamterene.

Decreased: Addison's disease, adrenal medulla unresponsiveness, alcoholism, carcinoma (adrenal gland, stomach, fibrosarcoma), cirrhosis, cretinism, diabetes mellitus (early), dumping syndrome, exercise, fever, Forbes' disease (type-III glycogen deposition disease), fructose intolerance, galactosemia, glucagon deficiency, hepatic phosphorylase deficiency (type-VI glycogen storage disease), hepatitis, hyperinsulinemia, hypopituitarism, hypothermia, hypothyroidism, infant of diabetic mother, insulin overdose (factitious hypoglycemia), insulinoma, kwashiorkor, leucine sensitivity, malnutrition, maple syrup urine disease, muscle phosphofructokinase deficiency (type-VII glycogen storage disease), myxedema, pancreatic islet cell tumor, pancreatitis, postoperatively (after gastrectomy or gastroenterostomy), postprandial hypoglycemia, Reye's syndrome, Simmonds' disease, vomiting, von Gierke's disease (type-I glycogen storage disease), Waterhouse-Friderichsen syndrome, and Zetterstrom's syndrome. Drugs include allopurinol, amphetamines, aspirin, beta-adrenergic blockers, caffeine, chlorpropamide, clofibrate, edetate disodium, ethanol, guanethidine sulfate, isoniazid, insulin, isocarboxazid, marijuana, nitrazepam, oral hypoglycemic agents, para-aminosalicylic acid, pargyline hydrochloride, phenacetin, phenazopyridine, phenelzine sulfate, phenformin, propranolol (in diabetics), and tranylcypromine sulfate.

Description: Glucose is a monosaccharide found naturally occurring in fruits. It is also formed from the digestion of carbohydrates and the conversion of glycogen by the liver and is the body's main source of cellular energy. Glucose is essential for brain and erythrocyte function. Excess glucose is stored as glycogen in the liver and muscle cells. Hormones influencing glucose metabolism include insulin, glucagon, thyroxine, somatostatin, cortisol, and epinephrine. Fasting glucose levels are used to help diagnose diabetes mellitus and hypoglycemia. A randomly timed test for glucose is usually performed for routine screening and nonspecific evaluation of carbohydrate metabolism.

Professional Considerations:

1. Consent form NOT required.
2. Preparation:
   A. *See Client and family teaching.*
   B. Tube: Red-top, red/gray-top, or gold-top or gray-top.
   B. Observe for signs of hypoglycemia (weakness, slurred speech, confusion, somnolence, pallor, palpitations, convulsions) in fasting clients.
3. Procedure:
   A. Draw a 1-ml blood sample.
4. Postprocedure care:
   A. Send the sample to the laboratory for immediate spinning. If transport is delayed, refrigerate the sample.
   B. The time of the client's last pretest meal, the sample collection time, and the time of the last pretest insulin or oral hypoglycemic agent (if applicable) should be noted on the laboratory requisition.
5. Client and family teaching:
   A. Fast (except for water) for 8–12 hours before collection for fasting specimen.
   B. Withhold morning insulin or oral hypoglycemic agent until after fasting blood sample has been drawn.
   C. Refer newly diagnosed diabetics for diabetic teaching and long-term medical follow-up care.
   D. Resume diet after the fasting specimen has been drawn.
   E. Watch for signs of hypoglycemia (listed on p. 565) and hyperglycemia (listed on p. 566). Teach appropriate intervention.
6. Factors that affect results:
   A. Reject specimens received more than 1 hour after collection to prevent falsely low results.
   B. Falsely decreased glucose values may occur when the glucose oxidase/peroxidase procedure is used or if the client has recently taken acetaminophen or oxycodone.
7. Other data:
   A. Spun samples are stable for 8 hours.
   B. In a client with diabetes, the blood specimen should be drawn prior to insulin treatment or administration of oral hypoglycemic drugs.

Bibliography:

Haheim LL, Holme I, Hjermann I, Leren P: Nonfasting serum glucose and the risk of fatal stroke in diabetic and nondiabetic subjects: 18-year follow-up of the Oslo Study. Stroke *26*(5):774–777, 1995.

Matsumoto K, Akazawa S, Abiru N, et al.: Insulin response after treatment depends on fasting plasma glucose level in NIDDM. Diabetes Res Clin Prac *26*(2):129–135, 1994.

Modan M, Harris MI: Fasting plasma glucose in screening for NIDDM in the U.S. and Israel. Diab Care *17*(5):436–439, 1994.

GLUCOSE, CEREBROSPINAL FLUID, SPECIMEN
(see Cerebrospinal Fluid, Glucose, Specimen)

GLUCOSE, QUALITATIVE, SEMIQUANTITATIVE, URINE

Norm: Negative.

Positive: Adrenal disorders, central nervous system disease, diabetes mellitus, eclampsia, Fanconi's syndrome, glomerulonephritis, glucose administration, heavy metal poisoning, hepatic disease, hyperalimentation, infections, nephrosis, pregnancy, presence of reducing substances and sugars other than glucose in the urine (copper-reduction method only), thyroid disorders, total parenteral nutrition, and toxic renal tubular disease. Drugs include ammonium chloride, asparaginase, carbamazepine, corticosteroids, dextrothyroxine sodium, indomethacin, isoniazid, lithium carbonate, nicotinic acid, phenothiazines, and thiazide diuretics.

Negative: Negative results occur with Clinistix when sugars other than glucose are present in the urine.

Description: A random urine specimen is tested by either copper reduction (Clinitest) or by the enzymatic glucose oxidase method (Clinistix) for the presence of glucose.

Clinitest is a copper reduction tablet test used to detect mellituria and to detect and monitor urine glucose and nonglucose sugar levels. Urine sugar up to 2% may be measured with the five-drop method, and up to 5% may be measured with the two-drop method. Copper-reduction methods are helpful when the test purpose is to detect both glucose and nonglucose sugars present in the urine, such as in metabolic disease, or parenteral nutrition administration.

Clinistix test is a qualitative dipstick method of urine glucose testing that involves an oxidation reaction between urine, impregnated enzymes, and a chromogen, resulting in a color change proportional to the amount of glucose present in the urine. Clinistix is classified as a glucose oxidase method of urine glucose testing. The advantage of glucose oxidase methods over copper-reduction tests is that this method is specific for glucose and unaffected by other sugars and reducing substances.

Professional Considerations:

1. Consent form NOT required.
2. Preparation:
   A. *Clinitest:*
      i. Obtain a 50-ml clean plastic container, a test tube, a dropper, and urine test tablets.
      ii. Dark blue tablets should be discarded. Use only fresh tablets, which are light blue and flecked with dark blue.
      iii. Avoid touching the tablets. To avoid burns, wash the affected area quickly if skin contact occurs.
      iv. A fresh-voided, postprandial specimen is recommended.
   B. *Clinistix:*
      i. For a Clinistix test, obtain a 50-ml clean plastic container and urine test strips.
      ii. Keep the Clinistix bottle tightly capped. Open the bottle to quickly remove a reagent strip and then recap it before performing test.
      iii. Light exposure and moisture speed degradation of Clinistix. Inspect the strip before use, even if the contents of bottle have not expired. If the strip is darkened, discard it as well as the bottle from which it was taken.
3. Procedure:
   A. Have the client completely empty the bladder and then drink at least 8 ounces of fluid; 30 minutes later, have him or her void at least 20 ml of urine into a clean plastic container. A fresh specimen may be taken from a urinary drainage bag. Refrigerate the specimen if it is not tested promptly.
   B. *Clinitest:*
      i. Five-drop method: Add five drops of urine to a clean test tube and rinse the dropper with water. Then add ten drops of water to a test tube.

   ii. Add one Clinitest tablet to this mixture.
   iii. Recap the Clinitest jar tightly.
   iv. Observe the color changes during the boiling phase. Be careful, because the tube is hot!
   v. Glucose >2 g/dl causes a rapid color change to orange during the boiling phase. If this occurs, the test should be repeated as above, using two drops instead of five drops of urine, and comparing results to the Clinitest color chart for the two-drop test.
   vi. 15 seconds after the boiling stops, agitate the test tube and immediately compare the mixture color to the Clinitest color chart. Record the results as shown in the table below.
   C. *Clinistix test:*
      i. Dip the Clinistix reagent strip into the urine, making sure to completely immerse the test pad for 2 seconds.
      ii. While removing the strip, slide the pad side against the edge of the container.
      iii. Exactly 30 seconds after removal of the strip from the urine, compare the color of the test pad to the colors on the bottle.
      iv. Record the results as either negative, light, medium, or dark.
4. Postprocedure care:
   A. Discard the specimen and the reagent strip, if used. Rinse the test tube, if used, with water.
5. Client and family teaching:
   A. New diabetics must learn home glucose testing, which may be with or without a machine.
   B. Do not contaminate the urine specimen with stool or toilet tissue.
   C. For home monitoring, provide the written instructions and a flow sheet so that the client can record the test results.
   D. Watch for signs of hyperglycemia and hypoglycemia (*see Glucose, Blood* for symptoms and treatment).
6. Factors that affect results:
   A. Failure to perform the test on a fresh or refrigerated specimen invalidates the results.

Five-Drop Method		Two-Drop Method	
Negative	blue-green	Negative	blue-green
¼%	green	Trace	dark green
½%	olive-green	½%	green
¾%	brown-green	1%	olive-green
1%	gold	2%	brown-green
2%	orange	3%	gold
		>5%	orange

B. *Copper reduction method (Clinitest):*
  i. The color charts for the two-drop and five-drop methods are different, and must be used with the appropriate test.
  ii. Failure to protect tablets from moisture can result in false findings and possibly an explosion.
  iii. Use of discolored or dark blue tablets invalidates the results.
  iv. The presence of radiographic contrast medium in the urine may cause false-negative results.
  v. Reducing substances that cause a false-positive test include aminosalicylic acid, ampicillin, ampicillin sodium, ascorbic acid, camphor, cephalosporins, chloral hydrate, chloramphenicol, chloroform, creatinine, formaldehyde, fructose, galactose, glucosamine, glucuronic acid, homogentisic acid, isoniazid, ketones, levodopa, maltose, menthol, metolazone, nitrofurantoin, nitrofurantoin sodium, penicillin G benzathine, penicillin G potassium, pentose, phenol, salicylates, streptomycin sulfate, tetracyclines, turpentine, and uric acid.

C. *Glucose oxidase method (Clinistix):*
  i. Clinistix strips must be compared with the color chart on the bottle from which they were taken.
  ii. Use of darkened strips, or those exposed to prolonged moisture or air, invalidates the results.
  iii. Drugs that may cause false-negative results with Clinistix include ascorbic acid, levodopa, methyldopa, methyldopate hydrochloride, phenazopyridine, and salicylates.

7. Other data:
  A. If the client is receiving ascorbic acid, hydrochlorites, levodopa, peroxides, phenazopyridine, or salicylates, use Clinitest tablets.
  B. Other available glucose oxidase urine testing strips include Diastix, n-Multistix, and Tes-Tape.
  C. These tests are now used less frequently to monitor urine glucose in clients with diabetes because of the availability of more precise techniques for blood glucose self-monitoring.
  D. *See also Benedict's Test, Diagnostic.*

Bibliography:

Tighe P: Urine testing with dipsticks [letter]. Lanc 344(8932):1295, 1994.

GLUCOSE, QUANTITATIVE, 24-HOUR, URINE

Norm: ≤100 mg/24 hours (≤5.6 mmol/day, SI units).

Increased: Adrenal disorders, central nervous system disease, diabetes mellitus, eclampsia, Fanconi's syndrome, glomerulonephritis, glucose administration, heavy-metal poisoning, hepatic disease, hyperalimentation, infections, nephrosis, pregnancy, thyroid disorders, and toxic renal tubular disease. Drugs include ammonium chloride, asparaginase, carbamazepine, corticosteroids, dextrothyroxine sodium, indomethacin, isoniazid, lithium carbonate, nicotinic acid, phenothiazines, and thiazide diuretics.

Description: A quantitative measurement of urine glucose may detect glucose spillage into the urine that occurs intermittently and thus may not be detected by random urine glucose measurement. The enzymatic glucose oxidase method is used to detect the presence and amount of glucose. However, the test is performed in the laboratory on an aliquot of a 24-hour urine collection, and the results are reported as numeric values.

Professional Considerations:

1. Consent form NOT required.
2. Preparation:
   A. Obtain a 3-L, 24-hour urine collection bottle containing toluene preservative.
   B. For pediatric collections, also obtain a pediatric urine collection device and tape.
   C. Write the beginning time of collection on the laboratory requisition.
3. Procedure:
   A. *Adult collection:*
      i. Discard the first morning urine specimen.
      ii. Save all the urine voided for 24 hours in a refrigerated, clean, 3-L container to which toluene preservative has been added. For catheterized clients, keep the drainage bag on ice and empty the urine into the refrigerated collection container hourly.
      iii. Document the quantity of urine output during the collection period. Include the urine voided at the end of the 24-hour period.
   B. *Pediatric collection:*
      i. Place the child in a supine position with the knees flexed and the hips externally rotated and abducted.
      ii. Cleanse, rinse, and thoroughly dry the perineal area.
      iii. To prevent the child from removing the collection device, a diaper may be placed over the genital area.
      iv. *Females:* Tape the pediatric collection device to the perineum. Start-

ing at the area between the anus and vagina, apply the device in the anterior direction.

v. *Males:* Place the pediatric collection device over the penis and scrotum and tape it to the perineal area.

vi. After each void, empty the collection device into a refrigerated, 3-L container to which toluene preservative has been added.

4. Postprocedure care:

A. Refrigerate the specimen until it is tested.

B. Compare the urine quantity in the specimen container with the urinary output record for the test. If the specimen contains less urine than was recorded as output, some of the sample may have been discarded, invalidating the test.

C. Document the quantity of urine output and the ending time on the laboratory requisition.

D. Send the specimen to the laboratory for measurement.

5. Client and family teaching:

A. Save all the urine voided in the 24-hour period and urinate before defecating to avoid loss of urine. If any urine is accidentally discarded, discard the entire specimen and restart the collection the next day.

6. Factors that affect results:

A. All the urine voided for the 24-hour period must be included to avoid a falsely low result.

B. Drugs that may cause false-negative results with Clinistix include ascorbic acid, levodopa, methyldopa, methyldopate hydrochloride, phenazopyridine, and salicylates.

C. Failure to refrigerate the specimen throughout the collection period decreases accuracy of the results, due to bacterial growth.

7. Other data:

A. This test aids in the regulation of diet and medication in clients with diabetes mellitus.

B. Because of the problem with incomplete urine collections, laboratories sometimes check the creatinine present in the urine to validate that the sample represents a full 24 hours.

Bibliography:

Korzeniowski PA: Assessment of proper collection in 24-hour urine samples [letter; comment]. Am J Obstet Gynecol *171*(1):281, 1994.

GLUCOSE, SEMIQUANTITATIVE, URINE

(see Glucose, Qualitative, Semiquantitative, Urine)

GLUCOSE MONITORING MACHINES, DIAGNOSTIC

Norm: Whole-blood glucose values are about 15% less than serum glucose values, due to greater dilution.

Whole Blood		SI Units
Adults	60–89 mg/dl	3.3–4.9 mmol/L
>Age 60	68–98 mg/dl	3.8–5.4 mmol/L
Children		
Cord blood	38–82 mg/dl	2.1–4.6 mmol/L
Premature infant	17–51 mg/dl	0.9–2.8 mmol/L
Neonate	25–51 mg/dl	1.4–2.8 mmol/L
Newborn–24 hours	34–51 mg/dl	1.9–2.8 mmol/L
Newborn >24 hours	42–68 mg/dl	2.3–3.8 mmol/L
Child	51–85 mg/dl	2.8–4.7 mmol/L

Usage: Chronic glucose monitoring for diabetes mellitus, monitoring for hypoglycemia in newborn, and bedside whole-blood glucose analysis.

Description: Blood glucose monitoring is generally considered to be more reliable for diabetic glucose monitoring than urine glucose levels. This is particularly true for clients with an abnormally low renal threshold for glucose reabsorption after glomerular filtration. The term *glucose monitoring machines* encompasses a variety of reflectance meters that can be used to quickly quantitate whole blood glucose levels. In general, the technique involves applying a drop of capillary or venous blood to a reagent strip, blotting the drop after a specific time period, inserting the strip into the reflectance meter, then following the manufacturer's recommended steps for processing. The result is generally obtained within 2–3 minutes, and has been estimated to cost as little as 1/20th of a "stat" laboratory glucose measurement.

Professional Considerations:

1. Consent form NOT required.
2. Preparation:
   A. Verify that the client's hematocrit level is within the range for which the specific brand of machine is designed to be accurate. If the hematocrit is outside the required range, perform the *Glucose, Blood* test instead of this test.
   B. Verify that the machine has been calibrated within the time requirements specified by the manufacturer.
   C. Obtain an alcohol wipe, a 2.5-mm lancet (or a needle and a syringe), a reagent strip, a cotton ball, a reflectance meter, sterile gauze, and a capillary tube if heelstick blood will be used.
   D. Read the instructions for the specific reflectance meter to be used.
3. Procedure:
   A. *Fingerstick capillary method:*
      i. Cleanse the lateral aspect of the pad of the finger with an alcohol wipe and allow the area to dry.
      ii. Using a 2.5-mm lancet, puncture the lateral aspect of the pad of the finger. Wipe the first drop of blood away with sterile gauze.
      iii. Holding the puncture site dependent, allow a second, large drop of blood to accumulate and drop onto the reagent strip, making sure there is enough blood to completely cover the pad of the reagent strip. The pad of the finger may be very gently and repeatedly pressed, to encourage blood flow, but avoid milking the finger.
      iv. Follow the directions for the specific reflectance meter being used.
   B. *Heelstick capillary method:*
      i. Prewarming the heel is not necessary.
      ii. Avoid puncturing over previous puncture sites or puncturing the posterior curvature of the heel.
      iii. Cleanse an area on the medial or lateral plantar surface of the heel with 70% alcohol and allow the area to dry.
      iv. Using a 2.5-mm lancet, puncture the heel until a free flow of blood is obtained. Wipe the first drop of blood away with sterile gauze.
      v. Holding the puncture site dependent, allow a second, large drop of blood to accumulate and drop onto

the reagent strip, making sure there is enough blood to completely cover the pad of the reagent strip. Avoid milking the heel.
      vi. Follow the directions for the specific reflectance meter being used.
   C. *Venous method:*
      i. Obtain a 1-ml venous blood sample in a syringe or green-top tube.
      ii. Completely cover the pad of the reagent strip with a drop of the blood specimen.
      iii. Follow the directions for the specific reflectance meter being used.
4. Postprocedure care:
   A. Hold pressure to the site until the bleeding stops. Leave puncture sites open to air, to heal.
5. Client and family teaching:
   A. Teach the newly diagnosed client with diabetes how to perform a fingerstick and use a reflectance meter.
   B. Watch for signs of hyperglycemia and hypoglycemia (*see Glucose, Blood* for symptoms and treatment).
   C. Bring a home reflectance meter to office appointments with the physician so that technique and machine calibration may be assessed.
6. Factors that affect results:
   A. After cleansing the skin with alcohol, the skin must be allowed to dry completely before the puncture is performed.
   B. Failure to completely cover the reagent area with blood may cause inaccurate results.
   C. Using too little or too much blood may cause inaccurate results. Cotton, rather than gauze, should be used for blotting the strip.
   D. Failure to follow timing instructions exactly as recommended by the manufacturer may cause inaccurate results.
   E. The most accurate and reliable results are obtained when the reflectance meter is calibrated according to the schedule recommended by the manufacturer.
   F. Instruments used for monitoring of hypoglycemia in newborns must have the calibration adjusted for this purpose.
   G. For glucose levels >400 mg/dl, accuracy of Chemstrip bG and the Accu-Check reflectance meter has been shown to improve when a 1-ml specimen of heparinized blood is diluted with 2 ml of 0.9% saline, and the corresponding result is multiplied by 3 to correct for dilution.
   H. Vigorous milking of the heel or finger may cause falsely low results due to dilution of the specimen with interstitial fluid.
   I. Many conditions and drugs affect glucose levels. (*See Glucose, Blood.*)
7. Other data:
   A. In normal clients, blood glucose levels

return to fasting levels within 2 hours postprandially.

B. Glucose monitoring machine: competency of the operator may be evaluated by assessing results of control solutions.

Bibliography:

Kestel F: Using blood glucose meters: What you and your patient need to know. Nurs 23(4):50–53, 1993.

Tomky D: Diabetes 2000: Advances in monitoring. RN 58(3):37–44, 1995.

GLUCOSE TOLERANCE TEST (GTT), BLOOD

Norm: (Serum levels):

		SI Units
Intravenous GTT		
Fasting	70–105 mg/dl	3.9–5.8 mmol/L
5 minutes	300–400 mg/dl	16.5–22.0 mmol/L
30 minutes	180–200 mg/dl	9.9–11.0 mmol/L
1 hour	160–180 mg/dl	8.8–9.9 mmol/L
2 hours	≤140 mg/dl	≤7.7 mmol/L
≥3 hours	70–105 mg/dl	3.9–5.8 mmol/L
Oral GTT		
Fasting	70–105 mg/dl	3.9–5.8 mmol/L
30 minutes	150–160 mg/dl	8.3–8.8 mmol/L
1 hour	160–170 mg/dl	8.8–9.4 mmol/L
1.5 hours	145–155 mg/dl	8.0–8.5 mmol/L
2 hours	≤120 mg/dl	≤6.6 mmol/L
≥3 hours	70–105 mg/dl	3.9–5.8 mmol/L

Usage: Evaluation of clients with symptoms of diabetic complications, but with fasting glucose levels <140 mg/dl; and screening during pregnancy for gestational diabetes.

Increased Results (Decreased Glucose Tolerance): Acromegaly, aldosteronism (primary), central nervous system lesions, Cushing's syndrome, cystic fibrosis, diabetes mellitus, Forbes' disease (type-III glycogen deposition disease, debrancher deficiency, limit dextrinosis), gigantism, hemochromatosis, hepatic damage (severe), hyperlipidemia types III, IV, V), hyperthyroidism, Louis-Bar syndrome, myocardial infarction, neoplasm, pancreatic tumor (islet cell), pancreatitis (chronic), pheochromocytoma, pregnancy, uremia, and von Gierke's disease (type-I glycogen storage disease, glucose-6-phosphatase deficiency). Drugs include anabolic steroids, androgens, arginine, ascorbic acid, asparaginase, aspirin, baclofen, benzodiazepines, bisacodyl (prolonged use), chlorpromazine, chlorthalidone, cimetidine, clonidine, corticosteroids, corticotropin, dextran, dextrothyroxine, diazoxide, disopyramide phosphate, epinephrine, epinephrine bitartrate, epinephrine borate, epinephrine hydrochloride, estrogens, ethacrynic acid, furosemide, glucose infusions, haloperidol, imipramine, isoproterenol hydrochloride, heparin calcium, heparin sodium, hydralazine hydrochloride, indomethacin, isoniazid, levodopa, levothyroxine sodium/T4, Lithium carbonate, magnesium hydroxide (prolonged high doses), mercaptopurine, methimazole, methyldopa, methyldopate hydrochloride), nalidixic acid, nicotine, nicotinic acid, oral contraceptives, oxazepam, para-aminosalicylic acid, phenolphthalein, phenytoin, phenytoin sodium, progestins, promethazine hydrochloride, propranolol (in diabetics), propylthiouracil, reserpine, ritodrine hydrochloride, terbutaline sulfate, tetracyclines, thiazides, thyroglobulin, thyroid, tolbutamide (SMA methodology), and triamterene.

Decreased Results (Increased Glucose Tolerance): Addison's disease (oral GTT only), celiac disease (oral GTT only), hepatic disease, hypoglycemia, hypoparathyroidism (oral GTT only), hypothyroidism (oral GTT only), islet cell adenoma, malabsorption (oral GTT only), narcotic addiction, pancreatic islet cell hyperplasia, and sprue (oral GTT only). Drugs include allopurinol, amphetamines, beta-adrenergic blockers, caffeine, chlorpropamide, clofibrate, edetate disodium, ethanol, guanethidine sulfate, isoniazid, insulin, isocarboxazid, marijuana, nitrazepam, oral hypoglycemic agents, *para*-aminosalicyclic acid, pargyline hydrochloride, phenacetin, phenazopyridine, phenelzine sulfate, phenformin, propranolol (in diabetics), and tranylcypromine sulfate.

Description: Glucose is a monosaccharide formed from the digestion of carbohydrates and the conversion of glycogen by the liver and is the body's main source of cellular energy. The glucose tolerance test is most commonly used to aid in the diagnosis of diabetes mellitus. If blood glucose levels peak at higher than normal levels at 1 and 2 hours (after injection or ingestion of glucose) and are slower than normal to return to fasting levels, then diabetes mellitus is confirmed.

Professional Considerations:

1. Consent form NOT required.
2. Preparation:
   A. *See Client and family teaching.*
   B. Tubes: Gray-top × 6–7.
   C. Label each tube as shown in the table below.
3. Procedure:
   A. Begin the test between 7 and 9 A.M.
   B. Draw a 1-ml venous blood sample.
   C. *Intravenous GTT:* Inject a standardized intravenous solution of 0.5 g/kg body weight of 50% glucose or 50 ml of 50% glucose intravenously over 4 minutes.
   D. *Oral GTT:* Adults should completely ingest a solution containing 75–100 g of glucose within 5 minutes.

For children, the dosages are as follows:

<18 months:	2.5 g/kg.
18 months–3 years:	2.0 g/kg.
3 years–12 years:	1.75 g/kg.
>12 years:	1.25 g/kg (100-g limit).

E. Repeat step 3B at the following precise time intervals after infusion or ingestion of glucose is started.
   i. *Intravenous GTT:* 5 minutes, 30 minutes, 1 hour, 2 hours, and 3 hours.
   ii. *Oral GTT:* 30 minutes, 1 hour, 1.5 hours, 2 hours, and 3 hours.
F. If evaluating for postprandial hypoglycemia, draw an additional sample at 4 hours.

4. Postprocedure care:
   A. Current administration of medications known to affect the test results should be noted on the laboratory requisition.
   B. Send blood samples to the laboratory immediately or refrigerate them.
5. Client and family teaching:
   A. Eat a high-carbohydrate (200–300 g) diet for 3 days before testing.
   B. Avoid alcohol, coffee, and smoking for 36 hours before testing.
   C. Fast (except for water) for 10–16 hours.
   D. When possible, drugs affecting results should be stopped 3–21 days prior to the test.
   E. Insulin and oral hypoglycemic agents should be withheld the morning of the test.
   F. Avoid strenuous exercise for 8 hours before and after the test.
   G. Because the test requires multiple blood samples, suggest bringing a book or other quiet diversion to the test, because it usually requires a minimum of 3 hours.
   H. Alert the client to the symptoms of hypoglycemia and tell him or her to report these symptoms immediately.
6. Factors that affect results:
   A. No eating, smoking, or exercise is permitted during the testing period. Caffeine interferes with the accuracy of the results.

Tube No.	Intravenous GTT	Oral GTT
1	Fasting	Fasting
2	5 minutes	30 minutes
3	30 minutes	1 hour
4	1 hour	1.5 hours
5	2 hours	2 hours
6	3 hours	3 hours
7	4 hours	4 hours

B. Water may be given to help ease the collection of urine specimens.

C. Failure to adhere to a high-carbohydrate diet for 3 days prior to the test may produce abnormally increased results.

D. Stresses due to acute illness, pregnancy, or surgery invalidate the results.

E. Slight increases are normal in clients over age 50 (up to 1 mg/dl per year of age over 50).

F. When the glucose oxidase/peroxidase procedure is used, falsely decreased glucose values may occur when the client has recently taken acetaminophen or oxycodone.

7. Other data:

A. This test usually takes 3–5 hours.

B. 10 ml of urine for glucose measurement may also be collected at the same time as the blood samples.

C. The intravenous glucose tolerance testing method is recommended for clients who may have impaired or erratic intestinal absorption of glucose.

D. The oral glucose tolerance test has been shown to be unreliable for use in the evaluation of reactive hypoglycemia.

E. In a client with non-insulin dependent diabetes (Type I), fasting serum glucose levels may be within normal range, but insufficient secretion of insulin after ingestion of carbohydrates causes serum glucose to increase sharply and return to normal slowly.

F. If a client develops severe hypoglycemia during the test, draw a blood sample, record the time on the laboratory requisition, and discontinue the test. Have the client ingest an oral form of glucose or administer intravenous glucose according to the physician's orders.

Bibliography:

Pettitt DJ, Bennett PH, Hanson RL, et al.: Comparison of World Health Organization and National Diabetes Data Group procedures to detect abnormalities of glucose tolerance during pregnancy. Diab Care 17(11):1264–1268, 1994.

Rowe RE, Leech NJ, Finegood DT, McCulloch DK: Retrograde versus antegrade cannulation in the intravenous glucose tolerance test. Diabetes Res Clin Prac 25(2):131–136, 1994.

GLUCOSE, 2-HOUR POSTPRANDIAL, SERUM

Norm:

		SI Units
Newborn–50 years	65–140 mg/dl	3.6–7.7 mmol/L
50–60 years	65–150 mg/dl	3.6–8.3 mmol/L
>60 years	65–160 mg/dl	3.6–8.8 mmol/L

Usage: Screening for diabetes mellitus and assessing control of hyperglycemia.

Increased: Acromegaly, anoxia, anxiety, brain tumor, cirrhosis, convulsive disorders, Cushing's disease, Cushing's syndrome, diabetes mellitus, dumping syndrome (following gastrectomy), hepatic disease (chronic), hyperlipoproteinemia, hyperthyroidism, infarction (myocardial, cerebral), lipoproteinemias, malnutrition, malignancy, nephrotic syndrome, pancreatitis, pheochromocytoma, preeclampsia, pregnancy, sepsis, and stress (physical, emotional). Drugs include: (*see Glucose, Blood*).

Decreased: Addison's disease, adrenal insufficiency, anterior pituitary insufficiency, congenital adrenal hyperplasia, hepatic insufficiency, hyperinsulinism, hypoglycemia, hypopituitarism, hypothyroidism, insulinoma, islet cell adenoma, malabsorption syndrome, myxedema, steatorrhea, and von Gierke's disease. Drugs include: (*see Glucose, Blood*).

Description: The 2-hour postprandial glucose test is the measurement of serum glucose 2 hours from the beginning of a meal containing a specific amount of carbohydrate. In normal clients, glucose should return to fasting levels within 2 hours after the ingestion of the test meal.

Professional Considerations:

1. Consent form NOT required.
2. Preparation:
   A. *See Client and family teaching.*
   B. Tube: Gray-top, and test meal.
3. Procedure:
   A. Draw a 5-ml blood sample 2 hours after beginning ingestion of the designated test meal.
4. Postprocedure care:
   A. Refrigerate specimens not sent to the laboratory within 1 hour.

5. Client and family teaching:
   A. Eat a high-carbohydrate (200–300 g) diet for 3 days prior to the test.
   B. Fast (except for water) for 8–12 hours and abstain from alcohol for 36 hours prior to the test.
   C. When possible, drugs affecting the results should be stopped 3–21 days prior to the test.
   D. Insulin and oral hypoglycemic agents should be withheld the morning of the test.
   E. Eat a meal containing 75–100 g of carbohydrate within 20 minutes during the testing period.
   F. Avoid strenuous activity, caffeine, and nicotine after the meal, until the sample is drawn.
6. Factors that affect results:
   A. Falsely increased values may occur with strenuous activity, inhalation of nicotine, or ingestion of caffeine during the test.
   B. Falsely decreased glucose values may occur with acetaminophen and oxycodone when the glucose oxidase/peroxidase procedure is used.
   C. Stresses due to acute illness, infection, pregnancy, or surgery invalidate the results.
7. Other data:
   A. An abnormally elevated test indicates the need for a glucose tolerance test.

Bibliography:

Anderson JW, O'Neal DS, Riddell-Mason S, et al.: Postprandial serum glucose, insulin, and lipoprotein responses to high- and low-fiber diets. Metab Clin Exp *44*(7):848–854, 1995.

GLUTETHIMIDE, BLOOD

Norm:

		SI Units
Therapeutic	2–6 µg/ml	9–28 µmol/L
Toxic level	>10 µg/ml	>45 µmol/L
Panic level	>30 µg/ml	>135 µmol/L

Overdose Symptoms and Treatment:

Symptoms: Central nervous system depression, cerebral edema, hypotension, paralysis, respiratory depression, spasticity, and tachycardia. Death may occur at doses over 30 µg/ml.

Treatment:

Gastric lavage of water and caster oil in a 1:1 mix, because glutethimide is soluble in lipids. Hemodialysis will NOT, but hemoperfusion WILL, remove glutethimide.

Usage: Glutethimide abuse and glutethimide overdose.

Description: Glutethimide is a schedule-III, piperidine derivative, nonbarbiturate sedative-hypnotic with actions similar to barbiturates used for temporary insomnia, preoperative sedation, and during stage 1 of labor. It is primarily stored in fat tissue, hydroxylized in the liver, and excreted primarily by the kidneys, with a biphasic half-life of 5–22 hours.

Professional Considerations:

1. Consent form NOT required.
2. Preparation:
   A. Tube: Red-top, red/gray-top, or gold-top, black-top, or lavender-top.
   B. MAY be drawn during hemodialysis.
3. Procedure:
   A. Draw a 7-ml blood sample.
4. Postprocedure care:
   A. Observe closely for symptoms of overdose. This includes continuous ECG and airway monitoring, frequent neurologic checks, and vital sign measurement every 15–60 minutes.
5. Client and family teaching:
   A. Be alert for symptoms of overdose (see 4A, above) and seek medical attention if they occur.
   B. Refer clients with intentional overdose for crisis intervention.
   C. Referrals to appropriate rehabilitation centers and therapeutic community programs should be offered to all addicted clients who may be interested.
6. Factors that affect results:
   A. Serial measurements for glutethimide are recommended due to the variable release of the drug from adipose tissue.
7. Other data:
   A. None.

Bibliography:

Pons G, Rey E, Matheson I: Excretion of psychoactive drugs into breast milk: Pharmacokinetic principles and recommendations. Clin Pharmacokinet *27*(4):270–289, 1994.

GLYCOSYLATED HEMOGLOBIN
(GHB, GLYCOHEMOGLOBIN, Hb A₁a, Hb A₁b, Hb A₁c), BLOOD

Norm:

	Percentage of Total Hb
Total of Hb A_1a, Hb A_1b, and Hb A_1c	5.5–8.8
Diabetes under control	7.5–11.4
Diabetes less well controlled	11.5–15
Diabetes out of control	>15
Ketoacidosis	14.3–20
High-performance liquid chromatography	
Hb A_1a	1.8
Hb A_1b	0.8
Hb A_1c	3.5–6.0

Increased: Diabetes mellitus, glycosuria, and hyperglycemia.

Decreased: See 6C, below, *Factors that affect results.*

Description: Glycosylated-hemoglobin is blood glucose bound to hemoglobin (Hb) and includes forms Hb A_1a, Hb A_1b, and Hb A_1c. Hb A_1c is formed as hemoglobin, is gradually glycosylated throughout the 120-day red blood cell lifespan, and forms the largest portion of the three glycosylated Hb fractions. The amount of glycosylated hemoglobin found and stored in erythrocytes depends on the amount of glucose available. Hb A_1c is a reflection of how well blood glucose levels have been controlled for up to the prior 4 months. Hyperglycemia in diabetics is usually a cause of an increase in Hb A_1c.

Professional Considerations:

1. Consent form NOT required.
2. Preparation:
   A. Tube: Lavender-top, green-top, or gray-top.
3. Procedure:
   A. Draw a 5-ml blood sample.
   B. Invert the tube gently several times to mix the sample.
4. Postprocedure care:
   A. Send the specimen to the laboratory for prompt spinning.
5. Client and family teaching:
   A. The test evaluates the effectiveness of diabetes therapy over a period of several months, so more samples will be needed in the future.
   B. The client should maintain his or her prescribed medication or diet regimen between physician visits.
6. Factors that affect results:
   A. Reject hemolyzed specimens.

B. Falsely increased values may be due to fetal-maternal transfusion, hemodialysis, hereditary persistence of fetal hemoglobin, neonates, and pregnancy.
C. Falsely decreased values may be due to anemia (hemolytic, pernicious, sickle cell); chronic loss of blood; effects of splenectomy; renal failure (chronic); and thalassemias.
7. Other data:
   A. Glycosylated hemoglobin *cannot* be used to monitor control of diabetic clients with chronic renal failure, as levels are significantly lower due to shortened erythrocyte survival.

Bibliography:

Anonymous: The relationship of glycemic exposure (Hb A_1c) to the risk of development and progression of retinopathy in the Diabetes Control and Complications Trial. Diabet *44*(8):968–983, 1995.

Boehm S, Sclenk EA, Raleigh E, et al.: Behavioral analysis and behavioral strategies to improve self-management of type II diabetes. Clin Nurs Res *2*(3):327–344, 1993.

Hamwi A, Schweiger CR, Veitl M, Schmid R: Quantitative measurement of Hb A_1c by an immunoturbidimetric assay compared to a standard HPLC method. Amer J Clin Path *104*(1):89–95, 1995.

GONORRHOEAE CULTURE
(see Genital, Neisseria Gonorrhoeae, Culture)

GRAM STAIN, DIAGNOSTIC

Norm:

Body fluid, drainage, or wound:
Interpretation required.
Urine: No organisms detected.

Usage:

Diagnostic: Cough (sputum sample), effusion (abdominal or pleural), empyema, gonorrhea, impetigo, legionella, tuberculosis, and wounds.

Sputum: Cough (productive), fever, infections, and pneumonia.

Urine: Cystitis and urethritis.

Description: Gram-staining divides bacteria into two groups according to their staining properties: gram-negative and gram-positive. The staining involves placing drops of crystal violet dye onto the specimen sample, washing off the violet stain, and flooding the smear with an iodine solution followed by a 95% alcohol solution. Gram-positive cells remain blue, and gram-negative cells are decolorized by the alcohol. The specimen is then stained with a red dye called safranin, which colors the gram-positive cells red and leaves the gram-negative cells appearing purple. The cell wall structure is the basis of the Gram reaction. Gram-staining of specimens aids in decision making for early, broad-spectrum antibiotic therapy.

Professional Considerations:

1. Consent form NOT required.
2. Preparation:
   A. *Diagnostic:* Obtain a sterile container or swab.
   B. *Sputum:* Obtain a sterile sputum container or suction tubing, suction source, and sputum trap.
   C. *Urine:* Obtain a sterile container and clean-catch urine specimen collection kit, or a straight catheter or a syringe and needle if the specimen will be collected from an indwelling catheter.
   D. *See Client and family teaching.*
3. Procedure:
   A. *Diagnostic:*
      i. Obtain the specimen using a sterile technique and a sterile container or swab.
      ii. Avoid contamination of the sample with surrounding tissue.
   B. *Sputum:*
      i. Collect an early-morning sputum sample into a sterile sputum container.
      ii. Specimens are of best quality when obtained by suctioning them directly into a sputum trap.
      iii. For expelled specimens, have the

client sit up, take two or three deep breaths without fully exhaling each, then cough expulsively to mobilize the sputum from the respiratory tract directly into the sterile specimen container.
   C. The clean-catch urine technique must be used to decrease the risk of specimen contamination. *See clean-catch collection instructions in the test Body Fluid, Routine, Culture.*
4. Postprocedure care:
   A. Write the specimen source, the diagnosis, and recent antibiotic therapy on the laboratory requisition.
   B. Place the specimen in the refrigerator if not delivered to microbiology immediately after collection.
5. Client and family teaching:
   A. *Sputum:* Cough the specimen directly into the container and avoid holding the sputum in the mouth. Deep coughs are necessary to produce sputum, rather than saliva. To produce the proper specimen, take several breaths in, without fully exhaling each, then expel sputum with a "cascade cough."
   B. *Urine: See clean-catch collection instructions in the test Body Fluid, Routine, Culture.*
6. Factors that affect results:
   A. Epithelial cells will appear in the specimen if it is contaminated with mucosal surfaces.
   B. Saliva contamination of sputum specimens invalidates the results.
7. Other data:
   A. Gram-staining is not useful for identifying species of bacteria, but can be suggestive of certain broad species.
   B. A culture and sensitivity study of the specimen should also be performed to confirm the diagnosis and proper choice of antibiotic.

Bibliography:

Sadeghi E, Matlow A, MacLusky I, et al.: Utility of gram stain in evaluation of sputa from patients with cystic fibrosis. J Clin Microbiol *32*(1):54–58, 1994.

Vincent MT, Goldman BS: Anaerobic lung infections. Am Fam Phys *49*(8):1815–1820, 1994.

GRANULOCYTE, BLOOD
(see Differential Leukocyte Count, Peripheral Blood)

GROWTH HORMONE (SOMATOTROPIN, GH), BLOOD

Norm:

		SI Units
Adults, female	<10 ng/ml	<440 pmol/L
>Age 60	1–14 ng/ml	44–616 pmol/L

		SI Units
Adults, male	≤5 ng/ml	≤220 pmol/L
>Age 60	0.4–10 ng/ml	18–440 pmol/L
Children		
Cord blood	10–50 ng/ml	440–2200 pmol/L
Newborn	15–40 ng/ml	660–1760 pmol/L
Child	<20 ng/ml	<880 pmol/L

Increased: Acromegaly, anorexia nervosa, deep sleep states, infants, gigantism, hypoglycemia, hyperpituitarism, starvation, and surgery. Drugs include arginine, beta blockers, estrogens, glucagon, levodopa, and oral contraceptives.

Decreased: Congenital growth hormone deficiency, congenital pituitary hypoplasia, dwarfism, failure to thrive, growth hormone deficiency, hyperglycemia, hypothalamic degeneration, hypopituitarism, lesion (pituitary or hypothalamus), and pituitary fibrosis or calcification. Drugs include corticosteroids and phenothiazines.

Description: Growth hormone (GH) is a polypeptide anterior pituitary hormone essential for bodily growth. GH synthesis and release is controlled by the hypothalamus through growth hormone releasing factor (GHRF) and growth hormone release-inhibiting hormone (GHRIH). GH stimulates the production of RNA, protein synthesis, and mobilizes fatty acids and insulin. It is influenced by several drugs, as well as exercise and stress.

Professional Considerations:

1. Consent form NOT required.
2. Preparation:
   A. *See Client and family teaching.*
   B. Tube: Red-top, red/gray-top, or gold-top.
   C. Have the client recline for 30 minutes prior to sampling.
3. Procedure:
   A. Draw a 1-ml blood sample.
4. Postprocedure care:
   A. Write the collection time and client's recent activity (sleeping, eating, resting, walking) on the laboratory requisition.
   B. Current administration of corticosteroids or phenothiazines should be noted on the laboratory requisition.
   C. Transport the specimen to the laboratory immediately. The serum should be separated into a plastic container and frozen until testing.

5. Client and family teaching:
   A. Fast and limit physical activity for 10–12 hours before the test.
   B. A second blood sample may have to be drawn the next day for comparison to the first sample.
6. Factors that affect results:
   A. Reject specimens if the client had a radioactive scan within the prior 48 hours.
   B. Growth hormone in serum samples is unstable at room temperature.
7. Other data:
   A. Serial measurements are recommended, due to the episodic release of growth hormone.
   B. This test may be performed as part of a GH-stimulation test, using arginine, glucose, glucagon, levodopa, insulin-induced hypoglycemia, or other methods.

Bibliography:

Procopio M, Invitti C, Maccario M, et al.: Effect of arginine and pyridostigmine on the GHRH-induced GH rise in obesity and Cushing's syndrome. Int J Obes Met Dis *19*(2):108–112, 1995.

Thakore JH, Dinan TG: Diurnal variation of growth hormone responses to acutely administered dexamethasone in healthy male volunteers. Horm Metab Res *27*(1):23–25, 1995.

Trumper BG, Reschke K, Molling J: Circadian variation of insulin requirement in insulin dependent diabetes mellitus: The relationship between circadian change in insulin demand and diurnal patterns of growth hormone, cortisol and glucagon during euglycemia. Horm Metab Res *27*(3):141–147, 1995.

GUTHRIE TEST FOR PHENYLKETONURIA, DIAGNOSTIC

Norm: Negative.

Usage: Diagnosis of phenylketonuria in newborn.

Description: Phenylketonuria (PKU) is an inherited metabolic disorder that results in mental retardation. Infants born with PKU lack the liver enzyme phenylalanine hydroxylase, which converts phenylalanine to tyrosine, an essential amino acid necessary for growth. As phenylalanine accumulates in the body, it is eventually spilled into the urine. If ingested, phenylalanine is not restricted and progressive mental retardation results.

PKU testing is mandatory in most states of the United States. The Guthrie test consists of placing several drops of the infant's blood on a special culture medium seeded with *Bacillus subtilis,* a bacteria that requires phenylalanine for growth. If colonies of the bacteria begin to grow around the blood samples, the test is positive for the possibility of PKU. Further serum and urine testing are necessary to confirm the diagnosis.

Professional Considerations:

1. Consent form NOT required.
2. Preparation:
   A. Obtain an identification card, an alcohol wipe, a lancet, filter paper, and a Band-Aid.
   B. Write the infant's name or identification number, date of birth, and date of first feeding on the identification card.
3. Procedure:
   A. Prewarming the heel is not necessary.
   B. Avoid puncturing over previous puncture sites or puncturing the posterior heel curvature.
   C. Cleanse an area on the medial or lateral plantar surface of the heel with 70% alcohol and allow it to dry.
   D. Using a 2.5-mm lancet, puncture the heel until a free flow of blood is obtained and collect 3 drops of blood (1 in each circle) on the filter paper.
4. Postprocedure care:
   A. Place pressure on the heel for 5–10 minutes and leave the site open to the air, to heal.
   B. Place the filter paper in a sealed, plastic bag and send it to the laboratory along with the completed identification card and laboratory requisition.
5. Client and family teaching:
   A. Inform the infant's parents immediately if positive results are obtained. Provide dietary counseling immediately.
6. Factors that affect results:
   A. The infant must have had 2–3 days of feedings of human or cow's milk. Inadequate protein intake by the infant can cause false-negative results.
   B. Avoid milking the heel.
   C. A positive test may also result from hepatic disease, galactosemia, or delayed development of certain enzyme systems.
7. Other data:
   A. If PKU blood testing is not performed prior to discharge from the hospital, a urine Phenistix test should be performed at the first well-baby checkup.

Bibliography:

Eisensmith RC, Goltsov AA, Woo SL: A simple, rapid, and highly informative PCR-based procedure for prenatal diagnosis and carrier screening of phenylketonuria. Prenat Diagn *14*(12):1113–1118, 1994.
Galloway A, Stevenson J: Audit improves neonatal (Guthrie) screening programme [letter; comment]. BMJ *309*(6958):878, 1994.

GYNECOLOGIC SONOGRAM (GYNECOLOGIC ECHOGRAM, GYNECOLOGIC SONOGRAM, PELVIC SONOGRAM, PELVIC ULTRASOUND), DIAGNOSTIC

Norm: Normal size, shape, and position of pelvic structures (uterus, ovaries, fallopian tubes); negative for cyst, foreign body, stones, or tumor.

Usage: Evaluation of the size, shape, and position of bladder, ovaries, vagina, and uterus; detection of pelvic cyst, ectopic pregnancy, endometrial abnormalities, foreign body (such as intrauterine device), hydatidiform mole, stones, or masses; differentiation of solid from liquid masses; infertility work-up (monitoring the ovarian follicle or screening for uterine cavity abnormalities); monitoring of pelvic tumor response to therapy; and transvaginal sonography has an added advantage of providing information regarding the cervical and uterine vascular supplies.

Description: Gynecologic sonography (ultrasound) is the evaluation of the pelvic structures via the creation of an oscilloscopic picture from the echoes of high-frequency sound waves passing over the pelvic area (acoustic imaging). The time required for the ultrasonic beam to be reflected back to the transducer from differing densities of tissue is converted by a computer to an electrical impulse displayed on an oscilloscopic screen to create a three-dimensional picture of the pelvic contents. Both transabdominal and transvaginal methods may be used. Traditional transabdominal methods are more helpful for the evaluation of large cysts and fibroids, while the newer, transvaginal method is more specific for ruling out ectopic pregnancy or evaluating endometrial abnormalities. Transvaginal methods have also been shown to provide better depictions of the fine structures and individual organs of the pelvic cavity, and are better tolerated by the subject, because a full bladder is not required. Gynecologic ultrasound may be used as an adjunct to the pelvic bimanual exam in women who are at risk for ovarian cancer.

Professional Considerations:

1. Consent form NOT required.
2. Preparation:
   A. This test should be performed before intestinal barium tests, or after the barium is cleared from the system.
   B. The client should disrobe below the waist or wear a gown.
   C. Obtain ultrasonic gel.
   D. *See Client and family teaching.*
3. Procedure:
   A. *Transabdominal method:*
      i. The client is positioned supine in bed, or on a procedure table.
      ii. The pelvic area is covered with ultrasonic gel and a lubricated transducer is passed slowly and firmly over the lower abdomen at a variety of angles and at 1- to 2-cm intervals.
      iii. The client may be repositioned to a right or slight left decubitus position in order to obtain better pictures of the ovaries or the adnexal area.
      iv. A water enema may be administered if more specific evaluation of the adnexal area is required.
      v. Photographs are taken of the oscilloscopic pictures.
      vi. The procedure takes less than 30 minutes.
   B. *Transvaginal method:*
      i. The client is positioned in the dorsal lithotomy position or on a conventional examination table, with a pillow supporting the hips.
      ii. A sterile, nonreservoir condom containing ultrasonic gel is placed over the transducer, and air bubbles are worked out of it. The condom is then coated with a sterile lubricant.
      iii. The client, or the examiner, may insert the transducer into the vagina until it touches the posterior or anterior walls.
      iv. The transducer is rotated 90 degrees against the vaginal vault to obtain sagittal and coronal scans of the uterus. The probe is pulled

back 2–3 cm to examine the cervix. Using identified landmarks, the ovaries and fallopian tubes are pictured. All possible angles are scanned. The client may be repositioned slightly to facilitate imaging.

4. Postprocedure care:
   A. Remove the lubricant from the skin.
   B. Allow the client to void.
   C. Disinfect the transducer probe by soaking in glutaraldehyde solution for 10 minutes.
5. Client and family teaching:
   A. The procedure is painless and carries no risks.
   B. If a transabdominal ultrasound is to be performed, drink 1 quart of water during the hour prior to the test, and refrain from voiding during this time. The full bladder provides an acoustic window for imaging.
   C. If a transvaginal ultrasound is to be performed, fast from fluids for 4 hours prior to the procedure, and void just prior to the procedure.
6. Factors that affect results:
   A. Dehydration interferes with adequate contrast between organs and body fluids.
   B. Intestinal barium or gas obscures results by preventing proper transmission and deflection of the high-frequency sound waves. This problem is particularly pronounced with pelvic sonogram, due to the proximity of the large bowel.
   C. The more abdominal fat present, the greater the attenuation (reduction in sound wave amplitude and intensity), which interferes with the clarity of the transabdominal picture.
   D. Transvaginal techniques are not adequate for very large masses.
7. Other data:
   A. Further studies may include tomography or other radiographic imaging.

Bibliography:

Fennell L: Midwives and ultrasound. Mod Midwifery *5*(1):36–37, 1995.
Gegor CL: Third-trimester ultrasound for nurse-midwives. J Nurse Midwifery *38*(2, Suppl):49S–61S, 1993.

HAGEMAN FACTOR, BLOOD

(see Factor XII, Blood)

HALOPERIDOL, SERUM

Norm: Negative.

Therapeutic level	3–20 µg/L
Panic level	>25 µg/L

Panic Level Symptoms and Treatment:

Symptoms: Hypotension, sedation with respiratory depression severe enough to cause a shocklike state, and severe extrapyramidal neuromuscular reactions (dystonia, hyperreflexia, and oculogyric crises).

Treatment:

Ipecac may be used to induce vomiting, with due regard for haloperidol's antiemetic properties and aspiration hazards. Induction of vomiting is contraindicated in clients with no gag reflex or with central nervous system depression or excitation. Gastric lavage may also be used, followed by activated charcoal and saline cathartics. Hemodialysis and peritoneal dialysis will NOT remove haloperidol.

B. Extrapyramidal effects occur frequently during the first few days and are dose related, although they can occur even with small doses.

C. Diphenhydramine may interfere with some methods used to measure haloperidol.

Bibliography:

Malt UF, Nystad R, Bache T, et al.: Effectiveness of zuclopenthixol compared with haloperidol in the treatment of behavioural disturbances in learning disabled patients. Br J Psychi *166*(3):374–377, 1995.

Stone CK, Garve DL, Griffith J, et al.: Further evidence of a dose-response threshold for haloperidol in psychosis. Amer J Psych *152*(8):1210–1212, 1995.

Usage: Periodic monitoring for therapeutic levels in clients receiving haloperidol. Screening for haloperidol toxicity or overdose.

Description: Haloperidol is a butyrophenone that acts as an antipsychotic, sedative, and antiemetic. It depresses the central nervous system, directly acts on the chemoreceptor trigger zone (CTZ), and inhibits catecholamines. This drug is used in agitation, schizophrenia, the manic phase of manic-depressive psychosis, and to manage vocal utterances in Gilles de la Tourette's syndrome. It is absorbed in the gastrointestinal tract, concentrates in the liver, and is excreted in the urine and in bile.

Professional Considerations:

1. Consent form NOT required.
2. Preparation:
   A. Tube: Red-top, red/gray-top, or gold-top.
   B. May require assistance if the client is uncooperative.
   C. MAY be drawn during hemodialysis.
3. Procedure:
   A. Obtain a 3-ml blood sample.
4. Postprocedure care:
   A. Refrigerate the specimen.
5. Client and family teaching:
   A. For periodic monitoring, it is not necessary to restrict food or fluids.
   B. If activated charcoal was given for elevated levels, the client should drink 4–6 glasses of water each day for 2 days to prevent constipation. The activated charcoal will also cause stools to be black for a few days.
6. Factors that affect results:
   A. Therapeutic norms are not well established; laboratory values vary among clients on equal doses.
7. Other data:
   A. For consistency, collect the specimen at least 12 hours after the last dose (trough level).

HAM TEST (ACIDIFIED SERUM TEST), BLOOD

Norm: Negative <5% lysis.

Usage: Paroxysmal nocturnal hemoglobinuria (PNH) or the PNH abnormality.

Description: For the Ham test, a blood sample is taken from the client, mixed with his or her own serum and with a sample of serum from an ABO-compatible donor, acidified, and examined for lysis. The presence of lysis in the client's own serum is definitive in the diagnosis of paroxysmal nocturnal hemoglobinuria (PNH). This rare condition, in which hemoglobin is found in the urine during and after sleep, is thought to be related to red blood cell hypersensitivity to higher levels of carbon dioxide and a resulting decrease in the plasma pH, although the cause of this disease is unknown.

Professional Considerations:

1. Consent form NOT required.
2. Preparation:
   A. Tube: Lavender-top.
3. Procedure:
   A. Draw a 7-ml blood sample.
4. Postprocedure care:
   A. Defibrinate the sample immediately.
5. Client and family teaching:
   A. Results are normally available within 24 hours.
6. Factors that affect results:
   A. Hemolysis of the specimen invalidates results.
   B. Transfusion of red blood cells within the last 3 weeks may cause false-negative results.
   C. False-positives may occur in dyserythropoietic anemia, spherocytosis, aplastic anemia, and leukemia.
7. Other data:
   A. PNH has been a candidate for myeloproliferative disease occurring in

55–65% of cases of myeloid metaplasia and primary myelofibrosis.

Bibliography:

Rafaloska J, Dziewulska D, Szyluk B, et al.: Morphological picture in paroxysmal nocturnal hemoglobinuria: Case report. Fol Neuro *32*(3):161–166, 1994.

Webb DI, Bundtzen JL: The effect of granulocyte-macrophage colony stimulating factor on paroxysmal nocturnal hemoglobinuria: A case report. Alaska Med *35*(3):216–217, 224, 1993.

HAPTOGLOBIN (Hp), SERUM

Norm:

			SI Units
Adult	40–240 mg/dl		0.4–2.40 g/L
Newborn	5–48 mg/dl		0.05–4.8 g/L

Usage: Serves as an index of hemolysis, investigates hemolytic transfusion reactions, identifies suspected ahaptoglobinemia, and helps establish proof of paternity.

Increased: Abscess, burns, acute rheumatic disease, arterial disease, biliary obstruction, infection, inflammation, malignancies, myocardial infarction, peptic ulcer, pneumonia, pregnancy tissue necrosis, tuberculosis, and ulcerative colitis. Drugs include corticosteroids and oral contraceptives.

Decreased: Ahaptoglobinemia, artificial heart valve implantation, G-6-PD deficiency, hemolysis (intravascular or extravascular), hemolytic anemia, liver disease, malarial infestation, megaloblastic anemia, mononucleosis (infectious), sickle cell anemia, systemic lupus erythematosus (SLE), thalassemia, tissue hemorrhage, and transfusion reaction (hemolytic). Drugs include estrogens.

Description: Haptoglobin is an alpha$_2$ globulin that combines with hemoglobin that has been released due to red blood cell destruction. Its primary function is to preserve the body's iron stores from being excreted in the urine. Haptoglobin can be depleted rapidly by any condition that destroys red blood cells.

Professional Considerations:

1. Consent form NOT required.
2. Preparation:
   A. Tube: Red-top, red/gray-top, or gold-top.
3. Procedure:
   A. Draw a 1-ml blood sample.
4. Postprocedure care:
   A. Report abnormal vital signs on the laboratory requisition.
   B. Deliver the specimen to the laboratory immediately, taking care not to shake it.
5. Client and family teaching:
   A. Results may not be available for several days.
   B. Call the physician if noting symptoms of hemolysis, which include back pain, chills, distended neck veins, fever, flushing, hypotension, tachycardia, and tachypnea.
6. Factors that affect results:
   A. Hemolysis of the specimen invalidates results.
   B. Specimen contact with peroxidase or other oxidants may falsely elevate the result.
7. Other data:
   A. Do not consider this test alone for diagnosing.
   B. Haptoglobin levels rise to normal by age 4 months.
   C. In about 1% of the population (4% of blacks), haptoglobin is permanently absent (congenital ahaptoglobinemia).

Bibliography:

Delanghe JR, Duprez DA, De Buyzere ML, et al.: Refractory hypertension is associated with the haptoglobin 2–2 phenotype. J Cardio Risk *2*(2):131–136, 1995.

Kajio H, Kobayashi T, Nakanishi K, et al.: Relationship between insulin-dependent diabetes mellitus (IDDM) and non-insulin-dependent diabetes mellitus: Beta-cell function, islet cell antibody, and haptoglobin in parents of IDDM patients. Metab Clin Exp *44*(7):869–875, 1995.

HB, BLOOD
(see Hemoglobin, Blood)

HBDH
(see Hydroxybutyrate Dehydrogenase, Blood)

HCO$_3$, SERUM
(see Bicarbonate, Serum)

HCT, BLOOD
(see Hematocrit, Blood)

HEAD-UP TILT TABLE TEST
(see Tilt Table Test, Diagnostic)

HEARING TEST FOR LOUDNESS—RECRUITMENT, DIAGNOSTIC
(see Audiometry Test, Diagnostic)

HEART SCAN, DIAGNOSTIC

Norm:

Technetium-99m Stannous Pyrophosphate (PYP): No evidence of myocardial ischemia.

Thallium-201: No evidence of myocardial ischemia or infarction.

Multigated Blood Pool Study (MUGA): Normal (55–65%) ejection fraction, symmetrical contraction of the left ventricle.

Nitroglycerin MUGA: Normal (55–65%) ejection fraction, symmetrical contraction of the left ventricle.

Sestamibi or Sestamibi-Dipyridamole Exercise Testing and Scan: No evidence of diminished perfusion, ischemia, or infarction.

Usage: Aneurysm, angina, cardiomegaly, coronary artery disease, myocardial infarction, and presurgical evaluation.

Dipyridamole Injection: Replaces the treadmill portion of the test for clients with chronic lung disease, peripheral vascular disease, impaired mobility, medication therapy that prevents demonstration of maximal exercise effort (calcium channel blockers, beta blockers) or post-myocardial infarction risk stratification.

Description: Heart scan encompasses any of several noninvasive scans that involve radiopharmaceutical injection.

The *PYP* scan is used to determine the occurrence, extent, and prognosis of myocardial infarction. Technetium-99m stannous pyrophosphate is thought to combine with the calcium in damaged myocardial cells, forming a spot on the scan. Such spots appear within 12 hours of infarction, are most prominent 48–72 hours postinfarction, and disappear within 1 week. A spot that does not disappear indicates continued myocardial damage.

The *Thallium-201* scan is used to show myocardial perfusion, location, and extent of acute or chronic myocardial infarction, coronary artery disease, or effectiveness of angioplasty, angina therapy, or grafted coronary arteries. An analogue of potassium, this radionuclide is absorbed in healthy tissue while avoiding damaged tissue forming spots on the scan. Ischemic areas (eventually absorb isotope) can be differentiated from infarcted areas (never absorb isotope) by repeating the scan within 5 minutes. May be performed under stress. Thallium scans are often combined with dipyridamole administration (described below), because this causes greater thallium uptake and improved quality of images and accuracy of diagnoses. The combination is used for clients who are unable to perform exercise treadmill or bicycle testing in conjunction with their scan.

The *MUGA* scan is used to assess the function of the left ventricle and show myocardial wall abnormalities. Once the isotope is injected, the heart appears as a map with all four chambers and the great vessels visualized simultaneously. A series of images are taken during systole (low isotope in left ventricle) and diastole (high isotope in left ventricle). These can be shown like a movie or superimposed to show the left ventricular function, and the ejection fraction can be calculated. May be performed under stress.

The *Nitroglycerin* scan is an additional feature of the MUGA scan. Another series of images is taken to evaluate the effectiveness of sublingual nitroglycerin administration. May be performed under stress.

The *Sestamibi exercise testing and scan* is used to evaluate cardiac perfusion before and after a treadmill exercise test. Injected radiopharmaceutical, technetium-99m pertechnetate (sestamibi), is taken up by ischemic or infarcted cardiac cells that did not improve in perfusion with exercise and is seen as a "hot spot" in nuclear imaging.

The *Sestamibi-Dipyridamole stress test and scan* is used in clients who can not walk on a treadmill or pedal a bicycle, because of physical mobility limitations. Dipyridamole is an antiplatelet drug used in nuclear medicine for its coronary artery vasodilatory action. It causes increased endogenous adenosine levels, which causes an effect on the perfusion of the heart muscle similar to that of an exercise test. For this test, the cardiac perfusion is compared in scans taken before and after the tracer and dipyridamole injections. Because the areas that vasodilate can draw blood flow from less-perfused areas, the test can cause ischemia and infarction. Thus, this test carries specific risks related to the radiopharmaceutical administered and requires a cardiologist to be present in many institutions.

The *single-photon emission computed tomography (SPECT)* scan is a newer nuclear medicine procedure in which the radiopharmaceutical technetium-99m hexamethyl propylenamine oxime is injected intravenously. This substance decomposes and remains for several hours in the heart and other tissues, where it can be detected with the SPECT camera. The camera sends images to a computer that can reproduce visual images or "slices" of the brain along several planes. Advantages of SPECT imaging over older nuclear medicine scans are that it can produce clear, more accurate images.

Professional Considerations:

1. Consent form IS required.

Risks:

Persantine (dipyridamole): chest pain/angina, ECG changes, ischemia, including infarction, bronchospasm, nausea, vomiting, hypotension, headache, dyspnea, facial flushing.
Radiopharmaceutical or radiolabeled albumin: allergic reaction (itching, hives, rash, tight feeling in the throat, shortness of breath, bronchospasm, anaphylaxis, death).
Treadmill testing: cardiac ischemia, including myocardial infarction, dysrhythmias, hypotension, hypertension, dizziness.

Contraindications:

Clients who are unable to lie motionless for the scan; during pregnancy or breast-feeding; previous allergic reaction to radiopharmaceutical or radiolabeled albumin, if use is planned.

A. *Dipyridamole:* Previous allergy to dipyridamole; unstable cardiac status; allergy to aminophylline (which is used as an antidote to adverse effects of dipyridamole); Aminophylline or pentoxifylline taken within the last 48 hours; severe asthma or bronchospasm.

B. *Relative contraindications, dipyridamole:* Congestive heart failure, status/post-heart transplant, bilateral carotid artery disease, days 1–3 after acute myocardial infarction.

C. *Treadmill testing:* Active unstable angina, recent significant changes in ECG, alcohol intoxication, uncontrolled dysrhythmias, chest pain, acute infection, cardiac inflammation (myocarditis, pericarditis), acute congestive heart failure, coronary insufficiency syndrome, digitalis toxicity, heart blocks (2°, 3°), thrombophlebitis, recent pulmonary embolism, inability to walk on a treadmill or pedal a bicycle.

2. Preparation:

A. Assess for history of hypersensitivity to radioactive dyes.

B. Have emergency equipment readily available. This includes aminophylline to counteract the side effects of dipyridamole, if the dipyridamole test will be performed.

C. For scans conducted in conjunction with stress testing, obtain a baseline 12-lead ECG.

D. *See Client and family teaching.*

3. Procedure:

A. *PYP:* Technetium-99m stannouspyrophosphate (20 mCi) is injected 2–3 hours prior to the test. Images are taken from different angles, taking a total of 30–60 minutes.

B. *Thallium-201:* Resting imaging takes place within the first few hours of cardiac symptoms. The radionuclide is injected and scanning begins within 5 minutes. For stress scanning, an intravenous line is started, and a blood pressure cuff and ECG leads are attached. After 15 minutes on a treadmill or bicycle, radioactive thallium is injected; 15 minutes later, imaging occurs for 1 hour, with a repeat scan performed within the next 24 hours. Thallium-201 dose is 1.5–3 mCi.

C. *Thallium-dipyridamole:* ECG and

blood pressure are monitored continuously throughout this scan. After the resting image is taken and the radionuclide is injected, dipyridamole is injected intravenously over 4 minutes. Some clients may be asked to perform mild exercise, which improves blood flow through the coronary arteries, increases uptake of the thallium, and reduces the side effects of the dipyridamole. Thallium is then injected about 4 minutes later, when peak coronary blood flow is expected and the final scan is taken. Aminophylline may be infused prophylactically or in response to adverse side effects of the dipyridamole. The client may then return for redistribution imaging in about 4 hours.

D. *MUGA:* 15–20 mCi of technetium-99m pertechnetate is tagged to serum albumin or red blood cells; 1 minute after injection, imaging begins. The client should be in a supine position, although he or she may be asked to exercise. The procedure takes 1 hour.

E. *Nitroglycerin:* A cardiologist assesses a baseline MUGA scan, injects nitroglycerin, takes another scan, and repeats this procedure until blood pressure reaches desired level.

F. *Sestamibi exercise testing and scan:* After a 12-lead ECG machine is attached to chest electrodes, the nuclear medicine technician injects the tracer and completes a resting scan, which lasts approximately 30 minutes. The ECG and blood pressure are then measured continuously as the client completes the exercise portion of the test on a treadmill. Heart rate, blood pressure, and ECG are recorded every 1–2 minutes during each 3-minute stage. If vital signs and ECG have remained stable, the nuclear medicine technician then injects additional tracer 1 minute before the client comes off the treadmill. The final scan of another 30 minutes is then completed.

G. *Sestamibi-dipyridamole stress test and scan:* After a 12-lead ECG machine is attached to chest electrodes, the nuclear medicine technician injects the tracer and completes a resting scan, which lasts approximately 30 minutes. The client is instructed to perform isometric hand grips until dipyridamole injection to help prevent the drug's side effects. The ECG and blood pressure are then measured continuously as a dose of dipyridamole is injected over 4 minutes. 2–7 minutes later, the nuclear medicine technician injects the sestamibi tracer. The side effects of persantine may include chest pain, dysrhythmias, nausea, vomiting, bronchospasm, headache, flushing, or dizziness and hypotension. The side effects may be treated with intravenous aminophylline, which acts as an adenosine receptor agonist. 30 minutes after the tracer injection, the final scan is completed.

H. *Single-photon emission computed tomography (SPECT) scan:* The client is transported to the nuclear medicine department, positioned supine on the scanning table, and left to rest quietly for approximately 10 minutes. A radiopharmaceutical is injected intravenously and allowed to circulate. The SPECT scan is then taken while the client lies motionless.

4. Postprocedure care:
   A. Monitor the pulse, blood pressure, and respirations every 15 minutes × 2.
   B. For scans that involved stress testing or administration of dipyridamole, the client is monitored until vital signs and/or ECG return to baseline.

5. Client and family teaching:
   A. Do not take drugs or drink caffeine-containing beverages for 6 hours prior to testing (24 hours for the SPECT scan).
   B. Some tests take several hours. Bring reading material or other diversional activity.
   C. *PYP, Thallium-201, dipyridamole:* Fast for 4 hours prior to the test.
   D. *Dipyridamole:* Do not take drugs containing aminophylline for 48 hours prior to the test.
   E. *Thallium-201, MUGA, nitroglycerin:* Report fatigue, pain, or shortness of breath immediately, particularly if stress (exercise) is used.
   F. You may be asked to move into different positions during the scan.
   G. Drink plenty of fluids for 24 hours after the procedure.

6. Factors that affect results:
   A. Digitalis and quinidine alter contractility. Notation should be made on the chart.
   B. Bundle branch block, left ventricular hypertrophy, or hypokalemia.
   C. Thallium-201 scans may produce false-negative results in clients with single-vessel disease.
   D. MUGA does not give positive results for 24 hours following myocardial infarction (MI), so it cannot be used to diagnose acute MI.
   E. Radionuclides or radioactive tracers with long half-lives from recent scans will interfere with the quality of the images.

7. Other data:
   A. The larger the perfusion defect, the poorer the prognosis.
   B. Abnormalities of the heart scan may

indicate the need for further studies or cardiac catheterization.

C. Health care professionals working in a nuclear medicine area should wear a film badge at waist level (the level closest to the client).

D. Technetium half-life is 6 hours. Thallium half-life is 73 hours.

E. Health care professionals working in a nuclear medicine area must follow federal standards set by the Nuclear Regulatory Commission. These standards include precautions for handling the radioactive material and monitoring of potential radiation exposure.

F. *See also Stress/Exercise Test, Diagnostic; and Stress Test, Pharmacologic, Diagnostic.*

Bibliography:

Hademenos GJ, Dahlbom M, Hoffman EJ: Simultaneous dual-isotope technetium-99m/thallium-201 cardiac SPET imaging using a projection-dependent spilldown correction factor. Eur J Nucl Med *22*(5):465–472, 1995.

Hnatowich DJ: Is technetium-99m the radioisotope of choice for radioimmunoscintigraphy? J Nucl Biol Med *38*(Suppl 1):22–32, 1994.

Schmidt DH, Grade IJ, Port SC: IV dipyridamole-thallium myocardial perfusion imaging. Cardio (Oct): 95–104, 1990.

HEART SHUNT SCAN, DIAGNOSTIC

Norm: Normal pulmonary transit time and chamber-filling sequence.

Usage: Determines improper shunting of blood in heart disorders, especially in children.

Description: The heart shunt scan is an angiography study to examine the transit of a bolus of technetium-99m into the jugular vein. Images are taken to follow the bolus on its journey through the heart chambers to visualize any abnormal shunting of blood between chambers.

Professional Considerations:

1. Consent form IS required.

Risks:
Infection.

Contraindications:
During pregnancy or breast-feeding.

2. Preparation:
   A. Have emergency equipment readily available.

3. Procedure:
   A. With the client positioned in a 20-degree Fowler's position, radionuclide is injected into the external jugular vein.
   B. Scanning is performed for approximately 45 minutes.

4. Postprocedure care:
   A. Assess the venipuncture site for bleeding, hematoma.
   B. Observe the client carefully for up to 60 minutes after the study for a possible (anaphylactic) reaction to the radionuclide.
   C. Wear rubber gloves when discarding urine for 24 hours after the procedure. Wash the gloved hands with soap and water before removing the gloves. Wash the ungloved hands after the gloves have been removed.

5. Client and family teaching:
   A. Meticulously wash the hands with soap and water after each void × 24 hours.

6. Factors that affect results:
   A. None.

7. Other data:
   A. This test is specific for left-to-right shunt and right-to-left shunt.
   B. Health care professionals working in a nuclear medicine area should wear a film badge at waist level (the level closest to the client).
   C. Health care professionals working in a nuclear medicine area must follow federal standards set by the Nuclear Regulatory Commission. These standards include precautions for handling the radioactive material and monitoring of potential radiation exposure.
   D. Technetium half-life is 6 hours.

Bibliography:

Davis LP, Fink-Bennett D: Nuclear medicine in the acutely ill patient: II. Crit Care Clin *10*(2):383–400, 1994.

HEART SONOGRAM, DIAGNOSTIC
(see Echocardiogram, Diagnostic)

HEART ULTRASOUND
(see Echocardiogram, Diagnostic)

HEAVY METALS, BLOOD AND 24-HOUR URINE

Norm:

	Blood	SI units
Antimony	0.052 ± 0.019 μg/dl	4.35 ± 1.6 nmol/L
Arsenic	2–23 μg/L	0.03–0.31 μmol/L
Chronic poisoning	100–500 μg/L	1.33–6.65 μmol/L
Acute poisoning	600–9300 μg/L	7.98–124 μmol/L
Bismuth	0.1–3.5 μg/L	0.5–16.7 nmol/L
Cadmium		
Smokers	0.6–3.9 μg/L	5.3–34.7 nmol/L
Nonsmokers	0.3–1.2 μg/L	2.7–10.7 nmol/L
Toxic	100–3000 μg/L	0.9–26.7 μmol/L
Cobalt	0.11–0.45 μg/L	1.9–7.6 nmol/L
Copper		
Infants	20–70 μg/dl	3.1–11 μmol/L
Child 6 years	90–190 μg/dl	14.1–29.8 μmol/L
Child 12 years	80–160 μg/dl	12.6–25.1 μmol/L
Adult male	70–140 μg/dl	11–22 μmol/L
Adult female	80–155 μg/dl	12.6–24.3 μmol/L
Pregnant	118–302 μg/dl	18.5–47.4 μmol/L
Lead		
Child	<25 μg/dl	<1.21 μmol/L
Adult	<40 μg/dl	<1.93 μmol/L
Industry exposure	<60 μg/dL	<2.90 μmol/L
Toxic concentration	≥100 μg/dl	≥4.83 μmol/L
Toxic concentration in children	≥25 μg/dl	1.21 μmol/L
Mercury	0.6–59 μg/L	3–294 nmol/L
Non-fish eaters	<5 μg/L	<25 nmol/L
Selenium	58–234 μg/L	0.74–2.97 μmol/L
Thallium	<0.5 μg/dl	<24.5 nmol/L
Toxic concentration	10–800 μg/dl	0.5–39.1 μmol/L
Zinc	70–150 μg/dl	10.7–23 μmol/L

	24-Hour Urine	SI Units
Antimony	<10 μg/L	<82.1 μmol/L
Toxic concentration	>10 μg/L	>82.1 μmol/L
Arsenic	5–50 μg/L	0.067–0.665 μmol/L
Chronic poison	50–5000 μg/L	0.67–66.5 μmol/L
Acute poison	1000–20,000 μg/L	13.3–266 mmol/L
Bismuth	0.3–4.6 μg/L	1.4–22 nmol/L
Cadmium	0.5–4.7 μg/L	4.4–41.8 nmol/L
Industrial exposure	10–580 μg/L	0.09–5.16 μmol/L
Cobalt	1–2 μg/L	17–34 nmol/L
Copper	2–80 μg/L	0.03–1.26 μmol/L
Lead	<80 μg/L	<0.39 μmol/L
Industrial exposure	<120 μg/L	<0.58 μmol/L
Mercury		
Adult	<20 μg/L	<0.10 μmol/L
Toxic concentration	>150 μg/L	>0.75 μmol/L
Lethal concentration	>800 μg/L	>4 μmol/L

(continued)	24-Hour Urine	SI Units
Selenium	7–160 µg/L	0.09–2.03 µmol/L
Toxic concentration	>400 µg/L	>5.08 µmol/L
Thallium	<2 µg/L	<9.8 nmol/L
Toxic concentration	1–20 mg/L	4.9–97.8 µmol/L
Zinc	150–1200 µg/L	2.3–18.4 µmol/L
Toxic concentration	>1200 µg/L	>18.4 µmol/L

Toxic/Poisoning Symptoms and Treatment:

Symptoms:

Antimony: Vomiting.

Arsenic: Gastric pain, vomiting, diarrhea, convulsions, coma, and death in acute poisoning; and diarrhea, scaling and pigmentation of skin, hair loss, and peripheral neuropathy in chronic poisoning.

Bismuth: Weakness, decreased appetite, fever, halitosis, black gum line, rheumatic type pain, and renal damage.

Cadmium: Pneumonia, pulmonary edema, and cardiovascular collapse from inhalation; violent gastrointestinal symptoms from acute ingestion; and osteomalacia and renal dysfunction from chronic ingestion.

Cobalt: Thyroid gland hyperplasia, cardiomyopathy, nerve damage, and myxedema.

Copper: Nausea, vomiting, headache, diarrhea, and abdominal pain.

Lead: Anorexia, abdominal pain, vomiting, irritability, and apathy.

Mercury: Fatigue, headache, loss of memory, apathy, emotional instability, paresthesia, ataxia, deafness, dysarthria, visual deterioration, dysphagia, coma, and death.

Selenium: Garlic smell in breath and urine, metallic taste, headaches, nausea, vomiting, pneumonia, and pulmonary edema.

Thallium: Ataxia, pulmonary edema, vomiting, constipation, restlessness, delirium, and coma.

Zinc: Cough, chest discomfort, tachycardia, hypertension, gastrointestinal irritation, nausea, vomiting, diarrhea, and metallic taste in mouth.

Treatment: Antidotes for heavy-metal poisoning include BAL (British antilewisite), deferoxamine, dimercaprol, and EDTA. Heavy metals respond to hemodialysis and/or hemoperfusion in varying degrees (poor to well).

Usage: Screening for heavy-metal toxicity from overexposure, ingestion, or occupational exposure. Disorders for individual metals found under test listings for individual metals. Drugs that may further increase some values include carbamazepine, estrogens, oral contraceptives, penicillamine, phenobarbital, phenytoin, and sodium salts.

Description: Heavy metals include antimony, arsenic, bismuth, cadmium, cobalt, copper, lead, mercury, selenium, thallium, and zinc.

Antimony exposure occurs in miners, smelters, and ore refinery workers.

Arsenic is found naturally in food and the environment as well as in pesticides.

Bismuth exposure occurs in workers in cosmetic, disinfectant, and pigment industries. It may also occur as a result of treatment for syphilis.

Cadmium accumulates in the lungs, liver, and kidneys via exposure to food, water, air, and cigarette smoke.

Cobalt, a component of vitamin B_{12}, is found in most foods. It is also used to treat some resistant anemias and some radiosensitive malignancies.

Copper is a trace element found in normal diets. It is one of the few heavy metals that are potentially harmful at low levels as well as at toxic levels. Toxic levels may be caused by the use of copper IUDs, ingestion of contaminated substances, or fungicide exposure.

Lead is absorbed into the body through the ingestion of lead-containing paint or through industrial exposure.

Mercury is found in fungicides, industrial processes, and in fish (polluted water). It can also be ingested in the form of mercury salts. High mercury levels have been noted among dental workers.

Selenium is a metal used for the activity of human glutathione peroxidase. Exposure occurs as a result of the manufacture of glass, paints, dyes, electronic equipment, fungicides, rubber, and semiconductors.

Thallium is present in cosmetics, pesticides, and in some medications. It is absorbed through intact skin and mucous membranes.

Zinc is a trace metal important for cellular growth and metabolism. Toxicity can occur from industrial exposure and consumption of acidic food or beverages from galvanized containers.

Professional Considerations:

1. Consent form NOT required.
2. Preparation:
   A. *Blood:*
      i. Tube: Metal-free tube containing EDTA anticoagulant.
      ii. Do NOT draw specimens during hemodialysis.
   B. *24-hour urine:*
      i. Obtain a 3-L, plastic, acid-washed collection container. Use a plastic bedpan or urinal for voided specimens.
      ii. Write the beginning date and the time of collection on the container and the laboratory requisition.
3. Procedure:
   A. *Blood:* Draw a 10-ml blood sample.
   B. *24-hour urine:* Save all the urine in a 3-L plastic, acid-washed container for 24 hours.
4. Postprocedure care:
   A. Do NOT spin blood.
   B. *24-hour urine:* Record the total volume and the ending time of collection on the specimen container and label the container with the client information.
   C. Refrigerate the specimen(s).
5. Client and family teaching:
   A. *24-hour urine:* Save all the urine voided for the next 24 hours and urinate before defecating to avoid contaminating the urine specimen with stool. If any urine is accidentally discarded, discard the entire specimen and restart the collection the next day.

6. Factors that affect results:
   A. A diet high in heavy metals may elevate results.
   B. Occupational exposure may elevate results.
   C. A recent seafood diet may cause increased arsenic values.
   D. A diurnal variation exists such that the highest copper levels are found in the morning.
   E. Copper levels are 8–12% higher in blacks.
   F. Drugs that may further increase some values include dimercaprol, loop diuretics (intravenous), naproxen, penicillamine, sodium chloride, and thiazide diuretics.
7. Other data:
   A. Make sure the specimen for the 24-hour urine is not voided into a metal bedpan or urinal.
   B. Urine is the preferred specimen for arsenic if symptoms are present, or in acute exposure.
   C. *See also Arsenic, Blood and Arsenic, Urine; Cadmium, Serum and 24-Hour Urine; Copper, Serum and Copper, Urine; Lead, Blood and Urine; Mercury, Blood and Mercury, 24-Hour Urine; Thallium, Serum and Thallium, 24-Hour Urine; and Zinc, Blood.*

Bibliography:

Aposhian HV, Maiorino RM, Gonzalez-Ramirez D, et al.: Mobilization of heavy metals by newer, therapeutically useful chelating agents. Toxicol 97(1–3):23–38, 1995.

Domingo JL: Prevention by chelating agents of metal-induced developmental toxicity. Repro Tox 9(2):105–113, 1995.

Lopez-Artiguez M, Camean A, Repetto M: Preconcentration of heavy metals in urine and quantification by inductively coupled plasma atomic emission spectrometry. J Anal Toxicol 17(1):18–22, 1993.

HEINZ BODY STAIN, DIAGNOSTIC

Norm: Negative.

Positive: G-6-PD deficiency, Heinz-body anemia, hemolytic anemia, homozygous B-thalassemia, and after splenectomy. Drugs include acetanilid, aminosalicylic acid, analgesics, aniline, antipyretics, chlorates, hydroxylamine, napthalene, nitrobenzene, phenol derivatives, phenolhydrazine, phenothiazines, phenylsemicarbazide, pyridine, resorcin, salicylazosulfidine, sodiumsulfoxone, sulfapyridine, sulfones, tolbutamide, and large doses of vitamin K.

Negative: No Heinz body identified.

Description: Heinz bodies are small, irregular particles of denatured hemoglobin within mature red blood cells. These appear when stained with methyl violet or cresyl blue but not under Wright-stained preparations. The presence of Heinz bodies in a stained specimen indicates an abnormal hemoglobin structure.

Professional Considerations:

1. Consent form NOT required.
2. Preparation:
   A. Tube: Lavender-top.
   B. Contact the laboratory to arrange for testing.
3. Procedure:
   A. Draw a 3.5-ml blood sample.
   B. Invert the tube gently several times to adequately mix the sample and the anticoagulant.
4. Postprocedure care:
   A. Refrigerate the specimen.
   B. Current administration of antimalarials, furazolidone, nitrofurantoin, phenacetin, procarbazine, or sulfonamides should be noted on the laboratory requisition.
5. Client and family teaching:
   A. Results are normally available within 24–48 hours.
6. Factors that affect results:
   A. Hemolysis or clotting of the specimen invalidates the results.
   B. Antimalarials, furazolidone (in infants), nitrofurantoin, phenacetin, procarbazine, and sulfonamides can cause false-positive results.
7. Other data:
   A. Heinz bodies per cell vary from 1 to 20.
   B. G-6-PD deficiency often affects Dutch, German, or French individuals.

Bibliography:

Hasegawa S, Rodgers GP, Shio H, et al.: Impaired deformability of Heinz body-forming red cells. Biorheol *30*(3–4):275–286, 1993.

Hinchliffe RF: Errors in automated reticulocyte counts due to Heinz bodies. J Clin Pathol *46*(9): 878–879, 1993.

HELICOBACTER PYLORI QUICK OFFICE SEROLOGY, SERUM AND TITER, BLOOD

Norm: Negative.

Usage: Duodenal ulcers, gastric cancer, gastric ulcers, gastritis (chronic), lymphoma (stomach), and peptic ulcers.

Description: *H. pylori* are *S*- or *C*-shaped, gram-negative bacilli with a smooth outer coat and two to four unipolar flagella. These organisms were first detected in the stomachs of clients with gastritis a decade ago and have now been shown to be the major cause of active chronic gastritis. In addition, the evidence that *H. pylori* plays a major role in the pathophysiology of duodenal and peptic ulcers and possibly gastric ulcers is compelling. An association between *H. pylori* and gastric cancer and lymphoma of the stomach may also exist. There is no known natural reservoir for *H. pylori* in the environment, but it is thought that these organisms are spread by the fecal-oral route. The Quick Office Serology test may be performed in the physician's office in 20 minutes on serum, providing a yes/no answer to the presence of IgA and IgG antibodies to *H. pylori*. Laboratory-based serology tests are more specific than office-based tests in that they quantitate antibody levels, providing titers so that antibody levels can be monitored following therapy. An elevated antibody level indicates active or recent infection.

Professional Considerations:

1. Consent form NOT required.
2. Preparation:
   A. Tube: Red-top, red/gray-top, or gold-top.
3. Procedure:
   A. Draw a 3-ml blood sample.
4. Postprocedure care:
   A. If shipping the sample to an off-site laboratory, keep the specimen cool with frozen coolant from April through October and with refrigerated coolant from November through March.
5. Client and family teaching:
   A. Because serologic tests may remain positive for many months after successful treatment for *H. pylori*, other tests are also recommended for evaluating progress (endoscopy or breath test).
6. Factors that affect results:
   A. Serology alone is associated with high false-positive rates due to past infection without active disease.
7. Other data:
   A. These tests require 1 ml of serum.
   B. *H. pylori* affects about 20% of clients younger than 40 years and 50% of those older than 60 years.
   C. *H. pylori* is uncommon in young children.
   D. More than 90% of duodenal ulcers are caused by *H. pylori*.

Bibliography:

Cerda JJ, Go MF, Loeb D, et al.: A revolution in peptic ulcer disease. Patient Care *28*(9):18–22, 24, 25–28, 1994.

Conwell CF, Lyell R, Rodney WM: Prevalence of *Helicobacter pylori* in family practice patients with refractory dyspepsia: A comparison of tests available in the office. J Fam Pract *41*(3):245–249, 1995.

Cutler AF, Havstad S, Ma CK, et al.: Accuracy of invasive and noninvasive tests to diagnose *Helicobacter pylori* infection. Gastroenterol *109*(1):313–315, 1995.

Fuchs PC: *Helicobacter pylori.* MLO *26*(12):10, 12, 1994.

Wallis J: *Helicobacter pylori* infection and growth retardation. Prof Nurse *10*(3):158, 1994.

HEMAGGLUTINATION TREPONEMAL TEST FOR SYPHILIS (HATTS), SERUM

Norm: Titer <1:160.

Usage: Serologic confirmation of syphilis when nontreponemal antibody tests are positive.

Description: Syphilis is a complex, sexually transmitted disease characterized by a wide range of symptoms that imitate other diseases and is caused by the organism *Treponema pallidum.* In this test, the client's serum is heat treated and mixed with *T. pallidum*-sensitized turkey red blood cells, incubated, and compared with a control. A positive result occurs when agglutination occurs in the test sample, but not in the control. Positive results will occur in treponemal diseases of bejel, pinta, syphilis, and yaws.

Professional Considerations:

1. Consent form NOT required.
2. Preparation:
   A. *See Client and family teaching.*
   B. Tube: Red-top, red/gray-top, or gold-top.
3. Procedure:
   A. Draw a 7-ml blood sample.
4. Postprocedure care:
   A. Send the specimen to the laboratory and refrigerate it until it is tested.
   B. All cases of syphilis should be reported to the Centers for Disease Control in Atlanta, Georgia.
   C. Sexual contacts should be notified in the event of positive results.

5. Client and family teaching:
   A. Fast overnight prior to the test.
   B. Refer clients with elevated titers for medical management, which is necessary to slow or prevent the sequelae of syphilis.
   C. If testing positive:
      i. Notify all sexual contacts from the last 90 days (if in the early stage) to be tested for syphilis.
      ii. Syphilis can be cured with antibiotics. These may worsen the symptoms for the first 24 hours.
      iii. Do not have sex for 2 months and until after repeat testing has confirmed that the syphilis is cured. Use condoms after that for 2 years. Return for repeat testing every 3–4 months for the next 2 years to make sure the disease is cured.
      iv. Do not become pregnant for 2 years, because syphilis can be transmitted to the fetus.
      v. If left untreated, syphilis can damage many body organs, including the brain, over several years' time.
6. Factors that affect results:
   A. False-positive results may be due to infectious mononucleosis, leprosy, or systemic lupus erythematosus.
   B. False-negative results may occur in clients with AIDS.
7. Other data:
   A. This test may remain positive indefinitely for clients previously infected with syphilis. Thus, it is not useful for monitoring clinical response to treatment for syphilis.
   B. Penicillin is the drug of choice to treat syphilis.

Bibliography:

Augenbraun MH, DeHovitz JA, Feldman J, et al.: Biological false-positive syphilis test results for women infected with human immunodeficiency virus. Clin Inf Dis *19*(6):1040–1044, 1994.

Larsen SA, Steiner BM, Rudolph AH: Laboratory diagnosis and interpretation of tests for syphilis. Clin Micro Rev *8*(1):1–21, 1995.

HEMATOCRIT (HCT), BLOOD
Norm:

		SI Units
Females		
Adult	35–47%	0.35–0.47
Pregnant	30–46%	0.30–0.46
Adult males	42–52%	0.42–0.52
Neonates	42–68%	0.42–0.68
3 months	29–54%	0.29–0.54
Children		
1–2 years	35–44%	0.35–0.44
6–10 years	31–43%	0.31–0.43
Panic levels	<15% or >60%	<0.15 or >0.60

Panic Level Symptoms and Treatment—Increased:

Cause	Symptoms	Possible Treatments
Hemoconcentration	Decreased pulse pressure and volume, decreased skin turgor, decreased venous filling, dry mucous membranes, low central venous pressure, orthostatic hypotension, tachycardia, thirst and weakness	Give IV fluids. Monitor hematocrit. Stop or reduce dose of diuretics if they are contributors to condition.
True polycythemia overtransfusion	Extremity pain and redness, facial flushing, irritability	Give IV fluids. Monitor hematocrit. Observe for signs of thrombosis. Perform bloodletting by venipuncture (phlebotomy).

Panic Level Symptoms and Treatment—Decreased:

Cause	Symptoms	Possible Treatments
Hemodilution	Rales, anxiety, edema, hypertension, jugular venous distention, restlessness, and shortness of breath	Administer diuretics. Restrict sodium. Restrict fluids. Monitor hematocrit and intake and output
Blood loss	Hypotension, bleeding, hypoxia	Identify and treat cause of bleeding. Give isotonic fluids. Perform blood transfusion. Administer vasopressin. Administer omeprazole. Protect airways.

Increased: Addison's disease, burns (severe), dehydration (severe), diarrhea, eclampsia, erythrocytosis, hemorrhage, hemoconcentration, pancreatitis (acute), polycythemia, shock, and tetralogy of Fallot. Any condition that increases red blood cells (RBCs).

Decreased: Anemia, bone marrow hyperplasia, burns (severe), cardiac decompensation, cirrhosis, congestive heart failure, cystic fibrosis, fatty liver, fluid overload, hemolytic reactions to chemicals or drugs or prosthetics, hemorrhage, hydremia of pregnancy, hyperthyroidism, hypothyroidism, idiopathic steatorrhea, intestinal obstruction (late), leukemia, overhydration, pancreatitis (hemorrhagic), pneumonia, and pregnancy. Also, conditions that decrease RBCs. Drugs include acetaminophen, acetohexamide, aminosalicylic acid, amphotericin, antimony potassium tartrate, antineoplastic agents, antibiotics, atabrine hydrochloride, chloramphenicol, chloroquine hydrochloride or phosphate, doxapram hydrochloride, ethosuximide, ethotoin, furazolidone, haloperidol, hydralazine hydrochloride, indomethacin, isocarboxazid, isoniazid, mefenamic acid, mephenytoin, mercurial diuretics, metaxalone, methaqualone, methisuximide, methyldopa, methyldopate hydrochloride, nitrates, nitrofurantoin, novobiocin sodium, oleandomycin, oxyphenbutazone, paramethadione, pargyline hydrochloride, penicillins, phenacemide, phenelzine sulfate, phenobarbital, phensuximide, phenylbutazone, phenytoin sodium, phytonadione, primidone, radioactive agents, rifampin, spectinomycin hydrochloride, sulfon-amides, tetracyclines, thiazide diuretics, thiocyanates, thiosemicarbazones, to-lazamide, tolbutamide, tranylcypromide sulfate, trimethadione, tripelennamine hydrochloride, troleandomycin, val-proic acid, and vitamin A.

Description: Hematocrit is the per-centage of red blood cells in a volume of whole blood.

Professional Considerations:

1. Consent form NOT required.
2. Preparation:
   A. Tube: Lavender-top or heparinized cap-illary tube with a red band on the anti-coagulant end.
   B. Do NOT draw during hemodialysis.
3. Procedure:
   A. Draw a 3.5-ml blood sample from an extremity that does not have intra-venous fluids infusing into it to avoid hemodiluted samples. Do not leave the tourniquet in place for longer than 1 minute during collection.
   B. For a capillary puncture (fingers, toes, heels), establish a free flow of blood to minimize dilution with tissue fluid. Fill the capillary tube from the red-banded end to about two-thirds capac-ity and seal this end with clay.
4. Postprocedure care:
   A. Invert the tube gently ten times to mix.
   B. Refrigerate the sample after 10 hours. Do not freeze it.

5. Client and family teaching:
   A. Results are normally available within less than 24 hours.
6. Factors that affect results:
   A. Hemolysis of the specimen invalidates results.
   B. Results are elevated with dehydration or leukocytosis over 100×10^9/L.
   C. False elevations occur with glucose >400 mg/dl.
   D. Obtain the specimen before bath, shower, or massage, as these can cause a temporary rise in the value.
   E. High altitude may increase the value.
7. Other data:
   A. The hematocrit value is approximately three times the value of the hemoglo-bin.
   B. Hematocrit does not detect iron defi-ciency in infants, but ferritin level will for ages 9–18 months.

Bibliography:

Kazal LA: Failure of hematocrit to detect iron defi-ciency in infants. J Fam Pract *41*(3):237–240, 1996.

Kelly ME, Luetkemeier MJ, Pantalos GM: A justifica-tion for high resolution hematocrit measure-ment. Med Sci Sports Exerc *26*(5):547–550, 1994.

McNulty SE, Sharkey SJ, Asam B, et al.: Evaluation of STAT-CRIT hematocrit determination in compar-ison to Coulter and centrifuge: the effects of iso-tonic hemodilution and albumin administration. Anesth Anal *76*(4):830–834, 1993.

HEMOCCULT, STOOL
(see Occult Blood, Stool)

HEMOGLOBIN (Hb, Hgb), BLOOD

Norm:

		SI Units
Females	12–15 g/dl	7.1–9.9 mmol/L
Pregnant	10–15 g/dl	6.3–9.3 mmol/L
Males	14–16.5 g/dl	8.7–11.2 mmol/L
Children		
Neonates	14–27 g/dl	9.6–15.5 mmol/L
3 months	10–17 g/dl	6.1–9.6 mmol/L
1–2 years	9–15 g/dl	5.6–9.0 mmol/L
6–10 years	11–16 g/dl	5.8–9.6 mmol/L
Panic levels	<5 g/dl	<3.1 mmol/L
	>20 g/dl	>11.2 mmol/L

Panic Level Symptoms and Treatment—Increased: *See Hematocrit, Blood.*

Panic Level Symptoms and Treatment—Decreased: *See Hematocrit, Blood.*

Increased: Burns (severe), congestive heart failure, chronic obstructive pul-monary disease (COPD), dehydration, diarrhea, erythrocytosis, hemorrhage, hemoconcentration, high altitudes, in-testinal obstruction (late), polycythemia vera, and thrombotic thrombocyto-penic purpura. Also, conditions that increase red blood cells (RBCs). Drugs include gentamicin and methyldopa.

Decreased: Andersen's disease, anemia (iron deficiency), carcinomatosis, cirrhosis, cystic fibrosis, fat emboli, fatty liver, fluid retention, hemorrhage, hemolysis, hemolytic reaction to chemicals or drugs or prosthetics, Hodgkin's disease, hydremia of pregnancy, hyperthyroidism, hypervitaminosis A, hypothyroidism, idiopathic steatorrhea, intravenous overload, leukemia, lymphoma, pregnancy, renal cortical necrosis, sarcoidosis, severe hemorrhage, systemic lupus erythematosus (SLE), tetralogy of Fallot, and transfusion of incompatible blood. Also, conditions that decrease RBCs. Drugs include antibiotics, antineoplastic agents, apresoline, aspirin, hydantoin derivatives, indocin, monoamine oxidase (MAO) inhibitors, primaquine, rifampin, sulfonamides, and tridione.

Description: Hemoglobin is the oxygen-carrying pigment of the RBCs. It is composed of amino acids that form a single protein called globin and a compound called heme. Heme contains iron atoms and the red pigment porphyrin. Each erythrocyte contains approximately 300 million molecules of hemoglobin.

Professional Considerations:
1. Consent form NOT required.
2. Preparation:
   A. Tube: Lavender-top or heparinized capillary tube with a red band on the anticoagulant end.
3. Procedure:
   A. Draw a 3.5-ml blood sample from an extremity that does not have intravenous fluids infusing into it. Do not leave the tourniquet in place for longer than 1 minute during collection.
   B. For capillary puncture (fingers, toes, heels), establish a free flow of blood to minimize dilution with tissue fluid. Fill the capillary tube from the red-banded end to about two-thirds capacity and seal this end with clay.
4. Postprocedure care:
   A. Invert the tube gently ten times to mix it.
   B. The specimen is stable at room temperature for 10 hours; then refrigerate it for up to 18 hours total.
5. Client and family teaching:
   A. Results are normally available within less than 24 hours.
6. Factors that affect results:
   A. Hemolysis of the specimen invalidates the results.
   B. Results are falsely elevated by lipemic samples and leukocytosis $>30 \times 10^9$/L.
   C. Obtain the specimen before bath, shower, or massage, as these can cause a temporary rise in value.
   D. High altitude may increase the value.
   E. The mean hemoglobin in blacks is 0.4–1.0 g/dl lower than in whites after the first decade of life.
7. Other data:
   A. The hemoglobin value is approximately one-third the value of the hematocrit.
   B. Recent animal studies of hemoglobin have suggested that it plays a role in blood pressure regulation by carrying and releasing "super nitric oxide," a form of gas that causes relaxation of muscle cells in peripheral blood vessels.

Bibliography:

Blakeslee S: Study finds major new task of hemoglobin in the blood. New York Times 3/21/96.

O'Connor G, Molloy AM, Daly L, et al.: Deriving a useful packed cell volume estimate from haemoglobin analysis. J Clin Pathol 47(1):78–79, 1994.

Patrinkarea A, Pierratos A, Mustata S, et al.: Pretreatment hemoglobin and response to erythropoietin in CAPD patients. Periton Dial Int 15(2):174–176, 1995.

HEMOGLOBIN A₁A
(see Glycosylated Hemoglobin, Blood)

HEMOGLOBIN A₁B
(see Glycosylated Hemoglobin, Blood)

HEMOGLOBIN A₁C
(see Glycosylated Hemoglobin, Blood)

HEMOGLOBIN A₂, BLOOD

Norm:

		SI Units (Mass Fraction)
Cord blood	0–1.8%	0–0.018
Birth–6 months	0–3.5%	0–0.035
>6 months	1.5–3.5%	0.015–0.035

		SI Units (Mass Fraction)
Beta-thalassemia		
Trait	3.7–6.5%	0.037–0.065
Sickle cell trait	1.7–4.5%	0.017–0.045

Increased: Anemia (megaloblastic) and beta-thalassemia (homozygous).

Decreased: Anemia (iron deficiency, microcytic, sideroblastic), δ-thalassemia, βδ-thalassemia, erythroleukemia, and hemoglobin H disease.

Description: Hemoglobin A_2 is a normally present hemoglobin component comprising 2–3% of the normally present hemoglobin. This test is used to help differentiate hemoglobin abnormalities.

Professional Considerations:

1. Consent form NOT required.
2. Preparation:
   A. Tube: Lavender-top.
3. Procedure:
   A. Draw a 2-ml blood sample, without hemolysis.
4. Postprocedure care:
   A. Invert the tube gently ten times to mix.
5. Client and family teaching:
   A. Results are normally available within 24–48 hours.

6. Factors that affect results:
   A. Hemolysis or clotting of the specimen invalidates the results.
   B. Clients with both beta-thalassemia and iron deficiency may demonstrate normal HbA_2 and may need to be retested after taking iron supplements.
   C. In clients who have received recent blood transfusions, the results may be unreliable.
7. Other data:
   A. HbA_2 cannot be measured in the presence of HbC, HbE, or HbO.

Bibliography:

Galanello R, Barella S, Ideo A, et al.: Genotype of subjects with borderline hemoglobin A_2 levels: Implication for beta-thalassemia carrier screening. Am J Hematol 46(2):79–81, 1994.

Ranney HM, Lam R, Rosenberg G: Some properties of hemoglobin A_2. Am J Hematol 42(1):107–111, 1993.

Routy JP, Monte M, Beaulieu R, et al.: Increase of hemoglobin A_2 in human immunodeficiency virus-1-infected patients treated with zidovudine. Am J Hematol 43(2):86–90, 1993.

HEMOGLOBIN ELECTROPHORESIS, BLOOD

Norm:

		SI Units (Hb Fraction)
Hemoglobin A	>95%	>0.95
Infants	10–30%	0.10–0.30
Hemoglobin A_2	3–4%	0.03–0.04
Hemoglobin F	<1%	<0.01
Neonates	70–80%	0.70–0.80
1 month	70%	0.70
2 months	50%	0.50
3 months	25%	0.25
6 months–1 year	3%	0.03
Hemoglobin C	Absent	
Hemoglobin D	Absent	
Hemoglobin E	Absent	
Hemoglobin H	Absent	
Hemoglobin S	Absent	

Usage: Heinz-body anemia, hemoglobin C disease (trait = 45%, disease >90%), hemolytic anemia (HbD and HbE), microcytic anemia, sickle cell anemia (HbS: trait = 20–40%, disease = 80–100%), and thalassemia minor (HbH).

Description: A screening procedure in which the hemoglobin molecules migrate in solution in response to electrical currents such that the different components and their percentages can be determined.

Hemoglobins A, A₂, and F are types of hemoglobin that are found normally in the body.

Hemoglobin C causes red blood cells to sickle, at times due to osmotic fragility. It occurs in 2–3% of the black population.

Hemoglobins D and E rarely occur by themselves, although the anemias are without symptoms. When either occurs in combination with sickle cell anemia or thalassemia, the disease takes a more serious form.

Hemoglobin H is known to develop many inclusion bodies within the red blood cell, resulting in a damaged cell membrane and premature (40 days) cell death. It also disrupts transport of oxygen to tissues by binding with, rather than releasing, the oxygen.

Hemoglobin S is the most common of the abnormal hemoglobin traits, occurring in 10% of the black population. Its presence results in a sickling distortion of the red blood cells in response to reduced oxygen levels.

Professional Considerations:
1. Consent form NOT required.
2. Preparation:
   A. Tube: Lavender-top.
3. Procedure:
   A. Draw a 2.5-ml blood sample.
4. Postprocedure care:
   A. Deliver the specimen to the laboratory immediately, as abnormal hemoglobins are unstable.
   B. Recent (within the past 4 months) blood transfusion(s) should be noted on the laboratory requisition.
5. Client and family teaching:
   A. The client should wear a medical identification tag if chronic anemia is present.
   B. If the sickle cell trait or the disease is present, offer genetic counseling.
6. Factors that affect results:
   A. Red blood cell transfusion within the last 4 months may mask or reduce the presence of abnormal hemoglobins.
   B. Hemoglobins A₂, C, and S may be decreased in iron deficiency.
   C. False-negative tests occur in hemoglobin S with clients with polycythemia or in those less than 3 months of age.
7. Other data:
   A. More than 350 variants of Hb have been recognized.
   B. Changes in the proportion of normal types of hemoglobin may imply a hemolytic disease.

Bibliography:

Fatunde Oj, Scott-Emuakpor AB: Haemoglobin F and A₂ in Nigerian children with sickle cell anaemia. J Trop Pediatr *39*(4):251–252, 1993.

Poillon WN, Kim BC, Rodgers GP, et al.: Sparing effect of hemoglobin F and hemoglobin A₂ on the polymerization of hemoglobin S at physiologic ligand saturations. Proc Nat Acad Sci (USA) *90*(11): 5039–5043, 1993.

HEMOGLOBIN (FREE), PLASMA AND QUALITATIVE, URINE

Norm:

Urine: Negative.

	Blood	SI Units
Normal	<3 mg/dl	<0.47 µmol/L
Hemoglobinemia	>10 mg/dl	>1.55 µmol/L
Intravascular hemolysis	>30 mg/dl	>4.65 µmol/L
Hemoglobinuria occurs at	>150 mg/dl	>23.25 µmol/L
Cherry-red plasma occurs at	>200 mg/dl	>31 µmol/L

Increased in Plasma: Autoimmune hemolytic anemia, burns, cold hemagglutins, disseminated intravascular coagulation, falciparum malaria, intravascular hemolysis, lupus erythematosus, paroxysmal nocturnal hemoglobinuria, septicemia, sickle cell anemia, thrombosis, transfusion reaction, and traumatic hemolysis. Drugs include analgesics, antimalarials, cinchona alkaloids, nitrofurantoins, sulfonamides, and sulfones.

Positive in Urine: Autoimmune hemolytic anemia, blackwater fever, bladder irrigation, burns, *Clostridium per-*

fringens infection, disseminated intravascular coagulation, hemolytic anemia, kidney infarctions, malaria, paroxysmal nocturnal hemoglobinuria, poisonings, pregnancy, transfusion reaction, and transurethral prostatectomy. Drugs include arsenic, bacitracin, ciprofloxacin, coumadin, cyclophosphamide, fenoprofen, gold salts, indomethacin, mebendazole, nitrofurantoin, phenacetin, phenothiazines, phenylbutazone, polymyxin B, quinine, and suprofen.

Description: Free hemoglobin is hemoglobin that escapes from erythrocytes during intravascular hemolysis. A small amount of hemoglobin is normally present, but it is raised in the bloodstream and urine after massive hemolysis.

Professional Considerations:

1. Consent form NOT required.
2. Preparation:
   A. Tube: Red-top, red/gray-top, or gold-top, and green-top for plasma sample.
   B. Obtain a sterile plastic specimen container for the urine sample.
   C. If the female client is menstruating, reschedule the urine test.
3. Procedure:
   A. *Plasma:* Do NOT draw from an extremity with intravenous solution infusing. Draw the blood sample using an 18-gauge needle with an attached infusion tubing as follows:
      i. Gently place the tourniquet around the upper arm. Follow this with venipuncture of the antecubital vein with as little trauma as possible.
      ii. Release the tourniquet and clamp the tubing as soon as flashback occurs.
      iii. Collect 3 ml of blood in the red-top tube. Remove the top from the green-top tube, and collect 5 ml of blood. Replace the top of the heparinized green-top tube.
      iv. Clamp the tubing, withdraw the needle, and apply pressure to the venipuncture site.
   B. *Urine:* Obtain a 20-ml random urine specimen in a sterile plastic container.
4. Postprocedure care:
   A. *Plasma:* Send the specimen to the laboratory immediately. The plasma must be separated from the cells within 1–2 hours.
   B. *Urine:*
      i. Do not shake the specimen.
      ii. Dip a commercial dipstick in the urine and match the stick with a color block or chart, or send the stick to the laboratory immediately.

      iii. Refrigerate the specimen if the test is not performed within 1 hour.
5. Client and family teaching:
   A. Urinate before defecating and avoid contaminating the urine with toilet tissue.
6. Factors that affect results:
   A. Hemolysis of blood specimens invalidates the results. The specimen collection procedure is critical because any damage to red blood cells can produce falsely elevated results.
   B. False-positive urine results may occur if the specimen is contaminated with menstrual blood.
   C. Ascorbic acid (or medications containing ascorbic acid as a preservative—e.g., antibiotics) may cause false-negative urine tests by inhibiting reagent activity.
   D. Bromides, copper, iodides, and oxidizing agents cause false-positive urine tests.
7. Other data:
   A. If plasma hemoglobin levels are increased, encourage periods of rest to preserve usable hemoglobin.
   B. Free hemoglobin can often be detected in the urine when red blood cells cannot, because they lyse in strongly alkaline or dilute urine.
   C. The urine test is often part of a routine analysis.

Bibliography:

Walls J: Haemoglobin: Is more better? Nephrol Dial Trans *10*(Suppl 2):56–61, 1995.

HEMOGLOBIN, UNSTABLE, HEAT LABILE TEST, BLOOD

Norm: <5% (<0.05 factor, SI units).

Increased: Heinz-body anemia and iron deficiency anemia.

Description: Unstable hemoglobin is a type of hemoglobin, normally absent, that precipitates faster than normal hemoglobin. After precipitation, unstable hemoglobin forms Heinz bodies, inclusions attached to erythrocyte membranes that increase the fragility of the red blood cell and lead to hemolysis. In Heinz-body and iron deficiency anemia, a small percentage of hemoglobin becomes denatured when subjected to acid and heated to 50°C.

Professional Considerations:

1. Consent form NOT required.
2. Preparation:
   A. Tube: *Two* (2) lavender-top.
3. Procedure:
   A. Draw a 3.5-ml blood sample in each of two tubes.

4. Postprocedure care:
   A. Invert the tube ten times gently to mix the specimen.
5. Client and family teaching:
   A. Results are normally available within 24 hours.
6. Factors that affect results:
   A. Reject specimens received more than 3 hours after collection.
7. Other data:
   A. The test should be run with a normal control.

Bibliography:

Ahluwalia N, Lammi-Keefe CJ, Bendel RB, et al.: Iron deficiency and anemia of chronic disease in elderly women: a discriminant-analysis approach for differentiation. Am J Clin Nutr 61(3):590–596, 1995.

HEMOGLOBIN, UNSTABLE, ISOPROPANOL PRECIPITATION TEST, BLOOD

Norm: Negative. No precipitation at 40 minutes.

Positive: Heinz-body anemia, and slight opacity at 10 minutes in the presence of hemoglobin H.

Description: Unstable hemoglobin is a type of hemoglobin, normally absent, that precipitates faster than normal hemoglobin. After precipitation, unstable hemoglobin forms Heinz bodies, inclusions attached to erythrocyte membranes that increase the fragility of the red blood cell and lead to hemolysis. Unstable hemoglobin is detectable when subjected to isopropanol.

Professional Considerations:

1. Consent form NOT required.
2. Preparation:
   A. Inform the laboratory of the time the specimen will be arriving.
   B. Tube: Lavender-top.
3. Procedure:
   A. Draw a 2-ml blood sample.
4. Postprocedure care:
   A. Invert the sample gently ten times to mix.
   B. Send the specimen to the laboratory immediately, since the test must be run on fresh blood.
5. Client and family teaching:
   A. Results are normally available within 24 hours.
6. Factors that affect results:
   A. The presence of hemoglobin F may cause a false-positive result.
7. Other data:
   A. More sensitive than heat denaturization.

Bibliography:

Sills MR, Zinkham WH: Methylene blue-induced Heinz body hemolytic anemia. Arch Pediatr Adolesc Med 148(3):306–310, 1994.

HEMOPHILIC FACTOR B, BLOOD
(see Factor IX, Blood)

HEMOSIDERIN STAIN (SIDEROCYTE STAIN), URINE

Norm: Negative.

Positive: Burns, cold hemagglutins, hemochromatosis, hemolytic anemia, hemosiderosis, megaloblastic anemia, paroxysmal nocturnal hemoglobinuria, pernicious anemia, renal tubular cell disintegration, sickle cell anemia, thalassemia major, and transfusions (multiple).

Description: Hemosiderin are iron-storage granules normally found in the liver cytoplasm, spleen, and bone marrow. Hemosiderin are not normally found in the urine, as they are absorbed by the renal tubules. They appear in hemolytic processes, iron overload, and renal tubular damage. This test involves the microscopic examination of urine sediment for coarse granules of hemosiderin, which stain blue when potassium ferrocyanide is added to the sample.

Professional Considerations:

1. Consent form NOT required.
2. Preparation:
   A. Obtain a sterile plastic specimen container.
3. Procedure:
   A. Collect the first 50 ml of the first morning void in a sterile plastic container.
4. Postprocedure care:
   A. Refrigerate the specimens.
5. Client and family teaching:
   A. There are no restrictions prior to the test.
6. Factors that affect results:
   A. Hemosiderin is not detected in alkaline urine.
7. Other data:
   A. Hemosiderin can also be present in pancreatitis with the breakdown of cells in the intraperitoneal cavity.
   B. A liver or bone marrow biopsy is necessary for confirmation of primary hemochromatosis.

Bibliography:

Eppley BL, Sadove AM: Systemic effects of photothermolysis of large port-wine stains in infants and children. Plast Reconstr Surg 93(6):1150–1153, 1994.

HEPATITIS A ANTIBODY, IgM AND IgG (HAV-ab), BLOOD

Norm: Negative.

Positive: Hepatitis A and jaundice.

Description: IgM is a marker for the hepatitis A virus that appears 2–4 weeks after exposure and is detectable for only 4–8 weeks. It does differentiate between an acute infection and a past or preexisting infection. IgG replaces IgM, and these antibodies persist for life, providing immunity from reinfection of hepatitis A. Hepatitis A is usually transmitted through the fecal-oral route.

Professional Considerations:

1. Consent form NOT required.
2. Preparation:
   A. *See Client and family teaching.*
   B. Tube: Red-top, red/gray-top, or gold-top.
3. Procedure:
   A. Draw a 2-ml blood sample.
4. Postprocedure care:
   A. Remove the serum and freeze it if the blood will not be tested within 7 days.
5. Client and family teaching:
   A. Results may not be available for several days.
   B. A person cannot be infected more than once with hepatitis A.
   C. Hepatitis A can be prevented by good handwashing. Wash your hands well with soap and water and with rapid scrubbing action after urinating or defecating.
   D. Do not drink alcohol, beer, or wine or take medicine that contains acetaminophen or paracetamol for 3 weeks, or as specified by your physician.
6. Factors that affect results:
   A. If using the radioimmunoassay technique, injection of radionuclides within the last week may falsely elevate results.
7. Other data:
   A. This test requires 2 ml of serum.
   B. The serum is stable at room temperature for 7 days and indefinitely if frozen.
   C. In the United States, although over 50% of the population is positive for anti-HAV IgG, it is clinically insignificant.
   D. The presence of anti-HAV IgG does not rule out acute hepatitis B or non-A, non-B hepatitis.

Bibliography:

Breningstall GN, Belani KK: Acute transverse myelitis and brainstem encephalitis associated with hepatitis A infection. Pediatr Neur 12(2):169–171, 1995.

Cohon O, Mevorach D, Ackerman Z, et al.: Thrombocytopenic purpura as a manifestation of acute hepatitis A. J Clin Gastroenterol 17(2):166–167, 1993.

Hirata R, Hoshino Y, Sakai H, et al.: Patients with hepatitis A with negative IgM-HA antibody at early stages. Am J Gastroenterol 90(7):1168–1169, 1995.

HEPATITIS B CORE ANTIBODY (ANTI-HBc), BLOOD

Norm: Negative.

Positive: Hepatitis B.

Description: Hepatitis B core antibody is the antibody marker that arises 1–2 weeks after contraction of the hepatitis B virus, rises during the chronic phase of the illness, and remains present for life. It is the most reliable test to determine the presence of hepatitis B infection in the absence of hepatitis B surface antibody and hepatitis B surface antigen.

Professional Considerations:

1. Consent form NOT required.
2. Preparation:
   A. Tube: Red-top, red/gray-top, or gold-top.
3. Procedure:
   A. Draw a 3-ml blood sample.
4. Postprocedure care:
   A. Remove the serum and freeze it if the blood will not be tested within 7 days.
5. Client and family teaching:
   A. Results may not be available for several days.
   B. Hepatitis B can be spread by blood and other body fluids, including the sharing of needles and sexual contact. An infected mother can pass the infection on to her baby.
   C. To help prevent spreading hepatitis B, wash your hands well with soap and water and use rapid scrubbing action after urinating or defecating.
   D. Do not drink alcohol, beer, or wine or take medicine that contains acetaminophen or paracetamol for 3 weeks, or as specified by your physician.
6. Factors that affect results:
   A. If using the radioimmunoassay technique, the injection of radionuclides within the last week may falsely elevate results.
7. Other data:
   A. The serum is stable at room temperature for 7 days and indefinitely if frozen.

Bibliography:

Adlassnig KP, Horak W: Development and retrospective evaluation of Hepaxpert-I: a routinely used expert system for interpretive analysis of hepatitis A and B serologic findings. Artif Intel Med 7(1):1–24, 1995.

Jackson MM, Rymer TE: Viral hepatitis: Anatomy of a diagnosis. Am J Nurs *94*(1):43–48, 1994.

McPherson RA: Laboratory diagnosis of human hepatitis viruses. J Clin Lab Anal *8*(6):369–377, 1994.

HEPATITIS B e ANTIBODY (ANTI-HBe, HBeAb), SERUM

Norm: Negative.

Positive: Hepatitis B.

Description: Hepatitis B e antibody is a serum marker for hepatitis B that appears 8–16 weeks after infection and indicates resolution of acute infection. The presence of this antibody in clients with chronic positive hepatitis B surface antigen indicates an asymptomatic, healthy carrier.

Professional Considerations:
1. Consent form NOT required.
2. Preparation:
   A. *See Client and family teaching.*
   B. Tube: Red-top, red/gray-top, or gold-top.
3. Procedure:
   A. Draw a 2-ml blood sample.
4. Postprocedure care:
   A. Remove the serum and freeze it if the blood will not be tested within 7 days.
5. Client and family teaching:
   A. Results may not be available for several days.
6. Factors that affect results:
   A. If using the radioimmunoassay technique, injection of radionuclides within the last week may falsely elevate results.
7. Other data:
   A. The serum is stable at room temperature for 7 days and indefinitely if frozen.
   B. The test is more meaningful when measured in conjunction with hepatitis B e antigen.
   C. The test should be prescribed only in clients with documented recent infection of hepatitis B.

Bibliography:

Sallberg M, Pushko P, Berzinsh I, et al.: Immunochemical structure of carboxy-terminal part of hepatitis B e antigen: identification of internal and surface-exposed sequences. J Gen Virol *74*(Pt 7):1335–1340, 1993.

HEPATITIS B e ANTIGEN (HBeAg), BLOOD

Norm: Negative.

Positive: Hepatitis B.

Description: Usually appearing within 4–12 weeks of infection, hepatitis B e antigen is one of the first indicators of hepatitis B infection, usually preceding symptoms and representing the greatest threat of transmission. It is usually present for only 3–6 weeks. Persistence of the antigen for greater than 3 months suggests chronic liver disease.

Professional Considerations:
1. Consent form NOT required.
2. Preparation:
   A. Tube: Red-top, red/gray-top, or gold-top.
3. Procedure:
   A. Draw a 2-ml blood sample.
4. Postprocedure care:
   A. Remove the serum and freeze it if the blood will not be tested within 7 days.
5. Client and family teaching:
   A. Results may not be available for several days.
6. Factors that affect results:
   A. If using the radioimmunoassay technique, injection of radionuclides within the last week may falsely elevate results.
7. Other data:
   A. The serum is stable at room temperature for 7 days and indefinitely if frozen.
   B. Clients with chronic positive tests should also be tested for the hepatitis B e core antibody, which indicates that the client is an asymptomatic, healthy carrier.
   C. A hepatitis B vaccine is available and recommended for health care workers who may come in contact with blood and body fluids.

Bibliography:

Wingfield PT, Stahl SJ, Williams RW, et al.: Hepatitis core antigen produced in *Escherichia coli:* Subunit composition, conformational analysis, and in vitro capsid assembly. Biochem *34*(15):4919–4932, 1995.

HEPATITIS B SURFACE ANTIBODY (HBsAB), BLOOD

Norm: Negative.

Positive: Hepatitis B.

Description: This marker appears 2–16 weeks after hepatitis B surface antigen has disappeared. It usually represents clinical recovery and immunity to the virus. It will also be present during passive transfer in blood by transfusion or by administration of hepatitis B immune globulin (HBIG). Presence of the hepatitis B surface antibody along with the hepatitis B surface antigen indicates a poor prognosis.

Professional Considerations:

1. Consent form NOT required.
2. Preparation:
   A. Tube: Red-top, red/gray-top, or gold-top.
3. Procedure:
   A. Draw a 3-ml blood sample.
4. Postprocedure care:
   A. Remove the serum and freeze it if the blood will not be tested within 7 days.
5. Client and family teaching:
   A. Results may not be available for several days.
6. Factors that affect results:
   A. If using the radioimmunoassay technique, injection of radionuclides within the last week may falsely elevate results.
7. Other data:
   A. The serum is stable at room temperature for 7 days and indefinitely if frozen.
   B. There is a high prevalence of positive tests among intravenous drug abusers.

Bibliography:

Petermann S, Ernest JM: Intrapartum hepatitis B screening. Am J Obstet Gynecol *173*(2):369–373, 1995.

HEPATITIS B SURFACE ANTIGEN (HBsAG:HAA), BLOOD

Norm: Negative.

Positive: Hepatitis B.

Description: The hepatitis B surface antigen usually appears between 4 and 12 weeks of infection. It is indicative of active hepatitis B, either acute or chronic. It is the earliest indicator of hepatitis B, often preceding clinical symptoms. Presence of the hepatitis B surface antibody along with the hepatitis B surface antigen indicates a poor prognosis.

This test, required by the Food and Drug Administration when clients wish to donate blood, has helped reduce the incidence of hepatitis.

Professional Considerations:

1. Consent form NOT required.
2. Preparation:
   A. Tube: Red-top, red/gray-top, or gold-top.
3. Procedure:
   A. Draw a 2-ml blood sample.
4. Postprocedure care:
   A. Remove the serum and freeze it if the blood will not be tested within 7 days.
5. Client and family teaching:
   A. If the client is giving blood, explain the donation procedure.

B. Results may not be available for several days.
6. Factors that affect results:
   A. If using the radioimmunoassay technique, injection of radionuclides within the last week may falsely elevate results.
7. Other data:
   A. The serum is stable at room temperature for 7 days and indefinitely if frozen.
   B. This test does not screen for hepatitis A, hepatitis C, or non-A, non-B viruses.
   C. HBsAG may also be present in more than 5% of clients with Down Syndrome, hemophilia, Hodgkin's disease, and leukemia.
   D. When HBsAG is found in donor blood, it must be discarded because it carries a 40–70% chance of transmitting hepatitis.
   E. Report confirmed viral hepatitis to public health authorities.

Bibliography:

Dyson MR, Murray K: Selection of peptide inhibitors of interactions involved in complex protein assemblies: Association of the core and surface antigens of hepatitis B virus. Proc Nat Acad Sci (USA) *92*(6):2194–2198, 1995.

Sheu SY, Lo SJ: Deletion or alteration of hydrophobic amino acids at the first and the third transmembrane domains of hepatitis B surface antigen enhances its production of *Escherichia coli.* Gene *160*(2):179–184, 1995.

Sonveaux N, Thines D, Ruysschaert JM: Characterization of the HBsAg particle lipid membrane. Res Virol *146*(1):43–51, 1995.

HEPATITIS C ANTIBODY, SERUM

Norm: Negative.

Positive: Hepatitis C and non-A, non-B hepatitis.

Description: An assay to identify antibodies of the IgG class to the hepatitis C virus, a newly identified gene to a ribonucleic acid (RNA) virus that does not have the qualities of either hepatitis A or hepatitis B; 20% of post-transfusion hepatitis falls into this category. Causes include intravenous drug use and abuse, transfusions, dialysis, and needlesticks.

Professional Considerations:

1. Consent form NOT required.
2. Preparation:
   A. Tube: Red-top, red/gray-top, or gold-top.
3. Procedure:
   A. Draw a 2-ml blood sample.
4. Postprocedure care:
   A. Remove the serum and freeze it if the blood will not be tested within 7 days.

5. Client and family teaching:
   A. If the client is giving blood, explain the donation procedure.
   B. Results may not be available for several days.
6. Factors that affect results:
   A. If using the radioimmunoassay technique, injection of radionuclides within the last week may falsely elevate results.
7. Other data:
   A. This test requires 0.5 ml of serum.
   B. The serum is stable at room temperature for 7 days and indefinitely if frozen.
   C. Notify public health authorities if the test results are positive.
   D. To date, there is no commercially available serologic test to detect hepatitis C antigen (HCAg).

Bibliography:

Haber MM, West AB, Haber AD, et al.: Relationship of aminotransferases to liver histological status in chronic hepatitis C. Am J Gastroenterol *90*(8): 1250–1257, 1995.

Hakozaki Y, Shirahama T, Katou M, et al.: A controlled study to determine the optimal dose regimen of interferon-alpha 2b in chronic hepatitis C. Am J Gastroenterol *90*(8):1246–1249, 1995.

Molinari JA: Hepatitis C: No longer a diagnosis by exclusion. Compend *15*(6):682, 684, 1994.

HEPATITIS DELTA ANTIBODY (TOTAL ANTI-HDV), SERUM

Norm: Negative.

Positive: Hepatitis D.

Description: An assay to identify total (that is, predominantly IgG) antibodies to the hepatitis D virus. Hepatitis D is an incomplete virus requiring the presence of HBsAg of the hepatitis B virus for replication and expression. It infects only clients concurrently infected with hepatitis B virus or those who have a pre-existing hepatitis B virus infection. Hepatitis D virus is most common among intravenous drug abusers, hemophiliacs, and clients who have received multiple blood transfusions. It is a more severe form of hepatitis than hepatitis B alone, accounting for a higher incidence of chronic hepatitis and cirrhosis.

Clinically, hepatitis D virus cannot be distinguished from other types of hepatitis. Serologic tests must be positive for hepatitis B virus and Total Anti-HDV to make a diagnosis of hepatitis D. Hepatitis D virus is not a reportable disease in most of the United States at the present time.

Professional Considerations:

1. Consent form NOT required.
2. Preparation:
   A. Tube: Red-top, red/gray-top, or gold-top.
3. Procedure:
   A. Draw a 3-ml blood sample.
4. Postprocedure care:
   A. Remove the serum and freeze it if the blood will not be tested within 7 days.
5. Client and family teaching:
   A. Results may not be available for several days.
6. Factors that affect results:
   A. If using the radioimmunoassay technique, injection of radionuclides within the last week may falsely elevate results.
   B. Clients with lipemia or high-titer rheumatoid factor may have false-positive results.
7. Other data:
   A. This test requires 2 ml of serum.
   B. Serum is stable at room temperature for 7 days and indefinitely if frozen.
   C. Blood is potentially infectious during all phases of active infection.
   D. Clients who test positive for HBsAg are at risk for hepatitis D; however, immunity to hepatitis B virus provides immunity to hepatitis D virus.
   E. Mortality is 30% in chronic cases.
   F. In rare cases, HBsAg may be transiently undetectable in serum, resulting in an erroneous diagnosis of non-A, non-B hepatitis, unless specific testing for hepatitis D is performed.
   G. To date, there is no commercially available serologic test to detect hepatitis D antigen (HDAg).

Bibliograp'hy:

Lai MM, Xia YP, Hwang SB, et al.: Functional domains of hepatitis delta antigen. Prog Clin Biol Res *382*:21–27, 1993.

Negro F, Rizzetto M: Diagnosis of hepatitis delta virus infection. J Hepatol *22*(Suppl 1):136–139, 1995.

Ryu WS, Netter HJ, Bayer M, et al.: Ribonucleoprotein complexes of hepatitis delta virus. J Virol *67*(6): 3281–3287, 1993.

Simpson LH, Battegay M, Hoofnagle JH, et al.: Hepatitis delta virus RNA in serum of patients with chronic delta hepatitis. Dig Dis Sci *39*(12):2650–2655, 1994.

Wang JG, Lemon SM: Hepatitis delta virus antigen forms dimers and multimeric complexes in vivo. J Virol *67*(1):446–454, 1993.

HEPATOBILIARY SCAN (HIDA SCAN), DIAGNOSTIC

Norm: Negative. Requires interpretation by a radiologist.

Normal anatomy and physiology of liver, spleen, and biliary tract as determined by a radiologist. Normal distribution of injectate: 86% in reticuloendothelial system (RES) of liver, 6% in spleen, 8% in RES of bone marrow.

Hepatobiliary (scan post-IV injection of Technetium 99m dimethy-acetic acid (IDA): First hour images show liver, cardiac, and vascular activity; gallbladder (GB) and common bile duct/bowel activity seen by 60 minutes. GB uptake should precede bowel visualization. An inflamed gallbladder will not take up radionuclide. In the presence of biliary tree obstruction, no radionuclide will be visualized beyond the point of obstruction.

Liver-spleen (scan post-IV injection of Technetium 99m radionuclide): Uniform uptake throughout liver and spleen. Decreased uptake or "cold spots" seen in areas with space-occupying lesions. Increased blood flow to the liver will be evidenced by increased radionuclide uptake or "hot spots."

Usage: Used to visualize biliary tract and to detect cholecystitis (due to obstruction of cystic ducts), hepatocellular disease, gallbladder disease, jaundice, liver cancer, liver metastasis, obstruction, and perihepatic abscess; used to study biliary kinetics (biliary dyskinesia, gallbladder ejection fraction); evaluates patency of biliary system and cystic duct, including postsurgically, and nonspecifically demonstrates focal disease as "cold spots" of nonuptake of the radionuclide. Evaluation of pediatric jaundice (choledocholecyst, biliary atresia versus neonatal hepatitis); conditions causing increased flow to the liver will appear as "hot spots."

Description: The hepatobiliary scan is a radionuclide study that demonstrates hepatic parenchyma, extrahepatic bile ducts, gallbladder, and normal passage into the intestines, as well as the position, size, and shape of the liver. Intravenously injected HIDA, a radionuclide, travels through the liver into the biliary system, enabling gamma camera imaging of the entire hepatobiliary system. The cells of the liver absorb the radionuclide within 30 minutes and can be observed on the scan before it is redeposited in the bloodstream and excreted. Dye is excreted in the bile, stored briefly in the gallbladder, and eliminated through the intestine, all within 4 hours. Failure of the dye to appear in the intestines is indicative of obstruction.

Professional Considerations:
1. Consent form IS required.

Risks:
Infection.

Contraindications:
During pregnancy or breast-feeding; in children.

2. Preparation:
   A. Establish intravenous access.
   B. Have emergency equipment readily available.
   C. *See Client and family teaching.*
3. Procedure:
   A. The client is injected with radionuclide (usually Technetium TC-99m IDA, the dose calculated by body weight) intravenously 30 minutes prior to the scan.
   B. Delay imaging for 6–48 hours after injection for clients known to have hepatocellular disease.
   C. The client is positioned supine on the scanning table during the scan.
   D. A gamma camera is placed over the right upper quadrant of the abdomen.
   E. Scintiphotos are obtained at 15, 30, 60, and 90 minutes after injection of the radiopharmaceutical.
   F. The procedure is repeated at 2–6 hours and 24 hours if obstruction is suspected or when the biliary system was not visualized.
4. Postprocedure care:
   A. Wear rubber gloves when discarding urine for 24 hours after the procedure. Wash the gloved hands with soap and water before removing the gloves. Wash the hands again after the gloves have been removed.
5. Client and family teaching:
   A. Fast from food and fluids for 4–6 hours prior to the scan.
   B. The scan takes 1.0–1.5 hours.
   C. Report any sensations that might indicate an allergic reaction such as itching or difficulty in breathing.
   D. Meticulously wash the hands with soap and water after each void for 24 hours after the procedure.
   E. Results are normally available from the physician within 24 hours.
6. Factors that affect results:
   A. The scan must be performed promptly after the injection, as radionuclides have a short transit time through the liver.
   B. Do not schedule any other radionuclear scans within 24 hours of this scan.
   C. Ingestion of food or liquids within 2–4 hours prior to the scan may result in impaired visualization of the gallbladder.
   D. Total parenteral nutrition may also result in impaired visualization of the gallbladder.

E. The presence of barium in the intestinal tract may inhibit gallbladder visualization.

7. Other data:

A. Health care professionals working in a nuclear medicine area must follow federal standards set by the Nuclear Regulatory Commission. These standards include precautions for handling the radioactive material and monitoring potential radiation exposure.

Bibliography:

Datz FL: Gastrointestinal and hepatobiliary imaging. *In* Datz, FL: Handbook of Nuclear Medicine. St. Louis, MO, CV Mosby 1993, pp 107–143.

Datz FL, Christian PE, Hutson WR, et al.: Physiological interventions in radionuclide imaging of the tubular gastrointestinal tract. Semin Nucl Med *28*:1204–1207, 1994.

Krug B, Harniscmacher, et al.: Digital luminescence radiography and conventional radiography in abdominal contrast examination. Acta Radiol *36*(3):284–289, 1995.

Malarkey LM, McMorrow ME: Nurse's Manual of Laboratory Tests and Diagnostic Procedures. Philadelphia, WB Saunders, 1996, pp 581–583, 587–589.

Shea JA, Berlin JA, Escarce JJ, et al.: Revised estimates of diagnostic test sensitivity and specificity in suspected biliary tract disease. Arch Intern Med *58*(4): 298–302, 1994.

Wexler RS, Greene GS, Scott M: Left hepatic and common hepatic ductal bile leaks demonstrated by Tc-99m HIDA scan and percutaneous transhepatic cholangiogram. Clin Nucl Med *19*(1):59–10, 1994.

HER-2 NEU ONCOGENE (C-ERB-S, HUMAN EPIDERMAL GROWTH FACTOR), SPECIMEN

Norm: Normally present in cell membranes as a single DNA copy. Must be interpreted by a pathologist.

Positive: Presence of either or both molecular genetic alterations:

Gene amplification	Multiple DNA copies, characterized by flourescence in situ hybridization
Gene overexpression	Characterized by membrane immunostaining by immunohistochemistry

Negative: Absence of gene amplification or overexpression.

Usage: Examination of cancer genetics to screen for identification of clients at highest risk, and as a general prognostic indicator for breast, endometrial, ovarian (adenocarcinomas), and salivary gland cancer (mucoepidermoid carcinoma).

Description: This proto-oncogene, located on chromosome 17, band q21, can mutate to become an oncogene by amplification. Amplification and/or overexpression in cancerous neoplasms is associated with a poor prognosis independent of histopathologic grade, tumor size, and regional lymph node involvement. Recent evidence suggests overexpression may have a direct role in the pathogenesis of ovarian cancer as well as being a prognosticator of poor disease outcome.

Professional Considerations: *(see Biopsy, Site-Specific* for technique steps for obtaining the tissue specimen). The considerations below are specific to the correct processing of tissue to maximize accurate results.

1. Consent form IS required for most specimens; institution-specific. See *Biopsy, Site-Specific, Specimen* for risks and contraindications.

2. Preparation:

A. Obtain sterile containers with the fixative appropriate to the antibody reagent that will be used in the testing (according to the recommendations of the histology/pathology departments of the institutions). Most often the fixative is 10% buffered formaldehyde.

3. Procedure:

A. Obtain an adequate amount of tissue (20–500mg depending on the site and the technique chosen), using an aseptic technique.

B. Place the sample in the fixative immediately and transport it to the laboratory immediately, noting the time the specimen was obtained on the requisition.

4. Postprocedure care:

A. Specific to site and procedure. Generally, dry, sterile dressing is applied to an external site. An internal site (such as a cervical site) may require packing.

B. Assess the site and vital signs for signs of bleeding. The frequency may vary with the physician. Generally, assess every 15 minutes the first hour, every 30 minutes the second hour, then every hour × 4.

C. Observe for signs of infection (fever,

chills, hypotension, tachycardia, inflammation at site) × 24–48 hours.

5. Client and family teaching:
   A. Provide emotional support to the client awaiting results.
   B. If biopsy confirms cancer, additional tests will be prescribed to determine appropriate treatment.

6. Factors that affect results:
   A. Dried specimens must be discarded.
   B. Reagents with a high degree of sensitivity and specificity to HER-2/neu in paraffin-embedded tissues should be selected for this test, or the sensitivity of the reagent used should be characterized to correctly interpret the significance of the test results. Studies have shown wide variability in the efficacy of the various antibody reagents currently in use. The use of more than one antibody (i.e., antibody "cocktails") may also improve immunostaining.

7. Other:
   A. The use and application of this test are still investigational, and the test is not yet routinely prescribed. Therefore, testing is likely to be performed on archival tissue samples, making the pre- and intraprocedural steps above not applicable.
   B. Clients showing amplification may qualify for clinical trials utilizing murine monoclonal antibodies, produced against the HER-2/neu receptor to inhibit tumor cell replication.
   C. Further studies of HER-2/neu amplification and overexpression promise to give insights into possible prevention, detection, and treatment strategies of cancers in which these genetic alterations occur.

Bibliography:

Karlan BY, Jones J, Slamon DJ, LaGasse LD: Glucocorticoids stabilize HER-2/neu messenger RNA in human epithelial ovarian carcinoma cells. Gynecol Oncol 53:70–77, 1994.

Leitzel K, Teramato Y, Konrad K, et al.: Elevated serum c-erbB-2 antigen levels and decreased response to hormone therapy of breast cancer. J Clin Oncol 13(5):1129–1135, 1995.

Loescher LJ: Genetics in cancer prediction, screening, and counseling: Part I, Genetics in cancer prediction and screening. Oncol Nurs Forum 22(Suppl 2):13, 1995.

Lydon J: Metastasis: Part I: Biology and prevention. Oncology Nursing: Patient treatment and support 2(5):3–4, 1995.

Press MF, Hung G, Godolphin W, Slamon DJ: Sensitivity of HER-2/neu antibodies in archival tissue samples: Potential source of error in immunohistochemical studies of oncogene expression. Cancer Res 54(10):2771–2777, 1994.

Press MF, Pike MC, Hung G, Zhou JY: et al: Amplification and overexpression of HER-2/neu in carcinomas of the salivary gland: Correlation with poor prognosis. Cancer Res 54:5675–5682, 1994.

Springhouse: Illustrated Guide to Diagnostic Tests, Springhouse, PA, Springhouse Corporation, 1994, pp 477, 479, 483.

HEROIN, URINE

Norm: Negative.

Positive: Drug abuse.

Overdose Symptoms and Treatment:

Symptoms: Bradycardia, euphoria, flushing, itching, hypotension, hypothermia, respiratory depression.

Treatment:
   Naloxone (Narcan).
   Hemodialysis will NOT remove heroin.

Description: Heroin (diacetyl-morphine), a drug of abuse, is made from morphine. The half-life is 1.7–4.5 hours. Heroin is rapidly metabolized back into morphine, and up to 67% of the dose is excreted in the urine as morphine or morphine glucuronides; 50% is excreted in the urine in the first 8 hours and 90% in the first 24 hours.

Professional Considerations:

1. Consent form NOT required unless results may be used as legal evidence.
2. Preparation:
   A. Obtain clean urine cup.
   B. If the specimen may be used as legal evidence, have the specimen collection witnessed.
3. Procedure:
   A. Obtain 50 ml of random urine in a clean container.
4. Postprocedure care:
   A. Store samples at –20°C.
   B. If the specimen may be used as legal evidence, write the client's name, date, exact time of collection, and specimen source on the laboratory requisition. Sign, and have the witness sign, the laboratory requisition. Transport the specimen to the laboratory immediately in a sealed plastic bag marked as legal evidence. All clients handling the specimen should sign and write the time of receipt on the laboratory requisition.
5. Client and family teaching:
   A. Offer information regarding drug rehab programs to facilitate treatment if desired.
6. Factors that affect results:
   A. False-positive results occur if the client ingested 20 mg of codeine cough syrup or 5–15 g of poppy seeds 24 hours before the sample was obtained.
   B. Heroin is eliminated from the system in 2 days, but quinine, which is a non-

narcotic used as a diluent, may stay in the system for up to 1 week.

7. Other data:
    A. Street heroin is generally 5–10% actual heroin, with the usual euphoric dose taken by abusers equivalent to 10–20 mg of morphine.
    B. Common complications of overdose are pulmonary edema, endocarditis, and septicemia.

Bibliography:

Bermejo BAM, Strano, Rossi S: Hair and urine analysis: relative distribution of drugs and their metabolites. Forensic Sci Int 70(1–3):203–210, 1995.

Goldberger BA, Loewenthal B, Darwin WD, Cone EJ: Clin Chem 41(1):116–117, 1995.

Wang WL, Darwin WD, Cone EJ: Simultaneous assay of cocaine, heroin, and metabolites in hair, plasma, saliva and urine by gas chromatography—mass spectometry. J Chromatogr Biomed Appl 660(2):279–290, 1994.

HERPES CULTURE, SPECIMEN

(see Viral Culture, Specimen)

HERPES CYTOLOGY, SPECIMEN

Norm: Negative.

Positive: Genital herpes, herpes virus infection, meningitis, and vaginitis.

Description: Herpes simplex 1 and 2 are two similar viruses, which differ slightly in structure. Herpes simplex 1 is generally found in the respiratory tract, eyes, or mouth (cold sores), and herpes simplex 2 is found in the genitourinary tract (transmitted by sexual contact, or during childbirth for infants). Both viruses have been isolated in both locations. Cytology is the examination of cells under a microscope to establish the presence of the virus, which is seen as multinucleated epithelial cells with enlarged atypical nuclei. This can be performed using a Papanicolaou test and has an average sensitivity of 45–50%.

Professional Considerations:

1. Consent form NOT required.
2. Preparation:
    A. Obtain a sterile tongue depressor or swab, slides, and a 95% alcohol fixative.
3. Procedure:
    A. Scrape the lesion with the sterile tongue depressor.
    B. Spread the scrapings evenly on the slide with the tongue depressor, or roll the specimen onto the slide using the swab.

4. Postprocedure care:
    A. Fix the slide with the 95% alcohol fixative.
    B. Deliver the specimen to the laboratory within 1 hour.
    C. The final report for a negative culture takes 5 days.
5. Client and family teaching:
    A. If the client is pregnant, a cesarean section may be required if the virus is still present at the time of delivery. The risk of miscarriage is higher than normal in women infected with genital herpes.
    B. Pain from sores may be treated with mild analgesics, warm baths, or wet tea bags held over the site.
    C. Safe sex practices to prevent transmission to partner(s):
        i. Notify all sexual partners to be tested for the virus.
        ii. Do not have sex when blisters or sores are present. These usually take about 4 weeks to clear up completely.
        iii. Use a condom during all sexual activity, even if sores are not present. Spermicides containing nonoxynol-9 help kill the herpes virus.
    D. Antivirals may reduce viral shedding and relieve skin discomfort.
    E. Lesions of confused clients should be covered with a dressing to prevent autoinoculation (spread from one site to another).
6. Factors that affect results:
    A. Air drying or improper fixative will cause the laboratory to reject the specimen.
    B. Smears with heavy inflammatory exudate are difficult to interpret because of the nonspecific staining technique.
7. Other data:
    A. Viral serology is more definitive, but serology in herpes simplex virus is of little practical importance in clients with HIV, since most are seropositive.
    B. 50% of active lesions may not demonstrate herpes inclusions.
    C. Lesions that are dry may be moistened with saline prior to scraping.

Bibliography:

Cohen PR: Tests for detecting herpes simplex virus and varicella-zoster virus infections. Rev Dermatol Clin 12(1):51–68, 1994.

Flaskerud JK, Ungvarski PJ: HIV/AIDS: A Guide to Nursing Care. Philadelphia, WB Saunders 1995, p 100.

HERPES SIMPLEX ANTIBODY, BLOOD

Norm: Negative, <0.25 by ELISA, or <1:10.

Positive: 1:10–1:100 indicates infection within 7 days, 1:100–1:500 Current-late infection, >1:500. Established latent infection.

Usage: Genital herpes, herpes simplex, and herpes zoster virus infection.

Description: See *Herpes Cytology, Specimen* for description of the virus characteristics. Peak antibody levels are reached 4–6 weeks after inoculation with the virus, and decline and stabilize thereafter. The serum sample is incubated onto a solid phase, and enzyme activity is quantitated and compared to a set of controls.

Professional Considerations:
1. Consent form NOT required.
2. Preparation:
   A. Tube: Red-top, red/gray-top, or gold-top.
3. Procedure:
   A. Draw a 10-ml blood sample.
4. Postprocedure care:
   A. Deliver the sample to the laboratory within 1 hour.
5. Client and family teaching:
   A. See *Herpes Cytology, Specimen.*
6. Factors that affect results:
   A. Hemolysis of the specimen invalidates the results.
   B. Herpes simplex 1, herpes simplex 2, and varicella zoster may cross-react, but the antibody rise in the infecting virus usually exceeds the other antibodies.
7. Other data:
   A. Diagnosis of a current infection should not be made based on the results of a single serum analysis. Two samples, 10–14 days apart, are recommended.

Bibliography:

Akron General Medical Center: Laboratory Users Guide. Akron, OH, Department of Pathology and Laboratory Medicine, 1991, p 244.

Cantin E, Chen J, Gaudulis L, et al.: Detection of herpes simplex virus DNA sequences in human blood and bone marrow cells. J Med Virol *42*(3):279–286, 1994.

Sivropoulou A, Vasilaki A, Asenakis M: Application of a transformed cell line constitutively expressing HSV-1 polypeptides for the detection of HSV antibodies in human sera by an enzyme immunoassay. Arch Virol *139*(1–2):183–188, 1994.

HERPES VIRUS ANTIGEN, DIRECT FLUORESCENT ANTIBODY, SPECIMEN

Norm: Negative.

Usage: Cervicitis, encephalitis, and herpes simplex.

Description: See *Herpes Cytology, Specimen* for description of the characteristics of the virus. If emergent diagnosis is necessary (e.g., encephalitis), this is the most rapid and sensitive test if cytology findings are negative. The specimen is examined by immunofluorescence or immunoperoxidase technique.

Professional Considerations:
1. Consent form NOT required.
2. Preparation:
   A. Obtain a sterile swab, and a sterile specimen container or Culturette.
3. Procedure:
   A. Collect the specimen from the infected site as described above.
   B. Do NOT place the specimen in a fixative.
4. Postprocedure care:
   A. Send the sample to the laboratory immediately or freeze it. This includes operative specimens and spinal fluid specimens.
   B. This test should be performed immediately, day or night, and the laboratory should be notified of arriving specimens.
5. Client and family teaching:
   A. See *Herpes Cytology, Specimen.*
   B. Results are normally available within 24 hours.
6. Factors that affect results:
   A. Specimens will be rejected if placed in fixative.
   B. Inflammatory exudate on specimens will cause nonspecific color development of the immunoperoxidase reagent.
7. Other data:
   A. None.

Bibliography:

Cohen PR: Tests for detecting herpes simplex virus and varicella-zoster virus infections. Dermatol Clin *12*(1):51–68, 1994.

Malarkey LN, McMorrow ME: Nurse's Manual of Laboratory Tests and Diagnostic Procedures. Philadelphia, WB Saunders, 1996, pp 151–155.

HETEROPHIL AGGLUTININS, BLOOD

Norm: Negative.

Positive: Cytomegalovirus, Epstein-Barr virus, infectious mononucleosis, serum sickness, and toxoplasmosis.

Description: A heterophil antibody is capable of reacting with an antigen that is completely unrelated to the antigen originally stimulating its formation. This infectious mononucleosis screening procedure tests for the presence of agglutinins (indicated by clumping) reacting to the red blood cells of horses or sheep. Infectious mononucleosis is a viral infection characterized by fatigue, anorexia, swollen glands, fever, and sore throat. Symptoms may continue for up to 6 weeks. Mode of transmission is through person-to-person transmission of saliva through kissing, sneezing, or coughing. Generally, this test is positive 3–10 days after infection, peaks within 3 weeks, and can remain elevated for up to 1 year.

Professional Considerations:

1. Consent form NOT required.
2. Preparation:
   A. Tube: Red-top, red/gray-top, or gold-top or lavender-top.
3. Procedure:
   A. Draw a 2.5-ml blood sample.
4. Postprocedure care:
   A. None.
5. Client and family teaching:
   A. For clients testing positive:
      i. Drink plenty of fluids and eat a balanced diet, even if not hungry or thirsty.
      ii. Use saltwater gargle for sore throat.
      iii. Use the antipyretic recommended by the physician for fever.
      iv. Get plenty of rest during the febrile period. Then limit physical activity for 5 weeks.
      v. Isolation is not necessary, but avoid coughing or sneezing on or near other persons, as well as kissing other persons until cleared by the physician.
6. Factors that affect results:
   A. Hemolysis of the specimen invalidates the results.
   B. This test may be falsely negative due to the occasional delay in the appearance of the agglutinins in the first 4 weeks after infection, despite the presence of clinical symptoms.
   C. False positives (<2%) have been reported with Hodgkin's disease, lymphoma, acute lymphocytic leukemia, infectious hepatitis, pancreatic cancer, cytomegalovirus, Burkitt's lymphoma, rheumatoid arthritis, malaria, and rubella.
7. Other data:
   A. With infectious mononucleosis, heterophil antibodies appear in 60% of clients within 2 weeks and in 90% within 4 weeks. Most titers decline in 3–6 months.
   B. 10% of true adult Epstein-Barr virus mononucleosis cases have negative heterophil agglutinins; the virus occurs more frequently in children. Epstein-Barr virus antibodies may occur in these cases.
   C. *See also Epstein-Barr Virus, Serology, Blood.*

Bibliography:

Aftercare instructions: infectious mononucleosis. Micromedx, Inc. *88,* 1996.

Akron General Medical Center: Laboratory Users Guide. Akron, Ohio. Department of Pathology and Laboratory Medicine, p 287, 1991.

Malarkey LM, McMorrow ME: Nurse's Manual of Laboratory and Diagnostic Procedures. Philadelphia: WB Saunders, 1996, p 162

HETEROPHIL SCREEN
(see Monospot Screen, Blood)

HIDA SCAN, DIAGNOSTIC
(see Hepatobiliary Scan, Diagnostic)

HIGH-DENSITY LIPOPROTEIN (HDL) CHOLESTEROL, BLOOD
Norm:

HIGH-DENSITY LIPOPROTEIN CHOLESTEROL

Age	Male		Female	
	mg/dl	SI Units mmol/L	mg/dl	SI Units mmol/L
20–24	30–63	0.78–1.63	33–79	0.85–2.04
25–29	31–63	0.80–1.63	37–83	0.96–2.15
30–34	28–63	0.72–1.63	36–77	0.93–1.99
35–39	29–62	0.75–1.60	34–82	0.88–2.12
40–44	27–67	0.70–1.73	34–88	0.88–2.28
45–49	30–64	0.78–1.66	34–87	0.88–2.25
50–54	28–63	0.72–1.63	37–92	0.96–2.38
55–59	28–71	0.72–1.84	37–91	0.96–2.35
60–64	30–74	0.78–1.91	38–92	0.98–2.38
65–69	30–75	0.78–1.94	35–96	0.91–2.48
>70	31–75	0.80–1.94	33–92	0.85–2.38

	Male		Female	
Age	mg/dl	SI Units mmol/L	mg/dl	SI Units mmol/L
Children				
Cord blood	6–53	0.16–1.37	13–56	0.34–1.45
5–9	38–75	0.98–1.94	36–73	0.93–1.89
10–14	37–74	0.96–1.91	37–70	0.96–1.81
15–19	30–63	0.78–1.63	35–74	0.91–1.91

Note: Levels for Afro-Americans are approximately 10 mg/dL higher than those listed.

Increased: Alcoholism, chronic hepatitis, biliary cirrhosis (primary), familial hyperalphalipoproteinemia. Drugs include chlorinated hydrocarbons, cimetidine, cyclofenil, estrogens, ethanol, lovastatin, nicotinic acid, phenytoin, and terbutaline.

Decreased: Arteriosclerosis, bacterial infections, cholestasis, coronary heart disease, hypercholesterolemia, hypertriglyceridemia, hypolipoproteinemia, liver disease, renal disease, Tangier's disease, type-IV hyperlipoproteinemia, and viral infections. Drugs include androgens and beta-blockers.

Description: High-density lipoprotein (HDL) is a type of cholesterol carried by alpha-lipoprotein. HDL is thought to help protect against the risk of coronary artery disease, and has been shown to be inversely related to the risk of coronary heart disease.

Professional Considerations:

1. Consent form NOT required.
2. Preparation:
   A. *See Client and family teaching.*
   B. Tube: Lavender-top (2 tubes for lipid profile).
3. Procedure:
   A. Draw a 7-ml blood sample.
4. Postprocedure care:
   A. Resume previous diet.
5. Client and family teaching:
   A. Fast for 12–14 hours prior to sampling. Water is permitted.
   B. For clients with low levels, provide information regarding the reduction of modifiable risk factors, i.e., smoking, obesity, and physical inactivity.
   C. A low cholesterol diet includes avoidance of butter, lard, palm oil, coconut oil, pastries, waffles, avocados, olives, liver, bacon, sausage, luncheon meats, hot dogs, red meat, whole milk, cream, ice cream, and chocolate.
6. Factors that affect results:
   A. A diet high in carbohydrates or polyunsaturated fats and/or smoking decreases the results.
7. Other data:
   A. For every 5 mg/dl decrease in HDL-C below the mean, the risk of coronary heart disease increases by 25%.
   B. *See also Cholesterol, Blood; and Low-Density Lipoprotein Cholesterol, Blood.*

Bibliography

Lemone P, Burke K: Menlo Park, Medical Surgical Nursing. Reading, MA, Addison-Wesley Nursing, 1996, pp 1054–1056.

Rainwater DL, Ludwig MJ, et al.: Lipid and lipoprotein factors associated with variation in Lp(a) density. Arteriosclerosis, Thromb Vasc Biol *15*(3):313–319, 1995.

Tall AR: Plasma cholesterol ester transfer protein and high-density lipoproteins: new insights from molecular genetic studies. J Med *237*(1):5–12, 1995.

HIGH MOLECULAR WEIGHT KININOGEN, PLASMA
(see Factor, Fitzgerald, Plasma)

HIS BUNDLE ELECTROGRAPHY, DIAGNOSTIC

Norm: Atrial-to-His (A–H) interval = 50–120 msec; His-to-ventricular (H–V) activation = 35–55 msec.

Usage: Antidysrhythmic drug evaluation, precise location of bundle branch block, bypass tract physiology evaluation, decision making about pacemaker implant, syncope evaluation, and differentiation of true AV block from concealed AV extrasystoles.

Description: His bundle electrography is the use of a bipolar catheter electrode system during right heart catheterization for recording activity of rhythm and conduction in the bundle of His located in the heart. This test provides information on intra-atrial and intraventricular conduction that is not available with regular electrocardiography.

Professional Considerations:

1. Consent form IS required.

Risks:

Dysrhythmias, phlebitis, pulmonary emboli, thromboemboli, and hemorrhage.

Contraindications:

Clients with coagulopathy and acute pulmonary embolism.

2. Preparation:
   A. Have emergency medication available for use in case a dysrhythmia develops.
   B. *See Client and family teaching.*
3. Procedure:
   A. A catheter is introduced through the femoral vein and guided by fluoroscopy to the right ventricle.
   B. Leads I, II, and III placed on the limbs are recorded simultaneously with two intracardiac bipolar electrograms. One is in the high right atrium (HRA) and the other is over the septal leaflet of the tricuspid valve to record the bundle of His (HBE). The first deflection of the HBE represents right atrial activity. The second deflection represents His bundle activity. The third deflection represents ventricular activation.
4. Postprocedure care:
   A. Monitor vital signs and lower extremity pulses and observe and palpate for hematoma at the catheter site every 15 minutes × 4, then hourly × 4.
   B. Maintain the extremity in extension until the frequent monitoring period has passed.
   C. Assess the catheter site for bleeding every 30 minutes × 4 hours.
5. Client and family teaching:
   A. Fast from food and fluids for at least 6 hours.
   B. The test takes 1–3 hours.
   C. Results are available immediately.
6. Factors that affect results:
   A. Poor catheter positioning.
7. Other data:
   A. *See also Cardiac Catheterization, Diagnostic* for other care required.

Bibliography:

Fleg JL, Das DN, Wright J, et al.: Age-associated changes in the components of atrioventricular conduction in apparently healthy volunteers. J Gerontol *45*(3):95–100, 1990.

Flowers NC, Horan LG, Yang WQ: Application of beat-to-beat techniques. PACE *13*:2148–2155, 1990.

HISTAMINE STIMULATION TEST, DIAGNOSTIC

(see Gastric Acid Secretion, Gastric Acid Stimulation, Diagnostic)

HISTOPATHOLOGY, SPECIMEN

Norm: Requires interpretation by pathologist.

Usage: Histologic diagnosis: Abortion, abscess, achlorhydria, acne vulgaris, actinomycosis, alcoholism, amenorrhea, amyloidosis, appendicitis, arthritis (osteo), brain tumors, cancers, cardiomyopathy, cervicitis, cholecystitis, cirrhosis, Crohn's disease, Cushing's syndrome, cystitis, cytomegalovirus, dermatitis, diverticulitis, diverticulosis, duodenal ulcer, echinococcosis, ectopic pregnancy, eczema, emphysema, endometritis, epididymitis, esophagitis, esophagoscopy, fever of undetermined origin, fibrocystic breast disease, G-cell hyperplasia, ganglioneuroblastoma, gangrene, gastric ulcer, gastritis, genital herpes, giardiasis, glycogen storage disease, gynecomastia, hairy-cell leukemia, Hashimoto's thyroiditis, hemochromatosis, hepatitis, Hirschsprung's disease, histoplasmosis, Hodgkin's disease, hyperaldosteronism, hydatidiform mole, hyperparathyroidism, idiopathic thrombocytopenic purpura, infertility, insulinoma, intraductal breast papilloma, jaundice, kidney stone, Legionnaires' disease, leprosy (Hansen's disease), lymphogranuloma venereum, melanoma, metastasis, myocarditis, necrotizing granulomas (histoplasmosis), nephrolithiasis, neuropathy, pancreatitis, pelvic inflammatory disease, pemphigus, peptic ulcer, pericarditis, peripheral neuropathy, peritonitis, pleurisy, psoriasis, Reye's syndrome, renal infarction, rubeola, sarcoidosis, scleroderma, sinusitis, Sjögren's syndrome, stress ulcers, tumors, ulcerative colitis, vasculitis, Whipple's disease, and xerostomia.

Description: Specimen or tissue pathology involving gross and microscopic examination of biopsy sample and diagnosis by a qualified pathologist.

Professional Considerations:

1. Consent form NOT required.
2. Preparation:
   A. Obtain a sterile container and fixative/formalin.
   B. The requisition must include the operative diagnosis and the site of the specimen.
3. Procedure:
   A. The tissue or fluid sample is obtained using local or general anesthesia.

B. Label the specimen with the client's name, age, sex, room number, and operative diagnosis; the source of the specimen; and the surgeon and other physicians desiring a copy of the pathology report.

4. Postprocedure care:
   A. Fresh tissue is fixed in phosphate-buffered formalin (5–20 times the bulk of the specimen), or submitted directly to a responsible party on saline-soaked sterile gauze.
   B. Deliver the specimen to the laboratory within 1 hour.

5. Client and family teaching:
   A. The diagnosis will take 1 day or more.
   B. See *Biopsy, Site-Specific, Specimen.*

6. Factors that affect results:
   A. Poor sampling technique or contamination.
   B. A sample that has become dried out will impair interpretation.

7. Other data:
   A. Tissue fixed in formalin CANNOT be used for bacteriology, electron microscopy, estrogen or progesterone receptors, or histochemistry.
   B. See also *Biopsy, Site-Specific, Specimen.*

Bibliography:

Devine SM, Larson RA: Acute leukemia in adults: Recent developments in diagnosis and treatment. CA *44*(5):326–352, 1994.

Mashberg A, Samit R: Early diagnosis of asymptomatic oral and oropharyngeal squamous cancers. CA *45*(6):328–351, 1996.

Maygarden SJ, McLendon WW: Pathology and laboratory medicine. JAMA *265*(23):3154–3156, 1991.

HISTOPLASMOSIS SEROLOGY, BLOOD

Norm:

Immunodiffusion test: negative.
Complement fixation titer: <1:4.

Positive: Histoplasmosis.

Complement fixation titer: Fourfold rise in titer indicates current infection.

Suspicious for infection: 1:8–1:16; diagnostic for active infection: >1:32.

Immunodiffusion test: Presence of H (active) and M (active, recent, or past) bands indicate infection.

Description: *Histoplasma capsulatum* is a soil saprobe fungus, which resides in the intestines of birds and bats that causes a common respiratory, noncommunicable, infection, histoplasmosis. *H. capsulatum* spores are inhaled, enter the bloodstream, and spread through the reticuloendothelial system, causing breathing difficulty and enlargement of the spleen and lymph nodes. The antibody titers are usually elevated 6 weeks after infection, last weeks or months, and decline quickly, although they may remain elevated for up to 1 year.

Professional Considerations:

1. Consent form NOT required.
2. Preparation:
   A. Tube: Red-top, red/gray-top, or gold-top.
   B. Obtain travel history to identify exposure to high-risk endemic areas.
   C. Ascertain if the client has been exposed to droppings of bats, chickens, pigeons, starlings, or blackbirds.
   D. The sample should be drawn prior to the histoplasmosis skin test.
3. Procedure:
   A. *Immunodiffusion:* Draw a 1-ml blood sample. Complement fixation: Draw a 2-ml blood sample.
4. Postprocedure care:
   A. No special care required.
5. Client and family teaching:
   A. Signs and symptoms of histoplasmosis include flulike symptoms, pleuritic pain, pericarditis, pancytopenia, and hepatosplenomegaly.
   B. HIV-positive clients should avoid travel to endemic areas (in the United States, these include the middle, central, and south central states).
   C. Follow-up specimens should be drawn at 2- to 3-week intervals to identify fluctuating antibody levels.
   D. A 3% solution of formalin sprayed on contaminated soil will destroy the fungi.
6. Factors that affect results:
   A. False-positive results can occur with aspergillosis, blastomycosis, and coccidioidomycosis.
   B. A recent histoplasmosis skin test may falsely elevate titer.
7. Other data:
   A. One-third of all cases are infants.
   B. Histoplasmosis can cause pleural effusion.

Bibliography:

Flaskerud JK, Ungvarski PJ: HIV/AIDS: A Guide to Nursing Care. Philadelphia, WB Saunders, 1995, pp 100–101.

Malarkey LM, and McMorrow ME: Nurse's Manual of Laboratory Tests and Diagnostic Procedures. Philadelphia, WB Saunders, 1996, pp 155–156.

Wheat J: Histoplasmosis: recognition and treatment. Clin Infect Dis *19*(Suppl 1):S19–S27, 1994.

Williams B, Fojtasek M, Connolly-Stringfield P, Wheat J: Diagnosis of histoplasmosis by antigen detection during an outbreak in Indianapolis. Arch Pathol Lab Med *118*(12):1205–1208, 1994.

HISTOPLASMOSIS SKIN TEST, DIAGNOSTIC

Norm: Negative as evidenced by no induration and erythema <5 mm in diameter.

Positive: Histoplasmosis.

Description: *(See Histoplasmosis, Serology).* Skin tests become positive 2–3 weeks after infection and remain positive in 90% of the infected population for life.

Professional Considerations:

1. Consent form NOT required.
2. Preparation:
   A. Travel history should be included as part of the client's health history to determine exposure to high-incidence endemic areas.
   B. Obtain an alcohol wipe; a needle; a syringe; and histoplasmin, an antigen prepared from culture (usually commercially prepared).
3. Procedure:
   A. Histoplasmin is injected intradermally.
   B. Record the location of the injection for reading.
   C. The injection should follow blood draw for serum titer.
4. Postprocedure care:
   A. Read the test in 24–48 hours. An area of erythema and induration of ≥5 mm diameter is indicative of a positive reaction.
5. Client and family teaching:
   A. *See Histoplasmosis Serology, Blood.*
6. Factors that affect results:
   A. Test may be falsely negative in 50% of people with disseminated histoplasmosis and 10% of people with cavitary histoplasmosis.
   B. False-negative results may occur due to depressed immunologic status or steroid therapy.
   C. False-positive results may occur in people with blastomycosis (30%) or coccidioidomycosis (40%).
7. Other data:
   A. Acutely ill clients may not have a positive skin reaction.
   B. This test is not recommended, because of the difficult interpretation and because it may cause the serology test to be falsely positive.

Bibliography:

Corbett JV: Laboratory Tests and Diagnostic Procedures with Nursing Diagnoses, 4th ed. Norwalk, CT, Appleton and Lange, 1996, p 381.

Hay RJ: Histoplasmosis [review]. Semin Dermatol *12*(4):310–314, 1993.

Wheat J: Histoplasmosis: recognition and treatment. Clinical infectious diseases. *19*(Suppl 1):S19–S27, 1994 (Aug).

HIV BATTERY

(see Acquired Immune Deficiency Syndrome Evaluation Battery, Diagnostic)

HIV P24 ANTIGEN

(see Acquired Immune Deficiency Syndrome Evaluation Battery, Diagnostic)

HLA

(see Human Leukocyte Antigen, Blood)

HLA-ANTIGEN B-27

(see Human Leukocyte Antigen B-27, Blood)

HOLLANDER (BASAL GASTRIC SECRETION) TEST, DIAGNOSTIC

Norm:

Complete Vagotomy: No acid secretion observed within 45 minutes of insulin-induced hypoglycemia.

Incomplete Vagotomy: Acid secretion is >20 mmol/L if total acid output is >2 mmol/hour.

Usage: Evaluate the effectiveness of a vagotomy.

Description: The Hollander test, usually performed 3–6 months after a surgical vagotomy, involves injecting insulin intravenously into a client with an otherwise normal blood sugar. The vagus nerve responds to hypoglycemia by stimulating gastric acid secretion. Thus, in the presence of hypoglycemia, increased acid production indicates an incomplete vagotomy, and absence of acid production indicates a complete vagotomy.

Professional Considerations:

1. Consent form IS required.

Risks:

Hypoglycemic seizures, strokes, myocardial infarction, and deaths have been reported during this test. Complications of nasogastric tube insertion include bleeding, dysrhythmias, esophageal perforation, laryngospasm, and decreased mean PO_2.

Contraindications:

Hypoglycemia, coronary artery disease, or cerebrovascular disease.

2. Preparation:
   A. The client should have patent intravenous access.
   B. Obtain regular insulin, a nasogastric tube and an irrigation syringe, a needle, a syringe, a fluoridated gray-top tube, and an ampule of dextrose 50.
   C. *See Client and family teaching.*
3. Procedure:
   A. Insert the nasogastric tube, aspirate gastric contents, and place these in a container to measure.
   B. Inject an intravenous bolus of 0.1–0.2 U/kg body weight of regular insulin. After the blood glucose falls to <50 mg/dl (usually within 30 minutes), the gastric contents should be aspirated.
   C. If postinsulin aspirate exceeds the preinjection amount of aspirate, then the vagotomy is likely incomplete.
4. Postprocedure care:
   A. Monitor vital signs every 15 minutes × 4, then every hour × 4. Monitor closely and treat for complications (listed in section 5C below).
   B. Monitor blood sugar every hour × 2. Provide food sources of glucose as needed if hypoglycemic symptoms appear.
5. Client and family teaching:
   A. Fast from food for 12 hours and from liquids for 8 hours prior to the test.
   B. Do not smoke for 8 hours prior to the test.
   C. A nasogastric tube will be inserted through your nose into your stomach. Insertion may be uncomfortable and cause a pressurelike feeling or cause you to gag and cough. You will be asked to take sips of water and swallow to make tube insertion easier.
6. Factors that affect results:
   A. None.
7. Other data:
   A. None.

Bibliography:

Huang YS, Huang TJ, et al.: Effect of vagotomy on cholecystokinin release and gallbladder contraction in patients with complicated duodenal ulcer. Eur Surg Res *26*(6):362–371, 1994.

Witte CL: Is vagotomy and gastrectomy still justified for gastroduodenal ulcer? [editorial]. J Clin Gastroenterol *20*(1):2–3, 1995.

HOLTER MONITOR, DIAGNOSTIC

Norm: No dysrhythmias.

Usage: Cardiomyopathy, cerebral ischemia, dysrhythmias (detection), mitral valve prolapse, pacemaker function, palpitations, and syncope.

Description: A Holter monitor is a portable, miniaturized electrocardiographic amplifier coupled to a magnetic recorder. It is used to obtain a permanent recording of continuous electrocardiographic activity of a client for an extended period of time, such as 24–48 hours. The client wears the monitor continuously, and must record all activity and symptoms experienced at the specific times of occurrence throughout the monitoring period. The resulting electrocardiographic recording is analyzed for abnormalities and correlated with the documented activities and symptoms to help diagnose or rule out abnormalities such as those listed under "Usage" (above).

Professional Considerations:

1. Consent form NOT required.
2. Preparation:
   A. Explain purpose to client/family.
   B. Obtain a diary and a pen or pencil, electrodes, and a Holter monitor.
   C. The electrodes must be applied to skin free of hair (shaved) that has been cleansed with acetone.
   D. *See Client and family teaching.*
3. Procedure:
   A. Assess for paper roll availability with each monitor.
   B. Maintain a diary of movements to assist the diagnostician in evaluating the heart rhythm.
4. Postprocedure care:
   A. Remove all electrodes.
5. Client and family teaching:
   A. This monitor is used to identify abnormal heart rhythms that may occur for brief periods of time. Keeping a complete diary of times, activities, and sensations throughout monitoring helps pinpoint the cause of symptoms and the effect of activities on the heart.
   B. Avoid bathing (other than sponge bath), magnets, metal detectors, high-voltage areas, and electric blankets, as these may interfere with recording.
6. Factors that affect results:
   A. An incomplete diary interferes with accurate interpretation of findings.
   B. Failure to apply electrodes correctly may cause an artifactual or incomplete signal.
7. Other data:
   A. None.

Bibliography:

Biederman J, Baldessarini RJ, Goldblatt A, et al.: A naturalistic study of 24-hour electrocardiographic recordings and echocardiographic findings in children and adolescents treated with desipramine. J Am Acad Child Adolesc Psychiatr 32(4):805–813, 1993.

Fernandez AR, Sequira RF, et al.: Tracking for rapid determination of patency of the infarct-related artery in acute myocardial infarction. J Am Coll Cardiol 26(3):675–683, 1995.

Jiang W, Blumenthal JA, Hanson MW, et al.: Relative importance of electrode placement over number of channels in transient myocardial ischemia detection by Holter monitoring. Am J Cardiol 76(5): 350–354, 1995.

HOMOVANILLIC ACID (HVA), 24-HOUR, URINE

Norm: Measures of HVA/measures of creatinine as follows:

		SI Units
Adults	0.25–2.5 µg/mg	1–14 µmol/mg
	or <8 mg/24 hours	10–35 mol/24 hours
Children		
<1 year	1.2–35 µg/mg	7–192 µmol/mg
1 year	4–23 µg/mg	22–126 µmol/mg
2–4 years	0.5–14 µg/mg	3–77 µmol/mg
5–9 years	0.5–9 µg/mg	3–49 µmol/mg
10–14 years	0.25–12 µg/mg	1–66 µmol/mg
15–18 years	0.5–2 µg/mg	3–11 µmol/mg

Increased: Brain tumor, ganglioneuroblastoma, neuroblastoma, and pheochromocytoma. Drugs include aminosalicylic acid, disulfiram, levodopa, methocarbamol, reserpine, and robaxin.

Decreased: Not clinically significant. Drugs include aminosalicylic acid, levodopa, methocarbamol, and monoamine oxidase inhibitors.

Description: Homovanillic acid is the major terminal metabolite of dopamine, one of the three catecholamines produced in the brain. Dopamine is broken down by the liver and excreted in the urine as homovanillic acid. Elevated levels can occur as a result of catecholamine-secreting tumors.

Professional Considerations:

1. Consent form NOT required.
2. Preparation:
   A. Obtain a clean, 3-L container without preservative.
   B. Write the beginning time of collection on the laboratory requisition.
   C. *See Client and family teaching.*
3. Procedure:
   A. Discard the first morning urine specimen.
   B. Save all urine voided for 24 hours in a refrigerated, clean, 3-L container to which 20 ml of hydrochloric acid (HCl) preservative has been added. Document the quantity of urine output during the collection period. Include the urine voided at the end of the 24-hour period. For catheterized clients, keep the drainage bag on ice and empty urine into the collection container hourly.
4. Postprocedure care:
   A. Compare the urine quantity in the specimen container with the urinary output record for the test. If the specimen contains less urine than was recorded as output, some of the sample may have been discarded, thus invalidating the test.
   B. Document the quantity of urine output and the ending time for the collection period on the laboratory requisition.
   C. Send the entire 24-hour urine specimen immediately to the laboratory for testing.
5. Client and family teaching:
   A. Avoid large doses of aspirin, coffee, tea, chocolate, caffeine, phenothiazine, antihypertension agents, fruit, and any vanilla-containing substances for 48 hours prior to urine collection.
   B. If taking levodopa medication, the physician may discontinue this medication for 2 weeks prior to the test.
   C. Save all the urine voided in the 24-hour period and urinate before defecating to avoid loss of urine. If any urine is accidentally discarded, discard the entire specimen and restart the collection the next day.
6. Factors that affect results:
   A. False elevation may occur with excessive physical exercise or emotional stress.

7. Other data:

A. Homovanillic acid is usually measured simultaneously with metanephrine, normetanephrine, and vanillylmandelic acid to assist in differential diagnosis.

Bibliography:

Cole M, Craft AW, Parker L, et al.: Urinary creatinine adjusted reference ranges for homovanillic and vanillylmandelic acid in children and adults. Clin Chim Acta 236(1):19–32, 1995.

Fitzgibbon MC, Tormey WP: Paediatric reference ranges for urinary catecholamines/metabolites and their relevance in neuroblastoma diagnosis. Ann Clin Biochem 31(Pt 1):1–11, 1994.

Kerbl R, Urban C, et al.: Neuroblastoma with N-myc amplification detected by urine: mass screening in infants after the sixth month of life. Med Pediatr Oncol 21(9):625–626, 1993.

HORMONAL EVALUATION, CYTOLOGIC, SPECIMEN

Norm: Requires interpretation based on clinical status. Maturation index is reported as percentages of parabasal/intermediate/superficial cells.

Usage: Amenorrhea, feminizing tumor, ovarian dysfunction, pituitary dysfunction, and virilizing tumor.

Description: Microscopic evaluation of cellular composition of the surface layers of the vaginal squamous epithelium, which reflects the balance of estrogen and progesterone.

Professional Considerations:

1. Consent form NOT required.
2. Preparation:
   A. Obtain drapes, a sterile wooden spatula, a glass slide, and a fixative spray or 95% alcohol.
   B. The client should disrobe below the waist.
   C. *See Client and family teaching.*

3. Procedure:
   A. Position the client in the dorsal lithotomy position, and drape her for privacy and comfort.
   B. Use lubricating gel sparingly, as excess will interfere with the cytology exam.
   C. Excess glove powder should be removed before handling the spatula, as starch granules make slide interpretation difficult.
   D. Scrape the lateral vaginal wall with a sterile wooden spatula.

4. Postprocedure care:
   A. Transfer the secretions to a glass slide and fix them with 95% alcohol or spray fixative.
   B. Include on the laboratory requisition the date of the last menstrual period, and history of radiation therapy or gynecologic surgery.

5. Client and family teaching:
   A. Do not douche for 24 hours prior to obtaining the smear.
   B. The test is painless and takes only a moment.

6. Factors that affect results:
   A. A dried specimen due to failure to apply fixative is cause for specimen rejection.
   B. Agents that cause misleading desquamation include cortisone, digitalis, estrogen, and tetracycline suppositories.

7. Other data:
   A. This test has limited value when applied to an individual, as there is a great variation in normal values and between counters.

Bibliography:

Akron General Medical Center: Laboratory Users Guide. Akron, OH, Department of Pathology and Laboratory Medicine, 1991, p 128.

Slagel DD, Zaleski S, Cohen MB: Efficacy of automated cervical cytology screening. Diagn Cytology 13(1):26–30, 1995.

HPV

(see Human Papillomavirus, Specimen)

HUMAN CHORIONIC GONADOTROPIN (HCG), BETA-SUBUNIT, SERUM

Norm:

		SI Units
Beta subunit	<2 ng/ml or <5 mIU/ml	<2 µg/L <5 IU/L

Increased: Choriocarcinoma, eclampsia, ectopic pregnancy, erythroblastosis fetalis, germ cell tumors gynecomastia, hydatidiform mole, insulinoma, neoplasms (colon, hepatoma, lung, pancreas, stomach), ovarian cancer, pregnancy, seminoma, and testicular cancer and possibly bladder cancer.

Decreased: Abortion and ectopic pregnancy.

Description: Human chorionic gonadotropin is a glycoprotein hormone with alpha- and beta-subunits, which are normally produced by a developing placenta and may be produced by some germ cell tumors. The alpha sequence is identical to the follicle-stimulating hormone, luteinizing hormone, and thyroid-stimulating hormone, which can cause a false-positive pregnancy test if not tested along with the beta-subunit. This test can detect pregnancy in as little as 1 week after conception. Serial monitoring is used to help determine gestational age. The beta-subunit is often used to follow the status of neoplasms after surgery or chemotherapy.

Professional Considerations:

1. Consent form NOT required.
2. Preparation:
   A. Tube: Red-top, red/gray-top, or gold-top.
   B. For females, write the date of the last menstrual cycle on the laboratory requisition.
3. Procedure:
   A. Obtain a 1-ml blood sample.
4. Postprocedure care:
   A. Send the sample to the laboratory immediately. The sample can be kept at 2–8°C for up to 24 hours. Additional delay in processing would require that the serum be frozen.
5. Client and family teaching:
   A. If the test is being used to determine pregnancy, results are normally available within 2 hours.
   B. Additional samples will be drawn periodically to help determine fetal gestational age.
6. Factors that affect results:
   A. False-positive tests result from hemolyzed, lipemic, or icteric serum.
   B. If the test is to be performed using radioimmunoassay, a radionuclide scan within 1 week of the test may falsely elevate results.
   C. EDTA (ethylenediaminetetraacetate) and heparin anticoagulants decrease plasma levels and may cause false-negative results.
   D. Values increase more slowly in ectopic than in normal pregnancies.
7. Other data:
   A. Does not eliminate the possibility of pregnancy if results are low or borderline.
   B. *See also Pregnancy Test, Routine, Serum.*

Bibliography:

Baltaci S, Kupeli S, Sak SD, et al.: Human chorionic gonadotropin in serum and neoplastic tissue from patients with bladder cancer. Int Urol Nephrol 27(3):289–295, 1995.

Kellner LH, Weiner Z, Weiss RR, et al.: Triple marker versus alpha-fetoprotein plus free-beta subunit in second-trimester maternal serum screening for fetal Down syndrome: a prospective comparison study. Am J Obstetr Gynecol 173(4):1306–1309, 1995.

Sancken U, Bahner D: The effect of thermal instability of intact human chorionic gonadotropin (ihCG) on the application of its free beta-subunit (free beta hCG) as a serum marker in Down syndrome screening. Prenat Diagn 15(8):731–738, 1995.

Springhouse, Illustrated Guide to Diagnostic Tests. Springhouse, PA, Springhouse Corporation, 1994, pp 189–191.

HUMAN CHORIONIC GONADOTROPIN (HCG, PREGNANCY TEST), SERUM

(see Pregnancy Test, Routine, Serum)

HUMAN EPIDERMAL GROWTH FACTOR

(see HER-2 Neu Oncogene, Specimen)

HUMAN IMMUNODEFICIENCY VIRUS

(see Acquired Immune Deficiency Syndrome Evaluation Battery, Diagnostic)

HUMAN LEUKOCYTE ANTIGEN (HLA) B-27, BLOOD

Norm: Requires clinical correlation.

Positive: Ankylosing spondylitis (Marie-Strumpell disease), arthritis (rheumatoid), congenital adrenal hyperplasia, Goodpasture's syndrome, narcolepsy, pemphigus, Reiter's syndrome, and thyroiditis (subacute).

Negative: Normal finding.

Description: *See Human Leukocyte Antigen Typing, Blood for description of the HLA antigen.* The presence of B-27 antigen is highly correlated with ankylosing spondylitis and rheumatoid arthritis.

Professional Considerations:

1. Consent form NOT required.
2. Preparation:
   A. Tube: Green-top.
   B. Preschedule this test with the laboratory.
3. Procedure:
   A. Draw a 10-ml blood sample.
4. Postprocedure care:
   A. Send the specimen to the laboratory immediately; do not freeze it.

5. Client and family teaching:
   A. Results are normally available within 24 hours.
6. Factors that affect results:
   A. The test must be performed on live lymphocytes. If the cells have died, a new sample must be drawn.
7. Other data:
   A. Clients who are HLA-B27-positive have a 120 times greater chance of developing ankylosing spondylitis than clients who are negative.

Bibliography:

Harley JB, Scofield RH: The spectrum of ankylosing spondylitis. Hosp Pract (Office Ed), *30*(7):37–43,46, 1995.

Hulstaert F, Albrecht J, Hannet I, et al.: An optimized method for routine HLA-B27 screening using flow cytometry. Cytometry *18*(1):21–29, 1994.

Paimela L, Leirisalo-Repo M, Helve T, Koskimies S: The prognostic value of HLA DR4 and B27 antigens in early rheumatoid arthritis. Scand J Rheumatol *22*(5):220–224, 1993.

HUMAN LEUKOCYTE ANTIGEN (HLA) TYPING (TISSUE TYPING), BLOOD

Norm: Interpretation required for tissue typing and determination of histocompatibility match or nonmatch.

Usage: Paternity testing and transplants (to determine histocompatibility); selection of platelet donors for immunized clients.

Description: Human leukocyte antigens (HLAs) are glycoproteins found on all nucleated cells. They result from four closely linked genes on chromosome 6 and are important to histocompatibility and complement and immune response. The antigens are divided into A, B, C (Class I, derived from T cells), D, and DR (D-related, Class II, derived from B cells). There are multiple antigens of each type, meaning that the combinations of antigens that identify any individual are infinite. The HLA antigens are inherited as two sets (one from each parent) of six antigens. This test is most commonly used in bone marrow and renal transplantation. The antigens must match in order for transplantation to occur without organ rejection.

Professional Considerations:

1. Consent form NOT required.
2. Preparation:
   A. Preschedule this test with the laboratory. The sample should be drawn be-

fore or 72 hours after a blood product transfusion.
   B. *For donor specimen:* Tube: Two green-top tubes.
   C. *For recipient specimen:* Tube: Red-top, red/gray-top, or gold-top.
3. Procedure:
   A. *Donor specimen:* Completely fill two green-top tubes with blood (7 ml each).
   B. *Recipient specimen:* Completely fill a red-top tube with 7 ml of blood.
4. Postprocedure care:
   A. Send the specimen to the laboratory for immediate testing.
   B. Do not refrigerate or freeze the specimen or place the specimen on ice.
5. Client and family teaching:
   A. Encourage the client to express concerns regarding illness (such as awaiting a suitable donor, symptom management).
6. Factors that affect results:
   A. Refrigeration of or delay in processing specimens may result in inadequate lymphocytes for accurate testing.
7. Other data:
   A. Samples that have been used for cross-matching should be frozen and stored for 1 year.
   B. *See also Human Leukocyte Antigen, B-27, Blood.*

Bibliography:

LeFever Kee J: Laboratory and Diagnostic Tests with Nursing Implications, 4th ed. Norwalk, CT, Appleton and Lange, 1995, pp 201–202.

Malarkey LM, McMorrow ME: Nurse's Manual of Laboratory Tests and Diagnostic Procedures. Philadelphia, WB Saunders, 1996, pp 410–411.

Springhouse: Illustrated Guide to Diagnostic Tests. Springhouse, PA, Springhouse Corporation, 1994, pp 312–313.

HUMAN PAPILLOMAVIRUS (HPV) IN SITU HYBRIDIZATION, SPECIMEN

Norm: Determination (by histopathologist) of absence of genetic changes consistent with the human-papillomavirus.

Usage: Determination of HPV type; confirmation of HPV infection; resolution of cases with definitive histology through the hybridization process that detects the presence of specific DNA sequences.

Description: A member of the Papoviridae family of viruses, HPV, associated with infection of surface epithelia, is the causative agent of sexually transmitted genital warts. It is important for its role as a major risk factor in the development of cervical cancer, and for cervical intraepithelial neoplasia (CIN). This virus may also have a role in the pathogenesis of Kaposi's sarcoma and progression to overt disease in the client with HIV infection. In situ hybridization is a variation of hybridization in which the cervical biopsy sample consists of the chromosomes within a cell arrested at metaphase. The metaphase chromosomes are spread out and partially denatured on a microscope slide, the probe is labeled with a fluorescent dye, and the bound probe is imaged with a flourescence microscope. The "probe" is a short stretch of single-stranded DNA whose sequence is identical or complementary to some unique portion of the segment of interest. Ideally, the probe hybridizes (binds) only to cloned fragment(s) containing the segment of interest, and the image of the bound probe is seen under a fluorescent microscope. Because in situ hybridization has poor sensitivity, it is most useful when viruses are present in the sample in large amounts.

Professional Considerations:

1. Consent form IS required for the procedure used to obtain the specimen.

Risks:

Bleeding, infection.

Contraindications:

Bleeding disorder or anticoagulated state.

2. Preparation:
   A. Schedule the client when she is not menstruating; the best time is 1 week postmenses (especially important if a PAP is also being obtained).
   B. Obtain a sterile speculum, 10% neutral buffered formalin, sterile punch biopsy forceps, a crushproof container for paraffin block, silver nitrate sticks or other hemostasis product, and a tampon. *For Detection and Typing, HPV PROBE*, it is necessary to use the HPV collection kit (supplied by Roche).
   C. Ask the client to void.
   D. Record the biopsy site and the client's and doctor's names on the laboratory requisition.
3. Procedure:
   A. *In situ hybridization:*
      i. Assist the client to the lithotomy position.

ii. A colposcope may be used to visualize the cervix, inserted, through the unlubricated speculum.
      iii. Tissue sample(s) removed from any visible lesion(s) or doctor-selected site(s); enough for a minimum of eight 5 micron sections.
   B. *DNA Probe:*
      i. *Male:* Collect cells from the urethra using a swab. Place the collection device in the HPV transport tube for shipment to the lab.
      ii. *Female:* Collect cervical cells from the endocervical canal and the exocervix using the HPV collection kit. Place a swab in the transport tube for shipment to the lab.
4. Postprocedure care:
   A. Tissue: Submit the biopsy (frozen), 3 mm in diameter, in an HPV collection tube. Biopsies must be shipped frozen at –20°C.
   B. Swab the cervix with silver nitrate to control bleeding postbiopsy, and the examiner may insert a tampon if bleeding persists.
   C. The tissue must be fixed with formalin solution immediately, then embedded in paraffin within 72 hours. Embed in paraffin in a way that the tissue section will fit into a 10-mm circle. The specimen may not remain in formalin beyond 72 hours.
   D. Complete the filling out of the requisition, noting the number and appearance of tissue samples.
5. Client and family teaching:
   A. Rest for 8–24 hours postprocedure, avoiding heavy lifting or strenuous exercise.
   B. Avoid douching and intercourse for 2 weeks or as directed by the physician.
   C. An odorous, gray-green vaginal discharge is normal, and may occur for up to 3 weeks postprocedure.
   D. Some bleeding will occur normally, but inform the doctor if heavy bleeding (heavier than menstrual, clots) occurs.
   E. Mild discomfort during and after the procedure is normal. Take a nonaspirin analgesic as needed.
6. Factors that affect results:
   A. Improperly fixed tissue cannot be used for this test.
   B. An inadequate amount of tissue would cause specimen rejection.
7. Other data:
   A. A DNA probe is used to aid in the diagnosis of sexually transmitted HPV infections, distinguishing between infections with types associated with low-grade squamous intraepithelial lesions (LSIL), types 6.11.42, 43, 44, and types associated with SIL of all grades, including high-grade (HSIL), types, 16, 18, 31, 33, 35, 45, 51, 52, and 56.
   B. The polymerase chain reaction test for HPV detection can identify 9 specific

types of the virus, but is currently *for investigational use only*. Specimen collection and pre- and postcare are essentially the same as for the in situ hybridization method.

Bibliography:

Borg AJ, Medley G, Garland SM: Polymerase chain reaction. A sensitive indicator of the prevalence of human papillomavirus DNA in a population with sexually transmitted disease. Acta Cytol *39*(4): 654–658, 1995.

Flaskerud JH, Ungvarski PJ: HIV/AIDS: A Guide to Nursing Care, 3rd ed. Philadelphia, WB Saunders, 1995, pp 35,71,85,86,71,103,116, 464, 465t.

Herrington CS, Anderson SM, Bauer HM, et al.: Comparative analysis of human papillomavirus detection by PCR and non-isotopic in situ hybridization. J Clin Pathol *48*(5):415–419, 1995.

Konya J, Veress G, Hernadi Z, et al.: Correlation of human papillomavirus 16 and 18 with prognostic factors in invasive cervical neoplasias. J Med Virol *46*(1):1–6, 1995.

Wagner RP: Understanding inheritance. *In* Cooper NG (ed): The Human Genome Project: Deciphering the Blueprint of Heredity. Mill Valley, CA, University Science Books, 1994, pp 60–64, 128–131.

HUMAN TUMOR STEM-CELL ASSAY, DIAGNOSTIC

Norm: Growth or inhibition of growth of tumor cells.

Usage: Determine the sensitivity or resistance of an individual's tumor cells to an anticancer drug.

Description: An in vitro test to determine responsiveness of tumor cells to specific drugs. A specimen of tumor is obtained from the individual. The cells are enzymatically dissociated, centrifuged, and placed into suspensions. Different anticancer drugs are added to each sample prior to being placed in agar plates. The plates are examined microscopically twice each week for at least 2–3 weeks when cell growth is likely to have occurred. Growth of the cells implies resistance to the drug or irradiation, and lack of growth indicates some anticancer effect.

Professional Considerations:

1. Consent form NOT required, but IS required for the procedure used to obtain the specimen. See individual procedure for risks and contraindications.
2. Preparation:
   A. Prepare surgical instruments for tissue removal.
3. Procedure:
   A. Cells from the tumor are obtained and enzymatically dissociated in the laboratory.

B. The cells are examined microscopically twice a week for 2–3 weeks.
4. Postprocedure care:
   A. Apply a sterile dressing to the incision site.
   B. Observe the site for bleeding and symptoms of infection for 24–48 hours.
   C. *See Biopsy, Site-Specific, Specimen.*
5. Client and family teaching:
   A. Results take approximately 3 weeks, but can help the physician select the treatment regimen most likely to be effective in destroying cancer cells.
6. Factors that affect results:
   A. Approximately 50% of tumors are unsuitable for in vitro growth, making the test difficult to interpret.
7. Other data:
   A. Prediction of drug sensitivity is 40–90% correct, and prediction of drug resistance is 90–95% correct.

Bibliography:

Aapro MS: Clonogenic assays for gynecologic malignancies: Methodology and results. EORTC Preclinical Therapeutic Models Group (PTMG) [review]. Contrib Gynecol Obstet *19*:24–29, 1994.

Bakerman S: ABC's of Interpretive Laboratory Data, 2nd ed. Greenville, NC, Interpretive Laboratory Data, Inc, 1984.

Casciari JJ, Hollingshead MG, Alley MC, et al.: Growth and chemotherapeutic response of cells in a hollow-fiber in vitro solid tumor model. Natl Cancer Inst *86*(24):1846–1852, 1994.

Lawton PA, Hodkiss RJ, Eyden BP, Joiner, MC: Growth of fibroblasts as a potential confounding factor in soft agar clonogenic assays for tumour cell radiosensitivity, Radiother Oncol *32*(3):218–225, 1994.

HYDROCEPHALUS RADIOLOGIC EVALUATION, DIAGNOSTIC

Norm: Absence of hydrocephalus.

Usage: Diagnosis of hydrocephalus and whether it is communicating or noncommunicating.

Description: Under computed tomography, radionuclide (usually technetium-99m) is tagged to albumin and injected into a lumbar puncture site. The radionuclide then travels upward into the brain, where it can be observed in terms of the amount of fluid and whether the fluid is able to travel into the ventricles (communicating). Noncommunicating hydrocephalus prevents the radionuclide from traveling into the ventricles.

Professional Considerations:

1. Consent form IS required.

Risks:

Increased intracranial pressure, allergic reaction to radiolabeled albumin (itching, hives, rash, tight feeling in the throat, shortness of breath, bronchospasm, anaphylaxis, death).

Contraindications:

Previous allergy to radiolabeled albumin; increased intracranial pressure; during pregnancy or breast-feeding.

2. Preparation:
   A. Remove all metal objects from the client's head.
   B. Obtain a lumbar puncture tray.
   C. A CT scan is typically performed to rule out increased intracranial pressure prior to lumbar puncture in critically ill clients or those with changed mental status.
3. Procedure:
   A. Radiolabeled human serum albumin is given to demonstrate the flow of CSF from the point of the lumbar puncture up to the cranium.
4. Postprocedure care:
   A. Assess vital signs every 15 minutes × 4.
   B. Observe the client carefully for up to 60 minutes after the study for a possible (anaphylactic) reaction to the radionuclide.
   C. Rubber gloves should be worn when discarding urine for 24 hours after the procedure. Wash the gloved hands with soap and water before removing the gloves. Wash the ungloved hands after gloves are removed.
5. Client and family teaching:
   A. The test takes 1–2 hours.
   B. Meticulously wash hands with soap and water after each void × 24 hours.
6. Factors that affect results:
   A. None.
7. Other data:
   A. Health care professionals working in a nuclear medicine area must follow federal standards set by the Nuclear Regulatory Commission. These standards include precautions for handling the radioactive material and monitoring of potential radiation exposure.
   B. Technetium half-life is 6 hours.

Bibliography:

Kang JK: Neuroimaging and functional examination in hydrocephalus: a comment [review]. Childs Nerv Syst *11*(8):478–482, 1995.

Maeder P, deTribolet N: Xenon CT measurement of cerebral blood flow in hydrocephalus. Childs Nerv Sys *11*(7):388–391, 1995.

Van Roost D, Solymosi L, Funke K: A characteristic ventricular shape in myelomeningocele-associated hydrocephalus? A CT stereology study. Neuroradiology *37*(5):412–417, 1995.

HYDROXYBUTYRATE DEHYDROGENASE (HBDH), BLOOD

Norm: 140–350 IU/L.

Increased: Anemia (hemolytic or megaloblastic), leukemia, lymphoma, malignant melanoma, muscular dystrophy, myocardial infarction, nephrotic syndrome, and orthopedic hip surgery, hepatic cellular damage.

Decreased: Not clinically significant.

Description: Enzyme similar to lactate dehydrogenase 1 (LD1) that is found in the brain, heart muscle, kidney, and red blood cells. It is most generally used to diagnose myocardial infarction, although levels may also be elevated when there is damage to other organs. HBDH levels are more specific and last longer than CK, AST, and total LD for diagnosing myocardial infarction. HBDH levels rise within 8–10 hours of infarction, peak in 48–96 hours, and remain abnormal for 16–18 days. This test is primarily used in small laboratories where the complete LD isoenzyme battery is unavailable, or because it is less costly and simpler to perform than LD electrophoresis.

Professional Considerations:

1. Consent form NOT required.
2. Preparation:
   A. Tube: Red-top, red/gray-top, or gold-top.
3. Procedure:
   A. Draw a 7-ml blood sample, without hemolysis.
4. Postprocedure care:
   A. Do not freeze the specimen.
5. Client and family teaching:
   A. Results are normally available within 24 hours.
6. Factors that affect results:
   A. Specimens may be falsely negative if frozen, because enzyme activity is lost.
   B. Traumatic venipuncture or hemolysis causes false-positive results.
7. Other data:
   A. HBDH is stable at room temperature for 5 days and for 10 days if refrigerated.

Bibliography:

Akenzua GI, Ihongbe JC, Asemota HN: Alpha-hydroxybutyrate dehydrogenase and the diagnosis of painful crisis in sickle cell disease. Afr J Med Med Sci *21*(2)a:13–17, 1992.

Kanok Ichimura T: Increased alpha-hydroxybutyrate dehydrogenase in serum from children with measles. Clin Chem.38(5):624–627, 1992.

Springhouse: Illustrated Guide to Diagnostic Tests., Springhouse, PA, Springhouse Corporation, 1994, pp 96–97.

17-HYDROXYCORTICOSTEROIDS (17-OHCS), 24-HOUR, URINE

Norm:

		SI Units
Adult female	2.5–10 mg/24 hours	6.9–27.6 μmol/24 hours
Adult male	4.5–12 mg/24 hours	12.4–33.1 μmol/24 hours
Child		
0–1 years	0.5–1 mg/24 hours	1.4–2.8 μmol/24 hours
<12 years	1–4.5 mg/24 hours	2.8–12.4 μmol/24 hours

Increased: Acetonuria, acromegaly, Cushing's syndrome, glucosuria, fructosuria, hirsutism, hypertension (severe), insomnia, obesity, pregnancy, stress, and virilization. Drugs include acetazolamide, ACTH, ascorbic acid, atarax, cephalothin, cefoxitin, chloral hydrate, chlordiazepoxide, chlorpromazine, colchisine, cortisone acetate, digitalis glycosides, doriden, erythromycin, etryptamine, glutethimide, gonadotropins, hydrocortisone, hydroxyzine, iodides, mandelamine, meprobamate, methenamine, methicillin, methyprylon, oleandomycin, paraldehyde, quinine, quinidine, spironolactone, and troleandomycin.

Decreased: Addison's disease, anorexia nervosa, congenital adrenal hyperplasia, hypopituitarism, and hypothyroidism. Drugs include apresoline, carbamazepine, corticosteroids, dextropropoxyphene, estrogens, medroxyprogesterone, meperidine, morphine, oral contraceptives, pentazocine, phenergan, phenothiazines, phenytoin, reserpine (high doses), salicylates, and thiazide diuretics.

Description: 17-hydroxycorticosteroids are carbon compounds that have a dihydroxyacetone group on the 17th carbon. In urine, the primary 17-OHCSs are breakdown products of cortisone and hydrocortisone, which can be used as a measure of their production (adrenal cortical function).

Professional Considerations:

1. Consent form NOT required.
2. Preparation:
   A. Obtain a 3-L plastic container with acetic, boric, or hydrochloric acid (HCl) additive.
   B. Write the beginning time of collection on the laboratory requisition.
   C. *See Client and family teaching.*
3. Procedure:
   A. Discard the first morning urine specimen.
   B. Save all the urine voided for 24 hours in a clean, 3-L container (on ice) to which acetic acid, boric acid, or HCl preservative has been added. Document the quantity of urine output during the collection period. Include the urine voided at the end of the 24-hour period. For catheterized clients, keep the drainage bag on ice and empty urine into the collection container hourly.
4. Postprocedure care:
   A. Compare the urine quantity in the specimen container with the urinary output record for the test. If the specimen contains less urine than was recorded as output, some of the sample may have been discarded, thus invalidating the test.
   B. Document the quantity of urine output and the ending time for the collection period on the laboratory requisition.
   C. Send the entire 24-hour urine specimen to the laboratory for testing. Refrigerate or freeze the specimen after collection.
5. Client and family teaching:
   A. Stop all medications 24 hours prior to the collection of urine (with physician's approval).
   B. Inform the physician ordering the test of any prescription or over-the-counter medications being taken.
   C. Save all urine voided in the 24-hour period and urinate before defecating to avoid loss of urine. If any urine is accidentally discarded, discard the entire specimen and restart the collection the next day.
   D. Resume medications after the 24-hour urine collection has been completed.
6. Factors that affect results:
   A. Increases in 17-OHCS can be caused by acute illness.

7. Other data:
   A. Urinary free cortisol and serum cortisol are more sensitive and specific tests.
   B. The specimen is stable up to 45 days if properly acidified and refrigerated.

Bibliography:

Barton RN, Horan MA, Weijers JW, et al.: Cortisol production rate and the urinary excretion of 17-hydroxycorticosteroids, free cortisol, and 6 beta-hydroxycirtisol in healthy elderly men and women. J Gerontol 49(1):8–35, 1994 [Published erratum appears in J Gerontol 49(1), following B35, 1994.]

Malarkey LM, McMorrow ME: Nurse's Manual of Laboratory Tests and Diagnostic Procedures. Philadelphia, WB Saunders, 1996, pp 659–661, 963t.

Mason BH, Holdaway IM, Skinner SJ, Kay RG: The relationship of urinary and plasma androgens to steroid receptors and menopausal status in breast cancer patients and their influence on survival. Breast Cancer Res Treat 32(2):202–212, 1994.

Sidha S, Balasubramanian K, et al.: Preliminary study of androgen, thyroid, and adrenal status in alcoholic men during deaddiction. Indian J Med Res 101:268–272, 1995.

Zilembo N, Bajetta E, Noberasco C, et al.: Formestane: an effective first-line endocrine treatment for advanced breast cancer. J Cancer Res Clin Oncol 121(6):378–382, 1995.

5-HYDROXYINDOLEACETIC ACID (5-HIAA), QUANTITATIVE, 24-HOUR, URINE

Norm:

Qualitative: Negative.

Quantitative: 1–10 mg/24 hours (5.2–52 μmol/24 hours, SI units).

Increased: Carcinoid tumors (foregut and midgut) (when dietary sources of 5-HIAA are eliminated before testing), celiac sprue, diarrhea, endocarditis, ganglioneuroblastoma, toxemia of pregnancy and tropical sprue. Drugs include acetaminophen, atenolol, cisplatin (peaks 6 hours after induction), diazepam, fluorouracil, glyceryl guaiacolate, melphalan, mephenesin, methenasin carbamate, methocarbamol, naproxen, oxprenolol, phenacetin, pindolol, and reserpine.

Decreased: Carcinoid tumors (rectal), depression, hartnup disease, mastocytosis, phenylketonuria, small intestine resection diarrhea, and nonmetastatic carcinoid tumors. Drugs include acetic acid; corticotropin; dihydroxyphenolacetic acid; ethanol; formaldehyde; gentisic acid; homogentisic acid; imipramine; isoniazid; levodopa; methenamine; methyldopa; monoamine oxidase (MAO) inhibitors; phenothiazines; salicylates; and sulfasalazine.

Description: 5-HIAA is a primary urinary metabolite of serotonin. Under normal conditions, serotonin is produced in the gastrointestinal tract and acts as a vasoconstrictor. Approximately 5% of serotonin is converted to 5-HIAA and excreted in the urine. Increased urinary 5-HIAA is reflective of overproduction of serotonin, which occurs with carcinoid tumors.

Professional Considerations:

1. Consent form NOT required.
2. Preparation:
   A. Obtain a 3-L plastic container to which 12 g of boric acid or 25 ml of hydrochloric acid (HCl) has been added.
   B. Write the beginning time of collection on the laboratory requisition.
   C. *See Client and family teaching.*
3. Procedure:
   A. Discard the first morning urine specimen.
   B. Save all the urine voided for 24 hours in a refrigerated, clean, 3-L container to which 12 g of boric acid or 24 ml of HCl has been added. Document the quantity of urine output during the collection period. Include the urine voided at the end of the 24-hour period. For catheterized clients, keep the drainage bag on ice and empty urine into the collection container hourly.
4. Postprocedure care:
   A. Compare the urine quantity in the specimen container with the urinary output record for the test. If the specimen contains less urine than was recorded as output, some of the sample may have been discarded, thus invalidating the test.
   B. Document the quantity of urine output and the ending time for the collection period on the laboratory requisition.
   C. Send the entire 24-hour urine specimen to the laboratory for testing.
5. Client and family teaching:
   A. Avoid the following foods 5 days prior to the test: bananas, avocados, plums, eggplant, tomatoes, plantain, pineapples, and walnuts. These are sources of 5-HIAA.
   B. Save all the urine voided in the 24-hour period and urinate before defecating to avoid loss of urine. If any urine is accidentally discarded, discard the entire specimen and restart the collection the next day.
6. Factors that affect results:
   A. Falsely elevated results may be caused by the ingestion of foods containing

serotonin within 48 hours prior to specimen collection. Examples are: avocados, bananas, eggplant, red plums, and tomatoes.

7. Other data:
   A. Carcinoid tumors may cause increased excretion of tryptophan, 5-hydroxytryptophan, and histamine.

Bibliography:

Coward S, Boa FG, Sherwood RA: Sulfasalazine interference with HPLC assay of 5-hydroxyindole-3-acetic acid [letter]. Clin Chem *41*(5):765–766, 1995.

Garvey MJ, Noyes, R Jr, Woodman C, et al.: Relationship of generalized anxiety symptoms to urinary 5-hydroxyindoleacetic acid and vanillylmandelic acid. Psychiatry Res *57*(1):1–5, 1995.

Garvey MJ, Noyes R Jr, Woodman C, et al.: The reliability of urinary 5-HIAA levels. Neuropsychobiology *29*(4):185–188, 1994.

Ishii Y, Kanai H, Maezawa A, et al.: Evaluation of intraplatelet and urinary 5-hydroxytryptamine, and HIAA levels in patients with toxemia of pregnancy. Res Commun Chem Pathol Pharmacol *80*(1):21–40, 1993.

Wilder-Smith OH, Borgeat A, et al.: Urinary serotonin metabolite excretion during cisplatin chemotherapy. Cancer *72*(7):2239–2242, 1993.

17-HYDROXYPROGESTERONE, BLOOD

Norm:

		SI Units
Adult male	50–250 ng/dl	1.5–7.5 nmol/L
Adult female		
Follicular phase	20–100 ng/dl	0.6–3.0 nmol/L
Midcycle peak	100–250 ng/dl	3.0–7.5 nmol/L
Luteal peak	100–500 ng/dl	3.0–15.5 nmol/L
Children		
Cord blood	900–5000 ng/dl	27.3–151.5 nmol/L
Newborn	7–77 ng/dl	0.2–2.3 nmol/L
Child	3–90 ng/dl	0.1–2.7 nmol/L
Puberty, male	3–175 ng/dl	0.1–5.3 nmol/L
Puberty, female	3–265 ng/dl	0.1–8.0 nmol/L

Increased: Congenital adrenal hyperplasia, hirsutism, ovarian tumors, and virilization.

Decreased: Not clinically significant.

Description: 17-Hydroxyprogesterone (17-OHP), which is derived from progesterone, is the metabolic precursor of 11-deoxycortisol in cortisol biosynthesis. Elevated levels generally occur as a result of 21-hydroxylase or 11-hydroxylase deficiency. 17-OHP is converted and excreted as pregnanetriol.

Professional Considerations:

1. Consent form NOT required.
2. Preparation:
   A. Tube: Red-top, red/gray-top, or gold-top; and ice.
3. Procedure:
   A. Draw a 1.5-ml blood sample. Place the sample immediately on ice.
4. Postprocedure care:
   A. Deliver the sample to the laboratory within 30 minutes for immediate testing.
5. Client and family teaching:
   A. Results are normally available within 24 hours.
6. Factors that affect results:
   A. Recent radionuclide administration (within 48 hours) may cause false-positive results if the test is performed using radioimmunoassay technique.
7. Other data:
   A. In clients with congenital adrenal hyperplasia, 17-ketosteroids may also be elevated.
   B. Measurement of 11-deoxycortisol may help differentiate between 11- and 21-hydroxylase deficiencies.

Bibliography:

al Saedi S, Dean H, Dent W, Cronin C: Reference ranges for serum cortisol and 17-hydroxyprogesterone levels in preterm infants. J Pediatr *126*(6):985–987, 1995.

Palonek E, Gottleib C, et al.: Serum and urinary markers of exogenous testosterone administration. J Steroid Biochem Mol Biol *55*(1):121–127, 1995.

Wudy SA, Wachter UA, Homoki J, et al.: 17- alpha-hydroxyprogesterone, r-androstenedione, and testosterone profiled by routine stable isotope dilution/gas chromatography-mass spectrometry in plasma of children. Pediatr Res *38*(1):76–80, 1995.

HYDROXYPROLINE, TOTAL, 24-HOUR, URINE
Norm:

		SI Units
Adults		
Age 18–21	20–55 mg/d	0.15–0.42 μmol/d
Age 22–40	15–42 mg/d	0.11–0.32 μmol/d
Age 41–55	15–43 mg/d	0.11–0.33 μmol/d
Children		
Age 1–5	20–65 mg/d	0.15–0.49 μmol/d
Age 6–10	35–99 mg/d	0.27–0.75 μmol/d
Age 11–14	63–180 mg/d	0.48–1.37 μmol/d

Increased: Acromegaly, Albright's syndrome, bone cancer, bone metastasis, burns, congenital hypophosphatasia, diabetes mellitus, growth spurts, healing fracture, hyperparathyroidism, hyperpituitarism, hyperthyroidism, Marfan's syndrome, multiple myeloma, osteomalacia, osteomyelitis, Paget's disease of the bone, psoriasis, and rickets. Drugs include growth hormone, parathyroid hormone, phenobarbital, and sulfonylureas.

Decreased: Hypoparathyroidism, hypopituitarism, hypothyroidism, malnutrition, and muscular dystrophy. Drugs include acetylsalicylic acid, antineoplastic agents, ascorbic acid, calcitonin, calcium gluconate, corticosteroids, diphosphonate, ergocalciferol, estradiol, estriol, glucocorticoids, mithramycin, and propranolol.

Description: Hydroxyproline is an amino acid found in collagen. Excretion of hydroxyproline in the urine is a useful measure of collagen turnover. It reflects bone resorption and is therefore a good test for monitoring the status of Paget's disease.

Professional Considerations:

1. Consent form NOT required.
2. Preparation:
   A. Obtain a clean, 3-L container without preservative.
   B. Write the beginning time of collection on the laboratory requisition.
   C. *See Client and family teaching.*
3. Procedure:
   A. Discard the first morning urine specimen.
   B. Save all the urine voided for 24 hours in a refrigerated, clean, 3-L container. Document the quantity of urine output during the collection period. Include the urine voided at the end of the 24-hour period. For catheterized clients, keep the drainage bag on ice and empty urine into the collection container hourly.
4. Postprocedure care:
   A. Compare the urine quantity in the specimen container with the urinary output record for the test. If the specimen contains less urine than was recorded as output, some of the sample may have been discarded, thus invalidating the test.
   B. Document the quantity of urine output and the ending time for the collection period on the laboratory requisition.
   C. Send the entire 24-hour urine specimen to the laboratory for testing and refrigerate it.
5. Client and family teaching:
   A. Avoid gelatin-containing foods and red meat, poultry, and fish 48 hours prior to urine collection.
   B. Save all the urine voided in the 24-hour period and urinate before defecating to avoid loss of urine. If any urine is accidentally discarded, discard the entire specimen and restart the collection the next day.
6. Factors that affect results:
   A. Meat and gelatin may produce false-positives.
7. Other data:
   A. Normal range is higher in infancy, childhood, and adolescence, especially during growth spurts.
   B. There is a diurnal variation in excretion, with higher levels excreted at night.

Bibliography:

Miyamoto KK, McSherry SA, Robins SP, et al.: Collagen cross-link metabolites in urine as markers of bone metastases in prostatic carcinoma. J Urol 151(4):909–1013, 1994.

Selby PL, Shearing PA, Marshall SM: Hydroxyproline excretion is increased in diabetes mellitus and related to the presence of microalbuminemia. Diabetic Med 12(3):241–243, 1995.

Thomas, CL (ed): Taber's Cyclopedic Medical Dictionary. Philadelphia, FA Davis, 1993, p 2204.

5-HYDROXYTRYPTAMINE, PLASMA

(see Serotonin, Plasma)

HYPERSENSITIVITY PNEUMONITIS SEROLOGY, BLOOD

Norm: Negative.

Positive: Asthma and farmer's lung.

Description: Hypersensitivity pneumonitis is an inflammatory, interstitial pneumonia that results from an immunologic reaction in response to a variety of inhaled antigens. These antigens usually include organisms such as *Aspergillus fumigatus, Micropolyspora faeni,* or *Thermoactinomyces vulgaris.*

Professional Considerations:

1. Consent form NOT required.
2. Preparation:
   A. Tube: Red-top, red/gray-top, or gold-top.
3. Procedure:
   A. Obtain a 7-ml blood sample.
4. Postprocedure care:
   A. None.
5. Client and family teaching:
   A. Results are normally available within 48 hours.
6. Factors that affect results:
   A. Reject hemolyzed, chylous, or contaminated samples.
7. Other data:
   A. A client with no symptoms may have a positive test, while a client with symptoms may have a negative test. Careful correlation of clinical symptoms and laboratory results is a must.

Bibliography:

Chiu A, Pegram PS Jr, Hponik EF: Hypersensitivity pneumonitis: a diagnostic dilemma. J Thorac Imaging *8*(1):69–78, 1993.

Krasnick J, Patterson R, Roberts M: Multifactorial immunologic lung disease: a case report. Ann Allergy, Asthma, Immunol *75*(3):239–241, 1995.

Sharma OP, Fujimura K: Hypersensitivity pnemonitis: a noninfectious granulomatosis [review]. Semin Resp Infect *10*(2):96–106, 1995.

HYSTEROSALPINGOGRAPHY (UTEROSALPINGOGRAPHY), DIAGNOSTIC

Norm: Normal uterine cavity and fallopian tubes.

Usage: Identification of adhesions of peritoneum, hydrosalpinx, infertility, pelvic abscess or infection, tubal abnormality, tubal pregnancy, tubal ligation, and uteroileal fistula confirmation.

Description: Using serial fluoroscopic radiographs, contrast media (usually water-soluble diatrizoate or iothalamate) is inserted via the cervix so that the uterus, and fallopian tubes, and lumens can be visualized. If laparoscopy is also used, the pelvic peritoneal space can be visualized. The test is used to identify malformations, foreign bodies, trauma, and fallopian tube patency as well as fistulas or adhesions.

Professional Considerations:

1. Consent form IS required.

Risks:

Allergic reaction to dye (itching, hives, rash, tight feeling in the throat, shortness of breath, bronchospasm, anaphylaxis, death); renal toxicity from contrast medium; uterine perforation; vascular injection of dye; and infection.

Contraindications:

Previous allergy to iodine, shellfish or radiographic dye; renal insufficiency; cervicitis; vaginal bleeding or infection; suspected pregnancy; and cardiopulmonary compromise.

2. Preparation:
   A. The test should be performed in the first part of the menstrual cycle.
   B. Administer cleansing enemas.
   C. Have emergency equipment readily available.
   D. The client should disrobe and wear a gown and void just prior to the procedure.
   E. Obtain a speculum, a uterine cannula, and dye (diatrizoate or iothalamate).
   F. Measure and document baseline vital signs.
   G. *See Client and family teaching.*
3. Procedure:
   A. The client is positioned in the lithotomy position on a tilt table or regular procedure table.
   B. A speculum is inserted into the vagina.
   C. Under fluoroscopy, 6–10 ml (in 3-ml increments) of dye is injected into the cervical opening with a uterine cannula to fill the uterine cavity and fallopian tubes. The table is tilted (or the client is moved) to various positions to

enable gravitational flow of the dye through the uterus and the fallopian tubes.

D. Radiographs are taken 8–24 hours later to help delineate delayed emptying when oily contrast medium is used.

4. Postprocedure care:
   A. Assess for signs of gross bleeding/vaginal discharge.
   B. Monitor vital signs every 15 minutes × 2, then every 30 minutes × 2.
   C. Small amounts of bloody, vaginal discharge may be present up to 2 days postoperatively.

5. Client and family teaching:
   A. Take the prescribed laxative the night before the procedure. Cleansing enemas will be given before the procedure.
   B. It is normal to experience cramping, similar to menstrual cramps, and dizziness during the procedure. Taking prostaglandin inhibitors such as ibuprofen before or after the procedure will lessen the cramping discomfort.
   C. The procedure lasts about 45 minutes.
   D. Avoid vaginal douching and sexual intercourse for 2 weeks after the procedure.

6. Factors that affect results:
   A. A normal fallopian tube may appear strictured if there is too much traction or if there is tubal spasm.
   B. Fallopian tubes may appear normal in the presence of adhesions if too much traction is applied.

7. Other data:
   A. *See also Rubin's Test, Diagnostic.*

Bibliography:

Confino E, Binor Z, Molo MW, et al.: Selective salpingography for the diagnosis and treatment of early tubal pregnancy. Fertil Steril *62*(2):286–288, 1994.

Hofmann GE, Scott RT, Rosenwaks Z: Common technical errors in hysterosalpingography. Int J Fertil *37*(1):41–43, 1992.

Snabes MC, Samaniego J, Poindexter AN: Hysterosalpingographic diagnosis of Crohn's disease. A case report. J Reprod Med *37*(3):285–288, 1995.

HYSTEROSCOPY, DIAGNOSTIC

Norm: Uterine cavity normal.

Usage: Asherman's syndrome, endocervical biopsy, fibroid removal, hysterectomy, infertility, intrauterine adhesions, IUD/foreign body removal, septate uteri, and uterine arterial bleeding location.

Description: A 4-mm hysteroscope (telescope-type instrument) is inserted vaginally into the uterus to view the pathology within the uterine cavity that is sometimes missed by hysterosalpingography or curettage.

Professional Considerations:

1. Consent form IS required.

Risks:

Allergic reaction to Hyskon (itching, hives, rash, tight feeling in the throat, shortness of breath, bronchospasm, anaphylaxis, death); renal toxicity from contrast medium. Risks include infection, perforation, and a 1–3% chance of developing PID. Possible life-threatening complications include disseminated intravascular coagulation (DIC) and acute respiratory distress syndrome (ARDS).

Contraindications:

Previous allergy to Hyskon (if use is planned). Hysteroscopy is contraindicated in pelvic inflammatory disease (PID), inflamed cervix, and purulent vaginal discharge.

2. Preparation:
   A. Schedule after menstrual bleeding has ceased and prior to ovulation.
   B. Have emergency equipment readily available.
   C. Have the client void before the procedure.

3. Procedure:
   A. A hysteroscope is inserted vaginally through the cervix, into the uterus following the use of a speculum.
   B. Carbon dioxide or Hyskon is instilled to distend the uterine cavity.
   C. The interior walls of the uterus are closely examined for abnormalities, lesions, or bleeding, and photographs or biopsies may be taken.

4. Postprocedure care:
   A. Assess for side effects from the use of carbon dioxide to distend the uterine cavity: shoulder pain, diaphoresis, nausea, and postoperative bleeding.
   B. Assess for side effects of Hyskon: pulmonary edema, coagulation defects, and anaphylaxis.

5. Client and family teaching:
   A. The procedure takes less than 30 minutes.
   B. It is normal to experience cramping, similar to menstrual cramps, and dizziness during the procedure. Taking prostaglandin inhibitors such as

ibuprofen before or after the procedure will lessen the cramping discomfort.

C. Carbon dioxide side effects (listed in section 4A above) may last for a few days. Use a mild analgesia to relieve discomfort.

D. Immediately report any nausea, pain, shortness of breath, or any other symptoms of discomfort after the procedure.

E. Avoid vaginal douching and sexual intercourse for 2 weeks after the procedure.

6. Factors that affect results:
   A. None found.
7. Other data:
   A. None.

Bibliography:

Jedeikin R, Olsfanger D, Kessler I: Disseminated intravascular coagulation and adult respiratory distress syndrome: Life-threatening complications of hysteroscopy. Am J Obstet Gynecol 162(1):44–45, 1990.

Levin H, Ben-David B: Transient blindness during hysteroscopy: a rare complication. Anesth Analg 81(4):880–881, 1995.

McLucas B: Hyskon complications in hysterscopic surgery. Obstet Gynecol Surg 46(4):196–200, 1991.

Nathanson MH, Ezeh U: Carbon dioxide embolism following diagnostic hysteroscopy [letter]. Br J Obstet Gynaecol 102(6):505, 1995.

Taylor PJ, Gomel V: Endometrial ablation: indications and preliminary diagnostic hysteroscopy. Bailleres Clin Obstet Gynecol 9(2):251–260, 1995.

IgA
(see Immunoglobulin A, Serum)

IgD
(see Immunoglobulin D, Serum)

IgE
(see Immunoglobulin E, Serum)

IgG
(see Immunoglobulin G, Serum)

IgM
(see Immunoglobulin M, Serum)

I-125-LABELED FIBRINOGEN (FIBRINOGEN UPTAKE) LEG SCAN, DIAGNOSTIC

Norm: No evidence of thrombi. No areas of abnormal concentration in the deep veins of the lower legs.

Usage: Used to monitor the development and progression of deep vein thromboses. Longitudinal screening for clients at risk for thrombotic processes.

Positive: Deep vein thrombosis, thrombophlebitis, and thrombosis.

Negative: Normal finding. Also negative after the active clotting process has stopped.

Description: Fibrinogen (Factor I) is a complex polypeptide that converts to the insoluble polymer of fibrin after thrombin enzymatic action and combines with platelets to clot the blood. The I-125-labeled fibrinogen leg scan is an invasive, nuclear medicine test involving the intravenous injection of radionuclide-labeled fibrinogen (fibrinogen labeled with radioactive iodine) and scanning with a well counter for subsequent incorporation of the radioactive material into a thrombus. The scan measures increased surface radioactivity (>20%), which indicates uptake by thrombi in the leg(s). The test is most useful in detecting actively forming thromboses of the calf. 85% of positive results are seen within the first 24 hours after being injected with iodine-125.

Professional Considerations:

1. Consent form IS required.

Risks:
Infection, allergic reaction to radiolabeled fibrinogen (itching, hives, rash, tight feeling in the throat, shortness of breath, bronchospasm, anaphylaxis, death).

Contraindications:
Anticoagulant therapy, bleeding disorders, thrombocytopenia, during pregnancy or breast-feeding, previous allergy radiolabeled albumin.

2. Preparation:
   A. Ten drops of Lugol's solution in juice are given to block thyroid gland uptake of the radioactive tracer.

B. Establish 18-gauge intravenous access.

C. Have emergency equipment readily available.

D. Assess for swelling in the calf, tenderness, and cyanosis of the skin.

E. Assess for Homans' sign. Once it is determined to be positive, do NOT repeat Homans' sign assessment.

F. Elevate the legs during the imaging procedure, which takes about 10 minutes.

3. Procedure:

A. The client's legs are elevated during scanning to prevent pooling of blood in the veins of the legs.

B. Iodine-125-labeled fibrinogen is injected intravenously and serial scans are performed on each leg 1, 4, 24, and 48 hours afterward. Surface radioactivity may be measured daily for as long as 2 days.

C. The extremity is marked in segments along the course of the vein tract.

D. Areas of fibrinogen incorporation into a thrombus are detected with the counter as areas exhibiting increased radioactivity, indicating increased concentration of radioactive tracer.

4. Postprocedure care:

A. Maintain bedrest if thrombi are detected.

B. Do not wash off markings on the extremity.

C. Assess the venipuncture site for infiltration.

D. Assess for swelling in the calf, tenderness, and cyanosis of the skin.

E. Observe the client carefully for up to 60 minutes after the study for a possible (anaphylactic) reaction to the radionuclide.

F. Rubber gloves should be worn when discarding urine for 24 hours after the procedure. Wash the gloved hands with soap and water before removing the gloves. Wash the ungloved hands after the gloves have been removed.

5. Client and family teaching:

A. This test involves several leg scans after the client receives an IV tracer that shows up on the scan. Scanning may continue for up to 2 days after the injection.

B. The test poses no risk of radioactive damage to the client.

C. Maintain bedrest until deep venous thrombosis (DVT) has been ruled out.

D. Meticulously wash hands with soap and water after each void × 24 hours.

6. Factors that affect results:

A. False-negative results may occur where active clot formation is completed, but the thrombus still remains.

B. Usually, 1–2 days are required for enough radiolabeled fibrinogen to be incorporated into the clot before the clot can be detected.

C. Thrombi of the pelvis are difficult to detect with this test.

D. False-positive results may occur in clients with bacterial inflammatory conditions of the lower extremities.

E. A radioactive test within the last 24 hours invalidates the results.

F. Up to 72 hours may elapse before the results become positive.

7. Other data:

A. Other tests to detect DVT are Doppler ultrasonography, venogram, thermography, perfusion lung scan, gas ventilation lung scan, and pulmonary angiography.

B. This test is insensitive to upper thigh and pelvic vein thrombosis.

C. Health care professionals working in a nuclear medicine area must follow federal standards set by the Nuclear Regulatory Commission. These standards include precautions for handling the radioactive material and monitoring of potential radiation exposure.

D. Iodine-125 half-life is 60 days.

Bibliography:

Hendolin H, Poikolainen E, Mattila MA, Alhava E, Hanninen A, Puttonen E, Kataja M: Effect of dihydroergotamine on leg blood flow during combined epidural and general anaesthesia and postoperative deep vein thrombosis after cholecystectomy. Acta Anaesthesiol Scand 37(3): 288–295, 1993.

Koopman MM, Buller HR, ten Cate JW: Diagnosis of recurrent deep vein thrombosis [review]. Haemostasis 25(1–2):49–57, 1995.

Wheeler HB, Anderson FA Jr: Diagnostic methods for deep vein thrombosis. Haemostasis 25(1–2):6–26, 1995.

IMIPRAMINE
(see Tricyclic Antidepressants, Plasma or Serum)

IMMUNE COMPLEX ASSAY, BLOOD

Norm:

Complexes not detected.
C1q binding: <13%.
Raji cell assay: <50 g aggregated human gamma globulin equivalents (AHG).

Positive: Arthritis (rheumatoid), biliary cirrhosis, dengue fever, disseminated gonorrhea, endocarditis, glomerulonephritis, Hansen's disease, Hodgkin's disease, leukemia, leprosy, malaria, malignant melanoma, pulmonary fibrosis, schistosomiasis, serum hepatitis, serum sickness, Sjögren's syndrome, and systemic lupus erythematosus (SLE).

Description: Complements are proteins, which when activated, assist the cell lysis function of antibodies. Activation of complement by an antigen-antibody response is called the classical pathway. Complement activation independent of antibody, initiated by complement binding to the surfaces of infectious organisms, is known as the alternate pathway. Both pathways ultimately result in the complement cascade's formation of the membrane attack complex (MAC). This radioimmunoassay (RIA) test is helpful in diagnosing autoimmune and infectious inflammatory disease processes.

Professional Considerations:

1. Consent form NOT required.
2. Preparation:
   A. Tube: Red-top, red/gray-top, or gold-top.
3. Procedure:
   A. Draw a 2-ml blood sample.
4. Postprocedure care:
   A. Write the collection time and date on the laboratory requisition.
5. Client and family teaching:
   A. Results are normally available with 2 days.
6. Factors that affect results:
   A. Reject specimens received more than 1 hour after collection.
   B. Certain cryoglobulins, cold agglutinins, rheumatoid factors, and paraproteins may cause false-positive results.
7. Other data:
   A. There are specific assays to measure different populations of immune complexes.
   B. Also see Raji cell and C1q binding assays.
   C. Clinical information and physical findings may be the first sign of an immune complex disorder.

Bibliography:

Abbas AK, Lichtman AH, Pober JS: Cellular and Molecular Immunology, 2nd ed. Philadelphia, WB Saunders, 1994, pp 56, 294–303.

Akron General Medical Center: Laboratory Users Manual. Akron, OH, Department of Pathology and Laboratory Medicine, 1991, pp 114, 341–342.

Corbett JV: Laboratory Tests and Diagnostic Procedures, 4th ed. Norwalk, CT, Appleton and Lange, 1996, pp 383–384.

Theofilopoulos AN, Dixon FJ: The biology and detection of immune complexes. Adv Immunol 28:89–220, 1979.

IMMUNOELECTROPHORESIS, SERUM AND URINE

Norm:

Serum: No abnormal proteins present.

Urine: No abnormal proteins present; requires pathologist's interpretation.

Usage: Dysproteinemia, Hodgkin's disease, humoral immune deficiency, multiple myeloma, renal failure, and Waldenström's macroglobulinemia.

Description: A sample of serum or urine is placed on a slide containing agar gel, and an electrical current is passed through the gel, causing separation according to different electrical charges in each immunoglobulin: IgG, IgA, IgM, IgD, and IgE. Each immunoglobulin develops a band that has a certain curvature, position, and intensity of color. Abnormalities in any immunoglobulin cause the band for that precipitation to be displaced, bowed, lighter in color, thicker, or absent. Following protein electrophoresis, antisera to immunoglobulins G, A, and M and to kappa and lambda light chains are applied to a urine sample to confirm and identify a suspected monoclonal protein or the presence of Bence-Jones proteins (free kappa or lambda light chains).

Professional Considerations:

1. Consent form NOT required.
2. Preparation:
   A. *For serum:* Tube: Red-top, red/gray-top, or gold-top.
      For urine: Sterile urine collection container.
   B. Record any vaccinations or immunizations within the last 6 months on the laboratory requisition.
   C. Record any blood or blood component therapy within the last 6 weeks on the laboratory requisition.
3. Procedure:
   A. *For serum test:* Draw a 1-ml blood sample.
   B. *For urine test:* Obtain a 12-ml urine sample in a sterile container.
4. Postprocedure care:
   A. Refrigerate the urine; send it to the laboratory within 2 hours.
5. Client and family teaching:
   A. Results are normally available within 24 hours.
6. Factors that affect results:
   A. Anticoagulants, anticonvulsants, hydralazine, oral contraceptives, and phenylbutazone affect the thickness of the bands, causing difficult interpretation in serum tests.
   B. Chemotherapy and radiation treatments affect color and thickness of the bands, adding difficulty to the interpretation of the serum test.

7. Other data:
   A. This is a valuable initial screening tool for identifying diseases with altered protein fractions.
   B. The urine test cannot be performed if urine protein is <60 mg/L or if urine protein electrophoresis is normal.

Bibliography:

Abbas AK, Lichtman AH, Pober JS: Cellular and Molecular Immunology, 2nd ed. Philadelphia, WB Saunders, 1994, p 61.

Akron General Medical Center: Laboratory Users Manual. Akron, OH, Department of Pathology and Laboratory Medicine, 1991, pp 356, 397.

Corbett JV: Laboratory Tests and Diagnostic Procedures, 4th ed. Norwalk, CT, Appleton and Lange, 1996, pp 255–256.

Sun T, Peng S, Narurkar L: Modified immunoselection technique for definitive diagnosis of heavy-chain disease. Clin Chem 40(4):664, 1994.

Wagner RP: Understanding inheritance. In Cooper NG (ed): The Human Genome Project: Deciphering the Blueprint of Heredity. Mill Valley, CA, University Science Books, 1994, pp 55–58.

IMMUNOFLUORESCENCE, SKIN BIOPSY, SPECIMEN

Norm: Requires interpretation by a pathologist.

Positive: Collagen disease, dermatitis herpetiformis, immune complex glomerulonephritis, immune disorders of the lung, lupus, Waldenström's macroglobunemia, malignant lymphoma, multiple myeloma, pemphigus.

Negative: Keratinized tissue.

Description: Identifies immune complexes, complement, and immunoglobulins by visualizing tissue antigenic activity and morphology with a fluorescent light.

Professional Considerations:

1. Consent form IS required for the procedure used to obtain the specimen. See *Biopsy, Site-Specific, Specimen* for procedure-specific risks and contraindications.
2. Preparation:
   A. Obtain covered saline-soaked gauze or filter paper, a punch biopsy instrument, ice or a Petri dish, and a local anesthetic.
   B. The container must be labeled with the client's identification information and the date.
3. Procedure:
   A. Local anesthetic may be injected into the biopsy site.
   B. A 3-mm punch biopsy of tissue is collected and placed on ice or in a Petri dish containing 0.9% saline.
4. Postprocedure care:
   A. Send the moistened tissue sample to the laboratory immediately to be quickly frozen in liquid nitrogen.
   B. The site may be left open to air or covered with a dry, sterile dressing.
5. Client and family teaching:
   A. Keep the site clean and dry and report any signs of infection, such as redness, pain (severe) for more than 24 hours, swelling, or purulent drainage.
   B. Keep the site covered with a Band-Aid or gauze for 2 days, then leave the site open to air.
   C. Call the physician if there is bleeding amounting to more than a small area on the dressing, or bleeding that won't stop after pressure is applied for 5–10 minutes.
   D. Use a mild analgesic as prescribed, if necessary, for site tenderness.
6. Factors that affect results:
   A. Reject specimens in a fixative or any that have dried out.
7. Other data:
   A. Failure to detect IgG may be due to an infectious or inflammatory process in the sampled tissue.
   B. Repeated biopsies may be necessary to diagnose dermatitis herpetiformis.
   C. Skin biopsy in combination with histopathology yields the best diagnostic results.
   D. Submit an additional specimen in formalin for light microscopy.

Bibliography:

Abbas AK, Lichtman AH, Pober JS: Cellular and Molecular Immunology, 2nd ed. Philadelphia, WB Saunders, 1994, pp 60–61.

Akron General Medical Center: Laboratory Users Manual. Akron, OH, Department of Pathology and Laboratory Medicine, 1992, pp 251–252.

al-Suwaid AR, Venkataram MN, Bhushnurmath SR: Cutaneous lupus erythematosus: comparison of direct immunofluorescence findings with histopathology. Int J Dermatology 34(7):480–482, 1995.

IMMUNOGLOBULIN A (IgA), SERUM

Norm:

		SI Units
Adults	90–400 mg/dl	0.9–4.00 g/L
Children		
Newborn	0–5 mg/dl	0–0.05 g/L
Infants 25% of adult	0–11 mg/dl	0–0.11 g/L

		SI Units
Children *(continued)*		
1–3 months	7–34 mg/dl	0.07–0.34 g/L
4–6 months	10–46 mg/dl	0.10–0.46 g/L
7–12 months	19–55 mg/dl	0.19–0.55 g/L
13–24 months	26–74 mg/dl	0.26–0.74 g/L
25–36 months	34–108 mg/dl	0.34–1.08 g/L
Age 3 50% of adult		
3–5 years	0.66–1.20 g/L	0.66–1.20 g/L
6–8 years	79–169 mg/dl	0.79–1.69 g/L
9–11 years	71–191 mg/dl	0.71–1.91 g/L
12–16 years	85–211 mg/dl	0.85–2.11 g/L
>Age 16	90–400 mg/dl	0.9–4.00 g/L

Increased: Arthritis (rheumatoid), autoimmune disorders, Berger's disease, carcinoma, cirrhosis, chronic infections, dysproteinemia, Henoch-Schönlein purpura, multiple myeloma, sinusitis, and Wiskott-Aldrich syndrome.

Decreased: Bruton's disease, burns, congenital IgA deficiency, hereditary ataxia telangiectasia, humoral immune deficiency, hypogammaglobulinemia, nephrotic syndrome, and protein-losing enteropathies. Drugs include carbamazepine, dextran, estrogens, gold, methylprednisolone, oral contraceptives, penicillamine, phenytoin, and valproic acid.

Description: Immunoglobulin A is the secretory antibody effective against viruses and certain bacteria such as *Clostridium tetani, Corynebacterium diphtheriae,* and *Escherichia coli.* With an area of response localized primarily to mucosal membranes, it is the main immunoglobulin in colostrum, saliva, tears, and secretions of the bronchial, genitourinary, and gastrointestinal tracts. Immunoglobulin A normally comprises 10–15% of client's total serum immunoglobulins.

Professional Considerations:
1. Consent form NOT required.
2. Preparation:
   A. Tube: Red-top, red/gray-top, or gold-top.
   B. Write the client's age on the laboratory requisition.
3. Procedure:
   A. Draw a 1-ml blood sample.
4. Postprocedure care:
   A. Refrigerate the specimen if it is not processed immediately.

5. Client and family teaching:
   A. Results are normally available within 24 hours.
6. Factors that affect results:
   A. Reject hemolyzed or turbid samples.
7. Other data:
   A. IgA does not cross the placenta.
   B. Clients with congenital IgA deficiency may develop anaphylaxis if transfused with blood products containing IgA.

Bibliography:

Corbett JV: Laboratory Tests and Diagnostic Procedures, 4th ed. Norwalk, CT, Appleton and Lange, 1996, pp 256–257.

Lewis, SM, Collier IC, Heitkemper MM. Medical-Surgical Nursing: Assessment and Management of Clinical Problems. St. Louis, MO, CV Mosby, 1996, p 2033.

IMMUNOGLOBULIN A (IgA) ANTIBODIES, SERUM

Norm: Antibody not present (i.e., negative).

Positive: Anaphylactic transfusion reaction in IgA-deficient individual.

Description: Antibody formed against immunoglobulin A (IgA) when IgA is introduced into the bloodstream of a client with a congenital IgA deficiency. The immunoglobulin A is recognized as a foreign antigen, with resultant action of IgG antibodies attacking it. Testing for IgA antibodies should be performed in all anaphylactic transfusion reactions.

Professional Considerations:
1. Consent form NOT required.
2. Preparation:
   A. Tube: Red-top, red/gray-top, or gold-top.
3. Procedure:
   A. Draw a 7-ml blood sample.
4. Postprocedure care:
   A. Give the client a wallet card, specifying the IgA deficiency.

5. Client and family teaching:
   A. If the test is positive, any future blood transfusions must be IgA deficient or else a severe allergic reaction will occur.
6. Factors that affect results:
   A. Temperature of specimen not held at 37°C.
7. Other data:
   A. None.

Bibliography:

Gompertz NR, Isenberg DA, Turner BM: Correlation between clinical features of systemic lupus erythematosus and levels of antihistone antibodies of the IgG, IgA, and IgM isotopes. Ann Rheum Dis 49(7):524–527, 1990.

Hill PG, Thompson SP, Holmes GK: IgA anti-gliadin antibodies in adult celiac disease. Clin Chem 37(5):647–650, 1991.

Knudtzon J, Fluge G, Aksnes J: Routine measurements of gluten antibodies in children of short stature. J Pediatr Gastroenterol Nutr 12(2):190–194, 1991.

IMMUNOGLOBULIN D (IgD), SERUM

Norm: Comprises <1% of client's serum immunoglobulins.

		SI Units
Adult	0–8.0 mg/dl	5–30 µg/L
Newborn	<1.0 mg/dl	<10 µg/L

Increased: Chronic infections, connective tissue disease, dysproteinemia, and IgD myeloma.

Decreased: Acquired immune deficiency syndromes. Drugs include phenytoin.

Description: Immunoglobulin D is a protein that may act as an autoimmune antibody in clients with collagen disease. The true biologic function of IgD is unknown but is suspected to play a role in the induction of humoral response and tolerance.

Professional Considerations:

1. Consent form NOT required.
2. Preparation:
   A. Tube: Red-top, red/gray-top, or gold-top.
   B. Write the client's age on the laboratory requisition.
3. Procedure:
   A. Draw a 1-ml blood sample.
4. Postprocedure care:
   A. None.

5. Client and family teaching:
   A. Results are normally available within 24 hours.
6. Factors that affect results:
   A. A chylous serum sample invalidates the results.
7. Other data:
   A. 75% of IgD is in the intravascular compartment.
   B. 90% of multiple myelomas are of the IgD type.

Bibliography:

Drenth JP, Haagsma CJ, van der Meer JW: Hyperimmunoglobulinemia D and periodic fever syndrome. The clinical spectrum in a series of 50 patients. International Hyper-IgD Study Group [review]. Medicine 73(3):133–144, 1994.

Haraldsson A, Weemaes CM, de Boer AW, Bakkeren JA: Clinical and immunological follow-up in children with hyper-IgD syndrome. Immunodeficiency 4(1–4):63–65, 1993.

Lio D, Candore G, Colucci AT, et al.: IgD serum levels are influenced by HLA-DR phenotype. Dis Markers 10(2):105–108, 1992.

Shimamoto Y: IgD myeloma: clinical characteristics and a new staging system based on analysis of Japanese patients [review]. Cancer Detect Prev 19(5):425–435, 1995.

IMMUNOGLOBULIN E (IgE), SERUM

Norm:

	IU/ml	U/ml	SI Units µg/L
Adults	3–423	4.2–592	10–1421
15–20 years	6.8–39.6	1.5–384	3.60–921.6
21–40 years	20.3–36.5	0.9–239	2.20–573.6
41–60 years	26–53	1.2–324	2.90–777.6
61–87 years	16.2–43.8	0.7–197	1.70–472.8

	IU/ml	U/ml	SI Units µg/L
Children			
Cord blood	0.1–1.5	0.1–2	0.24–4.8
6 weeks	0.1–2.8	0.1–4	0.24–9.6
6 months	0.9–28	0.1–56	0.24–134.4
1 year	1.1–10.2	0.1–83	0.24–199.2
4 years	2.4–34.8	0.4–144	0.96–345.6
10 years	0.3–215	1.9–421	4.56–1010.4
14 years	1.9–159	1.6–456	3.84–1094.4

Increased: Alcoholism, asthma, bronchopulmonary aspergillosis, dermatitis, eczema, food and drug allergies, hay fever, IgE myeloma, parasitic infections, pemphigoid, periarteritis nodosa, rhinitis, sinusitis, and Wiskott-Aldrich syndrome. Drugs include gold compounds.

Decreased: Advanced carcinoma, agammaglobulinemia, ataxia-telangiectasia, and IgE deficiency. Drugs include phenytoin sodium.

Description: Immunoglobulin E is the antibody protein primarily responsible for allergic reactions such as hay fever, asthma, and allergies to foods and drugs, as well as atopic reactions such as latex allergies. When inhaled or ingested, IgE comes in contact with and activates the mast cells in the respiratory and gastrointestinal tracts and causes a histamine response in the body.

Professional Considerations:

1. Consent form NOT required.
2. Preparation:
   A. Tube: Red-top, red/gray-top, or gold-top.
   B. Write the client's age on the laboratory requisition.
3. Procedure:
   A. Draw a 1-ml blood sample.
4. Postprocedure care:
   A. Handle the tube carefully, as hemolysis invalidates the test.
5. Client and family teaching:
   A. IgE is elevated in approximately half of the people with allergies.
6. Factors that affect results:
   A. The test should not be performed if the client has undergone a radionuclide scan within the last 72 hours.
7. Other data:
   A. 50% of IgE is intravascular.
   B. Normal IgE levels do not exclude allergic phenomena.
   C. IgE normally comprises <0.1% of the client's immunoglobulins.

Bibliography:

Ellaurie M, Rubinstein A, Rosenstreich DL: IgE levels in pediatric HIV-1 infection. Ann Allergy Asthma Immunol 75(4):332–336, 1995.

Gonzales-Quintela A, Vidal C, Gude F, et al.: Increased serum IgE in alcohol abusers. Clin Exper Allergy 25(8):756–764, 1995.

Niggemann B, Wahn U, Klinikum V: Latex-specific IgE in patients evaluated for allergy [letter]. American J Respir Crit Care Med 152(5, Pt 1):1497–1500, 1995.

Smith DL, Smith JG, Wong SW, deShazo RD: Netherton's syndrome: a syndrome of elevated IgE and characteristic skin and hair findings. J Allergy Clin Immunol 95(1, Pt 1):116–123, 1995.

IMMUNOGLOBULIN G (IgG), SERUM

Norm: Normally comprises 75% of client's total immunoglobulins.

		SI Units
Adults	565–1765 mg/dl	5.65–17.65 g/L
Children		
Cord	650–1600 mg/dl	6.5–16.0 g/L
1 month	250–900 mg/dl	2.5–9.0 g/L
2–5 months	200–700 mg/dl	2.0–7.0 g/L
6–9 months	220–900 mg/dl	2.2–9.0 g/L
10–12 months	290–1070 mg/dl	2.9–10.7 g/L
1 year	340–1200 mg/dl	3.4–12.0 g/L
2–3 years	420–1200 mg/dl	4.2–12.0 g/L
4–6 years	460–1240 mg/dl	4.6–12.4 g/L
>6 years	650–1600 mg/dl	6.5–16.0 g/L

Increased: Infections (chronic or recurrent), liver disease (chronic), malignancies (lymphomas), multiple myeloma, rheumatoid arthritis, sarcoidosis, Sjögren's syndrome, and systemic lupus erythematosus. The IgG titer is usually elevated in clients with *H. pylori,* indicating active infection.

Decreased: Acquired immune deficiency syndrome, bacterial infection, humoral immune deficiency, and Wiscott-Aldrich syndrome.

Description: Immunoglobulin G, comprising 75% of all immunoglobulins in the bloodstream, possesses antibody activity against viruses, some bacteria, and toxins. IgG is able to cross the placenta and provide immunity to a developing fetus. It also serves as an activator of the complement system. IgG levels increase in response to infection and remain elevated, even if the infection becomes chronic. IgG is also important in autoimmune diseases, because many of the autoantibodies belong in this class. This test evaluates humoral immunity and monitors therapy in IgG myeloma.

Professional Considerations:

1. Consent form NOT required.
2. Preparation:
   A. Tube: Red-top, red/gray-top, or gold-top.
   B. Write the client's age on the laboratory requisition.
3. Procedure:
   A. Draw a 1-ml blood sample.

4. Postprocedure care:
   A. None required.
5. Client and family teaching:
   A. Results are normally available within 24 hours.
6. Factors that affect results:
   A. Specimens should be stored at 37°C.
7. Other data:
   A. IgG is the only immunoglobulin that crosses the placenta.
   B. Laboratory-based serology titers should be obtained to quantitate the antibody level and establish a baseline when treatment for *H. pylori* is planned. This allows for follow-up after therapy, which if successful, will usually show a consistent fall in IgG titer levels.

Bibliography:

Haarbrink M, Terhell A, Abadi K, et al.: IgG4 antibody assay in the detection of filariasis [letter]. Lancet *346*(8978):853–854, 1995.

Jacquemin MG, Saint-Remy JM: Specific down-regulation of anti-allergen IgE and IgG antibodies in humans associated with injections of allergen-specific antibody complexes. Ther Immunol *2*(1):41–52, 1995.

Mascart-Lemone F, Gerard M, Libin M, et al.: Differential effect of human immunodeficiency virus infection on the IgA and IgG antibody responses to pneumococcal vaccine. J Infect Dis *172*(5):1253–1260, 1995.

IMMUNOGLOBULIN G (IgG) SYNTHESIS RATE, CEREBROSPINAL FLUID, SPECIMEN

(see Cerebrospinal Fluid, Immunoglobulin G, Immunoglobulin G Ratio and Immunoglobulin G Index, Immunoglobulin G Synthesis Rate, Specimen)

IMMUNOGLOBULIN M (IgM), SERUM

Norm: Normally comprises 5–10% of the client's total immunoglobulins.

		SI Units
Adults	35–375 mg/dl	0.35–3.75 g/L
Children		
Cord	0–19 mg/dl	0–0.19 g/L
1–3 months	7–78 mg/dl	0.07–0.78 g/L
3–6 months	19–72 mg/dl	0.19–0.72 g/L
6–12 months	21–104 mg/dl	0.21–1.04 g/L
1–2 years	19–148 mg/dl	0.19–1.48 g/L
2–3 years	40–151 mg/dl	0.40–1.51 g/L
3–5 years	28–142 mg/dl	0.28–1.42 g/L
5–8 years	30–162 mg/dl	0.30–1.62 g/L
8–12 years	24–161 mg/dl	0.24–1.61 g/L
12–16 years	26–221 mg/dl	0.26–2.21 g/L

Increased: Biliary cirrhosis, collagen vascular disease, dysproteinemia, Infection (bacterial, parasitic), Lyme disease, reticulosis, rheumatoid arthritis, sarcoidosis, toxoplasmosis, trypanoso-miasis parasite, and Waldenström's macroglobulinemia. Drugs include chlorpromazine.

Decreased: Humoral immune defi-ciency, hypogammaglobulinemia, multiple myeloma IgA or IgG, and protein-losing enteropathy. Drugs in-clude carbamazepine and dextran.

Description: Immunoglobulin M is the first antibody to appear after an antigen enters the body and is active against gram-negative organisms and rheumatoid factors. IgM forms the natural antibodies such as those to the ABO blood groups. The IgM molecule is too large to cross the placenta, thus it does not help provide fetal immu-nity to antigens. If levels are elevated in cord blood samples, it may indicate that the infant was infected prior to birth with organisms that can cause birth defects, such as *toxoplasma gondii,* cytomegalovirus, or rubella. This test is used to screen for congeni-tal infections and to help diagnose and monitor infections.

Professional Considerations:

1. Consent form NOT required.
2. Preparation:
   A. Tube: Red-top, red/gray-top, or gold-top.
3. Procedure:
   A. Draw a 1-ml blood sample.
4. Postprocedure care:
   A. None.
5. Client and family teaching:
   A. Results are normally available within 24 hours.
6. Factors that affect results:
   A. Specimen storage at a temperature other than 37°C may cause falsely de-creased results.
7. Other data:
   A. IgM development during pregnancy occurs at an increase of 0.5 mg/dl per week of gestation.

Bibliography:

Hadar T, Margalith M, Sagiv E, et al.: The significance of serum IgM IgA and IgG antibodies specific for Epstein-Barr virus as determined by immunoper-oxidase assay in the rapid diagnosis of infectious mononucleosis. Isr J Med Sci *31*(5):280–283, 1995.

Patniak M, Komaroff AL, Conley E, et al.: Prevalence of IgM antibodies to human herpesvirus 6 early antigen (p42/38) in patients with chronic fatigue syndrome. J Infect Dis *172*(5):1364–1367, 1995.

Vice DJ, Hogged WA, Normansell DE, et al.: Determi-nation of normal human fetal immunoglobulin M levels. Clin Diagn Lab Immunol *2*(1):115–117, 1995.

IMMUNOPEROXIDASE PROCEDURES (PAP), DIAGNOSTIC

Norm: Interpretation required.

Positive: Endocrine tumors, G-cell hyperplasia, Hodgkin's disease, Rocky Mountain spotted fever, splenomegaly, and tumors.

Description: A test using stain to lo-calize and recognize antigens in tis-sue. Includes the identification of cell origin, tissue-specific markers, and/or microorganism.

Professional Considerations:

1. Consent form IS required for sternal puncture or biopsy of tumor site. See *Biopsy, Site-Specific, Specimen* for proce-dure risks and contraindications.
2. Preparation:
   A. Obtain a sterile specimen jar.
   B. Preschedule this test with the patholo-gist/hematology laboratory.
3. Procedure:
   A. Obtain 5 ml of cell products or extra-cellular material by venipuncture or bone marrow biopsy.
   B. The blood or bone marrow smears are prepared by a laboratory technologist at bedside.
4. Postprocedure care:
   A. 6–10 bone marrow aspirate smears are prepared immediately.
   B. If the specimen is obtained via biopsy, *see Biopsy, Site-Specific, Specimen; or Bone Marrow Aspiration, Aspiration Analysis, Specimen.*
   C. Apply a pressure dressing to the biopsy site and monitor for bleeding.
5. Client and family teaching:
   A. See *Biopsy, Site-Specific, Specimen; or Bone Marrow Aspiration, Aspiration Analysis, Specimen.*
6. Factors that affect results:
   A. Tissue samples too small will invali-date the test.
7. Other data:
   A. Myoglobin is a marker for rhabdo-myosarcoma.

Bibliography:

Abbas AK, Lichtman AH, Pober JS: Cellular and Mole-cular Immunology, 2nd ed. Philadelphia, WB Saunders, 1994, pp 26, 61.

Akron General Medical Center: Laboratory Users Man-ual. Akron, OH, Department of Pathology and Laboratory Medicine, 1991, p 169.

Dumler JS, Gage WR, Pettis GL, et al.: Rapid im-munoperoxidase demonstration of *Rickettsia rickettsii* in fixed cutaneous specimens from pa-tients with Rocky Mountain spotted fever. Am J Clin Pathol *93*(3):410–414, 1995.

INDIA INK PREPARATION, SPECIMEN

Norm: No *Cryptococcus* present, or negative.

Usage: Fungal infections and meningitis.

Description: Special staining test of fluids for the diagnosis of fungal disorders from any site-specific specimen.

Professional Considerations:
1. Consent form NOT required.
2. Preparation:
   A. Obtain an adequate number of requisitions.
   B. Obtain a sterile specimen container.
3. Procedure:
   A. Send the specimen of cerebrospinal fluid, pleural fluid, or blood in a sterile container.
4. Postprocedure care:
   A. Specimens will be divided for fungal culture, mycobacteria culture and smear, and routine bacterial culture and Gram stain.
   B. Do not refrigerate specimens.
   C. List the site of specimen collection on the requisitions.
   D. Deliver the specimens to the laboratory within 4 hours.
5. Client and family teaching:
   A. Results are normally available within 24 hours.
6. Factors that affect results:
   A. If the specimens have not been totally enclosed within the containers, the results are invalid.
   B. Refrigeration of specimens invalidates the results.
7. Other data:
   A. This test is only positive in about half of cryptococcal meningitis cases.
   B. 24-hour turnaround time is routine; 2 hours is necessary for the entire test if it is prescribed to be run immediately.

Bibliography:
Flaskerud JH, Ungvarski PJ: HIV/AIDS: A Guide to Nursing Care. Philadelphia, WB Saunders, 1995, p 89.
McGinnis MR: Detection of fungi in cerebrospinal fluid. Am J Med 75(1B):129–137, 1983.
Rozenbaum R, Gioncalves AJ, Wanke B, et al.: Cryptococcus neoformans var. gattii in a Brazilian AIDS client. Mycopathologica 112(1):33–34, 1990.

INDICAN, URINE

Norm: <100 mg/dl in 24 hours, or negative.

Positive: Hartnup disease and ileal dysfunction.

Negative: Normal protein catabolism or intestinal absorption.

Description: Indican is a tryptophan metabolite that is excreted mostly in the feces, but also in small amounts in the urine as a result of absorption and detoxification of indole produced by bacterial action on tryptophan in the intestines. Normal urine will turn blue when 5 ml of urine is added to 5 ml of ferric chloride reagent.

Professional Considerations:
1. Consent form NOT required.
2. Preparation:
   A. Obtain a sterile plastic container.
3. Procedure:
   A. Collect a 50-ml random urine specimen in a sterile plastic container.
4. Postprocedure care:
   A. Transport the specimen to the laboratory within 1 hour after collection.
5. Client and family teaching:
   A. Results are normally available with 24 hours.
6. Factors that affect results:
   A. Results are invalid if the urine is not delivered to the laboratory within 1 hour after collection.
7. Other data:
   A. Increased indican may cause the urine specimen to blacken in color over time.

Bibliography:
Dealler SF, Belfield PW, Bedford M, et al.: Purple urine bags. J Urol 142(3):769–770, 1989.
Niwa T Ise M: Indoxyl sulfate, a circulating uremic toxin, stimulates the progression of glomerular sclerosis. J Lab Clin Med 124(1):96–104, 1994.

INDIRECT ANTIGLOBULIN TEST
(see Coombs', Indirect, Serum)

INFECTIOUS MONONUCLEOSIS SCREENING TEST, BLOOD
(see Heterophil Agglutinins, Blood)

INFERTILITY SCREEN, SPECIMEN

Norm: Negative for sperm agglutinating antibody.

Semen Analysis:

pH	7.12–8.00 (average 7.7).
Volume	2–6 ml (0.002–0.006 L SI units).
Count	50–200 million/ml.
Liquification time	Within 30 minutes of collection.
Motility	60–80% are motile.
Morphology	>70% are of normal shape.

Usage: Evaluation for possible causes of infertility.

Description: The infertility screen consists of two tests. Semen is analyzed for the presence, number, volume, motility, morphology, and liquification time of sperm, and both spermatozoa and serum are analyzed for the presence of sperm agglutinating antibodies. These antibodies may be present in seminal plasma, attached to spermatozoa, or circulating in the male or female bloodstream, and have been linked to infertility.

Professional Considerations:

1. Consent form NOT required.
2. Preparation:
   A. Obtain for each partner, a tube: Red-top, red/gray-top, or gold-top.
   B. Obtain a clean, plastic container.
   C. If the semen is to be collected on site, provide privacy for the male client.
   D. *See Client and family teaching.*
3. Procedure:
   A. Obtain a 7-ml blood sample from each partner.
   B. Obtain a fresh semen specimen from male. The specimen should be collected by masturbation, without using a condom or lubricants.
4. Postprocedure care:
   A. Explain that repeat testing may be necessary.
   B. Write the semen collection time on the laboratory requisition, and send the specimen to the laboratory within 2 hours of collection.
5. Client and family teaching:
   A. Do not have intercourse or masturbate for 48 hours before specimen collection.
   B. Collect a fresh semen specimen in a plastic cup. The specimen may be collected by masturbation at the institution or at home, but it must be collected by masturbation. Do not use a condom or a lubricant, other than saliva.
   C. Keep track of the time the semen was collected.
   D. After collecting the specimen, keep the container of semen warm by putting it in a pocket next to the body.
   E. If the specimen is collected at home, it must be delivered to the laboratory within 1 hour.
6. Factors that affect results:
   A. Reject semen specimens more than 2 hours old.
   B. Heavy tobacco smoking and heavy coffee consumption may decrease the number of motile spermatozoa.
7. Other data:
   A. Repeat testing may be necessary, as results vary with samples.

B. *See also Semen Analysis, Specimen.*

Bibliography:

Eggert-Kruse W, Probst S, Rohr G, et al.: Screening for subclinical inflammation in ejaculates. Fertil Steril 64(5):1012–1022, 1995.

Lewis SE, Boyle PM, McKinney KA, et al.: Total antioxidant capacity of seminal plasma is different in fertile and infertile men. Fertil Steril 64(4):868–870, 1995.

Oehinger S, Kruger T: The diagnosis of male infertility by semen quality. Clinical significance of sperm morphology assessment. Hum Reprod 10(5):1037–1038, 1995.

Seracchioli R, Porcu E, Flamigni C: The diagnosis of male infertility by semen quality. Sperm morphology is not the only criterion of male infertility. Hum Reprod 10(5):1039–1041, 1995.

INFLUENZA A AND B TITER, BLOOD

Norm: Less than a fourfold increase in titer in paired sera. Less than 1:8 titer indicates previous exposure.

Positive: Influenza.

Negative: Bacterial infections.

Description: Influenza viruses are typed for epidemiological surveys. Both viruses, A and B, cause major epidemics every 2–4 years, as antigenic shifts occur, leaving the population susceptible to reinfection by a different strain. Virus B usually is sporadic and local, whereas virus A spreads rapidly and to all population areas.

Professional Considerations:

1. Consent form NOT required.
2. Preparation:
   A. Tube: Red-top, red/gray-top, or gold-top.
3. Procedure:
   A. Draw a 7-ml blood sample at the onset of symptoms.
   B. Draw a convalescent sample 14 days later.
4. Postprocedure care:
   A. None.
5. Client and family teaching:
   A. Return in 2 weeks for a second sample to be drawn. This helps monitor recovery.
   B. Annual influenza vaccinations are recommended in the latter portions of each year for the elderly, health care workers, and others at high risk for exposure to the influenza virus.
6. Factors that affect results:
   A. Failure to collect a convalescent sample limits the value of the acute sample results.
7. Other data:
   A. Serologic diagnosis is not necessary during an epidemic, but is valuable for epidemiologic purposes.

Bibliography:

Levi R, Beeor-Tzahar T, Arnon R: Microculture virus titration—a simple colourimetric assay for influenza virus titration. J Virol Methods *52*(1–2): 55–64.

Ziegler T, Hal H, Sanchez-Fauquier A, et al.: Type- and subtype-specific detection of influenza viruses in clinical specimens by rapid culture assay. J Clin Microbiol *33*(2):318–321, 1995.

INHIBITION LEVEL, ANTIBIOTIC

(see Schlichter Test, Specimen)

INR

(see Prothrombin Time and International Normalized Ratio, Serum)

INSULIN, SERUM

Norm: Fasting: ≤25 µU/ml (≤179 pmol/L, SI units).

Panic Level Symptoms and Treatment: *See Insulin Assay, Blood.*

Increased: Acromegaly, Beckwith-Wiedemann syndrome, beta-cell adenoma, Cushing's syndrome, hyperinsulinism, nesidioblastosis, and pheochromocytoma. Drugs include quinine and insulin.

Decreased: Insulin-dependent diabetes mellitus and pancreatectomy-induced diabetes.

Description: A hormone produced in the pancreas by the beta cells of the Islets of Langerhans that regulates carbohydrate metabolism. Rate of secretion is determined by the level of blood glucose.

Professional Considerations:

1. Consent form NOT required.
2. Preparation:
   A. Tube: Red-top, red/gray-top, or gold-top. Also obtain ice.
   B. *See Client and family teaching.*
3. Procedure:
   A. Draw a 7-ml blood sample.
   B. Handle the specimen carefully, pack it in ice, and send it to the laboratory.
4. Postprocedure care:
   A. Assess the client for signs of hypoglycemia, which could occur as a response to fasting.
   B. Resume foods and any medications withheld prior to the test.
5. Client and family teaching:
   A. Fast from food and fluids (except water) for 8 hours prior to the test.

B. Review the procedure used to obtain the blood sample, including the fact that some discomfort may be experienced when the needle enters the skin.
6. Factors that affect results:
   A. Hemodialysis destroys insulin.
   B. Specimen hemolysis invalidates the results.
   C. Therapy with estrogen and progesterone may produce elevated levels of insulin.
   D. Failure to follow dietary restrictions before the test can lead to falsely elevated levels.
7. Other data:
   A. Serum insulin level is commonly prescribed in conjunction with serum glucose to confirm functional hypoglycemia, uncontrolled insulin-dependent diabetes mellitus, or fasting hypoglycemia of unknown etiology.
   B. The norms and standardization of the test method vary widely by laboratory.

Bibliography:

Moller LF, Jespersen J: Elevated insulin levels in men: an 11-year follow-up study. J Cardiovasc Risk *2*(4): 339–343, 1995.

INSULIN ANTIBODY, BLOOD

Norm: Interpretation required. Undetectable when using either bovine or porcine insulin as a reagent.

Positive: Factitious hypoglycemia.

Negative: Insulinoma.

Description: Insulin antibodies, also referred to as anti-insulin-Ab, are present in diabetics treated for several weeks or more with conventional insulin. This test may be used in combination with C-peptide to determine whether hypoglycemia is caused by insulin abuse. Insulin antibodies have been shown to occur more frequently with aging and more frequently in females than in males (Zimmet et al., 1994).

Professional Considerations:

1. Consent form NOT required.
2. Preparation:
   A. Tube: Red-top, red/gray-top, or gold-top.
   B. *See Client and family teaching.*
3. Procedure:
   A. Draw a 7-ml blood sample.
4. Postprocedure care:
   A. Assess the client for peripheral venipuncture complications.
   B. Assess the client for hypoglycemic reactions due to fasting.
5. Client and family teaching:
   A. Fast (except water) for 8 hours prior to the test.

6. Factors that affect results:
   A. Reject specimens if the client had a radioactive scan within 7 days prior to the test.
7. Other data:
   A. When insulin antibodies are present, the test of choice is C-peptide to determine whether exogenous insulin administration is being abused. If C-peptide levels are not elevated, endogenous insulin secretion has not increased.
   B. Insulin antibodies are transferred through the placenta.
   C. Anti-insulin antibodies are present in 30–50% of children at the time of diagnosis before beginning insulin therapy.

Bibliography:

Eguchi Y, Uchigata Y, Yao K, Yokoyama H, Hirata Y, Omori Y: Longitudinal changes of serum insulin concentration and insulin antibody features in persistent insulin autoimmune syndrome (Hirata's disease). Autoimmunity 19(4):279–284, 1994.

Shimizu T, Sasakuma F, Ishikawa O, Matsumiya K, Hasegawa K, Sasaki A: Assessment of immunoassays for insulin in diagnostic tests for insulinoma. Diabetes Res Clin Pract 26(2):149–154, 1994.

Zimmet PZ, Elliott RB, Mackay IR, Tuomi T, Rowley MJ, Pilcher CC, Knowles WJ: Autoantibodies to glutamic acid decarboxylase and insulin in islet cell antibody positive presymptomatic type 1 diabetes mellitus: frequency and segregation by age and gender. Diabet Med 1(9):866–871, 1994.

INSULIN ASSAY (RIA), BLOOD

Norm:

		SI Units
Adult		
Fasting level	<17 μU/ml	42–243 pmol/L or 1.00 mg/L
Newborn	3–20 μU/ml	21–139 pmol/L
Infant	<13 μU/ml	≤89 pmol/L
Prepubertal child	<13 μU/ml	≤89 pmol/L
Panic levels	>30 μU/ml	<290 pmol/L
Last trimester, amniotic fluid	11.3 μU/ml	78 pmol/L

Panic Level Symptoms and Treatment:

Symptoms: Diaphoresis, dizziness, faintness, pallor, weakness, progressing to stupor and seizures.

Treatment:

Administer 50% dextrose in water via 50-ml IV, followed by carbohydrate and protein foods.

Follow with D10%W infusion if NPH or other long-acting insulin was taken.

Administer glucagon IV if the client has normal liver function.

Take bedside or laboratory glucose measurement hourly.

If serum potassium level is low and/or cardiac dysrhythmias are present, give KCL infusion.

Hemodialysis and peritoneal dialysis will NOT remove insulin.

Increased: Acromegaly, Cushing's syndrome, dystrophia myotonica, familial fructose and galactose intolerance, hyperinsulinism, hypoglycemia, insulin-resistance syndromes, insulinoma, liver disease, non-insulin-dependent diabetes mellitus, obesity, overdose of insulin and pancreatic islet cell lesion. Drugs include albuterol, calcium gluconate in the newborn, fructose, glucagon, glucose, insulin, levodopa, medroxyprogesterone, oral contraceptives, prednisolone, quinidine, spironolactone, sucrose, terbutaline, tolazamide, and tolbutamide.

Decreased: Diabetes mellitus type I (with inadequate treatment), hyperglycemia, and hypopituitarism. Drugs include beta-adrenergic blockers, asparaginase, calcitonin, cimetidine, diazoxide, ethacrynic acid, ethanol, ether, furosemide, metformin, nifedipine, phenformin, phenobarbital, phenytoin, and thiazide diuretics.

Description: Measures endogenous insulin by using a series of tubes containing a fixed amount of antibody label, and an aliquot of standard, control, or unknown. The client's unlabeled antigen in the blood competes with labeled antigen for antibody binding sites. The percentage of antigen bound to antibody is related to the total antigen present and is reflected by the distribution of a radioactive label. Low immunoreactive insulin levels have been associated with a higher risk of developing degenerative diseases such as atherosclerosis, hypertension, and dyslipidemia. Levels have recently been shown to predict the development of diabetes mellitus.

Professional Considerations:

1. Consent form NOT required.
2. Preparation:
   A. Tube: Red-top, red/gray-top, lavender top, or gold-top. Obtain ice.
   B. Specimens MAY be drawn during hemodialysis.
   C. *See Client and family teaching.*
3. Procedure:
   A. Draw a 2-ml blood sample. Place the sample immediately on ice.
4. Postprocedure care:
   A. Client may resume diet.
5. Client and family teaching:
   A. This test is used to evaluate for insulin-producing neoplasm (islet cell tumor, insulinoma) or to evaluate insulin production in diabetes mellitus.
   B. Fast for 7 hours before sampling.
   C. Do not take insulin prior to the test.
6. Factors that affect results:
   A. Reject specimens if the client had a radioactive scan within 7 days prior to the test.
   B. Hemodialysis destroys insulin.
7. Other data:
   A. Undetectable in amniotic fluid <16 weeks.
   B. Complete absence of insulin during the last trimester of pregnancy is associated with intrauterine death.
   C. Values are higher in plasma samples than in serum.

Bibliography:

Department of Pathology, University of Michigan: Online Pathology Handbook: Insulin Assay, Adult or Pediatrics. Ann Arbor, August 1995.

Hoyer GL, Nolan PE Jr, LeDoux JH, Moore LA: Selective stability-indicating high-performance liquid chromatographic assay for recombinant human regular insulin. J Chromatogr A 699(1–2):383–388, 1995.

Robbins DC, Andersen L, Bowsher R, Chance R, Dinesen B, Frank B, Gingerich R, Goldstein D, Widemeyer HM, Haffner S, Hales CN, Jarett L, Polonsky K, Porte D, Skyler J, Webb G, Gallagher K: Report of the American Diabetes Association's Task Force on standardization of the insulin assay. Diabetes 45(2):242–256, 1996.

INSULIN-LIKE GROWTH FACTOR-I, BLOOD

Norm:

		SI Units
Adult females	24–253 ng/ml	24–253 m/L
	or 0.4–2 U/ml	or 400–2000 U/L
Adult males	43–178 ng/ml	43–178 m/L
	or 0.7–1.7 U/ml	700–1700 U/L
Children		
0–2 years		
Female	14–60 ng/ml	14–60 m/L
Male	14–56 ng/ml	14–56 m/L
3–5 years		
Female	18–97 ng/ml	18–97 m/L
Male	13–81 ng/ml	13–81 m/L
6–9 years		
Female	34–137 ng/ml	34–137 m/L
Male	29–108 ng/ml	29–108 m/L
10–12 years		
Female	66–215 ng/ml	66–215 m/L
Male	44–207 ng/ml	44–207 m/L
13–15 years		
Female	192–347 ng/ml	192–347 m/L
Male	98–319 ng/ml	98–319 m/L
16–18 years		
Female	132–305 ng/ml	132–305 m/L
Male	136–293 ng/ml	136–293 m/L

Increased: Acromegaly, diabetic retinopathy, hyperpituitarism, obesity, pituitary gigantism, precocious puberty, and pregnancy.

Decreased: Anorexia nervosa, cirrhosis, chronic illness, delayed puberty, diabetes mellitus, emotional deprivation syndrome, hepatoma, hypopituitarism, hypothyroidism, kwashiorkor, Laron dwarfs, liver disease, maternal deprivation syndrome, nutritional deficiency, and pituitary tumor.

Description: Insulin-like growth factor-I (IGF-I) is a small polypeptide produced primarily in the liver, transported in the plasma, and bound by carrier proteins. Acting via cell membrane receptors, IGF-I directly stimulates growth and proliferation of normal cells. It affects glucose metabolism and is affected by growth hormone activity. Thus, this test may be used when monitoring response to growth hormone treatment in pituitary dwarfism, as levels are highest during growth spurts. Insulinlike growth factor-I is also used to evaluate the severity of acromegaly.

Professional Considerations:

1. Consent form NOT required.
2. Preparation:
   A. Tube: Lavender-top.
   B. Specimens MAY be drawn during hemodialysis.
   C. *See Client and family teaching.*
3. Procedure:
   A. Draw a 2-ml blood sample.
4. Postprocedure care:
   A. Immediately separate and freeze serum. The specimen is stable for 30 days.
5. Client and family teaching:
   A. Fast from food and fluids from midnight prior to the test.
   B. Results may not be available for several days.
6. Factors that affect results:
   A. Decreased nutritional states.
   B. Results may be falsely elevated if the client received a radioactive scan within the past 7 days.
7. Other data:
   A. Norms in pregnant women are higher than in nonpregnant women.
   B. IGF-I is now produced by recombinant DNA technology and may be useful in the treatment of acromegaly and certain types of dwarfism.
   C. IGF-II is similar in structure to IGF-I and is thought to be an important regulator of embryonic and fetal growth. Its level remains fairly constant after an initial rise in the first year of life.
   D. The test was formerly known as Somatomedin C.

Bibliography:

Sassolas G: Acromegaly. *In* Bardin CW (ed): Current Therapy in Endocrinology and Metabolism, 5th ed. St. Louis, MO, CV Mosby, 1995, pp 44–52.

Strasser-Vogel B, Blum WF, Past R, et al.: Insulin-like growth factor (IGF)-I and -II and IGF-binding proteins -1, -2, and -3 in children and adolescents with diabetes mellitus: correlation with metabolic control and height attainment. J Clin Endocrinol Metab *80*(4):1207–1213, 1995.

INTERNATIONAL NORMALIZED RATIO, SERUM

(see Prothrombin Time and International Normalized Ratio, Serum)

INTRAVASCULAR COAGULATION SCREEN, BLOOD

Norm:

Fibrinogen	
Adult	200–400 mg/dl
Newborn	125–300 mg/dl
Fibrin breakdown products	<10 μg/ml
Platelet count	
Adult	150,000–400,000/mm³
Newborn	84,000–478,000/mm³
Activated partial thromboplastin time (APTT)	25–35 seconds
Prothrombin time	
Adult	11–15 seconds
Newborn	2–35 seconds
Premature	3–5 seconds
Thrombin time	200–400 mg/dl

Usage: Differentiation of acute disseminated intravascular coagulation (DIC) from chronic DIC.

Test	Acute DIC	Chronic DIC
Fibrinogen	Decreased	Normal or increased
Fibrin breakdown	Positive	Positive
Platelet count	Decreased	Normal or increased
APTT	Increased	Normal
Prothrombin time	Increased	Normal
Thrombin time	Increased	Increased

Description: Intravascular coagulation is a process whereby there are multiple fibrin thrombi with micro-infarctions and tissue and organ necrosis. This is caused by activation of the clotting mechanism and depletion of clotting factors and platelets with a secondary fibrinolysis that results in bleeding.

Professional Considerations:
1. Consent form NOT required.
2. Preparation:
   A. Tubes: Three red-top, red/gray-top, or gold-top.
3. Procedure:
   A. Draw three 5-ml blood samples in the three tubes.
4. Postprocedure care:
   A. Place a pressure dressing on the venipuncture site. Monitor closely for bleeding.
5. Client and family teaching:
   A. Clients with disseminated intravascular clotting syndrome (DIC) may be in acute crisis. Support the family; explain there may be a need for blood product therapy.
6. Factors that affect results:
   A. Heparin increases clotting time.
7. Other data:
   A. None.

Bibliography

Metz J, Cincotta R, Francis M, DeRosa L, Balloch A: Screening for consumptive coagulopathy in preeclampsia. Int J Gynaecol Obstet 46(1):3–9, 1994.

INTRAVASCULAR ULTRASOUND, DIAGNOSTIC
(see Coronary Intravascular Ultrasound, Diagnostic)

INTRAVENOUS CHOLANGIOGRAPHY

Norm: Even filling of the hepatic and biliary ducts. Complete filling of the gallbladder occurs. Negative for stones, stricture, or filling defects.

Usage: Alternative to oral cholecystography when client cannot tolerate oral iodopaque tablets or in clients with active intestinal inflammation; and detection of calculi (or their movement), strictures, or leaking anastamosis(es) in the biliary ductal system.

Description: Intravenous cholangiography involves taking a series of radiographs of the gallbladder and hepatobiliary duct systems over several hours after the intravenous administration of radiographic contrast media. The contrast media is allowed to circulate to the liver via the hepatic artery and empty into the biliary tree. Strictures or stones cause defects in the pattern of filling and can be visualized on the radiograph. Strictures occurring in the hepatobiliary ducts may be congenital; caused by ductal damage during exploratory or therapeutic biliary surgery; or caused by benign or malignant tumor or inflammation.

Professional Considerations:
1. Consent form IS required.

Risks:
Hypotension, infection, nausea, respiratory failure, tachycardia, vomiting, allergic reaction to dye (itching, hives, rash, tight feeling in the throat, shortness of breath, bronchospasm, anaphylaxis, death), renal toxicity from contrast medium.

Contraindications:
Respiratory failure; previous allergy to iodine, shellfish, or radiographic dye; renal insufficiency; during pregnancy or breast-feeding.

2. Preparation:
   A. A laxative or cathartic may be administered 24 hours prior to the procedure.
   B. A cleansing or tap-water enema may be given the morning of the procedure.
   C. Establish intravenous access.
   D. Have emergency equipment readily available.
   E. *See Client and family teaching.*
3. Procedure:
   A. The client is positioned supine on the scanning table.
   B. A radiographic contrast medium is injected intravenously or infused via drip and allowed at least 30 minutes to circulate to the liver and become excreted into the bile ducts. Radiographs of the hepatic and bile ducts are taken at this time.
   C. 2–3 hours are then allowed to pass, in order to allow the gallbladder to fill with contrast medium. Radiographs may be taken of the gallbladder and biliary system at intervals for up to 8 hours after injection.
4. Postprocedure care:
   A. Resume previous diet.
   B. Assess for allergy to contrast medium for 24 hours.
   C. Dysuria is not uncommon, because the contrast medium is excreted in the urine.
5. Client and family teaching:
   A. Fast from food and fluids overnight prior to the test.
   B. Morning insulin may be withheld for diabetics, because the test may take up to 8 hours.
   C. A burning or flushing sensation may be experienced when the dye is injected.
   D. Bring something to read, if desired, as the test may take several hours.
   E. Blockage of the gallbladder can be due to stones formed from natural bile salts and substances similar in nature to cholesterol. A low-fat diet is generally recommended for clients with gallbladder disease.
6. Factors that affect results:
   A. Hepatic failure with bilirubin >3.5 mg/dl (58 mmol/L, SI units) will interfere with gallbladder visualization. The dye must be processed in the liver before it passes into the gallbladder. The test will be cancelled for a high bilirubin level.
7. Other data:
   A. *See also Endoscopic Retrograde Cholangiopancreatography, Diagnostic; and Percutaneous Transhepatic Cholangiography, Diagnostic,* two tests that are used more commonly than intravenous cholangiography.

Bibliography:

Griscom NT, O'Conner JF: The rise and fall of radiologic technique. Am J Roentgenol *164*(4):1011–1012, 1995.

Reiger R, Sulzbacher H, Woisetschlager R, Schrenk P, Wayand W: Selective use of ERCP in clients undergoing laparoscopic cholecystectomy. World J Surg *18*(6):900–905, 1994.

Wigmore SJ, Wood K, Rainey JB, Macleod DA: Intravenous cholangiography in preoperative assessment of clients considered for laparoscopic cholecystectomy. Surg Laparoscopy Endoscopy *4*(4):254–257, 1994.

INTRAVENOUS PYELOGRAPHY (IVP, EXCRETORY UROGRAPHY), DIAGNOSTIC

Norm: Normal renal pelvis, ureters, and bladder. No obstruction or masses.

Usage: Berger's disease, glomerulonephritis, hydronephrosis, renal cell cancer, renal failure, renal hypertension, tubular necrosis, and Wilms' tumor.

Description: An invasive test that uses contrast radiopaque dye to assess the ability of the kidneys to excrete dye in the urine. Radiographs are taken following dye injection to visualize the kidneys, ureters, and bladder to assess for obstruction, hematuria, stones, bladder injury, and renal artery occlusion of the renal pelvis.

Professional Considerations:

1. Consent form IS required.

Risks:

Dysuria, nephrotoxicity, urinary tract infection, vasovagal response, allergic reaction to dye (itching, hives, rash, tight feeling in the throat, shortness of breath, bronchospasm, anaphylaxis, death), renal toxicity from contrast medium, weakness.

Contraindications:

Dehydration; previous allergy to radiographic dye; renal insufficiency.

2. Preparation:
   A. Bowel preparation of oral evacuation preparation 24 hours prior to the test and evacuation enema 8 hours prior to test.
   B. Assess for high-risk clients: dehydration, elderly, severe diabetes mellitus, renal insufficiency, or multiple myeloma.
   C. Have emergency equipment readily available.

3. Procedure:
  A. The client is placed in slight Trendelenburg position or supine.
  B. A venipuncture is performed and dye is injected into a vein.
  C. Serial radiographs are taken periodically for the next 30 minutes.
4. Postprocedure care:
  A. The client should drink at least three 8-ounce glasses of liquid to flush the kidneys of the dye (when not contraindicated).
  B. Assess for signs of allergic reaction to the dye (listed above) × 24 hours.
5. Client and family teaching:
  A. It is normal to feel flushed and warm and to notice a salty taste soon after the dye is injected. This will last only a few moments.
  B. Stress the importance of drinking water after the test to flush dye from the body, prevent osmotic diuresis from the dye, and protect the kidneys.
6. Factors that affect results:
  A. Poor bowel evacuation or poor renal perfusion will decrease the uptake of dye, leading to poor radiograph quality.
7. Other data:
  A. Dosages of radiation range from 1047 to 1465 mR (milliroentgens).

Bibliography:

Kessler O, Mukamel E, Hadar H, Gillon G, Kenechezky M, Servadio C: Effect of improved diagnosis of renal cell carcinoma on the course of the disease. J Surg Oncol 57(3):201–204, 1994.

Reiter L, Brown MA, Whitworth JA: Hypertension in pregnancy: the incidence of underlying renal disease and essential hypertension. Am J Kidney Dis 24(6):883–887, 1994.

INTRINSIC FACTOR ANTIBODY, BLOOD

Norm: Negative; none detected.

Positive: Graves' disease, insulin-dependent diabetes, megaloblastic anemia, and pernicious anemia.

Description: Intrinsic factor is produced by the parietal cells of the gastric mucosa and is required for the effective absorption of vitamin B_{12}. In some diseases, antibodies are produced that bind the cobalamin-intrinsic factor complex and prevent the complex from binding to receptors in the ileum.

Professional Considerations:

1. Consent form NOT required.
2. Preparation:
  A. Tube: Red-top, red/gray-top, or gold-top.
  B. Do not collect a sample if vitamin B_{12} was injected or ingested by client within 48 hours prior to the test.
3. Procedure:
  A. Draw a 3-ml blood sample.
4. Postprocedure care:
  A. None.
5. Client and family teaching:
  A. If the test results show the presence of antibodies and a positive diagnosis is made of pernicious anemia, the client requires regular injections of vitamin B_{12} due to the body's loss of ability to produce the intrinsic factor secreted by the parietal cells in the stomach lining.
6. Factors that affect results:
  A. Reject if the client had a radioactive scan within 7 days prior to the test.
7. Other data:
  A. Causes of vitamin B_{12} deficiency include pancreatic insufficiency, parasitic infestations of the small intestine, regional enteritis, malnutrition, or transcobalamin protein abnormalities.

Bibliography:

Altay C, Cetin M, Gumruk F, Irken G, Yetgin S, Laleli Y: Familial selective vitamin B12 malabsorption (Imerslund-Grasbeck syndrome). Pediatr Hematol Oncol 12(1):19–28, 1995.

Gordon MM, Howard T, Becich MJ, Alpers DH: Cathepsin L mediates intracellular ileal digestion of gastric intrinsic factor. Am J Physiol 268(1):G33–G40, 1995.

INULIN CLEARANCE TEST, DIAGNOSTIC

Norm:

Adults	90–130 ml/minute
>70 Years	Decreased clearance up to 45% of adult value
Children	
<11 years	82–122 ml/minute
11–20 years	86–126 ml/minute

Usage: Assessment of glomerular filtration rate.

Increased: Diuresis.

Decreased: Acute tubular necrosis, atherosclerosis (renal artery), congestive heart failure, decreased renal blood flow, dehydration, glomerulonephritis, malignancy (bilateral renal), nephrosclerosis, obstruction (renal artery), polycystic kidney disease, pyelonephritis (advanced bilateral chronic), renal lesions (bilateral), renal failure, shock (cardiogenic, hypovolemic), thrombosis (renal vein), tuberculosis (renal), and ureteral obstruction (bilateral). Drugs include aminoglycosides, amphotericin B, penicillins, and phenacetin.

Description: Inulin clearance is a very specific indicator of renal function. Inulin is a plant polysaccharide that, after intravenous injection, is freely and almost completely filtered by the glomeruli and is not readily absorbed from the tubules. Thus, with normal glomerular function, inulin clearance should equal the glomerular filtration rate, as all inulin that is filtered is excreted in the urine. This test measures both a blood sample and a urine sample for inulin to determine the rate at which inulin is being cleared from the blood by the kidneys. Specifically, "clearance" means the amount of blood that is cleared of inulin in 1 minute and that is independent of urine flow rate. Decreased results occur when over 50% of renal nephrons are damaged, thus indicating impaired glomerular filtration. The inulin clearance test may be included as one of four renal function studies, the others being the urine concentration test, phenosulfonphthalein test, and the creatinine clearance test.

Professional Considerations:

1. Consent form NOT required.
2. Preparation:
   A. The client should drink 32 ounces of water 30–60 minutes prior to the test.
   B. Insert an indwelling urinary catheter. Send a 50-ml baseline urine sample to the laboratory for inulin measurement.
   C. Obtain alcohol wipes, a tourniquet, five needles, five syringes, five green-top tubes, five clean specimen containers with lids, and a 500-ml bag of D5W with Y tubing.

D. Establish intravenous access, using 5% dextrose in water.
E. Number each set of tubes and specimen containers 1, 2, 3, 4, and 5, and use them sequentially throughout the test.
F. Obtain 25 ml of 10% inulin and 500 ml of 1.5% inulin along with an intravenous pump. Prepare the inulin by shaking the vial and heating it to promote crystal dissolution.
G. Use this test cautiously in clients with cardiac disease, as intravenous fluids given during the test may induce congestive heart failure.
H. *See Client and family teaching.*
3. Procedure:
   A. The client should drink water frequently throughout the test; 8 ounces of water every 15 minutes is desirable.
   B. Draw a 10-ml blood sample for inulin level, without hemolysis. Record the time of collection on each label.
   C. Infuse, intravenously, 10% inulin, 25 ml over 4 minutes.
   D. An hour later, begin an infusion of 1.5% inulin, 500 ml at 240 ml/hour.
   E. Obtain 10-ml urine samples in separate containers at 30, 50, 70, and 90 minutes after the initiation of the 1.5% inulin solution. This may be accomplished either by clamping the catheter between samples and drawing the sample from the catheter port, or by completely emptying the drainage bag after collecting each sample. Record the time of collection on each label.
   F. Draw a 10-ml blood sample for inulin level, without hemolysis, at 40, 60, 80, and 95 minutes after the initiation of the 1.5% inulin solution. Record the time of collection on each label.
   G. The test takes 2 hours.
4. Postprocedure care:
   A. Write the time and amount of each dose of inulin on the laboratory requisition.
   B. Each blood and urine sample should be sent immediately to the laboratory after being collected. If this is not possible, urine specimens should be refrigerated.
   C. Remove the urinary catheter and intravenous line.
   D. Resume previous diet.
5. Client and family teaching:
   A. Fast from food for 4 hours prior to the test, and refrain from exercise the morning of the test.
   B. A catheter will be placed in the bladder for this procedure, and blood will be drawn at intervals.
   C. The test takes 2 hours to complete.
6. Factors that affect results:
   A. Hemolysis of blood will falsely decrease results.
   B. Failure to infuse intravenous inulin at the prescribed rate will decrease results.

7. Other data:
   A. The initial bolus of inulin should be administered within 1 hour of preparation.

Bibliography:

Lindblad HG, Berg UB: Comparative evaluation of iohexol and inulin clearance for glomerular filtration rate determinations [see comments]. Acta Paediatr 83(4):418–422, 1994.

McFarland MB, Grant MM: Nursing Implications of Laboratory Tests. Albany, NY, Delmar Publishers, 1994.

Schmieder RE, Gatzka C, Schobel H, Schachinger H, Weihprecht H: Renal hemodynamic response to stress is influenced by ACE-inhibitors. Clin Nephrol 42(6):381–388, 1994.

van den Anker JN, de Groot R, Broerse HM, Sauer PJ, van der Heijden BJ, Hop WC, Lindemans J: Assessment of glomerular filtration rate in preterm infants by serum creatinine: comparison with inulin clearance. Pediatrics 96(6):1156–1158, 1995.

IRON (Fe), SERUM

Norm:

		SI Units
Adult female	40–150 µg/dl	7.2–26.9 µmol/L
Adult male	50–160 µg/dl	8.9–28.7 µmol/L
Newborn	100–250 µg/dl	17.9–44.8 µmol/L
Infant	40–100 µg/dl	7.2–17.9 µmol/L
Child	50–120 µg/dl	8.9–21.5 µmol/L

Increased: Acute hepatitis, aplastic anemia, blood transfusion, hemochromatosis, hemolytic anemia, hepatitis, lead poisoning, nephritis, pernicious anemia, polycythemia, sideroblastic anemia, thalassemia, and vitamin B_6 deficiency.

Decreased: Blood loss, burns, carcinoma, gastrectomy, infection, iron deficiency anemia, kwashiorkor, malabsorption, nephrosis, postoperative state, pregnancy, rheumatoid arthritis, schizophrenia (chronic), tetralogy of Fallot, and uremia.

Description: Iron is an inorganic ion, mostly found in hemoglobin, that acts as a carrier of oxygen from the lungs to the tissues and indirectly aids in the return of carbon dioxide to the lungs. Although the source for body iron is from food, only a small portion of that consumed from the diet is absorbed. Iron is stored in the liver and reticuloendothelial tissue in the form of ferritin and hemosiderin and is released from storage as needed to meet the body's demands.

Professional Considerations:

1. Consent form NOT required.
2. Preparation:
   A. Tube: Red-top, red/gray-top, or gold-top.
   B. Document the date of the last blood transfusion on the laboratory requisition.
   C. Do NOT draw specimens during hemodialysis.
3. Procedure:
   A. If using Vacutainer and venipuncture for multiple samples, draw this sample first to avoid mixing heparin with the sample. Draw a 7-ml blood sample.
4. Postprocedure care:
   A. None.
5. Client and family teaching:
   A. The basic role of iron in hemoglobin formation is to allow blood to efficiently carry oxygen to the tissues. Foods rich in iron include red meats and some green, leafy vegetables.
6. Factors that affect results:
   A. Hemolysis of the specimens invalidates the results.
   B. Vitamin B_{12} ingested within 48 hours may increase the results.
7. Other data:
   A. Adenocarcinoma of the gastrointestinal tract may be detected by iron deficiency.
   B. Increased serum iron concentrations of 300–500 mg/dl (53.7–89.6 mmol/L, SI units) can be the result of one ingested iron tablet.
   C. Increased ferritin levels frequently accompany neoplastic activity.
   D. See also Iron and Total Iron-Binding Capacity/Transferrin, Serum.

Bibliography:

Che P, Xu J, Shi H, Ma Y: Quantitative determination of serum iron in human blood by high-performance capillary electrophoresis. J Chromatogr B Biomed Appl 669(1):45–51, 1995.

Deehr MS, Dallal GE, Smith KT, et al.: Effects of different calcium sources on iron absorption in postmenopausal women. Am J Clin Nutr 51(1):95–99, 1990.

Litzman J, Dastych M, Hegar P: Analysis of zinc, iron and copper serum levels in patients with common variable immunodeficiency. Allergol Immunopathol (Madrid) 23(3):117–120, 1995.

SmithKline Beecham Clinical Laboratories: Directory of Services. Tucker, GA, 1993, p 87.

IRON (Fe) AND TOTAL IRON-BINDING CAPACITY (TIBC)/TRANSFERRIN, SERUM

Norm:

		SI Units
Iron		
Adult female	40–150 µg/dl	7.2–26.9 µmol/L
Adult male	50–160 µg/dl	8.9–28.7 µmol/L
Newborn	100–250 µg/dl	17.9–44.8 µmol/L
Infant	40–100 µg/dl	7.2–17.9 µmol/L
Child	50–120 µg/dl	8.9–21.5 µmol/L
TIBC		
Adult	250–400 µg/dl	44.8–71.6 µmol/L
Infant	100–400 µg/dl	17.9–71.6 µmol/L
Transferrin		
Adult	200–400 mg/dl	2–4.0 g/L
Maternal	305 mg/dl	3.0 g/L
(Term)		
Fetal	190 mg/dl	1.9 g/L
Newborn	130–275 mg/dl	1.3–2.8 g/L

Increased TIBC: Hepatitis, microcytic anemia, and pregnancy. Drugs include iron salts and oral contraceptives.

Decreased TIBC: Cirrhosis, dysmenorrhea, hemochromatosis, hemorrhage, hepatitis, hypothyroidism, kwashiorkor, microcytic anemia, myocardial infarction, neoplasm, nephrosis, pernicious anemia, thalassemia, and uremia. Drugs include ACTH, asparaginase, chloramphenicol, corticotropin, cortisone, dextran, steroids, and testosterone.

Description: This test differentiates anemia secondary to iron deficiency from other diseases associated with variations in cellular oxidation. Iron is an element necessary for many body processes, including the transport of oxygen to the tissues and for oxygen-carrying chromoproteins, hemoglobin, myoglobin, and enzymes such as xanthine oxidase and peroxidase. Transferrin is a plasma iron transport protein, also called siderophilin, formed in the liver, that has a half-life of 7–10 days. Transferrin is capable of binding more than its own weight in iron (i.e., 1 g of transferrin can carry 1.43 g of iron). In normal clients, iron saturation of transferrin is between 20% and 45%. Transferrin saturation by iron demonstrates a diurnal pattern, with a morning peak and an early evening trough. The formula for transferrin saturation by iron is:

(Serum iron/TIBC) × 100 = Transferrin saturation

TIBC is the maximum amount of iron that can be bound to transferrin. It is useful in distinguishing anemia (increased value) from chronic inflammatory disorders (normal value). In this test, iron is added to the client's serum until all transferrin binding sites are bound with iron. Then the excess iron is removed, and the total amount of remaining (bound) iron is measured, giving an assessment of the ability of the individual's transferrin to bind iron.

Professional Considerations:
1. Consent form NOT required.
2. Preparation:
   A. Tube: Red-top, red/gray-top, or gold-top; and 20-gauge or larger needle.
   B. Document the date of the last blood transfusion on the requisition.
   C. *See Client and family teaching.*
3. Procedure:
   A. Draw a 7-ml blood sample, without hemolysis.
4. Postprocedure care:
   A. None.

5. Client and family teaching:
   A. Fast 12 hours before sampling. Water is permitted.
   B. If the results indicate low iron, eat foods high in iron such as organ meats, eggs, and dried fruits.
6. Factors that affect results:
   A. Inflammatory states may decrease results below normal.
   B. Hemolysis may cause falsely elevated iron values.
7. Other data:
   A. A decrease in iron and an increase in TIBC is found in microcytic anemia.
   B. Serum transferrin may be calculated from TIBC using the formula $0.8 \times TIBC - 43$.

Bibliography:

Baynes RD, Cook JD, Bothwell TH, Friedman BM, Meyer TE: Serum transferrin receptor in hereditary hemochromatosis and African siderosis. Am J Hematol 45(40):288–292, 1994.

Bergstrom E, Hernell O, Lonnerdal B, Persson LA: Sex differences in iron stores of adolescents: what is normal? J Pediatr Gastroenterol Nutr 20(2):215–224, 1995.

Konijn AM: Iron metabolism in inflammation. Baillieres Clin Haematol 7(4):829–849, 1994.

IRON STAIN, BONE MARROW, SPECIMEN

(see Bone Marrow Aspiration Analysis, Specimen)

ISOCITRATE DEHYDROGENASE (ICD), BLOOD

Norm:

		SI Units
Adult	1.2–7.0 U/L	0.02–0.12 IU/L
Cord blood	2.4–14.0 U/L	0.04–0.23 IU/L
Newborn	4.8–28.0 U/L	0.08–0.47 IU/L
2 weeks	4.8–7.0 U/L	0.08–0.12 IU/L

Increased: Biliary tract (acute inflammation), cirrhosis, hepatic lesions that are bacterially infected, hepatitis (chronic), infectious mononucleosis, kwashiorkor, metastasis to the liver, pulmonary infarct (severe), and Reye's syndrome.

Decreased: Hepatocellular necrosis (massive).

Description: Isocitrate dehydrogenase (ICD) is an enzyme that catalyzes the conversion of isocitrate to oxalosuccinate and alpha-ketoglutarate in the Krebs cycle and is a sensitive indicator of parenchymal liver disease.

Professional Considerations:

1. Consent form NOT required.
2. Preparation:
   A. Tube: Red-top, red/gray-top, or gold-top.
3. Procedure:
   A. Draw a 7-ml blood sample.
4. Postprocedure care:
   A. Send the specimen to the laboratory immediately.
5. Client and family teaching:
   A. This test is used for diagnosing multiple diseases that affect the liver.
6. Factors that affect results:
   A. Hemolysis of the specimen invalidates the results.
7. Other data:
   A. This blood test is replaced by alanine aminotransferase.

Bibliography:

Suzuki M, Sahara T, Tsuruha J, Takada Y, Fukunaga N: Differential expression of *Escherichia coli* of the Vibrio Sp. Strain ABE-1 icdI and icdII genes encoding structurally different isocitrate dehydrogenase isozymes. J Bacteriol 177(8):2138–2142, 1995.

Yamamoto S, Atomi H, Ueda M, Tanaka A: Novel NADP-linked isocitrate dehydrogenase present in peroxisomes of n-alkaline-utilizing yeast, Candida tropicalis: comparison with mitochondrial NAD-linked isocitrate dehydrogenase. Arch Microbiol 163(2):104–111, 1995.

ISOPROPYL ALCOHOL, BLOOD

Norm: Negative.
Panic level: >340 mg/dl.

Panic Level Symptoms and Treatment:

Symptoms: Coma, confusion, dizziness, headache, nausea, oliguria initially followed by diuresis, respiratory depression, stupor, uncoordinated movement, vomiting. Death is possible.

Treatment:

Take aspiration precautions.
Administer activated charcoal and tap-water lavage.

Do gastric lavage.
Provide mechanical ventilation.
Give oxygen.
Administer stimulant medication.
Monitor electrolytes and treat imbalance.
Give IV NS and/or D_5W.
Monitor for hepatic or renal damage.
Hemodialysis WILL remove isopropyl alcohol. Peritoneal dialysis is minimally effective in removing isopropyl alcohol.

Increased: Alcoholism and poisoning.

Description: A portion of rubbing alcohol (70% isopropyl alcohol) that is metabolized to acetone, carbon dioxide, and water in the blood and urine. This alcohol is readily absorbed by the gastrointestinal tract, having a half-life of 30–180 minutes, and produces central nervous system depression. Isopropanol is often ingested in desperation by alcoholics.

Professional Considerations:

1. Consent form NOT required.
2. Preparation:
   A. Tube: Red-top, red/gray-top, or gold-top.
   B. Obtain povidone-iodine.
   C. Do NOT draw during hemodialysis.
3. Procedure:
   A. Cleanse the venipuncture site with povidone-iodine.
   B. Draw a 7-ml blood sample.
4. Postprocedure care:
   A. Monitor for panic level signs.
5. Client and family teaching:
   A. If the client tests positive, discuss the poisonous nature of isopropyl alcohol.
   B. Discuss avenues for crisis intervention should the ingestion be due to a suicide attempt.

C. If the client is having suicidal ideation, encourage him or her to participate in a contract to notify the caregiver.
D. If the client is being abused by an alcoholic, refer the client/family to alcoholic support programs.
E. If activated charcoal was given for elevated levels, the client should drink 4–6 glasses of water each day for 2 days to prevent constipation. The activated charcoal will cause stools to be black for a few days.
6. Factors that affect results:
   A. Cleansing the venipuncture site with alcohol may cause falsely elevated results.
7. Other data:
   A. A lethal dose is 8 ounces (240 ml).
   B. Positive acetone with a normal anion gap, bicarbonate, and plasma glucose suggests rubbing alcohol (isopropranol) intoxication.
   C. *See also Toxicology, Volatiles Group by GLC, Blood or Urine.*

Bibliography:

Ukai H, Takada S, Inui S, Imai Y, Kawai T, Shimbo S, Ikeda M: Occupational exposure to solvent mixtures: effects on health and metabolism. Occup Environ Med *51*(8):523–529, 1994 (Aug).
University of Michigan Department of Pathology: Online Handbook. Volatiles Group, Ann Arbor, 1995.
Vivier PM, Lewander WJ, Martin HF, Linakis JG: Isopropyl alcohol intoxication in a neonate through chronic dermal exposure: a complication of a culturally-based umbilical care practice. Pediatr Emerg Care *10*(2):91–93, 1994.

IVP
(see Intravenous Pyelography, Diagnostic)

IVY BLEEDING TIME, DIAGNOSTIC
(see Bleeding Time, Ivy, Blood; and Aspirin Tolerance Test, Diagnostic)

KETO-DIASTIX, DIAGNOSTIC

Norm: Negative.

Usage: Detection of ketones in the urine for carbohydrate deprivation, diabetes mellitus, diabetic ketoacidosis, or ketonuria.

Description: Ketones are the breakdown products resulting from fat metabolism. In a low-insulin state such as diabetes, fat and fatty acids are metabolized less efficiently, resulting in a build-up of serum ketones. Elevated serum ketones are excreted through the kidneys into the urine. In this test, semiquantitative screening is performed using a dipstick for determining ketones in the urine. The reagent strip correlates only moderately well with quantitative acetoacetate in plasma, and poorly with total blood ketones.

Professional Considerations:

1. Consent form NOT required.

2. Preparation:
   A. Obtain a clean specimen container.
3. Procedure:
   A. Instruct the client to void and then to drink a glass of water.
   B. 30 minutes later, ask the client to void into the specimen container.
   C. Dip the stick into the urine for 5 seconds.
   D. Tap the edge of the stick against the container of urine to remove excess urine.
   E. After 15 seconds, compare the color of the ketone section (buff or purple) with the appropriate color chart. Report the results of ketones that are positive as either small, moderate, or large.
4. Postprocedure care:
   A. Testing must occur within 60 minutes of the specimen being obtained for specimens kept at room temperature. Refrigerated urine may be tested later, but must first be returned to room temperature.
5. Client and family teaching:
   A. Keto-Diastix is often being replaced

with at-home blood test kits that are simple and more reliable indicators of blood levels of ketones.

6. Factors that affect results:
   A. Drugs that may cause false-positive results include levodopa, phenazopyridine, and sulfobromophthalein.
   B. Pentamidine therapy for AIDS may induce ketoacidosis in clients with diabetes mellitus.
7. Other data:
   A. Keto-Diastix assesses ketones only, not glucose. Read the dipstick after 15 seconds.

Bibliography:

Lott JA, Johnson WR, Luke KE: Evaluation of an automated urine chemistry reagent-strip analyzer. J Clin Lab Anal 9(3):212–217, 1995.

McClatchey KD: Clinical Laboratory Medicine. Baltimore, MD, Williams and Wilkins, 1994.

Pagana KD, Pagana TJ: Diagnostic Testing and Nursing Implications. St. Louis, MO, Mosby Year Book, 1993.

Patel JS, Leonard JV: Ketonuria and medium-chain acyl-CoA dehydrogenase deficiency. J Inherit Metab Dis 18(1):98–99, 1995.

17-KETOGENIC STEROIDS (17-KGS), 24-HOUR, URINE

Norm:

		SI Units
Adult female	3–15 mg/24 hours	8–41 µmol/day
Adult male	5–25 mg/24 hours	14–69 µmol/day
<1 year	<1 mg/24 hours	<3 µmol/day
<5 years	<2 mg/24 hours	<6µmol/day
5–10 years	3–6 mg/24 hours	8–17 µmol/day
>70 years	3–13 mg/24 hours	8–36 µmol/day

Increased: Adrenal carcinoma, adrenogenital syndrome, burns, Cushing's syndrome, hirsutism, hyperadrenalism, infectious disease, obesity, pregnancy, surgery, and virilization. Drugs include cephalothin, corticosteroids, digoxin, meprobamate, oral contraceptives, penicillin, phenothiazines, and spironolactone.

Decreased: Addison's disease, cretinism, hypoadrenalism, hypopituitarism, Simmonds' disease, and wasting-away diseases in general. Drugs include ampicillin, dexamethasone, estrogens, glucose, morphine, phenytoin, prednisone, and prednisolone.

Description: The 17-ketogenic steroids are hormones that are metabolites of glucocorticoids and pregnanetriol and are elevated when there is increased production by the adrenal gland and low if there is hypofunction of the adrenal cortex. This test may be used to help diagnose Cushing's syndrome or Addison's disease.

Professional Considerations:

1. Consent form NOT required.
2. Preparation:
   A. Obtain a 3-L, plastic urine container with boric acid or 33% acetic acid preservative.
   B. Whenever possible, withhold all medications for at least 24 hours before the specimen collection period, because many medications interfere with this test. These include chlordiazepoxide, dexamethasone, estrogens, methyprylon, phenazopyridine, piperidine, probenecid, pyrazinamide, quinidine, and secobarbital.
3. Procedure:
   A. Collect all the urine voided in a 24-

hour period in a 3-L, plastic specimen container to which boric acid or 33% acetic acid has been added.

4. Postprocedure care:
   A. Separate a 50-ml aliquot and refrigerate it.

5. Client and family teaching:
   A. Save all the urine voided in the 24-hour period and urinate before defecating to avoid contaminating urine with stool. If any urine is accidentally discarded, discard the entire specimen and restart the collection the next day.
   B. This 24-hour test indicates adrenal gland function.

6. Factors that affect results:
   A. ACTH or stress will increase results.
   B. Penicillin and radiographic dye interfere with test results.
   C. Drugs that may cause falsely decreased values include chlorothiazide, metyrapone, paraldehyde, quinine, reserpine, and thiazide.
   D. Drugs that may cause falsely elevated levels include acetazolamide, acetophenone, chlorpromazine, cortisone, ethinamate, glucuronide, hydralazine, meprobamate, oleandomycin, penicillin, phenothiazines, phenaglycodol, spironolactone, and triacetyloleandomycin.

7. Other data:
   A. Normally rises at puberty, levels off at age 25, then gradually decreases, more so in males.
   B. This test has been replaced by *Cortisol, Urine* in most laboratories.

Bibliography:

Ravel R: Clinical Laboratory Medicine: Clinical Application of Laboratory Data. St Louis, MO, Mosby Year Book, 1995.

KETONE (ACETONE) BODIES, BLOOD

Norm: Negative or 0.3–2.0 mg/dl (<0.17 mmol/L, SI units).

Panic Level: >20 mg/dl (>3.44 mmol/L, SI units).

Panic Level Symptoms and Treatment:

Symptoms: Fruity breath, acidosis, ketonuria, depressed level of consciousness.

Treatment:

Blood glucose measurement q 1 hour.
Insulin infusion.
Neurologic checks q 1 hour.

Positive: After anesthesia, alcoholism, carbohydrate deficiency, diabetes mellitus, eclampsia, glycogen storage disease, high-fat diet, hyperglycemia, isopropanol alcohol ingestion, ketoacidosis, pregnant diabetic, propranol poisoning, reducing diets, starvation, and von Gierke's disease.

Negative: Not applicable.

Description: Ketones are the intermediate breakdown products resulting from incomplete fat metabolism. In a low-insulin state such as diabetes, fat and fatty acids are metabolized less efficiently, resulting in a buildup of serum ketones. Ketone bodies consist of acetone, beta-hydroxybutyric acid, and acetoacetic acid. Extremely elevated levels in the bloodstream can lead to coma. This test is used to help differentiate coma due to a hyperosmotic state, in which a negative test would be expected, from coma due to ketoacidosis.

Professional Considerations:

1. Consent form NOT required.
2. Preparation:
   A. Tube: Red-top, red/gray-top, or gold-top; or capillary tubes.
3. Procedure:
   A. Draw a 1-ml blood sample in a tube or collect the specimen in capillary tubes, filling them as completely as possible.
4. Postprocedure care:
   A. None.
5. Client and family teaching:
   A. Ketone bodies, a natural byproduct of metabolism, can be dangerously elevated in some diseases.
   B. Coma caused by diabetic ketoacidosis is usually reversible.
6. Factors that affect results:
   A. Hemolysis of the specimen invalidates the results.
   B. A low-carbohydrate or low-fat diet may cause elevated results.
7. Other data:
   A. Elevated acetone with normal anion gap, bicarbonate, and plasma glucose suggests rubbing alcohol (isopropanol) intoxication.
   B. Ketones appear in the urine before there is a significant increase in the blood.

Bibliography:

Kabadi UM: Pancreatic ketoacidosis: ketonemia associated with acute pancreatitis. Postgrad Med J *71*(831):32–35, 1995.
Kawasaki S, Makuuchi M, Matsushita K, Urata K, Nakazawa Y, Ikegami T, Hashikura Y, Matsunami H, Miyagawa S: The arterial ketone body ratio in living-related donors. Transplantation *58*(12): 1412–1414, 1994.

KETONE, SEMIQUANTITATIVE, URINE

Norm: Negative or Keto-Diastix negative.

Positive: Alcoholism, diabetes mellitus, convulsions, eclampsia, Fanconi's syndrome, glycogen storage disease, ketoacidosis, and von Gierke's disease. Drugs include anesthesia, isopropyl alcohol, levodopa, and mesna.

Description: Ketone bodies consist of acetoacetic acid, beta-hydroxybutyric acid, and acetone, and are byproducts of fat and fatty acid metabolism. Semiquantitative results means testing several different dilutions of each urine specimen to obtain a better degree of differentiation of ketone body products that can be obtained from qualitative testing.

Professional Considerations:

1. Consent form NOT required.
2. Preparation:
   A. Obtain a clean, plastic specimen container.
3. Procedure:
   A. Collect a 12-ml random urine specimen in a clean, plastic specimen container.
4. Postprocedure care:
   A. Send the specimen to the laboratory immediately. If the specimen cannot be tested immediately, refrigerate it. Cap the container tightly.
5. Client and family teaching:
   A. Assess over-the-counter medications. If the client is taking large doses of vitamin C, this could cause false results.
6. Factors that affect results:
   A. Preservative in foods of 8-hydroxyquinoline may increase urine levels.
   B. Drugs that may cause false-positive results include ascorbic acid, levodopa, pyridium, phthalein compounds given for liver or kidney tests, and valproic acid.
   C. A low-carbohydrate or high-fat diet may cause elevated results.
7. Other data:
   A. Ketones appear in the urine before serum elevations are seen.

Bibliography:

Patel JS, Leonard JV: Ketonuria and medium-chain acyl-CoA dehydrogenase deficiency. J Inherit Metab Dis *18*(1):98–99, 1995.

Watson J, Jaffe MS: Nurse's Manual of Laboratory and Diagnostic Tests, 2nd ed. Philadelphia, FA Davis, 1995.

17-KETOSTEROID FRACTIONATION, 24-HOUR, URINE

Norm:

		SI Units
Adult		
Female	6–14 mg/24 hours	21–49 µmol/day
Male	10–25 mg/24 hours	35–87 µmol/day
Child		
1–4 years	<2 mg/day	<7 µmol/day
5–9 years	<3 mg/day	<10 µmol/day
10–12 years	1–5 mg/day	3–17 µmol/day
12–14 years	1–6 mg/day	3–21 µmol/day
14–16 years, female	2–8 mg/day	8–28 µmol/day
14–16 years, male	3–13 mg/day	10–45 µmol/day

Increased: Adrenal tumor, Cushing's syndrome, gynecomastia, ovarian tumor, pregnancy, testicular tumor, and virilization.

Decreased: Addison's disease, adrenalectomy, castration, and hypothyroidism.

Description: A test of adrenal function by measuring the excretion of urinary steroids. 17-ketosteroids are a group of steroid compounds that have a ketone at position C-17 of the steroid nucleus. Dividing the steroid compounds up (fractionation) is important when the need to assess androgenic properties is required. This test is useful in differentiating adrenal carcinoma, which causes a high level of dehydroepiandrosterone, from adrenal hyperplasia, which causes all ketosteroids to be elevated.

Professional Considerations:

1. Consent form NOT required.
2. Preparation:
   A. Obtain a 3-L, plastic specimen container with boric acid or 33% acetic acid preservative.
3. Procedure:
   A. Collect all the urine voided in a 24-hour period in a 3-L, plastic specimen container to which 20 ml of boric acid or 33% acetic acid preservative has been added. The container should be kept on ice throughout the collection period. Document the quantity of urinary output throughout the collection period.
4. Postprocedure care:
   A. Compare the documented urinary output with the urine quantity in the specimen container. If the container has less urine than was documented as output, some of the specimen may have been discarded, thus invalidating the test.
   B. Write the beginning and ending dates and times and the total urine voided during the 24 hours on the laboratory requisition and the container.
   C. Keep the specimen on ice until tested.
5. Client and family teaching:
   A. Urinate before defecating and avoid contaminating the urine with toilet tissue or stool. If any urine is accidentally discarded, discard the entire specimen and restart the collection the next day.
   B. Adrenal gland function is assessed with this test.
6. Factors that affect results:
   A. Age and sex are stratified for results.
   B. Contrast dyes decrease values.

C. Drugs that may cause falsely increased results include ACTH, ascorbic acid, cephalothin, clordiazepoxide, chlorpromazine cloxacillin, cortisone, digitoxin, erythromycin, hydralazine, meprobamate, methicillin, methyprylon, morphine, oxacillin, penicillin G, pyridium, phenothiazines, piperidine, quinine, salicylates, secobarbital, spironolactone, and testosterone.
D. Drugs that may cause falsely decreased results include aminoglutethimide, chlordiazepoxide, chlorpromazine, corticosteroids, dexamethasone, digoxin, diphenylhydantoin, estrogens, glucose, meprobamate, oral contraceptives, paraldehyde, penicillin, phenytoin, probenecid, promazine, propoxyphene, pyrazinamide, quinine, quinidine, reserpine, salicylates, secobarbital, and spironolactone.
7. Other data:
   A. This test is seldom used because serum levels of androgens are easily measured.

Bibliography:

Derksen J, Nagesser SK, Meinders AE, Haak HR, van-de-Velde CJ: Identification of virilizing adrenal tumors in hirsute women. New Engl J Med *331*(15):968–973, 1994.

Iwata J, Morita H, Yasuda K, Kuwayama A, Suzuki T, Demura H: Daily excretion levels of an unidentified ketosteroid in the urine of patients with Cushing's syndrome and healthy subjects measured by a new method. Endocr J *42*(3):449–453, 1995.

Remer T, Hintelmann A, Manz F: Measurement of urinary androgen sulfates without previous hydrolysis: a tool to investigate adrenarche. Determination of total 17-ketosteroid sulfates. Steroids *59*(1):16–21, 1994.

17-KETOSTEROIDS (17-KS), TOTAL, 24-HOUR, URINE

Norm:

		SI Units
Adult female	4–16 mg/24 hours	13–55 μmol/day
Adult male	6–21 mg/24 hours	21–72 μmol/day
>60 years	4–8 mg/24 hours	13–27 μmol/day
Infant	<1 mg/24 hours	<3 μmol/day
1–3 years	<2 mg/24 hours	<7 μmol/day
3–6 years	<3 mg/24 hours	<10 μmol/day
7–10 years	<4 mg/24 hours	<14 μmol/day
10–12 years		
Female	<5 mg/24 hours	<17 μmol/day
Male	<6 mg/24 hours	<21 μmol/day
Adolescent		
Female	3–12 mg/24 hours	10–41 μmol/day
Male	3–15 mg/24 hours	10–52 μmol/day

Increased: Adrenocortical tumors, adrenogenital syndrome, Cushing's syndrome, hirsutism, hyperplasia of adrenals, ovarian lutein cell tumor, Stein-Leventhal syndrome, and testicular interstitial cell tumor.

Decreased: Addison's disease, hypopituitarism, Klinefelter's syndrome, and menopause.

Description: 17-ketosteroids are composed of adrenal hormones and metabolites of testicular androgens. This test is becoming obsolete, because serum androgen measurement is readily available and involves less collection time.

Professional Considerations:

1. Consent form NOT required.
2. Preparation:
   A. Obtain a 3-L, plastic urine container with boric acid or 33% acetic acid preservative.
3. Procedure:
   A. Collect all the urine voided in a 24-hour period in a 3-L, plastic container to which boric acid or 33% acetic acid has been added. The specimen should be kept on ice throughout the collection period.
4. Postprocedure care:
   A. Compare the documented urinary output with the urine quantity in the specimen container. If the container has less urine than was documented as output, some of the specimen may have been discarded, thus invalidating the test.
   B. Write the beginning and ending dates and times and the total urine voided during the collection period on the laboratory requisition and container.
   C. Keep the specimen on ice until tested.
5. Client and family teaching:
   A. Urinate before defecating and avoid contaminating the urine specimen with stool or toilet tissue. If any urine is accidentally discarded, discard the entire specimen and restart the collection the next day.
   B. Avoid stressful situations prior to and during the 24-hour collection period.
6. Factors that affect results:
   A. Stress will increase the results.
   B. Drugs that may cause falsely increased results include ACTH, ascorbic acid, cephalothin, clordiazepoxide, chlorpromazine cloxacillin, cortisone, digitoxin, erythromycin, hydralazine, meprobamate, methicillin, methyprylon, morphine, oxacillin, penicillin G, pyridium, phenothiazines, piperidine, quinine, salicylates, secobarbital, spironolactone, and testosterone.
   C. Drugs that may cause falsely decreased results include aminoglutethimide, chlordiazepoxide, chlorpromazine, corticosteroids, dexamethasone, digoxin, diphenylhydantoin, estrogens, glucose, meprobamate, oral contraceptives, paraldehyde, penicillin, phenytoin, probenecid, promazine, propoxyphene, pyrazinamide, quinine, quinidine, reserpine, salicylates, secobarbital, and spironolactone.
   D. Contrast dyes interfere with the results.
7. Other data:
   A. This test does not detect the major androgen, testosterone.

Bibliography:

Higgins C: Laboratory backup. Nurs Times *90*(32): 44–48, 1994.

Wilson JD, Braunwald E, Isselbacher KJ, Petersdorf RG, Martin JB, Fauci AS, Root RK (eds): Harrison's Principles of Internal Medicine, 12th ed. New York, McGraw-Hill, 1991, pp 1637–1654.

KETOSTIX, DIAGNOSTIC
(see Keto-Diastix, Diagnostic)

17-KGS
(see 17-Ketogenic Steroids, 24-Hour, Urine)

Ki-67 PROLIFERATION MARKER (MIB 1–3), SPECIMEN

Norm: Rated from low proliferation index to high proliferation index. Varies with tumor type.

Usage: Determination of the proliferation index (PI) of a specific tumor type to provide prognostic information in predicting the clinical outcome of certain tumors. The Ki-67 monoclonal antibody is used to determine the proliferation state of breast cancer, bone cancer, brain tumors, cervical cancer, colorectal cancer, endometrial cancer, liver tumors, lymphomas, plasma cell tumors, smooth muscle tumors, and soft tissue tumors. Non-neoplastic conditions such as hemangiomas, inflammatory bowel disease, psoriasis, renal biopsy, and sarcoidosis also use the Ki-67 proliferation marker.

Description: Ki-67 is an IgG1 class, murine monoclonal antibody that reacts with a nuclear antigen expressed only by proliferating human cells. Expression of this antigen occurs during the late G1, S1, G2, and M phase of the cell cycle. The proliferation activity of a tumor tissue is determined by the growth fraction (number of cells in cell cycle) and the time taken to complete the cell cycle. A strong correlation exists between the proliferation rate of tumors and clinical outcome and there is an association between a high proliferation rate and the degree of tumor aggressiveness. The Ki-67 immunostaining, along with histopathologic evaluation, has been shown to be beneficial in correlating the proliferation state of cancers such as breast, lymphatic, lung, and brain with clinical prognosis. Results of Ki-67 immunostaining as a prognostic factor vary with each tumor type using quantitative analysis. MIB 1–3 are newer antibodies that recognize the Ki-67 antigen in both fixed and frozen tissue, whereas the Ki-67 antibody requires a fresh, frozen sample.

Professional Considerations:

1. Consent form IS required. See *Biopsy, Site-Specific-Specimen* for procedure-specific risks and complications.
2. Preparation:
   A. The client is prepared for surgical biopsy or resection.
3. Procedure:
   A. A fresh specimen, free of excess fat and blood and of at least 0.5–1.0 g, is obtained by surgical resection or needle biopsy.
   B. The specimen is cut into small pieces and quick-frozen on dry ice, cryostat, or liquid nitrogen within 20 minutes of excision.
   C. For Ki-67 immunostaining, do not place the specimen in formalin. Place the frozen specimen in a 60-ml solid-tumor biopsy bottle. The specimen must remain frozen ($-70°C$).
   D. For MIB-1(Ki-67) the specimen may be prepared using a formalin fixed paraffin block. Optimal fixation time is 12–24 hours, not to exceed 48 hours.
4. Postprocedure care:
   A. Apply a dry, sterile dressing to the biopsy or operative site.
   B. Assess the site for excessive bleeding, erythema, hematoma, or drainage.
5. Client and family teaching:
   A. Results will not be available for at least 2 days.
6. Factors that affect results:
   A. Thawed specimens will be rejected.
   B. Bronchial brushings are unacceptable because of tumor cell clumping and presence of mucus.

C. The Ki-67 antigen is very sensitive to chemical denaturation and is destroyed in weak solutions of formalin.
D. The Ki-67 antigen expression appears to be influenced by a cell's nutritional supply. Tissue taken from the central area of a large tumor may give an erroneously low value for the growth factor.
7. Other data:
   A. None.

Bibliography:

Brown DC, Gatter KC: Monoclonal antibody Ki-67: its use in histopathology. Histopathol *17*:489–503, 1990.

Colvin RB, Bhan AK, McCluskey RT: Diagnostic Immunopathology. New York, Raven Press, 1995, pp 673–693.

Hall PA, Levinson DA: Assessment of cell proliferation in histological material [review]. Am J Clin Pathol *34*:184–192, 1990.

Jordan PA, Kerns B-JM, Pence JC, et al.: Determination of proliferation index in advanced ovarian cancer using quantitative image analysis. Am J Clin Pathol *99*:736–740, 1993.

KIDNEY BIOPSY, SPECIMEN

Norm: Interpretation required.

Usage: Alport's syndrome, diabetic glomerulosclerosis, glomerulonephritis, Goodpasture's syndrome, hematuria, Kimmelstiel-Wilson disease, nephrosis, nephrotic syndrome, renal failure, and toxemia.

Description: The surgical or percutaneous needle biopsy resulting in the aseptic removal of a small quantity of kidney tissue.

Professional Considerations:

1. Consent form IS required.

Risks:

Bleeding, infection, pneumothorax.

Contraindications:

Percutaneous biopsy is contraindicated in uncooperative clients; in clients with bleeding diatheses, uncontrolled hypertension, or renal infection; or in clients with solitary functional kidney. Mendelssohn and Cole (1995) recommend conditions under which clients with solitary functional kidneys might be considered candidates for kidney biopsy.

2. Preparation:
   A. Prior to the biopsy, an intravenous pyelography test or renal scan should be performed to document bilateral renal function.
   B. Obtain a biopsy tray, including a needle, sponges, lidocaine (Xylocaine), and slides or a sterile specimen jar.
3. Procedure:
   A. A renal biopsy can be performed percutaneously with a special needle or under direct visualization during surgery.
4. Postprocedure care:
   A. Send the specimen to the laboratory immediately.
   B. Monitor vital signs every 15 minutes × 4.
   C. Monitor for blood in the urine 8 hours following the biopsy.
5. Client and family teaching:
   A. This examination of renal tissue can provide valuable details in diagnosing kidney disease.
   B. Report any pain in the flank or abdomen after the procedure.
6. Factors that affect results:
   A. None found.
7. Other data:
   A. Indications for a renal biopsy are not clear-cut or universally agreed upon.
   B. Histologic preparations using hematoxylin and eosin, periodic acid-Schiff, trichrome, and silver stains are also routinely performed on the tissue sample.
   C. Immunofluorescence and electron microscopic studies are routinely performed on biopsy specimens.

Bibliography:

Grenko RT, TenHave TR, Hartzel J, Sturtz KW, Savage CA: Percutaneous biopsy of the liver and kidney by using coaxial technique: adequacy of the specimen obtained with three different needles in vitro. Am J Roentgenol *164*(1):221–224, 1995.

Liu PI: Blue Book of Diagnostic Tests. Philadelphia, WB Saunders, 1986, p 181.

McClatchey KD: Clinical Laboratory Medicine. Baltimore, MD, Williams and Wilkins, 1994.

Mendelssohn DC, Cole EH: Outcomes of percutaneous kidney biopsy, including those of solitary native kidneys. Am J Kidney Dis *26*(4):580–585, 1995.

KIDNEY ECHOGRAM

(see Kidney Sonogram, Diagnostic)

KIDNEY PROFILE, BLOOD

(see SMA-7, Blood)

KIDNEY SCAN, DIAGNOSTIC

Norm: Normal renal vasculature and perfusion.

Usage: Renal transplants, trauma and urinary tract obstruction; examination of renal perfusion; helps diagnose renovascular hypertension.

Description: Radionuclide scanning to evaluate renal vascular supply, perfusion, and function. Less radiation exposure is required than for an IVP or CT scan. However, IVP is better for anatomic definition, and arteriography is better for assessing renal arterial anatomy.

Professional Considerations:
1. Consent form IS required.

Risks:
Infection.

Contraindications:
Open flank wounds.

---

2. Preparation:
   A. Establish intravenous access and infuse 500 ml of IV fluids (unless contraindicated).
   B. Have emergency equipment readily available.
   C. The client should empty the bladder. Insert an indwelling urinary catheter for pediatric clients.
3. Procedure:
   A. The client is positioned supine.
   B. A radionuclide analogue is injected intravenously, and multiple radiographs of the kidneys are taken over the next 45 minutes.
4. Postprocedure care:
   A. Assess the injection site for infiltration of radionuclide analogue.
5. Client and family teaching:
   A. This exam takes approximately 45 minutes and involves receiving an IV to administer the test material and some fluids.
   B. There will be a small amount of radiation exposure during testing.
6. Factors that affect results:
   A. None.
7. Other data:
   A. Useful in evaluating renal transplants for differentiating rejection from acute tubular necrosis.
   B. Spinal cord fractures may be noted in the scan.

Bibliography:

Aprile C, Saponaro R, Di Maio D, Beluffi G, Chiari G, Ruggiero R, Cannizzaro G, Avolio L: Cortical kidney scan evaluation in the follow-up of children with vesico-ureteric reflux. J Nucl Biol Med *38*(1): 89–95, 1994.

Doyle W: Renal scans. Shands Teaching Hospital, Department of Radiology, Nursing Procedure Manual. Gainesville, FL, 1995.

Liu PI: Blue Book of Diagnostic Tests. Philadelphia, WB Saunders, 1986, p 180.

Persuhn, PG: Nuclear Medicine: What exactly is it? Images *15*(1):11–14, 1996.

Wong JC, Rossleigh MA, Farnsworth RH: Utility of technetium-99m-MAG3 diuretic renography in the neonatal period. J Nucl Med 36(12):2214–2219, 1995.

KIDNEY SONOGRAM (KIDNEY ECHOGRAM, KIDNEY ULTRASOUND), DIAGNOSTIC

Norm: Bilateral kidneys are properly located and are of normal size and shape. The outer contour is smooth. Kidney is surrounded by echoes reflected from perirenal fat. Intense echoes are reflected by the renal sinus. Absence of calculi, cyst, hydronephrosis, obstruction, or tumor.

Usage: Alternative to renal dye imaging tests for clients with allergy to radiographic dyes; detection of hydronephrosis; diagnosis and localization of renal cysts, tumors, or calculi; evaluation of status following renal transplant; and guidance for antegrade pyelography biopsy, aspiration, or nephrostomy tube insertion.

Description: Evaluation of the kidney structure via the creation of an oscilloscopic picture from the echoes of high-frequency sound waves passing over the flank area (acoustic imaging). The time required for the ultrasonic beam to be reflected back to the transducer from differing densities of tissue is converted by a computer to an electrical impulse displayed on an oscilloscopic screen to create a three-dimensional picture of the kidney. The kidney is imaged by using the liver or spleen as an acoustic window. Renal cysts appear smooth, sonolucent, and spherical, with well-defined borders. In contrast, solid masses are of irregular shape, with poorly defined borders and higher attenuation. Inflammatory cysts have thicker walls, less well-defined borders, and contain low-level echoes. Early hematomas look like cysts and become more echogenic over time. Hydronephrosis is demonstrated by a large extrarenal pelvis, with renal parenchyma not detectable. In multicystic disease, the kidney is of smaller than normal size, and the renal pelvis can not be visualized. In polycystic disease, irregularly shaped cysts >1 mm diameter are present in variable shapes and sizes.

Professional Considerations:

1. Consent form NOT required.
2. Preparation:
   A. This test should be performed before intestinal barium tests, or else after the barium is cleared from the system.
   B. The client should disrobe below the waist or wear a gown.
   C. Obtain ultrasonic gel or paste.
3. Procedure:
   A. The client is positioned prone in bed or on a procedure table. Very young children are positioned supine.
   B. The flank area is covered with ultrasonic gel, and a lubricated transducer is passed slowly over the flank area at a variety of angles and at intervals about 1–2 cm apart.
   C. Photographs are taken of the oscilloscopic display.
4. Postprocedure care:
   A. Remove the lubricant from the skin.
   B. If a biopsy is performed, *see Biopsy, Site-Specific, Specimen.*
   C. If an antegrade pyelography or a nephrostomy tube insertion is performed in conjunction with this test, *see Antegrade Pyelography, Diagnostic.*
5. Client and family teaching:
   A. The procedure is painless and carries no risks (if a kidney sonogram is not performed in conjunction with invasive procedures).
   B. This procedure takes about 30 minutes.
6. Factors that affect results:
   A. Dehydration interferes with adequate contrast between organs and body fluids.
   B. Intestinal barium obscures results by preventing proper transmission and deflection of the high-frequency sound waves.
   C. A lower frequency transducer should be used if a great deal of fat surrounds the kidney.
   D. The more trunk fat present, the greater the attenuation (reduction in sound wave amplitude and intensity), which interferes with the clarity of the picture.
7. Other data:
   A. Further studies may include tomography or other radiographic imaging.
   B. *See also Antegrade Pyelography, Diagnostic.*

Bibliography:

Doyle W: Ultrasound procedures. Shands Teaching Hospital, Department of Radiology. Nursing Procedure Manual. Gainesville, FL, 1995.

Rudnick MR, Berns JS, Cohen RM, Goldfarb S: Nephrotoxic risks of renal angiography: contrast media-associated nephrotoxicity and atheroembolism: a critical review. Am J Kidney Dis 24(4):713–727, 1994.

KIDNEY STONE ANALYSIS, SPECIMEN

Norm: Interpretation required.

Usage: Hematuria, kidney stone, and nephrolithiasis.

Type of Stone	Condition
Calcium oxalate or phosphate	Hypercalcemia
	Hyperparathyroidism
	Hyperthyroidism
	Renal tubular acidosis
	Unknown etiology (common)
	Vitamin D intoxication
Cystine	Renal tubular defects
Magnesium ammonium phosphate (Struvite)	*Proteus* infection
	Urinary tract infection
Oxalate	Methoxyflurane anesthesia
	Vitamin B$_6$ deficiency
Uric acid	Gout
	Lymphoproliferative disorders

Description: Infrared spectroscopy examination of kidney stone after the specimen has been washed free of tissue and blood.

Professional Considerations:

1. Consent form NOT required but IS required for the procedure used to obtain the specimen. See the individual procedure for risks and contraindications.
2. Preparation:
   A. Obtain a clean specimen container.
3. Procedure:
   A. Send the stone in a plastic or glass container to the laboratory immediately.
4. Postprocedure care:
   A. Encourage the intake of fluids.
   B. A mild analgesic may be prescribed for use as needed.
5. Client and family teaching:
   A. Strain the urine for further stones if they are needed for analysis.
   B. If the stone can be removed and the infection stopped, the client has a low probability of the condition returning.
   C. A low-oxalate diet can help prevent kidney stones formed from calcium oxalate. A low-oxalate diet includes avoiding soybean products, wheat germ, grapefruit juice, strawberries, bananas, orange juice, canned pineapples or tomatoes, kidney beans, beets, spinach, carrots, celery, onions, sweet and white potatoes, green and waxed beans, cauliflower, cucumber, squash, broccoli, eggplant, cabbage, cashews, peanut butter and other nuts, cola beverages, and tea.
6. Factors that affect results:
   A. Do not apply tape to stones, as adhesives interfere with infrared spectroscopy.

7. Other data:
   A. Children commonly have stones from infection due to calcium phosphate and magnesium ammonium phosphate.

Bibliography:

Dussol B, Geider S, Lilova A, Leonetti F, Dupuy P, Daudon M, Berland Y, Dagorn JC, Verdier JM: Analysis of the soluble organic matrix of five morphologically different kidney stones. Evidence for a specific role of albumin in the constitution of the stone protein matrix. Urol Res *23*(1):45–51, 1995.

Flomenbaum N, Goldfrank L, Jacobson S: Emergency Diagnostic Testing, 2nd ed. St. Louis, MO, Mosby Year Book, 1995.

Gallegos C: Surgery for urinary tract stone disease. Practitioner *239*(1556):654–656, 1995.

Khatchadourian J, Preminger GM, Whitson PA, Adams-Huet B, Pak CY: Clinical and biochemical presentation of gouty diathesis: comparison of uric acid versus pure calcium stone formation. J Urol *154*(5):1665–1669, 1995.

Klugman V, Favus MJ: Diagnosis and treatment of calcium kidney stones. Adv Endocrinol Metab *6*:117–142, 1995.

Stephen M: University of Michigan Online Pathology Handbook: Stone Analysis. Ann Arbor, University of Michigan, 1995.

KIDNEY ULTRASOUND
(see Kidney Sonogram, Diagnostic)

KIDNEY-URETER-BLADDER, DIAGNOSTIC
(see Flat Plate X-Ray of Abdomen, Diagnostic)

KLEIHAUER-BETKE STAIN, DIAGNOSTIC
(see Betke-Kleihauer Stain, Diagnostic)

17-KS
(see 17-Ketosteroids,
Urine)

**KUB (KIDNEY, URETERS,
BLADDER), DIAGNOSTIC**
*(see Flat Plate X-Ray of Abdomen,
Diagnostic)*

LABILE FACTOR, BLOOD
(see Factor V, Blood)

LA CROSSE VIRUS TITER, SERUM
(see California Encephalitis Virus Titer, Serum)

LACTATE DEHYDROGENASE (LD), BLOOD
Norm:

		SI Units
Wroblewski method 30°C	150–450 U/L	72–217 IU/L
Adult		
≤Age 60	45–90 U/L	45–90 U/L
>Age 60	55–102 U/L	55–102 U/L
Newborn	160–500 U/L	160–500 U/L
Neonate	300–1500 U/L	300–1500 U/L
Infant	100–250 U/L	100–250 U/L
Child	60–170 U/L	60–170 U/L

Increased: Alcoholism, anemia (hemolytic, megaloblastic, pernicious), anoxia, burns (electric, thermal), cancer, cardiomyopathy, cerebrovascular accident, cirrhosis, congestive heart failure (with myocardial infarction), convulsions, delirium tremens, dysrhythmias (ventricular), folic acid anemia, hepatic neoplasm, hepatitis (acute, toxic), hypothyroidism, infectious mononucleosis, intracardiac prosthetic valves, jaundice (obstructive), lactic acidosis, leukemia (granulocytic, acute), lymphoma, malaria, megaloblastic anemia, mononucleosis (infectious), muscular dystrophy, myocardial infarction, myxedema, nephrectomy, nephritis, nephrotic syndrome, ovarian dysgerminoma, pain (muscle and bone), peritonitis, pernicious anemia, pheochromocytoma, pneumocystis carinii pneumonia, polymyositis, pulmonary embolism, pulmonary infarction, renal cortical infarction, renal infection, renal malignancy, sickle cell anemia, shock, skeletal muscle necrosis, splenomegaly, sprue, toxic shock syndrome, trauma, tumors (malignant), and ulcerative colitis. Drugs include chlorpromazine hydrochloride, clofibrate, codeine, floxuridine, lithium carbonate, lorazepam, meperidine, metoprolol tartrate, mithramycin, morphine, niacin, nifedipine, procainamide hydrochloride, propranolol, and thyroid hormone.

Decreased: Irradiation therapy. Drugs include oxalates.

Description: Lactate dehydrogenase (LD) is an intracellular enzyme found in almost all body tissues that is released after tissue damage. The highest concentrations are found in organs such as the heart, liver, kidneys, and skeletal muscle cells, as well as the red blood cells. When body tissue is damaged from trauma, ischemia, or acid/base imbalance, LD is released into the bloodstream. The results of this test indicate that tissue damage has occurred but cannot pinpoint the specific location of damage. When total LD is elevated to at least 130 IU/L, the *Lactate Dehydrogenase Isoenzymes* test should be performed to narrow down the source of tissue damage.

Professional Considerations:
1. Consent form NOT required.
2. Preparation:
   A. Tube: Red-top, red/gray-top, or gold-top.
   B. Do NOT draw during hemodialysis.

3. Procedure:
   A. Draw a 1-ml blood sample, without hemolysis.
4. Postprocedure care:
   A. None.
5. Client and family teaching:
   A. This test is used to look for compounds commonly found in the body after some type of damage to the tissue. If the results are elevated, another test is usually performed on the same blood specimen to help narrow down which type of tissue has been damaged.
6. Factors that affect results:
   A. Reject hemolyzed, frozen, or refrigerated samples. Hemolysis elevates the LD_1 isoenzyme, which will elevate total LD results.
   B. Heparin increases LD in one-third of all clients being treated with heparin.
7. Other data:
   A. LD is recommended as a prognostic factor in colorectal carcinoma. Clients with an initially normal level versus those with an abnormal level had median survivals of 16 and 7 months, respectively.
   B. *See also Lactate Dehydrogenase Isoenzymes, Blood.*

Bibliography:

Patel PS, Adhvaryu SG, Balar DB: Serum lactate dehydrogenase and its isoenzymes in leukemia patients: possible role in diagnosis and treatment monitoring. Neoplasma *41*(1):55–59, 1994.

Quist J, Hill AR: Serum lactate dehydrogenase (LDH) in Pneumocystis carinii pneumonia, tuberculosis, and bacterial pneumonia. Chest *108*(2):415–418, 1995.

Sulaiman ST, al-Najafi TS, Hamdon HS: Sensitive method for measuring lactate dehydrogenase activity in human serum by differential-pulse polarography. Analyst *119*(10):2199–2200, 1994.

Wallendal M, Stork L, Hollister JR: The discriminating value of serum lactate dehydrogenase levels in children with malignant neoplasms presenting as joint pain. Arch Pediatr Adolesc Med *150*(1):70–73, 1996.

LACTATE DEHYDROGENASE (LD) ISOENZYMES, BLOOD

Norm:

LD_1 = 22–36% cardiac and RBC origin.
LD_2 = 35–46% cardiac and RBC origin.
LD_3 = 13–26%.
LD_4 = 3–10% hepatic and skeletal muscle origin.
LD_5 = 2–9% hepatic and skeletal muscle origin.
$LD_2 > LD_1$.
$LD_1 : LD_2 \leq 1$.
$LD_4 > LD_5$.
$LD_5 : LD_4 \leq 1:3$.

Increased LD Total: Anemia (megaloblastic, hemolytic), cardiomyopathy, congestive heart failure, delirium tremens, hypothyroidism, inflammation, leukemia, muscle injury, myeloproliferative syndromes, myxedema, pulmonary infarction, and renal infarction. *See Lactate Dehydrogenase, Blood.*

Increased LD_1: Folic acid anemia, hepatitis, megaloblastic anemia, myocardial infarction (rises 24 hours after injury, peaks at 72 hours, and returns to baseline within 2 weeks), pernicious anemia, renal infarction, and testicular cancer.

Increased LD_2: Muscular dystrophy, pernicious anemia, and renal (cortex) infarction, rhabdomyolysis, tumor.

Increased LD_3: Advanced cancer, collagen disease, infection (viral), lymphocytosis, pancreatitis, pericarditis, platelet destruction, pulmonary embolism, pulmonary infarct with hepatic congestion, pulmonary pneumonia, and skeletal muscle injury.

Increased LD_4: Hepatitis, infectious mononucleosis, lymphoma, lymphocytic leukemia, and ovarian carcinoma, platelet destruction, pulmonary embolism, and skeletal muscle injury.

Increased LD_5: Alcoholism, cirrhosis, congestive heart failure, hepatitis, infectious mononucleosis, megaloblastic anemia, myocardial infarction, neonates, ovarian carcinoma, pulmonary infarct with hepatic congestion, and skeletal muscle injury.

Increased LD 1:2 Ratio: Inverted or "flipped" in anemia (hemolytic, megaloblastic, pernicious, sickle cell [acute]), cardiac hypoxia, folic acid deficiency, hemolysis, megaloblastic anemia, myocardial infarction, renal infarction.

Increased LD 5:4 Ratio: Alcoholism.

Decreased: LD_1 is normally decreased in neonates.

Description: *See Lactate Dehydrogenase, Blood.* This test is normally conducted when total LD levels are elevated. Electrophoresis is used to separate the five isoenzymes of lactate dehydrogenase (LD), an enzyme that catalyzes the reversible oxidation of lactic acid to pyruvic acid. LD isoenzymes help pinpoint whether tissue damage is of cardiac, red blood cell, hepatic, or skeletal muscle origin.

Professional Considerations:

1. Consent form NOT required.
2. Preparation:
   A. Tube: Red-top, red/gray-top, or gold-top.
3. Procedure:
   A. Draw a 1-ml blood sample, without hemolysis. The test may also be performed on the original specimen sent for total LD measurement.
4. Postprocedure care:
   A. Do not refrigerate or freeze the specimen.
5. Client and family teaching:
   A. This test is useful in diagnosing myocardial infarction, liver disease, tumors, and pulmonary embolus.

6. Factors that affect results:
   A. Reject hemolyzed specimens, as this elevates LD_1.
7. Other data:
   A. Isoenzymes should not be measured if total LD is <130 IU/L.

Bibliography:

Castaldo G, Oriani G, Cimino L, Topa M, Budillon G, Salvatore F, Sacchetti L: Discriminant function based on serum analytes differentiates hepatocarcinoma from secondary liver neoplasia. Clin Chem 41(3):439–443, 1995.

Rodrique F, Boyer O, Feillet F, Lemonnier A: Lactate dehydrogenase isoenzyme as an indicator of early graft function and complications following pediatric orthotopic liver transplantation. Transplant Proc 27(2):1871–1874, 1995.

LACTIC ACID, BLOOD

Norm:

		SI Units
Venous	0.5–2.2 mEq/L or 4.5–19.8 mg/dl	0.5–2.2 mmol/L
Arterial	0.5–1.6 mEq/L or 4.5–14.4 mg/dl	0.5–1.6 mmol/L

Increased: Alcoholism, diabetes mellitus, hepatic coma, hyperthermia, malignancy, peritonitis, and shock.

Decreased: Hypothermia.

Description: An acid derived from carbohydrate metabolism that is used for muscle contraction when energy needs exceed oxygen supply (anaerobic metabolism). One-fifth is oxidized through the citric acid cycle and the rest is synthesized in the muscle to glycogen. Elevated lactic acid levels indicate that hypoxia has occurred at the cellular level.

Professional Considerations:

1. Consent form NOT required.
2. Preparation:
   A. Tubes: Gray-top for the venous sample. Also obtain arterial puncture supplies and one heparinized tube.
   B. Draw the blood sample without a tourniquet if possible.
   C. Do NOT allow the client to clench/unclench the hand prior to blood drawing.
3. Procedure:
   A. Obtain a 1-ml venous blood sample in a gray-top tube containing a glycolytic inhibitor.
   B. Draw an arterial sample in a heparinized tube, place it on ice immediately, and transport it quickly to the laboratory.
4. Postprocedure care:
   A. Assess the arterial puncture site after holding pressure for 5 minutes.
   B. Send the specimen to the laboratory immediately.
5. Client and family teaching:
   A. Pressure will be maintained on the area where the artery was accessed to avoid unnecessary bruising.
6. Factors that affect results:
   A. Reject specimens received more than 15 minutes after collection.
   B. Intravenous infusions may affect acid-base balance.
7. Other data:
   A. Lactic acidosis is accompanied by an increase in the osmolar gap.
   B. Lactic acidosis has been successfully treated with dichloroacetate.

Bibliography:

Artuch R, Vilaseca MA, Farre C, Ramon F: Determination of lactate, pyruvate, beta-hydroxybutyrate and acetoacetate with a centrifugal analyser. Eur J Clin Chem Clin Biochem 33(8):529–533, 1995.

Barthelemy JC, Roche F, Gaspoz JM, Geyssant A, Minini P, Antoniadis A, Page E, Wolf JE, Wilner C, Isaaz K, Cavallaro C, Lacour JR: Maximal blood lactate level acts as a major discriminant variable in exercise testing for coronary artery disease detection in men. Circulation 93(2):246–252, 1996.

LACTIC ACID, CEREBROSPINAL FLUID, SPECIMEN
(see Cerebrospinal Fluid, Lactic Acid, Specimen)

LACTIC DEHYDROGENASE (LDH), BLOOD
(see Lactate Dehydrogenase, Blood)

LAPAROSCOPY (PERITONEOSCOPY), DIAGNOSTIC

Norm: Negative.

Usage: Ascites, biopsy, cholangiography, cirrhosis, dysmenorrhea, ectopic pregnancy, endometritis, fever of undetermined origin, gallbladder disease, identification of abdominal cavity adhesions, infertility, jaundice, lymphoma staging, malignancy staging, pancreatic disease, and pelvic inflammatory disease (PID).

Description: Direct inspection of the surfaces of the internal organs such as the liver, gallbladder, pancreas fallopian tubes, ovaries, uterus, and lymph nodes by use of a fiberoptic telescope inserted transabdominally into the abdominal cavity. Surgical procedures such as cholecystectomy, biopsy, or tubal ligation may be performed via laparoscopy.

Professional Considerations:

1. Consent form IS required.

Risks:
Acidosis, hemorrhage, infection, intestinal puncture, peritonitis, subcutaneous emphysema.

Contraindications:
Advanced abdominal wall malignancy, anticoagulant therapy, bleeding disorders, chronic tuberculosis, intra-abdominal hemorrhage, multiple surgical adhesions, peritonitis, thrombocytopenia.

2. Preparation:
   A. Assess for allergies.
   B. Prepare the surgical site with a shave.
   C. Insert an indwelling urinary catheter.
   D. Administer a cleansing enema 4 hours prior to the procedure.
   E. The client should void just prior to the procedure.
   F. Bandage inguinal and umbilical hernias.
   G. *See Client and family teaching.*
3. Procedure:
   A. Anesthesia may be given.
   B. A small surgical incision is made in the abdomen just below the umbilicus.
   C. Carbon dioxide is used to insufflate the abdominal cavity so that the organs are easily visualized.
   D. The laparoscope is inserted and visualization begins.
   E. The procedure takes about 30 minutes.
4. Postprocedure care:
   A. Assess the surgical incision area for signs of infection for 24 hours.
   B. Assess for signs/symptoms of hemorrhage as the major complication. Signs may include bleeding at the dressing site, increasing abdominal pain and firmness, and hypotension.
   C. Monitor vital signs q 30 minutes × 4 and PRN.
   D. Provide analgesia for incisional pain and for the pain caused by the carbon dioxide gas remaining in the peritoneal cavity.
5. Client and family teaching:
   A. Fast from food and fluids for 8–12 hours before the procedure.
   B. A common complaint after this procedure is shoulder, scapular, and general discomfort in the upper torso due to referred pain from the carbon dioxide gas remaining in the abdomen. This pain can last for several days, but should decrease in severity as each day passes. Pain medicine will be prescribed to help ease the pain.
   C. Avoid carbonated beverages for 1–2 days after the procedure, because this will add to the gas pains and may cause vomiting when added to the carbon dioxide left over from the procedure.
   D. Minimize physical activity for 3–7 days, as instructed by the physician.
   E. Notify the physician for increasing pain, redness, or drainage at the laparoscopy site.
6. Factors that affect results:
   A. Equipment should be in good working order.
7. Other data:
   A. Site-specific useful biopsy is a positive gain of this procedure.
   B. Nausea, puncture of the intestinal loop, infection, hemorrhage, and subcutaneous emphysema are possible complications of laparoscopy.

Bibliography:

Connor TJ, Garcha IS, Ramshaw BJ, Mitchell CW, Wilson JP, Mason EM, Duncan TD, Dozier FA, Lucas GW: Diagnostic laparoscopy for suspected appendicitis. Am Surg *61*(2):187–189, 1995.

Holcomb GW: Laparoscopic evaluation for a contralateral inguinal hernia or a nonpalpable testis. Pediatr Ann *22*(11):678–684, 1993.

Letterie GS, Haggerty M, Lindee G: A comparison of pelvic ultrasound and magnetic resonance imaging as diagnostic studies for mullerian tract abnormalities. Int J Fertil Menopausal Stud *40*(1): 34–38, 1995.

Liu PI: Blue Book of Diagnostic Tests. Philadelphia, WB Saunders, 1986, p 158.

LASA
(see Lipid-Associated Sialic Acid, Serum or Plasma)

LAXATIVE ABUSE TEST
(see Phenolphthalein Test, Diagnostic)

LD, BLOOD
(see Lactate Dehydrogenase, Blood)

LDH, BLOOD
(see Lactate Dehydrogenase, Blood)

LE CELL TEST
(see Lupus Test, Blood)

LE PREPARATION
(see Lupus Test, Blood)

LE SLIDE CELL TEST
(see Lupus Test, Blood)

LE TEST
(see Lupus Test, Blood)

LEAD, BLOOD AND URINE
Norm:

		SI Units
Whole Blood		
Adult	<20 µg/dl	<1.0 µmol/L
Child	<10 µg/dl	<1.5 µmol/L
Industrial exposure	<60 µg/dl	<2.9 µmol/L
Lead encephalopathy in children	>100 µg/dl	>4.8 µmol/L
Urine		
	0.08 mg/ml	0.39 mmol/L
	120 mg/24 hours	

The Centers for Disease Control defines *lead toxicity* in children as a blood level of ≥25 µg/dl combined with erythrocyte protoporphyrin ≥35 µg/dl.

Poisoning Level Symptoms and Treatment:

Symptoms: Early signs of lead poisoning include anorexia, apathy or irritability, headache, dizziness, sleep disturbances, fatigue, anemia, weight loss and abdominal "lead colic." Characteristic toxic effects include encephalopathy and peripheral neuropathy (wrist drop) and seizures. Elevated erythrocyte protoporphyrins in the blood is also suggestive of lead poisoning. Aminoaciduria, glycosuria, and Fanconi's syndrome have been demonstrated in children exposed to lead.

Treatment:
Lavage the stomach with magnesium sulfate or sodium sulfate.
Control seizures with valium.
Reduce cerebral edema with osmotic diuresis (mannitol) and corticosteroids.
Administer possible chelation therapy that includes several injections of calcium disodium EDTA and dimercaprol *(see Lead Mobilization Test, 24-Hour, Urine).*

Increased: Ataxia, metal poisoning, microcytic anemia from lead poisoning, and neuropathy.

Description: Lead is a heavy metal

that is used in paint, leaded gasoline, insecticides, pottery glaze, and illicit liquor and that is found in the fumes of old painted wood. It is an electropositive metal that has an affinity for the negatively charged sulfhydryl group and inhibits three enzymes in the body delta-aminolevulinic acid dehydrase, coproporphyrinogen oxidase, and ferrochelatase. These enzymes are necessary for the production of heme, the iron-containing portion of hemoglobin. The acceptable levels for blood lead content have been gradually lowered over time as new information on lead's detrimental effects is available. Lead measurements are performed on whole-blood specimens, because whole-blood concentrations are 75 times higher than those of serum or plasma. Exposure of children to low levels of lead has been associated with reduced intellectual and neuropsychological development. For this reason, many communities have in place routine screening for lead exposure of all schoolchildren. This test is the most appropriate test for screening for elevated lead levels in children and in workers in close contact with lead-containing substances.

Professional Considerations:

1. Consent form NOT required.
2. Preparation:
   A. Tube: Lead-free lavender-top or green-top for whole-blood sample. Samples MAY be drawn during hemodialysis.
   B. Obtain a 3-L, plastic, acid-washed urine collection container for the urine sample.
   C. *See Client and family teaching.*
3. Procedure:
   A. *Whole blood:* Draw a 3-ml blood sample.
   B. *Urine:* Collect all the urine voided in a 24-hour period in a 3-L plastic container that has been washed with 10% hydrochloric acid (HCl) solution.
4. Postprocedure care:
   A. *Urine:* Record starting and ending dates and times, as well as the total volume of urine, on the laboratory requisition.
5. Client and family teaching:
   A. Maintain on low-calcium diet for 3 days prior to collection of the 24-hour sample to mobilize lead from the bones and prevent false-positive results.
   B. Save all the urine voided in the container provided and avoid contaminating the urine with stool or toilet paper. If any urine is accidentally discarded, discard the entire specimen and restart the collection the next day.
   C. Avoid eating from old pottery bowls that may have been glazed with lead-base paint.
6. Factors that affect results:
   A. Anticoagulant other than heparin is found in the tube.
   B. A high-calcium diet creates false-positive results in the urine test.
7. Other data:
   A. Fingerstick specimens are not recommended. If they are used, positive results should be confirmed with venous whole-blood testing to rule out contamination of the fingerstick specimen.
   B. Urine levels for lead toxicity may be normal when serum levels indicate lead toxicity.
   C. Urine uric acid levels and blood erythropoietin levels may be elevated in lead exposure.

Bibliography:

Adult blood lead epidemiology and surveillance—United States, fourth quarter 1994. Morb Mortal Wkly Rep I(14):286–287, 1995.

Fels LM, Herbort C, Pergande M, Jung K, Hotter G, Rosello J, Gelpi E, Mutti A, De-Broe M, Stolte H: Nephron target sites in chronic exposure to lead. Nephrol Dial Transplant 9(12):1740–1746, 1994.

Schwartz J: Lead, blood pressure, and cardiovascular disease in men. Arch Environ Health 50(1):31–37, 1995.

LEAD MOBILIZATION TEST (CALCIUM DISODIUM EDTA MOBILIZATION TEST), 24-HOUR, URINE

Norm:

		SI Units
Normal lead level, before mobilization test		
Adult	<150 µg/day	<0.73 µmol/day
Child	<100 µg/day	<0.48 µmol/day
Normal lead level, after mobilization test		
Adult	<650 µg/day	<3.2 µmol/day
Child	<1 µgPb/mg CaNa$_2$ EDTA administered over a 24-hour period	

	SI Units

Lead level in clients with a higher than normal body burden of lead, after mobilization test

Adult	>1000 µg/day	>4.9 µmol/day
Child	>1 µgPb/mg CaNa$_2$ EDTA	
	administered over a 24-hour period	

Usage: Diagnosis and treatment of lead poisoning. Used when blood lead levels are >100 mg/dl.

Description: Lead is an environmental trace metal of which the average client takes in 150–250 mg/day. Only a small fraction of that taken in is absorbed. Lead poisoning occurs when clients frequently come into contact with items or industries that contain large amounts of lead. Some examples are paint, batteries, gasoline, pottery, bullets, and printing materials, and the mining, auto manufacturing, and welding industries. Lead affects many organs and tissues of the body, but most of it is stored in the bones. Symptoms of lead toxicity include gastrointestinal colic, vomiting, anorexia, anemia, and central nervous system abnormalities ranging from irritability, peripheral neuropathy, memory lapses, and impaired concentration, to severe lead encephalopathy.

Calcium disodium EDTA (calcium disodium edetate, CaNa$_2$ EDTA, calcium versenate) is one of three substances known to chelate lead or form tight complexes with lead, resulting in removal of lead from the body tissues and excretion of lead through the kidneys. The complex forms in which lead displaces calcium from the drug molecule. The test involves administering calcium disodium EDTA intravenously or intramuscularly and assessing the change in urinary lead excretion for 24 hours. Half-life of the drug is 20–60 minutes intravenously and 90 minutes intramuscularly. This test is currently the most reliable index of the body burden of lead.

Professional Considerations:

1. Consent form NOT required.

Risks and Precautions:

This procedure should be used with caution in clients with renal impairment.

Contraindications:

Severe lead encephalopathy, pregnancy, anuria, or severe renal disease.

2. Preparation:
   A. Assess for adequate urinary output.
   B. Obtain a baseline 24-hour urine collection for lead level in a refrigerated, lead-free (polyethylene), 4-L container that has been rinsed with hydrochloric acid (HCl).
   C. Obtain a baseline urinalysis; a urine coproporphyrin level; blood urea nitrogen; and serum creatinine, calcium, and phosphorus levels; and repeat daily throughout the test.
   D. Write the beginning time of the urine collection for the mobilization test on the laboratory requisition.
   E. Uncomfortable intramuscular injection site pain may be minimized by the addition of 1 ml of 1% procainamide to each milliliter of drug.

3. Procedure:
   A. Begin a 24-hour urine collection in a lead-free, 4-L container that has been washed with HCl.
   B. *Adults:* Perform the mobilization using one of the following three regimens:
      i. *Intravenous route:* Administer 1.0 g of CaNa$_2$ EDTA in 250–500 ml of 5% dextrose in water over 1–2 hours intravenously every 12 hours for no more than 5 days. Wait 2 full days before repeating the test, if necessary.
      ii. *Intramuscular route:* Administer 2 g of CaNa$_2$ EDTA per day intramuscularly in divided doses (i.e., 500 mg in each buttock, 12 hours apart).
      iii. *Long-term mobilization:* Administer 1 g of CaNa$_2$ EDTA three times a week until the urine collection shows normal levels of lead excretion.
   C. *Children:* Perform the mobilization using one of the following two regimens:
      i. *For mildly to moderately increased lead levels:* Administer CaNa$_2$ EDTA 500–1000 mg/m/24 hours intramuscularly (preferred) or intravenously every 12 hours for 3–5 days. Do not exceed 50 mg/kg/24 hours. Wait 4 full days before repeating the test, if necessary.

ii. *For severe lead intoxication:* Administer CaNa$_2$ EDTA 50 mg/kg/24 hours or 1500 mg/m/24 hours intravenously or intramuscularly in divided doses. Do not exceed 70 mg/kg/24 hours.

D. Continue urine collection for 24 hours. Encourage the oral intake of fluids throughout the collection period except for clients with lead encephalopathy (due to the risk of increasing intracranial pressure).

4. Postprocedure care:
A. Write the ending time and total urine output on the laboratory requisition.
B. Transport the entire specimen to the lab. The lead measurement is performed in a lead-free laboratory space on an aliquot of the 24-hour specimen.

5. Client and family teaching:
A. Save all the urine voided in the container provided and avoid contaminating the urine with stool or toilet paper. If any urine is accidentally discarded, discard the entire specimen and restart the collection the next day.
B. Outline environmental sources of lead.
C. *See also Lead, Blood and Urine.*

6. Factors that affect results:
A. Clients who have reached the point of lead encephalopathy may not show clinical improvement after this procedure.
B. The higher the blood lead level, the greater the excretable amount of lead.

7. Other data:
A. Intake and output must be monitored during this test. Diminished urine output may result in symptoms of lead toxicity.
B. Other substances used to chelate lead include dimercaprol (British antilewisite [BAL]) and *d*-penicillamine.
C. Dimercaprol (BAL) may be combined with CaNa$_2$ EDTA for clients with extremely severe lead intoxication.
D. As blood lead is chelated and excreted in the urine, levels may rise again as stored bone lead is mobilized. The mobilization test may be repeated in this circumstance.
E. There is some evidence that lead mobilized from the bones after chelation becomes redistributed to body organs, especially the brain and liver.
F. CaNa$_2$ EDTA is reported to also chelate some other heavy metals.

Bibliography:

Iniguez JL, et al.: Lead mobilization test in children with lead poisoning: validation of a 5-hour edetate calcium disodium provocation test. Arch Pediatr Adolesc Med *149*(3):338–340, 1995.

Lee BK, Schwartz BS, Stewart W, An KD: Provocative chelation with DMSA and EDTA: evidence for differential access to lead storage sites. Occup Environ Med *52*(1):13–19, 1995.

Wiley Jf, Bell LM, Rosenblum LS, Nussbaum J, Tobin R, Henretig FM: Lead poisoning: low rates of screening and high prevalence among children seen in inner-city emergency departments. J Pediatr *126*(3):392–395, 1995.

LEE-WHITE CLOTTING TIME (WHOLE BLOOD CLOTTING TIME), BLOOD

Norm:

Plain glass tube	5–15 minutes (reference range varies by laboratory)
Siliconized tube	24–45 minutes
Activated clotting time	<2 minutes and 10 seconds

Increased/Prolonged: Afibrinogenemia, dialysis (hemo), dysproteinemia, factor VIII and IX deficiency (<2% of normal), hypofibrinogenemia (<50 mg/dl), hypoprothrombinemia (<30% normal range), leukemia, and liver disorders. Drugs include carbenicillin, dicumarol, heparin, plicamycin, ticarcillin, and warfarin.

Decreased: Traumatic venipuncture. Drugs include oral contraceptives.

Description: Measurement of the time required for the interaction of all factors involved in the clotting process. The test is performed by timing the total amount of time required for 3 blood samples to clot. This test is not recommended for monitoring the effects of heparin therapy, because its reproducibility is poor. Sensitivity in detecting factor deficiencies is poor, because results will not be prolonged until factor levels fall below 1% of the normal levels, and this test cannot detect platelet Factor 3 deficiency.

Professional Considerations:

1. Consent form NOT required.
2. Preparation:
A. A plastic syringe, three glass tubes, and a stopwatch.
B. The client should not receive heparin therapy for 3 hours prior to specimen collection.

3. Procedure:
   A. Draw a 3-ml blood sample into a plastic syringe and place 1 ml in each of three glass tubes.
   B. The phlebotomist should start timing, using a stopwatch, after filling the third tube.
   C. Tube 1 is tilted once every 30 seconds until the blood is clotted. Then the procedure is repeated sequentially with the remaining tubes. The time from injection of the first specimen in tube 1 until a clot is noted in tube 3 is the clotting time for the sample.
   D. The timing and test are complete when the blood in the third tube is clotted.
4. Postprocedure care:
   A. None.
5. Client and family teaching:
   A. This test is used to time how long it takes for blood to clot. The doses of coumadin may be altered depending on the results.
6. Factors that affect results:
   A. The test is most reliable if the tubes are maintained at 37°C until clotting occurs.
   B. The test is prolonged by any anticoagulant therapy, tube agitation, or higher temperature changes.
   C. Contamination of the specimen with tissue thromboplastin from an inefficient venipuncture may cause false-normal results in hemophiliacs.
7. Other data:
   A. None.

Bibliography:

Janssen MJ, Huijgens PC, Bouman AA, van-der-Meulen J: Citrate anticoagulation and divalent cations in hemodialysis. Blood Purif *12*(6): 308–316, 1994.

Stephen M: Lee White Clotting Time. Online Handbook. Department of Pathology, University of Michigan, Ann Arbor, August 1995.

LEGIONELLA PNEUMOPHILIA, CULTURE

Norm: Negative. No growth.

A positive culture may be grown in 2–7 days.

Positive: Legionnaires' disease.

Description: A gram-negative, non-acid-fast bacillus that causes Legionnaires' disease, which causes symptoms of fever, headache, malaise, pneumonia, and diffuse alveolar damage. Concomitant symptoms of Legionnaires' disease may also include cardiac inflammation (endocarditis, pericarditis), pancreatitis, perirectal abscess, peritonitis, pyelonephritis, sinusitis, and wound infection. Two forms of this disease are a mild, self-limiting flulike syndrome of malaise and muscle aches, and a more severe form in which pneumonia is identified. Outbreaks of Legionnaires' disease have been attributed to community water supplies contaminated with *L. pneumophilia.* Symptoms develop 2–10 days after exposure to the organism. Clients at highest risk of developing this disease are smokers, those with pre-existing pulmonary disease, and those who have received cytotoxic chemotherapy or corticosteroids. This test includes culture and direct fluorescent antibody (FA) smear of a fresh specimen, which may be a biopsy of the lung; pleural fluid; washings or brushings from the bronchi; transtracheal aspirates; blood; pus; or sputum.

Professional Considerations:

1. Consent form NOT required for this test, but IS required when bronchoscopy, lung biopsy, or lung aspiration is used to obtain the specimen. See the individual procedure for risks and contraindications.
2. Preparation:
   A. Obtain a sterile specimen container.
3. Procedure:
   A. The physician obtains a sterile specimen of tissue by bronchoscopy or biopsy or pleural fluid by aspiration. Sterile collections of sputum, blood, or pus may also be collected.
   B. Send the specimen to the laboratory immediately.
   C. Expectorated sputum will NOT have an FA smear.
4. Postprocedure care:
   A. Reports take 1–2 weeks.
   B. Do not freeze the specimen.
5. Client and family teaching:
   A. Undue pain or shortness of breath should be reported.
   B. Legionnaires' disease is treated by erythromycin (drug of choice) or rifampin, if erythromycin does not eradicate the organism.
6. Factors that affect results:
   A. Contamination of the specimen will affect the results.
   B. The sensitivity of the sputum sample results is improved when the sample is treated with an acid wash prior to culturing.
7. Other data:
   A. Lung biopsy provides the highest rate of identification (>90%), followed by sputum (80–90%). The specificity of blood testing is only ≤30%.
   B. A negative culture does not rule out the presence of *Legionella,* as sensitivity of culturing methods may be 50%.

Bibliography:

Bhopal R: Source of infection for sporadic Legionnaires' disease: a review. J Infec *30*(1):9–12, 1995.
Hammerschlag MR: Atypical pneumonias in children. Adv Pediatr Infect Dis *10*:1–39, 1995.

LEGIONELLA PNEUMOPHILIA CULTURE, IgM TITER, BLOOD

Norm: Titer <1:256.

Increased: Legionnaires' disease and pneumonia.

Description: *See Legionella pneumophilia, Culture* for a description of Legionnaires' disease. IgM is the initial immunoglobulin produced in the immune response and is indicative of acute infections.

Professional Considerations:

1. Consent form NOT required.
2. Preparation:
   A. Tube: Red-top, red/gray-top, or gold-top.
3. Procedure:
   A. Draw a 7-ml blood sample.
4. Postprocedure care:
   A. Draw convalescent samples of blood 14 and 28 days after the onset of symptoms.
5. Client and family teaching:
   A. Legionnaires' disease is treated by erythromycin (drug of choice) or rifampin, if erythromycin does not eradicate the organism.
6. Factors that affect results:
   A. Gross contamination of specimen.
7. Other data:
   A. Use of indirect fluorescent antibody methodology may speed up the specific diagnosis of this disease.

Bibliography:

Abernathy-Carver KJ, Fan LL, Boguniewicz M, Larsen GL: Legionella and pneumocystis pneumonias in asthmatic children on high doses of systemic steroids. Pediatr Pulmonol *18*(3):135–138, 1994.
Byrd TF: Cytokines and Legionellosis. Biotherapy *7*(3–4):179–186, 1994.
Carratala J, Gudiol F, Pallares R, Dorca J, Verdaguer R, Ariza J, Manresa F: Risk factors for nosocomial Legionella pneumophila pneumonia. Am J Respir Crit Care Med *149*(3, Pt 1):625–629, 1994.

LEGIONELLA PNEUMOPHILIA, DIRECT FA SMEAR, SPECIMEN

Norm: Negative.

Positive: Legionnaires' disease.

Description: See *Legionella Pneumophilia, Culture* for a description of Legionnaire's disease. This test performs a direct fluorescent antibody microscopic examination of a specimen smear of lung tissue, pleural fluid, sputum, bronchial washing, or other body fluid. It provides rapid results (within 1–3 hours). The sensitivity of this test varies widely, from 24% to 80%, but has high specificity at >95%.

Professional Considerations:

1. Consent form NOT required for the test, but IS required for lung biopsy or lung aspiration by bronchial washing. See the individual procedure for risks and contraindications.
2. Preparation:
   A. Obtain the necessary sterile biopsy containers.
3. Procedure:
   A. Prepare for a lung biopsy, bronchial washing, pleural tap, or sterile sputum specimen.
4. Postprocedure care:
   A. Send the specimen to the laboratory in the sterile container immediately after collection.
5. Client and family teaching:
   A. Report undue pain or shortness of breath.
   B. Legionnaires' disease is treated by erythromycin (drug of choice) or rifampin, if erythromycin does not eradicate the organism.
6. Factors that affect results:
   A. False-positive results are seen with tularemic pneumonia.
   B. False-negative results may occur if a saliva specimen, rather than a sputum specimen, is sampled.
7. Other data:
   A. There are several subgroups of *Legionella: L. bozemanii, L. dumoffii, L. gormanii, L. jordanis, L. longbeachae,* and *L. micdadei.*

Bibliography:

Carratala J, Gudiol F, Pallares R, Dorca J, Verdaguer R, Ariza J, Manresa F: Risk factors for nosocomial Legionella pneumophila pneumonia. Am J Respir Crit Care Med *149*(3, Pt 1):625–629, 1994.
McClatchey KD: Clinical Laboratory Medicine. Baltimore, MD, Williams and Wilkins, 1994.
Stephen M: Online Pathology Handbook, University of Michigan, Ann Arbor, August 1995.

LEGIONNAIRES' DISEASE ANTIBODIES, BLOOD

Norm: Negative or less than a fourfold change in titer between acute and convalescent samples.

A fourfold rise in titer >1:128 from the acute to convalescent sample provides evidence of recent infection.

A single titer ≥1:256 is evidence of infection at an undetermined time.

Positive: Legionnaires' disease.

Negative: Normal.

Description: This test identifies specific antibodies produced after the body has been infected with the *Legionella* organism. In Legionnaires' disease, antibody titers rise and fall at a predictable rate. Levels are low the first week, rise steadily weeks 2–4 and peak during week 5 of the disease then drop slowly and remain elevated for many years.

Professional Considerations:

1. Consent form NOT required.
2. Preparation:
   A. Tube: Red-top, red/gray-top, or gold-top.
3. Procedure:
   A. Draw a 10-ml blood sample.
4. Postprocedure care:
   A. Draw convalescent samples of blood 4–6 weeks after the onset of symptoms.
5. Client and family teaching:
   A. Legionnaires' disease is treated by erythromycin (drug of choice) or rifampin, if erythromycin does not eradicate the organism.
6. Factors that affect results:
   A. Hemolysis of the specimen invalidates results.
   B. False-positive results may be caused when the client has tuberculosis.
   C. Clients with a past history of *Legionella pneumophilia* infection can have elevated titers for several years.
   D. 10–20% of clients with *L. pneumophilia* infection have false-negative results.
   E. False-positive results may occur in clients infected with gram-negative organisms and nonpneumophilia *Legionella* infections.
7. Other data:
   A. None.

Bibliography:

Carratala J, Gudiol F, Pallares R, Dorca J, Verdaguer R, Ariza J, Manresa F: Risk factors for nosocomial Legionella pneumonia pneumonia. Am J Respir Crit Care Med *149*(3, Pt 1):625–629, 1994.

Constantine CE, Wreghitt TG: A rapid micro-agglutination technique for the detection of antibody to *Legionella pneumophilia* serogroup 5. J Med Microbiol *34*(1):29–31, 1991.

Haraldsson A, Rechnitzer C, Friis-Moller A, et al.: Prevalence of IgM antibodies to nine *Legionella* species in Icelandic children. Scand J Infect Dis *22*(4): 445–449, 1990.

LEGIONNAIRES' DISEASE ANTIBODIES, IgM, BLOOD

(see Legionella pneumophilia Culture, IgM Titer, Blood)

LEPTOSPIRA CULTURE, URINE

Norm: Negative; no *Leptospira* isolated.

Positive: Leptospirosis.

Description: *Leptospira* is a pathogenic spirochete causing human infection (leptospirosis). Common hosts include cattle, dogs, foxes, mice, opossums, rats, raccoons, and skunks. This is an occupational disease for veterinarians, animal caretakers, butchers, fish handlers, and dog wardens, who contract the disease through direct skin contact with the urine or tissue of infected animals. Symptoms are flulike but may be as severe as meningitis, renal insufficiency, and hemolytic anemia. The infection is not transmitted from human to human except in unusual circumstances. Isolation of *Leptospira* in culture may occur in as little as 6–14 days or in as long as 28 days. Serum *Leptospira* serodiagnosis for antibody identification should always be performed concomitantly with urine culture.

Professional Considerations:

1. Consent form NOT required.
2. Preparation:
   A. Obtain a sterile urine specimen container.
   B. Alkalinization of the urine may reduce the chance of false-negative results.
3. Procedure:
   A. Collect a 50-ml midstream urine specimen in a sterile plastic container. *See clean-catch collection instructions in the test Body Fluid, Routine, Culture.*
4. Postprocedure care:
   A. Transport the specimen to the laboratory within 1 hour.
5. Client and family teaching:
   A. The clean-catch urine technique must be used to decrease the risk of specimen contamination. *See clean-catch collection instructions in the test Body Fluid, Routine, Culture.*
   B. Up to 4 weeks may be required for cultures to grow.
6. Factors that affect results:
   A. Repeat samples may be necessary if the sample is not tested immediately, as acidic urine destroys leptospiras.
7. Other data:
   A. Serum should always be obtained for antibody studies when the urine culture is obtained.
   B. Leptospirosis is treated with penicillin.
   C. Urine results are normally available in 4–8 weeks.
   D. *Leptospira* cultures are difficult to

grow and frequently give false-negative results when the specimen is not inoculated to medium within 30 minutes of its being obtained.

Bibliography:

Appassakij H, Silpapojakul K, Wansit R, Woodtayakorn J: Evaluation of the immunofluorescent antibody test for the diagnosis of human leptospirosis. Am J Trop Med Hyg *52*(4):340–343, 1995.

Gerritsen MA, Smits MA, Olyhoek T: Random amplified polymorphic DNA fingerprinting for rapid identification of leptospiras of serogroup Sejroe. J Med Microbiol *42*(5):336–339, 1995.

Heath SE, Johnson R: Leptospirosis. J Am Vet Med Assoc *205*(11):1518–1523, 1994.

Stephen M: Leptospira Culture. Online Handbook. Department of Pathology, University of Michigan, Ann Arbor, August 1995.

LEPTOSPIRA SERODIAGNOSIS, BLOOD

Norm: Negative.

Positive: Jaundice, leptospirosis (fourfold increase in titer between acute and convalescent specimens), meningitis, and renal failure (acute).

Description: *See Leptospira Culture, Urine* for a description of leptospirosis. This test is used to detect antibodies to Leptospira in the blood and can detect the antibodies when negative results are obtained from culture or darkfield examination for the *Leptospira* organism.

Professional Considerations:

1. Consent form NOT required.
2. Preparation:
   A. Tube: Red-top, red/gray-top, or gold-top.
3. Procedure:
   A. Draw a 7-ml blood sample.
4. Postprocedure care:
   A. Draw a convalescent sample of blood 14–21 days later.
5. Client and family teaching:
   A. Leptospirosis cannot be ruled out just because cultures were negative. This test can identify antibodies to the organism, even when cultures are negative. It is important to return for convalescent sampling in 2–3 weeks.
6. Factors that affect results:
   A. Hemolysis of the specimen invalidates the results.
7. Other data:
   A. None.

Bibliography:

Appassakij H, Silpapojakul K, Wansit R, Woodtayakorn J: Evaluation of the immunofluorescent antibody test for the diagnosis of human leptospirosis. Am J Trop Med Hyg *52*(4):340–343, 1995.

Gerritsen MA, Smits MA, Olyhoek T: Random amplified polymorphic DNA fingerprinting for rapid identification of leptospiras of serogroup Sejroe. J Med Microbiol *42*(5):336–339, 1995.

LEUCINE AMINOPEPTIDASE (LAP), BLOOD

Norm: <50 IU/L, or 12–33 IU/dl.

Increased: Cancer of the liver, pancreas, or head and neck; cholelithiasis; cirrhosis; jaundice (obstructive); liver dysfunction; and pancreatitis.

Description: Aminopeptidase is an enzyme present in blood, bile, and urine. This test is helpful in the differential diagnosis of elevated alkaline phosphatase, as the leucine aminopeptidase level is normal in clients with diseases of the bone.

Professional Considerations:

1. Consent form NOT required.
2. Preparation:
   A. Tube: Red-top, red/gray-top, or gold-top.
   B. *See Client and family teaching.*
3. Procedure:
   A. Draw a 7-ml blood sample.
4. Postprocedure care:
   A. None.
5. Client and family teaching:
   A. Fast, except for fluids, for 8 hours.
6. Factors that affect results:
   A. The last trimester of pregnancy increases the results.
7. Other data:
   A. None.

Bibliography:

Garg LN, Yadav SP, Lal H: Serum leucine aminopeptidase in head and neck cancer. J Laryngol Otol *108*(8):660–662, 1994.

Stephen M: Leucine Amino Peptidase. Online Pathology Handbook. University of Michigan, Ann Arbor, August 1995.

Volkmann A, Polzer M: Leucine aminopeptidase activity in adults of Pomphorhynchus laevis (Acanthocephala): a histochemical study. Parasitol Res *80*(6):502–504, 1994.

LEUKOCYTE, BLOOD
(see Differential Leukocyte Count, Peripheral Blood)

LEUKOCYTE ACID PHOSPHATASE, BLOOD
(see Tartrate-Resistant Acid Phosphatase, Blood)

LEUKOCYTE ALKALINE PHOSPHATASE (LAP, NEUTROPHIL ALKALINE PHOSPHATASE, NAP), BLOOD

Norm: Each laboratory establishes their own range. Score: 40–130. Score is based on a 0–4+ rating of 100 neutrophils.

Increased: Age ≤14 days, agnogenic myeloid metaplasia, aplastic anemia, burns, Down syndrome, Hodgkin's disease, immediately postoperatively, leukemia (acute lymphocytic or hairy cell), myelofibrosis with myeloid metaplasia, pregnancy and during lactation, polycythemia vera, stress, thrombocytopenia infection, tissue necrosis, trauma. Drugs include ACTH and oral contraceptives.

Decreased: Aplastic anemia, leukemia (acute monocytic or chronic myelogenous), cirrhosis, collagen disease, congestive heart failure, diabetes mellitus, erythroleukemia, gout, hereditary hypophosphatemia, hypophosphatasia, idiopathic thrombocytopenic purpura, infectious mononucleosis (early), and paroxysmal nocturnal hemoglobinuria.

Description: Leukocyte alkaline phosphatase (LAP) is an enzyme present in neutrophilic granules from the metamyelocyte to the segmented stage and represents intracellular metabolism. Dye is added to a smear of blood, and a color reaction occurs, enabling the stained neutrophils to be identified by the appearance of red, blue, or purple granules viewed in the cytoplasm of mature leukocytes. The neutrophils are given a rating of zero to four, based on the intensity of the color reaction. The score is the sum of the ratings for each neutrophil, with a total possible score of 400. This test helps differentiate between chronic myelogoneous leukemia, which produces low scores, from three other myeloproliferative diseases that produce higher scores: polycythemia vera, myelofibrosis, and essential thrombocytopenia. It also is useful for differentiating polycythemia vera from secondary polycythemia, in which normal scores would be found.

Professional Considerations:

1. Consent form NOT required.
2. Preparation:
   A. Preschedule the test with the laboratory.
   B. *For venous or arterial sample:* Tube: Green-top or black-top. Also obtain foil.
   C. *For capillary sample:* Obtain a lancet and 6 slides.

3. Procedure:
   A. Draw a 2-ml blood sample and wrap the tube in foil.
   B. Alternatively, obtain a peripheral fingerstick or earlobe capillary sample and smear it onto 6 slides.
4. Postprocedure care:
   A. Transport the specimen to the laboratory immediately. The slides must be fixed in formalin: methanol 1:9 for 30 seconds at 0–5°C, washed in running water, and air-dried within 30 minutes.
5. Client and family teaching:
   A. Results are normally available within 4 hours.
6. Factors that affect results:
   A. Reject specimens collected in EDTA-anticoagulated (lavender-top) tubes because EDTA inhibits the activity of LAP.
   B. Results are invalid if the client is neutropenic (i.e., <1000/mm³ neutrophils).
7. Other data:
   A. Values are normal in myelomonocytic leukemia, lymphosarcoma, multiple myeloma, relative polycythemia, sickle cell crisis, and viral infections.

Bibliography:

Gianni M, et al.: Tyrosine kinases but not cAMP-dependent protein kinase mediate the induction of leukocyte alkaline phosphatase by granulocyte colony stimulating factor and retinoic acid in acute promyelocytic leukemia cells. Biochem Biophys Res Commun 208(2):846–854, 1995.

Malarkey, LM, McMorrow, ME: Nurse's Manual of Laboratory Tests and Diagnostic Procedures. Philadelphia, WB Saunders, 1996, pp 422–423.

Wallach N, Gur Y: Leukocyte alkaline phosphatase as a probable predictor of the metastatic state in breast and colon cancer patients. Oncology 52(1):12–18, 1995.

LEUKOCYTE CYTOCHEMISTRY (CYTOCHEMICAL STAIN), SPECIMEN

Norm: Requires interpretation.

Increased: Cushing's disease, diphtheria, Down syndrome, eclampsia, hemolytic anemia, hemorrhage, Hodgkin's disease, leukemia (acute lymphocytic), lobar pneumonia, leukocytosis (15,000–50,000/mL) associated with infection, lymphoma, malaria, meningitis, mercury poisoning, myeloid metaplasia, multiple myeloma, polycythemia vera, pregnancy, stress, syphilis, tissue necrosis, tuberculosis, tumors, and trauma. Drugs include ACTH and oral contraceptives.

Decreased: Anemia (aplastic), collagen disease, hereditary hypophosphatasia, idiopathic thrombocytopenic purpura, leukemia (acute and chronic myelocytic, acute monocytic), myelosclerosis, paroxysmal nocturnal hemoglobinuria, and pernicious anemia.

Description: A staining of blood smears and bone marrow that estimates alkaline phosphatase enzyme activity in neutrophilic granules. This test helps differentiate types of leukemia.

Professional Considerations:

1. Consent form IS required for bone marrow biopsy. *See Bone Marrow Biopsy Aspiration Analysis, Specimen* for procedure risks and contraindications.
2. Preparation:
   A. Obtain a bone marrow biopsy tray, slides, a sterile container, an alcohol wipe, a tourniquet, a needle, a syringe, and a lavender-top tube.
3. Procedure:
   A. Draw a 2-ml or capillary (preferred) blood sample.
   B. Obtain a bone marrow biopsy and place it in a sterile container.
4. Postprocedure care:
   A. Apply a pressure dressing to the bone marrow site and assess it for bleeding every 5 minutes × 3.
   B. Transport the specimen to the laboratory immediately.
5. Client and family teaching:
   A. Bone marrow specimens are usually taken from the hip (iliac crest) or sternum. The procedure is transiently painful and has been described as extremely painful, but only for a short time.
6. Factors that affect results:
   A. Tubes containing EDTA inhibit the activity of leukocyte alkaline phosphatase.
7. Other data:
   A. Normal levels found in kwashiorkor, leukemia (chronic lymphocytic, acute and chronic myelomonocytic), lymphosarcoma, and viral infections.
   B. *See also Bone Marrow Aspiration Analysis, Specimen* for care implications for the bone marrow biopsy procedure.

Bibliography:

Brody JP, Allen S, Schulman P, et al.: Acute agranular CD4 positive natural killer cell leukemia. Comprehensive clincopathologic studies including virologic and in vitro culture with inducing agents. Cancer 75(10):2474–2483, 1995.

LEUKOCYTE DNA, SPECIMEN

Norm: DNA chain interpretation required.

Usage: Used in the establishment of genetic disorder, endocrinopathy,

leukemias, myotonic dystrophies, prion encephalopathies, and cellular alterations such as tumors.

Description: DNA studies of all specimens use a technique called polymerase chain reaction (PCR) to amplify the quantity of DNA being studied. The polymerase chain reaction technique has diverse applications in detecting mutations and rare sequences of DNA. The discovery of heat-stable polymerase led to the invention of the PCR machine. PCR has found its way into virtually all fields of biology, including medicine, evolutionary biology, and genetics.

Professional Considerations:

1. Consent MAY BE required, depending on the procedure used to obtain the specimen.
2. Preparation:
   A. Contact the laboratory for specific collection regimens, depending on the specimen required.
3. Procedure:
   A. For blood samples, obtain a 7-ml sample in a citrate-anticoagulated or EDTA-anticoagulated tube.
   B. A reaction mixture consisting of specimen DNA, primers, DNA polymerase, nucleotides, and buffer-containing magnesium is placed in the machine, which automatically runs through the cycles of heating and cooling. Generally 25–35 cycles are enough to amplify a single-copy genomic sequence by a factor of 10 million.
4. Postprocedure care:
   A. Care is specific to the procedure used to obtain the specimen. See each individual procedure for care implications.
5. Client and family teaching:
   A. Results may not be available for several days.
6. Factors that affect results:
   A. Anticoagulants mixed with samples invalidate the results.
7. Other data:
   A. This technique has the highest sensitivity of all molecular techniques to date.

Bibliography:

Endo K, Sato A, Sugawara T, et al.: A novel translocation involving chromosomes 2, 9, 14, and 22 in chronic myeloid leukemia. Cancer Genet Cytogenet 80(2):155–157, 1995.

Jiang G: In Situ Polymerase Chain Reaction and Related Technology. Natick, MA, Eaton Publishing, 1995.

Warren DJ, Andersen A, Slordal L: Quantitation of 6-thioguanine residues in peripheral blood leukocyte DNA obtained from patients receiving 6-mercaptopurine-based maintenance therapy. Cancer Res 55(8):1670–1674, 1995.

Williamson EA, Johnson SJ, Foster S, et al.: G protein

gene mutations in patients with multiple endocrinopathies. J Clin Endocrinol Metab *80*(5): 1702–1705, 1995.

L-FORM, CULTURE
(see Cell Wall Defective Bacteria, Culture)

LIDOCAINE (XYLOCAINE), SERUM

Norm:

		SI Units
	1.5–6.0 µg/ml	6.4–25.6 µmol/L
Panic level	6–8 µg/ml	25.6–34.2 µmol/L
Toxic level	>8 µg/ml	>34.2 µmol/L

Panic Level Symptoms and Treatment:

Symptoms:

Panic level: Slurred speech, central nervous system depression, cardiovascular depression.

Toxic level: coma, convulsions, decreased cardiac output, muscle twitching, obtundation.

Treatment:

Give continuous ECG monitoring for bradycardia, heart block, dysrhythmias, or cardiac arrest.

Support airway, breathing, and hemodynamic stability.

Monitor temperature q 1 hour for hyperthermia. Use cool room and/or hypothermia as needed.

Take seizure precautions.

Hemodialysis will NOT remove lidocaine.

Increased: Convulsions and drug abuse. Drugs include anesthetics, cimetidine, norepinephrine, propranolol. Dysrhythmias.

Decreased: Dysrhythmias. Drugs include anesthetics, norepinephrine, phenobarbital, phenytoin, and propranolol.

Description: Lidocaine is a drug used to suppress ventricular dysrhythmias, especially following an acute myocardial infarction in which the client is experiencing frequent ventricular ectopy or after ventricular tachycardia or defibrillation resistant to defibrillation. It is also used as a local anesthetic. Lidocaine suppresses automaticity of His-Purkinje system and elevates threshold of ventricle during diastole. Half-life is normally 70–140 minutes, but in uremia is 77 minutes, in cirrhosis is 296 minutes, and in cardiac failure is 115 minutes. Because the half-life increases after 24–48 hours, the dose should be reduced after 24 hours when prolonged infusions are given. Lidocaine is metabolized in the liver and excreted in the urine. Steady-state levels are reached after 5–10 hours.

Professional Considerations:

1. Consent form NOT required.
2. Preparation:
   A. Tube: Red-top, red/gray-top, or gold-top or lavender-top.
   B. Draw the first sample 12 hours after starting lidocaine.
   C. Specimens MAY be drawn during hemodialysis.
3. Procedure:
   A. Draw a 1-ml blood sample.
4. Postprocedure care:
   A. Observe for signs of lidocaine toxicity.
5. Client and family teaching:
   A. Toxic symptoms normally resolve within 12–24 hours after cessation of lidocaine therapy.
6. Factors that affect results:
   A. Cardiopulmonary bypass surgery decreases serum levels.
   B. Do not collect in a serum separator tube because the separator gel may extract the lidocaine and cause falsely low results.
7. Other data:
   A. Action of drug begins 10–90 seconds after intravenous administration.
   B. Due to the high incidence of side effects, the routine use of lidocaine after myocardial infarction is not recommended except in the conditions outlined above.

Bibliography:

Gandolfi L: Serum lidocaine and MEGX concentrations after pharyngeal anesthesia for gastroscopy. Gastrointest Endosc *42*(3):282–283, 1995.

Guidelines for cardiopulmonary resuscitation in emergency cardiac care. JAMA *268*(16):2206, 1992.

Lorec AM, Bruguerolle B, Attolini L, Roucoules X: Rapid simultaneous determination of lidocaine, bupivacaine, and their two main metabolites using capillary gas-liquid chromatography with nitrogen phosphorus detector. Ther Drug Monit *16*(6):592–595, 1994.

LIPASE, SERUM

Norm: <200 U/L with triolein; <160 U/L with olive oil.

		SI Units
Adults	13–141 U/L	0.22–2.40 µKat/L
Age 20–60	31–186 U/L	0.53–3.16 µKat/L
Over age 60	≤302 U/L	≤5.13 µKat/L
Over age 90	26–267 U/L	0.44–4.54 µKat/L
Children	20–136 IU/L	
Infants	9–105 IU/L	

Increased: Cholecystitis, cirrhosis, duodenal ulcers, fat embolism, gallstone colic, pain (abdominal), pancreatic carcinoma, pancreatic cholera, pancreatic trauma, pancreatitis, peritonitis, renal disease with impaired output, and strangulated bowel. Drugs include bethanechol, heparin, and narcotic analgesics.

Description: Lipase is a pancreatic enzyme that changes fats and triglycerides into fatty acids and glycerol. The pancreas is the only body organ that demonstrates significant lipase activity. In acute pancreatitis, serum lipase begins to increase in 2–6 hours, peaks at 12–30 hours, and remains elevated, but slowly decreases for 2–4 days. Lipase rises and falls in tandem with amylase in acute pancreatitis, but is a more specific marker for this condition.

Professional Considerations:

1. Consent form NOT required.
2. Preparation:
   A. Tube: Red-top, red/gray-top, or gold-top.
3. Procedure:
   A. Draw a 1-ml blood sample.
4. Postprocedure care:
   A. None.
5. Client and family teaching:
   A. Results are normally available within 12 hours.
6. Factors that affect results:
   A. Endoscopic retrograde cholangiopancreatography procedure (ERCP) may increase lipase activity.
   B. Traumatic venipuncture can inhibit lipase activity.
7. Other data:
   A. The sample is stable for several days at room temperature, longer if refrigerated or frozen.

Bibliography:

Cohen N, Golik A, Blatt A, et al.: Pancreatic enzyme elevation in measles. J Clin Gastroenterol *19*(4): 292–295, 1994.

King LD, Seelig CB, Ranney JE: The lipase to amylase ratio in acute pancreatitis. Am J Gastroenterol *90*(1):67–69, 1995.

LIPID-ASSOCIATED SIALIC ACID (LASA, LSA), SERUM OR PLASMA

Norm: Serum: <25mg/dl; plasma: <20 mg/dl.

Increased: Cancer: Breast, brain, cervical, colon, head and neck, leukemia, liver, lung, melanoma, metastatic, neuroblastoma, ovarian, pancreatic, renal, and uterine.

Decreased: Response in therapy from high tumor burden to low tumor burden.

Description: Lipid-associated sialic acid (LASA) is a derivative of neuraminic acid, a widely distributed sugar that attaches itself to proteins and lipids. This lipid-associated tumor marker is found in the serum of clients with malignant disease and is associated with higher tumor burdens as opposed to low and moderate tumor burdens. Theoretically, LASA levels are thought be increased in cancer because LASA has the ability to identify cells with altered surface properties, such as cancer cells, and bind to the surfaces, making the tumor cells more susceptible to metastasis and probable lysis by activated macrophages.

Professional Considerations:

1. Consent form NOT required.

2. Preparation:
   A. Tube: Lavender-top. Obtain ice.
3. Procedure:
   A. Draw a 5-ml blood sample.
4. Postprocedure care:
   A. Place the sample immediately on ice and deliver it to the laboratory for immediate spinning and freezing. The sample should be kept frozen until tested.
5. Client and family teaching:
   A. Results may take several days if the sample is sent off-site to be tested.
6. Factors that affect results:
   A. None found.
7. Other data:
   A. No significant difference has been found in LASA levels between survivors and nonsurvivors of persons with a myocardial infarction.
   B. No significant difference has been found in LASA levels in persons with low and those with moderate tumor burdens from melanoma.

C. The amount of sialic acid present on the surface of malignant cells has been correlated directly with the ability to metastasize.
D. The research findings of Petrick et al. (1994) suggest that sialic acid expression can change the binding of colorectal cancer cells. This binding is required for any cytotoxic effect to take place.

Bibliography:

Buzaid AC, Sandler AB, Hayden CL, Scinto J, Poo, WJ, Clark MB, Hotchkiss S: Correlation between lipid-associated sialic acid and tumor burden in melanoma. Int J Biol Markers 9(4):247–250, 1994.

Crook M, Haq M, Haq S, Tutt P: Plasma sialic acid and acute-phase proteins in patients with myocardial infarction. Angiology 45(8):709–715, 1994.

Petrick AT, Meterissian S, Steele GD, et al.: Desialylation of human colorectal carcinoma cells facilitates binding to Küpffer cells. Clin Exp Metastasis 12:108–116, 1994.

LIPID PROFILE, BLOOD

Norm: See individual test listings for age-specific norms, including norms for children.

		SI Units
Lipids, total	400–800 mg/dl	4.0–8.0 g/L
Triglycerides	10–190 mg/dl	0.2–4.8 mmol/L
HDL cholesterol		
Females	35–85 mg/dl	0.9–2.2 mmol/L
Males	30–65 mg/dl	0.8–1.7 mmol/L
LDL cholesterol	80–190 mg/dl	2.0–4.9 mmol/L

Condition	Triglycerides	Total Cholesterol	HDL	LDL
Alcoholism	Increase	Increase	Increase	Increase
Aortic aneurysm	Increase	Increase	Increase	Increase
Aortitis	Increase	Increase	Increase	Increase
Arteriosclerosis	Increase	Increase	Decrease	Increase
Diabetes mellitus	Increase	Increase	Increase	Increase
Glycogen storage	Increase	—	—	Increase
Hyperalimentation	Decrease	Decrease	Decrease	Decrease
Hypercholesterolemia	Increase	Increase	—	Increase
Hyperlipoproteinemia	Increase	Increase	Increase	Increase
Hypothyroid	Increase	—	Decrease	—
Malabsorption	Decrease	Decrease	Decrease	Decrease
Myxedema	Increase	Increase	Increase	Increase
Nephrotic syndrome	Increase	Increase	Increase	Increase
Pancreatitis	Increase	Increase	Increase	Increase

Description: Lipid profile is a battery of laboratory studies to help determine the risk factors in coronary artery disease. Blood lipids consist of cholesterol, triglycerides, and phospholipids. *See individual test sections for further descriptions of the components of the Lipid Profile.*

TOTAL CHOLESTEROL–CORONARY HEART DISEASE RISK

	Recommended mg/dl	SI Units mmol/L	Moderate Risk mg/dl	SI Units mmol/L	High Risk mg/dl	SI Units mmol/L
Adult	<200	<5.18	200–239	5.18–6.19	≥240	≥6.22
Child	<170	<4.40	170–199	4.40–5.15	≥200	≥5.18

HDL CHOLESTEROL–CORONARY HEART DISEASE RISK

High risk   ≤35 mg/dl (<0.91 mmol/L SI units)

TOTAL CHOLESTEROL/HIGH-DENSITY LIPOPROTEIN (MG/DL)

Coronary Heart Disease Risk	Average Risk	2× Average Risk	3× Average Risk
Male	5.0	9.6	23.4
Female	4.4	7.1	11.0

LDL CHOLESTEROL–CORONARY HEART DISEASE RISK

	Recommended mg/dl	SI Units mmol/L	Moderate Risk mg/dl	SI Units mmol/L	High Risk mg/dl	SI Units mmol/L
Adult	<130	<3.37	130–159	3.37–4.12	≥160	≥4.14
Child	<110	<2.85	110–129	2.85–3.36	≥130	≥3.37

Professional Considerations:

1. Consent form NOT required.
2. Preparation:
   A. Tubes: Two red-top, red/gray-top, or gold-top.
   B. *See Client and family teaching.*
3. Procedure:
   A. Draw two 7-ml blood samples.
4. Postprocedure care:
   A. None.
5. Client and family teaching:
   A. Maintain regular dietary habits for 2 weeks prior to the test.
   B. Fast from food and fluids for 12 hours prior to the test.
   C. Desirable levels and risk for coronary heart disease are shown in the table at top of the page.
6. Factors that affect results:
   A. Oral contraceptives may increase the levels of lipids in the serum.

7. Other data:
   A. Risk factors for heart disease include high-saturated-fat diet, cigarette smoking, hypertension, obesity, high salt intake, diabetes mellitus, and left ventricular hypertrophy.

Bibliography:

Keilani T, Schlueter W, Batlle D: Selected aspects of ACE inhibitor therapy for patients with renal disease: impact on proteinuria, lipids and potassium. J Clin Pharmacol 35(1):87–97, 1995.

Maki KC, Briones ER, Langbein WE, et al.: Associations between serum lipids and indicators of adiposity in men with spinal cord injury. Paraplegia 33(20):102–109, 1995.

Steinberger J, Moorhead C, Katch V, Rocchini AP: Relationship between insulin resistance and abnormal lipid profile in obese adolescents. J Pediatr 126(5, Pt 1):690–695, 1995.

LITHIUM, SERUM

Norm: Negative.

Therapeutic Levels		SI Units
Treatment of acute mania	0.8–1.3 mEq/L	0.8–1.3 mmol/L
Ongoing prophylaxis	0.5–1.0 mEq/L	0.5–1.0 mmol/L
Panic level	>1.6 mEq/L	>1.6 mmol/L

Panic Level Symptoms and Treatment:

Symptoms:

At levels = 1.5–2.5 mmol/L: Ataxia, coarse tremor, diarrhea, muscle weakness, sedation, and vomiting.

At levels = 2.5–4.0 mmol/L: Choreiform movements, confusion, convulsions, diminishing level of consciousness, increased deep tendon reflexes, muscle hypertonia, somnolence, stupor, T-wave flattening.

At levels >4.0 mmol/L: Coma, death possible.

Treatment:

Give activated charcoal.
Perform gastric lavage.
Administer intravenous fluids with diuresis.
Both hemodialysis and peritoneal dialysis WILL remove lithium.

Usage: Drug abuse, manic-depressive psychosis, metal poisoning, and monitoring for therapeutic levels during lithium therapy.

Increased: Lithium overdose. Drugs include thiazide diuretics.

Description: Lithium is an alkali metal salt used mostly in the treatment of bipolar disorder (manic-depressive illness) and shows promise in the treatment of cluster migraine headaches. This drug is absorbed in the gastrointestinal tract, has a half-life of 17–36 hours, an onset of 5–10 days, and is excreted in the urine. Lithium alters the sodium transport in nerve and muscle cells, which assists in stabilizing mood.

Professional Considerations:

1. Consent form NOT required.
2. Preparation:
   A. Tube: Green-top (not lithium-heparin).
   B. Do NOT draw during hemodialysis.
3. Procedure:
   A. Draw a 2-ml blood sample 8–12 hours after the last dose.
4. Postprocedure care:
   A. Sodium, lithium, and fluid balance must be assessed weekly.
5. Client and family teaching:
   A. Periodic lithium levels are necessary to identify and prevent lithium toxicity symptoms. Teach symptoms from the list above.

B. Clients with levels >2.5 mmol/L will require intensive care monitoring and intervention.
C. For intentional overdose, refer the client and family for crisis intervention.
D. If activated charcoal was given for elevated levels, the client should drink 4–6 glasses of water each day for 2 days to prevent constipation. The activated charcoal will cause stools to be black for a few days.

6. Factors that affect results:
   A. Reject the results if the specimen was collected in lithium-heparin.
7. Other data:
   A. The common side effects of lithium include elevated thyroid-stimulating hormone (TSH), decreased T_3 and T_4, polyuria, leukocytosis, and decreased urine osmolality.
   B. Levels correlate poorly with the appearance of toxic symptoms. Toxic symptoms may occur at normal lithium levels.

Bibliography:

Marken PA, McCrary KE, Lacombe S, et al.: Preliminary comparison of predictive and empiric lithium dosing: impact on patient outcome. Ann Pharmacother *28*(10):1148–1152, 1994.

Saxe A, Gibson G, Silveira E: Effects of long-term lithium infusion on normal parathyroid tissue. Surgery *117*(5):577–580, 1995.

Terao T, Oga T, Nozaki S, et al.: A further prospective evaluation of an equation to predict daily lithium dose. J Clin Psychiatr *56*(5):193–195, 1995.

LITHOTRIPSY (EXTRACORPOREAL SHOCK WAVE LITHOTRIPSY), DIAGNOSTIC

Norm: No stones present in the common bile duct, gallbladder, and kidney.

Usage: Destruction of common bile duct stones, gallstones, or kidney stones.

Description: The lithotripsy procedure is used to identify the presence and location of biliary system and renal stones, then remove them. This is done through use of a machine that generates shock waves, which focus on biliary stones, gallstones, or stones in the ureter or kidney. The shock waves mechanically stress and break apart the stones. This eliminates the need for manipulation or open procedure and results in shortened hospital stays for stone removal.

Professional Considerations:

1. Consent form IS required.

Risks:
Hydronephrosis, infection.

Contraindications:
Multiple stone recurrence. Sedatives are contraindicated in clients with central nervous system depression.

2. Preparation:
   A. Obtain vital signs and pulse oximetry reading.
   B. Apply topical anesthetic on intact skin, as prescribed, for minor procedures.
   C. Assist with the administration of anesthesia, as prescribed (e.g., fentanyl infusion, general and epidural anesthesia).
   D. Obtain sedatives for procedure as prescribed, such as fentanyl and Midazolam HCl.
   E. Have emergency equipment readily available if sedatives are used.
   F. *See Client and family teaching.*
3. Procedure:
   A. Place the client with gallstones in the prone position, so that the fundus of the gallbladder that contains the stones falls forward. Place the client with common bile duct stones or kidney stones in the supine position.
   B. After the stones are located by ultrasound, the physician aligns the stone in the focus area and the lithotripsy machine is activated slowly at first so that the client can feel and hear the shock wave. Then the shock waves are increased to Food and Drug Administration (FDA)-recommended standards of 1500 shocks at 16–23 kV until the stones are broken apart.
4. Postprocedure care:
   A. Monitor vital signs every 15 minutes × 2.
5. Client and family teaching:
   A. Fast from food and fluids from midnight before the test, except for prescribed medications, such as antihypertensives and cardiac medications.
   B. It is important to lie as still as possible during the procedure. Sedation will be used, which will cause the client to have no recollection of the procedure.
   C. The procedure takes 45–75 minutes.
   D. Hematuria is common up to 24 hours postoperatively.
   E. Nausea and vomiting may occur for up to 4 hours postoperatively.
   F. Biliary colic may occur for up to 24 hours postoperatively but is controlled by dicyclomine hydrochloride (Bentyl).
   G. Antibiotics to prevent infection symptoms may be prescribed postprocedure.
6. Factors that affect results:
   A. Movement by the client during the test may interfere with the results.
7. Other data:
   A. Studies have shown that EMLA cream, a topical anesthetic, is effective in dramatically decreasing or eliminating the pain of extracorporeal shock-wave lithotripsy (ESWL).
   B. Common bile duct lithotripsy must be performed under fluoroscopy, with the duct opacified with contrast dye.
   C. Clients who have had a higher frequency and number of urinary tract infections prior to the procedure, and who have larger stone sizes, are at higher risk for sepsis following urinary ESWL. These clients may be identified by a preprocedure evaluation and may require different prophylactic regimes and close postprocedure follow-up.

Bibliography:

Orenstein R, Bross JE, Dahlmann M: Risk factors for urinary lithotripsy-associated sepsis. Inf Control and Hosp Epid *14*(8):469–472, 1993.

Rowland GA, Marks DA, Torres WE: The new gallstone destroyers and dissolvers. Am J Nurs *89*(11): 1473–1476, 1989.

LIVER BATTERY (PROFILE), SERUM

Norm:

Alanine Aminotransferase (ALT or SGPT)

Adult female	4–35 U/L
Adult male	7–46 U/L
Children	
<12 months	≤54 U/L
Age 1–2	3–37 U/L
Age 2–8	3–30 U/L
Age 8–16	3–28 U/L

		SI Units

Alkaline Phosphatase (ALP)

Adults
  Age 20–60

Bodansky	2–4 U/dl	10.7–21.5 IU/L
King-Armstrong	4–13 U/dl	25.0–92.3 IU/L
Bessey-Lowry-Brock	0.8–2.3 U/dl	13.3–38.3 IU/L
Elderly	Slightly higher	
Newborn	1–4 times adult values	
Children	Values remain high until epiphyses close.	

Females	
Age 2–10	100–350 U/L
Age 10–13	110–400 U/L
Males	
Age 2–13	100–350 U/L
Age 13–15	125–500 U/L

Aspartate Aminotransferase

Adult females		
≤Age 60	8–20 U/L	8–20 U/L
>Age 60	10–20 U/L	10–20 U/L
Adult males		
≤Age 60	8–20 U/L	8–20 U/L
>Age 60	11–26 U/L	11–26 U/L
Children		
Newborn	16–72 U/L	16–72 U/L
Infant	15–60 U/L	15–60 U/L
Age 1 year	16–35 U/L	16–35 U/L
Age 5 years	19–28 U/L	19–28 U/L

Bilirubin

1 month–adult	<1.5 mg/dl	1.7–20.5 µmol/L
Premature infant		
Cord	<2.8 mg/dl	<48 µmol/L
24 hours	1–6 mg/dl	17–103 µmol/L
48 hours	6–8 mg/dl	103–137 µmol/L
3–5 days	10–12 mg/dl	171–205 µmol/L
Full-term infant		
Cord	<2.8 mg/dl	<48 µmol/L
24 hours	2–6 mg/dl	34–103 µmol/L
48 hours	6–7 mg/dl	103–120 µmol/L
3–5 days	4–6 mg/dl	68–103 µmol/L

Gamma-Glutamyl Transferase/Transpeptidase (GGT/GGTP)

Adult females	4–25 U
	9–31 mU/ml
	3.5–13 IU/L
	3–33 U/L >37°C
Adult males	7–40 U
	12–38 mU/ml
	4–23 IU/L
	9–69 U/L >37°C

		SI Units

Gamma-Glutamyl Transferase / Transpeptidase (GGT/GGTP) *(continued)*

Children

Cord blood	190–270 U/L >37°C	
Premature infant	<140 U/L >37°C	
1–3 days	56–233 U/L >37°C	
4–21 days	0–130 U/L >37°C	
3–12 weeks	4–120 U/L >37°C	
3–6 months, female	5–35 U/L >37°C	
3–6 months, male	5–65 U/L >37°C	
>6 months, female	15–85 IU/L	
>6 months, male	5–55 IU/L	
1–15 years	0–23 U/L >37°C	

Hepatitis B Surface Antigen

Negative

Lactate Dehydrogenase (LD/LDH)

Wroblewski method 30°C	150–450 U/L	72–217 IU/L
Adults		
≤Age 60	45–90 U/L	45–90 U/L
>Age 60	55–102 U/L	55–102 U/L
Children		
Newborn	160–500 U/L	160–500 U/L
Neonate	300–1500 U/L	300–1500 U/L
Infant	100–250 U/L	100–250 U/L
Child	60–170 U/L	60–170 U/L

Leucine Aminopeptidase (LAP)   12–33 IU/dl   <50 IU/L

5′Nucleotidase (5′NT or 5′N)

2–15 IU/L
0–17 U/L
0–1.6 U
0.3–3.2 Bodansky units

Protein Electrophoresis

Norms are dependent on laboratory procedure. Percentage values are for the Agarose method and represent the percentage of total protein:

Adult (Agarose method)		
Total protein		5.90–8.00
Albumin	58–74%	0.58–0.74
Alpha$_1$ globulin	2.0–3.5%	0.02–0.04
Alpha$_2$ globulin	5.4–10.6%	0.05–0.11
Beta globulin	7.0–14.0%	0.07–0.14
Gamma globulin	8.0–18.0%	0.08–0.18
Adult		
Total protein	6.0–8.0 g/dl	60–80 g/L
Albumin	3.3–5.0 g/dl	35–50 g/L
Alpha$_1$ globulin	0.1–0.4 g/dl	1–4 g/L
Alpha$_2$ globulin	0.5–1 g/dl	5–10 g/L
Beta globulin	0.7–1.2 g/dl	7–12 g/L
Gamma globulin	0.8–1.6 g/dl	8–16 g/L

		SI Units

Protein Electrophoresis (continued)

Premature infant

Total protein	4.4–6.3 g/dl	44–63 g/L
Albumin	3.0–4.2 g/dl	30–42 g/L
Alpha$_1$ globulin	0.11–0.5 g/dl	1.1–5 g/L
Alpha$_2$ globulin	0.3–0.7 g/dl	3–7 g/L
Beta globulin	0.3–1.2 g/dl	3–12 g/L
Gamma globulin	0.3–1.4 g/dl	3–14 g/L

Newborn

Total protein	4.6–7.4 g/dl	46–74 g/L
Albumin	3.5–5.4 g/dl	35–54 g/L
Alpha$_1$ globulin	0.1–0.3 g/dl	1–3 g/L
Alpha$_2$ globulin	0.3–0.5 g/dl	3–5 g/L
Beta globulin	0.2–0.6 g/dl	2–6 g/L
Gamma globulin	0.2–1.2 g/dl	2–12 g/L

Infant

Total protein	6.0–6.7 g/dl	60–67 g/L
Albumin	4.4–5.4 g/dl	44–54 g/L
Alpha$_1$ globulin	0.2–0.4 g/dl	2–4 g/L
Alpha$_2$ globulin	0.5–0.8 g/dl	5–8 g/L
Beta globulin	0.5–0.9 g/dl	5–9 g/L
Gamma globulin	0.3–0.8 g/dl	3–8 g/L

Child

Total protein	6.2–8.0 g/dl	62–80 g/L
Albumin	4.0–5.8 g/dl	40–58 g/L
Alpha$_1$ globulin	0.1–0.4 g/dl	1–4 g/L
Alpha$_2$ globulin	0.4–1.0 g/dl	4–10 g/L
Beta globulin	0.5–1.0 g/dl	5–10 g/L
Gamma globulin	0.3–1.0 g/dl	3–10 g/L

Prothrombin Time

Adult	10–15 seconds
Newborn	<17 seconds
Child	11–14 seconds

Usage: Work-up for liver disease, biliary disease; hepatoma; liver metastasis; chronic active hepatitis; cirrhosis, including biliary cirrhosis; hepatic complications associated with medications or TPN.

Increased: See individual test listings.

Decreased: See individual test listings.

Description: Liver battery includes testing for several blood levels that reflect hepatic function. In general, a liver battery includes the following: *Alanine Aminotransferase, Serum; Alkaline Phosphatase, Serum; Aspartate Aminotransferase, Serum; Bilirubin, Serum; Gamma-Glutamyl Transpeptidase, Blood; Hepatitis B Surface Antigen, Blood; Lactate Dehydrogenase, Blood; Leucine Aminopeptidase, Blood; 5' Nucleotidase, Blood; Protein, Electrophoresis, Serum; Prothrombin Time, Blood.* See individual test listings for specific descriptions.

Professional Considerations:

1. Consent form NOT required.
2. Preparation:
   A. Obtain foil or a paper bag.
   B. Tubes: two (2) red-top, red/gray-top, or gold-top, AND one blue-top.
3. Procedure:
   A. Completely fill all three tubes with blood. Cover one red-top, the red/gray-top, and the gold-top with foil, or place them in a paper bag to protect them from light.
4. Postprocedure care:
   A. Immediately spin the blue-top tube,

then refrigerate it. The testing should be performed within 4 hours.

5. Client and family teaching:
   A. *See individual test listings.*
6. Factors that affect results:
   A. *See individual test listings.*
7. Other data:
   A. *See individual test listings.*
   B. Interpretation of LFTs is an art, not a science. There are no absolute rules regarding how mild, moderate, or severe liver damage is defined. When identifying abnormalities, the client's clinical condition and other diagnostic testing must be considered.

Bibliography: *See also individual test listings.*

Herrera JL: Abnormal liver enzyme levels. Postgrad Med 9325(122):119–120, 125, 129–130, 1993.

Siconolf LA: Clarifying the complexity of liver function tests. Nursing *25*(5):39–44, 1995.

Walker JH: Commentary on the ABCs of pediatric LFTs. ENA's nursing scan. Emerg Care *3*(2):11, 1993.

LIVER BIOPSY (PERCUTANEOUS LIVER BIOPSY), DIAGNOSTIC

Norm: Normal liver cells and tissue. Negative for malignant or other abnormal cells and tissue.

Usage: Indicated for clients with unexplained hepatomegaly, unexplained jaundice, persistently elevated liver enzymes, and suspected liver disease. Used when the diagnosis or etiology cannot be established by other means. Confirm diagnosis of amyloidosis, benign tumor, drug reaction, hemochromatosis, hepatic cirrhosis, hepatic cysts, hepatic encephalopathy, hepatitis, jaundice, liver abscess, liver cancer or metastasis, liver dysfunction, metabolic disorders, Reye's syndrome, sarcoidosis, and schistosomiasis. Also indicated to assess client's response to therapy of chronic liver disease, monitor for hepatotoxicity of drug therapy, and evaluate liver transplant allografts.

Description: A liver biopsy is a safe, simple, and valuable method of diagnosing pathologic liver conditions. After the client is given local anesthetic, in using an aseptic technique, a needle is inserted through the abdominal wall to the liver. Liver tissue is obtained by the needle biopsy for microscopic examination.

Professional Considerations:

1. Consent form IS required.

Risks:
Pain, hemorrhage, bile peritonitis, penetration of abdominal viscera, pneumothorax, and death. Complications are reported in 0.06–0.32% of clients undergoing this procedure. Death, as a direct result of liver biopsy, is extremely rare (0.009–0.12%). Other risks include: minimal discomfort during injection of the local anesthetic and during needle insertion; hemorrhage caused by inadvertent puncture of intrahepatic blood vessel; also, intra-abdominal bleeding, bile peritonitis, and pneumothorax are small but possible risks.

Contraindications:
Prothrombin time in the anticoagulant range (2–3 seconds over control values); platelet count less than 50,000/mm^3; other bleeding disorders; anemia, and cannot tolerate major blood loss associated with inadvertent puncture of an intrahepatic blood vessel; marked ascites; obstructive jaundice caused by a possible bile leakage; infection of the biliary tract; infection in the right pleural space or right upper quadrant of the abdomen; a hemangioma; and/or an inability to cooperate during procedure (e.g., remain still and hold breath during sustained exhalation). Sedatives are contraindicated in clients with central nervous system depression.

2. Preparation:
   A. Obtain a biopsy tray, sterile gloves, slides, sterile sponges, and tape for dressing.
   B. Ensure that all coagulation tests are normal.
   C. Administer any sedative medications, as prescribed.
   D. A CT scan may need to be scheduled if the biopsy needle must to be inserted under CT guidance in order to obtain tissue from a specific area of the liver.
   E. *See Client and family teaching.*
3. Procedure:
   A. The area of the liver suspected of being abnormal is noted.
   B. The client is placed in the supine or left lateral position.

C. The skin area used for puncture is anesthetized locally.

D. The client is asked to exhale and hold the inhalation so that the liver descends and the possibility of a pneumothorax is decreased.

E. The biopsy needle is inserted by the physician into the liver during the client's sustained exhalation, and a liver tissue is obtained.

F. The needle is withdrawn from the liver.

G. A pressure dressing is applied.

H. The procedure takes approximately 30 minutes.

4. Postprocedure care:

A. Touch prints on glass slides may be made prior to fixation, and may be submitted for cytologic evaluation.

B. Needle rinses in 50% alcohol or saline may also provide helpful diagnostic material.

C. Direct slides from needle aspirates may be made, and the slides may be fixed immediately in 95% alcohol.

D. Tissue samples may be placed into a specimen bottle containing 10% formalin for fixation.

E. Send the specimens to the pathology department.

F. Assess vital signs frequently (every 15 minutes × 2) to determine evidence of hemorrhage (increased pulse and blood pressure) and peritonitis (increased temperature).

G. Assess the biopsy site for bleeding.

H. Place the client on the right side for 1–2 hours after the procedure. This position will compress the liver against the chest wall and will decrease the risk of hemorrhage or bile leak.

I. Bedrest with 24-hour observation after the biopsy is usually prescribed.

5. Client and family teaching:

A. Explain the purpose of the procedure.

B. Fast from food and fluids after midnight on the day of the test.

C. The procedure takes about 30 minutes. Local anesthetic is used to control pain.

6. Factors that affect results:

A. False-negatives may occur and localized liver disease may be missed, since a very small fragment of liver tissue, which is often partially destroyed, is taken in a random manner from a large organ. False-negatives may be due to (1) sampling error, since the detection rate of liver metastasis is approximately 60% with blind biopsy and about 85% using ultrasound guidance, and (2) degeneration or distortion, which has been caused by faulty preparation of the specimen.

B. False-positives may be due to incorrect interpretation of very reactive hepatocytes.

7. Other data:

A. An experienced physician should perform the procedure.

B. Specimens for histologic and cytologic examination may be obtained using ultrasound radiologic guidance and a tissue core biopsy needle, such as the Menghini needle. Specimens for cytologic examination only may be obtained using a fine aspirate needle.

C. Detection of portal vein tumor invasion in clients with hepatocellular carcinoma is important to determine therapy and prognosis. Fine-needle aspiration of a portal vein thrombus under ultrasound guidance helps to distinguish malignant from benign thrombus, without resorting to laparotomy.

Bibliography:

Berkovitch M: Hepatotoxicity of 6-mercaptopurine in childhood acute lymphocytic leukemia: pharmacokinetic characteristics. Med Ped Oncol 26(2): 85–89, 1996.

Chiu KW, Chang-Chien CS, Chen L, Liaw YF: Ultrasonically-guided needle aspiration with preparation of cell blocks in the diagnosis of liver tumors. Hepatogastroenterology 41(1):30–33, 1994.

Conn HO: Liver biopsy: Increased risks in patients with cancer. Hepatology 14(1):206–209, 1991

Dusenbery D, Dodd GD 3rd, Carr BI: Percutaneous fine-needle aspiration of portal vein thrombi as a staging technique for hepatocellular carcinoma. Cancer 75(8): 2057–2062, 1995.

Orlando R, Lirussi F, Okolicsanyi L: Laparoscopy and liver biopsy; further evidence that the two procedures improve the diagnosis of liver cirrhosis. A retrospective study of 1,003 consecutive examinations. J Clin Gastroenterol 12(1):47–52, 1990.

Tobkes AI: Liver biopsy: review of methodology and complications. Dig Dis 13(5):267–274, 1995.

Whitney JP: Liver enzymes and liver biopsy. Ann Intern Med 112(4):311, 1990.

LIVER ECHOGRAM

(see Liver Sonogram, Diagnostic)

LIVER I-131 (ROSE BENGAL) SCAN, DIAGNOSTIC

Norm: Normal size, shape, and position of liver.

Usage: Cirrhosis, diffuse infiltrating processes affecting the liver (e.g., amyloidosis, sarcoidosis), granulomas, hepatomas, hepatic abscesses or cysts, jaundice, tuberculosis, and tumors.

Description: A nuclear medicine scan in which radioactive iodine is used to determine the uptake in the liver in order to outline and detect structural changes in the liver.

Professional Considerations:

1. Consent form IS required.

Risks:

Allergic reaction to dye (itching, hives, rash, tight feeling in the throat, shortness of breath, bronchospasm, anaphylaxis, death).

Contraindications:

Previous allergy to iodine, shellfish or radiographic contrast medium; renal insufficiency; during pregnancy or breast-feeding.

2. Preparation:
   A. Have emergency equipment readily available.
3. Procedure:
   A. The client is transported to the nuclear medicine department. For inpatients, a nuclear medicine technologist may administer the radionuclide at the bedside.
   B. The client is injected intravenously with radioactive iodine-131.
   C. A gamma ray detector is placed over the right upper quadrant of the client's abdomen 30 minutes after the client has been injected.
   D. The client is placed in lateral, prone, and supine positions, so that all the surfaces of the liver may be visualized.
   E. Scans are taken of the liver at intervals.
   F. The radionuclide image of the distribution of radioactive particles in the liver is recorded on either x-ray or Polaroid film.
4. Postprocedure care:
   A. Assess vital signs every 15 minutes × 2.
   B. Observe the client carefully for up to 60 minutes after the study for a possible (anaphylactic) reaction to the radionuclide.
   C. Rubber gloves should be worn when discarding urine for 24 hours after the procedure. Wash the gloved hands with soap and water before removing the gloves. Wash the ungloved hands after the gloves have been removed.
5. Client and family teaching:
   A. No fasting or premedication is required.
   B. The IV injection of the radionuclide is the only discomfort associated with this procedure.
   C. You will not be exposed to large amounts of radiation, since only tracer doses of I-131 are used.
   D. This procedure is performed by a trained technologist in approximately 1 hour. A physician trained in nuclear medicine interprets the results.
   E. Meticulously wash your hands with soap and water after each void for 24 hours postprocedure.
   F. Family members must wear rubber gloves when discarding the client's urine for 24 hours postprocedure, if family will be providing this care.
   G. Follow-up diagnostic tests (e.g., ultrasound, CT scan, and/or biopsy) are needed to confirm the diagnosis.
6. Factors that affect results:
   A. Barium in the GI tract overlying the liver or spleen will produce defects on the scan, which may be mistaken for masses.
   B. False-negative results may occur in clients with space-occupying lesions (e.g., tumors, cysts, abscesses, etc.) smaller than 2 cm, because the scan can demonstrate only filling defects greater than 2 cm in diameter.
   C. False-positive results may occur in clients with cirrhosis. Due to the distortion of the client's liver parenchyma, the scan may be incorrectly interpreted as positive for filling defects.
7. Other data:
   A. Health care professionals working in a nuclear medicine area must follow federal standards set by the Nuclear Regulatory Commission. These standards include precautions for handling the radioactive material and monitoring of potential radiation exposure.
   B. If "cold spots" (areas that do not take up the radionuclide) appear, then cysts, abscesses, and tumors may be suspected.
   C. The half-life of iodine-131 is 8 days.
   D. The value of this test is related to its cost, and its potential benefit has been analyzed. In a study with a sample population size of 63 clients, 81% (51 clients) with elevated alkaline phosphatase levels had normal liver scans. Only 1 of the 63 clients had a liver scan suggestive of positive metastasis. Approximately $74,000 was spent on the liver and bone scans in this study.

Bibliography:

Brar HS: Value of preoperative bone and liver scans and alkaline phosphatase in the evaluation of breast cancer patients. Am J Surg *165*(2):221–223, 1993.

Rosenbaum RC, Johnston GS, Valente WA: Frequency of hepatic visualization during I-131 imaging for metastatic thyroid cancer. Clin Nucl Med *13*(9): 657–660, 1988.

Schober B, Cohen P, Lyster D, et al.: Diffuse liver uptake of iodine-131. J Nucl Med *31*(9):1575–1576, 1990.

Shah SM: Is radioisotope liver scan investigation obsolete? [editorial]. J Assoc Physicians India *42*(4): 279–280, 1994.

LIVER SCAN, DIAGNOSTIC

(see Computed Tomography of the Body, Diagnostic; or Liver I-131 Scan, Diagnostic)

LIVER SONOGRAM (LIVER ECHOGRAM, LIVER ULTRASOUND), DIAGNOSTIC

Norm: Liver is of proper size, shape, and position, with a homogenous soft echo pattern. Image indicates normal relationship to adjacent anatomic structures. Negative for intrahepatic duct dilation, abscess, cyst, hematoma, or tumor.

Usage: Determine the cause of jaundice; differentiate between obstructive and nonobstructive jaundice; detect cirrhosis, hepatic abscess, cyst, hematoma, and tumors; differentiate cysts and abscesses from tumors; examination of the shape and structure of intrahepatic ducts; visualize pleural effusion; evaluation of hepatic hemodynamic flow balance; evaluate ascites; and monitoring of hepatic metastasis response to cancer therapy. May be used before a liver biopsy, or can help differentiate the constitution of abnormalities identified during hepatobiliary nuclear medicine scanning. It is useful with liver scanning to define the "cold spots." Serial scans may be used to determine the volume of the liver. Is not reliable in detecting metastasis, especially when a client's liver is high, and primarily under the rib cage. Alternative to hepatic dye imaging tests for clients with allergy to radiographic dyes.

Description: This noninvasive diagnostic technique evaluates the liver, intrahepatic duct structure, and ancillary areas of the gallbladder and diaphragm. It creates an oscilloscopic picture from the echoes of high-frequency sound waves, which pass over the right upper quadrant of the abdomen (acoustic imaging). A computer converts the time required for the ultrasonic beam to be reflected back to the transducer from differing densities of tissue to an electrical impulse. This impulse is displayed on an oscilloscopic screen to create a three-dimensional picture of the liver. Hepatitis and fatty liver may be indicated by hepatomegaly. Fatty infiltration also causes brighter than normal echoes, with decreased amount of vascular structures. Hepatic fibrosis is demonstrated by a smaller than normal liver size and inhomogeneity of the liver tissue. Cysts appear sonolucent, with borders that are easily defined, and they have an echo-free nature. Abscesses may contain internal echoes. Malignant neoplasm (e.g., adenocarcinoma and other primary liver tumors) may appear as a diffusely distorted parenchymal area, where homogeneity of tissue would be expected. The image pattern, which is produced by malignant neoplasms, is called a "bull's eye." This is due to the dense central echo pattern, which is surrounded by the less-echo-producing halo.

Professional Considerations:

1. Consent form NOT required.
2. Preparation:
   A. This test should be performed before intestinal barium tests, or after the barium is cleared from the system.
   B. Obtain ultrasonic gel or paste.
   C. *See Client and family teaching.*
3. Procedure:
   A. The client is positioned supine in bed, or on a procedure table.
   B. The right upper quadrant of the abdomen is covered with ultrasonic gel and a lubricated transducer is passed slowly over the area along the transverse plane at intervals 1 cm apart with the client in deep inspiration. This is followed by longitudinal scanning in 0.5- to 2-cm increments, moving from the umbilicus to the xiphoid process, with the transducer angled so that the sound waves pass under the rib cage. The client may be changed to a left lateral decubitus position to obtain lateral views of the liver via coronal scanning. If the client is dehydrated, he or she may be asked to expand the abdomen to enhance the smoothness of the anterior abdominal wall. The final views taken are right anterior oblique.
   C. Photographs are taken of the oscilloscopic display.
   D. The procedure takes less than 30 minutes.
4. Postprocedure care:
   A. Remove the lubricant from the skin.
5. Client and family teaching:
   A. Fast from food and fluids, and refrain from tobacco smoking overnight prior to the test.
   B. The procedure is painless and carries no risk.
   C. Wear a gown during the test.
6. Factors that affect results:
   A. Dehydration interferes with the adequate contrast between the organs and body fluids.

B. Intestinal barium, gas, or food obscures results by preventing proper transmission and deflection of the high-frequency sound waves.

C. Fatty liver causes scattering in the attenuation of the ultrasonic beam.

D. The more abdominal fat present, the greater the attenuation (reduction in sound wave amplitude and intensity), which interferes with the clarity of the picture.

E. Lung tissue may interfere with visualization of the liver dome in transverse views.

F. Rib artifacts may obscure images of the right lobe of the liver.

7. Other data:
   A. *See also Gallbladder and Biliary System Sonogram, Diagnostic.*

Bibliography:

Bombelli L, Genitoni V, Biasi S, et al.: Liver hemodynamic flow balance by image-directed Doppler ultrasound evaluation in normal subjects. J Clin Ultrasound *19*(5):257–262, 1991.

Davies RJ, Saverymuttu SH, Fallowfield M, et al.: Paradoxical lack of ultrasound attenuation with gross fatty change in the liver. Clin Radiol *43*(6):393–396, 1991.

Hagen-Ansert SL: Textbook of Diagnostic Ultrasonography, 3rd ed. St Louis, MO, CV Mosby, 1989.

Lee RA, Charboneau JW: Cases of the day. Ultrasound.

Focal nodular hyperplasia of the liver. Radiographics *10*(5):954–956, 1990.

Lin BP, Chu JM, Rose RA: Ultrasound guided fine needle biopsy of the liver for cytology and histology. Australas Radiol *35*(1):33–37, 1991.

LIVER/SPLEEN SCAN, DIAGNOSTIC
(see Hepatobiliary Scan, Diagnostic)

LIVER Tc-99m SCAN OF BLOOD VESSELS, DIAGNOSTIC
(see Hepatobiliary Scan, Diagnostic)

LIVER ULTRASOUND
(see Liver Sonogram, Diagnostic)

LORAZEPAM
(see Benzodiazepines, Plasma and Urine)

LOW-DENSITY LIPOPROTEIN (LDL) CHOLESTEROL, BLOOD

Norm:

Age	Male mg/dl	Male SI Units mmol/L	Female mg/dl	Female SI Units mmol/L
Adults				
20–24	66–147	1.71–3.81	57–159	1.48–4.12
25–29	70–165	1.81–4.27	71–164	1.84–4.25
30–34	78–185	2.02–4.79	70–156	1.81–4.04
35–39	81–189	2.10–4.90	75–172	1.94–4.45
40–44	87–186	2.25–4.82	74–174	1.92–4.51
45–49	97–202	2.51–5.23	79–186	2.05–4.82
50–54	89–197	2.31–5.10	88–201	2.28–5.21
55–59	88–203	2.28–5.26	89–210	2.31–5.44
60–64	83–210	2.15–5.44	100–224	2.59–5.80
65–69	98–210	2.54–5.44	92–221	2.38–5.72
≥70	88–186	2.28–4.82	96–206	2.49–5.34
Children				
Cord blood	20–56	0.52–1.45	21–58	0.54–1.50
5–9	63–129	1.63–3.34	68–140	1.76–3.63
10–14	64–133	1.66–3.44	68–136	1.76–3.52
15–19	62–130	1.61–3.37	59–137	1.53–3.55

LDL CHOLESTEROL LEVELS AND RECOMMENDATIONS

	Desirable Level	Level for Diet Therapy and Increased Exercise	Level for Drug Consideration
Without CHD and with fewer than 2 risk factors	<160 mg/dl	160–190 mg/dl	≥190 mg/dl*
Without CHD and with 2 or more risk factors	<130 mg/dl	100–160 mg/dl	≥160 mg/dl
With CHD	≤100 mg/dl	100–130 mg/dl	≥130 mg/dl**

*In men <35 years of age and in premenopausal women with LDL cholesterol levels of 190 to 219 mg/dl, drug therapy should be delayed, except in high-risk clients (e.g., those with diabetes).

**In clients with CHD, with cholesterol levels of 100–129 mg/dl, the physician should exercise clinical judgment in deciding whether to initiate drug treatment.

Usage: Predict risk of coronary heart disease (CHD).

Increased: Acute myocardial infarction, anorexia nervosa, coronary arterial atherosclerosis, Cushing's disease, diabetes mellitus, diet high in cholesterol and saturated fats, dysglobulinemias, eclampsia, hepatic disease, type-II hyperlipoproteinemia, hyperlipidemia, hypothyroidism, Laennec's cirrhosis, multiple myeloma, nephrotic syndrome, porphyria, pregnancy, and renal failure. Drugs include androgens, aspirin, catecholamines, diuretics, glucogenic corticosteroids, oral contraceptives, phenothiazines, and sulfonamides.

Decreased: Arteriosclerosis, abetalipoproteinemia, chronic obstructive lung disease, type-I hyperlipoproteinemia, hyperthyroidism, hypoalbuminemia, inflammatory joint disease, malabsorption, malnutrition, multiple myeloma, pulmonary disease, Reye's syndrome, stress, and Tangier disease. Drugs include aspirin, cholestyramine, clofibrate, cortisone, estrogens, neomycin, nicotinic acid, probucol, and thyroxine.

Description: Low-density lipoproteins (LDLs), the "bad lipids," carry the body's cholesterol in plasma from the liver to other parts of the body, and deposit it in the peripheral tissues. LDL is associated with an increased risk of arteriosclerotic heart and peripheral vascular disease. High levels of LDL are atherogenic. Betalipoproteins, or LDLs, are moderately high in protein and cholesterol but low in triglycerides. LDL cholesterol is usually a calculation rather than a direct measurement. LDLs can be derived from the formula:

$$LDL = Cholesterol \times \frac{HDL + Triglycerides}{2}$$

Professional Considerations:

1. Consent form NOT required.
2. Preparation:
   A. Tube: Red-top, red/gray-top, or gold-top.
   B. Indicate on the laboratory requisition any drugs that may affect the test results.
   C. *See Client and family teaching.*
3. Procedure:
   A. Draw a 2-ml blood sample.
4. Postprocedure care:
   A. None.
5. Client and family teaching:
   A. Fast from food for 14 hours prior to the test. Only water is permitted.
   B. Follow a regular diet for 2 weeks prior to the test.
   C. For elevated levels, provide information regarding appropriate body weight, diet, and acarus.
   D. If cholesterol is still elevated after

lifestyle modifications, prescription medication may be an option to discuss with the physician.

6. Factors that affect results:
   A. Results are invalid if the client has undergone a radioactive scan within 7 days prior to this test.
   B. Consumption of alcoholic beverages within the last 24 hours will affect the results.
   C. Test results could be elevated by a diet high in saturated fats and sugar (e.g., butter, cream, fatty meats, bacon, and candy).
   D. Binge eating can also alter lipoprotein values.
7. Other data:
   A. Calculation is not valid for specimens over 400 mg/dl or clients with type-III hyperlipoproteinemia.

Bibliography:

National Cholesterol Education Program (US). Expert Panel on Detection, Evaluation, and Treatment of High Blood Cholesterol in Adults. The Second Report of the Expert Panel on Detection, Evaluation, and Treatment of High Blood Cholesterol in Adults (Adult Treatment Panel II). NIH, National Heart, Lung, and Blood Institute: 1405–1431, 1993.

Wilson PW: High-density lipoprotein, low-density lipoprotein and coronary artery disease. Am J Cardiol *66*(6):7A–10A, 1990.

LOWER GI, DIAGNOSTIC
(see Barium Enema, Diagnostic)

LP EXAMINATION
(see Lumbar Puncture, Diagnostic)

L-PHASE, CULTURE
(see Cell Wall–Defective Bacteria, Culture)

LSA
(see Lipid-Associated Sialic Acid, Serum or Plasma)

LSD (LYSERGIC ACID DIETHYLAMIDE), BLOOD OR URINE

Norm: Negative.

Positive: Drug abuse.

Description: A potent hallucinogen derived from ergot, a fungus that spoils rye grain. It is equally effective by intravenous route as by oral route; metabolized in the liver, excreted in the bile; and affects both parasympathetic and sympathetic nervous systems. May produce hallucinations years after ingestion, without warning.

Professional Considerations:

1. Consent form NOT required.
2. Preparation:
   A. Tube: Red-top, red/gray-top, or gold-top (for the blood sample).
   B. Obtain a sterile specimen container (for the urine sample).
3. Procedure:
   A. Draw a 7-ml blood sample or obtain 10 ml of urine.
4. Postprocedure care:
   A. None.
5. Client and family teaching:
   A. This drug may cause delirium, delusions, and hallucinations.
   B. Clients who experience palinopsia (prolonged afterimages) during LSD intoxication may continue to be symptomatic up to 3 years after they cease to ingest the drug.
   C. There is no systematic program of treatment for LSD ingestion. A quiet environment and diazepam may be effective in controlling the individual.
6. Factors that affect results:
   A. None.
7. Other data:
   A. Signs of toxicity include hypertension, tachycardia, piloerection, and suicidal tendency. LSD-related violent behavior includes suicide, homicide, and accidental death.
   B. Compared to the mean values during the years 1985–1990, there has been an increase in LSD-related arrests, LSD-related emergency room visits, and LSD-related violent behavior in adolescents in the 1990s.

Bibliography:

Kawasaki A: Persistent palinopsia following ingestion of lysergic acid diethylamide (LSD). Arch Ophthalmol *114*(1):47–50, 1996.

Kulig K: LSD. Emerg Med Clin North Am *8*(3):551–558, 1990.

McCarron MM, Walberg CB, Baselt RC: Confirmation of LSD intoxication by analysis of serum and urine. J Ann Toxicol *14*(3):165–167, 1990.

Schwartz RH: LSD: Its rise, fall, and renewed popularity among high school students. Pediatr Clin North Am *42*(2):403–413, 1995.

LUMBAR PUNCTURE, DIAGNOSTIC

Norm: *See Cerebrospinal Fluid, Glucose, Specimen; Cerebrospinal Fluid, Immunoglobulin G, Immunoglobulin G Ratios and Immunoglobulin G Index, Immunoglobulin G Synthesis Rate, Specimen; Cerebrospinal Fluid, Lactic Acid, Specimen; Cerebrospinal Fluid, Myelin Basic Protein, Oligoclonal Bands, Protein, and Protein*

Electrophoresis, Specimen; Cerebrospinal Fluid, Routine Analysis, Specimen; and Cerebrospinal Fluid Routine, Culture and Cytology.

Usage: To assist in the diagnosis of primary or metastatic brain or spinal cord neoplasm, cerebral hemorrhage, meningitis, encephalitis, degenerative brain disease, autoimmune diseases involving the central nervous system, neurosyphilis, and demyelinating disorders (e.g., multiple sclerosis, acute demyelinating polyneuropathy). Also, this procedure may be performed therapeutically to inject therapeutic or diagnostic agents, and to administer spinal anesthetics. *See individual test listings above for additional specific usage.*

Description: An invasive sterile procedure that can be performed at the bedside. A needle is placed into the subarachnoid space of the spinal column. Cerebrospinal fluid (CSF) pressure is measured, and CSF is obtained for examination. The spinal fluid is analyzed to diagnose spinal cord and brain diseases. CSF protects the brain and spinal column from injury and transports products of neurosecretion and cellular metabolism. Under special circumstances, CSF may be obtained from a ventriculotomy or from cisternal or lateral cervical punctures.

Professional Considerations:

1. Consent form IS required.

Risks:
Bleeding, dizziness, headache, hematoma, increased intracranial pressure, infection, meningitis, nausea.

Contraindications:
Degenerative joint disease affecting the spine; an agitated or uncooperative client; infection near the L2-S1 site, which could carry the infective process into the CSF and change cytologic results; and in clients with increased intracranial pressure (especially when papilledema or split cranial sutures are present), coagulation defects, low back pain, or spinal deformities.

2. Preparation:
   A. *See Client and family teaching.*
   B. Obtain a lumbar puncture or a spinal tap sterile tray, sterile drapes, 1–2% lidocaine (Xylocaine), and a dry, sterile dressing.
   C. If increased intracranial pressure is suspected, a computed tomographic scan of the brain should be performed to rule out this possibility prior to the lumbar puncture. Herniation of the brain may occur in such clients.
   D. Assess the client's vital signs. Perform a baseline neurologic assessment of the legs by assessing strength, sensation, and movement.
3. Procedure:
   A. Position the client in a lateral position with the knees drawn up to the abdomen, the chin placed on the chest, and hands clasped around the knees.
   B. Assist the client in relaxing during the procedure by using soothing words, and by instructing the client to breathe slowly and deeply with the mouth open. Give reassurance by using touch or holding the client's hand, unless this is opposed by the client.
   C. The puncture site is selected, usually in the lumbar sac at L3-L4 or at the L4-L5 site. A little bone at the L5-S interspace, the "surgeon's delight," facilitates selection of the puncture site.
   D. The site is thoroughly cleansed with an antiseptic solution.
   E. The surrounding area is draped carefully with sterile towels so that the towels do not obscure important landmarks.
   F. A local anesthetic (usually Xylocaine) is injected into the L3-L4 or L4-L5 spinal column area, creating a burning sensation.
   G. A spinal needle, which contains an inner obturator (stylet), is placed through the skin and into the spinal canal.
   H. The subarachnoid space is entered. The client may feel the entry ("pop") of the needle through the dura mater.
   I. The obturator is removed, and CSF will be seen slowly dripping from the needle.
   J. The needle is attached to a sterile manometer.
   K. Ask the client to relax and straighten the legs. This will reduce the intra-abdominal pressure, which will cause an increase in CSF pressure.
   L. The opening CSF pressure is recorded.
   M. Three numbered sterile test tubes are filled sequentially, with a total of 3–12 ml of CSF.
   N. The Queckenstedt procedure is performed during a lumbar puncture if blockage in the CSF circulation in the spinal subarachnoid space is suspected.

The jugular vein is temporarily occluded manually by digital pressure, or by a medium-sized blood pressure cuff inflated to approximately 20 mmHg. The CSF pressure should increase to 15–40 cm H_2O within 10 seconds of jugular occlusion. No rise after 10 seconds suggests a complete obstruction in the spinal canal. The pressure should return promptly to normal within 10 seconds of release of pressure. A sluggish rise or fall of CSF pressure suggests partial blockage of CSF circulation.

O. The closing pressure of CSF is measured.

P. The procedure takes 30 minutes.

4. Postprocedure care:
   A. Label all test tubes immediately with the proper number (1, 2, 3), the client's name, the date, and the room number.
   B. The first specimen may be discarded, as it is most likely to be contaminated with blood.
   C. Apply a dry, sterile dressing to the lumbar puncture site.
   D. Colored or very cloudy spinal fluid requires additional mixing with 0.5 ml sterile sodium citrate per 5 ml of CSF to prevent clotting.
   E. Transport the specimens to the laboratory immediately. Analysis must be performed promptly on freshly collected specimens.
   F. Monitor vital signs and for changes in level of consciousness, headache, and neurologic status every 15 minutes × 4, then every 30 minutes × 4, then hourly × 4.
   G. Place the client in a prone position with a pillow under the abdomen to increase the intra-abdominal pressure, or in a supine position, with the head of the bed elevated no more than 30 degrees. Allow the client to turn from side to side.
   H. Keep the client in a reclining position for 4–12 hours to prevent a spinal headache. (There is some debate as to whether this restriction is necessary.)
   I. Encourage the client to drink increased amounts of fluid with a straw to replace CSF removed during the lumbar puncture, unless this is contraindicated.
   J. Encourage women to use a "fracture bedpan" to help alleviate voiding problems.
   K. Administer analgesics and encourage a longer period of bedrest if a headache should occur.
   L. Assess the client for numbness, tingling, and movement of the lower extremities; irritability; change in level of consciousness; nonreactive eye pupils; and ability to void.
   M. Assess the puncture site for redness,

swelling, drainage, and pain every 4 hours × 24 hours.

N. Notify the physician of any unusual findings. Notify the physician immediately if there is a sign of leakage at the puncture site.

O. Refrigerate the CSF when prompt analysis is not possible. Store the specimens for culture in a bacteriologic incubator when prompt analysis is not possible.

5. Client and family teaching:
   A. Explain the procedure, potential risks and benefits, and postprocedural care. Allay the client's fears, and allow him or her time to verbalize concerns.
   B. There will be a burning sensation with the injection of local anesthetic, and transient pain or pressure may occur during the lumbar puncture.
   C. No fasting or sedation is required.
   D. Increase fluid intake to 6–8 glasses of water per day, unless contraindicated, in order to prevent and relieve possible headache.
   E. Empty the bladder and bowels prior to the procedure.
   F. You will have to lie on your side with your chin bent down onto your chest, and clasp your hands around your knees. The knees should be drawn up to, but not compress, the abdomen so that the back bows. (A sitting position, with the client straddling a straight-backed chair and flexing the head to the chest, can be used.)
   G. It is important to lie very still throughout this procedure, since movement may cause traumatic injury.
   H. Tell the client to refrain from holding his or her breath, straining, and talking during procedure.
   I. Notify the physician or nurse if you are having severe back pain, numbness or tingling in the lower extremities, more than minor bleeding, headache that lasts more than 1 day, or a fever of higher than 101°F (38.3°C).

6. Factors that affect results:
   A. Contamination of the specimen will cause inaccurate results. The first tube could be contaminated with blood from the spinal tap, and should not be used for protein determination, cell count, or culture.
   B. Cloudy specimens may be caused by elevated white blood cells. Yellow specimens may be caused by elevated protein >100 mg/dl. Pink or red specimens may be caused by red blood cells. Turbid specimens may be caused by the presence of fungi.
   C. Refrigeration will alter the test results if bacteriologic and fungal studies are done.
   D. Certain drugs could cause a false increased CSF protein level, such as anesthetics, acetophentidin (phenacetin),

chlorpromazine (Thorazine), salicylates (aspirin), streptomycin, and sulfonamides.

E. CSF chloride level determination may be invalidated by IV fluid containing chloride.

F. Hyperglycemia could increase the CSF glucose level.

7. Other data:

A. A traumatic spinal tap could cause blood to be present in the specimen, and this may be mistaken for a clinical problem.

B. Handle specimens cautiously to prevent self-contamination.

C. If the client is in an upright position after the procedure, headaches may occur due to spinal fluid leaking from the site of the lumbar puncture.

D. It is recommended that lumbar punctures continue to be performed in children with first febrile convulsions, especially if under the age of 18 months.

E. The total amyloid beta protein in CSF has not been found to be a useful marker for current diagnosis of Alzheimer's disease.

F. The role of routine lumbar puncture in the initial evaluation of symptom-free infants for congenital syphilis is not recommended, due to the low yield of reactive VDRL in CSF and to the similar CSF leukocyte and protein values in the syphilis group and control group.

Bibliography:

Beeram MR: Lumbar puncture in the evaluation of possible asymptomatic congenital syphilis in neonates. J Pediatr *128*(1):125–129, 1996.

Laditan AA: Analysis of the results of routine lumbar puncture after a first febrile convulsion in Hofuf, Al-Hassa, Saudi Arabia. East Afr Med J *72*(6):376–378, 1995.

Southwick PC: Assessment of amyloid beta protein in cerebrospinal fluid as an aid in the diagnosis of Alzheimer's disease. J Neurochem *66*(1):259–265, 1996.

LUMIAGGREGOMETRY, DIAGNOSTIC

Norm: Luminescence proportional to adenosine triphosphate (ATP) concentration.

Usage: Diagnose platelet dense granule storage pool disease (SPD), which is evidenced by reduced amounts of granule nucleotides, and platelet dense granule release defects, which is evidenced by abnormal release of granule nucleotides.

Description: Method for measuring platelet dense granule release and ag-

gregation simultaneously. This test quantifies ATP secreted during a platelet release reaction. It is based on the principle that the ATP secreted during the release reaction will react with luciferin, and will produce a luminescence that is measured with a photomultiplier tube. If the luminescence is low (decreased ATP), then the bleeding defect is in the storage pool, and is not in the release mechanism or prostaglandin pathway.

Professional Considerations:

1. Consent form NOT required.

2. Preparation:

A. Tube: Red-top, red/gray-top, or gold-top.

3. Procedure:

A. Draw a 3-ml blood sample.

4. Postprocedure care:

A. Assess the venipuncture site for bleeding every 5 minutes × 3.

5. Client and family teaching:

A. Results are normally available within 48 hours.

6. Factors that affect results:

A. Aspirin, heparin, and warfarin increase results.

7. Other data:

A. Flow cytometry is another method to study defects in platelet dense granule function.

Bibliography:

Liu PI: Blue Book of Diagnostic Tests. Philadelphia, WB Saunders, 1986.

Wall JE: A flow cytometric assay using mepacrine for study of uptake and release of platelet dense granule contents. Br J Haematol *89*(2):380–385, 1995.

White MM: Assessment of lumiaggregometry for research and clinical laboratories. Thromb Haemost *67*(5):572–577, 1992.

LUNG FUNCTION TEST
(see Pulmonary Function Test, Diagnostic)

LUNG SCAN, PERFUSION AND VENTILATION, DIAGNOSTIC

Norm: Negative for emboli/thrombus.

Perfusion scan	Uniform uptake of particles within the entire lung vasculature
Ventilation scan	Equal gas distribution in the pulmonary airways

Usage: Diagnosis of pulmonary embolism or thrombosis; determination of the percentage of lungs functioning normally; assessment of pulmonary vasculature supply, by providing an estimate of regional pulmonary blood flow and identifying areas of shunting and areas where capillaries are absent (i.e., emphysema); and diagnosis of atelectasis, asthma, bronchitis, chronic obstructive pulmonary disease, inflammatory fibrosis, lung cancer/tumors, and pneumonia.

Description: This is a nuclear medicine procedure. There are three types of lung scans: (1) the perfusion scan, (2) the ventilation scan, and (3) the inhalation scan. In the perfusion scan, blood flow to the lungs is evaluated using a macroaggregated albumin (MAA) tagged with technetium (Tc-99m). This is injected intravenously. The radiolabeled particles become temporarily lodged in the pulmonary vasculature, since the diameter of these particles is larger than that of the pulmonary capillaries. A gamma-ray detector scans the client, and a scintillation camera records the distribution of particles within the pulmonary vascular supply. Although the lung perfusion scan is sensitive, it is not specific, since a variety of pathologic conditions can cause the same abnormal results. Therefore, lung perfusion scans should be performed in conjunction with a lung ventilation scan. This scan determines the patency of the pulmonary airways and detects abnormalities in ventilation (e.g., pneumonia, pleural fluid, emphysema). Ventilation scans will show a normal wash-in and wash-out of radioactivity from the embolized lung area in embolic disorders. Conversely, the wash-in and wash-out will be abnormal in parenchymal disease (e.g., pneumonia). Finally, a normal inhalation scan looks much like a perfusion scan, except that the trachea and major airways are more visible.

Professional Considerations:

1. Consent form IS required.

Risks:
Allergic reaction to iodine-131, if use is planned (itching, hives, rash, tight feeling in the throat, shortness of breath, bronchospasm, anaphylaxis, death).

Contraindications:
In pregnant or lactating women. Lung perfusion scanning is contraindicated in clients with primary pulmonary hypertension or right-to-left heart shunts. During pregnancy or breastfeeding. Previous history of allergy to iodine, eggs or shellfish, if iodine-131 will be used.

2. Preparation:
   A. Have emergency equipment readily available.
   B. If iodine-131 is to be given (although this is rarely the case), give the client 10 drops of Lugol's solution several hours before the test. This will prevent iodine uptake by the thyroid gland.
   C. Sedation may be prescribed for very young children or those who are unable to lie still for the scan.
   D. Establish intravenous access.
   E. Breathing methods are reviewed with the client before injection and imaging.
   F. *See Client and family teaching.*
3. Procedure:
   A. Transport the client to the nuclear medicine department.
   B. In a perfusion scan, a radionuclide-tagged MAA is injected slowly intravenously over several respiratory cycles. Half is injected while the client is sitting up, and the other half while lying down. The client is placed in the supine, prone, and various lateral positions on the nuclear medicine table under the camera. Scanning with a gamma-ray detector is begun immediately. The scintillation camera takes several single stationary images of the anterior, posterior, and lateral chest. Perfusion imaging lasts about 45 minutes.
   C. In a ventilation scan, a client inhales a mixture of air and radioactive gas (xenon-133, krypton-85, krypton-81m, or Tc-diethylenetriamine pentaacetic acid [Tc-DTPA]) through the mouthpiece of a face mask. The radioactive gas follows the same pathway as the air in normal breathing. A nuclear scan is performed at three phases: during the buildup of gas, after the client rebreathes from a bag and the radioactivity reaches a steady level, and after removal of the radioactive gas from the lungs. Ventilation imaging lasts about 30 minutes.
   D. In an inhalation scan, droplets of radioactive material can be administered by a positive-pressure ventilator. The

aerosol is then inhaled through the mouthpiece of a face mask.

4. Postprocedure care:
   A. Observe the client carefully for up to 60 minutes after the study for a possible (anaphylactic) reaction to the radionuclide.
   B. When urine is being discarded, rubber gloves should be worn for 24 hours after the procedure. Wash the gloved hands with soap and water before removing the gloves. Wash the ungloved hands after the gloves have been removed.

5. Client and family teaching:
   A. Peripheral venipuncture is the only discomfort associated with this test.
   B. A physician trained in diagnostic nuclear medicine interprets the results.
   C. The total time for the procedure is approximately 2 hours.
   D. No fasting or premedication is required.
   E. The client will not be exposed to large amounts of radioactivity, because only tracer doses of isotopes are used.
   F. Remove jewelry around the chest area.
   G. Meticulously wash your hands with soap and water after each void for 24 hours postprocedure.
   H. Family members must wear rubber gloves when discarding the client's urine for 24 hours postprocedure, if the family will be providing this care.

6. Factors that affect results:
   A. Jewelry or metal objects in the x-ray field distort the results.
   B. The client must lie motionless throughout the scan for the most accurate results.
   C. Ventilation scans with Tc-DTPA require client cooperation with deep breathing and appropriate use of breathing equipment to prevent contamination with the radioactive gases.
   D. The scan results of clients with pulmonary parenchymal disease (e.g., pneumonia, emphysema, pleural effusion, tumors) will appear to demonstrate perfusion defect and simulate pulmonary embolism.
   E. False-positive scans occur in vasculitis, mitral stenosis, and pulmonary hypertension and when tumors obstruct a pulmonary artery with airway involvement.

7. Other data:
   A. In pulmonary emboli, perfusion is decreased but ventilation is maintained. Diagnosis of pulmonary embolus cannot be made on the basis of a lung perfusion scan alone.
   B. In pneumonia, ventilation is absent.
   C. "Hot spots" are areas of normal blood flow. "Cold spots" are areas of low radioactivity uptake, and indicate poor perfusion and emboli.
   D. A chest x-ray should be obtained prior to or after a lung perfusion scan. Comparison of the perfusion scan with a chest x-ray can detect infiltrating disease.
   E. The perfusion scan immediately follows the ventilation scan. However, ventilation scans using krypton can be performed before, during, or after perfusion scans.
   F. Long-term anticoagulant therapy can be safely withheld in symptomatic clients (e.g., suspected pulmonary embolus) with a normal perfusion scan.
   G. High-probability perfusion scans are usually diagnostic of pulmonary embolus.
   H. Less client cooperation is needed during a ventilation scan with a krypton tracer. It can even be performed on a comatose client.
   I. A pulmonary arteriogram is still necessary before an embolectomy can be attempted.
   J. Health care professionals working in a nuclear medicine area must follow federal standards set by the Nuclear Regulatory Commission. These standards include precautions for handling the radioactive material and monitoring of potential radiation exposure.
   K. Technetium half-life is 6 hours.
   L. *See also Gas Ventilation Lung Scan, Diagnostic.*

Bibliography:

Persuhn PG: Nuclear medicine: What exactly is it? Images *15*(1):11–14, 1996.

van Beek EJ: A normal perfusion lung scan in patients with clinically suspected pulmonary embolism. Frequency and clinical validity. Chest *108*(1):170–173, 1995.

Wells PS: DVT and pulmonary embolism: choosing the right diagnostic test for patients at risk. Geriatrics *50*(2):29–32, 35–36, 1995.

LUNG VOLUMES, DIAGNOSTIC
(see Pulmonary Function Test, Diagnostic)

LUPUS ANTICOAGULANT, BLOOD
(see Circulating Anticoagulant, Blood)

LUPUS ERYTHEMATOSUS CELL TEST
(see Lupus Test, Blood)

LUPUS PANEL, BLOOD
Norm:

		SI Units
Antinuclear antibody titer (ANA)	<1:20	
Anti-DNA titer	<1:10	
C3 complement, male	80–180 mg/dl	0.8–1.8 g/L
C3 complement, female	76–120 mg/dl	0.76–1.2 g/L
C4 complement, adult	15–45 mg/dl	0.15–0.45 g/L

Positive: Systemic lupus erythematosus (SLE), lupoid hepatitis, scleroderma, rheumatoid arthritis, discoid lupus, Sjögren's disease, dermatomyositis, polyarteritis, myasthenia gravis, and infectious mononucleosis.

Negative: Normal finding; lack of SLE.

Description: Three distinct laboratory tests are used to verify the diagnosis of SLE. First, antinuclear antibody (ANA), which assesses tissue-antigen antibodies, is frequently used for diagnosing SLE. Antinuclear antibodies, which are gamma globulins, react with the nuclei of all organs of people or animals. These ANAs usually belong to more than one immunoglobulin class. Immunofluorescence detects ANAs, and produces homogeneous and peripheral (RIM) staining patterns in clients with SLE. Second, anti-DNA, an antinuclear antibody, is almost always present in SLE and is present in lupus nephritis 95% of the time. Anti-DNA values may fluctuate according to the remission and exacerbation of the disease. Third, C_3 and C_4 complements are proteins that are activated into enzymes when IgG and IgM antibodies are combined with their specific antigens. These are measured during an acute and/or chronic inflammatory process. Both serum C_3 and C_4 complements will be decreased in clients with SLE.

Professional Considerations:
1. Consent form NOT required.
2. Preparation:
   A. Tube: Red-top, red/gray-top, or gold-top.
3. Procedure:
   A. Draw a 5-ml blood sample.
4. Postprocedure care:
   A. None.
5. Client and family teaching:
   A. Signs and symptoms of SLE include fatigue, fever, rash (butterfly over the nose), leukopenia, and thrombocytopenia.
   B. If positive for SLE, have daily rest periods, which will help to decrease the symptoms.
   C. Lupus Foundation of America, Inc. 4 Research Place, Suite 180 Rockville, MD 10850–3226 (800)558–0121
6. Factors that affect results:
   A. Hemolysis of the specimen invalidates the results.
   B. Several drugs may cause positive tests for ANAs. For example, clients who are receiving hydralazine or procainamide may demonstrate ANAs at increased titers, even though they do not exhibit any signs of SLE.
   C. Heat can destroy the complement components.
   D. The serum value of C3 may decrease if the sample is left standing for 1–2 hours at room temperature.
7. Other data:
   A. A positive (high) titer of ANAs does not necessarily indicate a disease process, since ANAs are present in some apparently normal clients.
   B. Some clients with connective tissue disease, or who may develop such a disease at a later time, have developed a positive titer of ANAs.
   C. A negative test for total antinuclear antibody is strong evidence that the client does not have SLE.
   D. Anti-DNA titer correlates with systemic lupus erythematosus and the occurrence of glomerulonephritis.
   E. Other tests to confirm the diagnosis of SLE include (1) anti-SM, (2) CH50, and (3) kidney and/or skin biopsy.

Bibliography:

Boackle RJ: The complement system. Immunol Serol 50:143–171, 1990.

Ginzler EM: Clinical features and complications of systemic lupus erythematosus and assessment of disease activity. Curr Opin Rheumatol 2(5):703–707, 1990.

Kamiyama M, Arkel YS, Chen K, et al.: Inhibition of platelet GP11b/IIIa binding to fibrinogen by serum factors: Studies of circulating immune complexes and platelet antibodies in platelets with hemophilia, immune thromboytopenic purpura, and systemic lupus erythematosus. J Lab Clin Med 117(3):209–217, 1991.

Lash AA: Systemic lupus erythematosus: diagnosis, treatment modalities, and nursing management, Pt 2. Dermatol Nurs 6(3):167–177, 220, 1994.

Pollard C: Lab quiz . . . systemic lupus erythematosus. Physician Assistant 17(5):72, 100–102, 1993.

Stevens MB: Systemic lupus erythematosus: the latest in diagnosis and management. J Am Acad Physician Assistants 6(4):275–282, 1993.

LUPUS TEST
(LE TEST, LE CELL TEST,
LE PREPARATION,
LE SLIDE CELL TEST,
LUPUS ERYTHEMATOSUS
CELL TEST,
LYMPHOCYTE
ERYTHEMATOUS CELL TEST),
BLOOD

Norm: Negative; no LE cells found.

Positive: Arthritis (rheumatoid), other rheumatic diseases, hepatitis, scleroderma, and systemic lupus erythematosus (SLE). Drugs include asulfidine, chlorpromazine, ethosuximide, hydralazine, isoniazid, methyldopa, penicillamine, phenytoin, practolol, primidone, procainamide, and thiouracils.

Description: This is a serologic test used to diagnose SLE and to monitor its treatment. Clients with SLE have antibodies against the components of nuclei within their own cells. This test is usually performed by traumatizing white blood cells and exposing the nuclear material within them. Then, the nuclear material is incubated with the client's serum. Neutrophils in the affected client's serum will phagocytize the traumatized nuclear material. The phagocytized complex appears as a blue-staining, amorphous mass in the neutrophil's cytoplasm, after the cells are stained with Wright's stain. When these neutrophils, which are now called LE cells, are seen, the test is considered positive.

Professional Considerations:

1. Consent form NOT required.
2. Preparation:
   A. Tube: Red-top, red/gray-top, or gold-top.
   B. Avoid heparin therapy for 2 days prior to the test.
3. Procedure:
   A. Draw a 5-ml blood sample.
   B. List on the laboratory requisition any drugs that may affect results (from the list above, under "Positive," and from the list below, section 6).
4. Postprocedure care:
   A. None.
5. Client and family teaching:
   A. No fasting is required.
   B. Discuss the signs of potential infection at the venipuncture site with the client, since clients with SLE are often immunocompromised.
6. Factors that affect results:
   A. Drugs that may cause false-negative results include heparin and steroids.
   B. Drugs that may cause false-positive results include acetazolamide, aminosalicylic acid, anticonvulsants (phenytoin [Dilantin], Mesantoin, Tridione), chlorprothixene, chlorothiazide, clofibrate, griseofluvin, isoniazid (INH), hydralazine (Apresoline), methyldopa (Aldomet), methysergide, oral contraceptives, penicillin, phenylbutazone, procainamide (Pronestyl), quinidine, reserpine, streptomycin, sulfonamides, and tetracyclines.
   C. This is a nonspecific test. False-positive results have been reported in those having rheumatoid arthritis, scleroderma, and drug-induced lupus, which was related to tetracycline, dilantin, and oral contraceptives.
   D. Reject clotted specimens. Hemolysis of the blood sample could affect the results.
7. Other data:
   A. The LE test is positive in only 60–80% of acutely ill cases.
   B. Use more sensitive tests, such as antinuclear antibodies or anti-DNA, to confirm SLE.

Bibliography: *(See also Lupus Panel.)*

Dubois EL: The lupus erythematosus cell test. *In* Dubois EL (ed): Lupus Erythematosus. A Review of the Current Status of Discoid and Systemic Lupus Erythematosus and Their Variants. Los Angeles, University of Southern California Press, 1974.

Jain A, Dash S, Marwaha N, et al.: Assays for lupus anticoagulant: The sensitivity of different assays. Med Lab Sci 48(1):31–35, 1991.

Keeling DM, Campbell SJ, Mackie IJ, et al.: Total and free protein S in systemic lupus erythematosus. Thromb Res 60(3):237–240, 1990.

Miale JB: Laboratory Medicine. Hematology, 6th ed. St Louis, MO, CV Mosby, 1982, pp 680–683, 912–913.

LUTEINIZING HORMONE, BLOOD

Norm: Ranges vary among laboratories.

		SI Units
Adult females		
Follicular phase	5–30 mIU/ml	5–30 Arb units
Midcycle	75–150 mIU/ml	75–150 Arb units
Luteal phase	3–40 mIU/ml	3–40 Arb units
Postmenopausal	30–200 mIU/ml	30–200 Arb units
Adult males	6–23 mIU/ml	6–23 Arb units
Female children		
1–3 months	7.8–27 mIU/ml	7.8–27 Arb units
3–5 months	5.6–20.8 mIU/ml	5.6–20.8 Arb units
5–7 months	5.4–21.4 mIU/ml	5.4–21.4 Arb units
7–12 months	2.1–4.7 mIU/ml	2.1–4.7 Arb units
10–13 years	2–14 mIU/ml	2–14 Arb units
14–18 years	2–29 mIU/ml	2–29 Arb units
Male children		
1–3 months	8.9–35.7 mIU/ml	8.9–35.7 Arb units
3–5 months	3.7–27.3 mIU/ml	3.7–27.3 Arb units
5–7 months	9.1–25.1 mIU/ml	9.1–25.1 Arb units
7–12 months	5.7–42.3 mIU/ml	5.7–42.3 Arb units
10–13 years	4–12 mIU/ml	4–12 Arb units
14–18 years	6–19 mIU/ml	6–19 Arb units

Usage: To evaluate infertility in women and men (high serum values of LH are related to gonadal dysfunction, and low values of LH are related to dysfunction or failure of the hypothalamus or pituitary gland); to evaluate hormonal therapy for inducing ovulation; and to evaluate endocrine problems related to precocious puberty in children.

Increased: Amenorrhea, endocrine problems related to precocious puberty in children, hyperpituitarism, Klinefelter's syndrome (e.g., sex chromosome disorder), liver disease, menopause, menstruation, ovarian or testicular failure (primary gonadal dysfunction), Stein-Leventhal syndrome (polycystic ovarian disease), tumors (pituitary, testicular), and Turner's syndrome (ovarian dysgenesis). Drugs include anticonvulsants, clomiphene, naloxone, and spironolactone.

Decreased: Adrenal hyperplasia or tumor, amenorrhea (pituitary failure; secondary gonadal insufficiency), anorexia nervosa, anovulation, hypophysectomy, hypopituitarism, hypothalamic disorder, malnutrition, pituitary disorder, and testicular failure (related to pituitary failure). Drugs include digoxin, estrogen compounds, oral contraceptives, phenothiazines, progesterone, stanozolol, and testosterone administration.

Description: Luteinizing hormone (LH), which is a gonadotropic hormone, is secreted by the anterior lobe of the pituitary gland. In women, LH initiates luteinization in the ovary, and LH and FSH induce ovulation together. A surge of LH in blood levels indicates that ovulation has occurred. The corpus luteum develops from the ruptured graafian follicle under the influence of LH. In men, LH stimulates the secretion of androgens and increases the production of testosterone. The testosterone, with FSH, influences the development and maturation of spermatozoa.

Professional Considerations:

1. Consent form NOT required.
2. Preparation:
   A. Tube: Red-top, red/gray-top, or gold-top.
   B. For females, write date of the last menstrual period on the laboratory requisition. Note if the woman is menopausal. For all clients, write their age on the laboratory requisition.
   C. Discuss with physician whether to

withhold medications that could inter-fere with the test results.

3. Procedure:
   A. Daily blood samples must be taken at the same time each day. A series of daily blood specimens can establish the presence or absence of a midcycle peak in women with anovulatory fertil-ity problems.
   B. Draw a 1-ml blood sample without he-molysis.
4. Postprocedure care:
   A. None.
5. Client and family teaching:
   A. Encourage the client to express con-cerns related to infertility or other health problems to the nurse or the physician.
   B. Episodic fluctuations in LH can be great; thus, multiple blood samples are more reliable than a single sample.
6. Factors that affect results:
   A. Hemolysis of the specimen invalidates the results.
   B. Results may be affected by the recent use of radioisotopes.
   C. Drugs that could increase or decrease plasma LH levels. (Refer to relevant sections above.)
   D. Women using oral contraceptives will have an absence of midcycle LH peak until the contraceptives are discontin-ued.
   E. Collection of the daily specimen at dif-ferent times in the day may cause inac-curate results.
7. Other data:
   A. Follicle-stimulating hormone (FSH) level may be requested from the same specimen.
   B. Progesterone, not luteinizing hor-mone, concentrations at the time of ovum transfer is a significant variable associated with miscarriage.
   C. There is no significant difference in LH levels between men who had a vasec-tomy 20 years ago and those who did not.

Bibliography:

Mo ZN: Early and late long-term effects of vasectomy on serum testosterone, dihydrotestosterone, luteinizing hormone and follicle-stimulating hor-mone levels. J Urol *154*(6):2065–2069, 1995.

Nunley WC, Urban RJ, Evans WS, et al.: Preservation of pulsatile luteinizing hormone release during postpartum lactational amenorrhea. J Clin En-docrinol Metab *73*(3):629–636, 1991.

Williams NI: Strenuous exercise with caloric restric-tion: effect on luteinizing hormone secretion. Med Sci Sports Excerc *27*(10):1390–1398, 1995.

LUTEINIZING HORMONE, URINE

Norm:

Adult female

Follicular phase	5–25 IU/24 hours
Midcycle	30–95 IU/ 24 hours
Luteal phase	2–24 IU/ 24 hours
Postmenopausal	40–100 IU/ 24 hours
Adult male	5–25 IU/ 24 hours

Increased: *See Luteinizing Hor-mone, Blood.*

Decreased: *See Luteinizing Hor-mone, Blood.*

Description: *See Luteinizing Hor-mone, Blood.* In addition, urine assays are used to monitor ovulatory cycles of clients undergoing in vitro fertiliza-tion.

Professional Considerations:

1. Consent form NOT required.
2. Preparation:
   A. Obtain a specimen container for 24-hour urine collection. (The presence of a preservative eliminates the need for refrigeration.)
   B. Label the container with the client's name, test, date, and time. For fe-males, write the date of last menstrual period on the laboratory requisition. Note if the woman is menopausal, and record her age.
3. Procedure:
   A. Discard the first morning-urine speci-men.
   B. Save all the urine voided for 24 hours in the collection container. Include the urine voided at the end of the 24-hour period. For catheterized clients, keep the drainage bag on ice and empty the urine into the collection container hourly.
   C. Refrigerate the urine, if the 24-hour container does not contain a preserva-tive.
4. Postprocedure care:
   A. Compare the urine quantity in the specimen container with the urinary output record for the test. If the speci-men contains less urine than was

recorded as output, some urine may have been discarded, thus invalidating the test.
B. Document the quantity of urine output for the collection period on the laboratory requisition.

5. Client and family teaching:
A. Save all the urine voided in the 24-hour period and urinate before defecating to avoid loss of urine. If any urine is accidentally discarded, discard the entire specimen and restart the collection the next day.

6. Factors that affect results:
A. Urine that is stored in a container without a preservative, or urine that is not refrigerated, will yield invalid results.

7. Other data:
A. The 24-hour urine collection will minimize the episodic "peak and valley" secretion of LH that may occur with blood serum specimens.
B. One or more blood samples of LH may be prescribed.

Bibliography:

Fischbach FT: A Manual of Laboratory and Diagnostic Tests, 4th ed. Philadelphia, JB Lippincott, 1992, pp 197–198.

Mo ZN: Early and late long-term effects of vasectomy on serum testosterone, dihydrotestosterone, luteinizing hormone and follicle-stimulating hormone levels. J Urol 154(6):2065–2069, 1995.

Nunley WC, Urban RJ, Evans WS, et al.: Preservation of pulsatile luteinizing hormone release during postpartum lactational amenorrhea. J Clin Endocrinol Metab 73(3):629–636, 1991.

Williams NI: Strenuous exercise with caloric restriction: effect on luteinizing hormone secretion. Med Sci Sports Excerc 27(10):1390–1398, 1995.

LYME DISEASE ANTIBODY, BLOOD

Norm: Negative.

Indirect fluorescent antibody titer: ≤1:256.
ELISA: Nonreactive.
Western blot assay: 5 bands (confirmatory test).

Increased: Indicative of recent infection or past exposure to Lyme disease.

Description: This blood test identifies antibodies to a spirochete, *Borrelia burgdorferi*. This spirochete, the agent of Lyme disease, is carried by several tick vectors, primarily the deer tick. This tick, usually Ixodes dammini, transmits Lyme disease, which is an inflammatory disorder, to humans. The ELISA is the best diagnostic test for Lyme disease. Levels of specific IgM antibodies peak during the third to sixth week after the onset of the disease and then gradually decline. Titers of specific IgG antibodies are usually low during the first several weeks of illness. The IgG antibodies will reach maximum levels months later and will often stay elevated for years. Lyme disease was first named because of its close geographic clustering in Lyme, Connecticut, in 1975. Today, it is found mostly in the northeastern, upper midwestern, and western United States.

Professional Considerations:

1. Consent form NOT required.
2. Preparation:
A. Tube: Red-top, red/gray-top, or gold-top.
B. Ask the client if there has been any recent history of a tick bite.
C. Assess for a reddish, macular lesion at the site of the tick bite and elsewhere.
3. Procedure:
A. Draw a 3-ml blood sample.
4. Postprocedure care:
A. None.
5. Client and family teaching:
A. No fasting or special preparation is required.
B. Return as prescribed for serial specimen collection.
C. A reddish, macular lesion usually occurs about 1 week after the tick bite.
D. The primary disease occurs 4–20 days after the initial bite. The secondary disease develops after 3–24 weeks of infection.
E. Arthritis (usually in the knees) is the most common complication of Lyme disease. Other complications include neuritis, meningitis, cardiac dysrhythmias, and carditis.
F. Wear clothing that covers the entire extremities when in areas infested by ticks and deer and when in the woods.
G. See a doctor immediately if bitten by a tick or if a macular lesion results from a tick bite. Antibiotic therapy will usually be started.
6. Factors that affect results:
A. False-positive results occur in 21% of clients with high rheumatoid factors.
B. There is considerable cross-reactivity in clients with treponemal disease (syphilis).
C. Reject specimens with low dilutions of serum.
7. Other data:
A. The organism may also be cultivated from cerebrospinal fluid (CSF) or skin biopsies.
B. Serial serum samples are the preferred method of measurement.
C. Seropositivity may indicate, but does not prove, infection with *Borrelia*

burgdorferi. Seronegativity usually rules out the diagnosis of Lyme disease.

Bibliography:

Luger SW, Krauss E: Serologic tests for Lyme disease. Interlaboratory variability. Arch Intern Med *158*(4):732–733, 761–763, 1990.

Newland JA: Nurse practitioner extra. Primary care protocol. Lyme disease. AJN *95*(7):160, 1995.

Powell MA: Lyme disease. J Am Acad Nurse Practitioners *5*(1):40–41, 1993.

Sigal LH: Lyme disease minus the mythology. J Musculoskeletal Med *12*(5):51–54, 57–58, 1995.

Sigal LH: Summary of the first 100 patients seen at a Lyme disease referral center. Am J Med *88*(6): 577–581, 1990.

LYMPH NODE BIOPSY, SPECIMEN

(see Biopsy, Site-Specific, Specimen)

LYMPH NODE AND RETROPERITONEAL SONOGRAM (LYMPH NODE AND RETROPERITONEAL ECHOGRAM, LYMPH NODE AND RETROPERITONEAL ULTRASOUND), DIAGNOSTIC

Norm: Lack of visualization of the lymph nodes by sonogram.

Usage: Detect retroperitoneal adenopathy or tumors, aortic or iliac lymph node enlargement from lymphoma, or other enlarged nodes, as with infection or in a nodal group. Determine retroperitoneal tumor response to therapy, without lymphangiography. Assist in planning radiation therapy treatment and in monitoring the effects of radiation treatment.

Description: Noninvasive procedure for visualizing lymph nodes and soft tissue of the retroperitoneum. An oscilloscopic picture is created from the echoes of high-frequency sound waves passing over the area (acoustic imaging). The time required for the ultrasonic beam to be reflected back to the transducer from differing densities of tissue is converted by a computer to an electrical impulse. This impulse is displayed on an oscilloscopic screen and creates a picture in transverse and longitudinal planes.

Professional Considerations:

1. Consent form NOT required.

2. Preparation:
   A. This test should be performed before intestinal barium tests, or else after the barium is cleared from the system.
   B. Obtain ultrasonic gel or paste.
   C. *See Client and family teaching.*
3. Procedure:
   A. The client is positioned supine.
   B. The area to be studied is covered with ultrasonic gel, and a lubricated transducer is passed slowly over the area in two planes: (1) The longitudinal plane is used to outline the aorta and to detect enlarged lymph nodes. The transducer is moved midline to right, then midline to left in small increments. Any abnormalities noted are marked with a grease pencil for further examination in the transverse plane. (2) The transverse plane is then scanned from the xiphoid process to the symphysis pubis.
   C. If the scan is below the umbilicus, the bladder should be full to push the bowel out of the pelvis.
   D. Photographs of the oscilloscopic display are taken.
4. Postprocedure care:
   A. Remove the lubricant from the skin.
   B. The client may void.
5. Client and family teaching:
   A. The procedure is painless and carries no risks.
   B. Ingest only clear liquids after midnight prior to the procedure. (A 12-hour fast from solid food before the test is usually required. Water is permitted.)
   C. Maintain a full bladder, if scanning is to be performed below the umbilicus. The presence of fluid in the bladder and a well-hydrated body improve the quality of the sonogram.
   D. The client must disrobe below the waist or wear a gown.
   E. The procedure takes less than 60 minutes.
6. Factors that affect results:
   A. Dehydration interferes with adequate contrast between organs and body fluids.
   B. A gas-filled, feces-filled, or barium-filled duodenum or bowel may interfere with results by preventing proper transmission and deflection of the high-frequency sound waves. This may cause confusion in diagnosing lymphadenopathy.
   C. Lymph nodes may be differentiated from the bowel by their constancy. The bowel has a changing pattern due to the movement of gas and air contents.
   D. If the study is inconclusive regarding the presence of enlarged lymph nodes, the scan should be repeated because enlarged lymph nodes are reproducible on subsequent scans.
7. Other data:
   A. Normal lymph nodes are smaller than

a fingertip (about 1.5 cm in diameter) and are not visible by sonogram.

B. Lymph nodes that are enlarged will be more homogeneous than surrounding structures.

C. Ultrasound studies of lymph nodes are often performed in conjunction with lymphangiography.

Bibliography:

Kuo CH: Sonographic features of retroperitoneal neurilemoma. J Clin Ultrasound *21*(5):309–312, 1993.

Wiener ES: Retroperitoneal node biopsy in paratesticular rhabdomyosarcoma. J Ped Surg *29*(2):171–177, 1994.

LYMPHANGIOGRAPHY (LYMPHOGRAPHY, LYMPHANGIOGRAM), DIAGNOSTIC

Norm: Normal-sized vessels and nodes containing no filling defects.

Usage: Indicated in clients with edema of lower extremities with unknown cause, Hodgkin's disease, lymphadenopathy, lymphoma, prostate cancer, tumor metastatic to the lymphatic system. Used to stage clients with lymphoma, demonstrate the extent and level of lymphatic metastasis, and evaluate the effectiveness of chemotherapy or radiation therapy.

Description: Radiographic test of the lymphatic vessels and lymph nodes. A radiopaque iodine contrast oil, such as Ethiodol, is injected into the lymphatics of the foot or hand. The dye remains in the lymph nodes for 6 months to 1 year; thus repeat plain x-rays films can be performed for follow-up of disease progression or to determine the effectiveness of the cancer treatment.

Professional Considerations:

1. Consent form IS required.

Risks:

Allergic reaction to dye (itching, hives, rash, tight feeling in the throat, shortness of breath, bronchospasm, anaphylaxis, death); renal toxicity from contrast medium; lipid pneumonia (e.g., contrast dye causes micropulmonary emboli); lymphangiitis; infection/cellulitis.

Contraindications:

Previous allergy to iodized oil, iodine preparations, contrast dye used in other x-ray tests, or shellfish are relative contraindications. If allergies exist, the radiologist may prescribe a diphenhydramine and steroid preparation, which may be given before the procedure. Then a hypoallergenic, nonionic contrast will be used during the test. Other contraindications: severe chronic lung diseases, pulmonary insufficiency, cardiac disease, and severe renal or hepatic disease.

2. Preparation:

A. Have emergency equipment readily available.

B. *See Client and family teaching.*

3. Procedure:

A. In the radiology department, the client is positioned supine on the examination table.

B. An oil-based dye is injected intradermally between each of the first three toes of each foot, in order to outline the lymphatic vessels. (The stain can also be injected into the web of the skin between the fingers.)

C. Under local anesthesia, a 1–2 inch incision is made in the dorsum of each foot (or hand) about 15–30 minutes later.

D. The lymphatic vessel is identified. This will be easily visualized after the stain is taken up.

E. A 30-gauge lymphangiographic needle with polyethylene tubing is carefully inserted into the identified lymphatic vessel. A low-rate infusion pump is used to administer an extremely low pressure, slow injection (1–1.5 hours) of iodine contrast material.

F. The flow of iodine dye is followed by fluoroscopy.

G. When the contrast material reaches the level of the third and fourth lumbar vertebra, the injection is stopped. This usually occurs in about 1½ hours.

H. Radiographs are then taken of the chest, abdomen, and pelvis. This will demonstrate the filling of the lymph nodes.

I. The cannula is removed and the incision is sutured closed after the injection of contrast is completed. The entire procedure takes about 3 hours.

J. A second set of x-ray films is often made in 24–48 hours.

4. Postprocedure care:
   A. Elevate legs to prevent swelling for 24 hours, if prescribed. Keep the client on bedrest for 24 hours, or as prescribed.
   B. Assess for signs of oil embolism every 4 hours × 24 hours (e.g., dyspnea, pain, and hypotension).
   C. Observe injection and incision sites for evidence of cellulitis (e.g., redness, drainage, swelling, pain). Monitor temperature every 4 hours × 48 hours after the procedure.
   D. The dressing is usually not changed for the first 48 hours.
   E. Allow the client to rest after the procedure.
   F. Monitor for complications, such as delayed wound healing or infection at the site of the incision or injection; edema of legs; allergic dermatitis; headache; sore mouth and throat; skin rashes; transient fever; lymphangitis; or oil embolism, which could occur if the contrast medium causes micropulmonary emboli and which could produce lipid pneumonia.
5. Client and family teaching:
   A. No fasting or sedation is required.
   B. Discomfort may be felt when the stain is injected and when the feet are anesthetized.
   C. It is important to lie very still during the injection of the contrast dye. X-ray filming usually takes about 30 minutes.
   D. The dye will turn the urine and stool blue for 48 hours. Also, IV administration of the lymphatic stain or excessive infiltration of the stain may impart a transient bluish tint to the entire skin surface.
   E. Inspect the injection and incision sites for redness, swelling, and pain, if the client will be returning home after the procedure.
   F. Sutures should be removed 7–10 days after the test.
6. Factors that affect results:
   A. Inability to cannulate lymphatic vessels.
7. Other data:
   A. To visualize axillary and supraclavicular nodes, injections are made in each hand.

Bibliography:

Athanasoulis CA, Kaufman JA, Roberts A, Struyven J, Yamada R, Zeitler E, Zollikofer CL: Controversies in vascular imaging and intervention: a panel discussion. Int Angiol 14(1):24–31, 1995.

Brader AH: Acute compartment syndrome of the thigh: Case report [letter]. Trauma 30(11):1420, 1990.

Griffith HJ, Sarno RC: Contemporary Radiology: Introduction to Imaging. Philadelphia, WB Saunders, 1979.

Whitehouse WM (ed): Diagnostic Radiology. Chicago, Year Book Medical Publishers, 1982.

LYMPHOCYTE, BLOOD

(see Differential Leukocyte Count, Peripheral Blood)

LYMPHOCYTE ERYTHEMATOUS CELL TEST

(see Lupus Test, Blood)

LYMPHOCYTE MARKER STUDIES

(see T and B Lymphocyte Subset Assay, Blood)

LYMPHOCYTE SUBSET ENUMERATION, BLOOD

(see Acquired Immune Deficiency Syndrome Evaluation Battery, Diagnostic)

LYMPHOCYTE SUBSET TYPING

(see T and B Lymphocyte Subset Assay, Blood)

LYMPHOCYTE (T & B) ASSAY

(see T and B Lymphocyte Subset Assay, Blood)

LYMPHOCYTE TRANSFORMATION TEST, BLOOD

Norm:

Mitogen: Phytohemagglutinin stimulation index: >130.
Pokeweed mitogen stimulation index: >20.
Concanavalin A stimulation index: >40.

Usage: Immunodeficiency and hypersensitivity (allergic) reactions.

Description: Blood is mixed with a plant protein (mitogen) that stimulates the transformation of lymphocytes into blast cells. A greater degree of cellular change (blastness) in a specified amount of time (up to 10 days) is indicative of poor lymphocyte production. In addition, if a substance (e.g., drug, antigen) induces a significant increase in 3H-thymidine (3H-TdR) incorporation into the lymphocytes, which have been stimulated by the mitogens, then the results indicate an immunoreactive process.

Professional Considerations:

1. Consent form NOT required.
2. Preparation:
   A. Tube: Green-top.
3. Procedure:
   A. Draw a 7-ml blood sample.
4. Postprocedure care:
   A. Write the collection time on the laboratory requisition.
   B. Send the specimen to the laboratory immediately.
5. Client and family teaching:
   A. Results are normally available within 48 hours.
6. Factors that affect results:
   A. Reject specimens received more than 2 hours after collection.
7. Other data:
   A. A large portion of normal lymphocytes undergo blastic transformation when exposed to plant proteins.
   B. Flow cytometry is a new method of performing this test, and it has been found to be more precise and reproducible and to reflect greater standardization.

Bibliography:

Bircher AJ: Lymphocyte transformation test in the diagnosis of immediate type hypersensitivity reactions to penicillins. Curr Probl Dermatol 9:31–37, 1995.

Bossa S: Evaluation of a new whole blood cytometric lymphocyte transformation test for immunologic screening. J Clin Lab Immunol 40(1):39–46, 1993.

Kristofferson A: Effect of zimeldine and its metabolites on [3H]thymidine incorporation in lymphocyte cultures from psychiatric patients with or without a hypersensitivity reaction during zimeldine therapy. Int Clin Psychopharmacol 9(3):179–185, 1994.

LYMPHOGRANULOMA VENEREUM TITER (LGV), BLOOD

Norm: Negative; indirect fluorescent antibody titer ≤1:64.

Usage: *Chlamydia psittaci* infections; and *Chlamydia trachomatis* infections, which are associated with *Lymphogranuloma venereum* (LGV). In women, chlamydia could cause pelvic inflammatory disease, endometriosis, or salpingitis. In men, chlamydia could cause Reiter's syndrome or epididymitis. Perihepatitis (Fitz-Hugh-Curtis syndrome) has also been linked to chlamydia.

Description: Indirect fluorescent antibody test, which is useful in identifying chlamydia antibodies. The bacterium *C. trachomatis* is associated with human diseases ranging from blinding trachoma to sexually acquired genital infections and the systemic disease LGV. LGV is a venereal infection caused by the L-1, L-2, or L-3 serotype of *C. trachomatis*. A primary lesion is followed by rapid swelling of regional lymph nodes.

Professional Considerations:

1. Consent form NOT required.
2. Preparation:
   A. Tube: Red-top, red/gray-top, or gold-top.
3. Procedure:
   A. Draw a 7-ml blood sample.
   B. Draw a convalescent sample in 10–14 days.
4. Postprocedure care:
   A. None.
5. Client and family teaching:
   A. Return in 2 weeks to have a follow-up sample drawn.
6. Factors that affect results:
   A. Failure to collect a convalescent sample may indicate that the disease has not been fully treated.
7. Other data:
   A. A fourfold increase in titer indicates acute infection.
   B. Clients being evaluated for LGV should also be tested for syphilis.
   C. Diagnosis of *C. psittaci* should include a record of prior contact with sick birds (parrots) or employment in pet shops.
   D. Direct fluorescent test or ELISA on clinical specimens is now preferred over chlamydia antibody titer.

Bibliography:

Bauwens JE: Infection with *Chlamydia trachomatis* lymphogranuloma venereum serovar L1 in homosexual men with proctitis: molecular analysis of an unusual case cluster. Clin Infect Dis 20(3):576–581, 1995.

Burgoyne RA: Lymphogranuloma venereum. Prim Care 17(1):153–157, 1990.

Fred HL: Case in point. Lymphogranuloma venereum. Hosp Pract 30(3):31, 1995.

Starnbach MN: Murine cytotoxic T lymphocytes induced following *Chlamydia trachomatis* intraperitoneal or genital tract infection respond to cells infected with multiple serovars. Infect Immun 63(9):3527–3530, 1995.

LYMPHOGRAPHY
(see Lymphangiography, Diagnostic)

LYMPHS
(see Differential Leukocyte Count, Peripheral Blood)

LYSOZYME, SERUM
(see Muramidase, Serum)

MAGNESIUM, SERUM

Norm:

		SI Units
Normal levels		
Newborn	1.2–2.9 mEq/L	0.6–1.45 mmol/L
Child	1.6–2.6 mEq/L	0.8–1.3 mmol/L
Adult	1.3–2.5 mEq/L	0.65–1.25 mmol/L
	or 1.8–3.0 mg/dl	
Panic level	>3.0 mg/dl or	
	<0.5 mEq/L	
Toxic level	>12.0 mEq/L	

Panic Level Symptoms and Treatment: High Magnesium

Symptoms: Lethargy, drowsiness, flushing, nausea, vomiting, slurred speech, hypotension, weak or absent deep tendon reflexes, electrocardiogram changes (e.g., prolonged PR and Q-T intervals, widened QRS, bradycardia), respiratory depression.

Treatment: Withholding source of magnesium excess, promoting excretion, giving calcium salts, hemodialysis.

Panic Level Symptoms and Treatment: Low Magnesium

Symptoms: Muscle tremors, twitching, tetany, hypocalcemia, hyperactive deep tendon reflexes, electrocardiogram changes (e.g., prolonged PR and Q-T intervals, broad flat T-waves, premature ventricular contractions, ventricular tachycardia, fibrillation), anorexia, nausea, vomiting, lethargy, insomnia.

Treatment:

Administer magnesium salts intravenously (8–16 mol magnesium sulfate in 10–100 ml D5W over 10–15 minutes, followed by 40 mmol magnesium sulfate in 500 ml D5W over 5 hours.

Reduce auditory, mechanical, and visual stimuli.

Monitor for respiratory depression and areflexia if intravenous magnesium sulfate is given.

Monitor for diarrhea and metabolic alkalosis if oral magnesium replacement is given.

Increased: Addison's disease, adrenalectomy, ataxia, dehydration (severe), diabetes (uncontrolled diabetes, diabetic acidosis before treatment, controlled diabetes in an older client), dysrhythmias, hypercalcemia, hypothyroidism, hypophosphatemia, kidney stone, leukemia (lymphocytic and myelocytic), nephrolithiasis, and renal insufficiency or failure. Drugs include antacids containing magnesium (e.g., Maalox, Mylanta, Aludrox, DiGel, milk of magnesium), calcium-containing medication, cathartics, ethacrynic acid, laxatives (e.g., epsom salts, magnesium citrate), loop diuretics, and thyroid medications.

Decreased: Acute tubular necrosis (diuretic phase), alcoholism (chronic), aldosteronism, Bartter's syndrome, bowel resection complications, convulsions, diabetic ketoacidosis, diarrhea (chronic), dysrhythmias, excessive lactation, excessive sweating, hepatitis, hepatic cirrhosis, hepatic insufficiency, hungry bone syndrome, hypokalemia, hypercalcemia, hyperthyroidism, hypoparathyroidism, hyperthyroidism, hypocalcemia, hypoparathyroidism, IV solutions without magnesium, ketoacidosis, kwashiorkor (severe malnutrition), laxative abuse, magnesium-deficiency tetany syndrome, pancreatitis (chronic, acute), phosphate depletion, postobstructive diuresis, postoperatively, primary hyperaldosteronism, prolonged gastric drainage, reduced magnesium intake, reduced magnesium absorption (specific magnesium malabsorption, generalized malabsorption syndrome, excessive bowel resections, diffuse bowel disease or injury), renal disease (chronic), renal defect of magnesium resorption, renal transplant, renal tubular acidosis, stress states with catecholamine excess, tetany, toxemia of pregnancy, ulcerative colitis, volume expansion (extracellular fluid). Drugs include alcohol, amphotericin B, some antibiotics (neomycin, aminoglycosides), calcium gluconate, cisplatinum, corticosteroids, cyclosporine, diuretics (e.g., mercurial, ethacrynic acid), glucose, insulin, mannitol, and urea.

Description: Measurement of magnesium levels is used as an index to (1) metabolic activity in the body (e.g., such as carbohydrate metabolism, protein synthesis, nucleic acid synthesis, contraction of muscular tissue), and (2) renal function, since 95% of magnesium that is filtered through the glomerulus is reabsorbed in the tubules. Most of the body's magnesium, which is an electrolyte, is concentrated in the bone, cartilage, and within the cell itself. In addition, magnesium is needed in the blood clotting mechanism, regulates neuromuscular irritability, acts as a cofactor that modifies the activity of many enzymes, and has a significant effect on the metabolism of calcium.

Professional Considerations:

1. Consent form NOT required.
2. Preparation:
   A. Tube: Red-top, red/gray-top, or gold-top or green-top.
   B. Do NOT draw during hemodialysis.
   C. *See Client and family teaching.*
3. Procedure:
   A. Draw a 1-ml blood sample without hemolysis.
4. Postprocedure care:
   A. Separate serum from the red blood cells within 6 hours.
   B. If storage is necessary, refrigerate the specimen.
   C. Serum separated from the cells is stable for 2–3 days.
5. Client and family teaching:
   A. No special diet or fasting is required before sampling.
   B. Eat foods rich in magnesium (e.g., seafood, meats, green vegetables, whole grains, and nuts) if magnesium level is low.
   C. Avoid constant use of antacids or laxatives containing magnesium, if magnesium level is high. Check drug labels to identify magnesium-containing formulations.
6. Factors that affect results:
   A. Hemolysis of the specimen will create falsely elevated levels of magnesium.
   B. Glucuronic acid therapy will interfere with the color reaction in some laboratory methods and will produce falsely decreased results.
   C. Prolonged intravenous fluid therapy, hyperalimentation, exchange blood transfusions, or prolonged nasogastric suctioning may yield falsely decreased results.
   D. Prolonged use of magnesium products (e.g., antacids, laxatives), lithium, or salicylate therapy will cause falsely increased levels, especially if renal damage is present.
   E. Hyperbilirubinemia interferes with serum magnesium, resulting in misleadingly low levels.
   F. High phosphate diet suppresses both magnesium and calcium absorption.
7. Other data:
   A. Nutritional status is important to the interpretation of the test results.
   B. If hypocalcemia is present, magnesium should also be measured. Magnesium deficiency may cause apparently unexplained hypocalcemia and hypokalemia.
   C. Respiratory failure and death are possible when magnesium levels exceed 12 mEq/L.
   D. Magnesium level may be decreased after surgery for hyperparathyroidism.

Bibliography:

Filos D, Okorodudu AO: A method for the measurement of ionized magnesium. Laboratory Medicine *26*(1):70–74, 1995.

Gaedeke MK: Lab test tips. Evaluating serum magnesium levels. Nursing *25*(8):75, 1995.

McCoy S, MacLaren NK, Gudat JC: Bilirubin interferes in the ACA determination of magnesium in serum. Clin Chem *29*:1309, 1983.

Ryan MF: The role of magnesium in clinical biochemistry: An overview. Ann Clin Biochem *28*(1): 19–26, 1991.

Toto KH, Yucha CB: Magnesium: homeostasis, imbalances, and therapeutic uses. Crit Care Nursing Clin North Am *6*(4):767–783, 1994.

MAGNESIUM, 24-HOUR, URINE

Norm:

	SI Units
5–16 mEq/24 hours	2.5–8.0 µmol/24 hours

Increased: Alcoholism, Bartter's syndrome, hypermagnesemia, and nephrolithiasis. Drugs include aldosterone, cisplatin, corticosteroids, diuretics (ethacrynic acid), and thiazide.

Decreased: Renal disease, kidney stone, magnesium deficit, osteoporosis, and syndrome of inappropriate antidiuretic hormone secretion (SIADHS).

Description: A 24-hour urine test, which is useful in the evaluation of renal disease and magnesium deficiency. In magnesium deficiency, urine magnesium decreases before serum magnesium. *See also Magnesium, Blood.*

Professional Considerations:

1. Consent form NOT required.
2. Preparation:
   A. Obtain a 3-L, acid-washed, metal-free urine collection container without preservatives.
3. Procedure:
   A. Instruct the client to void and discard the initial specimen.
   B. Collect all the urine voided in a 24-hour period in a 3-L, acid-washed, metal-free container without preservatives. The specimen should be maintained on wet ice throughout the collection period.
   C. Do not collect urine in a metal bedpan or urinal.
4. Postprocedure care:
   A. Record total 24-hour urine volume, and exact beginning and ending times of collection on the container and the laboratory requisition.
   B. Send the specimen to the laboratory on wet ice.
5. Client and family teaching:
   A. Save all the urine voided in the 24-hour period in the plastic, not metal, container provided. If any urine is accidentally discarded, throw out the entire specimen and restart the collection the next day.
6. Factors that affect results:
   A. Reject any urine specimen that has had contact with metal.
   B. Increased blood alcohol level increases urinary magnesium excretion.
7. Other data:
   A. Normal values may vary with different laboratory methods.
   B. Urinary excretion of magnesium is diet dependent.

Bibliography:

Alfrey AC: Disorders of magnesium metabolism. *In* Schrier RW (ed): Renal and Electrolyte Disorders, 2nd ed. Boston, Little, Brown, 1980, pp 299–319.

Flatman PW: Mechanisms of magnesium transport. Ann Rev Physiol *53*:259–271, 1991.

Ryan MF: The role of magnesium in clinical biochemistry: An overview. Ann Clin Biochem *28*(1):19–26, 1991.

Toto KH, Yucha CB: Magnesium: homeostasis, imbalances, and therapeutic uses. Crit Care Nursing Clin North Am *6*(4):767–783, 1994.

MAGNETIC RESONANCE ANGIOGRAPHY (MRA), DIAGNOSTIC

Norm: Anatomy of normal vessels are well visualized, and blood flow is unobstructed.

Usage: Evaluate vascular structure; evaluate blood flow, especially in the venous system, for possible aneurysms, stenosis, thromboses, or blockages; determine tumor vascularity; assess for evidence of direct tumor involvement of vascular structures; evaluate clients with carotid stenosis preoperatively so that the carotid artery endarterectomy is performed with decreased complication; assist in diagnosis of cerebrovascular disease, cardiovascular disease, cerebral arteriovenous malformations, congenital heart disease, renal or hepatic vasculature pathology, trigeminal neuralgia; assess effectiveness of various therapeutic interventions related to vascular structure and blood flow.

Description: Magnetic resonance angiography (MRA) is a recently developed, noninvasive vascular imaging technique. This procedure is performed using the magnetic resonance imaging (MRI) scanner equipment, and MRA may be performed in conjunction with MRI. MRA provides structural evaluation of arteries and veins, and image of blood flow. The two types of MRA are time-of-fight (TOF) and phase contrast (PC). TOF angiography uses a process described as "flow-related enhancement," which relies on the inflow of fully magnetized blood into the imaging plane. PC angiography directly measures flow by generating vascular images. These images detect changes in the phase of the blood's transverse magnetization as it moves along a magnetic field gradient. Therefore, it relies on alterations in spin phase for image contrast. Both of these methods emphasize the signals in the structures, which contain blood flow, and reconstruct only those structures with flow.

The computer subtracts images of other structures, which are of lesser interest, from the image. Both of these methods can obtain two- or three-dimensional images. MRA can be performed without injection of contrast or radiation exposure. However, some radiologists prefer using a contrast, such as gadolinium-chelate or gadolium-DTPA, to enhance the visualization of venous flow.

Professional Considerations:

1. Consent form IS required.

Risks:

Critical injury to the client could result from ferrous metal in the body (e.g., flecks of ferrous metal in eye could cause retinal hemorrhage).

Contraindications:

Intracranial aneurysm clips and intraocular metal foreign bodies; heart valves manufactured prior to 1964 and middle ear prosthetics (these can be tested by obtaining a duplicate, placing it into the bore, and if no torque is experienced, the test may be safely performed). Nerve-stimulating devices may be a contraindication.

Precautions:

Pregnant women should not be scanned unless absolutely necessary, although there is no evidence of teratogenic or developmental abnormalities associated with MRI or MRA imaging. Sedatives are contraindicated in clients with central nervous system depression.

2. Preparation:
   A. *See Preparation, MRI.*
3. Procedure:
   A. *See Procedure, MRI.*
4. Postprocedure care:
   A. If the client has been sedated for the procedure, make certain that he or she is fully awake before ambulating, and follow institutional protocol for postsedation monitoring.
5. Client and family teaching:
   A. This procedure may take 15–30 minutes to perform.
   B. *See Client and family teaching, MRI.*

6. Factors that affect results:
   A. *See Factors that affect results, MRI.*
7. Other data:
   A. The same MRI scanner equipment, with different software and pulse sequences, is used to perform MRA.
   B. The results of MRA are beginning to guide medical management and determine the extent of surgical intervention.
   C. The use of MRA versus conventional angiography remains controversial.

Bibliography:

Athanasoulis CA, Kaufman JA, Roberts A, et al.: Controversies in vascular imaging and interventions: a panel discussion. Int Angiol *14*(1):24–31, 1995.

Endres D, Manaligod J, Simonson T, Funk G, McCulloch T: The role of magnetic resonance angiography in head and neck surgery. Laryngoscope 105(10):1069–1076, 1995.

Hartnell GO, Hughes LA, Longmaid HE, Finn JP: Body magnetic resonance angiography and its effect on the use of alternative imaging—experience in 1026 patients. British J Radiol *68*(813):963–969, 1995.

Lamparello PJ, Riles TS: MR Angiography in carotid stenosis. A clinical perspective. Magn Reson Imaging Clin North Am *3*(3):455–465, 1995.

Lau F: Magnetic resonance angiography (MRA) . . . an applied radiology patient education chart. Appl Radiol *23*(8):21–22, 1994.

Turski P (ed): Vascular Magnetic Resonance Imaging: Signa Applications Guide, Vol 3. Milwaukee, WI, GE Medical Systems, 1990.

MAGNETIC RESONANCE IMAGING (MRI), DIAGNOSTIC

Norm: Description of normal tissue, structure, and blood flow.

Usage: To detect abscesses, abnormalities in blood flow through coronary branches and through extremities, acute tubular necrosis, adenopathy, aortic and ventricular aneurysm, atrial and ventricular septal defects, avascular necrosis, blood clots, cancer and tumors (brain, bone, extra-axial, head, intracardiac, hilar, mediastinal, neck, parenchymal, pericardiac, pituitary, pulmonary, renal, sarcoma, and spinal cord), cavernous hemangioma, cerebral infarction, congenital heart disease, cysts, dementia, demyelinating disease, edema, epilepsy, focal viral encephalitis, Gaucher's disease, glomerulonephritis, hemorrhage, hydronephrosis, hyperparathyroidism, infection, intervertebral disc abnormalities, knee abnormalities, Marfan's syndrome, myocardial infarction, multiple sclerosis, muscular disease, osteomyelitis, plaque formation, pulmonary atresia, renal transplants, renal vein thrombosis, seizures, shoulder abnormalities, skeletal abnormalities, soft tissue infections, spinal cord compression or injuries, subarachnoid hemorrhage, temporomandibular joint abnormalities, tumor invasion (inferior vena cava and seminal vesicles), and tumor staging (cervix, large hydronephroma, prostate, urinary bladder, and uterus).

Description: MRI is a noninvasive diagnostic tool that enables health care professionals to visualize the body's tissues, structure, and blood flow. It uses a strong magnetic field, in conjunction with radio frequency waves, to transmit signals from the body's cells to a computer. MRI actually stimulates the body to produce a signal of itself. The computer produces cross-sectional images of the body. The cell's nuclei react as tiny magnets in the presence of a strong external magnetic field (MRI). The multiple body plane images' signal density depends primarily on the tissue characteristics, pulse sequence, and timing parameters. It is painless and has no known side effects. MRI is the standard in the diagnosis of most abnormalities of the brain and spine (except trauma). The ability of MRI to support the diagnosis of multiple sclerosis declines with increasing age of the client. MRI eliminates the need for many knee arthroscopies and has virtually replaced arthrography. Unlike computerized axial tomographic (CAT) scans, MRI can evaluate cerebral infarction within hours of the event. MRI virtually eliminates the need for myelography. MRI is of limited use in the evaluation of ischemic heart disease.

Professional Considerations:
1. Consent form IS required. 1–2% of people refuse MRI due to claustrophobia.

Risks:
Critical injury to the client could result from ferrous metal in the body (e.g., flecks of ferrous metal in eye could cause retinal hemorrhage).

Contraindications:
Intracranial aneurysm clips and intraocular metal foreign bodies; heart valves manufactured prior to 1964 and middle ear prosthetics (these can be tested by obtaining a duplicate, placing it into the bore, and if no torque is experienced, the test may be safely performed); nerve-stimulating devices may be a contraindication.

Precautions:
Pregnant women should not be scanned unless absolutely necessary, although there is no evidence of teratogenic or developmental abnormalities associated with MRI. Radiologists and operators must be informed of the presence of cardiac pacemakers and implanted venous access devices, although they are rarely a contraindication. Most stainless steel orthopedic implants and prosthetic devices are not ferromagnetic and are not affected by MRI. Sedatives are contraindicated in clients with central nervous system depression.

2. Preparation:
   A. Screen the client for cardiac pacemaker, artificial heart valve, brain aneurysm clips, neurostimulate (TENS Unit), implanted insulin pump, implanted venous access infusion devices, bone growth stimulator, internal electrodes, embolic spring coil, eye implant surgery (with staples), cochlear implant, hearing aid, foil or metallic medication patches, pregnancy, shrapnel, metal fragments (in head, eye, skin), history of work in the machine tool industry, history of work with a metal lathe, or history of any accidents with metal or ferromagnetic objects (beebee guns, flecks of ferrous metal in eye). These items may be hazardous to the client's safety.
   B. Screen the accompanying adult for the above items, if the client undergoing the procedure is a pediatric client.
   C. Screen the client for a shunt, any type of surgical clip or staple, any orthopaedic item(s) (such as pins, wires, rods, screws, clips, plates, etc.), artificial limb or joint, dental braces, any type of removable dental item, IUD, eye makeup, clothing with metal snaps or zippers, metal hair barrettes or rubber bands, metal earrings, pen clip, or light-up shoes or steel-toed shoes. These items may interfere with the MR imaging.

D. Remove any loose metal objects (e.g., hairpins, barettes, watches, etc.), as they can become projectile in the magnetic force.

E. Inform the physician if the client is on an IV controller pump, or computerized equipment, since the magnets in the MRI can disrupt the function of the machine (e.g., IV flow).

F. Elicit any problems with claustrophobia. Relaxation techniques or a sedative may be used. Determine availability of an "open MRI."

G. If the client is very young or unable to follow directions, sedation may be indicated in order to complete the scan.

H. Start an IV line, if contrast is to be given.

3. Procedure:
A. The client is positioned on a padded table and moved into the cylinder-shaped scanner (e.g., magnet bore).

B. Contrast may be administered before the procedure, if prescribed.

C. The technologist will operate controls determining image signal density, pulse sequence, and timing parameters.

D. If blood flow is to be determined in an extremity, then the arm or leg to be examined is placed in a cradlelike support. The technologist will mark reference sites to be imaged on the arm or leg. Then the extremity is moved into a flow cylinder.

E. The MR image is interpreted by a radiologist, who is specially trained.

4. Postprocedure care:
A. Continue the assessment of respiratory status after receiving sedation. If deep sedation was used, follow institutional protocol for postsedation monitoring. Typical monitoring includes continuous ECG monitoring and pulse oximetry, with continual assessments (q 5–15 minutes) of airway, vital signs, and neurologic status until the client is lying quietly awake, is breathing independently, and responds to commands spoken in a normal tone.

B. Remove the IV, if one was inserted for injection of the contrast.

5. Client and family teaching:
A. You will lie on a flat, narrow, padded surface and will be rolled into a cylinder-shaped scanner. The scanner will be around the area of the body that is being scanned.

B. You will hear various noises from the test, including a muffled drumbeat sound. You may bring in earplugs for the test or use the earplugs that are available. In an open MRI machine, inform the client that there are no loud noises.

C. You can communicate with MRI personnel, who will be in another room, via an intercom system.

D. It is important to remain completely still during the scan.

E. Remove jewelry, watches, hairpins, glasses, and any metal objects. The magnetic field can damage watches.

F. Do not approach the MRI unit if you have a cardiac pacemaker.

G. You will not be exposed to radiation during this procedure. The contrast medium that may be used is not an iodinated contrast.

H. The procedure may take 45–90 minutes to scan the head or chest area, and approximately 15 minutes to scan an arm or leg.

6. Factors that affect results:
A. The image will be distorted by movement during the procedure.

B. Metal, whether ferrous or nonferrous, may produce artifacts that degrade the images, if the metal is in close proximity to the area of the body that is being scanned.

C. Because of the possibility of loss of data contained on magnetic recording media, MRI systems are normally contained within a restricted magnetic range, from 15 to 50 gauss.

D. MRI does not use ionizing radiation; therefore, there are none of the hazards found in x-rays.

7. Other data:
A. Intravenous gadolinium DTPA contrast, which is a commercially available contrast medium, may be necessary for some examinations at the discretion of the radiologist. This contrast is chemically unrelated to the iodinated contrast, which is used in conventional radiography.

B. Magnetophosphenes (flickering lights in the visual field) that can occur with MRI are completely reversible and have no known long-term health effects.

C. The Food and Drug Administration (FDA) has classified MRI devices into class II, which includes low-risk devices.

Bibliography:

Brand KP: How well is your patient prepared for an MRI? An insider's perspective. Cancer Nurs *17*(6):512–515, 1994.

Center for Devices and Radiological Health: Guidelines for Evaluating Electromagnetic Exposure Risk for Trials of Clinical NMR Systems. U.S. Food and Drug Administration, 1982.

Runge VM, Gelblum DY: Future directions in magnetic resonance contrast media. Top Magn Reson Imaging *3*(2):85–97, 1991.

Sharpe P: MRI review. Increase in units and interest. Radiography Today *61*(697):57, 1995.

Shellock FG, Croes JV III: Safety of MRI in patients with metallic implants or foreign bodies. Appl Radiol *21*(11):44–48, 1992.

Stark DD, Bradley WG: Magnetic Resonance Imaging. St Louis, MO, CV Mosby, 1988.

Tranter J: The use of magnetic resonance imaging in diagnosis. Nurs Times *91*(13):38–39, 1995.

Yamashita K, Hiroshima K, Kurata A: Gadolinium DTPA—enhanced magnetic resonance imaging of a sequestered lumbar intervertebral disc and its correlation with pathologic findings. Spine *19*(4):479–482, 1994.

MAGNETIC RESONANCE SPECTOGRAPHY (MRS), DIAGNOSTIC

Norm: Norms continue to be developed, since this is a very new diagnostic modality. Qualitative and quantitative cellular biochemical data, such as steady-state cellular concentrations of metabolites, are visible with MRS.

Usage: Provide follow-up and prognosis for clients with AIDS, cancer and tumors, diabetes mellitus, hepatic encephalopathy, intracranial mass, metabolic disorders, neurodegeneration, stroke, systemic lupus erythematosus (SLE); detect degeneration, inflammation, and necrosis in tissues; and monitoring and evaluation of therapeutic interventions, in conjunction with MRI. Future application may include detection of changes at the cellular level that precede morphologic changes detected with MRI or other radiologic imaging modalities.

Description: Magnetic resonance spectography (MRS) is a recently developed noninvasive vascular imaging technique. This procedure is performed using the magnetic resonance imaging (MRI) scanner equipment, and different software. Two types of MRS include the proton MRS and phosphorus-31 (P-31) MRS. The MRS describes the molecular state of water, the chemical environment of cells and tissues, and the qualitative and quantitative state of intermediary metabolism. It can produce specific metabolite profiles in various pathologies.

Professional Considerations:

1. Consent form IS required.

Risks:

Critical injury to the client could result from ferrous metal in the body (e.g., flecks of ferrous metal in eye could cause retinal hemorrhage).

Contraindications:

Intracranial aneurysm clips and intraocular metal foreign bodies; heart valves manufactured prior to 1964 and middle ear prosthetics (these can be tested by obtaining a duplicate, placing it into the bore, and if no torque is experienced, the test may be safely performed). Nerve-stimulating devices may be a contraindication.

---

2. Preparation:
   A. *See Preparation, MRI.*
3. Procedure:
   A. *See Procedure, MRI.*
   B. MRS always needs to be performed prior to contrast, since contrast may affect the expression of metabolites.
   C. In order to obtain the best image, the areas to be avoided in MRS include frontal and ethmoid sinuses; temporal bones, deep-in-posterior fossa; subcutaneous fat; and areas of high flow or hypervascular pathology.
4. Postprocedure care:
   A. *See Postprocedure care, MRI.*
5. Client and family teaching:
   A. *See Client and family teaching, MRI.*
6. Factors that affect results:
   A. *See Factors that affect results, MRI.*
   B. Many factors influence the profile of the MR spectra, including magnetic field uniformity, interclient variability, age, and developmental stage. Normal metabolite ratios change substantially during development, particularly from birth to 2 years of age. Quantification of metabolites is difficult due to the complexity of the spectra.
7. Other data:
   A. MRS may be performed in conjunction with MRI.

Bibliography:

Davie CA: Proton magnetic resonance spectoscopy of systemic lupus erythematosus involving the central nervous system. J Neurol 242(8):522–528, 1995.

Dunn RS: Proton Spectroscopy. [Copyrighted material]. Cincinnati, OH, Children's Hospital Medical Center, Imaging Research Center, 1994.

Karpen M: Using spectroscopy to predict clinical onset of AIDS. AIDS Patient Care 7(2):75–77, 1993.

Negendank W: Studies of human tumors by MRS: a review. NMR Biomed 5(5):303–324, 1992.

Ross BD: The biochemistry of living tissues: examination by MRS. Nucl Magn Reson Biochem 5(5): 215–219, 1992.

Tzika AA, Vigneron DB, Ball WS, Dunn RS, Kirks DR: Localized proton MR spectroscopy of the brain in children. JMRI 3:719–729, 1993.

Van Wassenaer-van Hall HN, van der Grond J, van Hattum J, Kooijman C, Hoogenraad TU, Mali WP: 31P magnetic resonance spectroscopy of the liver: correlation with standardized serum, clinical, and histological changes in diffuse liver disease. Hepatology 21(2):443–449, 1995.

MALARIA SMEAR, BLOOD

Norm: Negative.

Positive: Malaria (one of four plasmodium species: *P. falciparum, P. vivax, P. malariae, P. ovale*) and trypanosomiasis.

Description: Malaria is a contact disease caused by a plasmodia. The parasites, which are in the salivary glands of the anopheline mosquito, are introduced into the bloodstream of the human via mosquito bites. The parasites enter the cells of the liver, where they multiply without causing recognizable disease. A few days later, spores multiply asexually and fill red blood cells, destroying them and leading to fever and chills in the human.

Professional Considerations:

1. Consent form NOT required.
2. Preparation:
   A. Tube: Lavender-top.
   B. Obtain a lancet, six glass slides, and Giemsa's stain.
   C. Monitor the client's temperature every 4 hours, or as indicated.
   D. Report chills and fever to the physician.
   E. Obtaining specimens prior to fever spike is preferable.
   F. Include on the laboratory requisition any recent travel, including country and dates.
3. Procedure:
   A. Draw a 4-ml blood sample.
   B. Obtain fresh fingersticks (two or three each of thick and thin film on glass slides) stained with Giemsa's stain.
4. Postprocedure care:
   A. None.
5. Client and family teaching:
   A. Inform the nurse when having chills.
6. Factors that affect results:
   A. Hemolysis of the specimen invalidates the results.
   B. The level of parasitemia varies from hour to hour (especially for *Plasmodium falciparum* infections).
7. Other data:
   A. Blood samples are usually drawn when fever and chills are present daily for three days at specified times, such as every 6 or 12 hours.
   B. The smear is considered positive if ≥ 2–30% of the red blood cells are infected.
   C. Blood should be examined several times a day for 2–3 days because results are seldom greater than 2% of the total cells.
   D. In *P. falciparum* malaria, severe parasitemia is 10% total infected cells and may reach levels of 20–30% or more.
   E. Clinical signs and symptoms may include myalgias, arthralgias, chills, fever of unknown origin, drenching sweat, fatigue, nausea, vomiting, abdominal pain, diarrhea, splenomegaly, hepatomegaly, and jaundice.
   F. American trypanosomiasis (Chagas' disease) and African trypanosomiasis (sleeping disease) are two diseases caused by trypanosomes, which are flagellated protozoans.
   G. A new nonradioactive DNA diagnostic procedure is available to detect malaria infection, which may aid in determining the diagnosis.

Bibliography:

Ayyanathan K Datta S: A non-radioactive DNA diagnostic procedure for the detection of malarial infection: general application to genome with repetitive sequences. Mol Cell Probes *9*(2):83–89, 1995.

Hoffman SL: Diagnosis, treatment, and prevention of malaria. Med Clin North Am *76*(6):1327–1355, 1992.

Teglia MQ, Teglia O, Santiago S, Cunha BA: Falciparum malaria. Emergency Medicine *23*(11): 165–168, 172–173, 1991.

Waldman RH, Kluge RM (eds): Textbook of Infectious Diseases. New Hyde Park, NY, Medical Examination Publishing Company, 1984.

MAMMOGRAM
(see Mammography, Diagnostic)

MAMMOGRAPHY (MAMMOGRAM), DIAGNOSTIC

Norm: Radiographic image of normal breast tissue. Calcification, if present, is evenly distributed. Normal duct contrast with gradual narrowing of branches of the ductal system is evident.

Positive: Benign or malignant masses in the breast tissue or nipple. Radiographic signs of breast cancer include asymmetric density; a poorly defined spiculated mass; fine, stippled clustered calcifications, which are seen as white specks on the x-ray film; and skin thickening. Malignant cancers are irregular and poorly defined, and tend to be unilateral.

Negative: Normal finding.

Usage: Indicated to detect tumors, which are clinically nonpalpable, in women over age 40, as part of routine screening; to survey the opposite breast after mastectomy; to screen for breast cancer in clients at high risk (e.g., family history of breast cancer); to screen pendulous breasts, which are difficult to examine; to evaluate breasts when symptoms are present, such as skin changes, nipple or skin retraction, nipple discharge or erosion, breast pain, "lumpy" breast (e.g., multiple masses or nodules); to rule out breast cancer in a client with adenocarcinoma of undetermined site; to localize a mass before a biopsy is performed; to follow up after a previous breast biopsy; and to follow up after cancer treatment (e.g., surgery, radiation, chemotherapy) to determine its effectiveness. Used to diagnose benign breast masses, cysts, or abscesses; benign breast calcifications; breast cancer; fibrocystic breasts; intraductal papilloma of the breast; occult cancer (search in those with metastatic disease and unknown primary); suppurative mastitis; and Paget's disease of the breast.

Description: Mammography is a soft tissue radiographic examination of the breast. Careful interpretation of these x-ray films can detect cancer, even before they become palpable lesions. The accuracy of breast cancer detection with mammography is approximately 85%, and gives less than 10% false-positive diagnoses. It is believed that survival rates are improved with early detection of breast cancer. A "xeromammogram" provides the same information as a routine mammogram, and has the same risks and benefits. However, xeromammograms are positive prints, unlike regular x-rays which are negative prints. This test has four views: oblique, lateral, craniocaudal, and chest wall. At least two views of each breast should be performed, one of which should be the chest wall.

Professional Considerations:

1. Consent form IS required.

Risks:

The National Cancer Institute (United States) has estimated the risk of mammographically induced carcinogenesis to be 3.5 cancers per 1 million women per year per rad for Western women over the age of 30 years at the time of exposure after a latent period of about 10 years.

Contraindications:

In clients who are pregnant, due to the potential risk of fetal damage.

2. Preparation:
   A. Ask client to identify areas of lumps or thickening, if any.
   B. Ask the client if she is pregnant.

C. Be supportive. Allow time for questions and for verbalization of feelings.
D. *See Client and family teaching.*

3. Procedure:
   A. The client is taken to the radiology department and is seated in front of the mammography machine.
   B. The breast(s) is/are exposed, and one breast is placed on the x-ray plate.
   C. The x-ray cone is brought down on top of the breast to compress it gently between the broadened cone and the x-ray plate.
   D. The x-ray film is exposed. This creates the craniocaudal view.
   E. The x-ray plate is turned perpendicular to the floor, and then it is placed laterally on the outer aspect of the breast.
   F. The broadened cone is brought in medially, and the breast is gently compressed. This is the lateral, or axillary, view.
   G. Occasionally, a third view, the oblique view, is required. At least two views of each breast should be performed.
   H. This procedure is performed in 10–20 minutes by a radiologic technician.

4. Postprocedure care:
   A. Inform client that the x-ray films must be interpreted by a radiologist.
   B. Often the technologist or radiologist will palpate the breasts.

5. Client and family teaching:
   A. The mammogram takes 10–20 minutes for both breasts to be x-rayed.
   B. Fasting is not required. Mammography is the single best method for detecting breast cancer in a curable stage.
   C. Some discomfort is experienced when the breast is compressed. Compression allows better visualization of the breast tissue. The breast will not be harmed in any way.
   D. Do not use any powder, deodorant, perfume, or ointments in the underarm area on the day of the test. Residue on the skin from these agents can obscure the visualization of the mammogram.
   E. A minimal radiation dose will be used during the test.
   F. Wear a blouse with a skirt or slacks, rather than a dress, since you will need to remove clothing from the upper half of the body.
   G. If experiencing painful breasts, refrain from coffee, tea, cola, and chocolate 5–7 days before testing.
   H. American Cancer Society mammography screening guidelines: screening mammogram by age 40; mammogram every 1 to 2 years if client is 40–49 years old; mammogram annually at age 50 and older.
   I. An annual clinical breast examination by a health professional is recommended every 3 years if the client is

20–40 years old, and annually if the client is 40 years old or older.

J. Perform a monthly breast self-examination if 20 years old or older. Breast self-examination should be performed after each menstrual period.

K. 80% of lumps found by a mammogram are benign.

6. Factors that affect results:

A. False-positive mammograms may result from calcifications of fibrocystic changes, calcific-like deposits in the skin secondary to tattoos, sebaceous gland secretions, and talcum powder.

B. Postoperative and postradiotherapy changes may be mistaken for carcinomas.

C. The principal cause of false-negative mammograms is dense parenchymal tissue, because masses show up more clearly in fatty breasts.

D. Jewelry worn around the neck can preclude total visualization of the breast(s).

E. Breast augmentation implants prevent total visualization of the breast(s).

7. Other data:

A. Mammography is the only imaging modality effective for the early detection of breast cancer. Mammography can detect nonpalpable lesions <0.5 cm diameter 2 years before reaching a palpable size.

B. Magnification mammography is limited due to its higher radiation doses, but can be useful in postoperative and postradiotherapy examinations, possibly preventing unnecessary biopsy.

C. Mammography immediately after stereotaxic breast biopsy is suboptimal for establishment of a new baseline due to the frequent finding of hematoma.

D. According to one study, women undergoing mammography preferred to have their doctor call them with the result, if the results were normal. If the results were abnormal, the subjects preferred to be told by their own physician in the office.

Bibliography:

Bassett LW, Manjikian V, Gold RH: Mammography and breast cancer screening. Surg Clin North Am *70*(4):775–800, 1990.

Feig SA: Assessment of the hypothetical risk from mammography and evaluation of the potential benefit. Radiol Clin North Am *21*:173–191, 1983.

Hann LE, Liberman L, Dershaw DD, Cohen MA, Abramson AF: Mammography immediately after stereotaxic breast biopsy: is it necessary? Am J Roentgenol *165*(1):59–62, 1995.

Lind SE, Kopans D, Good MJ: Patients' preferences for learning the results of mammographic examinations. Breast Cancer Res Treat *23*(3):223–232, 1992.

Richardson JD, Cigtay OS, Grant EG, et al.: Imaging of the breast. Med Clin North Am *68*(6):1481–1514, 1984.

Taylor VM, Montano DE, Koepsell T: Use of screening mammography by general internist. Cancer Detect Prev *18*(6):455–462, 1994.

MAMMOTHERMOGRAPHY
(see Thermography, Diagnostic)

MANTOUX SKIN TEST (PPD-PURIFIED PROTEIN DERIVATIVE TEST, TB TEST, TUBERCULOSIS TEST), DIAGNOSTIC

Norm: Negative.

Positive: Localized erythema and induration of skin (>10 mm) at site of skin test is indicative of tuberculosis (pulmonary).

Negative: Normal finding; lack of redness or induration of skin at site of skin test; zone of redness and induration ≤5- mm.

Usage: Indicated for clients with signs (e.g., abnormality in mediastinum on x-ray) or symptoms (e.g., cough, hemoptysis, weight loss, etc.). Suggestive of current tuberculosis (TB) disease; recent contact with clients with confirmed or suspected cases of TB; clients with abnormal chest x-rays compatible with past TB; clients with medical conditions that increase the risk of TB (e.g., diabetes, immunosuppressive therapy, AIDS, etc.); groups at high risk for developing TB.

Description: An intradermal skin test to detect tuberculosis infection (active or dormant). Tuberculin, a protein fraction of tubercle bacilli, is injected intradermally in the human. A localized thickening with redness indicates an accumulation of small, sensitized lymphocytes, which occurs due to active or dormant tuberculosis. Clients with human immunodeficiency virus infection are at increased risk for developing tuberculosis infection and should be screened with the tuberculin skin test. Other clients at high risk for becoming infected with *Mycobacterium tuberculosis* include the very young and the very old, those who are malnourished, alcohol and drug abusers, and the chronically ill.

Professional Considerations:

1. Consent form IS required.

Risks:

It is not known whether the test can cause fetal harm or affect reproductive capacity.

Contraindications:

The test should be given to pregnant women only if clearly indicated. The test should not be given if the client has had a previous positive test.

2. Preparation:
   A. Assess for previous history of positive purified protein derivative (PPD) reaction. (The test should not be administered in this case.)
   B. Obtain a tuberculin syringe and PPD.
   C. Draw up PPD in a tuberculin syringe, following the manufacturer's directions. Use a ½-inch 26- or 27-gauge needle.
3. Procedure:
   A. Cleanse the injection site on the lower, dorsal aspect of the forearm with alcohol, and allow the area to dry.
   B. Stretch the skin taut.
   C. Inject intradermally 0.1 ml of a solution containing 0.5 tuberculin units of PPD. A wheal of 6–10 mm in diameter should be produced when the test is administered accurately.
4. Postprocedure care:
   A. Mark the test area to locate it for reading.
   B. Read the test area 48–72 hours later. Examine the site, using good light. Inspect the skin for induration. Induration >5 mm diameter generally indicates infection. Rub lightly from the area of normal skin to the indurated area. Circle the induration with a pencil.
   C. An induration of ≤5 mm diameter should be interpreted as a positive reaction if the client has known contact with an individual with active tuberculosis or if there is a chest x-ray with findings consistent with tuberculosis. Isoniazid therapy is recommended to decrease the risk of developing the disease in positive reactors.
   D. A chest x-ray is necessary with all positive reactions.
   E. Epinephrine hydrochloride solution (1:1000) should be readily available for use in the event of anaphylaxis.
5. Client and family teaching:
   A. The skin test does not distinguish between current disease or past infection.
   B. The skin test should not be administered to known tuberculin-positive reactors because of the possibility of severe reactions (vesiculation, ulceration, and necrosis).
6. Factors that affect results:
   A. Tuberculin must be stored as recommended by the manufacturer. Tuberculin solution should be stored between 2° and 8°C (35–46°F). It should be exposed to light only when being withdrawn and administered. An open vial may be used only for 1 month.
   B. Subcutaneous rather than intradermal injection will nullify the test.
   C. Cross-reactions with nontuberculous mycobacteria may cause false-positive results.
   D. Serial testing may cause false-positive results.
   E. Vaccination with the bacille Calmette-Guérin (BCG) has a variable effect on the skin test reaction. However, a history of BCG vaccination should not alter interpretation of the skin test.
   F. False-negative reactions may occur in the following instances: bacterial infections, immunologic defects, immunosuppressive agents, live virus vaccinations (BCG, measles, mumps, polio, and rubella), malnutrition, old age, overwhelming tuberculosis, renal failure, and viral infections (chickenpox, measles, and mumps).
   G. False-negative results can occur, even in the presence of active TB, whenever sensitized T lymphocytes are temporarily depleted in the body.
7. Other data:
   A. None.

Bibliography:

Khan J, Akhtar M, von Sinner WN, Bouchama A, Bazarbashi M: CT-guided fine needle aspiration biopsy in the diagnosis of mediastinal tuberculosis. Chest *106*(5):1329–1332, 1994.

Rodnick JE: New guidelines for tuberculin skin test interpretation. West J Med *154*(3):322–323, 1991.

Sokal JE: The tuberculin skin test. Am Rev Respir Dis *124*:356–363, 1981.

MAPROTILINE
(see Tricyclic Antidepressants, Plasma or Serum)

MARIJUANA, BLOOD OR URINE
(see Cannabinoids, Qualitative, Blood or Urine)

MCA
(see Mucin-Like Carcinoma-Associated Antigen, Blood)

MCH, BLOOD
(see Blood Indices, Blood)

MCHC, BLOOD
(see Blood Indices, Blood)

MCV, BLOOD
(see Blood Indices, Blood)

MEAN CORPUSCULAR HEMOGLOBIN, BLOOD

(see Blood Indices, Blood)

MEAN CORPUSCULAR HEMOGLOBIN CONCENTRATION, BLOOD

(see Blood Indices, Blood)

MEAN CORPUSCULAR VOLUME, BLOOD

(see Blood Indices, Blood)

MEAN PLATELET VOLUME, BLOOD

Norm:

Preterm infants	7.5–9.5 fl
Term infants	
(0–1 month)	7.6–9.9 fl
1 month–48 months	6.3–8.9 fl
48 months–adult	7.0–9.0 fl

Usage: Evaluates platelet abnormalities; improves detection of platelet-related diseases when the platelet count is normal; determines the platelet changes associated with exercise and hyperthyroidism; predicts hypertensive crisis in pregnancy; predicts the presence of sepsis in neonates; and predicts hemorrhage in clients with rheumatoid arthritis, who are experiencing thrombocytopenia as a side effect of parental gold therapy.

Increased: Acute poststreptococcal glomerulonephritis (APSGN), arterial disease (angina, atherosclerotic disease), coagulase-negative staphylococcal sepsis in neonates, cyanotic congenital heart disease, diabetes, hyperthyroidism, iron-deficiency anemia, ITP (idiopathic thrombocytopenic purpura), myeloproliferative disorders, myocardial infarction, pregnant women with preeclampsia, renal failure, rheumatic heart disease, smokers, splenomegaly, states of increased platelet production, and thrombocytopenia.

Decreased: Clients with rheumatoid arthritis, who are receiving parental gold therapy.

Description: The MPV is an automated measurement of the average volume of platelets. It is the arithmetic mean volume of the platelet population derived from the platelet histogram on automated Coulter counters. A high MPV indicates the presence of generally larger platelets. When the MPV is low, the platelets are generally smaller. The MPV is expressed in femtoliters (fl).

Professional Considerations:

1. Consent form NOT required.
2. Preparation:
   A. Tube: Lavender-top.
3. Procedure:
   A. Leaving a tourniquet in place less than 1 minute, draw a 5-ml blood sample.
   B. Gently invert the tube two or three times.
4. Postprocedure care:
   A. Send the specimen to the laboratory within 1 hour.
5. Client and family teaching:
   A. Results are normally available within 4 hours.
6. Factors that affect results:
   A. When potassium EDTA is used as an anticoagulant, platelets demonstrate a progressive increase in mean platelet volume with storage, as measured by the Coulter counter. This increase is most marked within the first 2 hours, but continues at a slower rate subsequently.
7. Other data:
   A. The mean platelet volume (MPV) is comparable to the mean corpuscular volume (MCV) of red blood cells.
   B. Increased MPV may reflect either increased platelet activation or increased numbers of large, hyperaggregable platelets.
   C. The MPV increases during conditions of rapid platelet turnover, probably signifying the release of larger, younger platelets into the circulation.
   D. Younger platelets are larger than older platelets. Larger platelets are functionally and metabolically more active than smaller ones, contain more granules, and express more enzymatic activity in vitro.
   E. Increases in MPV can occur, although thrombocytopenia has developed.
   F. The mean MPV may be normal in central thrombocytopenic diseases, such as aplastic anemia and acute leukemia.

Bibliography:

Kim KY, Kim KE, Kim KH: Mean platelet volume in the normal state and in various clinical disorders. Yonsei Med J *27*(3):219–226, 1986.

Martin JF, Bath PMW, Burr ML: Mean platelet volume and myocardial infarction. Lancet *339*:1000–1001, 1992.

O'Connor TA, Ringer KM, Gaddis ML: Mean platelet volume during coagulase-negative staphylococcal sepsis in neonates. Am J Clin Pathol *99*(1):69–71, 1993.

Patrick CH, Lazarchick J, Stubbs T, Pittard WB: Mean platelet volume and platelet distribution width in the neonate. Am J Pediatr Hematol Oncol *9*(2): 130–132, 1987.

Vukelja SJ, Krishnan J, Diehl LF: Mean platelet volume improves upon the megathrombocyte index but cannot replace the blood film examination in the evaluation of thrombocytopenia Am J Hematol *44*(2):89–94, 1993.

MEAT FIBERS, STOOL

Norm: Negative.

Positive: Gastroenteritis, intestinal lymphoma, malabsorption syndrome, pancreatic insufficiency, severe ulcerative colitis, surgical removal of section of intestine, and Whipple's disease.

Description: Examination of stool for yield of meat fibers correlates with the amount of fat secretion in the stool. Meat fibers found in stool result from multiple abnormalities in absorption of nutrients. These include defects in the intestinal lumen that result in inadequate fat hydrolysis; inadequate proteolysis; altered bile salt metabolism; and defects in mucosal epithelial cells or intestinal lymphatics, which affect absorbing surfaces and interfere with the transport of nutrients.

Professional Considerations:

1. Consent form NOT required.
2. Preparation:
   A. Barium procedures or laxatives should be avoided for 1 week prior to specimen collection.
   B. Obtain an enema apparatus and warm saline, or a prepackaged enema; and a sterile plastic specimen container
   C. *See Client and family teaching.*
3. Procedure:
   A. Obtain a stool specimen by giving the client a warm saline enema or a prepackaged enema.
   B. Collect the stool specimen in a sterile plastic container.
4. Postprocedure care:
   A. None.
5. Client and family teaching:
   A. Include at least 3 ounces of red meat per day for 24–72 hours prior to the test.
   B. Results are normally available after 24 hours.
6. Factors that affect results:
   A. Reject specimens collected with enemas other than saline or Fleets (e.g., mineral oil, bismuth, or magnesium compounds).
7. Other data:
   A. Serum protein level should be determined as hypoproteinemia is the major clinical feature of protein-losing enteropathy.

B. Biopsy of the intestinal mucosa is more useful for definitive diagnosis of intestinal mucosal abnormalities.

Bibliography:

Reddy BS: Effect of types of dietary fiber on fecal mutagens and bacterial enzymes in relation to colon cancer. Adv Exp Med Biol *270*:159–167, 1990.

Zierdt WS: Occult blood testing using tetramethylbenzidine in an extraction procedure for patients on restricted diets. Am J Clin Pathol *83*(4):486–488, 1985.

MECKEL SCAN, DIAGNOSTIC

Norm: Negative; no increased uptake of radionuclide in the right lower quadrant of the abdomen.

Usage: Detection of Meckel's diverticulum, which contains ectopic gastric mucosa, in clients with abdominal pain or occult gastrointestinal bleeding.

Description: A nuclear medicine scan in which a radioisotope, Tc-99m (technetium) pertechnetate is injected intravenously. The radioisotope is concentrated in the normal gastric mucosa within the stomach, and in the ectopic gastric mucosa in the Meckel's diverticulum. This is a very sensitive and specific test for this congenital abnormality.

Professional Considerations:

1. Consent form IS required.

Risks:
Hematoma, infection.

Contraindications:
During pregnancy or breast-feeding.

2. Preparation:
   A. Assure the client that nuclear medicine personnel will remain within hearing range and will be able to see the client throughout the study.
   B. A histamine H_2-receptor antagonist (e.g., Cimetidine orally every 6 hours for 24 hours) is usually administered for 1–2 days before the test. This drug inhibits acid secretion and allows for improved visualization of the Meckel's diverticulum.
   C. *See Client and family teaching.*
3. Procedure:
   A. In the nuclear medicine department, the client lies in a supine position.
   B. Tc-99m pertechnetate is administered intravenously 15 minutes prior to imaging.

C. An anterior body image view is obtained with a rectilinear scanner or scintillation (gamma) camera. Images are taken at 5-minute intervals for 1 hour.

D. During the scan, the client may be asked to lie on the left side to increase the amount of radioisotope to the intestines.

E. Total examining time is 60 minutes.

4. Postprocedure care:

A. Observe the client carefully for up to 60 minutes after the study for a possible (anaphylactic) reaction to the radionuclide.

B. Ask the client to void after the procedure, and a repeat image may be obtained.

C. Rubber gloves should be worn for 24 hours after the procedure when urine is being discarded. Wash the gloved hands with soap and water before removing the gloves. Wash the ungloved hands after the gloves are removed.

5. Client and family teaching:

A. It is necessary to lie still for 60 minutes for this scan. There is no pain associated with this test.

B. Refrain from eating or drinking anything for 6–12 hours before the test.

C. Void prior to the study to increase the visibility of the intestines.

D. Meticulously wash your hands with soap and water after each void for 24 hours postprocedure.

E. Family members must wear rubber gloves for 24 hours postprocedure when discarding the client's urine, if the family will be providing this care.

6. Factors that affect results:

A. A positive scan is dependent on an adequate amount of gastric mucosa within a Meckel's diverticulum. Only 25% of clients with Meckel's diverticulum will have sufficient ectopic gastric mucosa to produce a positive scan.

B. The literature reports several cases of a false-positive Meckel's scan revealing the true source of gastrointestinal bleeding: a carcinoid tumor.

C. Other radionuclide studies performed within the prior 24 hours will interfere with this test.

D. A waiting period that is either too short or too long following the radionuclide injection will alter the results.

E. Premedication with pentagastrin and histamine H_2-receptor blocker (Zantac) may increase the sensitivity of the test.

F. Barium in the small or large bowel may mask the radionuclide concentration.

7. Other data:

A. Health care professionals working in a nuclear medicine area must follow federal standards set by the Nuclear Regulatory Commission. These standards include precautions for handling the radioactive material and monitoring of potential radiation exposure.

B. The half-life of technetium is 6 hours.

Bibliography:

Heyman S: Meckel's diverticulum: possible detection by combining pentagastrin with histamine H2 receptor blocker. J Nucl Med 35(10):1656–1658, 1994.

Spieth ME: False-positive Meckel's imaging and true positive imaging of a gastrointestinal bleed and surgical lesion. Clin Nucl Med 19(4):298–301, 1994.

MEDIASTINOSCOPY, DIAGNOSTIC

Norm: Normal mediastinal structure and lymph nodes; lack of disease process.

Usage: To detect lymphoma (e.g., Hodgkin's disease), lung metastasis to mediastinal lymph nodes, granulomatous infection, mediastinal tuberculosis, sarcoidosis; to obtain biopsy of mediastinal lymph nodes or intrathoracic lesions; to determine staging of bronchogenic carcinoma; and to evaluate tumor spread or intrathoracic diseases.

Description: Surgical endoscopic procedure that is performed under general anesthesia. A small incision is made at the suprasternal notch, and a mediastinoscope is inserted into the mediastinum. The purpose of this procedure is to visualize the mediastinal structure and lymph nodes, and to obtain biopsy of lymph nodes or other lesions. The lymph nodes in the mediastinum receive lymphatic drainage from the lungs. A mediastinoscopy is usually performed when x-rays, sputum cytology, and lung scans (CT and nuclear) have not confirmed a diagnosis. Mediastinoscopy is an invasive procedure and is performed under general anesthesia, due to the pain and coughing that result from the manipulation of the trachea.

Professional Considerations:

1. Consent form IS required.

Risks:

Blood vessel, esophageal, or tracheal puncture or rupture.

Contraindications:

Previous mediastinoscopy (due to adhesions); clients who are not candidates for general anesthesia.

2. Preparation:
   A. *See Client and family teaching.*
   B. Complete pre-op checklist, and perform routine pre-op care, which is the same as with any other surgical procedure. Check if the client's blood needs to be typed and cross-matched.
   C. Measure and record baseline vital signs.
   D. Ask the client if he or she is allergic to any anesthetic medicine.
   E. Encourage the client and family members to express concerns about the procedure. Answer questions and refer those that you cannot answer to appropriate health care professionals.
   F. Administer preprocedural medication approximately 1 hour before the test, as prescribed.
3. Procedure:
   A. The client is transported to the operating room.
   B. General anesthesia is administered.
   C. A small incision is made in the suprasternal fossa.
   D. A mediastinoscope is passed through this neck incision, along the anterior course of the trachea, and into the superior mediastinum.
   E. The area is visualized. Photographs of specific areas and structures may be taken. Biopsies of the lymph nodes may also be performed.
   F. The mediastinoscope is withdrawn, and the incision is sutured closed.
4. Postprocedure care:
   A. Assess vital signs every 15 minutes × 2, then every 30 minutes × 2, then hourly × 4, then every 4 hours until 24 hours after the procedure. Report changes in vital signs (e.g., increase in pulse rate or respiratory rate, decrease in blood pressure).
   B. Auscultate lung sounds, and assess for any respiratory abnormalities, such as dyspnea.
   C. Check for bright red blood or increased blood on the dressing. Observe the wound for symptoms of infection.
   D. Provide comfort measures as needed (e.g., position change, medication, etc.).
   E. Send biopsy specimens to the pathology laboratory immediately.
5. Client and family teaching:
   A. Refrain from eating or drinking for 8–12 hours prior to the procedure.
   B. Void prior to the surgical procedure.
   C. This procedure will take approximately 1 hour and is performed by a surgeon.
   D. You will be asleep during the procedure.
6. Factors that affect results:
   A. Phenytoin hypersensitivity may result in a "pseudolymphoma," causing false-positive cytology.
7. Other data:
   A. Complications may include perforation of the trachea, esophagus, aorta,

or other blood vessels; pneumothorax; laryngeal nerve damage; and infection.
   B. Thoracotomy is advisable in the instance of negative cytology in lesions likely to be malignant.

Bibliography:

Gephardt GN, Rice TW: Utility of frozen-section evaluation of lymph nodes in the staging of bronchogenic carcinoma at mediastinoscopy and thoracotomy. J Thorac Cardiovasc Surg *100*(6): 853–859, 1990.

Heilo A: Tumors in the mediastinum: US guided histologic core-needle biopsy. Radiology *189*(1):143–146, 1993.

Puhakka HJ, Liippo K, Tala E: Mediastinoscopy in relation to clinical evaluation. Scand J Thorac Cardiovasc Surg *24*(1):43–45, 1990.

MELANIN, URINE

Norm: Negative.

Positive: Malignant melanoma.

Description: Urine test to detect biochemical markers of melanoma progression. Melanin, which is the main pigment in the body, is synthesized by the melanocyte primarily in the skin and eyes. It is highly elevated in malignant melanoma. Both eumelanin (brown/black pigment) and pheomelanin (yellow/red pigment) are produced, with dihyroxyindole (DHI) and cyseinyldopa (CD) being the major precursors. Melanin metabolites are often released in the urine of clients with disseminated melanoma metastasis (melanuria). These metabolites include a pheomelanin metabolite, 5-S-CD, and a eumelanin metabolite, 6-hydroxy-5-methoxyindole-2-carboxylic acid (6H5MI2C). Melanogen, a colorless precursor of melanin, is also excreted in the urine of 25% of people with melanin-producing tumors.

Professional Considerations:

1. Consent form NOT required.
2. Preparation:
   A. Obtain a sterile, plastic specimen container.
3. Procedure:
   A. Obtain a freshly voided urine specimen in a sterile, plastic container.
4. Postprocedure care:
   A. None.
5. Client and family teaching:
   A. Results are normally available within 24 hours.
6. Factors that affect results:
   A. Drugs that may cause false-positive results include salicylates.
7. Other data:
   A. The test is more frequently positive in people with hepatic metastasis.

B. Urine exposed to room temperature for 24 hours will turn dark brown and later black as the melanogens oxidize to melanin.

C. Plasma 6H5MI2C levels are usually high (>1.75 ng/ml) in clients with metastatic malignant melanoma, and is a more sensitive and reliable test than melanin (5-S-CD) urine test.

D. Elevated urine melanin test results is a high risk factor for metastatic malignant melanoma.

Bibliography:

Hara H: High plasma level of a eumelanin precursor, 6-hydroxy-5-methoxy indole-2-carboxylic acid, as a prognostic marker for malignant melanoma. J Invest Dermatol *102*(4):501–505, 1994.

Hegedus ZL: Homogentisic acid and structurally related compounds as intermediates in plasma soluble melanin formation and in tissue toxicities. Arch Int Physiol Biochem Biophys *102*(3):175–181, 1994.

Horikoshi T: Evaluation of melanin-related metabolites as markers of melanoma progression. Cancer *73*(3):629–636, 1994.

MELANOCYTE-STIMULATING HORMONE (MSH), URINE

Norm: Negative for melanin.

Positive: Addison's disease, hyperpituitarism, melanoma, and liver metastasis.

Description: Hormone secreted by the anterior lobe of the pituitary gland that affects pigment metabolism by promoting the synthesis of melanin.

Professional Considerations:

1. Consent form NOT required.
2. Preparation:
   A. Obtain a sterile, plastic specimen container.
3. Procedure:
   A. Obtain a freshly voided urine specimen in a sterile, plastic container.
4. Postprocedure care:
   A. None.
5. Client and family teaching:
   A. Results are normally available after 24 hours.
6. Factors that affect results:
   A. The secretion of MSH is increased when levels of circulating cortisol are low.
7. Other data:
   A. MSH secretion is closely linked to ACTH secretion.

Bibliography:

Cieszka KA: Growth and pigmentation in genetically related Cloudman S91 melanoma cell lines treated with 3-isobutyl-1-methylxanthine and beta-melanocyte stimulating hormone. Exp Dermatol (Aug 4):192–198, 1995.

MENDELIAN INHERITANCE IN GENETIC DISORDERS, DIAGNOSTIC

Norm: Negative for genetic disorders.

Usage: Genetic counseling and mendelian inheritance.

Description: This procedure is an analysis of the presence of genetic disorders in the family history. It is performed to identify the likelihood that inherited genes, which obey statistical laws, exist in a family. There are over 4000 Mendelian diseases such as breast cancer, colon cancer, color blindness, congenital malformations, cystic fibrosis, hemophilia, Marfan's syndrome, and sickle cell anemia.

Professional Considerations:

1. Consent form NOT required.
2. Preparation:
   A. Provide teaching.
3. Procedure:
   A. A family pedigree analysis is performed, including generational continuity of the disorder, sex relationship, and segregation ration.
4. Postprocedure care:
   A. Genetic counseling and referral for follow-up.
5. Client and family teaching:
   A. Inform the client about the reasons for genetic counseling.
6. Factors that affect results:
   A. Accuracy of the analysis.
7. Other data:
   A. Other disorders can mimic Mendelian disorders, such as chromosomal disorders, congenital infections, and mental retardation.

Bibliography:

Aminoff M: Selective intestinal malabsorption of vitamin B$_{12}$ displays recessive Mendelian inheritance: assignment of a locus to chromosome 10 by linkage. Am J Hum Genet *57*(4):824–831, 1995.

McLellan DL: Hereditary aspects of prostate cancer. Can Med Assoc J *157*(7):895–900, 1995.

Rashbass J: Online Mendelian inheritance in man. Trends Genet *11*(7):291–292, 1995.

Wilkie AO: A gene map of congenital malformations. J Med Genet *31*(7):507–517, 1994.

MEPHENYTOIN, BLOOD

Norm:

Therapeutic level	5–16 µg/ml
Toxic level	>20 µg/ml
Panic level	>50 µg/ml

Overdose Symptoms and Treatment:

Symptoms: Ataxia, blood dyscrasias, coma, drowsiness, dysarthria, hypotension, nystagmus, and unresponsive pupils may be seen.

Treatment: There is no specific treatment. Refer to a physician. Give general supportive care: lavage and maintenance of airway and blood pressure. Hemodialysis WILL remove mephenytoin and is utilized, especially with drug toxicity in children.

Increased: Overdose. Drugs include mephenytoin (Mesantoin) chloramphenicol.

Decreased: Convulsions, inadequate dosage, and noncompliance with therapeutic regimen.

Description: Mephenytoin (Mesantoin) is an anticonvulsant used to treat grand mal, tonic-clonic, psychomotor, temporal lobe, focal, and Jacksonian seizures. It is metabolized in the liver and excreted in the urine.

Professional Considerations:
1. Consent form NOT required.
2. Preparation:
   A. Tube: Red-top, red/gray-top, or gold-top.
   B. Do NOT draw during hemodialysis.
3. Procedure:
   A. Draw a 5-ml blood sample.
4. Postprocedure care:
   A. None.
5. Client and family teaching:
   A. Explain overdose symptoms and treatment (see above), as appropriate.
   B. Drug levels should be monitored routinely during therapy.
6. Factors that affect results:
   A. Compliance with administration.
7. Other data:
   A. Trade name is Mesantoin.

Bibliography:
Balian JD: The hydroxylation of omeprazole correlates with S-mephenytoin metabolism: a population study. Clin Pharmacol Ther 57(6):662–669, 1995.

MEPROBAMATE, BLOOD

Norm:

Therapeutic level	16–27 µg/ml
Toxic level	>35 µg/ml
Panic level	>50 µg/ml
Lethal level	>200 µg/ml

Death has been reported with as little as 12 gm, and survival with as much as 40 gm.

Overdose Symptoms and Treatment:

Symptoms: Drowsiness, lethargy, stupor, ataxia, hemolytic toxicity symptoms (fever, sore throat, bruising, bleeding), coma, shock, vasomotor and respiratory collapse, and death may occur.

Treatment:
   Administer gastric lavage and supportive therapy as needed.
   Both hemodialysis and peritoneal dialysis WILL remove meprobamate.
   Osmotic diuresis with mannitol has also been effective.
   Avoid dehydration.

Increased: Drug abuse and overdose.

Decreased: Noncompliance with therapeutic regimen.

Description: A sedative hypnotic used to treat anxiety disorders. A central nervous system depressant, metabolized in the liver, excreted in urine and feces.

Professional Considerations:
1. Consent form NOT required.
2. Preparation:
   A. Tube: Red-top, red/gray-top, or gold-top.
   B. Do NOT draw during hemodialysis.
3. Procedure:
   A. Draw 5-ml blood sample.
4. Postprocedure care:
   A. None.
5. Client and family teaching:
   A. For intentional overdose, refer for cri-

sis intervention and counseling. Referrals to appropriate rehabilitation centers and therapeutic community programs should be offered to all clients who may be interested.

B. Explain overdose symptoms and treatment (see above), as appropriate.

6. Factors that affect results:
   A. Onset of action is within 1 hour after oral dosage. Peak concentration is 2 hours from dosage, half-life is 6–17 hours, steady-state levels occur in 1.5–4.0 days.

7. Other data:
   A. An alternative method of determining meprobamate levels is by gas chromatography. This method is accurate and precise, and is particularly suitable for toxicology studies.

Bibliography:

Trenque T, Lamiable D, Millart H, Vistelle R, Choisy H: Gas chromatographic determination of meprobamate in human plasma. J Chromatogr *615*(2): 343–346, 1993.

MERCURY, BLOOD AND URINE

Norm:

Blood: ≤5 μg/ml

Urine: <20 μg/24 hours

Increased: Mercury poisoning.

Description: Mercury is the only metal that is liquid at ordinary temperatures. Mercury is primarily absorbed by inhalation, but can also be absorbed through the skin and gastrointestinal tract. It is then distributed to the central nervous system and kidneys and excreted in the urine.

Professional Considerations:

1. Consent form NOT required.
2. Preparation:
   A. *For blood sample:* Tube: Lavender-top.
   B. *For urine specimen:* Obtain a 3-L, acid washed plastic specimen container without preservative.
   C. Assess the possible causes of mercury poisoning: occupational activities, hobbies (e.g., painting ceramics), target shooting, home renovation, and auto repair.
3. Procedure:
   A. *Blood:* Draw a 5-ml blood sample.
   B. *Urine:* Collect all the urine voided in a 24-hour period in a 3-L, acid-washed plastic container without preservative.
4. Postprocedure care:
   A. For increased levels, encourage fluids and monitor urine output, because mercury is nephrotoxic.
5. Client and family teaching:
   A. *Urine:* Save all the urine voided in the 24-hour period and urinate before defecating to avoid loss of urine. If any urine is accidentally discarded, discard the entire specimen and restart the collection the next day.
6. Factors that affect results:
   A. Drugs that may cause falsely low levels include iodine-containing medications.
7. Other data:
   A. Blood is the recommended specimen for measuring organic mercury.
   B. Urine is the recommended specimen for measuring inorganic mercury.

Bibliography:

Ash KO: CE Update—toxicology III. Trace elements: when essential nutrients become poisonous: separating fact from fiction. Lab Med *26*(4):266–272, 1995.

Sandborgh EG, Dahlqvist R, Lindelof B, et al.: DMSA administration to patients with alleged mercury poisoning from dental amalgams: a placebo-controlled study. J Dent Res *73*(3):620–628, 1994.

METANEPHRINES, TOTAL, 24-HOUR, URINE

Norm:

		SI Units
Adults	<1 mg/d	<5 μmol/d
	0.05–1.20 μg/mg creatinine[2]	0.03–0.69 mmol/mol creatinine
Children		
<12 months	0.001–4.60 μg/mg creatinine[2]	0.0006–2.64 mmol/mol creatinine
12–24 months	0.24–5.38 μg/mg creatinine[2]	0.15–3.09 mmol/mol creatinine
24 months–5 years	0.35–2.99 μg/mg creatinine[2]	0.21–1.72 mmol/mol creatinine

	SI Units
Children *(continued)*	
5–10 years	0.43–2.70 μg/mg creatinine[2]	0.25–1.55 mmol/mol creatinine
10–15 years	0.001–1.87	0.0006–1.07
15–18 years	0.001–0.67	0.0006–0.38

Increased: Brain tumors, chemodectomas, ganglioneuroblastoma, ganglioneuroma, hypertension with pheochromocytoma, malignant pheochromocytoma, metastasis (widespread), myasthenia gravis, neuroblastoma, pheochromocytoma, progressive muscular dystrophy, sepsis, and severe stress.

Description: 24-hour urine test of adrenomedullar function. It is usually performed when a client with hypertension is suspected of having pheochromocytoma, which is a tumor of the chromaffin cells of the adrenal medulla. (Less than 1% of clients with hypertension have pheochromocytoma.) Metanephrines (e.g., normetanephrine and metanephrine) are one of the principle substances formed by the adrenal medulla, released into the bloodstream, and excreted into the urine. These substances contain a catechol nucleus and an amine group; therefore, they are referred to as *catecholamines*. The release of metanephrines into the urine is indicative of pathology, such as hypertension and pheochromocytoma, which are associated with excessive catecholamine secretion.

Professional Considerations:

1. Consent form NOT required.
2. Preparation:
   A. Obtain a 3-L, plastic container with 20–25 ml of hydrochloric acid (HCl) preservative.
   B. Label the container with the client's name, the test, and the date.
   C. Discuss with the physician if any drugs are to be discontinued 3–7 days before the testing.
   D. *See Client and family teaching.*
3. Procedure:
   A. Collect all the urine voided in a 24-hour period in a refrigerated, 3-L, plastic container to which 20–25 ml of HCl preservative has been added. For specimens collected from an indwelling urinary catheter, keep the drainage bag on ice, and empty urine into the refrigerated collection container hourly.

Document urinary output throughout the collection period.

4. Postprocedure care:
   A. Send the urine specimen to the laboratory refrigerator after the 24-hour collection is completed. Metanephrines are stable for at least 1 week.
   B. Write the beginning and ending times of collection and total urinary output (container quantity should match output record) on the laboratory requisition and on the specimen container.
5. Client and family teaching:
   A. Save all the urine voided in the 24-hour period and urinate before defecating to avoid loss of urine. If any urine is accidentally discarded, discard the entire specimen and restart the collection the next day.
   B. Avoid caffeine, coffee, tea, cocoa products, bananas, vanilla products, aspirin, and phenothiazine-containing medications for 48 hours prior to collecting urine and during the urine collection.
   C. Encourage the client to rest, take in adequate food and fluids, and avoid stress during the test.
6. Factors that affect results:
   A. Drugs that may cause false-positive results include chlorpromazine, dopamine, guanethidine, hydralazine, hydrocortisone, imipramine, isoetharine, levodopa, monoamine oxidase (MAO) inhibitors, nalidixic acid, phenacetin, phenobarbital, phenylephrine, tetracycline, and unipramine.
   B. Drugs that may cause false-negative results include clonidine, guanethidine, propranolol, reserpine, and theophylline.
   C. Dietary intake high in bananas may cause falsely increased results.
   D. Vigorous exercise may cause an increase in catecholamine levels.
   E. The 24-hour urine collection is problematic for practical reasons and for client compliance.
7. Other data:
   A. Urinary catecholamines and vanillylmandelic acid (VMA) are often measured with urinary metanephrines.
   B. A major disadvantage of this test is that there is variability in the excretion of metanephrines during illness.
   C. Tests for plasma metanephrines are more sensitive than urinary meta-

nephrines for the diagnosis of pheochromocytoma. Sensitivities for the tests for urinary metanephrines vary from 89% to 100%.

D. This test is recommended for clients in whom an adrenal mass is found.

Bibliography:

Gerlo EA: Urinary and plasma catecholamines metabolites in pheochromocytoma: diagnostic value in 19 cases. Clin Chem *40*(2):250–256, 1994.

Lenders JW: Plasma metanephrines in the diagnosis of pheochromocytoma. Ann Intern Med *123*(2):101–109, 1995.

Marini M: Determination of serum metanephrines in the diagnosis of pheochromocytoma. Ann Endocrinol (Paris) *54*(5):337–342, 1994.

METHACHOLINE CHALLENGE TEST (BRONCHIAL CHALLENGE TEST), DIAGNOSTIC

Norm: Negative.

Usage: Diagnosis of asthma when the diagnosis cannot be made with certainty from the history, physical examination, and conventional pulmonary function tests.

Description: The methacholine challenge test involves measurement of lung volumes before and after inhalation of methacholine chloride, a bronchial constrictor. This test is useful in demonstrating bronchial hyperreactivity (BHR), which is a defining characteristic of asthma. Clients with symptoms suggestive of asthma often have normal resting pulmonary function test results but are more sensitive to the bronchoconstrictive effects of methacholine than are healthy people.

Professional Considerations:

1. Consent form NOT required.

2. Preparation:
   A. Obtain nebulizer and methacholine chloride.

3. Procedure:
   A. The client performs a forced vital capacity (FVC), and the forced expiratory volume (FEV) is measured.
   B. The client then inhales 3.12 mg of methacholine chloride via nebulizer, waits 5 minutes, and performs the FVC and FEV. A 20% reduction in the FEV is a positive response.
   C. If there is no response, the test is repeated using 6.25 mg, 12.5 mg, and 25 mg of methacholine, respectively. Failure to achieve a 20% reduction in the FEV is considered a negative test.

4. Postprocedure care:
   A. Monitor respiratory status.

5. Client and family teaching:
   A. Symptoms suggestive of asthma include cough, chest tightness, and dyspnea.

6. Factors that affect results:
   A. Inability to follow directions and comply with instructions yields invalid results.
   B. Inhaled heparin may have an inhibitory role on methacholine bronchial challenge, possibly through a direct effect on smooth muscle.

7. Other data:
   A. None.

Bibliography:

Basir R: Lack of significant bronchial reactivity to inhaled normal saline in subjects with a positive methacholine challenge test. J Asthma *32*(1): 63–67, 1995.

Ceyhan B: Effect of inhaled heparin on methacholine-induced bronchial hyperreactivity. Chest *107*(4): 1009–1012, 1995.

Paoletti P: Distribution of bronchial responsiveness in a general population: effect of sex, age, smoking, and level of pulmonary function. Am J Respir Crit Care Med *151*(6):1770–1777, 1995.

METHANOL, BLOOD
(see Toxicology, Volatiles Group by GLC, Blood or Urine)

METHAQUALONE, BLOOD

Norm: Negative.

		SI Units
Therapeutic level	2–3 µg/ml	8–12 µmol/L
Panic level	>8 µg/ml	>32 µmol/L
Toxic level	>10 µg/ml	>40µmol/L

Panic Level Symptoms and Treatment:

Symptoms: Marked drowsiness, confusion, dilated pupils, delirium, coma, restlessness, hyperexcitability, hypertonia, convulsions, shock, and cardiopulmonary failure may occur. Spontaneous vomiting with increased secretions may cause aspiration pneumonia or respiratory obstruction. Swelling, fluid retention, and abnormal bleeding may also occur. Death may occur from doses >5 gm (20 mmol).

Treatment:

Maintain patent airway.

Support blood pressure.

Perform gastric lavage and evaluation of gastric contents by lavage after airway has been ensured.

Monitor neurologic, cardiac, and respiratory status closely.

Be prepared to mechanically ventilate and to treat bradycardia or cardiac arrest.

Analeptics are contraindicated.

Hemodialysis and peritoneal dialysis will NOT remove methaqualone. Hemoperfusion WILL remove methaqualone.

Usage: Drug abuse and therapeutic monitoring.

Description: Methaqualone (Quaalude) is a nonbarbiturate, sedative-hypnotic agent with unknown mechanism of action. It is absorbed from the gastrointestinal tract, metabolized in the liver, and excreted in the urine, bile, and feces. This drug has a high abuse potential. The minimum lethal dose of methaqualone is 5g (20 mmol).

Professional Considerations:

1. Consent form NOT required.

2. Preparation:
   A. Tube: Red-top, red/gray-top, or gold-top or lavender-top.
   B. If the client may also have taken diazepam or chlordiazepoxide, indicate so on the laboratory requisition.
   C. Specimens MAY be drawn during hemodialysis.
3. Procedure:
   A. Draw a 5-ml blood sample.
4. Postprocedure care:
   A. None.
5. Client and family teaching:
   A. Explain the procedure and the reason for drawing the specimen.
   B. Explain the overdose symptoms and treatment (see above), as appropriate.
   C. Withdrawal symptoms may not appear for 2–3 days, and convulsions may occur on the eighth or ninth day after cessation of the drug.
   D. Referrals to appropriate rehabilitation centers and therapeutic community programs should be offered to all clients who may be interested.
6. Factors that affect results:
   A. The peak level of methaqualone is 2 hours after dose. Half-life is 33–38 hours, and steady-state levels occur in 7–8 days.
   B. Results are unreliable with concurrent administration of diazepam or chlordiazepoxide when the spectrophotometric method is used.
7. Other data:
   A. Monitor coagulation studies carefully if the client is taking an anticoagulant.
   B. Methaqualone can be detected in the urine for up to 7 days.

Bibliography:

Kauert G, Herrle I, Wermeille M: Quantification of dimethindene in plasma by gas chromatography—mass fragmentography using ammonia chemical ionization. J Chromatogr *617*(2):318–323, 1993.

METHEMOGLOBIN, BLOOD

Norm: Up to 2% (0.02) of total hemoglobin.

	SI Units
0.06–0.24 g/dl	9.3–37.2 μmol/L

Methemoglobinemia Symptoms and Treatment:

Symptoms:

Normal pO_2 with decreased pCO_2: Decreased *calculated* oxygen saturation; decreased HCO_3.

>15% methemoglobin: Chocolate cyanosis (pale blue-gray skin, brownish lips, and mucous membranes).

>30% methemoglobin: Dizziness, fatigue, headache, tachycardia, weakness.

>45% methemoglobin: Signs of CNS depression.

>55% methemoglobin: Acidemia, bradycardia, dysrhythmias, respiratory compromise.

>70% methemoglobin: Death may occur secondary to hypoxia. Fatal dose of nitroglycerin or sodium nitrite is reported to be 2 g.

Treatment:

1. Support symptoms: Protect airway, administer 100% oxygen, neurologic status q 1 hour.
2. Perform continuous pulse oximetry.
3. Do NOT induce emesis in clients with no gag reflex, or with central nervous system depression or excitation.
4. Do gastric lavage if it can be done soon after ingestion.
5. Give activated charcoal if soon after ingestion.
6. Administer arterial blood gas with measured oxygen saturation.
7. Methylene blue must be administered with caution when methemoglobin level is >30%. Methylene blue reverses the process of methemoglobin formation by reducing methemoglobin back to hemoglobin. This treatment should not be used in the presence of G-6-PD deficiency.
8. Give blood exchange transfusion(s).
9. Administer hyperbaric oxygen therapy.
10. Forced diuresis and urine alkalinization are NOT helpful.
11. Do NOT acidify urine.

Increased: Acquired or hereditary methemoglobinemia, carbon monoxide poisoning, ionizing radiation, smoking. Drugs include acetanilid, aniline dyes, benzene derivatives, benzocaine, Bromo-Seltzer, chlorates, chloroquine, dapsone, isoniazid, lidocaine, metoclopramide, nitrates, nitrites (including silver nitrate topical ointment), phenacetin, resorcinol, and sulfonamides.

Decreased: Pancreatitis.

Description: This test is used to help detect the adverse effects of drugs containing nitrates or nitrites, such as nitroglycerine. Methemoglobin is formed when the iron in the heme portion of deoxygenated hemoglobin is oxidized to a ferric form due to a hereditary deficiency of nicotinamide adenine dinucleotide-diaphorase or due to exposures to chemicals and drugs. In the ferric form, oxygen and iron cannot combine. This is a normal process, and it is balanced by the reduction of methemoglobin to hemoglobin. However, when a high concentration of methemoglobin is produced in the red blood cells (RBCs), then the capacity of RBCs to combine with oxygen is reduced, and anoxia and

cyanosis result. Methemoglobinemia occurs when greater than 1% of the blood hemoglobin has been oxidized to the ferric form and is a rare, but potentially dangerous, condition in which the oxygen-carrying capacity of the blood is compromised.

Professional Considerations:

1. Consent form NOT required.
2. Preparation:
   A. Tube: Green-top. Also obtain ice.
3. Procedure:
   A. Draw a 7-ml blood sample.
4. Postprocedure care:
   A. Place the specimen on ice and deliver immediately to the laboratory. Specimens must be tested within 1 hour of collection.
5. Client and family teaching:
   A. If activated charcoal was given for elevated levels, the client should drink 4–6 glasses of water each day for 2 days to prevent constipation. Activated charcoal will cause stools to be black for a few days.
   B. Review with the client and family potential sources that may have caused methemoglobinemia and identify corrective measures for removal of the exposure.
6. Factors that affect results:
   A. The intestinal flora of nursing infants is capable of converting significant amounts of inorganic nitrate (e.g., well water) to the nitrite ion, which can produce serious toxicity.
   B. Amyl nitrite ingestion increases methemoglobinemia.
   C. Falsely elevated results occur when there is a delay of more than 1 hour after collection before the test is measured.
   D. Falsely low results may occur when the sample is not kept on ice until testing.
   E. Symptoms will appear at lower than the above scale in clients who are anemic.
7. Other data:
   A. Clients suspected of having methemoglobinemia may experience symptoms of anoxia or cyanosis, without evidence of cardiovascular or pulmonary disease.
   B. Hidden sources of nitrates, which could cause methemoglobinemia, include spinach and Polish sausage, which is rich in nitrite and nitrate, and drinking well water, which contains nitrites.
   C. Nitrate can be absorbed from topical applications, such as silver nitrate (used to treat serious burns). It must be used sparingly when applied to infants, in order to avoid serous conversion of nitrate to nitrite.
   D. Infants are more susceptible to methemoglobinemia than adults, since fetal hemoglobin is more easily converted

to methemoglobin than adult hemoglobin.

E. Poisoning is reportable to public health authorities if secondary to occupational or environmental causes.

Bibliography:

Forsyth RJ, Moulden A: Methaemoglobinaemia after ingestion of amyl nitrite. Arch Dis Child 66(1): 152, 1991.

Gonzalez-Aller de Solis M, Hendrix LY: Acute methemoglobinemia: a nursing perspective. Crit Care Nurs 15(3):33–38, 1995.

Micromedx, Inc: Methemoglobinemia, 82, 1994.

Uchida I, Tashiro C, Koo YH, et al.: Carboxyhemoglobin and methemoglobin levels in banked blood. J Clin Anesth 2(2):86–90, 1990.

Bibliography:

American Hospital Association: Methicillin-Resistant Staphylococcus Aureus Task Force. Methicillin-resistant Staphylococcus aureus (MRSA): a briefing for acute care hospitals and nursing facilities. Infect Control Hosp Epidemiol 15(2):105–115, 1994.

Chambers HF: Detection of methicillin-resistant staphylococci. Infect Dis Clin North Am 7(2): 425–433, 1993.

Hartstein AI, Denny MA, Morthland VH, LeMonte AM, Pfaller MA: Control of methicillin-resistant Staphylococcus aureus in a hospital and an intensive care unit. Infect Control Hosp Epidemiol 16(7):405–411, 1995.

Zafar AB, Butler RC, Reese DJ, Gaydos LA, Mennonna PA: Use of 0.3% triclosan (BACTI-STAT) to eradicate an outbreak of methicillin-resistant Staphylococcus aureus in a neonatal nursery. Am J Infect Control 23(3):200–208, 1995.

METHICILLIN-RESISTANT *STAPHYLOCOCCUS AUREUS* (MRSA), CULTURE

Norm: Negative.

Usage: Infections.

Description: MRSA is a strain of *Staphylococcus aureus* that is resistant to methicillin, the antibiotic most commonly used to treat staphylococcal infections. This organism is most commonly acquired in hospitals.

Professional Considerations:

1. Consent form NOT required.
2. Preparations:
   A. Obtain a sterile cotton-tip Culturette swab with sodium chloride medium.
3. Procedure:
   A. Culture a specific site, using a rotating motion for 10 seconds, using one swab per site.
   B. Place the swab in the sodium chloride medium.
4. Postprocedure care:
   A. Transport the sample to the laboratory within 8 hours.
5. Client and family teaching:
   A. Results are normally available within a few days.
6. Factors that affect results:
   A. Methicillin-resistant staphylococci are considered resistant to all cephalosporins and imipenem.
   B. Detection is enhanced by incubation at 30–35°C and the use of sodium chloride medium.
7. Other data:
   A. Methicillin resistance occurs in up to 40% of isolated *Staphylococcus epidermidis* and is increasing as an isolate of *S. aureus* in hospitals and extended care facilities.
   B. 0.3% triclosan (BACTI-STAT), used as a hand-washing soap, has eradicated MRSA outbreaks.

METHOTREXATE (MTX), SERUM

Norm: Levels for therapeutic maintenance are variable.

High dose MTX for cancer treatment: 10^{-6} M and 10^{-7} M at 24–72 hours after drug infused.

Panic Level: At 48 hours after high-dose MTX: 454 mg/ml or 1000 μmol/L.

Panic Level Symptoms and Treatment:

Symptoms: Increased severity of expected side effects, including stomatitis, nausea, vomiting, anorexia, diarrhea, infection, bleeding, bone marrow depression, gastrointestinal ulceration, and, with prolonged use, pneumonitis and serious hepatotoxicity. Drugs that increase toxicity include chloramphenicol, *para*-amino benzoic acid phenytoin, probenecid, salicylates, sulfonamides, and tetracycline.

Treatment:

Perform leucovorin calcium rescue. Continued monitoring of blood levels is necessary.
Hemodialysis WILL, but peritoneal dialysis will NOT, remove methotrexate.

Usage: Monitor for therapeutic levels of methotrexate, which is used to treat cancer, cholangitis, rheumatoid arthritis, and sarcoidosis.

Description: A blood test for monitoring the serum levels of methotrexate. MTX is a protein-bound, folic acid antagonist and antimetabolite, and its action is specific in the cell cycle S-phase. It is used primarily in the treatment of cancer, including acute leukemias. MTX interferes with normal biosynthesis of nucleic acids, which are necessary for synthesis of deoxyribonucleic acid (DNA) and ribonucleic acid (RNA). Intravenous methotrexate may be given in low doses (10–50 mg/m^2), medium doses (100–500 mg/m^2), or high doses (500 mg/m^2 or more). MTX is absorbed by the gastrointestinal tract and cleared by the kidneys, with a half-life of 1.5–15 hours, and peak blood levels occurring 1–2 hours after dose.

Professional Considerations:

1. Consent form NOT required.
2. Preparation:
   A. Tube: Red-top, red/gray-top, or gold-top.
   B. Renal and hepatic function must be assessed prior to the administration of MTX.

  C. Do NOT draw specimens during hemodialysis.
3. Procedure:
   A. Draw a 1-ml blood sample.
4. Postprocedure care:
   A. Observe for symptoms of methotrexate toxicity.
5. Client and family teaching:
   A. Results are normally available within 24 hours.
6. Factors that affect results:
   A. Drugs that displace MTX from plasma proteins include chloral hydrate, phenytoin, salicylates, sulfonamides, and tetracyclines.
7. Other data:
   A. Leucovorin rescue is essential following high-dose MTX administration. It is generally administered 24 hours after the first methotrexate dose is begun, and it is dosed every 6 hours for up to 12 doses.

Bibliography:

Anonymous. Drug watch. Folic acid for Methotrexate toxicity. Am J Nurs *95*(2):55–56, 1995.
Burke MB, Wilkes GM, Berg D, Bean CK, Ingwerson K: Cancer Chemotherapy: A Nursing Process Approach. Boston, MA, Jones and Bartlett, 1991, pp 290–294.

METHSUXIMIDE, SERUM

Norm: Negative.

Therapeutic range of metabolite n-desmethyl methsuximide	10–40 µg/ml
Toxic level (of metabolite)	>40 µg/ml
Panic level (of metabolite)	>150 µg/ml

Panic Level Symptoms and Treatment:

Symptoms: CNS symptoms (ataxia, dizziness, drowsiness) and GI symptoms (anorexia, abdominal pain, diarrhea, nausea, vomiting) are most common. Other symptoms include severe depression, skin rash, periorbital edema, urinary frequency, vaginal bleeding, pancytopenia, hepatotoxicity, neuropathy.

Treatment:

Give activated charcoal slurry.
Administer saline cathartic unless client has an ileus.
Administer Sorbitol.
Do gastric lavage if possible soon after ingestion.
Protect airway and support breathing.
Perform neurologic checks q 1 hour.
Forced diuresis is not helpful.

Charcoal hemoperfusion may be helpful in removing the methsuximide metabolite in comatose clients. No information was found on the effectiveness of hemodialysis in removing methsuximide.

Increased: Overdose.

Decreased: Convulsions and epilepsy.

Description: Anticonvulsant for petit mal seizures that depresses nerve transmission to the motor cortex, thereby decreasing paroxysmal spike and wave patterns. Plasma half-life is 2–4 hours. Methsuximide is metabolized in the liver and excreted in urine.

Professional Considerations:

1. Consent form NOT required.
2. Preparation:
   A. Tube: Red-top, red/gray-top, or gold-top.

B. Do NOT draw specimens during hemodialysis.
3. Procedure:
   A. Draw a 7-ml blood sample prior to the next dose of medication.
4. Postprocedure care:
   A. None.
5. Client and family teaching:
   A. Explain overdose symptoms and treatment (see above), as appropriate.
   B. For an intentional overdose, refer the client and family for crisis intervention and counseling.
6. Factors that affect results:
   A. Obtaining specimens after medication has been ingested will cause increased results.
   B. Hepatic or renal dysfunction may cause increased results.
7. Other data:
   A. This drug may cause a positive albumin in the urine and an elevated BUN.
   B. In pediatric clients, the C/D ratio (plasma concentration and dose per kg) is less sensitive to both age and associated therapy.

Bibliography:

Battino D: Clinical pharmokinetics of antiepileptic drugs in paediatric patients. Pt I: Phenobarbital, primidone, valproic acid, ethosuximide and mesuximide (methsuximide). Clin Pharmacokinet *29*(4):257–286, 1995.
Hacobs DS, Kasten BL Jr, Demott WR, et al.: Laboratory Test Handbook with DRG Index. St Louis, MO, Mosby/Lexi-Comp, 1984, p 515.
Tennison MB: Methsuximide for intractable childhood seizures. Pediatrics *87*(2):186–189, 1991.

METHYLENE BLUE STAIN, STOOL

Norm: No predominance of yeast, gram-positive cocci in clusters, or leukocytes.

Positive: Amebiasis, antibiotic-associated colitis, *Campylobacter,* Crohn's disease, dysentery, enteric fever, gastroenteritis of bacterial origin, *Helicobacter pylori,* salmonellosis, shigellosis, ulcerative colitis, and *Yersinia* infection.

Negative: Toxigenic bacterial infection (*Escherichia coli, Vibrio cholerae,* or *Clostridium difficile*), giardiasis, and viral gastroenteritis.

Description: Microscopic examination of feces for leukocytes. White blood cells are microscopically identified in the stool with either Wright's staining or methylene blue staining in diarrheal diseases. In dysentery and ulcerative colitis, there are increased leukocytes; in viral gastroenteritis, leukocytes are absent.

Professional Considerations:
1. Consent form NOT required.
2. Preparation:
   A. Collect specimens prior to the barium procedure.
   B. Obtain a Culturette or bedpan or a plastic specimen hat for use with a toilet seat, a wooden tongue blade, and a sterile container with lid.
3. Procedure:
   A. Stool samples from 3 consecutive days are recommended.
   B. *Rectal swab:* Collect a fresh random stool on a Culturette swab, allowing the swab to remain in the rectum for 15–30 seconds. Insert the swab into the tube and crush the distal end to release an ampule of media.
   C. *Stool sample:*
      i. Instruct the client to defecate in a bedpan or toilet seat specimen hat, and to avoid contaminating the stool with urine, toilet paper, soap, or water.
      ii. Using a wooden tongue blade, place a 1-inch diameter, fresh stool sample into a sterile container and cap tightly.
4. Postprocedure care:
   A. Document the specimen collection time on the laboratory requisition.
   B. Send the specimen to microbiology within 6 hours.
   C. Refrigerate the specimen until testing.
5. Client and family teaching:
   A. Explain the collection procedure if the client will be collecting the sample.
6. Factors that affect results:
   A. Reject specimens contaminated with urine or >6 hours old.
   B. Reject stools mixed with barium, castor oil, or bulk laxatives, all of which inhibit leukocyte growth.
7. Other data:
   A. *Salmonella typhi* may evoke a monocyte response.
   B. In utero methylene blue exposure may relate to fetal intestinal obstruction.
   C. Detection of salmonella and shigellosis is most likely during the first 3 days of infection.
   D. Testing stool specimens for fecal leukocytes is not useful for predicting the presence of C. difficile toxin, because 72% of stool specimens positive for C. difficile toxin are negative for fecal leukocytes, despite their stability.
   E. *Entamoeba histolytica* amebiasis is a reportable disease in most areas.

Bibliography:

Jacobs DS, Kasten BL Jr, Demott WR, et al.: Laboratory Test Handbook with DRG Index. St Louis, MO, Mosby/Lexi-Comp, 1984, pp 460–461.
Marx CE: Fecal leukocytes in stool specimens submit-

ted for *Clostridium difficile* toxin assay. Diagn Microbiol Infect Dis *16*(4):313–315, 1993.

Misra V: The Loeffler's methylene blue stain: an inexpensive way for detection of *Helicobacter pylori*. J Gastroenterol Hepatol *9*(5):512–513, 1994.

METHYLENEDIOXY-AMPHETAMINE

(see Amphetamines, Blood)

METHYLPHENIDATE, SERUM

Norm: Negative.

Therapeutic Level: 0.01–0.04 µg/ml (0.04–0.17 µmol/L, SI units).

Overdose Symptoms and Treatment:

Symptoms: Agitation, hyperactive, talkative, sleepless for days, paranoia, hallucinations, violent behavior possible, confusion, dryness of mucous membranes, headache, mydriasis, hypertension, rapid and irregular pulse, sweating, vomiting, cerebral hemorrhage, seizures, convulsions, and coma.

Treatment:

Do gastric lavage.
Give activated charcoal.
Perform forced diuresis.
Acid urine hastens excretion.
Administer cathartic.
Acidify urine.
Support symptoms.
Take precautions to prevent self-injury.
Treatments administered outside a health care facility should be used as directed by a poison control center.
No information on the effectiveness of dialysis is known.

Usage: Monitor levels of methylphenidate, which is used in the treatment of hyperkinetic disorders (e.g., ADHD, hyperactivity associated with minimal brain dysfunction), nar-colepsy, mild depression, senile behavior, and children with perceptual problems; and methylphenidote also counteracts overdosage from depressant drugs.

Increased: Overdose and stimulant drug abuse.

Decreased: Subtherapeutic dose.

Description: Methylphenidate (Ritalin) is a central nervous system (CNS) stimulant and antidepressant that presumably activates brainstem and cortex arousal. Methylphenidate is well absorbed from the gastrointestinal tract and is distributed throughout the body. Its actions appear in about 1 hour after ingestion and last up to 6 hours. The drug is completely metabolized in the liver to inactive products that are excreted in urine. Tolerance to the CNS and peripheral effects develops with continued use.

Professional Considerations:

1. Consent form NOT required.
2. Preparation:
   A. Tube: Lavender-top.
   B. Do NOT draw specimens during hemodialysis.
3. Procedure:
   A. Draw a 7-ml blood sample.
4. Postprocedure care:
   A. None.
5. Client and family teaching:
   A. If activated charcoal was given for elevated levels, the client should drink 4–6 glasses of water each day for two days to prevent constipation. The activated charcoal will cause stools to be black for a few days.
6. Factors that affect results:
   A. None found.
7. Other data:
   A. None.

Bibliography:

Lazarus LW, Moberg PJ, Langsley PR, Lingam VR: Methylphenidate and nortriptyline in the treatment of poststroke depression: a retrospective comparison. Arch Phys Med Rehab *75*(4):403–406, 1994.

Scahill L, Lynch KA: The use of methylphenidate in children with attention-deficit hyperactivity disorder. J Child Adolescent Psychiatr Nurs *7*(4):44–47, 1994.

METHYPRYLON, SERUM

Norm: Negative.

		SI Units
Therapeutic level	8–10 µg/ml	44–55 µmol/L
Panic level	>50 µg/ml	>273 µmol/L

Panic Level Symptoms and Treatment:

Symptoms: Apnea, central nervous system depression, hypotension, pulmonary edema, shock, coma. Death has occurred after ingestion of 6 g.

Treament:
Perform diuresis with IV fluids.
Give gastric lavage if possible soon after ingestion.
Give activated charcoal.
Give supportive therapy.
Hemodialysis, peritoneal dialysis, and hemoperfusion WILL remove methyprylon.

Usage: Monitoring for therapeutic drug level.

Description: Methyprylon is a sedative-hypnotic that induces sleep within 45 minutes by increasing the threshold of the arousal centers of the brain. Plasma half-life is 3–6 hours. It is conjugated in the liver and excreted in the urine. Addiction and physical dependence can occur.

Professional Considerations:

1. Consent form NOT required.
2. Preparation:
   A. Tube: Red-top or red/gray-top or gold-top.
   B. Do NOT draw specimens during hemodialysis.
3. Procedure:
   A. Draw a 7-ml blood sample.
4. Postprocedure care:
   A. None.
5. Client and family teaching:
   A. If activated charcoal was given for elevated levels, the client should drink 4–6 glasses of water each day for two days to prevent constipation. The activated charcoal will cause stools to be black for a few days.
6. Factors that affect results:
   A. Interferes with urine diagnostics for 17-KS and 17-OHCS.
7. Other data:
   A. The trade name is Noludar.

Bibliography:

Contos DA: Nonlinear elimination of methyprylon (noludar) in an overdosed patient: correlation of clinical effects with plasma concentration. J Pharm Sci 80(8):768–771, 1991.

Gwilt PR: Pharmokinetics of methyprylon following a single oral dose. J Pharm Sci 74(9):1001–1003, 1985.

Kleeman WP: Thermodynamic evaluation of activated charcoal as a poison antidote by high-performance liquid chromatography. II: In vitro method for the evaluation of activated charcoal as a poison antidote. J Pharm Sci 77(6):506–510, 1988.

Pancorbo AS, Palagi PA, Piecoro JJ, Wilson HD: Hemodialysis in methyprylon overdose. Some pharmacokinetic considerations. JAMA 237:470–471, 1977.

Rall TW: Hypnotics and sedatives. In Gillman AG, Rall TW, Niles AS, Taylor P (eds): Goodman and Gillman's The Pharmacological Basis of Therapeutics, 8th ed. New York, Pergamon Press, 1990, p 366.

METYRAPONE (CORTISOL) TEST, SERUM

Norm:

		SI Units
11-Deoxycortisol	>7 µg/dl	>202 nmol/L
Cortisol	<3 µg/dl	<83 nmol/L

Increased: Adrenal carcinoma, Cushing's syndrome, diabetic acidosis, fever, hepatic disease, hyperthyroidism, hypoalbuminemia, obesity, pain, pregnancy, renal disease, and stress. Drugs include estrogens, oral contraceptives, and spironolactone.

Decreased: Addison's disease, fungal invasion, hemorrhage, hepatic disease, hypopituitarism, hypothyroidism, low birth weight infants, respiratory distress syndrome, and tuberculosis. Drugs include amitriptyline, androgens, chlordiazepoxide, glucocorticoids, methysergide, oral contraceptives, phenobarbital, phenothiazines, phenytoin, progestins, rifampin, and steroids.

Description: The metyrapone test is a diagnostic test for secondary adrenal insufficiency. Metyrapone is an inhibitor of 11-betahydroxylase that prevents the conversion of 11-deoxycortisol to cortisol in the adrenal glands. The diminished level of cortisol stimulates the pituitary to produce adrenocorticotropic hormone (ACTH) in a negative feedback mechanism. In normal individuals, more ACTH is produced.

Professional Considerations:

1. Consent form NOT required.
2. Preparation:
   A. Tube: Red-top, red/gray-top, or gold-top or green-top. Also obtain ice.
   B. Metyrapone, 30 mg/kg (range 2–3 g), is given orally, usually with milk, at 11 P.M.
   C. Assess for a history of heroin addiction or use and methadone maintenance, as this test may induce a narcotic withdrawal-like syndrome.
3. Procedure:
   A. Draw a 1-ml blood sample at 8 A.M. the following morning.
4. Postprocedure care:
   A. Specimens should be placed on ice.
5. Client and family teaching:
   A. Return tomorrow at approximately 8 A.M. for a repeat blood draw.
6. Factors that affect results:
   A. Reject the specimen if the client had a radioactive scan within 7 days of the test.
   B. Specimens should be frozen if the test is not performed within 24 hours.
   C. Results are highly dependent on the time of day the specimen is obtained (circadian variation).
7. Other data:
   A. Do NOT perform this test if primary adrenal insufficiency is likely.
   B. Long-term treatment with metyrapone can cause hypertension.
   C. See also Cortisol, Serum or Plasma; and Metyrapone (Cortisol), 24-Hour, Urine.

Bibliography:

Kodama C, Nakada T, Sasagawa I, et al.: An unusual profile of endocrine study in a patient with pre-Cushing's syndrome. Int Urol Nephrol 25(6): 517–524, 1993.

Lieberman SA, Eccleshall TR, Feldman D: ACTH-independent massive bilateral adrenal disease (AIMBAD): A subtype of Cushing's syndrome with major diagnostic and therapeutic implications. Eur J Endocrinol 131(1):67–73, 1994.

Touitou Y: Effects of ageing on endocrine and neuroendocrine rhythms in humans. Horm Res 43:12–19, 1995.

Yu J, Zolle I, Mertens J, et al.: Synthesis of 2-[131 I] Iodophenyl-metyrapone using Cu(I)-assisted nucleophilic exchange labeling: Study of the reaction conditions. Nucl Med Biol 22(2):257–262, 1995.

METYRAPONE (CORTISOL), 24-HOUR, URINE

Norm:

17-Hydroxycorticosteroids (17-OHCS): 2–4 times base level.

17-Ketogenic steroids (17-KGS): 2.5–3.0-fold rise, but at least 10 mg/dl (35 μmol/day, SI units).

17-Ketosteroids (17-KS): >2 times base level.

Increased: Acute alcohol intoxication, Cushing's syndrome, ectopic ACTH syndrome, hepatic disease, hyperthyroidism, obesity, and stress. Drugs include amphetamines, corticosteroids, morphine, phenothiazines, and reserpine.

Decreased: Addison's disease, adrenogenital syndrome, and pituitary insufficiency.

Description: Diagnostic test for secondary adrenal insufficiency. An inhibitor of 11-betahydroxylase that prevents the conversion of 11-deoxy-cortisol to cortisol. The diminished levels of cortisol stimulate the pituitary to produce more adrenocorticotropic hormone (ACTH) in a negative feedback mechanism. In normal individuals, more ACTH is produced, which results in an increase in urinary hydroxysteroids and ketosteroids.

Professional Considerations:

1. Consent form NOT required.
2. Preparation:
   A. Assess for history of heroin addiction/use or methadone maintenance, as this test may cause narcotic withdrawal-like symptoms.
   B. Administer metyrapone to adults in doses of 750 mg every 4 hours × 6 doses. In the child, the dose is 300 mg/m².
   C. Begin administration at 11 P.M.
3. Procedure:
   A. Begin a 24-hour urine collection at 8 A.M. the morning after the drug was ingested.
   B. Collection container must be acidified with either hydrochloric or acetic acid as a preservative.
4. Postprocedure care:
   A. Write the beginning and ending date and time, as well as total urine voided in the 24-hour period, on the laboratory requisition.
   B. Record the total dose and the time metyrapone was given on the laboratory requisition.
5. Client and family teaching:
   A. Minimize stress levels prior to urine collection.
   B. Save all the urine voided in the 24-hour period and urinate before defecating to avoid loss of urine. Keep the specimen on ice or refrigerate it during the collection period. If any urine is accidentally discarded, discard the entire specimen and restart the collection the next day.

6. Factors that affect results:
   A. Inaccurate collection of urine.
   B. When possible, hold all medications for several days prior to testing. Drugs that may interfere with results include estrogens, glucose, meprobamate, penicillin, and radiographic contrast materials.
   C. Obesity, pregnancy, and stress may affect results.
7. Other data:
   A. Hospitalization may be required to ensure accuracy of the 24-hour urine collection.
   B. Long-term treatment with metyrapone can cause hypertension.
   C. The 24-hour urine specimen reflects cumulative levels rather than circadian variation.
   D. *See also Cortisol, Urine; Metyrapone (Cortisol) Test, Serum; 17-OHCS, Urine; 17-KGS, Urine; and 17-KS, Urine.*

Bibliography:

Kodama C, Nakada T, Sasagawa I, et al.: An unusual profile of endocrine study in a patient with pre-Cushing's syndrome. Int Urol Nephrol 25(6): 517–524, 1993.

Lieberman SA, Eccleshall TR, Feldman D: ACTH-independent massive bilateral adrenal disease (AIM-BAD): A subtype of Cushing's syndrome with major diagnostic and therapeutic implications. Eur J Endocrinol 131(1):67–73, 1994.

Touitou Y: Effects of ageing on endocrine and neuroendocrine rhythms in humans. Horm Res 43: 12–19, 1995.

Yu J, Zolle I, Mertens J, et al.: Synthesis of 2-[131 I] Iodophenyl-metyrapone using Cu(I)-assisted nucleophilic exchange labeling: Study of the reaction conditions. Nucl Med Biol 22(2):257–262, 1995.

MIB 1–3

(see Ki-67 Proliferation Marker, Specimen)

MICROALBUMIN, SPOT URINE

(see Albumin, Serum, Urine, and 24-Hour Urine)

MICROFILARIA, PERIPHERAL BLOOD

Norm: Negative or no parasite identified. An indirect hemagglutination titer of 1:128 as well as a bentonite flocculation titer of 1:5 are considered minimally significant titers.

Positive: *Brugia, Dipetalonema, Loa loa, Mansonella,* and *Wuchereria.*

Description: Filaria make up a large group of parasitic worms that produce embryos known as microfilaria (intermediate stage between egg and larvae). These parasites invade the lymphatics, causing lymphedema and elephantiasis. Microfilaria are the smallest forms of filaria.

Professional Considerations:
1. Consent form NOT required.
2. Preparation:
   A. Tube: Green-top.
   B. Include the client's recent travel history on the laboratory requisition.
3. Procedure:
   A. Draw a 4-ml blood sample.
   B. Repeat the test to obtain daytime and nighttime specimens.
4. Postprocedure care:
   A. Transport specimens to the laboratory immediately. Specimens should NOT be clotted.
5. Client and family teaching:
   A. Two specimens, preferably 12 hours apart, are necessary.
6. Factors that affect results:
   A. One negative result does not rule out a parasitic infection.
   B. Circulating microfilaria may NOT be detected in blood for 6–12 months after transmission occurs.
7. Other data:
   A. Because *Wuchereria* and *Brugia* are nocturnal, the optimal blood sample time would be 10 P.M. to 2 A.M.
   B. Because *Loa loa* is diurnal, the optimum time for the blood sample would be 12 P.M. (noon).

Bibliography:

Anosike JC, Onwuliri COE, Abanobi OC: A case of probable transplacental transmission of *Wuchereria bancrofti microfilariae.* Appl Parasitol 35(4):294–296, 1994.

El Bassiouny AEI, El Gammal NE, Mahmoud AM: Isolation and concentration of microfilariae from peripheral blood of *Wuchereria bancrofti* infected patients by density gradient centrifugation. J Egypt Soc Parasitol 23(1):255–261, 1993.

Harbut CL, Orihel TC: *Brugia beaveri:* Microscopic morphology in host tissues and observations on its life history. J Parasitol 81(2):239–243, 1995.

Rawlins SC, Chailett P, Ragoonanansingh RN: Microscopical and serological diagnosis of *Wuchereria bancrofti.* West Indian Med J 43:75–79, 1994.

MICROHEMAGGLUTINATION *TREPONEMA PALLIDUM* (MHA-TP) TEST, SERUM

Norm: Titer <1:160 or nonreactive.

Usage: Serologic confirmation of syphilis when nontreponemal antibody tests (RPR or VDRL) are positive.

Description: Syphilis is a complex, sexually transmitted disease characterized by a wide range of symptoms that imitate other diseases and that is caused by the organism *Treponema pallidum*. In this test, the client's serum is heat treated and mixed with *Treponema pallidum*-sensitized sheep red blood cells, incubated, and compared with a control. A positive result occurs when agglutination occurs in the test sample, but not in the control. This test is less sensitive than the fluorescent treponemal antibody-absorption (FTA-ABS) DS for primary syphilis. Positive results will occur in treponemal diseases of bejel, pinta, syphilis, or yaws.

Professional Considerations:

1. Consent form NOT required.
2. Preparation:
   A. *See Client and family teaching.*
   B. Tube: Red-top.
3. Procedure:
   A. Draw a 1-ml blood sample.
4. Postprocedure care:
   A. Send the specimen to the laboratory and refrigerate them until tested.
5. Client and family teaching:
   A. Fast overnight prior to the test.
   B. The use of condoms significantly reduces the risk of sexually transmitted diseases.
   C. A referral for HIV testing may be indicated and should be discussed and offered to interested clients.
   D. If testing is positive:
      i. Notify all sexual contacts from the last 90 days (if early stage) to be tested for syphilis.
      ii. Syphilis can be cured with antibiotics. These may worsen the symptoms for the first 24 hours.
      iii. Do not have sex for 2 months and until after repeat testing has confirmed that the syphilis is cured. Use condoms after that for 2 years. Return for repeat testing every 3–4 months for the next 2 years to make sure the disease is cured.
      iv. Do not become pregnant for 2 years, because syphilis can be transmitted to the fetus.
      v. If left untreated, syphilis can damage many body organs, including the brain, over several years' time.
6. Factors that affect results:
   A. False-positive results may be due to autoimmune disorders, connective tissue diseases, infectious mononucleosis, leprosy, or systemic lupus erythematosus.
   B. Testing errors may be associated with dusty or improper plates and pipetting errors.
7. Other data:
   A. This test may remain positive indefinitely for clients previously infected

with syphilis. Thus, it is not useful for monitoring clinical response to treatment for syphilis.
   B. Test results may become negative after treatment. Therefore, negative results do NOT necessarily exclude a past history of syphilis.
   C. There is a significant correlation between the diagnosis of syphilis and seropositive HIV.
   D. *See also FTA-ABS DS, Serum; RPR, Diagnostic; and VDRL, Serum.*

Bibliography:

Anderson MD, Kennedy CA, Lewis AW, et al.: Retrobulbar neuritis complicating acute Epstein-Barr virus infection. CID *18*:799–801, 1994.

Augenbraun MH, DeHovitz JA, Feldman J, et al.: Biological false-positive syphilis test results for women infected with human immunodeficiency virus. CID *19*:1040–1044, 1994.

Larsen SA, Steiner BM, Rudolph AH: Laboratory diagnosis and interpretation of tests for syphilis. Clin Microbiol Rev *8*(1):1–21, 1995.

Marra CM, Critchlow CW, Hook EW III, et al.: Cerebrospinal fluid treponemal antibodies in untreated early syphilis. Arch Neurol *52*:68–72, 1995.

MIDAZOLAM

(see Benzodiazepines, Plasma and Urine)

MIGRATION INHIBITION TEST, BLOOD

Norm: Requires interpretation.

Increased: Allergic reactions, Hodgkin's disease, immunodeficiency, lymphoma, nephritis, and sarcoidosis. Drugs include chemotherapeutics.

Decreased: Not applicable.

Description: The lymphokine, migration inhibition factor, is released from sensitized lymphocytes for up to 4 days in the presence of stimulation by a specific type of antigen. Migration inhibition factor causes a change in the macrophage membrane so that clumping of macrophages occurs, thus preventing normal macrophage motility and phagocytic activity. The presence of migration inhibition factor is a sign of the body's impaired ability to fight off foreign antigens and may be used to evaluate cell mediated immunity.

Professional Considerations:

1. Consent form NOT required.
2. Preparation:
   A. Tube: Red-top, red/gray-top, gold-top, or green-top.

B. Preschedule the test with the laboratory.
3. Procedure:
   A. Draw a 7-ml blood sample.
4. Postprocedure care:
   A. Send the specimen to the laboratory
   promptly. Blood must be processed on
   the same day it is collected.
5. Client and family teaching:
   A. Results are normally available within
   24 hours.
6. Factors that affect results:
   A. Results are invalidated if the specimen
   is not fresh (i.e., was not collected the
   same day, resulting in nonviable lymphocytes).
7. Other data:
   A. The use of the migration inhibition test
   is questionable due to its expense and
   to the subjectivity of interpretation.

Bibliography:

Amichai B, Grunwald MH, Halevy S: Allergic vasculitis
induced by ecapepptyl-r: Confirmation by
macrophage migration inhibition factor (MIF)
test. Eur J Obstet Gynecol Reprod Biol 52(3):
217–218, 1993.
Brenner S, Halevy S, Livni E, et al.: Macrophage migration inhibition test in patients with drug-induced pemphigus. Isr J Med Sci 29:44–46, 1993.
Garty BZ, Offer I, Livni E, et al.: Erythema multiforme
and hypersensitivity myocarditis caused by ampicillin. Ann Pharmacother 28(6):730–731, 1994.
Mirecka J, Gil K: Influence of initial medium content
(pH, serum and Ca++ concentration) on leukocyte
migration test. Materia Med Pol 25(3–4):137–141,
1993.

MILK PRECIPITINS, BLOOD

Norm: Negative.

Increased: IgA deficiency, celiac disease, infantile diarrhea, mongolism,
pulmonary hemosiderosis, and
Wiskoff-Aldrich syndrome.

Description: Milk precipitins are antibodies found occasionally in children
who are sensitive to milk. This test involves adding blood to an agar gel and
waiting for a specific antibody concentration to develop in a line formation.
The distance of the precipitin line
from the point of application of the
blood is directly proportional to the
concentration of antigens in the
client's bloodstream.

Professional Considerations:

1. Consent form NOT required.
2. Preparation:
   A. Tube: Red-top, red/gray-top, or gold-
   top.
3. Procedure:
   A. Draw a 7-ml blood sample.
4. Postprocedure care:
   A. Results are normally available within

48 hours, but may take several days if
the test is performed off-site.
5. Client and family teaching:
   A. The test does not differentiate between
   sensitivity and allergy.
6. Factors that affect results:
   A. Gross contamination.
7. Other data:
   A. A positive test does not necessarily
   mean that the child is allergic to milk,
   as milk sensitivity may also cause a
   positive test.

Bibliography:

Halsey JF: Telephone interview, October 30, 1995. Lab-
oratory director, IBT Reference Laboratory, Spe-
cializing in Allergy and Clinical Immunology.
Lenexa, KS.
Jacobs DS, Kasten BL Jr, Demott WR, Wolfson WL:
Laboratory Test Handbook with DRG Index. St
Louis, MO, Mosby/Lexi-Comp, 1984, p 403.
Simickova M, Lang BA, Slepicka L: Polyclonal antibod-
ies to human milk caseins. J Dairy Res 58(1):
115–125, 1991.

MINIMUM BACTERICIDAL CONCENTRATION (MBC), CULTURE

Norm: >99% of colonies killed.

Increased: Not applicable.

Decreased: Endocarditis, leukopenia, and osteomyelitis.

Description: Also known as "minimum lethal concentration." Minimum
bactericidal concentration (MBC)
refers to the smallest concentration of
a specific antibiotic needed to cause
the death of a specific microorganism.
The MBC is performed routinely as
part of antibiotic susceptibility testing.
The test is performed by inoculating
the organism into media containing
serial dilutions of the antibiotic, incubating them, and then subculturing
them into antibiotic-free media and
incubating again. The MBC is the lowest antibiotic concentration that
causes death of at least 99.9% of the
organism on the first inoculum. The
test is especially important in infected
clients with impaired hepatic or renal
function, as many antibiotics can
worsen these conditions. Knowing the
MBC enables the physician to adjust
the antibiotic dose to the lowest effective level.

Professional Considerations:

1. Consent form NOT required.
2. Preparation:
   A. The physician must specify the culture
   source, culture date, specific bacterial

isolate to be tested, and antimicrobial agent to be tested.

3. Procedure:
   A. Culture the site, using a sterile Culturette.
4. Postprocedure care:
   A. Transport the culture to microbiology within 30 minutes of collection.
   B. Results are normally available in 2–4 days.
5. Client and family teaching:
   A. Results are normally available within 2–4 days.
6. Factors that affect results:
   A. Bacterium isolate from the client not available.
   B. Bacterium isolate fails to grow for testing.
7. Other data:
   A. Results are accurate to plus or minus one dilution, although the value to clinical practice is uncertain.
   B. Tolerance, inhibition of growth without killing, has been observed with *Staphylococcus aureus* and other gram-positive cocci.

Bibliography:

Butts JD: Intracellular concentrations of antibacterial agents and related clinical implications. Clin Pharmacokinet 27(1):63–84, 1994.

Corpet DE: Current status of models for testing antibiotic residues. Vet Human Toxicol 35(Suppl 1): 37–46, 1993.

Costerton JW, Khoury AE, Ward KH, et al.: Practical measures to control device-related bacterial infections. Int J Artif Organs 16(11):765–770, 1993.

Lee CK, Rubin LG, Moldwin RM: Synergy between protamine and vancomycin in the treatment of staphylococcus epidermidis biofilms. Urology 45(4):720–724, 1995.

MIXED LEUKOCYTE CULTURE (MIXED LYMPHOCYTE CULTURE), SPECIMEN

Norm: Requires interpretation.

Usage: Aplastic anemia, immunodeficiency (detection of T-lymphocyte abnormalities), transplants, and tuberculosis.

Description: Mixed leukocyte culture is performed to determine whether a prospective tissue transplant recipient's mononuclear cells will react against a potential donor's leukocyte antigens. This histocompatibility test may be performed in two ways. In a one-way test, the potential donor sample is irradiated or treated with mitomycin C, which prevents the sample from blast formation in reaction to mixture with the prospective recipient sample. This allows mea-

surement of prospective recipient blast formation only. In a two-way test, blast formation of both samples is monitored by comparing the amount of blast formation in the combined sample with that of each separate sample in combination with controls.

Professional Considerations:

1. Consent form NOT required.
2. Preparation:
   A. Preschedule the test with the laboratory.
   B. Tube: Two (2) green-top tubes.
3. Procedure:
   A. Draw a 7-ml blood sample from the prospective transplant donor. Label the tube as the "donor sample."
   B. Repeat the test for the prospective recipient. Label the tube as the "recipient sample."
4. Postprocedure care:
   A. Send the specimens to the laboratory within 2 hours.
   B. Specimens must be tested the same day.
5. Client and family teaching:
   A. Results are normally available in 7–10 days.
6. Factors that affect results:
   A. Reject any specimen that was not collected using a sterile procedure, not drawn in a heparinized tube, or arrives in the laboratory more than 2 hours after collection.
   B. False-negative results may occur if the prospective recipient is severely immunocompromised.
7. Other data:
   A. May be helpful in predicting graft survival.
   B. This test should be repeated for several days.

Bibliography:

Casper J, Camitta B, Truitt R, et al.: Unrelated bone marrow donor transplants for children with leukemia or myelodysplasia. Blood 85(9):2354–2363, 1995.

Rivas A, Ruegg CL, Zeitung J, et al.: V7, A novel leukocyte surface protein that participates in T cell activation. J Immunol 154(9):4423–4433, 1995.

Tanaka J, Imamura M, Kasai M, et al.: Cytokine gene expression after allogeneic bone marrow transplantation. Leukemia Lymphoma 16(5–6):413–418, 1995.

MIXING STUDY (CIRCULATING ANTICOAGULANTS), PLASMA

Norm: Requires interpretation.

Usage: To determine if prolonged coagulation studies (prothrombin time [PT] or partial thromboplastin time [PTT]) are resulting from circulating anticoagulants or Factor deficiencies.

Description: The coagulation system involves a number of reactions (clotting cascade) that are initiated when bleeding occurs. The clotting cascade requires clotting proteins (Factors I-XII, except Factor IV), fibrinogen, lymphocytes, macrophage, neutrophils, platelets, and prothrombin. These substances are naturally circulating and awaiting activation. There are also naturally occurring anticoagulants that circulate and inhibit the clotting process. Examples of anticoagulants include antithrombin, antithromboplastin, and heparin. When prolonged clotting studies are discovered (prolonged PT and or PTT), bleeding tendencies may arise. These prolonged studies may result from either Factor deficiencies or circulating anticoagulants. To determine which problem is occurring, a MIXING study may be performed. A mixing study involves mixing the plasma sample from a specimen with a prolonged PT and or PTT with a fresh plasma specimen having normal PT and/or PTT findings. Once the specimens are mixed, a repeat PT and PTT are performed to determine if a change or correction has occurred. If the cause of the prolonged coagulation study or studies is due to a circulating anticoagulant, the circulating anticoagulant will also alter the normal specimen it was mixed with and the PT and/or PTT will remain prolonged. If the problem is from a Factor deficiency or from Factor deficiencies, mixing the specimen with a normal specimen will correct the deficiency resulting in a corrected or normal PT and or PTT. Disorders associated with Factor deficiencies may include hemophilias (Hemophilia A and B and Von Willebrand's disease), hypoprothrombinemia and disseminated intravascular coagulation. Identifying circulating anticoagulants, such as the lupus anticoagulant, may assist in the diagnosis of systemic lupus erythematosus (SLE) or identify clients with lymphoproliferative disorders and thrombotic tendencies.

Professional Considerations:

1. Consent form NOT required.
2. Preparation:
   A. Preschedule this test with the laboratory.
   B. Tube: Four (4) 5-ml blue-top tubes.
   C. History of present or recent use of an-

ticoagulant therapy or medications that may cause inhibitory effects must be documented on the laboratory requisition.
   D. *See Client and family teaching.*
3. Procedure:
   A. Venipuncture should be performed as nontraumatically as possible. The time the tourniquet is applied should be minimized.
   B. Draw 4 blood samples, completely filling each tube with 5 ml of blood.
   C. If multiple blood tests are to be drawn, the mixing study specimens should be obtained LAST. If no other tests are to be drawn, discard at least 2 ml of blood before collecting the mixing study specimens.
   D. If hematocrit is >55%, special collection tubes, without vacuum, must be used when obtaining the specimens.
4. Postprocedure care:
   A. Promptly send the specimens to the laboratory. If the mixing study is not performed immediately, the specimens should be refrigerated. If testing is delayed >48 hours, the specimens should be double-spun and the plasma frozen.
   B. Specimens should be centrifuged for 10–15 minutes to produce platelet-poor plasma.
5. Client and family teaching:
   A. Fast for 8 hours prior to testing to minimize interference by lipemia.
   B. To minimize bleeding or injury, refrain from dental flossing or using a hard toothbrush. Do not receive intramuscular injections, aspirin, or nonsteroidal medications, and minimize activity that may produce physical injury when possible.
   C. Bleeding may not be unusual due to bleeding tendencies. An ice bag may be applied to the bruise, but excessive bruising should be reported to a physician.
6. Factors that affect results:
   A. Reject specimens if they are hemolyzed, their blood volume is insufficient, they are clotted, any processing error has occurred, or the specimens taken were from a heparinized intravenous line or arterial line site.
   B. Plasma not free of platelets (before freezing) or lipemia may affect results.
   C. Drugs that may affect results include antibiotics, chlorpromazine, phenytoin, procainamide, and quinidine.
7. Other data:
   A. Lupus anticoagulant is present in approximately 30% of clients with SLE and in those with lymphoproliferative disorders, recurrent abortions, and thrombotic phenomena.
   B. The more platelet-free the specimen, the greater the sensitivity in identifying the lupus anticoagulant.
   C. Fresh normal plasma should be ob-

tained from a specimen received no longer than 1 hour prior to performing the mixing study.

D. Acquired Factor V inhibitors may occur transiently postoperatively or post-blood transfusion.

E. *See also Prothrombin Time (PT), Serum and Partial Thromboplastin Time (PTT), Plasma.*

Bibliography:

Clyne LP, Fimls MS, Yen Y, et al.: The lupus anticoagulant: High incidence of "negative" mixing studies in a human immunodeficiency virus-positive population. Arch Pathol Lab Med *117*(6):595–601, 1993.

Robert A: Two different incubation times for the activated partial thromboplastin time (APTT): A new criterion for diagnosis of lupus anticoagulant. Thromb Haemost *71*(2):220–224, 1994.

Suehisa E, Toku M, Akita N, et al.: Study of an antibody against F1F2 fragment of human factor V in a patient with Hashimoto's disease and bullous pemphigoid. Thromb Res *77*(1):63–68, 1995.

Working Group on Hemostasis of the Société Française de Biologie Clinique: Comparison of a standardized procedure with current laboratory practices for the detection of lupus anticoagulant in France. Thromb Haemost *70*(5):781–786, 1993.

MONOCYTES, BLOOD

(see Differential Leukocyte Count, Peripheral Blood)

MONOS, BLOOD

(see Differential Leukocyte Count, Peripheral Blood)

MONOSPOT SCREEN (HETEROPHIL SCREEN), BLOOD

Norm: Negative.

Positive: Adenovirus, Burkitt's lymphoma, cytomegalovirus, Epstein-Barr virus, herpes simplex virus, HIV, Hodgkin's disease, infectious mononucleosis, Izumi fever, leukemia, malaria, pancreatic cancer, rubella virus, rheumatoid arthritis, sarcoidosis, serum sickness, systemic lupus erythematosus, and viral or infectious hepatitis.

Negative: Normal finding or infection of bacterial etiology.

Description: The monospot screen, a screening test that rapidly detects

heterophil agglutinins, is performed on two slides, each containing serum and horse red cells, with one slide also containing guinea pig kidney and the other slide containing beef red cell stroma. Agglutination that occurs on only the slide with guinea pig kidney is diagnostic of infectious mononucleosis. Heterophil agglutinins can appear in serum approximately 6–10 days after contact. Detection may remain for up to 1 year and peaks between 4 and 8 weeks after exposure.

Professional Considerations:

1. Consent form NOT required.
2. Preparation:
   A. Tube: Red-top, red/gray-top, or gold-top or lavender-top.
3. Procedure:
   A. Draw a 2-ml blood sample (red-top, red/gray-top, or gold-top) or a 3-ml blood sample (lavender-top).
4. Postprocedure care:
   A. Specimens should be refrigerated before testing.
5. Client and family teaching:
   A. Results are normally available within 72 hours.
6. Factors that affect results:
   A. A hemolyzed or chylous sample invalidates the results.
   B. About 10% of adults (more for children) produce false-positive or false-negative results.
7. Other data:
   A. The monospot screen has a 99% specificity and an 86% sensitivity in diagnosing infectious mononucleosis.
   B. In the presence of infectious mononucleosis, 10–25% atypical lymphocytes may be observed in the differential cell count.
   C. If mononucleosis is suspected based on clinical symptoms but the screening test is negative, more sensitive tests, such as heterophil antibody, cytomegalovirus, or toxoplasmosis antibodies, should be considered.
   D. *See also Heterophil Agglutinins, Blood.*

Bibliography:

Bailey RE: Diagnosis and treatment of infectious mononucleosis. Am Fam Physician *94*(4):879–885, 1994.

Markin RS: Manifestations of Epstein-Barr virus-associated disorders in liver. Liver *14*:1–13, 1994.

Weisenthal RW, Streeten BW, Dubansky AS, et al.: Burkitt lymphoma presenting as a conjunctival mass. Ophthalmology *102*(1):129–143, 1995.

MORPHINE, BLOOD

(see Toxicology, Drug Screen, Blood)

MORPHINE, URINE

Norm: Negative.

Panic Levels:

		SI Units
Hydromorphone	>0.1 mg/dl	>0.2 μmol/L
Methadone	>0.2 mg/dl	>10 μmol/L
Morphine	>0.005 mg/dl	>0.2 μmol/L

Panic Level Symptoms and Treatment:

Symptoms: Bradycardia, itching, hypotension, bradypnea, hypoxia, muscle spasms, pinpoint (miotic) pupils, dilated pupils in mixed drug overdose or severe acidosis, coma.

Treatment:

Administer naloxone 0.4 to 2 mg IV q 2–3 minutes in adults.
Administer naloxone 0.01 mg/kg IV q 2–3 minutes in children.
Provide respiratory support.
Hemodialysis will NOT remove morphine.

Increased or Positive: Drug use/abuse (especially heroin).

Description: Morphine is a narcotic analgesic used for pain relief. It relieves anxiety and tension, and causes sedation. It is habit forming and addictive. Overdose may cause bradycardia, hypotension, and severe respiratory and central nervous system depression. Ninety percent of a morphine dose is excreted in the urine within 24 hours of administration. Although morphine may be a potentially addictive or abused narcotic, two derivatives of morphine (heroin and codeine) are more commonly abused.

Professional Considerations:

1. Consent form NOT required unless the specimen is collected as legal evidence.
2. Preparation:
   A. Supervise the client when obtaining the sample if results may be used as medicolegal evidence.
   B. Obtain a sterile, preservative-free plastic or silanized-glass specimen container.
3. Procedure:
   A. Obtain a 25-ml random urine specimen.

4. Postprocedure care:
   A. If the results are to be used as legal evidence, the chain of possession must remain unbroken from the time the specimen is collected until court testimony.
5. Client and family teaching:
   A. Referrals to appropriate rehabilitation centers and therapeutic community programs should be offered to all addicted clients who may be interested.
   B. Behavior and level of consciousness may be significantly altered under the influence of opiates.
   C. Signs and symptoms of withdrawal may include agitation, anorexia, anxiety, diaphoresis, disorientation, hallucinations, insomnia, seizures, and tremors.
6. Factors that affect results:
   A. Poppy seed ingestion may produce false-positive results with the immunoassay method for up to 60 hours after ingestion.
   B. Morphine, 10 mg intravenously, is detectable in the urine for up to 84 hours.
7. Other data:
   A. Heroin is rapidly deacetylated to morphine in the human body.
   B. Hydromorphone is a semisynthetic phenanthrene derivative structurally similar to morphine. Hydromorphone has an 8–10 times more potent analgesic effect compared to morphine.
   C. Codeine is a phenanthrene derivative of opium made by methylation of morphine.
   D. Methadone is a synthetic diphenylheptane derivative similar to morphine. Oral methadone has a superior analgesic effect and a longer duration of action when compared to morphine.
   E. Phenothiazines prolong the depressant effect of morphine.
   F. Morphine will not dialyze out of the blood.
   G. *See also Toxicology, Drug Screen, Urine.*

Bibliography:

Ferrara SD, Tedeschi L, Frison G, et al.: Drugs-of-abuse testing in urine: Statistical approach and experimental comparison of immunochemical and chromatographic techniques. J Anal Toxicol *18*:278–291, 1994.

Molteni S, Caslavska J, Alleman D, et al.: Determination of methadone and its primary metabolite in human urine by capillary electrophoretic techniques. J Chromatogr B *658*:355–367, 1994.

Storrow AB, Wians FH, Mikkelsen SL, et al.: Does naloxone cause a positive urine opiate screen? Ann Emerg Med *24*(6):1151–1153, 1994.

MOTILE SPERM, WET MOUNT, DIAGNOSTIC

Norm: Negative.

Usage: Reported sexual assault.

Description: Fresh vaginal specimen examined microscopically for presence of sperm.

Professional Considerations:

1. Consent form or verbal consent IS usually required, because specimens may be used as legal evidence.
2. Preparation:
   A. Obtain a speculum, a wooden Pap-smear stick, normal saline with a 60-ml syringe, a sterile specimen cup, and slides with frosted tips on which to label client information.
   B. *See Client and family teaching.*
3. Procedure:
   A. Have the specimen collection witnessed, if the specimen may be used as legal evidence.
   B. Do NOT lubricate the speculum; this may inhibit sperm mobility.
   C. Obtain a vaginal specimen by vaginal wash with normal saline or a Pap-smear stick.
   D. Avoid cotton applicators.
4. Postprocedure care:
   A. Write the client's name, the date, exact time of collection, and specimen source on the laboratory requisition. Sign, and have the witness sign, the laboratory requisition.
   B. Transport the specimen to the laboratory immediately in a sealed plastic bag marked as legal evidence. All clients handling the specimen should sign and mark the time of receipt on the laboratory requisition.
5. Client and family teaching:
   A. The client may urinate before the procedure but should not wipe the vulva afterward; this may eliminate sperm.
   B. Survivors of sexual assault should be referred to appropriate crisis counseling agencies as well as for gynecologic follow-up.
   C. Referral for HIV testing should be reviewed and offered to all sexual assault victims.
   D. Preventive treatment for *Chlamydia*, gonorrhea, and syphilis should be provided to all survivors of sexual assault.
   E. The option of a postcoital contraceptive should be reviewed with all survivors of sexual assault.
6. Factors that affect results:
   A. Avoid extreme temperature change or direct sunlight on slides when en route to the laboratory or a legal agency.
   B. Delayed delivery of the specimen or use of a condom may decrease the number of viable sperm.
7. Other data:
   A. The presence of sperm is not proof of rape, as the definition of rape is a legal matter. Low levels do not exclude intercourse.
   B. Normal postcoital cervical mucosa reveal at least 10 motile sperm per high-power field.
   C. Federal/local laws, regulations, customs, and procedures must be known.

Bibliography:

Blain TMH, Warner CG: Rape and sexual assault. *In* Kravis TC, Warner CG, Jacobs LM (eds): Emergency Medicine, 3rd ed. New York, Raven Press, 1993, pp 1241–1257.

Gresham R, Rench J, Helbling-Sirinek L: Sexual Assault Protocol for the Treatment of Adult Sexual Assault Survivors. Columbus, Ohio Department of Health, 1992.

Guidi F, Revelli A, Soldati G, et al.: Influence of peritoneal fluid from spontaneous and stimulated cycles on sperm motility in vitro. Andrologia *25*:71–76, 1993.

MPV

(see Mean Platelet Volume, Blood)

MRI

(see Magnetic Resonance Imaging, Diagnostic)

MRSA

(see Methicillin-Resistant Staphylococcus Aureus, Culture)

MUCIN CLOT TEST, SPECIMEN

Norm: Firm clot formation with surrounding fluid appearing clear.

Usage: Helps differentiate the types of joint diseases.

Description: The mucin clot test reflects the polymerization of synovial fluid hyaluronate and correlates with viscosity except in acute effusions. Test is normal with degenerative joint disease, rheumatic fever, and systemic lupus erythematosus. An abnormal test demonstrated by a friable clot and turbid surrounding fluid occurs in a wide variety of inflammatory joint diseases such as arthritis of acute bacterial, rheumatoid, septic, or tuberculous origin, and gout. The addition of acetic acid to synovial fluid causes a mucin clot that is graded good, fair, or poor.

Professional Considerations:

1. Consent form IS required for synovial fluid aspiration. See *Biopsy, Site-Specific, Specimen* for procedure-specific risks and contraindications.
2. Preparation:
   A. Obtain a sterile aspiration tray.
   B. Tube: Lavender-top or any sterile tube containing 20 ml of 5% acetic acid.
   C. A local anesthetic should be considered prior to aspiration of synovial fluid.
3. Procedure:
   A. Aspirate the synovial fluid into a sterile tube while using a sterile technique.
   B. Add 5 ml of fluid into 20 ml of 5% acetic acid; normally, a clot will form in 60 seconds.
4. Postprocedure care:
   A. Refrigerate specimens if not tested within 5 hours.
5. Client and family teaching:
   A. Monitor the site for bleeding, drainage, or inflammation for 24–48 hours.
   B. A mild analgesic may be required for pain control.
   C. Call the physician for signs of infection at the procedure site: increasing pain, redness, swelling, purulent drainage, or fever >101°F (38.3°C).
6. Factors that affect results:
   A. Lack of synovial fluid aspirate.
7. Other data:
   A. Results are nonspecific alone and are not diagnostic of a single pathologic entity.

Bibliography:

McCarty DJ: Synovial fluid. *In* Bussy RK, Rondinelli SA, Hunsberger SL (eds): Arthritis and Allied Conditions, 12th ed, Vol 1. Philadelphia, Lea and Febiger, 1993, pp 63–84.

Schumacher HR: Synovial fluid analysis and synovial biopsy. *In* Kelley WN, Harris ED, Ruddy S, Sledge CB (eds): Textbook of Rheumatology, 4th ed. Philadelphia, WB Saunders, 1993, pp 562–578.

Wilson DG, Cooley AJ, MacWilliams PS, et al.: Effects of 0.05% chlorhexidine lavage on the tarsocrural joints of horses. Vet Surg *23*:442–447, 1994.

MUCIN-LIKE CARCINOMA-ASSOCIATED ANTIGEN (MCA), BLOOD

Norm: <11 U/ml.

Increased: Breast cancer, cirrhosis of the liver, gastrointestinal cancer, hepatitis, lung cancer, mammary dysplasia, metastasis, and ovarian cancer.

Decreased: Not clinically significant.

Description: Mucin-like carcinoma-associated antigen (MCA) is a high molecular weight glycoprotein. Small amounts of MCA are normally produced by epithelial cells that line the respiratory, gastrointestinal, and genitourinary tracts. Exocrine tissues such as mammary, salivary, and sweat glands will also produce small amounts of MCA. MCA can be useful as a serial marker for metastasis, in monitoring therapeutic responses to cancer treatment, in detecting relapse metastasis, enhancing specificity of bone scintigraphy, and for tumor staging.

Professional Considerations:

1. Consent form NOT required.
2. Preparation:
   A. Tube: Red-top, red/gray-top, or gold-top for serum samples.
   B. Tube: Lavender-top for plasma samples.
3. Procedure:
   A. Draw a 0.5-ml blood sample.
4. Postprocedure care:
   A. If the specimen is not tested immediately, it can be refrigerated for up to 48 hours. If testing is delayed beyond 48 hours, the specimen should be frozen.
5. Client and family teaching:
   A. Results are normally available within 72 hours.
6. Factors that affect results:
   A. MCA is normally elevated in the second trimester of pregnancy and will steadily rise until postpartum.
   B. When using MCA to monitor therapeutic response to cancer treatment, it is necessary to consistently measure either serum or plasma samples; they should not be interchanged.
   C. Specimens should be rejected if testing was >48 hours and specimens were not frozen.
7. Other data:
   A. Performance characteristics of testing have NOT been established.
   B. Two-thirds of all clients with breast or ovarian cancer have elevated MCA levels.
   C. Single MCA levels are NOT helpful when screening women for breast cancer.
   D. MCA has a 72% sensitivity in detecting reoccurrence of cancer in high-risk populations.

Bibliography:

Frenette PS, Thirlwell MP, Trudeau M, et al.: The diagnostic value of CA 27–29, CA 15–3, mucin-like carcinoma antigen, carcinoembryonic antigen, and CA 19–9 in breast and gastrointestinal malignancies. Tumor Biol *15*:247–254, 1994.

Lamerz R, Stieber P, Fateh-Moghadam A: Serum marker combinations in human breast cancer. In Vivo 7(68):607–613, 1993.

Sell S: Detection of cancer by tumor markers in the blood: A view to the future. Crit Rev Oncogen 4(4):419–433, 1993.

Werner M, Faser C, Silverberg M: Clinical utility and validation of emerging biochemical markers for mammary adenocarcinoma. Clin Chem 39(11, Pt 2):2386–2396, 1993.

MUCOPOLYSACCHARIDES, QUALITATIVE, URINE

Norm: Negative.

Positive: Beta-glucuronidase syndrome, Hunter's syndrome, Hurler syndrome, Maroteaux-Lamy syndrome, Morquio syndrome, Sanfilippo's syndrome, and Scheie syndrome. Drugs include heparin.

Description: Mucopolysaccharidoses are a group of inherited, autosomal recessive diseases. These inborn errors of metabolism result in an increased excretion of urinary mucopolysaccharides due to a lysosomal enzyme deficiency of either alpha-L-iduronidase, sulfoiduronate sulfatase, chondroitin sulfate, or arylsulfatase B.

Professional Considerations:

1. Consent form NOT required.
2. Preparation:
   A. Obtain a sterile specimen container.
3. Procedure:
   A. Obtain a 20-ml random urine specimen in a sterile container without preservative.
4. Postprocedure care:
   A. The specimen is stable for 1 week at 4°C.
5. Client and family teaching:
   A. Results are normally available within 72 hours.
6. Factors that affect results:
   A. Increased turbidity of urine causes positive results.
7. Other data:
   A. False-negative results can be as high as 32%.

Bibliography:

Beaudet AL: Lysosomal storage diseases. In Isselbacher KJ, Braunwald E, Wilson JD, Martin JB, Fauci AS, Kasper DL (eds): Harrison's Principals of Internal Medicine, 13th ed. New York, McGraw-Hill, 1994, pp 2090–2099.

Duran M, Dorland L, Wadman SK, et al.: Group tests for selective screening of inborn errors of metabolism. Eur J Pediatr 153(7, Suppl 1):S27–S32, 1994.

Gitzelmann R, Bosshard NU, Superti-Furga A, et al.: Feline mucopolysaccaridosis VII due to B-glucuronidase deficiency. Vet Pathol 31:435–443, 1994.

MULTIGATED EQUILIBRIUM HEART SCAN (MUGA), DIAGNOSTIC

(see Heart Scan, Diagnostic)

MUMPS ANTIBODY, BLOOD

Norm: Negative or titer <1:8.

Positive: Viral mumps. Recent infection with the virus is indicated by a fourfold rise in titer between the acute and convalescent specimens, with ration of viral (V) to soluble (S) titer increasing.

Description: Mumps (infectious parotitis) is an acute, contagious, febrile disease that causes inflammation of the parotid glands and other salivary glands. Symptoms include fever, malaise, chills, headache, pain below the ear, and swelling of the parotid glands. In clients who have passed puberty, it may cause orchitis, oophoritis, and inflammation of many vital organs. It is caused by the paramyxovirus mumps virus that is spread from client to client through droplet spray or direct contact with the saliva of an infected client. This test supports recent mumps virus infection or previous exposure to it. Besides mumps, this virus has been known to cause meningitis and encephalitis.

Professional Considerations:

1. Consent form NOT required.
2. Preparation:
   A. Tube: Red-top, red/gray-top, or gold-top.
3. Procedure:
   A. Draw a 5-ml blood sample. Label the tube as the acute sample.
   B. Repeat the test in 7–14 days, and label the tube as the convalescent sample.
4. Postprocedure care:
   A. Place the specimens on ice.
5. Client and family teaching:
   A. Return in 1–2 weeks for drawing of a convalescent sample.
   B. If mumps is suspected, the client should be isolated for 9 days after parotid gland swelling appears, until the period of communicability has passed. The incubation period is between 16 and 18 days.
   C. Infection confers lifelong immunity.
   D. There is no specific treatment for mumps after it has been acquired. Vaccination is available for clients who have not had the infection.

6. Factors that affect results:
    A. Reject hemolyzed or chylous serum specimens.
    B. Failure to collect a convalescent sample limits the value of the acute sample results.
7. Other data:
    A. Increased hemagglutination inhibition titer indicates either mumps or another parainfluenza virus.
    B. Peak infection rates occur in the winter and spring months.

C. Mumps virus contracted in the first trimester of pregnancy may be associated with a higher risk of congenital anomalies.

Bibliography:

Gut JP, Lablache C, Behr S, et al.: Symptomatic mumps virus reinfections. J Med Virol *45*:17–23, 1995.

Srikanth S, Ravi V, Shenoy Poornima K, et al.: Viral antibodies in recent onset, nonorganic psychoses: Correspondence with symptomatic severity. Biol Psychiatry *36*:517–521, 1994.

MURAMIDASE (LYSOZYME), SERUM

Norm:

		SI Units
Gel diffusion assay	0.4–1.3 mg/dl	4–13 mg/L
Nephelometric	0.36–0.78 mg/dl	3.6–7.8 mg/L
Radioimmunoassay	0.46 ± 0.08 mg/dl	4.6 ± 0.8 mg/L
Turbidimetric	0.27–0.93 mg/dl	2.7–9.3 mg/L

Increased: Crohn's disease, histiocytic medullary reticulosis, Hodgkin's disease, human immunodeficiency virus, leukemia (myelogenous, monocytic), otitis media, polycythemia vera, sarcoidosis, and tuberculosis.

Decreased: Not clinically significant.

Description: Muramidase (lysozyme) is an enzyme present in numerous body fluids (saliva, sweat, tears) and renal cells that is released into the bloodstream as a result of degradation of granulocytes and monocytes. It normally functions in the process of gram-positive bacterial destruction. In renal damage, serum levels may be normal in the presence of elevated urine levels.

Professional Considerations:

1. Consent form NOT required.
2. Preparation:
    A. Tube: Red-top, red/gray-top, or gold-top or lavender-top.
3. Procedure:
    A. Draw a 1-ml blood sample.
4. Postprocedure care:
    A. Separate the serum and freeze it immediately in a plastic vial on dry ice.
5. Client and family teaching:
    A. Results are normally available within 1 week.
6. Factors that affect results:
    A. Inability to separate the serum and freeze the sample.
7. Other data:
    A. The level of serum lysozyme has been used as an indicator of central nervous system involvement associated with leukemia.
    B. *See also Muramidase, Urine.*

Bibliography:

Hiemstra PS, VanFurth R: Antimicrobial mechanisms: Anti-microbial polypeptides of mononuclear phagocytes. Immunol Ser *60*:197–202, 1994.

Johannsen L: Biological properties of bacterial peptidoglycan. APMIS *101*(5):337–344, 1993.

Kikuchi M, Ikehara M: From genesis to function of proteins: Investigation of general principles by engineering human lysozyme. Protein Engin *7*(6):735–742, 1994.

Sugai S, Ikeguchi M: Conformational comparison between alpha-lactalbumin and lysozyme. Adv Biophys *30*:37–84, 1994.

Valdes L, SanJose E, Alvarez D, et al.: Diagnosis of tuberculous pleurisy using the biologic parameters adenosine deaminase, lysozyme, and interferon gamma. Chest *103*(2):458–465, 1993.

MURAMIDASE, URINE

Norm: <3 µg/ml, 0–2.9 mg/L (1.3–3.6 mg/24 hours, SI units).

Increased: Crohn's disease, histiocytic medullary reticulosis, Hodgkin's disease, human immunodeficiency virus, leukemia (granulocytic, myelogenous, monocytic), nephrotic syndrome, otitis media, polycythemia vera, pyelonephritis (acute), renal transplant rejection, sarcoidosis, and tuberculosis.

Decreased: Not clinically significant.

Description: Muramidase (lysozyme) is an enzyme present in numerous body fluids and renal cells that is released into the bloodstream as a result of degradation of granulocytes and monocytes. It normally functions in the process of gram-positive bacterial destruction. In renal damage, serum levels may be normal in the presence of elevated urine levels. The proximal tubule of the kidney is the site of catabolism and reabsorption.

Professional Considerations:
1. Consent form NOT required.
2. Preparation:
   A. Preschedule this test with the laboratory.
   B. Obtain a sterile, preservative-free plastic specimen container.
3. Procedure:
   A. Collect a 5-ml random urine specimen.
4. Postprocedure care:
   A. Freeze the specimen on dry ice if the specimen is not tested immediately.
5. Client and family teaching:
   A. Results are normally available within 72 hours.
6. Factors that affect results:
   A. Urine not maintained on ice after collection invalidates the results.
   B. Clients who are menstruating should be rescheduled for this test. Blood in the urine may produce falsely elevated results.
   C. Bacteria in the urine may produce falsely low results.
7. Other data:
   A. Muramidase is excreted in renal tubular disease but not in glomerular disease.
   B. Serum levels must exceed three times the normal range before the enzyme will appear in the urine.
   C. *See also Muramidase (Lysozyme), Serum.*

Bibliography:
Hiemstra PS, VanFurth R: Antimicrobial mechanisms: Antimicrobial polypeptides of mononuclear phagocytes. Immunology Series *60*:197–202, 1994.

Johannsen L: Biological properties of bacterial peptidoglycan. APMIS *101*(5):337–344, 1993.

Kikuchi M, Ikehara M: From genesis to function of proteins: Investigation of general principles by engineering human lysozyme. Protein Engin *7*(6):735–742, 1994.

Sugai S, Ikeguchi M: Conformational comparison between alpha-lactalbumin and lysozyme. Adv Biophys *30*:37–84, 1994.

Valdes L, SanJose E, Alvarez D, et al.: Diagnosis of tuberculous pleurisy using the biologic parameters adenosine deaminase, lysozyme, and interferon gamma. Chest *103*(2):458–465, 1993.

MUSCLE BIOPSY, SPECIMEN

Norm: Interpretation by a pathologist is required.

Usage: Dermatomyositis, Duchenne's muscular dystrophy, muscular dystrophy, myositis, neurogenic atrophy, pain (muscle and bone), and trichinosis.

Description: Microscopic examination of a piece of muscle for evaluation, diagnosis, or classification of muscular disease.

Professional Considerations:
1. Consent form IS required.

Risks:
Bruising, infection.

Contraindications:
Anticoagulant therapy, bleeding disorders, thrombocytopenia.

2. Preparation:
   A. Serum CK, 24-hour urine for creatine and serum creatinine, sedimentation rate, erythrocyte (ESR), serum aldolase, and thyroid profile may be desirable before biopsy.
   B. Obtain a biopsy tray, sterile drapes, a sterile jar of sterile 0.9% saline, a sterile specimen container of formalin, and a sterile container of glutaraldehyde.
3. Procedure:
   A. Obtain a biopsy, using a sterile procedure.
   B. If histochemistry is desired, do not use epinephrine with lidocaine or procaine in securing the biopsy.
4. Postprocedure care:
   A. Place the biopsy in a sterile jar containing sterile saline. For histopathology, place the specimen in formalin, and for electron microscopy, submit a small or minced specimen that is placed into glutaraldehyde.
   B. Label the container with the client's name, the room number, date, and site of specimen collection.
   C. The specimen should be delivered to the pathology department within 30 minutes. If the specimen cannot be delivered within 30 minutes, freeze it quickly, using liquid nitrogen.
   D. Turnaround time is between 48 hours and 3 weeks.
5. Client and family teaching:
   A. Call a physician for signs of infection at the biopsy site over the next 24–48 hours: increasing pain, redness, swelling, purulent drainage, or for fever >101°F (38.3°C).
   B. Mild pain should be expected at the biopsy site. Severe pain should be reported to a physician.

C. A mild analgesic may be required for pain control.

D. Monitor for signs and symptoms of infection until the site is healed.

6. Factors that affect results:

A. Use of wrong fixative.

B. The specimen dries out.

C. Unlabeled specimen container.

D. Muscle that has been recently injected or undergone electromyographic studies may not be suitable for microscopic examination.

7. Other data:

A. The quadriceps femoris is recommended for generalized diseases, and the gastrocnemius is suggested as a distal muscle for biopsy.

B. The deltoid is not suitable for enzyme histochemistry.

C. Tissue should be obtained from a relaxed, noncontracted isometric muscle.

D. Optimally, a specimen should be taken from a muscle with known disease that has NOT reached end-stage atrophy.

E. Specimens for histologic examination are commonly stained with hematoxylin-eosin. This allows for the assessment of inflammatory processes.

Bibliography:

Goebel HH, Husmann G, Voit T, et al.: Special techniques in diagnostic myopathology. Turk J Pediatr 36:223–237, 1994.

Leff RL, Kurent JE, Dickoff DJ: Polymyositis and dermatomyositis: Meeting the diagnostic challenge. J Musculoskel Med 11(4):57–68, 1994.

Pearson AM, Young RB: Diseases and disorders of muscle. Adv Food Nutr Res 37:339–423, 1993.

Tollback A, Borg J, Borg K, et al.: Isokinetic strength, marco EMG and muscle biopsy of paretic foot dorsiflexors in chronic neurogenic paresis. Scand J Rehab Med 25:183–187, 1993.

MUSCLE PROFILE, SPECIMEN

(see Aldolase, Serum; Aspartate Aminotransferase, Serum; Creatine Kinase, Serum; Differential Leukocyte Count, Peripheral Blood (Eosinophils); Lactate Dehydrogenase, Blood; Myoglobin, Serum; Thyroid Test: Thyroxin (T) by RIA, Blood; Thyroid Test: Thyroxin (T) Free, Serum; Thyroid Test: Triiodothyronine (T) Uptake, Blood; and Thyroid Test: Free Thyroxin Index, Serum)

MYCOBACTERIA, CEREBROSPINAL FLUID, CULTURE

(see Cerebrospinal Fluid, Routine, Culture and Cytology, Specimen)

MYCOPLASMA TITER, BLOOD

Norm: Negative or complement fixation (CF) <1:64 and seradyn color vue (SCV) agglutination <1:320.

Positive: Diarrhea and mycoplasmal pneumonia.

Description: *Mycoplasma* are pleuropneumonia-type organisms that can pass through bacteriologic filters, the smallest ranging from 125 to 250 mm. *Mycoplasma* are the smallest free living organisms and characteristically have no cell wall.

Professional Considerations:

1. Consent form NOT required.

2. Preparation:

A. Tube: Red-top, red/gray-top, or gold-top.

3. Procedure:

A. Draw a 3-ml blood sample.

4. Postprocedure care:

A. Draw a convalescent sample of blood 10–14 days later.

5. Client and family teaching:

A. Return in 10–14 days to have another blood sample drawn from the vein in order to have accurate results.

6. Factors that affect results:

A. False-positive results may occur in clients with acute pancreatitis or streptococci infection.

B. A diet of green, leafy vegetables may produce false-positive results.

7. Other data:

A. High titers are not significant for recent infection, since antibodies may persist >1 year and repeated infections occur.

B. Mycoplasmal pneumonia is treated with tetracycline or erythromycin.

C. Serologic confirmation is desirable, since mycoplasma is difficult to culture.

Bibliography:

Kaku M, Kohno S, Koga H, et al.: Efficacy of roxithromycin in the treatment of *Mycoplasma* pneumonia. Chemotherapy 41:149–152, 1995.

Leland DS, Barth KA, Cunningham EB: Comparison of the seradyn color vue passive agglutination test and complement fixation for detection of *Mycoplasma pneumoniae* antibodies. J Clin Microbiol 31(4):1013–1015, 1993.

Prabhakar K, Subramanian S, Thyagarajan SP: *Mycoplasma hominis* in pelvic inflammatory disease. Indian J Pathol Microbiol 37(3):293–298, 1994.

MYELIN BASIC PROTEIN (MBP), SPECIMEN

(see Cerebrospinal Fluid, Myelin Basic Protein, Oligoclonal Bands, Protein, and Protein Electrophoresis, Specimen)

MYELOGRAM, DIAGNOSTIC

Norm: Normal cervical, lumbar, or thoracic myelogram. Normal spinal subarachnoid space with no obstructions.

Usage: Arachnoiditis, back pain, disk rupture, spinal problems, traumatic injury, and tumors of the spine.

Description: Radiographic study of the spinal cord and nerve roots by using contrast dye or air injected, by way of spinal needle, into the spinal subarachnoid space.

Professional Considerations:

1. Consent form IS required.

Risks:

Allergic reaction to dye (itching, hives, rash, tight feeling in the throat, shortness of breath, bronchospasm, anaphylaxis, death); renal toxicity from contrast medium.

Contraindications:

Previous allergy to dye, iodine, or shellfish; renal insufficiency; bleeding abnormalities or clients receiving anticoagulants; increased intracranial pressure, low back pain, spinal deformities, or infections near the puncture site.

2. Preparation:
   A. Sedation or narcotic analgesia should be considered prior to this procedure.
   B. Shave the lumbar area if necessary.
   C. Obtain a lumbar puncture tray, sterile drapes, 1–2% lidocaine (Xylocaine), iodized Pantopaque oil or water-soluble iodine metrizamide contrast medium, antiseptic, and sterile gauze.
   D. If metrizamide is to be used as a contrast dye, discontinue the use of phenothiazines 48 hours prior to the procedure.
   E. Obtain baseline vital signs.
   F. Have emergency equipment readily available.
   G. If increased intracranial pressure is suspected, a CT of the brain should be performed prior to lumbar puncture to rule out this condition.
   H. *See Client and family teaching.*
3. Procedure:
   A. The client is positioned on the side with the knees drawn up toward the abdomen and the chin on the chest for the lumbar puncture.
   B. The lumbar puncture is verified by fluoroscopy.
   C. Spinal fluid is generally obtained for analysis.
   D. 5–15 ml of iodized Pantopaque oil dye or water-soluble iodine metrizamide contrast is injected into the subarachnoid space in the lumbar area or into the cisterna magna.
   E. The client is tilted to maneuver oil up and down the spine.
   F. Radiographic films are taken.
   G. Oil is removed by aspiration after the procedure.
4. Postprocedure care:
   A. Cleanse the puncture site with antiseptic and cover with a dry, sterile dressing.
   B. Prescribe bedrest for 6–8 hours, with the head of the bed elevated no more than 30–45 degrees during the last 6 hours.
   C. Assess vital signs every 30 minutes × 4.
   D. Do not administer phenothiazines for nausea or vomiting if water-soluble contrast was used.
   E. Results are normally available within 48 hours.
5. Client and family teaching:
   A. The client should fast from food and fluids for 4–8 hours prior to the procedure.
   B. The procedure takes 1 hour.
   C. Review activity limitations.
   D. Drink 6–8 glasses of water or other fluids each day for 2 days (when not contraindicated) to hasten removal of any contrast medium.
   E. Potential side effects/complications include arachnoiditis, headache, nausea and vomiting, seizures, spinal infection, subarachnoid bleeding, and tingling at the puncture site.
   F. Observe the puncture site for bleeding, hematoma, or swelling for 24–48 hours following the procedure.
   G. A mild analgesic may be required for pain control.
   H. Monitor the lumbar puncture site for signs and symptoms of infection until the site is healed.
6. Factors that affect results:
   A. Complications such as convulsions, pain, stiffness of the neck, and stupor may interfere with the procedure.
   B. Severe kyphosis or scoliosis may prohibit completion of this procedure.
7. Other data:
   A. Dye usage affects preparation and postprocedure care.
   B. Use of oil contrast has the disadvantage of tissue irritation and poor absorption by the subarachnoid spaces.
   C. Air contrast may be used instead of oil, but tomography is essential to improve visualization.
   D. Potential complication: Multiple sclerosis may be worsened by this procedure.

Bibliography:

Casey Laizure S, Miller JH, Stevens RC, et al.: The disposition and cerebrospinal fluid penetration of morphine and its two major glucuronidated metabolites in adults undergoing lumbar myelogram. Pharmacotherapy *13*(5):471–475, 1993.

Janssen ME, Bertrand SL, Joe C, et al.: Lumbar herniated disk disease: Comparison of MRI, myelography, and post-myelographic CT scan with surgical findings. Lumbar Herniated Disk Dis *17*(2):121–127, 1994.

Trojaborg W: Clinical, electrophysiological, and myelographic studies of 9 patients with cervical spinal root avulsions: Discrepancies between EMG and x-ray findings. Muscle Nerve *17*:913–922, 1994.

MYOGLOBIN ASSAY, SERUM

(see Myoglobin, Serum)

MYOGLOBIN, QUALITATIVE, URINE

Norm: Negative or <20 ng/ml.

Positive: Acute alcohol intoxication with delirium tremens, acute or chronic muscular disease, barbiturate toxicity, burns (severe), diabetic acidosis, glycogen and lipid storage diseases, hyperthermia, hypothermia, hypokalemia, hypophosphatemia, muscular dystrophy, myocardial infarction, poisoning, polymyositis, renal failure, surgical procedure, trauma, and viral or bacterial infection.

Description: Myoglobin is a heme-containing, oxygen-binding protein similar to hemoglobin that is exclusive to striated and nonstriated skeletal or cardiac muscle. It serves as a short-term oxygen store, carrying the muscle from one contraction to the next. It is released into the interstitial fluid as early as 3 hours following any muscle injury including a myocardial infarct and remains detected in the urine for up to 7 days later.

Professional Considerations:

1. Consent form NOT required.
2. Preparation:
   A. Obtain a sterile specimen container.
3. Procedure:
   A. Collect a 10-ml random urine specimen in a sterile plastic container without preservatives.
   B. Collection time should be early morning when possible.
4. Postprocedure care:
   A. Specimens should be refrigerated.
5. Client and family teaching:
   A. Results are normally available within 72 hours.

6. Factors that affect results:
   A. False-negative results are likely if the test is used for screening.
   B. The presence of hypochlorite or microbial peroxidase or other oxidizing contaminants may cause false-positive results.
   C. Clients should not receive isotopes 7 days prior to testing.
   D. High concentrations of vitamin C decrease the sensitivity of this test.
7. Other data:
   A. Because myoglobin is excreted by the kidney, renal function should be assessed.
   B. Serum levels are preferred to urine levels when obtaining myoglobin values.
   C. *See also Myoglobin, Serum.*

Bibliography:

Chen-Levy Z, Daum P, Wener M, et al.: Urine myoglobin: Evaluation of the Behring NA latex myoglobin method reveals instability of myoglobin in urine. Am J Clin Pathol *100*:178, 1993.

Laios I, Green S, Wu A: Evaluation of immunoassays for serum and urine myoglobin. Am J Clin Pathol *100*:178, 1993.

Nakamura RM: Urine myoglobin. MLO *26*(3):11, 14, 1994.

MYOGLOBIN, SERUM

Norm: RIA <85 ng/ml OR (5–70 μg/L, SI units).

Increased: Acute alcohol intoxication with delirium tremens, after cardioversion (possible increase), after open heart surgery, angina (possible increase), burns (severe), congestive heart failure (possible increase), dermatomyositis, dysrhythmias (possible increase), glycogen and lipid storage diseases, hyperthermia, hypothermia, muscular dystrophy, myocardial infarction (increased levels detected 2–3 hours after injury, peaks at 6–9 hours and returns to baseline within 36 hours), polymyositis, renal failure, shock, skeletal muscle injury or extreme skeletal muscle exertion, surgical procedure, systemic lupus erythematosus (SLE), trauma, and viral or bacterial infection. Drugs include ethanol (heavy use).

Description: Myoglobin is a heme-containing, oxygen-binding protein similar to hemoglobin that is exclusive to striated and nonstriated skeletal or cardiac muscle. It serves as a short-term oxygen store, carrying the muscle from one contraction to the next. It is released into the interstitial fluid with elevated serum levels detected as early as 30–60 minutes following a myocardial infarct or damage to any muscle tissue. Serum myoglobin is generally detected earlier than traditional cardiac enzymes (total creatinine kinase [CK] or isoenzyme creatinine kinase-MB [CK-MB]). Serum myoglobin has been used to monitor for reinfarct, success of thrombolytic treatment, and myocardial injury during open heart surgery.

Professional Considerations:

1. Consent form NOT required.
2. Preparation:
   A. Tube: Red-top, red/gray-top, or gold-top.
3. Procedure:
   A. Draw a 2-ml blood sample.
4. Postprocedure care:
   A. Specimens should be refrigerated.
   B. Specimens may be frozen and stored for up to 2 years.
5. Client and family teaching:
   A. Results are normally available within 48 hours.
6. Factors that affect results:
   A. Hemolysis of the specimen invalidates the results.
   B. False-negative results are likely if the test is used for screening.
   C. Clients should have no isotopes 7 days prior to testing.
   D. Serum levels must be obtained within 2–12 hours of the onset of symptoms of a myocardial infarct to be useful in assessing myocardial injury.
   E. Normal levels may be higher in men compared to women, but increase in both sexes with age.
   F. Hypertriglyceridemia or postprandial specimens may affect the results.
   G. Serum myoglobin has been found to increase proportionally with the size of muscle damage.
7. Other data:
   A. Serum myoglobin may lack specificity in the diagnosis of myocardial infarct.

Elevated levels are also observed following angina, chest trauma, cocaine use, electrical accidents, exercise, intramuscular injection, muscular injury of any type, and renal failure. Within 8 hours of symptoms, myoglobin specificity is 97.9% for acute MI, as opposed to CK-MB, which has 100% specificity.

B. Increased levels should be correlated with client signs and symptoms.
C. Myoglobin can be measured using a variety of approaches, including fluorometric measurement, latex agglutination, and nephelometric and turbidimetric assay. Each approach has its own reference range.
D. IM injections, bicycle exercise, and cardiac catheterization should NOT increase levels.
E. *See also Myoglobin, Qualitative, Urine.*

Bibliography:

Baum H, Booksteegers P, Steinbeck G, et al.: A rapid assay for the quantification of myoglobin: Evaluation and diagnostic relevance in the diagnosis of acute myocardial infarction. Eur J Clin Chem Clin Biochem 32(11):853–858, 1994.

Bhayana V, Henderson AR: Biochemical markers of myocardial damage. Clin Biochem 28(1):1–29, 1995.

Rider LG, Miller FW: Laboratory evaluation of the inflammatory myopathies. Clin Diagn Lab Immunol 2(1):1–9, 1995.

Woo J, Lacbawan FL, Sunheimer R, et al.: Is myoglobin useful in the diagnosis of acute myocardial infarction in the emergency department setting. Am J Clin Pathol 103(6):725–729, 1995.

Yamashita T, Abe S, Arima S, et al.: Myocardial infarct size can be estimated from serial plasma myoglobin measurements within 4 hours of reperfusion. Circulation 87(6):1840–1849, 1993.

MYOGLOBIN, URINE
(see Myoglobin, Qualitative, Urine)

MYSOLINE
(see Primidone, Serum)

NAP
(see Leukocyte Alkaline Phosphatase, Blood)

NARCOTICS DRUG SCREEN, URINE
(see Toxicology, Drug Screen, Urine)

NASAL CULTURE, SWAB, DIAGNOSTIC
(see Culture, Routine, Specimen)

NASOPHARYNGEAL CULTURE, SWAB, DIAGNOSTIC
(see Culture, Routine, Specimen)

NEEDLE ASPIRATION, DIAGNOSTIC

Norm: Nonmalignant, or negative.

Usage: Essential to diagnosing malignancies and benign growths. Also used to evaluate tissue for reaction to hormones; these results assist in selecting appropriate therapy for cancer.

Description: Surgical procedure in which a sample of body tissue or fluid is removed transcutaneously through a needle, then examined microscopically for abnormal cells or tested in a hormone receptor assay. This procedure can be performed on an ambulatory surgery basis under local anesthesia.

Professional Considerations:

1. Consent form IS required.

Risks:

Infection at needle aspiration site.

Contraindications:

Cutaneous infection at site.

2. Preparation:
   A. Obtain 1–2% lidocaine (Xylocaine) for local anesthesia, a cutting needle, a sterile cup with normal saline, and a heparinized tube.
3. Procedure:
   A. Position the client supine.
   B. Under local anesthesia, a cutting needle such as the Cope's or Vim-Silverman is inserted into the suspected area and a core of tissue is removed and placed in normal saline, or fluid is aspirated and placed in a heparinized tube.
4. Postprocedure care:
   A. Apply a dry, sterile dressing to the site.
   B. Label the specimens and transport them to the laboratory promptly.
   C. Assess vital signs every 15 minutes × 2.
   D. Monitor the site every 2 hours × 3 for bleeding, inflammation, or drainage.
   E. Results are normally available in 48–72 hours.
5. Client and family teaching:
   A. Monitor for drainage and inflammation for 24–48 hours.
   B. A mild analgesic may be required for pain control.
   C. Call the physician for signs of infection at the procedure site: increasing pain, redness, swelling, purulent drainage, or for fever >101°F (38.3°C).
6. Factors that affect results:
   A. Failure to obtain adequate sample(s) or a sample from a nonsuspect site.
7. Other data:
   A. Permanent microscopic sections are preferred to frozen sections, as permanent sections have more clarity.
   B. A negative result does not always exclude the diagnosis of cancer.
   C. *See also Needle Aspiration Cytology, Specimen.*

Bibliography:

Andersson L, Hagmar B, Ljung BM, et al.: Fine needle aspiration biopsy for diagnosis and follow-up of prostate cancer. Scand J Urol Nephrol *162* (Suppl): 43–49, 1994.

Choe W, McDougall IR: Thyroid cancer in pregnant women: Diagnostic and therapeutic management. Thyroid *4*(4):433–435, 1994.

Gharib H: Fine-needle aspiration biopsy of thyroid nodules: Advantages, limitations, and effect. Mayo Clin Proc *69*:44–49, 1994.

Wong MP, Yuen ST, Collins RJ: Fine-needle aspiration biopsy of pilomatrixoma: Still a diagnostic trap for the unwary. Diagn Cytopathol *10*(4):365–370, 1994.

NEEDLE ASPIRATION CYTOLOGY, SPECIMEN

Norm: Interpretation required.

Usage: Hashimoto's thyroiditis, histoplasmosis, Hodgkin's disease, and metastasis from malignancy.

Description: Surgical procedure in which a sample of body tissue or fluid is removed transcutaneously through a needle and then examined microscopically for origin, structure, function, and pathology of cells. This procedure can be performed on an ambulatory surgery basis under local anesthesia.

Professional Considerations:

1. Consent form IS required for the procedure used to obtain the specimen.

Risks:

Bruising, infection.

Contraindications:

Anticoagulant therapy, bleeding disorders, thrombocytopenia. Sedatives are contraindicated in clients with central nervous system depression.

2. Preparation:
   A. Obtain 1–2% lidocaine (Xylocaine) for local anesthesia, a cutting needle, slides, and 95% ethyl alcohol as fixative.
   B. Consider sedation or narcotic analgesic.
3. Procedure:
   A. The client is positioned supine.
   B. Under local anesthesia, a cutting needle such as Cope's or Vim-Silverman is inserted into the suspected area, and fluid is aspirated.
   C. The fluid is placed onto a glass slide.
   D. Another slide is placed on top of the specimen, and the two slides are gently pulled apart for even distribution of cells.
   E. Both slides are fixed immediately with 95% ethyl alcohol.
4. Postprocedure care:
   A. Label the specimens and transport them to the laboratory promptly.
   B. Monitor vital signs every 15 minutes × 2.
   C. Monitor the site every 2 hours × 3 for bleeding, inflammation, and drainage.

D. Results are normally available in 24–72 hours but can be as early as 30 minutes.
5. Client and family teaching:
  A. Monitor for drainage and inflammation for 24–48 hours.
  B. A mild analgesic may be required for pain control.
  C. Call the physician for signs of infection at the procedure site: increasing pain, redness, swelling, purulent drainage, or for fever >101°F (38.3°C).
6. Factors that affect results:
  A. Failure to obtain adequate samples or samples from a nonsuspect site.
7. Other data:
  A. Aspirations of the thyroid cannot distinguish follicular adenoma from follicular carcinoma.
  B. European laboratories prefer air-dried smears.
  C. The location in which this procedure is performed should be equipped to handle medical emergencies.
  D. *See also Cerebrospinal Fluid, Routine, Culture and Cytology, Specimen; or Cytologic Study of Breast Cyst, Effusions, Gastrointestinal Tract, Needle Aspiration, Diagnostic; Nipple Discharge, Respiratory Tract or Urine, Diagnostic.*

Bibliography:

Huvos AG: Fine-needle aspiration cytology of tumors: Diagnostic accuracy and potential pitfalls. Cancer Invest *12*(5):505–515, 1994.

Layfield LJ, Berek JS: Fine-needle aspiration cytology in the management of gynecologic oncology patients. *In* Rothenberg, ML (ed): Gynecologic Oncology: Controversies and New Developments. Boston, MA, Kluwer Academic Publishers, 1994, pp 1–13.

Paksoy N, Lilleng R, Hagmar B, et al.: Diagnostic accuracy of fine needle aspiration cytology in pancreatic lesions. Acta Cytol *37*(6):889–893, 1993.

NEISSERIA GONORRHOEAE SMEAR, SPECIMEN

Norm: Negative.

Positive: Gonorrhea.

Description: *Neisseria gonorrhoeae* is a pyogenic, gram-negative, oxidase-positive cocci that is an obligate parasite of humans. *N. gonorrhoeae* inhabits the mucous membranes of the genital tract, causing gonorrhea. Symptoms include dysuria, fever, pharyngitis, peripheral skin lesions, proctitis, and purulent urethral discharge. It may also cause inflammation of any of the mucous membranes of the body. Females are often asymptomatic. Left untreated, gonorrhea leads to skin lesions, arthritis, meningitis, and reproductive problems. *N.*

gonorrhoeae is most often found in the urethra of males and the endocervical canal of females.

Professional Considerations:

1. Consent form NOT required.
2. Preparation:
  A. Determine the potential infected area(s): anus, cervix, conjunctiva, endocervix, skin lesion, throat, and urethra.
  B. Wait 1 hour after urination to collect urethral specimens.
  C. Obtain a wooden scraper or swab and a glass slide with frosted edges.
3. Procedure:
  A. Obtain a sterile microbiologic smear. With a swab, swab the potential infected area for 10 seconds.
  B. Apply to a glass slide and allow to air-dry.
  C. Label the slide.
4. Postprocedure care:
  A. Place the air-dried slide in a sterile container and send it to the laboratory.
  B. Results are normally available immediately or within 24 hours.
5. Client and family teaching:
  A. The client should be referred for medical follow-up after the treatment is concluded. Repeat cultures or smears may be necessary to assess response to treatment.
  B. The use of condoms significantly reduces the risk of sexually transmitted diseases.
  C. Gonorrhea infection is treatable with antibiotics.
  D. If results are positive, provide the client with the appropriate information on sexually transmitted diseases.
    i. Notify all sexual partners from the last 90 days to be tested for gonorrhea infection.
    ii. Do not have sexual relations until the physician confirms that the infection is gone.
    iii. Referral for HIV testing should be reviewed and offered to all clients.
  E. Do not use feminine hygiene sprays or douche during treatment.
  F. Wear underpants and pantyhose that have a cotton lining in the crotch.
  G. Take showers instead of tub baths until the infection is gone.
6. Factors that affect results:
  A. False-positives occur in 50% of endocervical specimens, as normal flora have similar morphologic appearance.
  B. Insufficient specimen volume.
7. Other data:
  A. DNA probe assay (gen-probe) is an alternative test that can be used to diagnosis *N. gonorrhoeae.*
  B. A culture is necessary to confirm diagnosis.
  C. *See also Genital, Neisseria Gonorrhoeae, Culture.*

Bibliography:

Chapin-Robertson K: Use of molecular diagnostics in sexually transmitted diseases. Diagn Microbiol Infect Dis *16*:173–184, 1993.

Kihlstrom E, Danielsson D: Advances in biology, management and prevention of infections caused by *Chlamydia trachomatis* and *Neisseria gonorrhoeae.* Curr Opin Infect Dis *7*:25–33, 1994.

Vlaspolder F, Mutsaers JAEM, Blog F, et al.: Value of a DNA probe assay (gen-probe) compared with that of culture for diagnosis of gonococcal infection. J Clin Microbiol *31*(1):107–110, 1993.

NEPHROTOMOGRAPHY, DIAGNOSTIC

Norm: Normal kidney size, shape, and position.

Usage: Adrenal tumor, carcinoma of the kidney, cyst on the kidney, and renal laceration.

Description: Radiographic examination of a single plane of renal tissue. May be performed in conjunction with excretory urography (intravenous pyelography). Delineates renal borders and aids in distinguishing cystic from solid lesions.

Professional Considerations:

1. Consent form IS required.

Risks:

Radiation exposure, allergic reaction to contrast media (itching, hives, rash, tight feeling in the throat, shortness of breath, bronchospasm, anaphylaxis, death), renal toxicity from contrast medium.

Contraindications:

Pregnancy, previous allergy to dye, iodine, or shellfish, renal insufficiency.

2. Preparation:
   A. Have emergency equipment readily available.
   B. Residual barium from prior studies should be completely cleared from the gastrointestinal tract prior to performing this test.
   C. *See Client and family teaching.*
3. Procedure:
   A. A plain film of the kidneys is taken.
   B. Contrast medium is injected intravenously, the first half in 5 minutes (rapid phase) and the next half in 10 minutes (slow phase).
   C. Serial tomograms are initiated as soon as the slow phase begins.

D. The procedure takes 1 hour.
4. Postprocedure care:
   A. Monitor vital signs and urinary output every 4 hours × 24 hours.
5. Client and family teaching:
   A. Fast from food and fluids for 8 hours before the procedure.
   B. Be alert for an allergic reaction to the dye × 24 hours (itching, hives, shortness of breath). Call the physician immediately if these symptoms occur or go to the nearest emergency room.
6. Factors that affect results:
   A. Residual barium interferes with visualization.
7. Other data:
   A. Perform this procedure with caution on individuals who have severe cardiovascular disease or multiple myeloma.
   B. This test is often performed in conjunction with an intravenous pyelogram (IVP).
   C. *See also Intravenous Pyelography (IVP, Excretory Urography), Diagnostic.*

Bibliography:

Webb JAW, Britton KE: Intravenous urography, ultrasonography, and radionuclide studies. *In* Schrier RW, Gottschalk RW (eds): Diseases of the Kidney, 5th ed. Boston, MA, Little, Brown, 1993, pp 407–447.

NERVE BIOPSY, DIAGNOSTIC

Norm: Negative.

Usage: Amyloid infiltration, demyelination, hypertrophic polyneuropathy, inflammation anoxal degeneration, lepromatous leprosy lesions, metachromatic leukodystrophy, sarcoidosis, and vasculitis.

Description: Removal of peripheral nerve tissue for electromicroscopic, biochemical, histochemical, or virologic examination to establish a diagnosis for neuropathies when radiology and direct inspection have been inconclusive.

Professional Considerations:

1. Consent form IS required.

Risks:

Bruising, infection.

Contraindications:

Anticoagulant therapy, bleeding disorders, thrombocytopenia.

2. Preparation:
   A. Prepare for local anesthesia and obtain

biopsy instruments and a 3 × 5-inch index card.

B. Consult laboratory personnel for special handling of the specimen if electron microscopic examination is required.

3. Procedure:

A. Place a 1.5-cm portion of nerve on cardboard with the firmness of a 3 × 5-inch index card, then straighten and slightly stretch it.

B. Allow the specimen to adhere to the cardboard for 1 minute.

C. Keep the handling of specimens to a minimum.

D. Submerge the specimen in 0.05 mol/L phosphate-buffered glutaraldehyde.

4. Postprocedure care:

A. Transport specimens to the laboratory immediately.

5. Client and family teaching:

A. Monitor for drainage and inflammation for 24–48 hours.

B. A mild analgesic may be required for pain control.

C. Call the physician for signs of infection at the procedure site: increasing pain, redness, swelling, purulent drainage, or for fever >101°F (38.3°C).

6. Factors that affect results:

A. Drying out of samples invalidates the results.

7. Other data:

A. The nerve where the biopsy was taken will not regenerate.

B. The most common nerve used for biopsy is the superficial peroneal sensory nerve.

Bibliography:

Mackin GA: Diagnosis of patients with peripheral nerve disease. Clin Podiatr Med Surg *11*(4):545–569, 1994.

Raps EC, Bird SJ, Hansen-Flaschen J: Prolonged muscle weakness after neuromuscular blockage in the intensive care unit. Crit Care Clin *10*(4): 799–813, 1994.

NERVE CONDUCTION STUDIES, DIAGNOSTIC

Norm: Maximum conduction velocity = 40–80 ms for ages 3 years and older. Distal latency <4 msec and amplitude 13.2 mV. Values decreased by half for infants and elderly. Equipment and technique varies, thus, laboratories establish their own norms.

Usage: Carpal tunnel syndrome, peripheral entrapment neuropathies, tarsal tunnel syndrome, and thoracic outlet syndrome.

Description: Percutaneous stimulation of peripheral, sensory, or mixed sensory motor nerve fibers. Recording of muscle and sensory action potentials distinguishes between disease processes that cause both segmental demyelinative lesions and axonal losses.

Professional Considerations:

1. Consent form IS required.

Risks:

Pain at needle electrode sites.

Contraindications:

Nicotine patch drug users.

2. Preparation:

A. Shave the area for better conduction if needed.

3. Procedure:

A. An electrode is applied to the specific nerve area.

B. Electrical current is passed through and read distally to determine nerve conduction time.

4. Postprocedure care:

A. Assess the skin area for irritation.

5. Client and family teaching:

A. Results are normally available within 48 hours.

6. Factors that affect results:

A. Poor conduction of electrodes.

7. Other data:

A. Professional interpretation must follow the results of the study.

B. Supplements electromyographic studies.

Bibliography:

Buch-Jaeger N, Foucher G: Correlation of clinical signs with nerve conduction tests in the diagnosis of carpal tunnel syndrome. J Hand Sur *19B*(6):720–724, 1994.

Espino P: Neurogenic impotence: Diagnostic value of nerve conduction studies, bulbocavernosus reflex, and heart rate variability. Electromyogr Clin Neurophysiol *34*:373–376, 1994.

Hennessey WJ, Falco FJE, Braddom RL: Median and ulnar nerve conduction studies: Normative data for young adults. Arch Phys Med Rehabil *75:* 259–264, 1994.

Raynor EM, Shefner JM, Preston DC, et al.: Sensory and mixed nerve conduction studies in the evaluation of ulnar neuropathy at the elbow. Muscle Nerve *17*:785–792, 1994.

NEUROLOGIC EXAMINATION, DIAGNOSTIC

Norm: Negative.

Usage: Alzheimer's disease, brain tumors, cerebral palsy, motor and sensory disorders, and trauma.

Description: An examination designed to identify and distinguish between disorders of mentation; cranial nerves; and motor, sensory, or autonomic function.

Professional Considerations:

1. Consent form NOT required.
2. Preparation:
   A. Plan for uninterrupted time and privacy for the examination.
3. Procedure: A thorough, systematic examination, including history, physical exam, functional assessment, and diagnostic tests:
   A. The history.
      i. Chief complaint.
      ii. Biographic data.
      iii. Past medical history, including medication usage.
   B. The physical exam.
      i. *Vital signs:* Common changes secondary to neurologic disorders include bradycardia, hypotension, hypothermia, and increased pulse pressure.
      ii. *Pupils:* The optic nerve, intracranial pressure, ability to follow commands, response to light, extraocular movements, and nystagmus can be assessed by fundoscopic and visual examination of the pupils.
      iii. *Mental status:*
         a. State of consciousness.
         b. Orientation to person, place, and time.
         c. Memory of past and recent events.
         d. Tests of memory, attention, and clarity of thought such as serial addition or subtraction by 3's, recall of three items after 3 minutes, or interpretation of a proverb.
      iv. *Head and neck:* Palpate for lumps and lesions, assess for neck rigidity, and auscultate for bruits. Note the physical findings suggestive of a head injury or trauma.
      v. *Motor function:*
         a. Upper extremities:
            1. Finger-to-nose test.
            2. Patting test.
            3. Power of grip.
            4. Abduction/adduction of fingers.
            5. Extension/flexion of forearm and arm.
            6. Muscle bulk and tone.
            7. Reflexes: triceps, biceps, and brachioradialis.
            8. Sensation: position sense, vibration, and pain.
         b. Lower extremities:
            1. Heel-to-knee test.
            2. Extension/flexion of knee, toe, and foot.
            3. Muscle bulk and tone.
            4. Reflexes: patellar, achillea, and plantar response.
            5. Sensation: position, vibratory, and pain.
      c. Gait and posture: Observe stance, posture, gait, ability to stand on each foot alone, and ability to walk on heels or toes.
      d. Sensory function.
      e. Reflexes.
      vi. *Cranial nerves:*
         a. *Olfactory:* Check the ability to detect and identify common odors such as lemon, peppermint, or coffee, and whether impairment is unilateral or bilateral.
         b. *Optic:* Check visual acuity, visual fields, pupil size and response to light, and fundoscopic examinations.
         c. *Oculomotor, trochlear, and abducens:* Check palpebral fissures; observe for extraocular movements or nystagmus.
         d. *Trigeminal:* Check corneal reflex; sensation of face with pain, temperature, and light touch; and jaw muscle power.
         e. *Facial:* Check facial muscle power, assessing for twitching, tremors, and drooping.
         f. *Auditory:* Rinne's test and Weber's test.
         g. *Glossopharyngeal and vagus:* Observe the pharynx and uvula during phonation for symmetry; check the gag reflex.
         h. *Accessory:* Check trapezius power and bulk.
         i. *Hypoglossal:* Check lingual power and bulk.
   C. Functional assessment: Assess for changes in the ability to carry out activities of daily living and coping skills.
   D. Diagnostic tests: A variety of diagnostic tests may be useful:
      i. Skull and spinal radiologic x-ray studies.
      ii. Computed tomography (CT scan).
      iii. Magnetic resonance imaging (MRI).
      iv. Electroencephalogram (EEG).
      v. Lumbar puncture (LP).
      vi. Myelography.
4. Postprocedure care:
   A. Assess for fatigue.
5. Client and family teaching:
   A. Examination may take up to 2 hours.
6. Factors that affect results:
   A. Actual head injury, Alzheimer's disease, and sedative or narcotic medications.
7. Other data:
   A. None.

Bibliography:

Adams RD, Victor M: The clinical method of neurology. *In* Lamsback WJ, Navrozov M (eds): Principles of Neurology, 5th ed. New York, McGraw-Hill, 1993, pp 3–10.

Davids JR, Wenger DR: Back pain in children and adolescents: An algorithmic approach. J Musculoskel Med *11*(3):19–32, 1994.

Kumar KL, Reuler JB: Uncommon headaches: Diagnosis and treatment. J Gen Intern Med *8*:333–341, 1993.

NEURON-SPECIFIC ENOLASE (NSE), SERUM

Norm: 0–12.5 ng/ml.

Method:

RIA 6.0 ± 5.0 (SE) ng/ml
EIA 3.45 ± 1.6 ng/ml (2SD)

Increased: Medullary carcinoma of the thyroid, neuroblastoma that is metastatic, small cell carcinoma of the lung and uremia.

Decreased: Not applicable.

Description: Isoenzyme of a glycolytic enzyme found in neuronal and neuroendocrine cells of the central and peripheral nervous system. A sensitive tumor marker used to monitor response to therapy or detect neuroendocrine cell destruction disease progression, as there is a strong correlation between disease state and concentration.

Professional Considerations:

1. Consent form NOT required.
2. Preparation:
   A. Tube: Red-top, red/gray-top, or gold-top. Also obtain ice.
3. Procedure:
   A. Collect a 1-ml blood sample. Place the specimen in a container of ice.
4. Postprocedure care:
   A. Send the specimen to the laboratory immediately. Serum must be separated and refrigerated within 45 minutes of collection. The specimen should be frozen at –70°C if not tested the same day.
5. Client and family teaching:
   A. Results may not be available for as long as 7 days.
6. Factors that affect results:
   A. Serum is not separated after collection.
7. Other data:
   A. One study found a significant relation between elevated NSE and cerebral ischemia and how NSE may be a useful indicator in detecting cerebral ischemia.
   B. This test is not useful in screening for early stages of neoplasms.

Bibliography:

Collazos J, Esteban C, Fernandez A, et al.: Measurement of the serum tumor marker neuron-specific enolase in patients with benign pulmonary disease. Am J Respir Crit Care Med *150:*143–145, 1994.

Horn M, Seger F, Schlote W: Neuron-specific enolase in gerbil brain and serum after transient cerebral ischemia. Stroke *26*(2):290–297, 1995.

Maurea S, Lastoria S, Caraco C, et al.: Iodine-131-MIBG imaging to monitor chemotherapy response in advanced neuroblastoma: Comparison with laboratory analysis. J Nucl Med *35*(9): 1429–1435, 1994.

O'Shea P, Cassidy M, Freaney R, et al.: Serum neuron-specific enolase and immunohistochemical markers of neuroendocrine differentiation in lung cancer. Irish J Med Sci *164*(1):31–36, 1995.

NEUT, BLOOD
(see Differential Leukocyte Count, Peripheral Blood)

NEUTROPHIL ALKALINE PHOSPHATASE
(see Leukocyte Alkaline Phosphatase, Blood)

NEUTROPHILS, BLOOD
(see Differential Leukocyte Count, Peripheral Blood)

NH₃ BLOOD
(see Ammonia, Blood and Urine)

NIPPLE DISCHARGE CYTOLOGY, SPECIMEN
(see Cytologic Study of Nipple Discharge, Diagnostic)

NITRITE, BACTERIA SCREEN, URINE

Norm: <0.1 mg/dl, <100,000 organisms/ml, or negative.

Usage: Cystitis, differentiation between acute bacterial infections and viral or tuberculosis (TB) infections, dysuria, pyelonephritis, and urinary tract infection.

Description: Humans normally oxidize ingested nitrite and excrete it as nitrate. The presence of nitrite in urine indicates a urinary tract infection caused by organisms that reduce nitrate back to nitrite.

Professional Considerations:

1. Consent form NOT required.

2. Preparation:
   A. Cleanse the urethral orifice with a sterile wipe.
   B. Obtain a sterile plastic container.
3. Procedure:
   A. Collect a first morning void of 12 ml of urine, or a specimen collected at least 4 hours after the client last voided, in a sterile plastic container.
4. Postprocedure care:
   A. Refrigerate the sample within 2 hours.
5. Client and family teaching:
   A. Results are normally available within 72 hours.
6. Factors that affect results:
   A. Incidence of false-positives is 12–34% due to age less than 2 months, *Candida albicans* and *Nocardia* infections, echovirus, hemophilia A, Hodgkin's disease, lymphoma, malaria, and parasitic infections.
   B. Drugs that may cause false-positive results include oral contraceptives and phenazopyridine.
   C. Incidence of false-negatives is 5–9% due to agammaglobulinemia, diabetes mellitus, localized infection, sickle cell anemia, and systemic lupus erythematosus.
   D. Drugs that may cause false-negative results include antibiotics, anti-inflammatories (corticosteroids and phenylbutazone), and ascorbic acid concentration >25 mg/dl in specimens containing <0.03 mg/dl of nitrite ions.
   E. Diuresis, delay of several hours without refrigeration of specimen, and contamination in obtaining specimen invalidate the results.
   F. Dipsticks stored in ambient humidity may produce false-negative results.
7. Other data:
   A. Another degree of color development on the reagent test strip is NOT proportional to the number of bacteria present.
   B. Bacteria infections are less likely to be detected when the output is high.
   C. An increased urine specific gravity will decrease the sensitivity of this test.
   D. Urinary tract infections may be caused from organisms that will not produce a positive nitrite test.
   E. If nitrites are positive on the dipstick or are negative but the client is symptomatic, a urine culture should be performed.

Bibliography:

Bartlett RC, Zern DA, Ratkiewicz I, et al.: Reagent strip screening for sediment abnormalities identified by automated microscopy in urine from patients suspected to have urinary tract disease. Arch Pathol Lab Med *118*:1096–1101, 1994.

Kovach CR, Puetzer M, Gretzinger P: A descriptive study of nosocomial urinary tract infection in a rehabilitation patient population. Rehab Nurs Res *2*(2):81–86, 1993.

Lohr JA, Portilla MG, Geuder TG, et al.: Making a presumptive diagnosis of urinary tract infection by using a urinalysis performed in an on-site laboratory. J Pediatr *122*(1):22–25, 1993.

Smith SD, Wheeler MA, Weiss RM: Nitric oxide synthase: An endogenous source of elevated nitrite in infected urine. Kidney Int *45*:586–591, 1994.

NITROBLUE TETRAZOLIUM TEST (NBT), DIAGNOSTIC

Norm: 2–8% segmented neutrophils reduce the dye.

Usage: Chronic granulomatous disease in childhood.

Description: This demanding test uses different reagents to differentiate bacterial from nonbacterial infections. Nitroblue tetrazolium is a yellow compound that turns blue when reduced by an increase in the hexose monophosphate shunt generated by phagocytic activity. In granulomatous disease, neutrophil phagocytic activity is absent, thus resulting in absence of blue dye formation. This test is often replaced by the formazan test, which depends on the reduction of nitroblue tetrazolium to insoluble formazan. The formazan test is simpler to perform and more cost effective.

Professional Considerations:

1. Consent form NOT required.
2. Preparation:
   A. Preschedule this test with the laboratory.
   B. Tube: Green-top (heparinized) tube.
3. Procedure:
   A. Draw a 4-ml blood sample.
4. Postprocedure care:
   A. Write the collection time on the laboratory requisition.
   B. Transport the specimen to the laboratory immediately.
5. Client and family teaching:
   A. Results are normally available in 72 hours.
6. Factors that affect results:
   A. Reject clotted specimens or specimens received more than 1 hour after collection.
   B. False-negative results may occur in clients with solid cancerous nonlymphomatous tumors.
   C. Specificity is poor, as many secondary diseases cause false-positive results.
   D. Diets high in fats may affect the results.
7. Other data:
   A. Neutrophils reduce the dye to dark blue-black upon phagocytosis.
   B. Unreliable in differentiating bacterial from viral infections.

Bibliography:

Bellinati-Pires R, Waitzberg DL, Salgado MM, et al.: Functional alterations of human neutrophils by medium-chain triglyceride emulsions: Evaluation of phagocytosis, bacterial killing, and oxidative activity. J Leukoc Biol 53:404–410, 1993.

Liel Y, Rudich A, Nagauker-Shriker O, et al.: Monocyte dysfunction in patients with Gaucher disease: Evidence for interference of glucocerebroside with superoxide generation. Blood 83(9):2646–2653, 1994.

Matsuda J, Tsukamoto M, Saitoh N, et al.: Polymorphonuclear leukocyte function tests: A comparison of cytochrome C reduction and flow cytometric analysis. Br J Biomed Sci 50(1):60–63, 1993.

Sedel D, Huguet P, Lebbe C, et al.: Sweet syndrome as the presenting manifestation of chronic granulomatous disease in an infant. Pediatr Dermatol 11(3):237–240, 1994.

NITROGLYCERIN SCAN
(see Heart Scan, Diagnostic)

NOCARDIA CULTURE, ALL SITES, SPECIMEN

Norm: Negative.

Positive: Human immunodeficiency virus, immunodeficiency, leukemia, lymphoma, lymphoreticular malignancy, pulmonary alveolar proteinosis, tuberculosis, and wounds. Drugs include corticosteroids and chemotherapeutic agents.

Description: Microscopic examination to detect gram-positive filamentous branching bacteria that may segment into reproductive bacillary fragments. *Nocardia* is found in soil, grass, grain, straw, and decaying matter. The human infections produced are primary skin lesions (rare), lung (60–80%), and brain (20–40%).

Professional Considerations:

1. Consent form NOT required.
2. Preparation:
   A. Preschedule the test with the laboratory.
   B. Obtain a sterile Culturette or a sterile plastic container.
3. Procedure:
   A. Obtain a sterile culture from a suspected site.
4. Postprocedure care:
   A. Send the specimen to the laboratory within 1 hour.
5. Client and family teaching:
   A. Results are normally available from 72 hours to 30 days.
6. Factors that affect results:
   A. A contaminated culture invalidates the results.

7. Other data:
   A. *Nocardia* grows on various media, but may take 3–30 days or more to appear.
   B. *Nocardia* is extremely difficult to culture. A modified acid-fast stain is helpful in the diagnosis of *Nocardia*.
   C. *Nocardia* infections are uncommon, with approximately 500–1000 reported cases annually in the United States.
   D. Respiratory symptoms appear first because the lung is the most common portal of entry.
   E. Brain abscess is the most fatal complication of *Nocardia*.
   F. Sulfonamides or minocycline is the treatment of choice.

Bibliography:

LeBlang SD, Hansman Whiteman ML, Donovan Post MJ, et al.: CNS *Nocardia* in AIDS patients: CT and MRI with pathologic correlation. J Computer Assist Tomogr 19(1):15–22, 1995.

Lungu O, Della Latta PD, Weitzman I, et al.: Differentiation of *Nocardia* from rapidly growing *Mycobacterium* species by PCR-RFLP analysis. Diagn Microbiol Infect Dis 18:13–18, 1994.

Salinas-Carmona MC, Welsh O, Casillas SM: Enzyme-linked immunosorbent assay for serological diagnosis of *Nocardia brasiliensis* and clinical correlation with mycetoma infections. J Clin Microbiol 31(11):2901–2906, 1993.

Yoon HK, Im JG, Ahn JM, et al.: Pulmonary nocardiosis: CT findings. J Comp Assist Tomogr 19(1):52–55, 1995.

NOREPINEPHRINE, SERUM
(see Catecholamines, Plasma)

NORPACE, SERUM
(see Disopyramide, Serum)

NORTRIPTYLINE, BLOOD
(see Tricyclic Antidepressants, Plasma or Serum)

NOSE, ROUTINE, CULTURE
(see Culture, Routine, Specimen)

5'-NUCLEOTIDASE, SERUM

Norm: 2–15 IU/L, 0–17 U/L, 0–1.6 U, or 0.3–3.2 Bodanzky units.

Increased: Alcoholism, cirrhosis, drug-induced cholestasis, extrahepatic obstruction, granulomatous infiltrative disease, liver dysfunction, liver failure, liver metastasis, sickle cell anemia, and surgery. Drugs include acetaminophen, aspirin, narcotics, phenothiazines, and phenytoin.

Decreased: Hepatitis.

Description: A plasma membrane enzyme that is an isozyme of alkaline phosphatase that is found in hepatic parenchyma and bile ductal cells. This test aids differential diagnosis between bone and liver cancer, as 5'-nucleotidase is rarely elevated in bone cancer. When coupled with elevated alkaline phosphatase, the levels are indicative of liver metastasis.

Professional Considerations:

1. Consent form NOT required.
2. Preparation:
   A. Tube: Red-top, red/gray-top, or gold-top or blue-top.
3. Procedure:
   A. Draw a 2-ml blood sample.
4. Postprocedure care:
   A. The sample remains stable for 5 days at room temperature, 1 week when refrigerated, and 1 month when frozen.

5. Client and family teaching:
   A. Results are normally available within 72 hours.
6. Factors that affect results:
   A. Contaminated sample and hemolysis.
7. Other data:
   A. Liver enzyme studies should be evaluated with results.
   B. One study found elevated 5'-nucleotidase to be a useful indicator in predicting liver metastasis secondary to breast cancer.

Bibliography:

Mohamed AO, Jansson A, Ronquist G: Increased activity of 5' nucleotidase in serum of patients with sickle cell anaemia. Scand J Clin Lab Invest 53: 701–704, 1993.

Ramalingam V, Krishnamoorthy G, Govindarajulu P: Plasma membrane enzymes in human breast carcinoma: Relationship with serum hormones. J Exper Clin Oncol 40(5):363–367, 1993.

O₂ SAT, BLOOD

(see Blood Gases, Arterial, Blood)

O-BANDING (CSF PROTEIN), PLASMA

Norm: Negative.

Usage: Burkitt's lymphoma, cryptococcal meningitis, multiple sclerosis, neurosyphilis, polyneuropathy, rubella panencephalitis of progressive nature, and subacute sclerosing panencephalitis.

Description: Serum electrophoresis to diagnose inflammatory and autoimmune central nervous system (CNS) diseases that produce quantitative changes in oligoclonal proteins in the serum. O-Banding can also be performed on cerebrospinal fluid (CSF) by electrophoresis. Two or more definite bands with no counterparts is considered positive identification.

Professional Considerations:

1. Consent form NOT required.
2. Preparation:
   A. Tube: Red-top, red/gray-top, or gold-top.
   B. *See also Lumbar Puncture, Diagnostic.*
3. Procedure:
   A. Draw a 1-ml blood sample.
   B. Draw a 5-ml CSF sample.
4. Postprocedure care:
   A. Plasma or CSF specimens should be frozen if testing is delayed.
   B. *See also Lumbar Puncture, Diagnostic.*

5. Client and family teaching:
   A. Results are normally available within 72 hours.
   B. *See also Lumbar Puncture, Diagnostic.*
6. Factors that affect results:
   A. Unlabeled specimens.
7. Other data:
   A. These bands are not seen in vascular disease, brain tumors, or other nonimmunologic brain disorders.
   B. O-banding is not a significant prognostic factor in heart transplant recipients, HIV infections, or multiple sclerosis.
   C. This test has a 90% sensitivity level.
   D. If both plasma and CSF are being evaluated, they should be drawn at approximately the same time.

Bibliography:

Filippini G, Comi GC, Cosi V, et al.: Sensitivities and predictive values of paraclinical tests for diagnosing multiple sclerosis. J Neurol 241:132–137, 1994.

Frankel EB, Greenberg ML, Makuku S, et al.: Oligoclonal banding in AIDS and hemophilia. Mt Sinai J Med 60(3):232–237, 1993.

Prabhakar S, Kurien E, Gupta RS, et al.: Heat shock protein immunoreactivity in CSF: Correlation with oligoclonal banding and demyelinating disease. Neurology 44:1644–1648, 1994.

OBSTETRIC SONOGRAM (OBSTETRIC ECHOGRAM, OBSTETRIC ULTRASOUND), DIAGNOSTIC

Norm: Fetus(es) and sac are of normal size for gestational date. No fetal abnormality detected.

Usage: Evaluate amniotic fluid volume, fetal age, position, size, or viability for proper timing of induced or cesarean delivery; fetal abnormality detection; and multiple gestation determination. Helps diagnose ectopic tubal pregnancy, fetal death, placenta previa, or abruptio placentae; and provides guidance for amniocentesis, cervical cerclage placement, fetoscopy, or intrauterine procedures.

Description: Evaluation of size, status, and location of fetus, fetal sac, and pelvic organs via the creation of an oscilloscopic picture from the echoes of high-frequency sound waves passing over the pregnant abdomen (acoustic imaging). The time required for the ultrasonic beam to be reflected back to the transducer from differing densities of tissue is converted by a computer to an electrical impulse displayed on an oscilloscopic screen to create a three-dimensional picture of the pelvic contents.

Professional Considerations:

1. Consent form NOT required.
2. Preparation:
   A. This test should be performed before intestinal barium tests, or else after the barium is cleared from the system.
   B. The client should disrobe below the waist or wear a gown.
   C. Obtain water-soluble gel, a transducer for the ultrasound machine, a camera and videotape, and/or an oscilloscope.
   D. *See Client and family teaching.*
3. Procedure:
   A. The client is positioned supine.
   B. The pelvic and abdominal areas are coated with water-soluble gel.
   C. A lubricated transducer is passed slowly and firmly over the abdominal and pelvic area at a variety of angles.
   D. Photographs are taken of the images transmitted to the oscilloscopic screen.
   E. The procedure should take approximately 30–60 minutes.
4. Postprocedure care:
   A. Wipe the gel off the abdominal/pelvic area.
   B. Instruct the client to empty her bladder immediately.
5. Client and family teaching:
   A. The client should drink 1 quart of water 1 hour before the procedure, as a full bladder is needed to define pelvic organs by serving as an acoustic window for transmission of the sound waves. The full bladder also properly positions the uterus so that it is perpendicular to the transducer. Do not void until the test is completed.

B. Lying supine may cause shortness of breath. This may be relieved by elevating the upper body or by lying on either side.
6. Factors that affect results:
   A. Miscalculation of the conception date.
   B. Dehydration interferes with adequate contrast between the organs and body fluids.
   C. Intestinal barium or gas obscures the results by preventing the proper transmission and deflection of the high-frequency sound waves.
   D. Although a full bladder is recommended, during the first trimester, one that is overfilled may compress the uterus, making it difficult to obtain adequate pictures of the early embryonic and extra-embryonic structures.
7. Other data:
   A. An abnormal echo pattern may indicate a multiple pregnancy.
   B. This procedure has a 98% accuracy rate for identifying the placental site.
   C. In the first trimester of pregnancy, a transvaginal approach to sonography may be preferred. This method requires an empty bladder and the passage of a small transducer gently into the vagina. This process eliminates the interference of transverse abdominal tissue, allowing for more detailed visualization.
   D. A chaperone should be present during a transvaginal sonogram.

Bibliography:

Confino E, Binor Z, Wood Molo M, et al.: Selective salpingography for the diagnosis and treatment of early tubal pregnancy. Fertil Steril 62(2):286–288, 1994.

Dell'Agnola CA, Tomaselli V, Teruzzi E, et al.: Prenatal diagnosis of gastrointestinal obstruction: A correlation between prenatal ultrasonic findings and postnatal operative findings. Prenat Diagn 13: 629–632, 1993.

Emanuel MH, Verdel MJ, Wamsteker K, et al.: A prospective comparison of transvaginal sonography and diagnostic hysteroscopy in the evaluation of patients with abnormal uterine bleeding: Clinical implications. Am J Obstet Gynecol 172(2, Pt 1):547–552, 1995.

Willems JJ, Sandler DE: Obstetric and gynecological emergencies. In Kravis TC, Warner CG, Jacobs LM (eds): Emergency Medicine, 3rd ed. New York, Raven Press, 1993, pp 1229–1240.

OBSTETRIC ULTRASOUND
(see Obstetric Sonogram, Diagnostic)

OCA-125 ANTIGEN, SERUM
(see CA-125, Blood)

OCCULT BLOOD, GASTRIC CONTENTS, DIAGNOSTIC
(see Gastric Analysis, Specimen)

OCCULT BLOOD, STOOL

Norm: Negative.

Positive: Alcohol abuse, colon cancer, Crohn's disease, diverticulitis, esophageal varices, gastric ulcer, gastritis, gastrointestinal bleeding, hemorrhage, intussusception, pancreatic carcinoma, peptic ulcer, stress ulcers, tumors, and ulcerative colitis. Drugs include aspirin, boric acid, bromides, colchicine, indomethacin, iodine, iron preparations, potassium preparations, reserpine, salicylates, steroids, and thiazide diuretics.

Description: Rapid method for qualitative detection of red blood cells in stool, based on pseudoperoxidase reaction between hemoglobin, the developer (hydrogen peroxide and denatured ethanol), and guaiac.

Professional Considerations:

1. Consent form NOT required.
2. Preparation:
   A. *See Client and family teaching.*
   B. Obtain a guaiac-impregnated card for occult blood testing and a wooden applicator.
3. Procedure:
   A. Obtain a stool sample.
   B. Open the front flap of the guaiac-impregnated slide.
   C. Using the applicator provided, apply a thin smear of stool in each box. Use a separate sample from a different part of the stool specimen for each smear.
   D. Close the slide cover.
   E. Open the flap on the back of the slide.
   F. Apply two drops of developer to each box and to the quality control monitor.
   G. Read the results after 30 seconds and within 2 minutes. Any trace of blue color is positive for occult blood.
   H. Repeat for three consecutive bowel movements.
   I. Test stools within 48 hours of collection.
4. Postprocedure care:
   A. Assess the rectal area for irritation.
5. Client and family teaching:
   A. Follow a meat-free, high-residue diet for 24–48 hours prior to the test. The diet should also be free of vegetables with high peroxidase activity (including bananas, beets, broccoli, cantaloupe, cauliflower, grapes, horseradish, mushrooms, parsnips, and turnips).
   B. The client may perform this test at home following the same procedure stated above. Slides should be mailed to the physician's office or to the laboratory, as instructed.
   C. Factors that may interfere with results

should be reviewed with the client and avoided prior to testing.
6. Factors that affect results:
   A. Specimens will be positive if contaminated by menstrual or hemorrhoidal blood or povidone-iodine.
   B. Diets rich in meats, green leafy vegetables, poultry, and fish may produce false-positive results. Drugs include alcohol, anti-inflammatory agents, ascorbic acid (vitamin C), and nonsteroidal agents.
   C. Inadequate stool on the slide may produce false-negative results.
7. Other data:
   A. False-positives occur in about 10% of tests.
   B. Check the developer and the slides for expiration dates.
   C. Occult stool testing is an easy, inexpensive test in screening for colorectal cancer, specifically, in asymptomatic clients.

Bibliography:

Fric P, Zavoral M, Dvorakova H, et al.: An adapted program of colorectal cancer screening—7 years experience and cost-benefit analysis. Hepato-Gastroenterol *41*:413–416, 1994.

Hynam KA, Hart AR, Gay SP, et al.: Screening for colorectal cancer: Reasons for refusal of faecal occult blood testing in a general practice in England. J Epidemiol Community Health *49*:84–86, 1995.

Weinrich SP, Weinrich MC, Boyd MD, et al.: Teaching older adults by adapting for aging changes. Cancer Nurs *17*(6):494–500, 1994.

OCCULT BLOOD, URINE

Norm: Negative, <5000–10,000 RBC/ml or 2–3 RBCs per high power field.

Positive: Bladder cancer, benign familial hematuria, benign prostatic hypertrophy, burns, cystitis, dysuria, glomerulonephritis, Goodpasture's syndrome, heavy exercise, hematuria, hemophilia, nephrolithiasis, thrombocytopenia, transfusion reaction, trauma, and urinary tract infection. Drugs include heparin, salicylates, and warfarin.

Description: Screening by dipstick or examination of urine sediment for asymptomatic hematuria, which may be associated with a serious urologic disease, or the presence of active bleeding with a hematologic disorder.

Professional Considerations:

1. Consent form NOT required.
2. Preparation:
   A. Obtain a plastic specimen container and a centrifuge tube. If testing is to be performed immediately, obtain

reagent strips with the manufacturer's instructions.

3. Procedure:
   A. Cleanse the genital area with soap and water.
   B. Collect a 10-ml random urine specimen in a centrifuge tube and send the tube to the laboratory, or collect a specimen in a clean plastic cup for dipstick usage as directed by the manufacturer.
4. Postprocedure care:
   A. Perform a dipstick reading according to the manufacturer's directions immediately, or send the specimen to the laboratory within 2 hours.
   B. Write the collection time on the laboratory requisition.
5. Client and family teaching:
   A. Results are normally available within 24 hours.
6. Factors that affect results:
   A. Reject specimens received more than 2 hours after collection, as standing destroys red cells.
   B. The presence of urinary bacteria may cause false-positive results, as will large amounts of ascorbic acid or formaldehyde in urine.
   C. False-positives may also be caused by contact of the specimen with povidone-iodine, bleach, menstrual blood, or hemorrhoidal blood.
   D. Failure to mix the sample, resulting in no RBCs in supernatant and high levels of nitrite, may cause false-negative results.
   E. Do NOT use a reagent strip to test urine if the client is receiving tetracycline, terramycin, panmycin, bromides, or copper, as these create false-positive results.
7. Other data:
   A. Sensitivity of reagent strips decreases with age and if urine contains high protein or high specific gravities.
   B. Reagent strips are more sensitive to free hemoglobin than to intact red blood cells.

Bibliography:

Baer DM: Confirmation of urine screening tests. Med Lab Observer *25*(8):14, 16, 1993.

Brigden ML, Leadbeater A: Stick 'em up: Optimizing results with urinalysis dipsticks. Med Lab Observer *26*(6):32–36, 1994.

OCULAR CYTOLOGY, SPECIMEN

Norm: Negative.

Usage: Adenovirus infection, *Chlamydia,* conjunctivitis, dry eye conditions, Kaposi's sarcoma, keratitis, and metastatic cancer from the breast or melanoma.

Description: An ocular smear is evaluated for the presence of polymorphs or other inflammatory cells. Test commonly includes staining by either Papanicolaou or Giemsa stain.

Professional Considerations:
1. Consent form IS required.

Risks:
Infection, unilateral blindness.

Contraindications:
Central retinal artery occlusion.

2. Preparation:
   A. Obtain a sterile fine-needle aspiration tray, a sterile plastic container, and a sterile 2-×-2-inch gauze or sterile cotton-tipped applicator approved for microbiologic use.
   B. Obtain two glass slides and spray the fixative.
3. Procedure:
   A. A fine-needle biopsy is taken from the eye or a cotton-tipped application, or a scrape is obtained.
   B. Place the smears on two clean glass slides, and immediately fix one slide with the spray and let the other slide air-dry.
4. Postprocedure care:
   A. Assess the aspiration area every 5 minutes × 4 for bleeding, edema, or redness.
   B. Results are normally available in 24 hours.
5. Client and family teaching:
   A. Monitor ocular site for inflammation or redness for 24–48 hours.
   B. A mild analgesic may be required for pain control.
   C. Monitor ocular site for signs and symptoms of infection until the site is healed.
6. Factors that affect results:
   A. A contaminated sample of the aspirate invalidates results.
7. Other data:
   A. Impression cytology is an alternative to biopsy in detecting mucus deficiency. A filter paper is applied to the conjunctiva and viewed microscopically. Topical anesthesia must NOT be used when obtaining this specimen.

Bibliography:

Holly FJ: Diagnostic methods and treatment modalities of dry eye conditions. Int Ophthalmol *17:* 113–125, 1993.

Obata H, Horiuchi H, Tsuru T: Clinical application of new membrane filter for cytopathological diagnosis in ophthalmology. Jpn J Ophthalmol *37*(3): 344–351, 1993.

OCULOPLETHYSMOGRAPHY (OPG), DIAGNOSTIC

Norm: Negative, or all pulses should occur simultaneously.

Usage: Ataxia, carotid occlusive disease, following carotid endarterectomy, syncope, and transient ischemic attacks.

Description: Noninvasive test that measures ocular artery pressure by comparing pulse arrival times in the eyes with the ears, which reflects the adequacy of cerebrovascular blood flow in the carotid arteries.

Professional Considerations:

1. Consent form IS required.

Risks:

Corneal abrasion.

Contraindications:

Clients who have had eye surgery within 2–6 months, cataract, conjunctivitis, diabetes mellitus, uncontrolled glaucoma, enucleation, history of retinal detachment or lens implantation, or in those who are hypersensitive to local anesthetic or uncooperative and combative clients.

2. Preparation:
   A. Obtain anesthetic eye drops, an eyecup, and photoelectric cells.
3. Procedure:
   A. Instill the anesthetic eye drops and apply the eyecup to the corneas with light suction (40–50 mmHg).
   B. Apply the photoelectric cells to earlobes.
   C. Record the cyclic changes in volume on a graphic machine.
4. Postprocedure care:
   A. Observe for ocular pain or photophobia, which may indicate corneal abrasion.
5. Client and family teaching:
   A. Do not rub the eyes or insert contact lenses for 30 minutes after the test.
   B. Anesthetic eye drops may cause slight temporary burning.
   C. It is not unusual to experience blurred vision for a short period following this procedure.
   D. Continued blurred vision or pain should be reported to the physician.
   E. The procedure takes a few minutes.
6. Factors that affect results:
   A. Constant blinking, nystagmus, or poor cooperation prevent accurate measurement.

7. Other data:
   A. A 20-ms or greater delay in the pulse wave in the ophthalmic artery is abnormal, signifying stenosis.
   B. Delayed arrival of the ocular pulse is associated with ipsilateral carotid stenosis.
   C. This test does NOT distinguish between a completely occluded internal carotid artery and one that is nearly occluded.
   D. This procedure is extremely useful for evaluating deep orbital circulation.
   E. *See also Carotid Phonoangiography and Oculopneumoplethysmography (OPPG), Diagnostic.*

Bibliography:

Loeb S, Lewis JA, Ambrose MW: Illustrated Guide to Diagnostic Tests. Springhouse, PA, Springhouse Corporation, 1994, pp 782–785.

Wray SH: The management of acute visual failure. J Neurol Neurosurg Psychiatry 56:234–240, 1993.

OCULOPNEUMOPLETHYS-MOGRAPHY (OPPG), DIAGNOSTIC

Norm: Difference between ophthalmic artery pressures should be <5 mmHg. Ophthalmic artery pressure divided by the higher brachial systolic pressure should be >0.67.

Usage: Ataxia, carotid bruits of asymptomatic origin, carotid endarterectomy monitoring, carotid occlusive disease, syncope, and transient ischemic attacks.

Description: A vacuum applied to the sclera allows adjustment of intraocular pressure and a recording of ocular pressure waveform. Ophthalmic artery pressures are compared with the higher brachial pressure and with each other.

Professional Considerations:

1. Consent form IS required.

Risks:

Corneal abrasion, erythema, hematoma (sclerae).

Contraindications:

Anticoagulant therapy, conjunctivitis, enucleation, retinal detachment or history, uncontrolled glaucoma, eye surgery within the previous 2–6 months, increased intracranial pressure.

2. Preparation:
   A. Obtain anesthetic eye drops such as 0.5% proparacaine, an eyecup, suction vacuum apparatus, a plethysmograph, a sphygmomanometer, and a stethoscope.
3. Procedure:
   A. Instill the anesthetic eye drops.
   B. Attach the eyecup to the scleras of the eyes.
   C. Apply a vacuum of 300 mmHg to each eye so that the pulse disappears. Then gradually release the suction until the pulse returns.
   D. Take both brachial pressures.
   E. The higher systolic brachial pressure is compared with the ophthalmic artery pressures.
4. Postprocedure care:
   A. Observe for ocular pain or photophobia, which may indicate corneal abrasion.
5. Client and family teaching:
   A. Transient loss of vision when suction is applied is not unusual.
   B. Anesthetic eye drops may cause slight temporary burning.
   C. Do not rub the eyes or insert contact lenses for 2 hours after the test.
   D. Continued pain should be reported to the physician.
6. Factors that affect results:
   A. Constant blinking, hypertension, nystagmus, and poor cooperation prevent accurate measurement.
   B. Results may be difficult to interpret if the client has a history of hypertension.
   C. Cardiac dysrhythmias may alter the results.
7. Other data:
   A. This method is more accurate than oculoplethysmography.
   B. See also Oculoplethysmography (OPG), Diagnostic.

Bibliography:

Loeb S, Lewis JA, Ambrose MW: Illustrated Guide to Diagnostic Tests. Springhouse, PA, Springhouse Corporation, 1994, pp 782–785.

OKT3 CELLS, OKT4 CELLS, OKT8 CELLS

(see Acquired Immune Deficiency Syndrome Evaluation Battery, Diagnostic)

OLIGOCLONAL BANDS, CEREBROSPINAL FLUID, SPECIMEN

(see Cerebrospinal Fluid, Myelin Basic Protein, Oligoclonal Bands, Protein, and Protein Electrophoresis, Specimen)

OLIGOCLONAL BANDS, DIAGNOSTIC

(see O-Banding, Serum)

ONE-STEP, DIAGNOSTIC

(see Glucose Monitoring Machines, Diagnostic)

ONE TOUCH, DIAGNOSTIC

(see Glucose Monitoring Machines, Diagnostic)

OPHTHALMODYNAMOMETRY, DIAGNOSTIC

Norm: No difference in pressure of both eyes.

Usage: Carotid occlusive disease, extracranial vascular disease, and transient ischemic attacks.

Description: Compares the retinal artery pressures in both eyes in the supine and upright positions. A decrease in retinal arterial pressure with a normal brachial pressure when the client moves from a supine position to an upright position indicates carotid occlusive disease.

Professional Considerations:

1. Consent form NOT required.

Risks:
Corneal abrasion.

Contraindications:
In thrombocytopenia and for clients receiving anticoagulants.

2. Preparation:
   A. Obtain an ophthalmoscope, a blood pressure cuff, a stethoscope, and a sphygmomanometer.
3. Procedure:
   A. The ophthalmoscope is pressed gradually against the eye to measure arterial systolic pressure and diastolic pressures in supine and upright positions.
   B. Brachial blood pressures are also measured in the arm.
4. Postprocedure care:
   A. Assess for ocular photophobia or pain that may indicate corneal abrasion.

5. Client and family teaching:
   A. Results are normally available within 24 hours, interpretation to follow.
6. Factors that affect results:
   A. Constant blinking, nystagmus, and poor cooperation.
7. Other data:
   A. The oculoplethysmography test is the preferred test when evaluating carotid arteries when compared to the ophthalmodynamometry test.
   B. A 20% difference in diastolic pressure between eyes suggests insufficient carotid artery flow on the side with the lower finding.
   C. See also Oculoplethysmography (OPG), Diagnostic.

Bibliography:

Barnes RW: Other noninvasive techniques in cerebrovascular disease. In Bernstein EF (ed): Vascular Diagnosis, 4th ed. St. Louis, MO, Mosby Year Book, 1993, pp 398–402.

ORAL CAVITY CYTOLOGY, SPECIMEN

Norm: Negative.

Usage: Cancers of the tongue, gum, or mouth; *Candida albicans;* herpes virus infection; human immunodeficiency virus; Klinefelter's syndrome; pemphigus; trisomy 13, 18, and 21; and Turner's syndrome.

Description: Microscopic examination of cells scraped from the oral cavity surface.

Professional Considerations:

1. Consent form NOT required.
2. Preparation:
   A. Obtain a glass of water, a spatula or tongue blade, a glass slide, a specimen container of 95% ethyl alcohol or spray fixative, and a light source.
   B. Label the slide with the client's name and the specimen source.
3. Procedure:
   A. The client should rinse the mouth vigorously with water several times before the scraping is performed.
   B. The lesion or oral surface is scraped with a spatula or tongue blade.
   C. Smear the scraping on a labeled glass slide and fix it immediately in 95% alcohol or spray fixative.
4. Postprocedure care:
   A. The requisition should include age, physical findings, history of smoking, dentures, skin lesions, and reverse smoking; and history of chemotherapy, immunotherapy, or radiation therapy.

5. Client and family teaching:
   A. Results are normally available in 24–48 hours.
6. Factors that affect results:
   A. Failure to fix specimens invalidates the results.
7. Other data:
   A. Occasional diagnosis of palatal salivary gland neoplasm occurs.
   B. *Candida albicans* can spread to the esophagus and down to the intestines.

Bibliography:

Gunhan O, Dogan N, Celasun B, et al.: Fine needle aspiration cytology of oral cavity and jaw bone lesions. Acta Cytol *37*(2):135–141, 1993.

Koss LG: Cytologic diagnosis of oral, esophageal, and peripheral lung cancer. J Cell Biochem Suppl 7F:66–81, 1993.

ORNITHINE CARBAMOYLTRANSFERASE (OCT), BLOOD

Norm: 0–500 sigma units/ml, or 0–16 U/L.

Increased: Acute viral hepatitis, cholecystitis, cirrhosis, enteritis, hepatic necrosis, hepatotoxicity due to drugs or alcoholism (rare), infectious mononucleosis, liver dysfunction, obstructive jaundice, metastatic liver carcinoma, and prolonged exercise. Drugs include all hepatotoxic drugs, heavy alcohol, and oral contraceptives.

Decreased: Congenital hyperammonemia. Drugs include mercuric salts, *p*-chloromercuribenzoate, and 2,3-dimercaptopropanol.

Description: OCT is an enzyme found in the liver and to a lesser extent in the intestinal mucosa that is involved in urea metabolism of the Krebs' cycle. An elevation specifically and sensitively indicates liver cell disease. Insufficient production of OCT is an inherited x-linked dominant genetic defect.

Professional Considerations:

1. Consent form NOT required.
2. Preparation:
   A. Tube: Red-top, red/gray-top, or gold-top.
3. Procedure:
   A. Draw a 7-ml blood sample.
4. Postprocedure care:
   A. None.
5. Client and family teaching:
   A. Results are normally available within 72 hours to 1 week.

6. Factors that affect results:
   A. Hemolysis of the specimen invalidates the results.
7. Other data:
   A. The test is more sensitive than AST (SGOT) or ALT (SGPT) in assessing liver function.
   B. The test does not distinguish between hepatic and biliary diseases.
   C. The exact occupance of the inherited X-linked genetic defect is unknown but has been estimated to be 1:80,000, with males more affected.

Bibliography:

Harbrecht BG, DiSilvio M, Demetris AJ, et al.: Tumor necrosis factor—regulates in vivo nitric oxide synthesis and induces liver injury during endotoxemia. Hepatology 20(4):1055–1060, 1994.

Kamoun P, Fensom AH, Shin YS, et al.: Prenatal diagnosis of the urea cycle disease: A survey of the European cases. Am J Med Genet 55(2):247–250, 1995.

Ping Lim S, Andrews FJ, O'Brien PE: Misoprostol protection against acetaminophen-induced hepatotoxicity in the rat. Dig Dis Sci 39(6):1249–1256, 1994.

Tuchman M: Mutations and polymorphisms in the human ornithine transcarbamylase gene. Hum Mutation 2(3):174–178, 1993.

OSMOLALITY, CALCULATED TEST (OSMOLAR GAP), BLOOD

Norm:

Serum osmolality	280–300 mOsm/kg H_2O
Osmolar gap	<10 mOsm/kg H_2O

Increased: Alcoholism, azotemia, burns, convulsions, dehydration, diabetes insipidus, diarrhea, hyperaldosteronism, hyperlipidemia, hyperproteinemia, presence of hyperosmolar substances such as ethanol or methanol or lactic acid, syndrome of inappropriate antidiuretic hormone secretion (SIADHS), and uremia. Drugs include mannitol.

Decreased: Hyponatremia and overhydration.

Description: Osmolality refers to a solution's concentration of solute particles per kilogram of solvent and is expressed in mOsm/kg. In the laboratory, it is measured by an osmometer. However, it is possible to calculate serum osmolality using serum measurements of sodium, glucose, and urea (BUN) according to the formula(s) listed under *Procedure*, below. The osmolar gap is the difference between the laboratory serum osmolarity value and the calculated osmolar value. Assessing this gap is most important in the diagnosis of ethanol or methanol poisoning.

Professional Considerations:

1. Consent form NOT required.
2. Preparation:
   A. None, other than locating the results of serum sodium, glucose, and BUN levels.
3. Procedure:
   A. Calculate osmolality as follows:

$[(1.86) \times (Sodium)] + (Glucose/18) + (BUN/2.8)$

B. Rounded formula:

$[(2) \times (Sodium)] + (Glucose/18) + (BUN/2.8)$

C. Dr. Weisberg's formula:

$[(2) \times (Sodium)] + (Glucose/20) + (BUN/3)$

4. Postprocedure care:
   A. Calculated osmolality may be compared to laboratory-measured osmolality.
5. Client and family teaching:
   A. Results are normally available within 72 hours.
6. Factors that affect results:
   A. Hemolysis of specimens used to obtain sodium, glucose, and BUN values invalidates results.
7. Other data:
   A. A difference between measured and calculated serum osmolality (osmolal gap) of >10 mOsm/kg H_2O may indicate pseudohyponatremia caused by severe hyperlipidemia or hyperproteinemia.
   B. Abnormal calculated results should be confirmed by a serum osmolality test.
   C. *See also Osmolality, Serum.*

Bibliography:

Hirschl MM, Derfler K, Bieglmayer C, et al.: Hormonal derangements in patients with severe alcohol intoxication. Alcohol Clin Exp Res 18(3):761–766, 1994.

Hoffman RS, Smilkstein MJ, Howland MA, et al.: Osmol gaps revisited: Normal values and limitations. Clin Toxicol 31(1):81–93, 1993.

Rose, BD: Clinical Physiology of Acid Base and Electrolyte Disorders. New York, McGraw-Hill, 1994.

OSMOLALITY, SERUM
Norm:

		SI Units
Adult	280–300 mOsm/kg H_2O	285–293 mmol/kg H_2O
Child	270–290 mOsm/kg H_2O	270–290 mmol/kg H_2O
Panic levels:	<240 mOsm/kg H_2O	<240 mmol/kg H_2O
	>320 mOsm/kg H_2O	>320 mmol/kg H_2O

Panic Level Symptoms and Treatment:

Symptoms: Poor skin turgor or interstitial edema, listlessness, acidosis by decreased pH, shock, seizures, coma, cardiopulmonary arrest. Respiratory arrest may occur when value exceeds 360 mOsm/kg.

Treatment:

1. Assess electrolytes.
2. Administer IV fluids in specific osmotic concentrations to shift fluid into or out of the intravascular space, as appropriate.
3. Add corrected electrolytes as needed.
4. Monitor for side effects of fluid and electrolyte imbalance.
5. Possibly conduct cardiac monitoring, depending on electrolyte values.
6. Perform neurologic checks q 1–4 hours.
7. Take seizure precautions (the client is at risk for intracerebral edema or brain cell dehydration, depending on the relative serum osmolality in comparison with intracellular osmolality).
8. Treat gastrointestinal symptoms supportively.
9. Identify and correct cause.

Increased: Acidosis, advanced liver disease, alcoholism, burns, dehydration (associated with diabetes insipidus as too much antidiuretic hormone causes the kidney to excrete large amounts of water), diabetic ketoacidosis, hyperbilirubinemia, hypercalcemia, hyperglycemia, hyperglycemic hyperosmolar nonketotic coma, hypernatremia, high-protein diet, hypovolemic shock, methanol poisoning, nephrogenic diabetes insipidus.

Decreased: Acute renal failure; Addison's disease; hyponatremia; overhydration; syndrome of inappropriate antidiuretic hormone secretion (SIADHS), which is often associated with cancers (especially oat cell of the lung) or medications such as chemotherapy, oral agents for diabetes mellitus and tricyclic antidepressants, and narcotics; and disorders of the posterior pituitary.

Description: Osmolality is a measure of the concentration of particles in the serum per kilogram of water. Osmolarity is nearly the same but measures said concentration per liter of water. Used to assess the fluid state of the client and determine the cause of fluid and electrolyte imbalances, particularly in endocrine disorders. The normally functioning osmoregulation system maintains the serum osmolality (the concentration of the blood) within a tight normal range. Receptors in the hypothalamus adjust the level of antidiuretic hormone from the posterior pituitary, which affects the free water excreted from the kidney. Disorders of the hypothalamus, the posterior pituitary, or the kidney, may alter serum osmolality. Dehydration from any cause increases osmolality. Overhydration decreases serum osmolality. Either is dangerous to the client. Urine osmolarity is usually obtained with serum osmolality, because the comparison gives the true picture of the fluid balance state. The set of serum electrolytes (especially sodium and glucose) will also be assessed.

Professional Considerations:

1. Consent form NOT required.
2. Preparation:
   A. Tube: Red-top, red/gray-top, or gold-top.
   B. Do NOT draw samples during hemodialysis.

3. Procedure:
   A. Draw a 1-ml blood sample.
4. Postprocedure care:
   A. Measure the intake and output q 1 hour until the results are within normal limits.
5. Client and family teaching:
   A. Results are normally available within 4 hours.
   B. Clients with adrenocortical insufficiency should consult a physician about the continuation of steroid therapy.
6. Factors that affect results:
   A. The specimen is stable for only 10 hours if refrigerated.
   B. The use of mineralocorticoids, osmotic diuretics, insulin, or mannitol may increase values due to the effect on fluid balance.

C. Hemolysis of specimens invalidates the results.
D. Lipemic serum may alter the results.
7. Other data:
   A. None.

Bibliography:

Batcheller J: Syndrome of inappropriate antidiuretic hormone secretion. Crit Care Nurs Clin North Am 6(4):687–692, 1994.

Blevins LS, Wand GS: Diabetes insipidus. Crit Care Med 22(1):69–80, 1992.

Rose BD: Clinical Physiology of Acid-Base and Electrolyte Disorders, 4th ed. New York, McGraw-Hill, 1994.

Trivedi HS, Nolph KD: Nephrogenic diabetes insipidus presenting after head trauma. Am J Nephrol 14(2):145–147, 1994.

OSMOLALITY, URINE

Norm: *See range below; the concentration of the urine has a wide range as the body adjusts to varying fluid intake and requirements.*

		SI Units
13 months–adult	200–1200 mOsm/kg H2O	200–1200 mmol/kg H_2O
0–12 months	50–600 mOsm/kg H2O	50–600 mmol/kg H_2O

The comparison of urine osmolality to serum osmolality is important for determining the significance of the urine osmolality.

Increased: Acidosis; Addison's disease; congestive heart failure; high-protein diet; hyperglycemia; hypernatremia; hypovolemia; intracellular dehydration; renal disease; shock, and syndrome of inappropriate antidiuretic hormone secretion (SIADHS), in which the serum osmolality will be decreased.

Decreased: Aldosterone insufficiency, diabetic ketoacidosis, diabetes insipidus, diuretic therapy, hypokalemia, hyponatremia, nephrogenic diabetes insipidus, overhydration with intravenous D5W, psychogenic polydipsia, renal disease that affects the kidneys' ability to concentrate urine.

Description: Measure of the number of osmotically active particles in a given urine volume, which reflects the kidney's concentrating ability. Normal fluid balance is achieved by the action of the posterior pituitary (ADH secretion) and properly functioning kidneys. Fine adjustments are made continuously to maintain normal fluid and electrolyte balance. The kidney is able to adjust the urine concentration over a wide range to maintain a normal serum concentration or osmolality. Normally, when the client becomes even slightly dehydrated, the urine will become more highly concentrated. Therefore, if there is high fluid intake, the urine will become more dilute in ridding the body of the excess fluid.

Professional Considerations:

1. Consent form NOT required.
2. Preparation:
   A. The collection may be random, or the client may be required to fast from food and fluids from midnight before the collection the next day.
   B. Obtain a sterile, plastic specimen container.
3. Procedure:
   A. Collect a 10-ml random or morning urine specimen in a sterile, plastic container without preservatives.
4. Postprocedure care:
   A. Send the specimen to the laboratory for immediate processing.
   B. Intake and output (I&O) until the results are normal.
5. Client and family teaching:
   A. Results are normally available within 24 hours.

B. Clients with adrenocortical insufficiency should consult a physician about the continuation of steroid therapy.

6. Factors that affect results:
   A. Anesthetics, antibiotics, carbamazepine, chlorpropamide, detergent, dextran, diuretics, glucose, Mannitol, and radiographic contrast agents affect the urine volume and therefore cause abnormal results.

7. Other data:
   A. Urine osmolality is considered a better measurement than specific gravity to assess for the state of hydration.

Bibliography:

Batcheller, J: Syndrome of inappropriate antidiuretic hormone secretion. Crit Care Clin North Am 6(4):687–692, 1994.

Blevins LS, Wand GS: Diabetes insipidus. Crit Care Med 25(1):69–80, 1992.

Diamond JR, McLaughlin ML: Urinary parameters to assess renal function. Clin Lab Med 8:493–506, 1988.

Trivedi HS, Nolph KD: Nephrogenic diabetes insipidus presenting after head trauma. Am J Nephrol 14(2):145–147, 1994.

OTOSCOPY, VIDEO, DIAGNOSTIC

Norm: Normal structure, absence of inflammation, infection, growths or obstruction.

Usage: Anatomy and physiology of the ear canal, visualization of the tympanic membrane. Any trauma causing bleeding may be diagnosed, as well as vascular tumors of the middle ear. Using pneumatic video-otoscopy, the mobility of the tympanic membrane is observed. Video recordings can be made during surgery.

Description: This technique combines the standard methods of ENT endoscopy with a small, hand-held, video camera for viewing and recording the examination and ENT procedure. It can be used with the ears, nose, or larynx. The advantage of the video is in the visual record of the anatomy and physiology, which can be carefully studied at a later time without further discomfort to the client adding to the increased means of physician consultation and as an excellent teaching tool. The recording is stored as part of the client record.

Professional Considerations:

1. Consent form IS required.

Risks:
Infection.

Contraindications:
Sedatives are contraindicated in clients with central nervous system depression.

2. Preparation:
   A. Obtain a video camera; a light source; a video cassette recorder 3/4"; a video printer; a monitor and an enhancer; and film.
   B. Obtain an endoscope: Hopkins 4.0 mm for adults and Hopkins 2.7 mm for children.
   C. Anesthetic spray and sedation, as prescribed. Monitor respiratory status closely throughout the procedure if sedation is given.
   D. Obtain instruments to remove wax and superficial hairs from the ear.
   E. *See Client and family teaching.*

3. Procedure:
   A. Wax and hair are removed.
   B. A topical anesthetic is applied to the canal.
   C. Sedatives may be given intravenously.
   D. The client is placed in an upright or supine position and the endoscope is inserted.
   E. The video recording may begin at the time of insertion.

4. Postprocedure care:
   A. Continue the assessment of the respiratory status. If deep sedation was used, follow institutional protocol for postsedation monitoring. Typical monitoring includes continuous ECG monitoring and pulse oximetry, with continual assessments (q 5–15 minutes) of airway, vital signs, and neurologic status until the client is lying quietly awake, is breathing independently, and responds to commands spoken in a normal tone.
   B. Assess for postoperative complications, including bleeding and pain.

5. Client and family teaching:
   A. The procedure should take less than 1 hour.
   B. Hold very still during the procedure.

6. Factors that affect results:
   A. The client must be able to sit still for an extended length of time.

7. Other data:
   A. Videos are also used in rhinoscopy and laryngoscopy.

Bibliography:

Newby HA, Popelka GR: Audiology, 6th ed. Englewood Cliffs, NJ, Prentice Hall, 1992.

Yanagisawa E: The use of video in ENT endoscopy: its value in teaching. Ear Nose Throat J 73(10): 754–763, 1994.

OVA AND PARASITES (O & P), STOOL

(see Parasite Screen, Stool)

OVARIAN CANCER ANTIGEN-125, SERUM

(see CA-125, Blood)

OXALATE, 24-HOUR, URINE

Norm: 8–40 mg/24 hours (92–456 mmol/24 hours, SI units).

Increased: Celiac disease, cirrhosis, Crohn's disease, ethylene glycol poisoning, diabetes mellitus, hyperoxalauria (primary), kidney stone, nephrolithiasis, pancreatic insufficiency, sarcoidosis, vitamin B-6 deficiency. Drugs include megadoses of ascorbic acid and calcium. Also, ingestion of certain foods—see *Client and family teaching* below.

Decreased: Gastrointestinal disease or surgery that affects absorption; renal failure.

Description: Oxalate is an end product of metabolism that is excreted through the urine. It may accumulate in the soft and connective tissues of the kidneys and bladder and cause renal calculi and chronic inflammation and fibrosis.

Professional Considerations:

1. Consent form NOT required.
2. Preparation:
   A. Obtain a 3-L plastic container to which 30 ml of 6N hydrochloric acid (HCl) has been added.
   B. *See Client and family teaching.*
3. Procedure:
   A. Collect all the urine voided in a 24-hour period in a refrigerated, 3-L plastic container to which 30 ml of 6N HCl has been added. For specimens collected from an indwelling urinary catheter, keep the drainage bag on ice and empty the urine into the collection container hourly. Document the quantity of the urinary output throughout the collection period. Not all laboratories require refrigeration.
4. Postprocedure care:
   A. Write the beginning and ending dates and times as well as the total 24-hour urine output on the collection container and the laboratory requisition.
   B. Transport the specimen to the laboratory and refrigerate it until testing.
5. Client and family teaching:
   A. For 48 hours before testing, maintain a diet that avoids increasing oxalate by avoiding soybean products, wheat germ, grapefruit juice, strawberries, rhubarb, bananas, orange juice, canned pineapples or tomatoes, kidney beans, beets, spinach, carrots, tomatoes, celery, onions, sweet and white potatoes, green and waxed beans, cauliflower, cucumber, squash, broccoli, eggplant, cabbage, spinach, cashews, chocolate, cocoa, gelatin, peanut butter and other nuts, cola beverages, and tea.
   B. Urinate before defecating, and avoid contaminating the urine with the stool or toilet tissue. If any urine is accidentally discarded, discard the entire specimen and restart the collection the next day.
   C. A high-calcium diet may promote the development of kidney stones. Consult a dietician.
   D. Results are normally available within 24 hours.
6. Factors that affect results:
   A. Failure to include all urine voided in the 24-hour period invalidates the results.
   B. Ascorbic acid may interfere with the testing process. It does not affect the level of oxalate excretion.
   C. Certain foods need to be avoided, as they raise oxalate levels (see above, section 5A).
7. Other data:
   A. Studies show that stone formation is not age specific or gender specific.

Bibliography:

Grover PK, Ryall RL: Urate and calcium oxalate stones: from repute to rhetoric to reality. Miner Electrolyte Metab *20*(6):361–370, 1994.

Massey LK, Roman-Smith H, Sutton RA: Effect of dietary oxalate and calcium on urinary oxalate and risk of calcium oxalate renal stones. J Am Dietetic Assoc *93*(8):901–906, 1993.

Pierratos AE, Khalaff H, Cheng PT, Psihramis K, Jewett MA: Clinical and biochemical differences in patients with pure calcium oxalate monohydrates and calcium oxalate dihydrate kidney stones. J Urol *151*(3):571–574, 1994.

Wandzilak TR, D'Andre SD, Davis PA, Willians HE: Effect of high dose vitamin C on urinary oxalate levels. J Urol *151*(4):834–837, 1994.

OXAZEPAM

(see Benzodiazepines, Plasma and Urine)

OXIMETRY (PULSE OXIMETRY), DIAGNOSTIC

Norm: Adult arterial blood saturation is 95–100%; newborn arterial blood saturation, 40–92%, is dependent on lung development.

Usage: Any clinical situation in which adequate oxygenation is potentially compromised. Particularly helpful when used between arterial blood gas (ABG) determinations, to reduce both the number of blood draws and costs when the accuracy and correlation is known to the clinicians. Advantages: quick, noninvasive, and continuous, and can detect variations in saturation that may not be noted with ABGs. Disadvantage: only provides one of the determinants of the ABG and may be of only limited value when single readings are obtained if carefully correlated with the clinical situation. Conditions when it is used include acute myocardial infarction, acute respiratory distress syndrome (ARDS), anesthesia monitoring, asthma, cerebrovascular accident, chronic obstructive pulmonary disease, congenital heart defects, congestive heart failure, cor pulmonale, cystic fibrosis, emphysema, head trauma, intraoperatively, lung cancer, oxygen therapy, postoperatively, premature infant monitoring, pulmonary edema, pulmonary emboli, sickle cell anemia, tuberculosis, and ventilator dependence and weaning.

Description: Pulse oximetry involves the spectrophotometric estimate of functional oxygen saturation on hemoglobin. This is a noninvasive measurement of the SaO *(see Arterial Blood Gases),* a percentage representing the ratio of arterial hemoglobin saturated with oxygen. Measurement is performed via a spectrophotometer probe connected to the adult's finger, temporal area, or bridge of the nose, or to an infant's foot or toe. The probe emits red and infrared light that passes through the body part directed at a photo detector that determines the amplitude of the transmitted light and isolates the blood's pulsatile flow. This enables calculation of SaO through measurement of light absorption based on known amounts absorbed by saturated and reduced hemoglobin.

Professional Considerations:

1. Consent form NOT required.
2. Preparation:
   A. Cleanse the area with water and dry it prior to attaching the probe.
   B. For clients with impaired tissue perfusion, use a nasal probe or a temporal

probe. If a finger probe must be used, apply a warm pack around the hand and the extremity for 10 minutes before the probe application.
   C. Earlobe probes provide only a reflection of capillary blood unless the earlobe is rubbed vigorously prior to placement to arterialize the capillary blood. Ear oximetry should not be used for continuous monitoring. Intermittent ear oximetry monitoring of arterialized capillary blood is acceptable.
3. Procedure:
   A. The skin should be clean and dry prior to placement. If the ear is used, blood should be arterialized as described above. Attach the probe to the toe or foot for infants; the finger, temporal area, bridge of the nose, or earlobe for adults; and the bridge of the nose for obese clients. Nasal probes should be placed over cartilage for best results.
   B. Activate the pulse oximeter and set low and high alarm limits according to the manufacturer's instructions.
   C. Note SaO after allowing at least 30 seconds for the reading to stabilize.
   D. For continuous or periodic oximetry, observe for downward trends in SaO. Generally, decreased SaO below 90–92% must be addressed by thorough assessment of the client and clinical status.
4. Postprocedure care:
   A. Remove the probe. Clean nondisposable probes according to the manufacturer's instructions.
   B. Wash the area with soap and water.
5. Client and family teaching:
   A. Results are normally available immediately.
   B. Alarms are normally set to sound for a trend downward in values. Keeping the probe covered with a cloth improves signal clarity.
   C. In cases of lung disease, discuss smoking cessation programs/strategies, if applicable.
6. Factors that affect results:
   A. Hyperbilirubinemia, hypotension, hypothermia, use of vasopressor medications, impaired tissue perfusion, or cold extremities may result in no reading or a falsely low reading, necessitating use of ABG SaO. Desaturation by pulse oximetry may be used as a sign of severe hypotension requiring evaluation.
   B. Failure to place the probe properly may result in no reading or a falsely low or high reading.
   C. Very bright light surrounding the probe may make obtaining a reading difficult. If so, cover the probe with a sheet or other opaque material.
   D. Falsely elevated results may occur in the presence of dyshemoglobins (carboxyhemoglobin, >3%; methemoglobin, 1.5/dl; sulfhemoglobin, 0.5 g/dl),

necessitating periodic validation with ABG SaO.

E. Falsely decreased results may be caused by hyperbilirubinemia >20 mg%, necessitating periodic validation with ABG SaO.

F. Unreliable results may occur with the injection of radiographic dyes, necessitating periodic validation with ABG SaO.

G. Use of ear oximetry for continuous pulse oximetry monitory is unreliable and may produce falsely normal results. This is because it is impossible to keep the earlobe capillary blood arterialized on a continuous basis without continuous intervention.

H. Clients who are anemic may have misleadingly high saturation of hemoglobin and still be hypoxemic due to decreased oxygen-carrying capacity.

7. Other data:
A. Accurate between SaO levels of 85 and 100%.
B. Some pulse oximeters give slightly false higher readings in dark-skinned clients, but use after validation with ABG is not affected.

Bibliography:

Barker SJ, Tremper KK: Pulse oximetry: applications and limitations. Int Anesthesiol Clin 25(3):155–175, 1987.

Cahan C, Decer MJ, Hoekje Pl, Strohl, KP: Agreement between noninvasive oximetric values for oxygen saturation. Chest 97(4):814–819, 1990.

Decker MJ, Arnold JL, Haney D, Masny J, Strohl KP: Extended monitoring of oxygen saturation in chronic lung disease. Chest 102(4):1075–1079, 1992.

Schroeder CH: Pulse oximetry: A nursing care plan. Crit Care Nurs 8(8):50–68, 1988.

Tasota FJ, Wesmiller SW: Assessing ABG's. Maintaining the delicate balance. Nursing 94(May):34–49.

Webb RK, Ralston AC, Runciman WB: Potential error in pulse oximetry. II. Effects of changes in saturation and signal quality. Anaesthesia 46(3):207–212, 1991.

OXYGEN SATURATION (O₂ Sat, SO₂, SaO₂), BLOOD
(see Blood Gases, Arterial, Blood; Blood Gases, Venous, Blood; Blood Gases, Capillary, Blood; and Oxyhemoglobin Dissociation Curve, Diagnostic)

OXYHEMOGLOBIN DISSOCIATION CURVE (P-50), DIAGNOSTIC
(see Blood Gas, Arterial, Blood)

P-50
(see Blood Gas, Arterial, Blood)

PA
(see Transthyretin, Serum)

PANCREAS SONOGRAM (PANCREAS ECHOGRAM, PANCREAS ULTRASOUND), DIAGNOSTIC

Norm: The pancreas is properly located and positioned, and is of normal size and shape, with a regular border, and homogenous pattern that is of finer texture than the peritoneum, more intense than area soft tissue, and less intense than the liver. Major supporting arteries and veins as well as the pancreatic duct are visible and normal.

Usage: Aids diagnosis of pancreatic inflammation, pseudocyst, or tumor; guidance for needle biopsy of pancreas; and ongoing monitoring of pancreatic carcinoma response to therapy (i.e., change in the size of a tumor). Work-up of abdominal pain, particularly in clients with alcoholism, blunt abdominal trauma, gallbladder stones, and known hyperlipidemia, as they are more prone to pancreatitis.

Description: Evaluation of pancreatic structure via the creation of an oscilloscopic picture from the echoes of high-frequency sound waves passing over the epigastric area (acoustic imaging). The time required for the ultrasonic beam to be reflected back to the transducer from differing densities of tissue is converted by a computer to an electrical impulse displayed on an oscilloscopic screen to create a three-dimensional picture of the pancreas. An advantage of this test is that it can help diagnose acute pancreatitis retrospectively. In acute pancreatitis, the pancreas appears larger than normal, and is less echogenic than the liver. The edema may cause compression of the inferior vena cava, and the pancreatic duct may appear enlarged. In chronic pancreatitis, calculi, shadows, strictures, or stenoses may be viewed in the pancreatic duct, as well as calcified areas in the body of the pancreas. An abscess may appear as an irregular-shaped, highly echogenic structure with thick walls. Adenocarcinoma may cause the gland to appear enlarged, with an irregular border and absence of normal parenchymal echo pattern. True cysts may be differentiated from pseudocysts by their spherical, sonolucent appearance. Pseudocysts are non-spherical and may contain scattered echoes caused by debris contained within them.

Professional Considerations:

1. Consent form NOT required.
2. Preparation:
   A. *See Client and family teaching.*
   B. This test should be performed before intestinal barium tests, or after the barium is cleared from the system.
   C. If the pancreas alone will be studied, a full stomach improves visualization of the posterior portion of the pancreas. The client should drink 500–1000 ml of tomato or orange juice to distend the stomach. Alternatively, glucagon (1 mg) may be administered intravenously, with 500 ml of water ingested a few minutes later to reduce stomach peristalsis. This causes the stomach to function as a fluid-filled window for scanning for up to 60 minutes.
   D. The client should wear a gown.
   E. Obtain ultrasonic gel or paste.
3. Procedure:
   A. The client is positioned supine in bed or on a procedure table.
   B. The area of the abdomen overlying the pancreas is covered with conductive gel, and a lubricated transducer is passed slowly and repeatedly over the pancreas. Scanning begins with transverse views taken at 1-cm intervals with the client in full inspiration. Scanning is started at the level of the xiphoid process and proceeds until the presence of intestinal gas hinders the view. The client may then be changed to a sitting position, which moves gastric air to the fundus and distends the abdominal veins to provide landmarks for identifying the pancreas. This is followed by sagittal scanning, which alternates moving from midline to the right, then midline to the left, at 1-cm intervals.
   C. Photographs of the oscilloscopic display are taken.
4. Postprocedure care:
   A. Remove the gel from the skin.
   B. If a biopsy is performed, *see Biopsy, Site-Specific, Specimen.*

5. Client and family teaching:
   A. The procedure is painless and carries no risks.
   B. If the biliary system will also be examined, a fast from food and fluids for 8 hours before the test is required.
   C. Oral ingestion of fluids prior to the procedure is for stomach distension that aids in the visualization of the pancreas.
   D. It is important to lie still during the procedure.
   E. The procedure takes less than 60 minutes.
   F. Results are normally available within 48 hours.
6. Factors that affect results:
   A. Dehydration interferes with adequate contrast between the organs and body fluids. Dehydration may cause the duodenum to be mistaken for the pancreas.
   B. Intestinal barium, gas, or food obscures the results by preventing proper transmission and deflection of the high-frequency sound waves.
   C. The more abdominal fat present, the greater the attenuation (reduction in sound wave amplitude and intensity), which interferes with the clarity of the picture. Abdominal muscles and cartilage may have the same effect, necessitating repositioning of the client.
   D. The stomach may interfere with views of the pancreatic anatomy in transverse scans.
   E. If the left lobe of the liver is very small (<2 cm), it will function poorly as an acoustic window.
7. Other data:
   A. Severe dehydration, especially when combined with obesity, has the potential to impair visualization of the pancreas and the surrounding area.

Bibliography:

Bernier DR, Christion PE, Langan JK: Nuclear Medicine Technology and Techniques. St. Louis, MO, CV Mosby, 1994.

Sanders RC (ed): Clinical Sonography. A Practical Guide. Boston, MA, Little, Brown, 1991.

PANCREAS ULTRASOUND
(see Pancreas Sonogram, Diagnostic)

PANCREATIC SECRETORY TRYPSIN INHIBITOR (PTSI), SERUM (TATI)

Norm: $3–20 \ \mu g/L^{-1}$.

Increased: Crohn's disease, pancreatitis, and with severe infection of the GI tract or with cell destruction in the mucosal layers of the GI tract. The related TATI tumor-associated trypsin inhibitor is considered a marker for certain cancers such as lung and ovarian. Levels may increase with rejection of transplanted pancreas. It is considered a marker for threatened organ rejection. Drugs: misoprostol (Cytotec).

Decreased: None.

Description: A new clinical study, which may be valuable as a marker for inflammatory disease of the bowel, as in Crohn's disease and other diseases of the gut. Pancreatic secretory trypsin inhibitor (PSTI) is a naturally occurring substance produced by the pancreas that is thought to have its action in the gut, because it protects the mucosal cells from proteolytic breakdown. PSTI is a potent protease inhibitor. It may also be capable of promoting growth activity. It is found in the gut and the stomach. It is absorbed into the blood stream and therefore can be measured by immunoradioassay. Absorbed PTSI is excreted in the urine. The test is performed by radioimmunoassay.

Professional Considerations:
1. Consent form NOT required.
2. Preparation:
   A. Tube: Red-top, red/gray-top, or gold-top.
   B. No fasting required.
3. Procedure:
   A. Draw 5 ml of blood.
4. Postprocedure care:
   A. No special handling of the specimen is known.
5. Client and family teaching:
   A. Results will not be available for up to 5 days.
6. Factors that affect results:
   A. Radioisotope testing within the last week invalidates the results.
   B. Hemolysis of blood samples invalidates the results.
   C. Oral contraceptives and steroids have a possibility of interfering with test results.
7. Other data:
   A. None.

Bibliography:
Halme L, von Smitten K, Stenman S, Turpeinen U, Stenman UH: Concentrations of pancreatic secretory trypsin inhibitor (PTSI), acute phase proteins, and noepterin in Crohn's disease. Comparison with clinical disease activity and endoscopical findings. Scand J Clin Lab Invest *53*(4): 359–366, 1993.

Higashiyama M, Doi O, Kodmam K, Tateishi R, Matsuura N, Murata A, Tomita N, Monden T, Ogawa M: Immunohistochemical analysis of pancreatic secretory trypsin inhibitor expression in pulmonary adenocarcinoma: its possible participation in scar formation of the tumor tissues. Tumor Biol *13*(5–6):299–307, 1992.

Playford RJ, Batten JJ, Freeman TC, Beardshall K, Vesey DA, Fenn GC, Baron JH, Calam J: Gastric output of pancreatic secretory trypsin inhibitor is increased by misoprostol. Gut *32*(11):1392–1400, 1991.

Suzuki Y, Kuroda Y, Sollinger HW, Reed AI, Hullett DA, Saitoh Y: Plasma pancreatic secetory trypsin inhibitor as a marker of pancreas graft rejection after combined pancreas-kidney transplantation. Transplantation *52*(3):504–507, 1991.

PAP
(see Prostatic Acid Phosphatase by RIA, Blood)

PAP SMEAR, DIAGNOSTIC
Norm:

Previous Terminology:

Class I	Normal
Class II	Probably normal
Class III	Doubtful (may be malignant)
Class IV	Probably malignant
Class V	Malignant

Newer Terminology: Results reported in a descriptive statement regarding the adequacy of the sample, followed by a descriptive diagnosis. Abnormalities are described as either benign, low-grade squamous, high-grade squamous, glandular, or severe dysplasia with carcinoma in situ.

Positive: Abnormal cells indicative of endocrine disorders, cancer (uterine), endometriosis, lymphogranuloma venereum, tumors (cervical), and vaginal adenosis or inflammation that could lead to cancer.

Negative: Normal cervical cells.

Description: Cytologic examination of desquamated epithelial tissue to differentiate normal from anaplastic cells. Smears are prepared by scraping or aspirating cells from the tissue to be examined (i.e., cervix) and fixing them on glass slides, using ether and 95% ethyl alcohol solution. Slides are then dried, stained, and examined under a microscope by a pathologist or cytotechnologist. This test is primarily used in the early detection of cervical and vaginal carcinomas and scrapings from the uterus. The *smear technique* can also used to detect cancerous cells of the breast (aspiration of mammary gland tissue), lung (bronchial brushing and washing from bronchoscopy or coughed-up sputum), stomach (aspirated gastric secretions), and renal system (urine sediment). It is indicated as routine screening and for work-up of disorders of reproduction function.

Professional Considerations:

1. Consent form NOT required.
2. Preparation:
   A. *See Client and family teaching.*
   B. Obtain a glass slide, a sterile ayre spatula, a tongue blade, a pipette, a sterile cotton swab, sterile gloves, ether/95% alcohol solution (1:1), spray fixative for use as fixative, a graphite pencil, and a speculum. Using the graphite pencil, label the frosted ends of the slide with the client's name and the collection site.
   C. The client should disrobe below the waist.
   D. Position the client recumbent on a gynecologic examination table in the lithotomy position and drape for comfort and privacy.
3. Procedure:
   A. *Note:* Fixative must be applied to the slide before any drying of the specimen occurs.
   B. *Endocervical smear:*
      i. Aspirate endocervical secretions from the cervical os as through a pipette. Spread the secretions onto a glass slide. Dip or spray the slide with the prepared fixative and dry it.

      OR

      ii. Insert a sterile spatula into the cervical os and rotate it 360 degrees. Smear the scrapings onto a glass slide. Fix immediately as described above.

      OR

      iii. Lightly brush the cervical os circumference and secretions with a tapered synthetic fiber brush. Gently roll the brushings onto the slide and fix as above immediately.

      OR

      iv. Insert a sterile cotton swab into the cervical os and rotate it 360 degrees. Leave the swab in place for 10–20 seconds. Remove the swab and smear onto a glass slide. Fix it immediately as described above.
      v. *Ectocervical scraping:* Using a wooden tongue blade or the blunt side of a wooden ayre spatula inserted into the cervical os, rotate or scrape the entire surface at the squamocolumnar junction. Re-

move the tongue blade and smear onto a glass slide. Fix immediately as described above.
   C. *Cervical scraping:* Insert the pointed edge of a wooden ayre spatula into the cervical os and rotate the spatula 360 degrees. Spread the cervical scrapings on a glass slide, fix it with an ether/95% ethyl alcohol solution, and dry the slide. A Cervex-Brush sampling device may be used, which is recommended to be rotated a full 1800 degrees to improve the sampling for abnormal cervical cells.
   D. *Vaginal pool:* Using the blunt side of a wooden ayre spatula, scrape the vaginal floor behind the cervix. Spread the vaginal pool secretions on a glass slide, spray or soak them in fixative, and dry the slide. Vaginal fluid is obtained for suspected endometrial cancer or for a hormonal evaluation.
   E. *Vulva smear:* Using the blunt side of a wooden ayre spatula, directly scrape the vulvar lesion. Spread the scraping on a glass slide and fix it immediately with spray fixative.
4. Postprocedure care:
   A. Write the client's age; the reason for the study; the date of the last menstrual period; any chemotherapy or hormonal medications; and history, including any previous abnormal Pap smears, and treatment for cancer and/or abnormal vaginal bleeding on the laboratory requisition.
   B. Send the slides to the cytology laboratory.
5. Client and family teaching:
   A. Do NOT douche for 18–72 hours before the procedure.
   B. It is customary practice for the client to be informed of the results, either positive or negative. The method of information exchange needs to be arranged with the client's physician.
   C. Results are normally available within 1 week.
   D. Further testing may be needed, including a repeat Pap, endometrial biopsy, or colposcopy. This decision will be made when the results of the test are received.
   E. Pap smears should be performed yearly after age 18. If the client is sexually active, has a family history of cervical or uterine cancer, has venereal disease, or has a mother who took diethylstilbestrol during pregnancy, a Pap smear should be performed before age 18 and yearly thereafter.
6. Factors that affect results:
   A. Do not lubricate the speculum; such lubrication distorts cells.
   B. Use of formalin as a fixative invalidates the results.
   C. Water or lubricant on the specimen can distort the cells.

D. A smear taken any time other than in the mid-menstrual cycle can result in abnormal findings. The best time for a cervical cytology study is 5–6 days after menses.

E. Inadequate specimens may require retesting.

F. Tetracycline or digitalis preparations can affect the look of squamous epithelium.

7. Other data:

A. False-positive Pap smear results requiring a repeat in 6–12 weeks, as is standard, may be avoided if a culture for *Chlamydia* and *Neisseria gonorrhoeae* and wet mount slides are examined at the time of the exam.

B. False-negative results can be minimized by obtaining double scrapings and smear cultures.

Bibliography:

Brotzman GL, Julian TM: The minimally abnormal Papanicolaou smear. Am Fam Physician 53(4): 1154–1162, 1996.

Eltabbakh GH, Eltabbakh GD, Broekhuizen FF, Griner BT: Value of wet mount and cervical cultures at the time of cervical cytology in asymptomatic women. Obstet Gynecol 85(4):499–503, 1995.

Ferris DG, Berrey MM, Ellis KE, Petry LJ, Voxaes J, Beatie RT: The optimal technique for obtaining a Papanicolaou smear with the Cervex-Brush. J Fam Pract 34(3):276–280, 1992.

Germain M, Heaton R, Erickson D. Henry M, Nash J, O'Connor D: A comparison of the three most common Papanicolaou smear collection techniques. Obstet Gynecol 84(2):168–173, 1994.

Solomon D: The 1988 Bethesda system for reporting cervical/vaginal cytologic diagnoses. Developed and approved at the national cancer institute workshop, Bethesda, Maryland, USA Acta Cytol 33(5):567–574, 1989.

PAPANICOLAOU SMEAR, ULTRAFAST, AND FINE-NEEDLE ASPIRATION, DIAGNOSTIC

Norm: Normal cell and structure for the area biopsied. Absence of tumor cells or abnormalities of the cell nucleus.

Usage: Fine-needle aspiration for cytology; particularly when a quick turnaround time of results is important. This includes ambulatory care biopsies and intraoperative specimens. The method is particularly advantageous for looking at the cell nucleus as it provides the cytologist/histologist with a clear, stained view of the cell and organelles. Adenocarcinoma, of various organs; squamous cell carcinoma; neuroendocrine carcinomas; clear cell type renal cell carcinoma; schwannoma; noram lymphocytes; lymphoid hyperplasia, with small round lymphocytes, small cleaved lymphocytes, large noncleaved lymphocytes, and histocytes. Breast tissue lesions, thyroid lesions, hurthle cell carcinoma, and colloid nodule with hemorrhagic degeneration.

Professional Considerations:

1. Consent form IS required for all fine-needle aspiration biopsy procedures. For specimens taken during surgery, the client gives consent for the surgical procedure.

2. Preparation:

A. Obtain clear glass slides, a syringe, and 18-gauge needles; Choplin jars; normal saline, and ethanol 95% for storage and transport to the laboratory.

B. Notify the laboratory for on-site processing, staining, handling, and consultative interpretation of the specimen.

3. Procedure:

A. Depends on the body site and location of the area for biopsy. Some clients will be prepared for surgery and taken to the operating room.

B. Ambulatory care and ward procedures may require local anesthesia.

C. The skin is prepared for the procedure.

D. Needle aspiration of the tissue is obtained; sometimes special procedures such as fluoroscopy or isolation of a nodule are required. The specimen is taken with a sterile technique and smears made on the clear microscope slides. It is air-dried and processed for 30 seconds in normal saline and then in 95% ethanol and sent immediately to the laboratory for processing. Or the cytologist at the procedure handles the specimen.

4. Postprocedure care:

A. The specimen is carefully labeled and transported immediately to the cytology laboratory.

B. Apply a dry, sterile dressing over the site.

C. Monitor for bleeding at the site.

D. Give postsurgical care as appropriate.

5. Client and family teaching:

A. Call the physician for signs of infection at the procedure site: increasing pain, redness, swelling, purulent drainage, or for fever >101°F (38.3°C).

B. Results are normally available within 24 hours.

6. Factors that affect results:

A. Inappropriate processing.

7. Other data:

A. Total turn-around time for these specimens may be as little as 30 minutes.

B. The developers suggest that fine-needle aspirations for cytology follow this procedure: Prepare several clear glass slides and air-dry. Stain and process the Ultra fast slide; save the other slides for laboratory use for other methods such as Diff-Quik Stain, which has other advantages for final diagnosis.

Bibliography:

Yang GC: Fine-needle aspiration cytology of low grade endometrial stromal sarcomas. Acta Cytol 39(4): 701–705, 1995.

Yang GC, Alvarez II: Ultrafast Papanicolaou stain: an alternative preparation for fine-needle aspiration cytology. Acta Cytol.39(1):5–60, 1995.

Yang GC, Coleman B, Daly JM, Gupta PK: Presacral myelolipoma. Report of a case with fine-needle aspiration cytology and immunohistochemical and histochemical studies. Acta Cytol 36(6):932–936, 1992.

PARACENTESIS (PERITONEAL FLUID ANALYSIS), DIAGNOSTIC

Norm:

Appearance	Clear, serous, light yellow
Amount	<50 ml
Protein	<4.1 g/dl
Glucose	70–100 mg/dl (equals serum)
Amylase	140–400 U/L (equals serum)
Ammonia	<50 mg/dl
Alkaline phosphatase	
Adult female	45–250 U/L
Adult male	90–240 U/L
Red blood cells	Negative
White blood cells	<300/ml
Culture	Negative
Cytology	No malignant cells
CEA and CA-125	Negative
Fungus	Negative

Usage: Effusion, abdominal, and ascites due to hepatic encephalopathy or other causes. Trauma.

Abnormal Appearance:

Bloody: Trauma (or traumatic tap). Turbid (cloudy): Infection, pancreatitis, intestinal perforation, and cirrhosis. Milky: Chylous ascites.

Increased Protein: Cancer, tuberculosis, peritoneal carcinomatosis, and peritonitis.

Increased Amylase: Pancreatitis and intestinal strangulation, necrosis (intestinal), pancreatic pseudocyst, pancreatic trauma.

Increased Alkaline Phosphatase: Intestinal strangulation and ruptured intestine.

Increased Red Blood Cells: Intra-abdominal trauma, neoplasm, and tuberculosis.

Increased White Blood Cells: Infection and chylous ascites, cirrhosis, and peritonitis. Granulocyte count of >250 cells/ml is diagnostic for infection.

Increased CEA and CA125: Malignancy. *Note:* an elevated CA125 without elevation in CEA indicates primary malignancy is ovarian or endometrial.

Decreased Glucose: Below serum: malignancy or TB peritonitis.

Description: Paracentesis is the transabdominal removal of fluid from the peritoneal cavity for analysis of electrolytes, red blood cells, white blood cells, bacterial and viral cultures, and cytology studies. It may be used in trauma cases, as part of a standard acute work-up to assess for the presence of intestinal injury and/or bleeding, especially if blunt trauma to the chest and abdomen is suspected. The procedure listed below is followed except that a small volume of normal saline lavage may be instilled and aspirated and examined as below.

Paracentesis removal of peritoneal fluid may be therapeutic as well as diagnostic when the volume of ascites is such that it interferes with venous return, normal breathing, appetite, and the activities of daily living.

Professional Considerations:
1. Consent form IS required.

Risks:
Abdominal wall infection, hemorrhage, perforated bowel, increased peritonitis.

Contraindications:
This procedure should be used with caution during pregnancy and in clients with coagulation abnormalities or bleeding tendencies.

2. Preparation:
   A. Have the client urinate or empty the bladder by catheterization. This will help prevent accidental bladder trauma.
   B. Measure abdominal girth, weight, and baseline vital signs. Monitor vital signs every 10–15 minutes during the procedure.
   C. Obtain povidone-iodine, sterile gauze sponges, 1–2% lidocaine (Xylocaine), 10- and 30-ml syringes, 22- and 24-gauge needles, sterile gloves, sterile drapes, a trochar with a cannula, a sterile vacuum collection bottle, plastic tubing, a scalpel, a suture, a needle holder, and tape.
3. Procedure:
   A. Position the client sitting on the edge of a bed or examination table with the back supported and the feet resting on a stool. The procedure may also be performed with the client lying prone.
   B. Cleanse the client's abdomen with povidone-iodine and allow it to dry; then cover the areas surrounding the site with a sterile drape.
   C. Numb the area with 1–2% lidocaine (Xylocaine), first using a 22-gauge needle locally and then changing to a 24-gauge needle and anesthetizing the area deeper.
   D. A scalpel is used to make a stab wound into the peritoneal cavity midway between the umbilicus and the symphysis pubis. Alternatively, the insertion may be through the iliac fossa, through the flank, or in each abdominal quadrant. The trochar/cannula is threaded through the incision. An audible sound may be heard when the needle pierces the peritoneum. The trochar is removed, and plastic tubing is attached to the cannula; the other end of the tubing is placed in the collection receptacle (usually a 500- to 1000-ml vacuum bottle). The fluid is slowly drained from the abdominal cavity. The client may need to be repositioned to improve drainage.

E. Do not drain more than 1000 ml at a time. If hypovolemia occurs due to rapid drainage, raise the bottle to slow the drainage rate or clamp the drainage tube.
   F. When the fluid collection is complete, remove the cannula, and suture the incision if necessary.
4. Postprocedure care:
   A. Apply a dry, sterile dressing to the site.
   B. Observe the site for bleeding or drainage.
   C. Measure abdominal girth and weight.
   D. Monitor vital signs for evidence of hemodynamic changes every 30 minutes × 2 hours, every hour × 4 hours, then every 4 hours × 24 hours.
   E. Write any recent antibiotic therapy on the laboratory requisition. Send the samples to the laboratory for analysis immediately.
   F. Document in the client's record the time of the procedure; the name of the physician; the color, consistency, and amount of fluid withdrawn; and the client's response to the procedure.
   G. Monitor daily sequential multiple analyzer (SMA7).
   H. Observe for hematuria due to bladder trauma. If this is suspected at the time of the procedure, a BUN and creatinine obtained on the paracentesis fluid should be sent to confirm the condition.
5. Client and family teaching:
   A. Notify the physician immediately if you notice bloody, pink, or red urine.
   B. Results are normally available within 72 hours.
6. Factors that affect results:
   A. Inadvertent internal organ injury, including female organs, may contaminate the sample with bile, blood, urine, or feces or with bacterial flora.
   B. Delay in analysis may cause inaccurate results.
   C. Care must be taken to ensure a sterile technique, especially in handling specimens for culture and gram stain.
7. Other data:
   A. Frequently, salt-poor albumin is infused for 24 hours after paracentesis for clients with ascites and poor nutrition, which increase the third spacing of fluid into this cavity.
   B. Transient initial bloody fluid may result from a traumatic tap.

Bibliography:
Garcia-Tsao G: Cirrhotic ascites: pathogenesis and management. Gastroenterologist 3(1):41–54, 1995.

Kellerman PS, Linas SL: Large volume paracentesis in treatment of ascites. Ann Intern Med 112(12): 889–891, 1990.

Labovich TM: Selected complications in the patient with cancer: spinal cord compression, malignant bowel obstruction, malignant ascites and gastrointestinal bleeding. Semin Oncol Nurs 10(3): 189–197, 1994.

Runyon BA: Malignancy-related ascites and ascitic fluid "humoral tests of malignancy." J Clin Gastroenterol *18*(2):94–98, 1994.

Sivit CJ, Taylor GA, Bulas DI, et al.: Blunt trauma in children: Significance of peritoneal fluid. Radiology *178*(1):185–188, 1991.

PARACENTESIS, FLUID ANALYSIS, SPECIMEN

(see Paracentesis, Diagnostic)

PARASITE SCREEN, BLOOD

Norm: Negative. Acute parasitic infection is strongly indicated when titers increase fourfold (for most organisms) between acute and convalescent sera.

Usage: Nonspecific detection of parasitic infection.

Positive: Chagas' disease, small protozoans malaria (*Plasmodium falciparum, P. malariae, P. ovale,* and *P. vivax*), cysticercosis, babesia, Echinococcus, *Entamoeba histolytica, Fasciola hepatica,* filariasis (*Wuchereria bancrofti*), giardia, kala-azar (leishmaniasis), *Paragonimus, Strongyloides, Taenia solium, T. saginata,* toxoplasmosis (*Toxoplasma gondii*), trichinosis, trypanosomiasis (*Trypanosoma brucei,* and *T. brucei rhodesiense*), and VLM (*Ascaris* and *Toxocara*).

Description: Parasites are organisms that must live in or on a host to survive and often require different hosts at different stages of development. Parasitic infections in humans may be acquired from the fecal-oral route, contaminated food, animals, and some arthropods. Some parasites survive on the host by changing antigenic characteristics or becoming coated with host immunoglobulins, so that they are no longer recognized as foreign by the immune system. The most accurate method of diagnosing a blood-borne parasitic infection is to identify the actual parasite in a Giemsa-stained thick or thin film of blood. This is not always easy, however, as the amount of blood-borne parasites present at any given time may vary depending on the parasitic stages and cycles. The parasite screen is used when the presence of the actual parasite cannot be established. This screen involves several laboratory procedures that help to detect the presence of parasite antigen-antibody complexes in a sample of blood. Three of the methods typically used to identify parasitic infection are complement fixation, hemagglutination inhibition, and immunodiffusion. Results are reported in titers as the highest dilution of serum that tests positive for parasitic antibodies.

Professional Considerations:

1. Consent form NOT required.
2. Preparation:
   A. Tube: Red-top, red/gray-top, or gold-top or pink-top, or Corvac tube.
3. Procedure:
   A. Parasite screen-fresh blood for filaria and trypanosomiasis should be collected between 2200 (10 P.M.) and 2400 (12 A.M.) hours.
   B. Draw a 5-ml blood sample.
   C. Avoid causing hemolysis.
   D. An acute sample should be drawn as soon as possible after a parasitic infection is suspected.
   E. Draw a convalescent sample in 2–4 weeks.
4. Postprocedure care:
   A. None.
5. Client and family teaching:
   A. Return in 2–4 weeks to have a follow-up sample drawn.
   B. Avoid donating blood until the results are known.
6. Factors that affect results:
   A. Hemolysis of the specimen may cause false-negative results.
   B. A single test has little significance unless the results are extremely high.
   C. For several of the parasites, false-negative results may be caused by the presence of antibodies from past infection.
7. Other data:
   A. Even with positive results, diagnosis of a parasitic infection cannot be confirmed without recovery of the parasite.

Bibliography:

Araujo FG: Diagnosis of parasitic disease. Mem Inst Oswaldo Cruz *83*(Suppl 1):464–465, 1988.

Germain BF: Mycobacterial, fungal and parasitic infections. Curr Op Rheumatol *1*(2):178–184, 1989.

Kehl KS, Cicirella H, Havens PL: Comparison of four different methods for detection of Cryptosporidium species. J Clin Microbiol *33*(2):416–418, 1995.

Markill E, Vogi M, John DT: Medical Parasitology. Philadelphia, WB Saunders, 1992.

PARASITE SCREEN (OVA AND PARASITES), STOOL

Norm: Negative. No parasite, ova, or larvae identified.

Usage: Diagnosis of parasitic infestation of the intestinal tract.

Positive: *Ancylostoma duodenale* (hookworm), *Ascaris lumbricoides* (roundworm), *Balantidium coli, Blastocystis hominis, Capillaria philippinensis, Chilomastix mesnili, Chlonorchis-Opisthorchis, Cryptosporidium* spp., *Dientamoeba fragilis, Diphyllobothrium latum* (fish tapeworm), *Dipylidium caninum* (tapeworm), *Endolimax nana, Entamoeba histolytica, E. hartmanni, E. coli, E. polecki, Enterobius vermicularis* (pinworm) *Enteromonas hominis, Fasciola hepatica, Fasciolopsis buski, Giardia lamblia*, Helminths and protozoa, *Hymenolepis diminuta* (tapeworm), *Hymenolepis nana* (dwarf tapeworm), *Iodamoeba butschlii, Isospora belli, Metagonimus yokogawai, Necator americanus* (hookworm), *Paragonimus westermani* (long fluke), *Retortamonas intestinalis, Sarcocystis* sp., *Schistosoma mansoni (ova), Strongyloides stercoralis* (threadworm), *Taenia saginata* (beef tapeworm), *T. solium* (pork tapeworm), *Trichinella spiralis, Trichomonas hominis, Trichostrongylus* sp., and *Trichuris trichiura* (whipworm).

Description: Microscopic examination of stool to detect parasites at various stages of development from ova through mature or motile forms. A parasite screen is performed on a stool sample when a parasitic infection is suspected as evidenced (usually) by diarrhea of unknown origin. A parasite is an organism that survives at the expense of a host organism. Frequently, protozoa, amebas, and worms infect the gastrointestinal tract from contaminated food and water sources. Parasites, larvae, or ova may not be continuously present in fecal specimens; thus, at least three samples, spaced 2–3 days apart, or as prescribed, are taken. For a screen the laboratory will need to know travel information and will likely perform screens based on the parasites usually found in that location. Laboratory preparations for each parasite to be identified may vary.

Professional Considerations:

1. Consent form NOT required.
2. Preparation:
   A. Question the client carefully about any recent travel and about hygiene practices.
   B. Clarify whether a preservative is needed by contacting the laboratory that will be performing the test. If a preservative is to be used, stools for ova and parasite examination should be preserved in 5% formalin or polyvinyl alcohol solutions. Specimens should be diluted in a 3:1 stool-to-preservative ratio.
   C. Obtain a clean plastic, waxed cardboard, or glass container and a tongue blade; or obtain clear cellophane tape, a tongue blade, a glass slide, and a clean container. If protozoa, amebas, or flagella are suspected, the specimen must be taken STAT to the laboratory for examination.
   D. *See Client and family teaching.*
3. Procedure:
   A. *Stool collection:* Collect three random stool samples, each 2–3 days apart. The specimens should be collected in a plastic, waxed cardboard, or glass container with a tight-fitting lid. The client should defecate directly into the container or into a clean, sterile bedpan. If a bedpan is used, lift 2 tablespoons of stool into the container with a wooden tongue blade, being cautious not to contaminate the outside of the container. Apply the lid tightly.
   B. *Collection of pinworm or tapeworm eggs:* Collect the specimen between 2200 (10 P.M.) and 2300 (11 P.M.) hours or early in the morning before bath or bowel movement. Wrap clear cellulose tape around the end of a tongue blade and firmly press it against three or four separate portions of the perianal area, close to the anus. Do not insert the tongue blade in the anus. Remove the tape and, using a cotton ball, press it lightly onto a glass slide with the gummed side against the glass. Place the slide in a clean container for transport to the laboratory.
   C. *Collection of tapeworm:* If tapeworm is suspected, send the entire stool so that the head of the tapeworm can be identified.
4. Postprocedure care:
   A. Write the collection time, travel history, and suspected diagnosis on the laboratory requisition.
   B. Send the specimen to the laboratory within 1 hour of collection. Unformed stools should have a preservative added.
   C. Several specimens are usually prescribed: three is a standard number.
5. Client and family teaching:
   A. Collect the stool specimen according to the procedure described above and avoid contaminating it with urine.
   B. Cook food properly, boil water, and wash hands thoroughly if contamination is suspected.
   C. Have water analyzed, especially well water.

D. With diarrhea, avoid milk, milk products, greasy foods, and spicy foods. Drink clear fluids with electrolytes.

6. Factors that affect results:
   A. Fresh, room-temperature stool samples provide the best specimens. Do not incubate, refrigerate, or freeze the specimens.
   B. Reject specimens contaminated with urine, toilet paper, diapers, or toilet water.
   C. Mineral oil or magnesium antacids, MOM, Kaolin, anti-malarial drugs, or bismuth may interfere with accuracy.
   D. Specimens obtained by using saline or phosphosoda enemas are acceptable. Often the first stool after the enema is discarded and the subsequent stools are examined.
   E. Stool samples should be collected during laboratory hours so that they can be promptly examined.
   F. Antimicrobial or antiamebic therapy within 5–10 days prior to specimen collection may cause false-negative results.
   G. Residual barium from recent gastrointestinal studies may interfere with microscopic examination. Wait 1 week after barium procedures or laxative administration before collecting stool samples.
   H. Drugs and other substances that interfere with microscopic examination of fecal samples include antacids, antibiotics, barium, bismuth, castor oil, enemas, iron, magnesia, Metamucil, and tetracyclines.

7. Other data:
   A. Use with caution when handling the sample, as some parasitic infections are very contagious.
   B. One negative result does not rule out a parasitic infection.
   C. A 24-hour stool collection may be requested to obtain an estimated egg count in known parasitic infestation.
   D. Information about travel is of utmost importance to the laboratory in detecting the suspected parasite, because different techniques are used to analyze stool in looking for specific parasites or ova.

Bibliography:

Kokoskin E, Gyorkos TW, Camus A Cedilotte L, Purtill T, Ward B: Modified technique for efficient detection of microsporidia. J Clin Microbiol 32(4): 1074–1075, 1994.

Markill E, Vogi M, John DT: Medical Parasitology. Philadelphia, WB Saunders, 1992.

Nazer H, Greer W, Donnelly K, Mohamed AE, Yaish H, Kagalwalla A, Pavillard R: The need for three stool specimens in routine laboratory examinations for intestinal parasites. Br J Clin Pract 47(2):76–80, 1993.

Parija SC, Prabhakar PK: Evaluation of lacto-phenol cotton blue for wet mount preparation of feces. J Clin Microbiol 33(4):1019–1021, 1995.

PARATHYROID HORMONE (PTH), BLOOD

Norm:

		SI Units
Serum	11–54 pg/mL laboratory specific	
Cord	≤3 pg/mL	≤3 ng/L
2–20 years	9–52 pg/mL	9–52 ng/L
Adults	10–65 pg/mL	10–65 ng/L
Plasma	1.0–5.0 pmol/L	
Mid-molecule and C terminal: Also check laboratory specific norms.		
Serum		
1–16 years	51–217 pg/mL	51–217 ng/L
Adults	50–330 pg/mL	50–330 ng/L
Plasma	<50 µLEq/ml	<50 mLEq/L
N-terminal: Also check laboratory specific norms.		
Serum		
2–13 years	14–21 pg/mL	14–21 ng/L
Adults	8–24 pg/mL	8–24 ng/L
Plasma	< 6.1 pmol/L	

Usage: Primarily in the evaluation of abnormal calcium states to assist with the diagnosis of hyperparathyroid or hypothyroid disease. An ionized calcium is usually drawn with the parathyroid hormone (PTH) sample. Levels are also followed in chronic renal clients to identify the development of hyperthyroid function due to phosphate retention and to monitor clients treated for same.

Increased: As a response to low serum calcium levels due to calcium malabsorption, chronic renal failure, dietary vitamin D deficiency, osteomalacia, and renal dialysis. Also, ectopic production of PTH, lactation, primary hyperparathyroidism, parathyroid adenoma, parathyroid carcinoma, parathyroid hyperplasia, pregnancy, pseudohypoparathyroidism (sometimes), renal hypercalciuria, rickets (vitamin D-dependent, vitamin D-deficient), secondary hyperparathyroidism, and squamous cell carcinoma (kidney, lung, ovary, pancreas). PTH levels increase with the aging process.

Decreased: As a response to high calcium levels, autoimmune disease or cancer, Graves' disease, hypomagnesemia, hypoparathyroidism, parathyroidectomy (transient decrease), sarcoidosis, and vitamin A and D intoxication. Drugs include thiazide diuretics.

Description: Parathyroid hormone (PTH) is measured by radioassay using competitive protein-binding agents to identify and measure several molecular forms of PTH: intact and midmolecule fragments. N-terminal fragments, and C-terminal fragments may be tested in some laboratories. Intact PTH is secreted by the parathyroid gland and is metabolized by the liver and kidneys into N-terminal fragments and C-terminal fragments. The intact and N-terminal fragments are helpful in identifying acute conditions, while C-terminal fragments indicate chronic disturbances of PTH metabolism. Parathyroid hormone is directly responsible for the plasma regulation of calcium and phosphorus. When the body's normal autoregulatory mechanism senses a decrease in serum calcium, the parathyroid gland is stimulated to secrete PTH. The elevated serum PTH triggers the release of calcium from bone and stimulates the renal tubules to increase reabsorption of calcium ions in the distal convoluted tubules and to decrease reabsorption of phosphorus in the proximal convoluted tubules. When the serum calcium concentra-

tion again becomes adequate, the parathyroid gland decreases PTH secretion. In the presence of primary parathyroid tumor or hyperplasia, the PTH-calcium autoregulation fails. As PTH secretion increases, so does the serum calcium level, ultimately resulting in a hypercalcemic condition that can be life threatening. Assessment of radioassayed PTH is helpful in differentiating parathyroid causes from nonparathyroid causes of hypercalcemia. Other etiologies of hypercalcemia generally display normal to slightly high or low PTH secretion. Thus, PTH should always be evaluated in conjunction with serum ionized calcium levels.

Professional Considerations:

1. Consent form NOT required.
2. Preparation:
   A. Tube: Red-top, red/gray-top, or gold-top or lavender-top; and ice.
   B. A morning fasting sample is recommended, as there is a diurnal variation in PTH levels.
   C. *See Client and family teaching.*
3. Procedure:
   A. Completely fill the red-top, red/gray-top, or gold-top tube with blood.
   B. Some laboratories require that the sample be packed in ice.
   C. Some laboratories request 7 ml of blood in a lavender-top tube as well.
4. Postprocedure care:
   A. Send the specimen to the laboratory immediately.
   B. Resume previous diet.
   C. Assess for signs of hypercalcemia: lethargy, headache, thirst, increased urinary output, decreased muscle tone, nausea, thirst, and flank pain.
   D. Assess for signs of hypocalcemia: lethargy, nausea, cramps, dysrhythmias, shallow breathing, tetany, and Chvostek's and Trousseau's signs.
5. Client and family teaching:
   A. Fast overnight before sampling.
   B. A change in diet may be needed, based on results. A diet either low or high in calcium may be indicated. Consider consulting a dietician.
   C. Calcium is important to your body. It helps with blood clotting, bone strength, and heart contraction.
6. Factors that affect results:
   A. Reject lipemic specimens or specimens not received on ice.
   B. Ingestion of milk prior to the test may cause falsely low values.
   C. Radioisotope testing within the last 7 days may alter the results.
7. Other data:
   A. A neck venipuncture PTH level should

be compared to a peripheral venipuncture PTH level if the test is performed to rule out parathyroid adenoma. The neck vein technique may help to confirm the diagnosis of hyperparathyroidism, if the PTH level is much higher than that from a peripheral site.

Bibliography:

Avioli LV: Hormonal alterations and osteoporotic syndromes. J Bone Min Res 8(Suppl 2):S511–S514 1993.

Hellman P, Albert J, Gidlund M, Klareskog L, et al.: Impaired parathyroid hormone release in human immunodeficiency virus infection. AIDS Res Hum Retroviruses 10(4):391–394, 1994.

Neer M, Slovik DM, Daly M, Potts T Jr, Nussbaum SR: Treatment of postmenopausal osteoporosis with daily parathyroid hormone plus calcitriol. Osteopor Int 3(Suppl 1):204–205, 1993.

PARATHYROID HORMONE RADIOIMMUNOASSAY, DIAGNOSTIC

(see Parathyroid Hormone, Blood)

PARIETAL CELL ANTIBODY, BLOOD

Norm: Negative, none detected, or titer <1:120.

Abnormal: Weakly positive, titer 1:120–1:140.

Positive: Titer >1:180.

Usage: Aids in differential diagnosis of autoimmune gastritis and pernicious anemia. Not as widely accepted as in the past for the diagnosis of pernicious anemia.

Positive: Autoimmune atrophic gastritis or pernicious anemia and thyroiditis. Parietal cell antibodies are also found in (but are not diagnostic of) Addison's disease, gastric ulcer, juvenile diabetes mellitus, iron deficiency anemia, myasthenia gravis, and Sjögren's syndrome.

Description: Parietal cells are located among the epithelial cells of the stomach and secrete hydrochloric acid (HCl) that is essential for protein breakdown. Many adults who suffer from alterations in gastric acid stimulation (e.g., pernicious anemia) have an autoimmune response with circulating parietal cell antibodies or other antibodies. The antibodies can be detected with indirect immunofluorescence and have been associated with pernicious anemia and other gastric disorders. They have no connection to the client's ability to absorb vitamin B. The presence of parietal cell antibodies is used in the differential diagnosis of pernicious anemia. However, newer research has shown that parietal cell antibodies may not be a valid diagnostic tool for pernicious anemia.

Professional Considerations:

1. Consent form NOT required.
2. Preparation:
   A. Tube: Red-top, red/gray-top, or gold-top.
3. Procedure:
   A. Draw a 10-ml blood sample.
4. Postprocedure care:
   A. None.
5. Client and family teaching:
   A. Results are normally available within 72 hours.
6. Factors that affect results:
   A. None.
7. Other data:
   A. Parietal cell antibodies are present in 20–30% of people who have other autoimmune disorders. They are occasionally present in people who have gastric cancer or ulcers and are also found in up to 2% of normal children and 20% of older adults, particularly the siblings of clients with pernicious anemia. Some researchers believe that there may be a genetic component to pernicious anemia or gastric ulcer with parietal cell antibody activity.

Bibliography:

Carmel R: Reassessment of the relative prevalence of antibodies to gastric parietal cell and to intrinsic factor in patients with pernicious anaemias: influence of patient age and race. Clin Exper Immunol 89(1):74–77, 1992.

Davidson RJ, Atrah HI, Sewell HF: Longitudinal study of circulating gastric antibodies in pernicious anemia. J Clin Pathol 42(10):1092–1095, 1989.

Gleeson PA, Toh BH: Molecular targets in pernicious anaemia. Immunol Today 12(7):233–238, 1992.

Kohlstadt IC, Antunez de Mayolo EA, Ramirez-Icaza C: Parietal cell antibodies among Peruvians with gastric pathologic changes. Scand J Gastroenterol 28(11):973–977, 1993.

PAROTID (SALIVARY GLAND) SCAN, DIAGNOSTIC

Norm: Rapid, simultaneous, symmetrical uptake of the Tc pertchnetate with radio-tagged saliva are present in the oral cavity within 2 minutes. Parotid gland images shown are smooth, symmetrical, equal in size and no mass or irregularity is noted.

Usage: To determine the size, location, and function of the salivary glands. For diagnosis of Warthin's tumor, Sjögren's syndrome, and as part of an evaluation of dry mouth (Xerostomia) with no other systemic cause. May be useful in the diagnosis of accessory parotid gland masses.

Description: A parotid gland nuclear medicine scan provides a measurable assessment of the parotid gland anatomy and function by intravenously injecting the client with technetium-99m pertechnetate. This is a nuclear medicine test in which a scintillation camera is used to take sequential images of the oral cavity over 10–15 minutes. Circulation to the glands is also evaluated.

Professional Considerations:

1. Consent form IS required.

Risks:
Hematoma, infection.

Contraindications:
During pregnancy or breast-feeding.

2. Preparation:
   A. *See Client and family teaching.*
   B. Have emergency equipment available.
   C. Obtain a radionuclide.
3. Procedure:
   A. A radionuclide is injected intravenously.
   B. Images of the oral cavity are obtained at set intervals after injection.
   C. Anterior and bilateral anterior-oblique views should be obtained.
   D. The client is provided with a citrus meal (lemon drop, orange, grapefruit slices) to stimulate salivation.
   E. The imaging is repeated.
4. Postprocedure care:
   A. No special handling of respiratory or oral secretions is required.
   B. Observe the client carefully for up to 60 minutes after the study for a possible (anaphylactic) reaction to the radionuclide.

C. When urine is being discarded, rubber gloves should be worn for 24 hours after the procedure. Wash the gloved hands with soap and water before removing the gloves. Wash the ungloved hands after the gloves are removed.
5. Client and family teaching:
   A. Scanning will be performed before and after salivation is stimulated.
   B. Results are normally available within 24 hours.
   C. There is no radiation danger to the client or others after the procedure.
6. Factors that affect results:
   A. Rinsing the mouth with water between images may cause a decrease in the radioactivity of the saliva.
7. Other data:
   A. Health care professionals working in a nuclear medicine area must follow federal standards set by the Nuclear Regulatory Commission. These standards include precautions for handling the radioactive material and monitoring of potential radiation exposure.
   B. Technetium half-life is 6 hours.

Bibliography:

Nemecek JR, Marzek PA, Young VL: Diagnosis and treatment of accessory parotid gland masses. Ann Plast Surg *33*(1):75–79, 1994.

Shikhani AH, Shikhani LT, Kuhajuda, FP, Allam, CK: Warthin's tumor-associated neoplasms: report of two cases and review of the literature. Ear Nose Throat J *72*(4):264–269, 273–275, 1993.

PARTIAL THROMBOPLASTIN TIME (PTT), PLASMA

Note: Activated Partial Thromboplastin Time (APTT) is the current method of this test: it is still commonly referred to as PTT.

Norm: Standardized times should be reported by each laboratory because results depend on the type of activator used. In general, standards are less than 35 seconds and vary 20–36 seconds.

THERAPEUTIC HEPARIN THERAPY LEVELS	
Acute coronary artery disease	60–70 seconds
Peripheral vascular disease with embolism	60–80 seconds
Premature infants	<120 seconds
Newborn	<90 seconds
Infants	24–40 seconds
Children	24–40 seconds
Adult panic level	>70 seconds

Panic Level Symptoms and Treatment:

Symptoms: Prolonged bleeding, hematoma at venipuncture site, cerebrovascular accident, hemorrhage, shock.

Treatment:

Assess heparin therapy.
Administer protamine sulfate (usual dose of 1 g of protamine sulfate for every 100 units of heparin).
Monitor vital signs.
Monitor for neurologic changes q 1 hour until levels are within desired range.

Increased: Major causes: genetic or acquired deficiency of blood clotting Factors IX, X, XI, or XII and with Factor V or II deficiencies. Deficiencies are usually below 30–40% normal levels for clotting factors to produce increased APTT and bleeding tendencies as seen in hemophilia A. Associated with deficiencies of HMW-kininogen and Fletcher factor, prekallikrein. Also occurs with Abruptio placentae, afibrinogenemia, cardiac surgery, hypothermia, cirrhosis, disseminated intravascular coagulation, dysfibrinogenemia, fibrinolysis, Fitzgerald factor deficiency (severe), in clients on hemodialysis, hemorrhagic disease of the newborn, hypofibrinogenemia, liver disease, hypoprothrombinemia, presence of circulating anticoagulants, lupus anticoagulant, and von Willebrand's disease. Drugs include alcohol, antistreplase (a thrombolytic agent) bishydroxycoumarin (excess therapy), chlorpromazine, codeine, heparin calcium, heparin sodium, phenothiazines, salicylates, Warfarin administration, and valproic acid.

Decreased: May occur with abnormalities of Fletcher factor, which are not associated with bleeding and in which thromboemboli may occur.

Description: Partial thromboplastin time (PTT) evaluates how well the coagulation sequence is functioning by measuring the amount of time it takes for recalcified, citrated plasma to clot after partial thromboplastin is added to it. The PTT is abnormal in 90% of coagulation defects and screens for deficiencies and inhibitors of all factors except VII and XIII. Most commonly used to monitor effectiveness of heparin therapy and to screen for disorders of coagulation. When commercial activating materials are used to standardize the test, the PTT is called the APTT, or activated partial thromboplastin time.

Professional Considerations:

1. Consent form NOT required.
2. Preparation:
   A. For intermittent heparin dosing, the sample should be drawn 1 hour prior to the next dose. A baseline APTT may not be needed prior to heparin therapy unless disease is suspected.
   B. Tube: 2.7-ml or 4.5-ml blue-top and a control tube and a waste tube or syringe.
   C. Do NOT draw specimens during hemodialysis.
3. Procedure:
   A. Withdraw 2 ml of blood into a syringe or vacuum tube. Remove the syringe or tube, leaving the needle in place. Attach a second syringe, and draw a blood sample quantity of 2.4 ml for a 2.7-ml tube or 4.0 ml for a 4.5-ml tube. Collect the sample without trauma.
4. Postprocedure care:
   A. If the test cannot be performed within 2 hours after specimen collection, separate and freeze the plasma.
   B. Transport the specimen to the laboratory immediately.
5. Client and family teaching:
   A. Surgery may need to be postponed if the results are prolonged.
   B. Bleeding precautions for prolonged values include: use a soft toothbrush; use an electric razor; avoid aspirin/aspirin products; avoid constipation; wear loose clothing; avoid intramuscular injections.
   C. Watch for and report signs of bleeding: bruising, petechiae, blood in stool/urine/sputum, bleeding from invasive lines, bleeding gums, abnormal/excessive vaginal bleeding.
6. Factors that affect results:
   A. Do NOT draw samples from an arm into which heparin is infusing.
   B. Failure to completely fill the tube will alter the results.
   C. If drawing samples from an arterial line with a heparin-flush pressure bag, at least 10 ml of blood must be withdrawn before the PTT sample is drawn.
   D. Failure to discard the first 1–2 ml or traumatic venous draw may result in a falsely decreased APTT.
   E. A false-normal PTT may occur if factor levels are deficient, but not less than 25–30% of normal.

F. Factor I (fibrinogen) deficiency may not be detectable unless levels are <100 mg/dl.

G. Hematocrit >55% may cause falsely prolonged results. The test should be redrawn in a tube furnished by the laboratory that has had the concentration or amount of citrate adjusted for the elevated hematocrit level.

H. Freezing the sample will decrease the test sensitivity to lupus anticoagulant and to deficiencies of XII, XI, HMW-K and prekallirein.

7. Other data:

A. Protamine sulfate, 1 mg, will reverse the effects of 100 U of heparin.

B. Hemophilia A has increased APTT, with normal PT and bleeding time.

C. Hemophilia B is diagnosed by increased APTT with normal or increased PT and direct assay of levels of Factor IX.

D. APTT is not helpful in the diagnosis of hemophilia type.

E. APTT and PT are both increased with prothrombin and HMW-K and prekallikrein deficiencies.

F. Age, sex, and ABO blood group may have an influence on the APTT in normal clients.

Bibliography:

Becker RC, Cyr J, Corrao JM, Ball SP: Bedside coagulation monitoring in heparin treated patients with active thromboembolic disease: a coronary care unit experience. Am Heart J *128*(4):719–723, 1994.

Levine MN, Hirsh J, Gent M, Turpie AG, Cruickshank M, Weitz J, Anderson D, Johnson M: A randomized trial comparing activated thromboplastin time with heparin assay in patients with acute venous thrombembolism requiring large daily doses of heparin. Arch Int Med *154*(1):49–56, 1994.

McKinnley L, Wren K: Are baseline prothrombin/partial thromboplastin time values necessary before instituting anticoagulation? Ann Emerg Med *22*(4):697–702, 1993.

PCG, DIAGNOSTIC

(see Phonocardiography, Diagnostic)

PCHE, PLASMA

(see Pseudocholinesterase, Plasma)

PCO, BLOOD

(see Carbon Dioxide, Partial Pressure, Blood and Arterial Blood Gases)

PCP, URINE

(see Phencyclidine, Qualitative, Urine)

PELVIC ECHOGRAM

(see Gynecologic Sonogram, Diagnostic)

PELVIC SONOGRAM

(see Gynecologic Sonogram, Diagnostic)

PELVIC X-RAY FOR FLAT ILEUM, DIAGNOSTIC

Norm: Iliac index >60%.

Usage: Seldom used but can give indications for Down syndrome (trisomy 21). Cytogenetic analysis is a must for the diagnosis of trisomy 21.

Description: Down syndrome (trisomy 21) is a chromosomal abnormality of gene pair 21. An extra chromosome is present on the genes, resulting in mental retardation and multiple congenital abnormalities. Pelvic x-ray for flat ileum can provide suspicion of Down syndrome as 65% of infants have these abnormalities. Infants who have Down syndrome will have a characteristic widening and flaring of the pelvic ileum, sometimes called "elephant ears." The acetabular roof of the ileum will appear flat, with a narrow elongation of the ischium.

Professional Considerations:

1. Consent form NOT required.

2. Preparation:

A. Obtain a lead shield, to be worn by personnel.

3. Procedure:

A. The film is placed behind the client's pelvis.

B. The camera is positioned 14–17 inches above the film, anteriorly, and a short exposure film is taken.

4. Postprocedure care:

A. None.

5. Client and family teaching:

A. Results are normally available within 24 hours.

B. The client is not radioactive after undergoing x-ray.

6. Factors that affect results:

A. In infants, the radiograph should be taken between the ages of 6 and 12 months.

7. Other data:

A. Other abnormalities that may be noted on the x-ray are:

i. Shortening of the middle phalanx of the fifth finger.

ii. Lateral chest x-ray reveals an ossification of the manubrium stem in two or three centers, instead of the normal one center.

iii. The anteroposterior diameters of the lumbar vertebrae are decreased, while the vertebrae are lengthened in height.

iv. Facial and skull changes include delayed cranial suture closure; high, short-arched oral palate; small nasal sinuses; dental defects with delayed tooth eruption; sphenoid bones are rotated up and back; and calvarian bones are thinner than normal.

B. Genetic karyotyping is the definitive method of diagnosis for any genetic disease.

Bibliography:

De Luca B, Massimino R, Materazzo S, et al.: Skeletal alterations in Down syndrome: Bibliographic review and case study contribution. Rays *13*(3): 49–59, 1988.

Nora JJ, Fraser FC, Bear J, Greenberg CR, Patterson D, Warburton H: Medical Genetics: Principles and Practice. Philadelphia, Lea and Febiger, 1993, pp 43–49.

PELVIMETRY AND PELVICEPHALOGRAPHY, DIAGNOSTIC

Norm:

Pelvic inlet (anteroposterior diameters)

Diagonal conjugate	12.5 cm
Obstetric conjugate	11.0 cm
True conjugate	11.5 cm

Pelvic cavity (midpelvis)

Midplane	12.75 cm
Anteroposterior diameter	11.5–12.0 cm
Posterior sagittal diameter	4.5–5.0 cm
Transverse diameter	10.5 cm

Pelvic outlet

Anteroposterior diameter	9.5 cm
Obstetric anteroposterior diameter	11.5 cm
Transverse diameter	8.0 cm
Suprapubic angle	85–90 degrees

Usage: Evaluation of pelvic adequacy for vaginal delivery when any of the following conditions are present: labor has been dysfunctional or slow; fetal positioning is breech, the fetal head fails to engage, or other abnormal positioning in labor occurs, especially in primigravidae, when maternal pelvic adequacy is questioned; history of pelvic fracture or injury or congenital deformity or disease, such as Rickets, polio, or hip dysplasia, may affect the bony pelvis or hips. Examination of very small women or those with kyphoscoliosis or dwarfism. May be indicated when the physician is considering oxytocin administration. It is not the pelvic measurements alone but the pelvic measurements in relation to the size of the fetal head that are important to ensure safe delivery for these indicators. Pelvimetry measurements may be used when previous deliveries have been difficult or have produced large infants or in previous deliveries with an unplanned forceps delivery or nonelective cesarean section, prior to another pregnancy. The x-ray tests are not performed as often as a decade ago.

Description: Pelvimetry is measurement of the internal dimensions of the bony pelvis, usually to determine the adequacy and shape of the maternal pelvis in relationship to fetal size and positioning for or during vaginal delivery. Estimates of pelvic measurements may be performed digitally during the physical exam by an obstetrician, nurse midwife, or trained obstetrical nurse *(see Pelvic measurements)*. Other methods for more specific measurements of the pelvic outlet capacity and the fatal head size may be performed by x-ray, CT scan, or MRI. Ultrasound pelvimetry is not considered accurate at this time. Pelvicephalography is a measurement of the fetal head diameters via a radiologic measurement. It is performed with special methods used to correct for radiographic distortion and magnification. Pelvimetry by radiography, ultrasonography, or computed tomography requires a physician's prescription.

Professional Considerations:

1. Consent form NOT required.
2. Preparation:
   A. Prepare the client for transport to the appropriate radiology department.
3. Procedure:
   A. *Radiographic pelvimetry* is completed in the x-ray department. The client is positioned carefully for an erect lateral view of the pelvis and a supine AP view of the pelvis. It is important that exact measurement of the woman's position and distance from the film at the time of x-ray be taken for a correction factor used in the computation of pelvic measurements. The disadvantages include radiation hazards to the fetus and the fact that x-ray alone is no longer considered reliable as a tool to diagnose problems with labor and delivery.
   B. *Computed tomograph pelvimetry* is considered more accurate and easier to perform. There is less x-ray exposure to the fetus and less chance of distortion if the woman is positioned correctly on the table. Three views are taken: anterior, lateral, and axial. Electronic calipers are used to take the numerical pelvic measurements. CT is particularly useful in women with a history of pelvic fractures and prior to delivery for any situation except those in which a cesarean section is already planned.
   C. *Ultrasound* is not yet clinically helpful. An x-ray is also required, and a fetal pelvic index must be computed that estimates proportion or disproportion for vaginal delivery.
   D. *MRI* is considered quite accurate and allows for imagery of the complete fetus as well as the mother's pelvis and pelvic measurements. The MRI has the advantage of evaluation of the soft tissues of the pelvic region as reasons for dystocia and uses NO radiation to the fetus. MRI is costly and difficult to access in emergency situations.
   E. *Cephalopelvic proportion:* Use of the above radiographic techniques late in the pregnancy or during a difficult labor, to assess the mother's pelvic dimensions as relates specifically to the size of the fetal head and position.
   F. Knowledge of the course of normal labor and delivery and full understanding of the correction factors for radiographic pelvimetry are essential.
   G. For digital examination, the lengths of the first two fingers on either hand of the examiner are measured in centimeters. These fingers should be used for obtaining all measurements.

4. Postprocedure care:
   A. Assist the woman to a position of comfort.
   B. Assess the parents' readiness for new roles; include information on feeding, supplies, safety, and referral agencies.
5. Client and family teaching:
   A. The procedure takes 15 minutes.
   B. The client must remove clothes and put on a gown.
   C. Explain the relationship of the results to the type of delivery—vaginal versus cesarean.
6. Factors that affect results:
   A. None.
7. Other data:
   A. Emotional support is more likely needed during this test than at other times during pregnancy.

Bibliography:

Crowley P, Elbourne D, Ashurst J, Garcia J, Murphy D, Duigan N: Delivery in an obstetric birth chair: A randomized controlled trial. Br J Gynecol 53:677, 1991.

Cunningham FG, MacDonald PC, Gant NF, Leverno KJ, Gilstrap LC: Williams Obstetrics, 19th ed. Norwalk, CT, Appleton and Lange, 1992.

Gupta JK, Glanville JN, Johnson N, Lilford RJ, Dunahn RJ, Walters JK: The effect of squatting in pelvic dimensions. Eur J Gynecol Reprod Biol 42(19): 19–22, 1991.

Hanzal E, Kainz C, Hoffman G, Deutinger J: An analysis of prediction of cephalopelvic disproportion. Arch Gynecol Obstet 253(4):161–166, 1993.

Morris CW, Heggie JC, Acton CM: Computed tomography pelvimetry: accuracy and radiation dose compared with conventional pelvimetry. Australas Radiol 37(2):186–191, 1993.

Wright DJ, Godding L, Kirkpatrick C: Technical note: digital radiographic pelvimetry—a novel, low dose accurate technique. Br J Radiol 68(809): 528–530, 1995.

PELVIMETRY, DIAGNOSTIC (PELVIC EXAMINATION, DIGITAL)

Norm:

Pelvic inlet: 11.0 cm.
Pelvic outlet: 8.0 cm.

Usage: Evaluation of the pelvic adequacy for vaginal delivery. Clinical, noninvasive estimations of the important pelvic measurements in pregnancy. If there have been pelvic injuries, known bony abnormalities, or a previous difficult labor, an x-ray or a CT scan is needed to fully assess the adequacy for vaginal delivery.

Description: Digital pelvimetry may be preformed by the physician or nurse midwife during pregnancy or nearing delivery to estimate the adequacy of the woman's pelvic measurements for vaginal delivery. Any abnormality noted with this method is confirmed by other methods, and pelvicephalography is utilized to fully assess the prospects of normal delivery.

Professional Considerations:

1. Consent form NOT required.
2. Preparation:
   A. Obtain rubber gloves, lubricant, and a ruler or Thom's pelvimeters.
   B. Position the woman on the examination table in the dorsal lithotomy position with her feet supported in stirrups.
3. Procedure:
   A. The lengths of the first two fingers on either hand of the examiner are measured in centimeters. These fingers should be used for obtaining all measurements.
   B. *Pelvic inlet measurement:* The examiner inserts these fingers into the vagina, using the middle finger to locate the lower border of the symphysis pubis and the sacral promontory. To measure the diagonal conjugate, the other hand is used to indicate where the pubis makes contact with the proximal part of the hand. This distance is calculated in centimeters. The obstetric conjugate is calculated by subtracting 1.5 cm from the length of the diagonal conjugate. The true conjugate is calculated by subtracting 1.0 cm from the diagonal conjugate. Since the obstetric conjugate is the narrowest anteroposterior diameter through which the fetus must travel, radiographic examination for accurate measurement is helpful. To measure the obstetric conjugate on radiographic film, locate the inner point of the symphysis and measure back to the sacral promontory. This distance should be approximately 11.0 cm.
   C. *Pelvic capacity measurement:* The sagittal posterior diameter is the only midpelvis diameter that can be palpated. The fingers are inserted into the vagina, locating the sacrospinous ligament. This ligament is traced by palpation from the ischial spines to the sacrum. The sacrospinous ligament is usually three finger breadths long, or 4–5 cm. The capacity of the midpelvis, particularly the midplane, will give the examiner an idea of how labor will progress, if at all.
   D. *Pelvic outlet measurement:* The pelvic outlet is the area in which the fetal head crowns and extends for delivery. The pelvic outlet measurements can be obtained by palpation. The most important diameter is the obstetric anteroposterior outlet diameter. The flexibility and mobility of this diameter are usually assessed by palpating the coccyx. With the finger inserted into the

rectum while the thumb externally grasps the coccyx, the examiner attempts to move the coccyx downward. An immobile coccyx indicates a decreased outlet diameter. The anteroposterior outlet diameter is obtained by inserting two fingers into the vagina and locating the tip of the sacrum and externally locating the symphysis pubis with the other hand. The distance between the fingers is marked. The suprapubic angle is estimated by placing the thumbs, side by side, at the symphysis border. The fingers are then separated from the thumbs and placed flat against the thighs. The angle at which the fingers are able to separate from the thumbs is the suprapubic angle. If the suprapubic angle is narrow, minimal finger-thumb separation will occur. Another way to measure the suprapubic angle is to insert one finger into the vagina, locating the internal margin while the other hand externally palpates the top of the symphysis pubis. An imaginary line is drawn between the two points and assessments of the depth and bend of the symphysis pubis are made. From these calculations, an estimate of the angle is made. Preferably, the symphysis pubis is short and continues inward, allowing for an adequate obstetric conjugate. If it were bony and elongated, the fetus might have difficulty extending the head during delivery. The transverse outlet diameter is measured with the fist on Thom's pelvimetry position between the ischial tuberosities. Pelvimetry outlet measurements are important in the assessment of the potential for fetal head injuries and perineal tearing during the final stages of labor.

4. Postprocedure care:
   A. Assist the woman to a position of comfort.
5. Client and family teaching:
   A. The procedure takes 15 minutes.
   B. Explain the implications of the findings in relation to the type of delivery anticipated.
6. Factors that affect results:
   A. The accuracy of the results depends on the skill and performance technique of the examiner.
7. Other data:
   A. Outlet dystocia is a narrowing of the pubic arch and may make it difficult for the fetus to extend its head, resulting in the need for a forceps delivery.

Bibliography:

Mahmood TA: The influence of maternal height, obstetrical conjugate and fetal birth-weight in the management of patients with breech presentation. Aust NZ J Obstet Gynaecol *30*(1):10–14, 1990.

Olds SB, London ML, Ludiwig PA, et al.: Obstetric Nursing. Menlo Park, CA, Addison-Wesley, 1980.

PEMPHIGUS ANTIBODIES, BLOOD

Norm: Negative.

Usage: Confirmation of diagnosis and management of pemphigus and pemphigoid. Diagnosis is usually made by clinical findings and biopsy with findings of a histologic picture of disruption of the epidermal intercellular connections (this is called acantholysis) and microscopic deposits of IgG.

Description: Pemphigus and pemphigoid are autoimmune blistering diseases of the skin and mucus membranes. Its cause is unknown and it occurs in middle-age or older adults. Initial lesions are located in the mouth and/or on the scalp. After the blisters break, secondary infections may occur in the raw, eroded areas. Before the discovery of steroid therapy, the disease was fatal in 95% of cases. Pemphigus is an autoimmune disease, cause unknown, in which the autoantibodies cause a separation of the epidermal cells, especially after even mild trauma to a specific area. The circulating IgG antibodies can be detected by indirect immunofluorescence.

Professional Considerations:
1. Consent form NOT required.
2. Preparation:
   A. Tube: Red-top, red/gray-top, or gold-top.
3. Procedure:
   A. Draw a 3-ml blood sample.
4. Postprocedure care:
   A. None.
5. Client and family teaching:
   A. Pemphigus is treatable with immunosuppressive and steroid drugs. These drugs can cause side effects that include slow healing, weight redistribution, and psychoses. It is important to watch for signs of these changes and tell the doctor about them.
   B. Bedrest and attention to nutrition are important.
   C. Anesthetic mouth rinses may reduce oral pain, especially prior to eating.
   D. Secondary infection and fluid and electrolyte losses are the most common complications and causes of mortality.
6. Factors that affect results:
   A. False-positive results may occur in the presence of lupus, burns, or drug reactions.
7. Other data:
   A. In pemphigoid, antibody titer levels may provide a correlate for disease activity and may be used to follow management or predict a relapse.
   B. Pemphigus may be drug induced by penicillamine or captopril.

Bibliography:
Brenner S, Wolf R: Possible nutritional factors in induced pemphigus. Dermatology *189*(4):337–339, 1994.
Lyde CB, Cox SE, Cruz PD Jr: Pemphigus erythematosus in a five year old child. J Am Acad Dermatol *31*(5, Pt 2):906–909, 1994.
Tierney LM, McPhee SJ, Papadakis MA, Schroeder SA: Current Medical Diagnosis and Treatment. Norwalk, CT, Appleton and Lange, 1994.

PENICILLIN SKIN TEST, DIAGNOSTIC

Norm: Absence of immediate wheal and flare.

Usage: Determination of hypersensitivity to penicillin after previous history of allergic sensitivity.

Description: After a period of time, many people stop expressing IgE sensitivity to beta-lactam antibiotics (i.e.: penicillin), particularly if the reaction occurred during childhood or while taking the drug orally. This test is used for individuals with a previous history of hypersensitivity to penicillin and who require the drug to treat a particular infection. By injecting small amounts of PrePen (Kremer-Urban), benzylpenicilloyl polylysine, or benzylpenicillin G intradermally and examining for evidence of an enlarged wheal with erythema, many individuals at risk for developing anaphylaxis can be identified.

Professional Considerations:
1. Consent form NOT required.

Risks:
Allergic reaction to intradermal injection (itching, hives, rash, tight feeling in the throat, shortness of breath, bronchospasm, anaphylaxis, death).

Contraindications:
Previous anaphylactic reaction to penicillin.

2. Preparation:
   A. Withhold antihistamines for 24–48 hours prior to the test.
   B. Emergency readiness: The test should be completed in an area where appropriately trained ACLS personnel and emergency medical equipment are

available, due to the possibility of anaphylactic reaction.

C. Obtain 0.9% saline for the injection, PrePen or benzylpenicillin G, alcohol, tuberculin syringes, and 25-gauge ½-inch needles for intradermal injection.

3. Procedure:

A. Initially, prick or scratch the skin on a distal extremity with PrePen or benzylpenicillin G.

B. Wait 15 minutes to examine the area for evidence of wheal and flare.

C. If these are not evident, proceed with one of the following procedures:

  i. *PrePen test:* Inject 0.02–0.04 ml of PrePen reagent intradermally to make a 3-mm bleb on the forearm. At the same time, inject the same amount of 0.9% saline intradermally near the same area, making the same size bleb for use as a control site. After 15–20 minutes, examine the forearm for wheals. Measure the wheals, if present, in millimeters. A positive result will be >5 mm in diameter, with or without a surrounding erythematous area.

  ii. *Benzylpenicillin G test:* Inject a small bleb of benzylpenicillin G, 100 U/ml, intradermally in the forearm. At the same time, inject the same amount of 0.9% saline intradermally near the same area, making the same size bleb for use as a control site. If no reaction occurs after 15–30 minutes, repeat the procedure, using benzylpenicillin G, 1000 U/ml. If no reaction occurs after 15–30 minutes, repeat the procedure using benzylpenicillin G, 10,000 U/ml. A 0.9% saline control should be administered with each successive dose. After 15–20 minutes, examine the forearm for wheals. Measure the wheals, if present, in millimeters. A positive result will be >5 mm in diameter, with or without a surrounding erythematous area.

  iii. If the procedure is to be repeated using several strengths of penicillin, start with the lowest concentration.

4. Postprocedure care:

A. Keep the area uncovered and open to air.

5. Client and family teaching:

A. Call the physician immediately if symptoms of a delayed allergic reaction (listed above, under *Risks*) occur, and seek immediate medical attention if any difficulty in swallowing or breathing occurs.

B. The penicillin skin test assesses only for immediate or accelerated hypersensitivity reactions. There is no test to assess for risk of delayed reactions.

C. Clients with a positive skin test to penicillin are also generally reactive to first-generation cephalosporins.

6. Factors that affect results:

A. Recent administration of antihistamines may cause false-negative results.

7. Other data:

A. A positive skin test indicates a 67–73% risk of immediate to accelerated reaction to penicillin therapy.

B. 2–6% of clients with negative penicillin skin tests have anaphylactic reactions with the administration of penicillin.

C. Repeat skin testing should be performed before reinitiation of penicillin therapy if the initial test was negative and the first course of the drug has been completed.

D. It is not necessary to withhold corticosteroids prior to penicillin skin testing.

E. Clients with a negative skin test should still be given penicillin cautiously; IV administration may quickly resensitize the client to the drug.

Bibliography:

Redelmeier DA, Sox HC Jr: The role of skin testing for penicillin allergy. Arch Intern Med *150*(9):1939–1945, 1990.

Tierney, LM, McPhee SJ, Papadakis MA, Schroeder SA (eds): Current Medical Diagnosis and Treatment. Norwalk, CT, Appleton and Lange, 1994.

PENICILLINASE TEST (BETA-LACTAMASE PRODUCTION TEST), DIAGNOSTIC

Norm: Negative for penicillinase.

Usage: Client on antibiotic therapy for bacterial infections, especially *Haemophilus influenzae, Staphylococcus aureus,* and *Moraxella cularhales.* To test for bacterial strains that may be resistant to penicillin-type antibiotics.

Description: Penicillin and some cephalosporin antibiotics work by attaching to a receptor in the cell membrane of bacteria and inhibiting bacteria cell synthesis. As the receptor/penicillin bond is broken, the bacteria is destroyed. Penicillin's bonding ring is a beta-lactam ring. Certain strains of bacteria may have penicillinase (also called beta-lactamase), an enzyme that destroys the beta-lactam ring of penicillin, making it ineffective against the bacteria. When certain strains of bacteria, including *Staphylococcus, Neisseria gonorrhoeae,*

Haemophilus influenzae, and others produce penicillinase, drugs such as penicillins and first- and second-generation cephalosporins are rendered ineffective against them. This test is performed on isolates of body substances when penicillin treatment shows no improvement in clinical condition. If test results are positive, the treatment is changed to a penicillinase-resistant penicillin or a cephalosporin such as Augmentin, Unasyn, or Timentin.

Professional Considerations:

1. Consent form NOT required.
2. Preparation:
   A. For sputum samples, obtain a suction catheter and tubing, a sputum trap, and a suction source.
   B. For wounds or abscesses, obtain a sterile needle, a syringe, and a red-top tube.
   C. For urine, obtain a straight catheter and a sterile container; or a syringe, a needle, and alcohol wipes; or a clean-catch urine collection kit.
3. Procedure:
   A. Using a sterile technique, collect at least a 1-ml sample of the particular body substance to be tested.
   B. For sputum, collect the sample directly into a sputum trap, via suction.
   C. For wounds or abscesses, aspirate 1 ml through a needle into a syringe and inject it into a red-top tube.
   D. For urine, obtain the sample via straight catheterization by aspirating through the collection port of an indwelling urinary catheter or by a voided clean-catch technique. *See clean-catch collection instructions in the test Body Fluid, Routine, Culture.*
4. Postprocedure care:
   A. Write the specimen source, collection time, and recent antibiotic therapy on the laboratory requisition.
   B. Send specimens to the laboratory immediately.
5. Client and family teaching:
   A. Deep coughs are necessary to produce sputum rather than saliva. To produce the proper specimen, take in several breaths without fully exhaling each. Then expel sputum with a "cascade cough."
   B. The necessity of the test is associated with the choice of antibiotic to treat the infectious organism.
   C. Results are normally available within 48 hours.
6. Factors that affect results:
   A. Do not contaminate the specimen with surrounding tissue.
7. Other data:
   A. This test is not routinely performed before penicillin therapy is initiated.
   B. Recent development of a fluorescent developer for use in the laboratory has increased the sensitivity of the test.

Bibliography:

Chen KC, Chen L Lin JY: Fluorescent spot test method for specific detection of beta-lactamases. Analyt Biochem *219*(1):53–60, 1994.

Cohen M: Epidemiology of drug resistance: Implications for a post-antimicrobial era. Science *257*:1050–1055, 1992.

Nichols WW: Beta-lactamases: A new twist to an old problem. Microbiol Sci *4*(5):143–146, 1987.

PEPSINOGEN I, BLOOD

Norm:

		SI Units
Adults	124–142 ng/ml	124–142 µg/L
Women at delivery	116–138 ng/ml	116–138 µg/L
Premature infants	20–24 ng/ml	20–24 µg/L
Cord blood	24–28 ng/ml	24–28 µg/L
Children		
<12 months	72–82 ng/ml	72–82 µg/L
12 months–<2 years	90–106 ng/ml	90–106 µg/L
3–6 years	80–104 ng/ml	80–104 µg/L
7–10 years	77–103 ng/ml	77–103 µg/L
11–14 years	96–118 ng/ml	96–118 µg/L

Increased: Diseases or situations in which gastric acid is increased: duodenal ulcer (30–50% of clients with duodenal ulcer have increased pepsinogen levels); gastrinomas; gastritis, acute and chronic; hypergastrinemia; hypertrophic gastropathy; and, associated with chronic renal failure, Zollinger-Ellison syndrome. Drugs include omeprazole, which may cause an increase.

Decreased: Diseases or conditions in which there is a decrease in the mass of chief cells: Addison's disease, atrophic gastritis, gastric cancer, hypopituitarism, myxedema, pernicious anemia, and after vagotomy. Absence of pepsinogen I is seen with achlorhydria with pernicious anemia. Drugs include GIP, anticholinergics, and histamine H_2 antagonists.

Description: The term *pepsinogen I* encompasses five of the eight fractions of pepsinogen found in the bloodstream. It may also be called pepsinogen A. The remaining related pepsinogens are pepsinogen II. It is an inactive precursor of the proteolytic enzyme pepsin and is produced by the chief cells of the gastric glands. When the pH of the stomach is acidic, pepsinogen I is converted to pepsin. Activated pepsin is capable of converting additional pepsinogen(s) to active enzymes. Pepsin activity on amino acids within the chains is the first step in the digestion of proteins. A small amount of pepsinogen (1%) is absorbed into the bloodstream and can be assayed. Serum concentration of pepsinogen I reflects the parietal cell mass and the acid-secreting capacity for the client. Pepsinogen secretion is stimulated by the vagus nerve, as well as hormonal activity of gastrin, secretin, and CCK.

Professional Considerations:

1. Consent form NOT required.
2. Preparation:
   A. Preschedule this test with the laboratory.
   B. Tube: Red-top, red/gray-top, or gold-top.
   C. *See Client and family teaching.*
3. Procedure:
   A. Draw a 10-ml blood sample.
4. Postprocedure care:
   A. Begin meals as prescribed.
5. Client and family teaching:
   A. Fast overnight prior to the test.
   B. High pepsinogen is considered a risk factor for duodenal ulcer.
   C. High pepsinogen I levels and low pepsinogen I:II ratios are associated with *Helicobacter pylori* infection, which is now associated with ulcer disease.
6. Factors that affect results:
   A. Impaired renal function causes elevated results.
   B. Newer laboratory methods of pepsinogen analysis by immunofluorescence are not available.
7. Other data:
   A. Endoscopy is considered of more use in diagnosing gastric abnormalities than is the pepsinogen I level.
   B. Pepsinogen levels may increase with age.
   C. Pepsinogen levels, especially pepsinogen II, may be useful as a clinical monitor efficacy of the treatment of gastric ulcer disease.
   D. Low pepsinogen I and low pepsinogen I:II ratio is considered to be indicative of gastric neoplasm.
   E. *See also Pepsinogen I Antibody, Blood.*

Bibliography:

Biasco G, Paganelli GM, Vaira D, Holton J, Brillanti S, Miglioli M, Barbara L, Samloff IM: Serum pepsinogen I and II concentrations and IgG antibody to Helicobacter pylori in dyspeptic patients. J Clin Pathol 46(9):826–828, 1993.

Hunter, FM, Correa P, Fontham E, Ruiz B, Sobhan M, Samloff IM: Serum pepsinogens as markers of response to therapy for Helicobacter pylori gastritis. Dig Dis Sci 38(11):2081–2086, 1993.

Konish N, Natsumoto K, Hiasa Y, Kitahori Y, Hayashi I, Matsuda H: Tissue and serum pepsinogen I and II in gastric cancer identified using immunohistochemistry and rapid ELISA. J Clin Pathol 48(4): 364–347, 1995.

Webb PM, Hengels KJ, Moller H, Newell DG, Palli D, Elder JB, Coleman MP, De Backer G, Forman D: The epidemiology of low serum pepsinogen A levels and an international association with gastric cancer rates. EUROGAST Study Group. Gastroenterology 107(5):1335–1344, 1994.

PEPSINOGEN II, BLOOD

Norm: 3–19 ng/mL (3–19 µg/L SI units).

Increased: Acute and chronic superficial gastritis, gastric and duodenal ulcers, Zollinger-Ellison syndrome. Drugs include Omeprazole.

Decreased: Addison's disease, gastric neoplasia, gastric resection, gastritis, myxedema, postgastrectomy.

Description: Pepsinogens group II (there are two identified) are related to the pepsinogen I group, but are found in Brunner's glands and pyloric glands in the gastric antrum and proximal duodenum. Pepsinogen II is normal in pernicious anemia. They are not found in the urine.

Professional Considerations:

1. Consent form NOT required.
2. Preparation:
   A. Tube: Red-top, red/gray-top, or gold-top.
   B. The sample should be a fasting morning specimen.
   C. *See Client and family teaching.*
3. Procedure:
   A. Draw a 10-ml blood sample.

B. Send the sample to the laboratory for evaluation or storage (frozen) immediately.

4. Postprocedure care:
   A. None.
5. Client and family teaching:
   A. Fast overnight before sampling.
   B. High serum pepsinogen II is a risk factor for developing gastric ulcers.
   C. Results are normally available within 48 hours.
6. Factors that affect results:
   A. Renal failure may enhance positive results.
   B. There is a diurnal pattern to pepsinogen II secretion; failure to obtain an early-morning specimen may affect the interpretation of results.
7. Other data:
   A. Endoscopy may be a more accurate diagnostic test.
   B. May be used as a marker in clients with ulcer tendencies.
   C. May be useful as a clinical indicator of the efficacy of ulcer treatment.

Bibliography:

Biasco G, Paganelli GM, Vaira D Holton J, DiFebo G, Brillianti S, Miglioli M, Barbara, L, Samloff IM: Serum pepsinogen I and II concentrations and IgG antibody to *Helicobacter pylori* in dyspeptic patients. J Clin Pathol 46(9):826–828, 1993.

Biemond I, Kreuning J, Jansen JB, Lamers CB: Diagnostic value of serum pepsinogen C in patients with raised serum concentrations of pepsinogen A. Gut 34(10):1315–1318, 1993.

Konishi N, Matsumoto K, Hiasa Y, Kitahori Y, Hayashi I, Matsuda H: Tissue and serum pepsinogen I and II in gastric cancer identified using immunohistochemistry and rapid ELISA. J Clin Pathol 48(4): 364–367, 1995.

PEPSINOGEN I ANTIBODY, BLOOD

Norm: Negative.

Usage: Method of detection of autoantibodies of pepsinogen I in the serum.

Positive: Pernicious anemia (some gastric lesions and some duodenal lesions).

Description: This test is performed by using the enzyme-linked immunosorbent assay to detect the occurrence of autoantibodies against pepsinogen. Pepsinogen I antibody has been shown to be a major chief cell antigen. Its presence may indicate the presence of a gastric and/or duodenal lesion that destroys the mucosa of the surrounding area. This destruction is thought to trigger the production of autoantibodies against the pepsinogen cell contents not recognized as self by the immune system.

Professional Considerations:

1. Consent form NOT required.
2. Preparation:
   A. Tube: Red-top, red/gray-top, or gold-top.
3. Procedure:
   A. Draw a 7-ml blood sample.
4. Postprocedure care:
   A. None.
5. Client and family teaching:
   A. Results are normally available within 48 hours.
6. Factors that affect results:
   A. Renal failure may enhance positive results.
7. Other data:
   A. This test may serve as a subclinical marker of clients with ulcer tendencies.
   B. *See also Pepsinogen I, Blood.*

Bibliography:

Mardh S, Song YH: The occurrence of auto-antibodies in patients with gastroduodenal lesions. J Intern Med 732 (Suppl):77–82, 1990.

PEPTAVLON STIMULATION TEST
(see Gastric Acid Analysis Test, Diagnostic)

PERCUTANEOUS LIVER BIOPSY
(see Liver Biopsy, Diagnostic)

PERCUTANEOUS TRANSHEPATIC CHOLANGIOGRAPHY (PTHC, PTC), DIAGNOSTIC

Norm: Normal diameter and filling of the cystic, hepatic, and common bile ducts. Normal-shape gallbladder; no masses or irregular borders.

Usage: Identification and determination of obstructive jaundice. The procedure may also be completed as part of a work-up for continued pain following cholecystectomy.

Description: Fluoroscopic examination of the biliary ducts using an iodine-based contrast dye, performed in the radiology department by a radiologist under IV sedation or local anesthesia. This allows visualization of all of the bile ducts and biliary flow. These ducts will appear dilated if there is an obstruction. Biliary obstruction causes that can be identified may be filling defects, spasms of the sphincter of Oddi, strictures, tumors, and stones, particularly those located in the common bile duct.

Professional Considerations:

1. Consent form IS required.

Risks:

Allergic reaction to dye (itching, hives, rash, tight feeling in the throat, shortness of breath, bronchospasm, anaphylaxis, death); renal toxicity from contrast medium.

Contraindications:

Previous allergy to iodine, shellfish, or radiographic dye. (Relative contraindication: Client may be premedicated with Benadryl to prevent reaction.) Contraindicated in clients with massive ascites or uncontrolled coagulopathies; renal insufficiency; sedatives are contraindicated in clients with central nervous system depression.

2. Preparation:
   A. *See Client and family teaching.*
   B. Notify the physician and the radiologist of any known or possible allergy to determine if premedication will be prescribed.
   C. Obtain baseline prothrombin time, clotting time, and platelet counts. Notify the physician and the radiologist of any abnormalities. Transfusion to normalize coagulation may be prescribed just prior to the study.
   D. A sedative may be prescribed, especially for children. Monitor the respiratory status continually if sedation is given.
   E. Obtain a surgical scrub and povidone-iodine solutions, 2% lidocaine (Xylocaine), a 23-gauge flexible needle, sterile gloves and drapes, and contrast medium.
   F. Have emergency equipment readily available.
3. Procedure:
   A. The client is secured in a supine position on the fluoroscopy tilt table.
   B. The upper right quadrant of the abdomen is cleansed with surgical scrub solution and prepared with povidone-iodine solution. The entire abdomen is covered with sterile drapes.
   C. The skin is anesthetized with 2% Xylocaine.
   D. Using a long, flexible, 23-gauge needle, the liver is punctured, and the needle is advanced under fluoroscopy until bile is aspirated from the duct. A small amount of contrast dye is injected, and placement is visualized via fluoroscopy. Once the needle is located in the biliary tract, the remaining contrast dye is injected. If the bile ducts appear dilated, the contrast material will be diluted to allow for full visualization to the biliary tract without additional contrast medium dose.
   E. Fluoroscopy is used to observe the flow of contrast media through the ducts into the small intestine. It may be necessary to gently rotate the scanning table vertically and horizontally, or the client may be asked to change to a side-lying position. Erect or decubitus films may be required to visualize the complete system.
4. Postprocedure care:
   A. Apply a dry, sterile dressing to the injection site.
   B. Assess the injection site for bleeding, swelling, or tenderness every hour × 4, then every 8 hours until 24 hours after the procedure.
   C. Continue postsedation assessment of the respiratory status. If deep sedation was used, follow institutional protocol for postsedation monitoring. Typical monitoring includes continuous ECG monitoring and pulse oximetry, with continual assessments (q 5–15 minutes) of airway, vital signs, and neurologic status until the client is lying quietly awake, is breathing independently, and responds to commands spoken in a normal tone.
   D. Maintain bedrest for several hours as prescribed. A right-side lying position may be prescribed.
   E. Resume previous diet.
   F. Analgesics may be prescribed for pain.
   G. Observe for signs of septicemia, peritonitis, hemorrhage, and tension pneumothorax.
   H. Antibiotics may be continued for 2–3 days.
5. Client and family teaching:
   A. Fast from food and fluids for 8–12 hours prior to the procedure.
   B. A mild laxative such as magnesium citrate may be prescribed the night before the procedure.
   C. Antibiotics may be prescribed during the 24–48 hours prior to the procedure.
   D. Transient pain may be experienced during the injection of the dye.
   E. It is important to lie still for the study to avoid injury to internal organs. Sedation may be used to help you lie still.
   F. There should be a responsible adult

available to take you home and care for you for 24 hours.

G. Surgical intervention may be required if obstruction is diagnosed.

H. The procedure takes up to 1 hour.

6. Factors that affect results:

A. Gas overlying the biliary ducts or obesity can interfere with radiograph clarity.

B. Barium, from previous studies, may interfere with the fluoroscopy.

7. Other data:

A. Potential complications include bleeding, septicemia, peritonitis, extravasation of contrast dye into the peritoneal cavity, and subcapsular injection.

B. With the small, flexible needle, surgical backup is no longer considered necessary. If a large-bore needle is used, this procedure should have surgical backup.

Bibliography:

Chen MF, Jan YY, Jeng LB, Hwang CS, Chen SC: Obstructive jaundice secondary to ruptured hepatocellular carcinoma into the common bile duct. Surgical experiences in 20 cases. Cancer 73(5):1335–1340, 1994.

Dudley SL, Starin RB: Cholelithiasis: Diagnostic and current therapeutic options. Nurs Pract 16(3):18–8, 23–24, 1991.

Goodacre B, vanSonnenberg E, D'Agostino MH, Sanchez R: Interventional radiology in gallstone disease. Gastroenterol Clin North Am 20(1):209–224, 1991.

Shamsi Z, Anwar MA, Khan MN: Fine needle percutaneous transhepatic cholangiogram (PTC). JAMA 39(8):219–221, 1989.

PERFUSION LUNG SCAN, DIAGNOSTIC

(see Lung Scan, Perfusion and Ventilation, Diagnostic)

PERICARDIOCENTESIS, DIAGNOSTIC

Norm:

Quantity of fluid	10–50 ml
Appearance	Clear, straw-colored
Bacteria	Absent
Glucose	Approximates blood glucose level
Erythrocytes	Absent
Leukocytes	Absent

Abnormal Findings:

Appearance:

Blood streaks	Tuberculosis or tumors
Turbid	Infection, pericarditis, or malignancy
Grossly bloody	Traumatic tap, cardiac rupture, or bleeding disorders
Blood obtained on pericardiocentesis	If it clots, this indicates entering the heart. If it does not clot, it is from the pericardium.
Milky	Lymphatic drained into the pericardium, chylopericardium

Chemistry:

Low glucose compared to serum levels	Bacterial infection or malignancy
CEA levels	Tumor—correlate with cytology studies

Usage: Effusion (pericardial), emergency treatment for pericardial tamponade, and removal of pericardial fluid for diagnostic testing.

Description: Pericardiocentesis is the aspiration of fluid surrounding the heart and contained within the pericardial sac. Excess fluid may accumulate due to pericarditis, post-cardiac surgery, heart transplant rejection, cardiac trauma, myocardial rupture, acute rheumatic fever, metabolic diseases (fluid will likely be clear), or tumor. If the amount is greater than 50 ml or accumulates rapidly, it may result in restricted ventricular filling and stroke volume, which progresses to elevated venous blood pressure, tachycardia, and, eventually, cardiac tamponade. Other less common causes of pericardial effusion are blunt chest trauma in children, sarcoidosis and other connective tissue disorders, and AIDS. Cases of chylopericardium following aortic valve surgery or CABG have been recorded.

Professional Considerations:

1. Consent form IS required unless the procedure is performed as an emergency.

Risks:

Cardiac arrest, cardiac tamponade, dysrhythmias, hemorrhage, hemothorax, infection, laceration of coronary artery, peritoneal puncture, pneumothorax, puncture of cardiac chamber, ventricular fibrillation.

Contraindications:

Anticoagulant therapy, bleeding disorders, thrombocytopenia.

2. Preparation:
   A. Obtain baseline vital signs and neurologic check, and monitor closely throughout the procedure. The procedure will likely be performed in the cardiac catheterization laboratory or an intensive care unit.
   B. Have an emergency cart, a defibrillator, and a 12-lead ECG machine at the bedside, with appropriate personnel trained in ACLS.
   C. Establish intravenous access.
   D. Obtain 1–2% lidocaine (Xylocaine), sterile gloves, povidone-iodine solution, and a sterile pericardiocentesis tray. The tray should include a short-bevel, 14- to 18-gauge, 4- to 5-inch cardiac needle or cath-over needle (spinal needle); a 25-gauge needle; a 35- to 50-ml syringe; a three-way stopcock; red-top, green-top, and lavender-top tubes; sterile gauze; a Kelly clamp; ground wire; and an alligator clip.
   E. Perform continuous ECG monitoring prior to, during, and after the procedure. Observe for development of potentially life-threatening dysrhythmias.
   F. *See Client and family teaching.*
3. Procedure:
   A. Position the client semirecumbent with the head of the bed elevated between 30 and 60°.
   B. Cleanse the skin of the chest from the xiphoid process to the left costal margin with povidone-iodine solution.
   C. The subxiphoid insertion site is injected with 1–2% Xylocaine.

D. A sterile alligator clip is used to attach the ECG lead V to the aspiration needle, or an echocardiogram is utilized to guide the needle insertion. In emergency situations, in cardiac arrest, the needle insertion is performed "blind."
E. An open three-way stopcock with a 50-ml syringe attached is connected to the cardiac needle. The needle is then inserted into the subxiphoid area, between the xiphoid and the costal margin.
F. The ECG (grounded) is used to monitor and to guide the needle insertion as follows: The appearance of an acute increase in the QRS complex indicates pericardial penetration. Epicardial ventricular contact by the needle is indicated by elevation of the ST segment and ventricular ectopy, and atrial contact by the needle is indicated by elevation of the PR segment. An abnormally shaped QRS complex may indicate myocardial perforation. Echocardiography is increasingly used, especially in the nonemergency situation to guide pericardiocentesis.
G. When the pericardium is penetrated, pericardial fluid should appear in the syringe. Grossly bloody aspirate will occur if a cardiac chamber is perforated. At this point, a Kelly clamp applied to the needle at the point of insertion stabilizes the position. The remainder of the pericardial fluid is aspirated.
H. The Kelly clamp and syringe are then removed, and a gauze pad is applied with pressure to the site for 3–5 minutes.
I. The pericardial fluid is measured and injected into the red-top, green-top, and lavender-top tubes.
4. Postprocedure care:
   A. Label the specimen tubes with the site and time of collection. Write the diagnosis and any recent antibiotic therapy on the laboratory requisition. Send the specimens to the laboratory.
   B. The client is usually maintained in the intensive care unit to monitor continuous ECG for 24 hours after the procedure.
   C. Assess vital signs every 15 minutes × 4, then every 30–60 minutes × 2 hours, then every 4 hours × 24 hours, if the client is hemodynamically stable.
   D. Monitor for symptoms of cardiac tamponade for at least 24 hours. Beck's triad, the classic symptoms of cardiac tamponade, includes neck vein distention, hypotension, and heart sounds that are muffled and distant. The narrowing of pulse pressure (when the systolic and diastolic blood pressure numbers begin to go toward one another) may also be a sign of cardiac tamponade.

5. Client and family teaching:
   A. Inform the client and family about the procedure and the seriousness of the condition. They should, if possible, understand the procedure and the need for ICU care prior to consent.
   B. It is important to lie motionless throughout the procedure.
   C. Assure that the client and family fully understand the condition related to the pericardiocentesis.
   D. Signs and symptoms to report to the physician include chest pain, shortness of breath, and dizziness or lightheadedness.
   E. The catheter may be left in place if there is a need for further fluid drainage.
   F. The family should be approached on CPR readiness and given resources on how to learn CPR.
6. Factors that affect results:
   A. Prepericardiocentesis echocardiographic localization of the effusion helps to minimize the chance of complications from the procedure.
7. Other data:
   A. Potential complications of pericardiocentesis include air embolism, cardiac arrest, cardiac tamponade, coronary artery laceration, dysrhythmias, gastric puncture, hepatic puncture, hydropneumothorax, infection, pleural puncture, vasovagal arrest, and ventricular perforation.

Bibliography:

Bowers P, Harris P, Truesdell S, Stewart S: Delayed hemopericardium and cardiac tamponade after unrecognized chest trauma. Pediatr Emerg Care 10(4):222–224, 1994.

Eisenburg MJ, Gordon, AS, Schiller NB: HIV-associated pericardial effusions. Chest 102(3):956–958, 1992.

Israel RH, Poe RH: Massive pericardial effusion in sarcoidosis. Respiration 61(3):176–180, 1994.

Langley RL, Treadwell EL: Cardiac tamponade and pericardial disorders in connective tissue diseases: case report and literature review. J Nat Med Assoc 86(2):149–153, 1994.

Schactman M, Scott C, Glibbery-Fiesel DR, Murello M, Kerr P: Chylopericardium following aortic valve replacement and coronary artery bypass surgery: a case report and discussion. Am J Crit Care 3(4):313–315, 1994.

Wheelock KL: Pericardiocentesis. American Association of Critical Care Nurses (AACN) Procedure Manual for Critical Care. Philadelphia, WB Saunders, 1985.

PERIODIC ACID-SCHIFF STAIN (PAS), SPECIMEN

Norm: No abnormal findings.

Usage: Limited clinical use includes:

1. Whole blood or bone marrow indicative for leukemia diagnosis, although phenotyping for the markers of the various forms of leukemia are more accurate and more widely used.

2. PAS may also be utilized to identify a fungus infection. The polysaccharide cell walls of fungus are stained by PAS so that a fungal infection is suspected when exudate, body fluids, or tissue homogenates are stained with PAS and the cell walls or portions of the cell wall identified. The test is nonspecific for the type of fungus.

Description: The agent stains glycogen, whole-blood and bone marrow specimens, and gives a pattern when positive that is indicative for several forms of leukemia. PAS does not stain normal lymphocytes, myeloblasts normoblasts, or megakarioblasts. It stains granulocytes, platelets, megakaryocytes, fungus, and some bacteria.

Professional Considerations:

1. Consent form NOT required for whole-blood specimens or for swabs of most body fluids and exudates. Consent IS required for bone marrow aspiration. Consent IS required for tissue sampling for PAS for fungus or for sampling of exudates, which requires an invasive procedure. See individual procedures for risks and contraindications.

2. Preparation:
   A. Obtain a sterile swab approved for microbiologic use, a glass slide, and a sterile container. Obtain sterile saline if the conjunctiva will be swabbed.
   B. Determine the specimen source and equipment required for the specimen.

3. Procedure:
   A. Obtain 10 ml of whole blood in a nonheparinized tube.
   B. See Bone Marrow Aspiration Analysis, Diagnostic, if the test is to be performed on bone marrow.

4. Postprocedure care:
   A. Write the specimen source, the collection time, and the client's diagnosis on the laboratory requisition.
   B. Send the specimen to the laboratory within 2 hours.

5. Client and family teaching:
   A. Results are normally available within 5 days.
   B. This test does not identify specific funguses, nor can it distinguish between ALL and AML.

6. Factors that affect results:
   A. Contamination of specimens invalidates the results.

7. Other data:
   A. The smears of blood or bone marrow of clients with acute lymphatic leukemia show coarse granules or blocks of PAS+ material in 67% of cases.

B. The smears of blood or bone marrow of clients with acute monocytic leukemia have PAS+ discrete granules.
C. The "hairy" appearance of cells in hairy cell leukemia are PAS+.
D. PAS cannot be used to distinguish between acute lymphatic leukemia and acute myeloid leukemia. Nor can it be used to determine benign or malignant lymphatic disorders.
E. PAS does not identify the type of fungal infection, only that fungal infection is present.

Bibliography:

Campana D, Freitas RO, Coustan-Smith E: Detection of residual leukemia with immunologic methods: Technical developments and clinical implications. Leukemia Lymphoma (13, Suppl) *1*:31–34, 1994.
Potter MN: The detection of minimal residual disease in acute lymphoblastic leukemia. Blood Review *6*(2):68–82, 1992.

PERITONEAL FLUID ANALYSIS, SPECIMEN
(see Paracentesis, Diagnostic)

PERITONEOSCOPY, DIAGNOSTIC
(see Laparoscopy, Diagnostic)

PERSANTINE-SESTAMIBI STRESS TEST AND SCAN, DIAGNOSTIC
(see Heart Scan, Diagnostic)

PET SCAN
(see Positron Emission Tomography, Diagnostic)

PFT
(see Pulmonary Function Test, Diagnostic)

PH, BLOOD
(see Blood Gases, Arterial, Blood, Blood Gases, Capillary, Blood, or Blood Gases, Venous, Blood)

PH, STOOL

Norm:

Adult	7.0–7.5
Newborn	5.0–7.0
Bottle-fed infants	neutral to slightly alkaline pH of 7.0–8.0
Breast-fed infants	slightly acidic

Increased: Colitis, protein breakdown, and villous adenoma.

Decreased: Breast-fed infants, celiac disease, disaccharidase deficiency, diabetes mellitus, lactose intolerance, malabsorption (carbohydrates, fats), malnutrition, nontropical sprue (adult celiac disease), and tropical sprue. Drugs include antibiotics.

Description: pH of stool is used to screen clients with gastrointestinal tract disorders for malabsorption of carbohydrates and fats and disaccharide intolerance. Stools with pH >6.0 are indicative of disaccharide intolerance, while those <6.0 indicate malabsorption of sugars and fats.

Professional Considerations:

1. Consent form NOT required.
2. Preparation:
   A. The client should not have undergone barium procedures or taken laxatives for 1 week prior to specimen collection.
   B. Obtain a bedpan, a stool specimen container with a lid, a tongue blade, and pH paper.
3. Procedure:
   A. Collect a random stool specimen in a bedpan or collection container. Mix the specimen with water to make a suspension. Test it with commercially prepared pH paper as directed.
4. Postprocedure care:
   A. Refrigerate the specimen if the test cannot be performed promptly.
5. Client and family teaching:
   A. Results are normally available within 24 hours.
   B. Do not contaminate the stool with urine or other secretions or with toilet paper.
6. Factors that affect results:
   A. Reject specimens mixed with urine, toilet paper, or toilet water.
7. Other data:
   A. Acidic stools will have a sickly sweet odor in both adults and children.
   B. Stool pH may be one factor related to the development of cancers of the GI tract.

Bibliography:

Gibson FR, Cummings JH, Macfarlane GT, et al.: Alternative pathways for hydrogen disposal during fermentation in the human colon. Gut *31*(6):679–683, 1990.

Klurfeld DM: Dietary fiber-mediated mechanisms in carcinogenesis. Cancer Res *52*(7, Suppl):2055S–2059S, 1992.

Strassinger SK: Urinalysis and Body Fluids. Philadelphia, FA Davis, 1994.

PH, URINE

Norm: Normal values have a wide range because the renal system acts as a buffer for the body and adjustments in urine pH provide homeostasis. Urine pH should be evaluated with other data and client information.

Adult
Early-morning specimen	pH 5–6
Random	4.5–8.0 as the body adjusts acid base
Average	5–6
Newborn	5.0–7.0

Increased: As a response to alkali overdose, a diet high in vegetables and fruits (especially citrus) and after meals. Also occurs with metabolic alkalosis without potassium loss, Fanconi's syndrome, prolonged gastric suction or vomiting, hyperaldosteronism, hypokalemia, renal insufficiency, respiratory alkalosis, and urinary tract infection with *Proteus* or *Pseudomonas*. Drugs include acetazolamide, aldosterone, amiloride, amphotericin B, carbenoxolone, epinephrine, mafenide acetate, niacinamide, phenacetin, potassium citrate, and sodium bicarbonate. Increased pH levels may be associated with renal calculi.

Decreased: Diets high in meat protein and cranberries or starvation diets; achlorhydria, alkaptonuria, diabetes, or other metabolic acidosis; severe diarrhea due to potassium depletion; methyl alcohol poisoning; phenylketonuria; respiratory acidosis; and renal tuberculosis. Drugs include acid phosphate, ascorbic acid, ammonium chloride, corticotropin, diazoxide, hippuric acid, methiomine, mandelate, and methenamine.

Description: Measurement of free hydrogen ion excretion in urine. Urine pH is reflective of plasma pH and is an indicator of renal tubular function. Playing a role in acid-based balance, normally functioning kidneys will excrete excess hydrogen ions in the urine.

Professional Considerations:

1. Consent form NOT required.

2. Preparation:
   A. Obtain a clean specimen container with a lid.
3. Procedure:
   A. Have the client urinate into a 50- to 100-ml collection container. A fresh specimen may be taken from a urinary drainage bag.
   B. If urine is to be tested with a commercially prepared test reagent, follow the manufacturer's directions.
4. Postprocedure care:
   A. Cover the container tightly and send the specimen to the laboratory if it is not tested immediately with a commercially prepared test reagent.
5. Client and family teaching:
   A. Notify the nurse immediately after you have collected the sample.
   B. Results are normally available within 24 hours.
6. Factors that affect results:
   A. Urine pH testing must be performed on a freshly collected specimen. Urine left to stand will falsely raise the pH.
   B. Urine with glucose may have falsely low pH due to bacterial activity.
   C. Bacterial infections can alter the pH in either direction.
7. Other data:
   A. Early-morning voids are preferred for urine pH testing.
   B. pH results should be read immediately.
   C. Urine pH is related to diet and may be one factor in the development of renal stones.

Bibliography:

Carlisle EJ, Donnelly SM, Halperin ML: Renal tubular acidosis (RTA): recognize the ammonium defect and pH or get the urine pH. Pediatr Nephrol *5*(2):242–248, 1991.

Preisig P: Renal physiology series: Part 7 of 8: Renal Acidification. ANNA J *21*(5):251–257, 1994.

Smith LH: Dietary management of urolithiasis. Curr Opinion Nephrol Hypertension *3*(2):189–194, 1994.

PHENCYCLIDINE (PCP, ANGEL DUST), QUALITATIVE, URINE

Norm: Negative.

		SI Units
Nonfatal level	0.4–40 mg/L	21–397 µmol/L
Fatal level	5–120 mg/L	21–493 µmol/L

Overdose Symptoms and Treatment:

Symptoms of Phencyclidine Use Include:

Stage I Psychiatric signs: drunken or euphoric with possible ataxia, muscle spasms, fever, tachycardia, flushing, small pupils, diaphoresis, salivation, nausea and vomiting.

Stage II Stupor, convulsions especially following stimulation, hallucinations, and progressive increases in heart rate, fever, and blood pressure. CNS stimulation or depression may occur.

Stage III Increases in heart rate and metabolism progress to cardiac and respiratory failure.

Treatment:

1. Provide respiratory support if needed.
2. Administer activated charcoal with a cathartic such as sorbitol, followed by gastric lavage and suction for oral ingestion.
3. Administer benzodiazapines or haloperidol for severe agitation.
4. Treat seizures as needed.
5. Give IV nutrition and fluid and electrolyte support as needed. Acidification of urine will increase the rate of phencyclidine excretion.
6. If rhabdomyolysis occurs, then IV fluids, mannitol, and diuretics are required.
7. Close observation of electrolytes, respiratory, and circulatory status until the client returns to baseline.
8. Chronic abusers may become increasingly psychotic after the drug wears off.
9. Drug counseling and psychiatric counseling are advised.

Usage: Screening for drug abuse or PCP toxicity, and psychosis or coma (unexplained), which may be related to PCP use. Metabolites of abused drugs are excreted and can be detected in the urine for several days following ingestion. PCP is just one of the drugs tested for in urine toxicology screening as recommended by the National Institute of Drug Abuse (NIDA) for new-job physicals, criminals, and after industrial accidents.

Description: Phencyclidine is a highly addictive, illegal, hallucinative drug designed for use as an anesthetic and a veterinary tranquilizer. It causes euphoria by accelerating the metabolism of the body. Phencyclidine is available in powder or capsule form and can be smoked, snuffed, injected, or swallowed. It is excreted by the kidneys and is detectable in the urine for 7 days.

Professional Considerations:

1. Consent form NOT required.
2. Preparation:
   A. Obtain a clean plastic container.
3. Procedure:
   A. Obtain a 100- to 125-ml random urine sample in a clean plastic container. A fresh specimen may be taken from a urinary drainage bag.
4. Postprocedure care:
   A. Send the specimen to the laboratory. For screening for known drug abusers: Special care MUST be taken in obtaining the specimen and in specimen handling to avoid falsification of results. Documentation of observed collection and handling may be required.
5. Client and family teaching:
   A. Obtain a past and recent history of drug abuse.
   B. Referrals to appropriate rehabilitation centers and therapeutic community programs should be offered to all addicted clients who may be interested.
   C. If activated charcoal was given for elevated levels, the client should drink 4–6 glasses of water each day for 2 days to prevent constipation. Activated charcoal will cause stools to be black for a few days.

6. Factors that affect results:
   A. Peak serum concentrations occur within 15 minutes after smoking phencyclidine. Half-life is 11 hours.
   B. Drugs that may cause decreased levels include ketamine hydrochloride.
7. Other data:
   A. Qualitative urine testing identifies the presence of phencyclidine, but does not indicate toxic levels.

Bibliography:

Burst JC: Other agents. Phencyclidine, marijuana, hallucinogens, inhalants and anticholinergics. Neurol Clin *11*(3):555–561, 1993.

Goldfrank LR, Flomenbaum NE, Lewin NA, Weisman RS, Howland MA, Hoffman RS: Goldfrank's Toxicologic Emergencies. Norwalk, CT, Appleton and Lange, 1994.

Milton HT: Diagnosis and management of phencyclidine intoxication. Am Fam Physician *43*(4): 1293–1302, 1991.

PHENDIMETRAZINE
(see Amphetamines, Blood)

PHENISTIX TEST, DIAGNOSTIC

Norm: Negative.

Usage: Screening for phenylketonuria (PKU) disease. Other screening methods are Guthrie test and serum phenylalanine, which are more often utilized. Serum phenylalanine levels can detect PKU much earlier after birth. Phenostix also turns brown with salicylate and phenothiazine ingestion.

Description: Use of Phenistix is a simple method of screening infant urine for phenylketonuria. Blood tests for pheylketonuria are more accurate. Phenistix are seldom utilized today. Phenistix are strips impregnated with ferric chloride that turn green when saturated with urine containing phenylalanine.

Professional Considerations:

1. Consent form NOT required.
2. Preparation:
   A. Obtain Phenistix and a urine-soaked diaper of the infant.
3. Procedure:
   A. Place the Phenistix on a urine-soaked diaper until it is saturated with urine. Observe it for color changes.
4. Postprocedure care:
   A. Discard the diaper.
5. Client and family teaching:
   A. If this test is positive, a Guthrie test and/or serum phenylalanine should be performed to confirm the diagnosis.
   B. PKU testing is required in most of the United States.
6. Factors that affect results:
   A. None found.
7. Other data:
   A. *See also Phenylalanine, Blood, and Guthrie Test for Phenylketonuria, Diagnostic.*

Bibliography:

Ris MD, Williams Se, Hunt MM, Berry HK, Leslie N: Early-treated Phenylketonuria: Adult neuropsychological outcome. J Pediatr *124*(3):388–392, 1994.

Smith I, Cook B, Beasley M: Review of neonatal screening programs for phenylketonuria. Br Med J *303*(6798):333–335, 1991.

PHENMETRAZINE, BLOOD

Norm: Negative.

		SI Units
Therapeutic level (single dose)	0.06–0.25 mg/L	0.34–1.41 µmol/L
Levels in abuse	0.5–4.0 mg/L	
Panic level		>28.20 µmol/L

Overdose Symptoms and Treatment:

Symptoms: Acute intoxication includes blood pressure extremes, hallucinations, panic, dysrhythmias, and delirium. At higher levels phenmetrazine can cause hyperventilation, convulsions, and hypertension.

Treatment:
Do gastric lavage.
Give activated charcoal.
Sedate with barbiturate.
Severe hypertension may be treated with intravenous phentolamine (Regitene).
Acid urine tends to increase the rate of excretion.

Usage: Monitor obesity treatment and for suspected stimulant drug abuse or overdose.

Description: Phenmetrazine is a schedule-II, CNS stimulant, anorexiant agent that was frequently used for obesity treatment but has a high instance of abuse. The drug is seldom used because of its central catecholamine action. The drug is most commonly abused by those hoping that a higher dose will increase the weight loss rate. There have been cases of accidental ingestion by children and abuse by teenagers hoping for a "high." The adverse effects (without toxicity levels) include nervousness, agitation, hyperthermia and insomnia, and elevated blood pressure. It is metabolized in the liver and excreted by the kidneys, with duration of effects lasting 4–12 hours. The half-life is 8 hours.

Professional Considerations:

1. Consent form NOT required.
2. Preparation:
   A. Tube: Red-top, red/gray-top, or gold-top.
3. Procedure:
   A. Draw a 7-ml blood sample.
4. Postprocedure care:
   A. None.
5. Client and family teaching:
   A. Discuss the need for rehabilitation and/or counseling. Referrals to appropriate rehabilitation centers and therapeutic community programs should be offered to all clients who may be interested.
   B. If activated charcoal was given for elevated levels, the client should drink 4–6 glasses of water each day for 2 days to prevent constipation. The activated charcoal will cause stools to be black for a few days.
6. Factors that affect results:
   A. Peak serum concentration occurs 2 hours after ingestion.
7. Other data:
   A. Many OTC weight loss and cold medications contain amphetamines or their analogs and may falsely elevate results, although the significance is not well established.

Bibliography:

Chait LD, Ohlenhuth EH, Johanson CE: Reinforcing and subjective effects of several anorectics in normal human volunteers. J Pharmacol Exp Ther *242*(3): 777–783, 1987.

Hood I, Monforte J, Gault R, et al.: Fatality from illicit phendimetrazine use. J Toxicol Clin Toxicol *26* (3–4):249–255, 1988.

Kay JM: Dietary pulmonary hypertension. Thorax *49*(Suppl):S33–S38, 1994.

PHENOBARBITAL, PLASMA OR SERUM

Norm: Negative. Therapeutic levels are relative. For control of seizures the clinical picture is important.

Therapeutic Levels		SI Units
Adults	15–40 µg/ml	86–72 µmol/L
Infants	15–30 µg/ml	65–129 µmol/L
Children	15–30 µg/ml	65–129 µmol/L
Toxic level	>40 µg/ml	>172 µmol/L
Panic levels		
Coma with reflexes	65–117 µg/ml	280–504 µmol/L
Coma without reflexes	>90 µg/ml	>430 µmol/L

Panic Level Symptoms and Treatment:

Symptoms: Cold/clammy skin, ataxia, CNS depression, hypothermia, hypotension, cyanosis, Cheyne Stokes respirations, tachycardia, coma. Toxicity may cause severe renal impairment.

Treatment:

Do gastric lavage, followed by a slurry of activated charcoal with cathartic.
Measure urine alkalinization (to pH>7.5) with bicarbonate and hydration. Measure urine pH q 1 hour.
Protect the airway.
The client may require intubation and mechanical ventilation, especially

Treatment (*continued*)

during gastric lavage if the gag reflex has been affected by the barbiturates.
Monitor closely for hypotension.
Hemodialysis, peritoneal dialysis, and hemoperfusion all WILL remove phenobarbital. Charcoal hemoperfusion is very effective in removing phenobarbital.

Usage: Suspected drug toxicity or abuse in clients with symptoms of lethargy, dizziness, ataxia, and diplopia. Monitoring therapeutic levels of phenobarbital especially for seizure disorders during puberty, after weight gain or loss, and if renal failure develops.

Increased: Drug (barbiturate) abuse and renal failure in clients treated with phenobarbital. Drugs that can increase levels for clients taking phenobarbital include monamine oxidase (MAO) inhibitors, sodium valproate, and valproic acid.

Decreased: (Below therapeutic range) Inadequate therapy, noncompliance, and malabsorption (oral doses).

Description: A long-acting, schedule-IV barbiturate most commonly used for its anticonvulsant effect and occasionally used as a sedative. It is widely distributed throughout the body, metabolized by the liver, and 50% is excreted unchanged in the urine. The half-life is normally 50–120 hours in adults and 40–70 hours in children. Allowance of time for steady-state levels after changes in dosage should be considered, with monitoring of therapeutic blood levels.

Professional Considerations:

1. Consent form NOT required.
2. Preparation:
   A. Tube: Red-top, red/gray-top, or gold-top or black-top.
   B. Do NOT draw specimens during hemodialysis.
3. Procedure:
   A. Draw a 1-ml blood sample.
4. Postprocedure care:
   A. None.
5. Client and family teaching:
   A. Discuss the schedule and dose of taking medication.
   B. Results are normally available within 24 hours.

C. Return for serum re-evaluation within 7 days for long-term phenobarbital therapy.
D. If activated charcoal was given for elevated levels, the client should drink 4–6 glasses of water each day for 2 days to prevent constipation. Activated charcoal will cause stools to be black for a few days.
6. Factors that affect results:
   A. Draw the specimen within 1 hour prior to the next dose for ongoing monitoring.
   B. Remeasure the phenobarbital level 7 days after dosage change for long-term therapy.
7. Other data:
   A. Mephobarbital is metabolized to phenobarbital.
   B. Peak levels occur 6–18 hours after dose.

Bibliography:

Fairchild L, Wong E, Li TM, Litman DJ: Phenobarbital monitoring in whole blood with a quantitative noninstrument test. Ther Drug Monit *13*(5): 425–427, 1991.
Hardoin RA, Henslee JA, Christenson CP, Christensen PJ, White M: Colic medication and apparent life threatening events. Clin Pediatr *30*(5):281–285, 1991.
Lindberg MC, Cunningham A, Lindberg NH: Acute phenobarbital intoxication. South Med J *85*(8): 803–807, 1992.

PHENOLPHTHALEIN TEST (LAXATIVE ABUSE TEST), DIAGNOSTIC

Norm: Negative.

Usage: Anorexia nervosa (laxative use for weight loss), chronic self-prescribed laxative use, and unexplained diarrhea.

Description: The phenolphthalein test is a toxicologic screening for evidence of recent laxative use. Phenolphthalein is the active ingredient of many over-the-counter laxative preparations. It causes stool evacuation by enhancing fluid and electrolyte accumulation in the intestines. After ingestion, phenolphthalein is excreted in both the feces and the urine and is detectable for up to 32 hours. It may also have laxative effects for up to 4 days and cause fluid and electrolyte abnormalities. This test is performed on an aliquot of a 24-hour urine sample to detect the presence of phenolphthalein via thin-layer chromatography.

Professional Considerations:

1. Consent form NOT required.

2. Preparation:
   A. Preschedule this test with the laboratory.
   B. Obtain a clean, 3-L container without preservative.
   C. Write the beginning time of collection on the laboratory requisition.
3. Procedure:
   A. Discard the first morning-urine specimen.
   B. Begin to time a 24-hour urine collection.
   C. Save all the urine voided for 24 hours in a refrigerated, clean, 3-L container. Document the quantity of urine output during the specimen collection period. Include the urine voided at the end of the 24-hour period. For catheterized clients, keep the drainage bag on ice and empty the urine into the collection container hourly.
4. Postprocedure care:
   A. Compare the urine quantity in the specimen container with the urinary output record for the test. If the specimen contains less urine than was recorded as output, some of the sample may have been discarded, thus invalidating the test.
   B. Document the quantity of urine output and the ending time for the 24-hour collection period on the laboratory requisition.
   C. Send the entire 24-hour urine specimen to the laboratory for testing. The test is performed on a 20-ml aliquot of the 24-hour specimen.
5. Client and family teaching:
   A. Save all the urine voided in the 24-hour period and urinate before defecating to avoid loss of urine. If any urine is accidentally discarded, discard the entire specimen and restart the collection the next day.
   B. Results are normally available within 24 hours.
   C. Discuss psychological and rehabilitation services if laxative abuse is determined.
6. Factors that affect results:
   A. Repeating the collection on consecutive days for a total of three 24-hour specimens increases the likelihood of detecting laxative abuse.
7. Other data:
   A. Methods are available to test for a wide range of laxative ingredients in urine.
   B. Complications of laxative abuse may include diarrhea, abdominal pain, hypokalemia, hypermagnesemia, cathartic colon, and the development of ammonium urate renal calculi.

Bibliography:

Bytzer P, Stokholm, M, Andersen I, et al.: Prevalence of surreptitious laxative abuse in patients with diarrhea of uncertain origin: a cost benefit analysis of a screening procedure. Gut 30(10):1379–1384, 1989.

de Wolf FA, de Haas EJM, Verweij M: A screening method for establishing laxative abuse. Clin Chem 27(6):914–917, 1981.

Mrvos R, Swanson-Biearman B, Deam BS, Drenzelok EP: Acute phenolphthalein ingestion in children. A retrospective review. J Pediatr Health Care 5(3):147–151, 1991.

Zanolli MD, McAlvany J, Krowchuk DP: Phenolphthalein-induced fixed drug eruption: a cutaneous complication of laxative use in a child. Pediatrics 91(6):1199–1201, 1993

PHENOLSULFONPHTHALEIN TEST, DIAGNOSTIC

Note: This test is seldom performed because there are newer, more precise tests for measuring glomerular flow rate and renal function.

Norm:

Excretion Time Intervals	
Adults	
15-minute specimen	25% of injected dye
30-minute specimen	50–60%
60-minute specimen	60–70%
120-minute specimen	70–80%
Children	

Excretion percentages are increased by 5–10% at the same time intervals.

Decreased: Less PSP dye is excreted by the kidneys at the various time intervals signaling impaired renal tubular function and/or plasma flow with renal vascular disease:

Slight	15-minute results of 15–25% excretion
Mild	15-minute results of 10–15% excretion
Moderate	15-minute results of 5–10% excretion
Marked impairment	15-minute results of less than 5% excretion

Also: Amyloidosis, cirrhosis (*with normal renal function*), congestive heart failure, cystitis, elevated serum protein levels, essential hypertension, nephritis (chronic), nephrosclerosis, nephrosis (lower nephron), polycystic kidney disease (congenital), prostatic or other urinary tract obstruction, and pyelonephritis. Drugs include BSP dye, chlorothiazide and other diuretics, penicillin G benzathine, penicillin G potassium, penicillin G procaine, probenecid, radiographic contrast media (intravenous dyes), salicylates, sulfinpyrazone, and sulfonamides.

Increased: Increased rate of excretion of PAS is associated with hepatic disease (severe), hyperalbuminemia, and multiple myeloma.

Description: The phenolsulfonphthalein (PSP) test measures proximal renal tubular function as a reflection of renal circulation through excretion of PSP, the plasma albumin-binding dye. Normally, PSP dye is quickly excreted by the kidneys. In renal impairment, excretion is slowed. PSP dye excretion measured in four serial urine collections correlates with renal blood flow and imparts a pinkish color to alkaline urine. A spectrophotometer measures the excreted dye; thus, any substance that affects the color of the urine will alter the results. The results correlate with the GFR.

Professional Considerations:

1. Consent form IS required.

Risks:

Allergic reaction to dye (itching, hives, rash, tight feeling in the throat, shortness of breath, bronchospasm, anaphylaxis, death).

Contraindications:

Previous allergy to phenolsulfonphthalein dye or to shellfish; dysphagia; conditions that preclude large-volume intake, such as acute renal insufficiency; congestive heart failure; clients with elevated blood urea nitrogen (BUN) level.

2. Preparation:
   A. *See Client and family teaching.*
   B. The client must be well hydrated to produce alkaline urine and is encouraged to drink 4 or 5 glasses of water 30 minutes prior to the test. Ingestion of a glass of water every 20 minutes for the duration of the test is required to assure adequate renal blood flow and brisk urine flow.
   C. Record any allergies to shellfish on the laboratory requisition and notify the physician performing the test of allergies.
   D. Establish intravenous access.
   E. Obtain phenolsulfonphthalein dye and four clean, dry, 1-L plastic urine containers.
   F. Have an emergency cart readily available.
3. Procedure:
   A. Administer the phenolsulfonphthalein dye intravenously and record the exact time of administration.
   B. Instruct the client to void and discard the entire sample.
   C. Obtain serial urine samples of at least 50 ml at exactly 15, 30, 60, and 120 minutes after injection.
   D. The bladder should be emptied completely with each void.
   E. Collect each sample separately in a clean, dry plastic container.
   F. Label each container sequentially, and include the exact time of collection.
   G. If the client is unable to void at the prescribed times, a straight catheter may be inserted to obtain the urine samples.
4. Postprocedure care:
   A. Remove the intravenous access.
   B. Write the exact time of each urine specimen collection on the laboratory requisition, as well as the time and dose of phenolsulfonphthalein administered.
   C. Urine samples must be transported to the laboratory immediately or be refrigerated.
5. Client and family teaching:
   A. Avoid food and medications that impart color to the urine for 24 hours before testing. *See Factors that affect results,* below.
   B. It is important to comply with timed urine samples.
   C. The urine will be red with the excretion of the test material.
6. Factors that affect results:
   A. Reject urine specimens obtained at improper time intervals.
   B. Impaired circulation and cardiac and vascular disease obscure the results.
   C. Inconclusive results have been reported in clients with edematous states and urinary retention disorders.
   D. Inadequate urinary output (less than 40 ml) may alter test results.
   E. Foods that may alter urine color include beets, carrots, and rhubarb.
   F. Substances that may alter urine color

include bilirubin, biliverdin, hemoglobin, homogentisic acid, indicans, melanin, methylene blue, myoglobin, porphobilinogen, porphyrins, and urobilinogen.

G. Drugs that may alter urine color include aminosalicylic acid, amitriptyline hydrochloride, anisindione, anthraquinones, anticoagulants (oral), cascara sagrada, chloroquine hydrochloride, chloroquine phosphate, chlorzoxazone, chlorpromazine, cinchophen, dihydroxyanthraquinone, diuretics, emodin, ethanol, ethoxazene hydrochloride, fuscin, indomethacin, iron complexes, levodopa, methocarbamol, methyldopa, methyldopate hydrochloride, metronidazole, nitrofurazone, nitrofurantoin, pamaquine, phenacetin, phenazopyridine hydrochloride, phenindione, phenols, phenothiazines, phensuximide, primaquine phosphate, quinacrine hydrochloride, quinine sulfate, riboflavin, rifampin, salicylates, salicylazosulfapyridine, senna, sulfasalazine, sulfonamides, thiazolsulfone, tolonium, triamterene, and vitamins.

7. Other data:
A. Acute glomerulonephritis shows a specific result to the PSP test in which the excretion test is normal but the BUN and creatinine are elevated.

Bibliography:

Flynn FV: Assessment of renal function: Selected developments. Clin Biochem 23(1):49–54, 1990.

Murry DJ, Synold TW, Pui CH, Rodman JH: Renal function and methotrexate clearance in children with newly diagnosed leukemia. Pharmacotherapy 15(2):144–149, 1995.

Van Lente F, Suit P: Assessment of renal function by serum creatinine and creatinine clearance: Glomerular filtration rate estimated by four procedures. Clin Chem 35(12):2326–2330, 1989.

PHENOTHIAZINES, BLOOD

Norm: Negative.

		SI Units
Quantitative Test		
Chlorpromazine (Thorazine)		
Adults	50–300 ng/ml	157–942 nmol/L
Children	40–80 ng/ml	126–251 nmol/L
Panic level	>750 ng/ml	>2355 nmol/L
Fluphenazine	0.2–4.9 ng/ml	0.4–8.4 nmol/L
Prochlorperazine (Compazine)	<0.5 µg/ml	
Panic level	>1.0 µg/ml	
Thioridazine (Mellaril)	1.0–1.5 µg/ml	2.7–4.1 µmol/L
Panic level	>10 µg/ml	>27 µmol/L
Trifluoperazine (Stelazine)	<500 ng/ml	<1040 nmol/L
Panic level	>1000 ng/ml	>2080 nmol/L

Overdose Symptoms and Treatment:

Symptoms: Extrapyramidal symptoms, central nervous system (CNS) depression, respiratory depression. CNS and respiratory depressive effects are worse when alcohol or antihypertensives are concomitantly ingested.

Treatment:
Monitor for CNS and cardiac depression.
ECG monitoring.
Do gastric lavage for oral doses or a saline cathartic for oral spansules.
Give activated charcoal.
Do not induce vomiting.

Hemodialysis and peritoneal dialysis will NOT remove chlorpromazine. No information was found on prochlorperazine, thioridazine, and trifluoperazine regarding dialysis effect on blood levels.

Increased: Phenothiazine abuse and phenothiazine overdose. Drugs that may increase levels above therapeutic for clients on various phenothiazines include monoamine oxidase (MAO) inhibitors.

Decreased: Inadequate therapy. Drugs include antacids, antidiarrheals, anticholinergics, barbiturates, CNS depressants, and lithium carbonate. Thorazine absorption from the gut is pH-dependent, so H_2 antagonists may decrease steady-state levels for client on thorazine therapy.

Description: A group of drugs with antipsychotic, antihistaminic, antipruritic, and antiemetic effects that act centrally on the reticular activating system and peripherally with anticholinergic and alpha-adrenergic blocking effects. Phenothiazines are widely distributed in body tissues, metabolized by the liver, and excreted by the kidney, with a half-life of 20–40 hours. Correlation of therapeutic effectiveness with blood levels is poor. This test is mainly used to determine whether or not the phenothiazine is being taken or for the diagnosis of possible overdose. Fatalities from large doses are rare.

Professional Considerations:

1. Consent form NOT required.
2. Preparation:
   A. Tube: Red-top, red/gray-top, or gold-top.
   B. Chlorpromazine levels MAY be drawn during hemodialysis.
3. Procedure:
   A. Draw a 7-ml blood sample.
4. Postprocedure care:
   A. Send the specimen to the laboratory immediately and refrigerate it until tested.
5. Client and family teaching:
   A. Evaluate the need for psychological

and rehabilitation support if an overdose is involved. Referrals to appropriate rehabilitation centers and therapeutic community programs should be offered to all addicted clients who are interested.

   B. If activated charcoal was given for elevated levels, the client should drink 4–6 glasses of water each day for 2 days to prevent constipation. The activated charcoal will cause stools to be black for a few days.
6. Factors that affect results:
   A. For therapeutic monitoring, draw samples within 1 hour prior to the next dose and at least 3 hours after the last dose.
7. Other data:
   A. Newer phenothiazines include trifluopromazine (Vesprin), perphenazine (Trilafon), Fluphenazine (Prolixin), and mesoridazine (Serentil).

Bibliography:

Dani SG: Pharmacokinetics of antipsychotic drugs in man. Acta Psychiatr Scand 358(Suppl):37–40, 1990.

Goldfrank LR, Flomenbaum NE, Lewin NA, Weisman RS, Howland MA, Hoffman RS: Goldfrank's Toxicologic Emergencies. Norwalk, CT, Appleton and Lange, 1994.

Remy AJ, Larrey D, Pageaux GP, Ribstein J, Michel H: Cross hepatotoxicity between tricyclic antidepressants and phenothiazines. Eur J Gastroenterol Hepatol 7(4):373–376, 1995.

PHENTERMINE
(see Amphetamines, Blood)

PHENYLALANINE, BLOOD

Norm:

		SI Units
Infants	<4 mg/dl	<272 µmol/L
Newborn	1.2–3.4 mg/dl	73–206 µmol/L
Premature	2.0–7.5 mg/dl	121–454 µmol/L
Low birth weight	2.0–7.5 mg/dl	121–454 µmol/L
Adult	0.8–1.8 mg/dl	48–109 µmol/L
Adult—monitoring for diet compliance	1.3–3.4 mg/dl	78–204 µmol/L

Positive Test (increased result): Phenylketonuria (PKU) is diagnosed and confirmed by:

1. Greater than 4 mg/dl serum phenylalanine.
2. Associated with low tyrosine < than 0.6 mg/dl.
3. Urinary excretion of phenylpyruvic acid.

Description: PKU is caused by an autosomal recessive gene. The infant (client) lacks the ability to produce the enzyme phenylalanine hydroxylase, which converts phenylalanine to tyrosine. The resulting buildup of phenylalanine leads to severe mental retardation. The carrier rate for PKU is 2% in the United States. This test is performed when either a urine screening or Guthrie test screening for PKU has been positive or as the PKU screening test in newborns.

Professional Considerations:

1. Consent form NOT required.

2. Preparation:
   A. Mark the birth date and the date of initiation of feedings on the laboratory requisition.
   B. Tube: Green-top.
3. Procedure:
   A. Draw a 0.5-ml blood sample. Do not use cord blood.
4. Postprocedure care:
   A. None.
5. Client and family teaching:
   A. Refer parents with PKU infants for genetic counseling.
   B. Clients with PKU may be monitored for serum phenylalanine levels for life. The client must follow a low-protein diet, which is effective treatment but not a cure.
   C. Level of mental capacity has been shown to be related to serum levels. Range is 1.3–3.4 mg/dl for best control.
   D. Results are normally available within 48 hours.
6. Factors that affect results:
   A. False-negative results may occur with other tests for PKU prior to the third day of feeding, but the serum phenylalanine test for PKU has the advantage that it is usually accurate in the first 24 hours of life—especially in breast-fed babies because colostrum has a high protein content.
   B. Phenylalanine clearance has been shown to be delayed in elderly males.

C. Do not use cord blood.
D. Fasting is not needed even for monitoring of older PKU clients.
E. The presence of antibiotics in the sample make results uninterpretable.

7. Other data:
   A. Diagnosis of PKU may be made with concomitant urine testing and a plasma level >2 mg/dl (121 μmol/L, SI units) on consecutive tests.
   B. Male infants with PKU increase levels of phenylalanine at a faster rate than affected females.
   C. *See also Guthrie test for Phenylketonuria, Diagnostic (Filter Paper Test); and Phenistix Test, Diagnostic.*

Bibliography:

Doherty LB, Rohr FJ, Levy HL: Detection of phenylketonuria in the very early newborn blood specimen. Pediatrics 87(2):240–244, 1991.

Lee C: Enzymatic Ddetermination of L-phenylalanine in serum. Lab Med 24(5):301–304, 1993.

Ris MD, Williams SE, Hunt MM, Berry HK, Leslie N: Early-treated phenylketonuria: Adult neuropsychologic outcome. J Pediatr 124(3):388–392, 1994.

van Spronsen FJ, van Rin M, van Dijk T, Smit GP, Reijngoud DJ, Berger R, Heymans HS: Plasma phenylalanine and tyrosine response to different nutritional conditions (fasting/postprandial) in patients with phenylketonuria. Pediatrics 92(4): 570–573, 1993.

PHENYLPROPANOLAMINE
(see Amphetamines, Blood)

PHENYTOIN, SERUM

Norm:

		SI Units
Therapeutic range	10–20 μg/ml	40–79 μmol/L
Toxic level	45–112 μg/ml	177–442 μmol/L
Panic level	>60 μg/ml	>237 μmol/L

Panic Level Symptoms and Treatment:

Symptoms: Double vision, nystagmus, lethargy. Central nervous system depression: drowsiness, confusion, slurred speech, coma, respiratory depression.

Treatment:
   ECG monitoring.
   Phenytoin levels q 4 hours.
   Support airway and breathing.
   Gastric lavage with warm saline or tap water.
   Activated charcoal (multiple dose).
   Saline or sorbitol cathartic.
   Hemodialysis and peritoneal dialysis will NOT remove phenytoin.

Increased: Phenytoin abuse, phenytoin overdose, and renal disease in clients on maintenance dilantin. Drugs that may increase phenytoin levels for clients on chronic treatment include allopurinol, amiodarone, anticoagulants (oral), benzodiazepines, chloramphenicol, chlordiazepoxide, cimetidine, diazepam, H_2 antagonists, disulfiram, estrogens, ethanol (acute intake), ethosuximide, isoniazid, methylphenidate, phenacemide, phenothiazines, phenylbutazone, propoxyphene, salicylates, sulfonamides, thiazides, trazodone, tolbutamide, trimethoprim, and vinblastine sulfate.

Decreased: Inadequate phenytoin therapy; noncompliance. Drugs that may alter (speed up) metabolism of phenytoin leading to lower serum levels for clients on dilantin include carbamazepine, diazoxide, ethanol (chronic intake), folic acid, loxapine, methotrexate, sulfonylureas, theophylline, reserpine, sucrafate, and calcium-containing medications. Enteral tube feedings may decrease absorption of oral phenytoin. Drugs that may *either increase or decrease* levels: phenobarbital, sodium valproate, and valproic acid.

Description: A hydantoin derivative anticonvulsant also used as an antidysrhythmic. Phenytoin is widely distributed throughout the body, metabolized by the liver, and excreted in bile and urine, with a half-life of approximately 22 hours for oral administration. Five to 6 days of therapy are required to reach steady-state levels in adults, and 2–5 days are necessary in children.

Professional Considerations:

1. Consent form NOT required.
2. Preparation:
   A. Tube: Red-top, red/gray-top, or gold-top.
   B. Specimens MAY be drawn during hemodialysis.
3. Procedure:
   A. Draw a 1-ml blood sample.
4. Postprocedure care:
   A. None.
5. Client and family teaching:
   A. Explore the reasons for inappropriate ingestion of phenytoin, if appropriate.
   B. If activated charcoal was given for elevated levels, the client should drink 4–6 glasses of water each day for 2 days to prevent constipation. The activated charcoal will cause stools to be black for a few days.
6. Factors that affect results:
   A. Tube feedings should be held prior to and up to 2 hours after oral phenytoin administration.
   B. Peak levels should be drawn 3–9 hours after administration of oral phenytoin. Trough levels should be drawn just prior to the administration of the next dose.
   C. Five days should be allowed before measurement of phenytoin level after a change in dose.
7. Other data:
   A. Susceptibility to side effects and toxic effects, including Steven's-Johnson syndrome, may be increased in clients with head injuries or those with intracranial lesions, especially if irradiation is used as a treatment modality.
   B. High levels of dilantin may be associated with head and neck symptoms.

Bibliography:

Estoup M: Approaches and limitations of medication delivery in patients with enteral feeding tubes. Crit Care Nurs *14*(1):68–72, 77–81, 1994.

Massagli TL: Neurobehavioral effects of phenytoin, carbamazepine, and valproic acid: implications for use in traumatic brain injury. Arch Phys Med Rehabil *72*(3):219–226, 1991.

Pryka RD, Rodvold KA, Erdman SM: An updated comparison of drug dosing methods. Part I: Phenytoin. Clin Pharmacokinet *20*(3):209–217, 1991.

Rees TD, Levine RA: Systematic drugs as a risk factor for periodontal disease initiation and progression. Compendium *16*(1):20, 22, 26, 1995.

PHLEBOGRAPHY
(see Venography, Diagnostic)

PHONOCARDIOGRAPHY (PCG), DIAGNOSTIC

Norm: Normal S_1 and S_2 appear as spikes above the baseline on phonocardiograph paper. Absence of abnormal heart sounds as recorded by the phonocardiogram.

Usage: Aids diagnosis of cardiac valve abnormalities, hypertrophic cardiomyopathy, and left ventricular failure. May be performed and retained for reference as part of the client's permanent record as a visual representation of the intensity and loudness of murmurs and other abnormal heart sounds. Excellent teaching tool because it allows the learner to visualize the different heart sounds.

Description: A pictorial recording of the cardiac sounds heard on auscultation. A phonocardiogram uses microphones to transduce and amplify the sound into electrical impulses that are graphically recorded as a waveform by a high-speed recording apparatus. Generally, PCG is performed simultaneously with an electrocardiograph (ECG); The S_1, S_2, and any additional sounds, including S_3, S_4, murmurs, and clicks, are recorded. By comparing the ECG and PCG, normal and abnormal heart sounds and cardiac events can be located and timed during the cardiac cycle. Phonocardiography with the addition of echocardiography is becoming a valuable noninvasive diagnostic tool. Newer phonocardiography technology may soon be available to noninvasively study coronary artery flow as well as estimate great vessel pressures, provide more reliable diagnosis, and stratify the severity of cardiac value disfunction.

Professional Considerations:

1. Consent form NOT required.
2. Preparation:
   A. Obtain electrodes and alcohol.
   B. Clip the hair from the electrode sites prior to placement.
3. Procedure:
   A. The client is positioned supine. The electrode sites should be cleansed with alcohol and lightly scraped with the edge of an electrode prior to placement.
   B. After the heart apex and base are located with a stethoscope, a microphone is strapped (or secured with suction cups) in place over each site.
   C. Both an ECG and PCG are recorded simultaneously for four complete cardiac cycles of sinus rhythm. For dysrhythmias, seven to ten cardiac cycles are recorded. The procedure is repeated with the client changed to upright and left-lateral oblique positions. The client may be asked to change his or her breathing patterns (i.e., hold breath or perform deep inspiration and expiration).
4. Postprocedure care:
   A. Remove the electrodes and the residual electrode gel.
5. Client and family teaching:
   A. Cooperation is imperative throughout the procedure.
   B. Phonocardiography is noninvasive and takes about 30 minutes.
6. Factors that affect results:
   A. Failure to obtain secure electrode placement causes an artifact in the electrocardiographic recording.
   B. Careful calibration is needed for the results to be diagnostic and generalizable.
7. Other data:
   A. Phonocardiography with esophageal echocardiography provides a valuable permanent and comparable record of cardiac valve murmurs. The progress of the disease process can be followed using serial recordings.

Bibliography:

Akay M, Akay YM, Welkowitz W, Semmlow JL, Kostis J,: Application of adaptive FTF/FAEST zero tracking filters to noninvasive characterization of the sound pattern caused by coronary artery stenosis before and after angioplasty. Ann Biomed Eng *21*(1):9–17, 1993.

Hahn AW, Knowles MJ, Klimczak JC: A "listener/viewer" for phonocardiograms. Proc Ann Symp Computer Appl Med Care *1039*, 1994.

Longhini C, Baracca E, Brunazzi C, Vaccari M, Longhini L, Barbaresi F: A new noninvasive method for estimation of pulmonary arterial pressure in mitral stenosis. Am J Cardiol *68*(4):398–401, 1991.

Van Vollenhovca E, Chen JG: Phonocardiography, past, present and future. Acta Cardiol *48*(4):337–344, 1993.

PHOSPHOLIPIDS, SERUM

Norm: 180–320 mg/dl.
Males > females except during pregnancy.

Adults ≤age 65	125–275 mg/dl
Adults >age 65	196–366 mg/dl
Birth	75–170 mg/dl
Infant	100–275 mg/dl
Child	180–295 mg/dl

Usage: Evaluation of fat metabolism. Less used today because there are other specific tests for the plasma phospholipids. Levels are increased or decreased in the diseases listed below with more specific diagnostic tests available for most. Amniotic fluid levels of phospholipids reflect the surfactant level and give an indication of fetal lung maturity.

Increased: Diabetes mellitus, biliary cirrhosis, cholestasis, LCAT deficiency, hypothyroidism, ETOH cirrhosis, obstructive jaundice, and nephrotic syndrome with breast cancer, and chronic pancreatitis. Drugs include estrogens, epinephrine, and some phenothiazine.

Decreased: Primary hypolipoproteinemia, Tangiers disease, abetalipaprotenemia, and a dietary restriction of fat intake. Drugs include antilipemic agents such as Clofibrate.

Description: Phospholipids, the largest and most soluble of the lipid elements of the blood, contain phosphorus, fatty acids, and nitrogen and are needed for lipid transport. Phospholipids are essential in cellular membranes. Serum phospholipid determinations may be monitored when disorders in lipid metabolism are suspected. Cholesterol levels are more often prescribed and evaluated.

Professional Considerations:

1. Consent form NOT required.
2. Preparation:
   A. Tube: Red-top, red/gray-top, or gold-top.
   B. *See Client and family teaching.*
3. Procedure:
   A. Draw a 5-ml fasting blood sample in the morning before any medications are administered.
4. Postprocedure care:
   A. Note any medications taken on the laboratory requisition.
   B. Specimens should be taken to the laboratory immediately.

5. Client and family teaching:
   A. Do NOT drink alcohol for 24–48 hours before sampling.
   B. Consume a low- to moderate-fat evening meal on the day prior to the test.
   C. Fast from midnight prior to sampling.
6. Factors that affect results:
   A. Hemolysis of the specimen invalidates results.
   B. Recent intravenous injection of radiographic dye invalidates results.
   C. Significant weight changes within 2 weeks prior to the test invalidate results.

7. Other data:
   A. This test is not included in a routine assay of a "lipid profile."

Bibliography:

Almog R, Anderson-Samsonoff C, Berns DS, et al.: A methodology for determination of phospholipids. Ann Biochem *188*(1):237–242, 1990.

Lloyd-Still JD, Johnson SB, Holman RT: Essential fatty acids and fluidity of plasma phospholipids in cystic fibrosis infants. Am J Clin Nutr 54(6):1029–1035, 1991.

Musil J: Metabolism and function of phospholipids. Acta Univ Carol [Med] (Praha) *32*(1–2):59–74, 1986.

PHOSPHORUS, SERUM

Norm:

		SI Units
Adults ≤age 60	2.7–4.5 mg/dl	0.87–1.45 mmol/L
Females >age 60	2.8–4.1 mg/dl	0.90–1.30 mmol/L
Males >age 60	2.3–3.7 mg/dl	0.74–1.20 mmol/L
Cord blood	3.7–8.1 mg/dl	1.20–2.62 mmol/L
Premature infant	5.4–10.9 mg/dl	1.74–3.52 mmol/L
Newborn	4.5–9 mg/dl	1.45–2.91 mmol/L
Infant (10 days–24 months)	4.5–6.7 mg/dl	1.45–2.16 mmol/L
Child (24 months–12 years)	4.5–5.5 mg/dl	1.45–1.78 mmol/L

Increased: >4.7 mg/dl or 1.3 mmol/L fasting: acromegaly, acute or chronic renal disease, bone tumors, diabetic ketoacidosis, healing bone fractures, hyperthyroidism, hypoparathyroidism, lactic and respiratory acidosis, leukemia (myelogenous), magnesium deficiency, malignant hyperpyrexia following anesthesia, massive blood transfusions, metastatic bone tumors, milk-alkali (Burnett's) syndrome, multiple blood transfusions, multiple myeloma, portal cirrhosis, pseudohypoparathyroidism, pulmonary embolism, sarcoidosis, sickle cell, renal failure, sarcoidosis, secondary hypoparathyroidism, uremia, vitamin D toxicity. Drugs include androgens, beta blockers, chemotherapy, dyphosphates, steroids, ethanol, growth hormone, hydroclorothiazide, lasix, methicillin, phenytoin, phosphate enemas or infusions, phosphate laxative abuse, and tetracycline (nephrotoxicity).

Decreased: <0.8 mg/dl, panic <0.3 mg/dl: acute alcoholism, burns (diuretic phase), Crohn's disease (due to vomiting and diarrhea), diabetic ketoacidosis, dialysis, Fanconi's syndrome (renal tubular defects), gout, hyperalimentation (without phosphorus supplement), hypercalcemia (severe), hyperparathyroidism, hypokalemia, hypomagnesemia, hypothermia, hypovolemia, malabsorption, malnutrition, nasogastric suction, osteomalacia, respiratory alkalosis, rickets (primary or familial hypophosphatemia), salicylate poisoning, septicemia (gram-negative bacterial), sprue, vitamin D deficiency. Drugs include albuterol, acetazolamide, amino acids, anesthetic agents, antacids (aluminum-containing and phosphate-binding), carbamazepine, calcitonin, diuretics, epinephrine, estrogens, glucagon, glucocorticoids, glucose IV, insulin, isoniazid, oral contraceptives, phenytoin.

Description: Total plasma phosphate level is 39 mmol/L. Two thirds of this is in organic form of phospholipids and not measured as inorganic phosphorus. The inorganic element is important for bone formation, energy storage and release, urinary acid-base buffering, and carbohydrate metabolism. Only a portion is able to be measured in the serum; high concentrations are stored in bone and skeletal muscle. Phosphorus is absorbed from food and excreted by the kidneys.

Professional Considerations:

1. Consent form NOT required.
2. Preparation:
   A. The client must fast for 8–12 hours.
   B. Tube: Red-top, red/gray-top, or gold-top.
   C. Do NOT draw samples during hemodialysis.
   D. *See Client and family teaching.*
3. Procedure:
   A. Draw a 1-ml blood sample.
4. Postprocedure care:
   A. Send the specimen to the laboratory for immediate spinning.
5. Client and family teaching:
   A. Foods high in phosphorus include beans, chicken, eggs, fish, milk, and milk products.
   B. Avoid excessive antacid intake and laxatives/enemas containing sodium phosphate.
   C. For low-phosphorus levels, avoid other persons with infections because low phosphorus interferes with the functioning of the white blood cells.

6. Factors that affect results:
   A. Hemolysis of the specimen causes falsely elevated results.
   B. Serum levels vary throughout the day and are lowest in the morning.
   C. Eating before the test may falsely lower the phosphate level.
7. Other data:
   A. Calcium levels should also be prescribed to aid interpretation of results.
   B. Hyperphosphatemia is related to LOW calcium levels and associated symptoms: tetany, dyshythmias, seizures.
   C. Hypophosphatemia is associated with muscle weakness, difficult-to-wean chronic ventilator clients, encephalopathy, poor platelet function, decreased cardiac contractility, and paraesthesias.
   D. A 24-hour urine test for phosphate may be helpful in the work-up of low phosphate levels.

Bibliography:

Bourke E, Yanagawa N: Assessment of hyperphosphatemia and hypophosphatemia. Clin Lab Med *13*(1):183–207, 1993.

Crook M: Phosphate: an abnormal anion? Br J Hosp Med *52*(5):200–203, 1994.

Gertner JM: Disorders of calcium and phosphorus homeostasis. Pediatr Clin North Am *37*(6):1441–1465, 1990.

PHOSPHORUS, URINE

Norm:

		SI Units
Adults	0.4–1.3 g/24 hours	13–42 mmol/day
Restricted diet	<1.0 g/24 hours	<32 mmol/day

Note: Restricted diet contains 0.9–1.5 g (29–48 mmol) phosphorus and 10 mg (0.25 mmol) calcium per day.

Increased: Bone fractures (transiently), Fanconi's syndrome (renal tubular damage), familial hypophosphatemia, hyperparathyroidism, nonrenal acidosis because phosphate excretion is a buffering mechanism, paraplegia, vitamin D-resistant rickets, and vitamin D toxicity. Drugs include acetazolamide, asparagine, bicarbonate, bismuth salts, calcitonin, corticosteroids, dihydrotachysterl, diuretics, hydrochlorothiazide, metolazone, phosphates (increased intake), PTH, valine, and vitamin D.

Decreased: Hypoparathyroidism or parathyroidectomy, pseudohypoparathyroidism. Drugs include aluminum-containing antacids. Alanine in the obese fasting client.

Description: An inorganic element important for bone formation, energy storage and release, urinary acid-base buffering, and carbohydrate metabolism. Much is stored in bone and skeletal muscle. Phosphorus is absorbed from food and excreted by the kidneys. Phosphorus absorption is enhanced by the presence of vitamin D. Excretion is a renal buffering mechanism.

Professional Considerations:

1. Consent form NOT required.
2. Preparation:
   A. Obtain a clean, detergent-free, 3-L urine container to which acetic acid wash has been added.
   B. Write the beginning time of collection on the laboratory requisition.

3. Procedure:
   A. Discard the first morning-urine specimen.
   B. Save all the urine voided for 24 hours in a clean, refrigerated, 3-L container. Document the quantity of urine output during the specimen-collection period. Include urine voided at the end of the 24-hour period. For catheterized clients, keep the drainage bag on ice and empty the urine into the collection container hourly.
4. Postprocedure care:
   A. Compare the urine quantity in the specimen container with the urinary output record for the test. If the specimen contains less urine than was recorded as output, some of the sample may have been discarded, invalidating the test.
   B. Document the quantity of urine output and the ending time on the laboratory requisition.
   C. HCl acid is added in the laboratory on arrival for preservation.
5. Client and family teaching:
   A. Save all the urine voided in the 24-hour period and urinate before defecating to avoid loss of urine and to avoid contaminating the urine with stool. If any urine is accidentally discarded, discard the entire specimen and restart the collection.
6. Factors that affect results:
   A. All urine voided for the 24-hour period must be included to avoid a falsely low result.
7. Other data:
   A. Because phosphorus levels vary throughout the day, this test is most informative if performed on a 24-hour urine sample.
   B. Poor creatinine clearance will invalidate the results.

Bibliography:

Bourke E, Yanagawa N: Assessment of hyperphosphatemia and hypophosphatemia. Clin Lab Med *13*(1):183–207, 1993.

Crook M: Phosphate: an abnormal anion? Br J Hosp Med *52*(5):200–203, 1994.

Lobaugh B, Neelon FA, Oyama H, et al.: Circadian rhythms for calcium, inorganic phosphorus, and parathyroid hormone in primary hyperparathyroidism: Functional and practical considerations. Surgery *106*(6):1009–1016, 1989.

PHYTANIC ACID, SERUM

Norm:

		SI Units
Normal	<0.3% of total serum fatty acids	<0.003 fraction of total serum fatty acids
Borderline	0.3–0.5% total of serum fatty acids	0.003–0.005 fraction of total serum fatty acids
Suggestive of disease	>0.5% of total serum fatty acids	>0.005 fraction of total serum fatty acids

Increased: Refsum's disease. May also be elevated in Zellweger syndrome and infantile Refsum disease.

Decreased: None.

Description: The phytanic acid portion of serum fatty acids is elevated in Refsum's disease. Refsum's is a rare hereditary disease caused by a recessive gene, which causes a deficiency in phytanic acid alpha-oxidase, resulting in higher phytanic acid in serum. The disease is characterized by the eventual development of retinitis pigmentosa, peripheral neuropathy, cerebellar ataxia, nerve deafness, and ichthyosis due to lipidosis of the nervous system. Mental retardation is common. Hyperglycemia may also be present.

Professional Considerations:

1. Consent form NOT required.
2. Preparation:
   A. No fasting is required.
   B. Tube: Red-top, red/gray-top, or gold-top.
   C. Check the local laboratory for special collection instructions because different analysis techniques may require a different tube or a different amount of blood.
3. Procedure:
   A. Draw a 3–5-ml blood sample.
4. Postprocedure care:
   A. Send the specimen to the laboratory immediately; the specimen needs special handling and freezing.
5. Client and family teaching:
   A. Results are normally available within 5 days.
6. Factors that affect results:
   A. None found.

7. Other data:
   A. In Refsum's disease the CSF has a characteristic normal cell count with a high CSF protein level (100–700 mg/dl). There is no cure, and health management consists of supportive treatment for symptoms.

Bibliography:

Herbert MA, Clayton PT: Phytanic acid alpha-oxidase deficiency (Refsum's disease) presenting in infancy. J Inherited Metabol Dis *17*(2):211–214, 1994.

Singh I, Pahan K, Singh AK, Barbosa E: Refsum disease: a defect in the alpha-oxidation of phytanic acid in peroxisomes. J Lipid Res *34*(10):1755–1764, 1993.

Tranchant C, Aubourg P, Mohr M, Rocchiccioli F, Zaenker C, Warter JM: A new peroxisomal disease with impaired phytanic and pipecolic acid oxidation. Neurology *43*(10):2044–2048, 1993.

PINWORM, CULTURE

(see Parasite Screen, Stool)

PKU

(see Phenylalanine, Blood)

PLASMA RECALCIFICATION TIME, PLASMA

Norm: 75–90 seconds, or control clotting time.

Usage: Primarily used in research. Detection of abnormalities in hemostasis: procoagulation abnormalities and the procoagulation effects of drugs and diseases. Nonspecific.

Increased: In the presence of circulating anticoagulants or deficiencies of the important clotting factors: II, V, VII, X, XII.

Decreased: Shortened clotting time after recalcification. Clients with gram-negative septicemia, leukemia, malignancies, thromboembolic and hemorrhagic complications of diseases (thought to be related to some procoagulation process that consumes the usual coagulation factors, causing clot formation, and leaving the client without sufficient coagulation factors for normal clotting function). Procoagulation is thought to be increased by certain drugs such as dyes utilized for cardiac catheterization.

Description: Plasma recalcification time involves the addition of calcium in the from of Ca$^+$ citrate or CaCL$_2$ to blood and measurement of the time required for clotting to occur. Deficiencies in the plasma, platelets, or clotting factors will cause clot formation to be prolonged. The procoagulation factors such as the effects of malignancies or systemic disease may cause the recalcified plasma clotting time to be shortened. In these diseases, increased thrombus formation and may lead to emboli or to Disseminated intravascular coagulation (DIC). In this test, a blood sample is drawn into an anticoagulated tube. The specimen is slowly centrifuged to separate the cells from the plasma. With the exception of calcium, the separated plasma normally contains all of the clotting factors and blood components necessary for fibrin clot formation. Calcium is then added to the plasma (hence the name, plasma recalcification) and clot formation is timed. If the time is decreased there is some factor in the client which puts them at risk for accelerated coagulation. If the time required for clot formation to occur is over 150 seconds, a deficiency exists and further studies are indicated to identify the specific cause of prolonged clotting.

Professional Considerations:

1. Consent form NOT required.
2. Preparation:
   A. Obtain a plastic syringe and a blue-top tube.
3. Procedure:
   A. Draw a 5-ml blood sample in a plastic syringe or a blue-top tube.
4. Postprocedure care:
   A. Send the specimen to the laboratory immediately.
5. Client and family teaching:
   A. This test is nonspecific as to the cause of hemostasis.
   B. Results are normally available within 48 hours.
6. Factors that affect results:
   A. Heparin therapy will increase the recalcification time to 130–150 seconds.
   B. A delay in testing after specimen collection will cause a prolonged test.
7. Other data:
   A. This test is nonspecific for the cause of the abnormality in hemostasis. It shows enhanced coagulation states, NOT the actual causative factor.

Bibliography:

Falanga A, Alessio MG, Donati MB, Barbui T: A new procoagulant in acute leukemia. Blood *71*(4): 870–875, 1988.

Jungi TW: A turbidimetric assay in an ELISA reader for the determination of mononuclear phagocyte

procoagulant activity. J Immunol Methods
133(1):21–29, 1990.

Oshima G: Anticoagulant effect of inositol hexasulfate
as measurable by clotting times of fibrinogen and
recalcified plasma. Thromb Res *58*(3):243–250,
1990.

Parvez Z, Vik H: Intravascular contrast media and
thrombin generation. Acta Radiol *35*(2):172–175,
1994.

PLASMA RENIN ACTIVITY, PLASMA

(see Renin, Plasma)

PLASMINOGEN ASSAY, BLOOD

Norm: 20 mg/dl, 2.5–5.2 U/ml or
3.8–8.4 CTA (Council on Thrombolytic Agents) U/ml.

Increased: Anxiety, congenital defect
in the release of plasminogen inhibitors, deep-vein thrombosis, infancy,
infection, inflammation, malignancy,
myocardial infarction, pregnancy,
stress, and surgery. Drugs include oral
contraceptives.

Decreased: Cirrhosis, congenital defect in the release of plasminogen acti-
vators, disseminated intravascular coagulation, fibrinolysis, hyaline membrane
disease, hypofibrinogenemia (acquired),
liver disease, nephrosis, surgery (coronary artery bypass graft, postoperatively), and thrombosis. Drugs include
atelplase, L-asparaginase, streptokinase,
and urokinase.

Description: Plasminogen is a beta
globulin protein found in fibrin clots
of blood vessels, soft tissue, and any
body cavity lined with endothelial
cells. When healing or cellular repair
has occurred, endothelial cell enzymes trigger the conversion of plasminogen to the fibrinolytic enzyme
plasmin, and lysis of the fibrin clot begins. Plasminogen has a biologic half-
life of 2 days. Plasminogen assays are
used in the evaluation of fibrinolysis,
increased fibrin-fibrinogen degradation products, and to diagnose the
source of hypofibrinogenemia.

Professional Considerations:

1. Consent form NOT required.
2. Preparation:
   A. Clarify with the laboratory whether
      this test must be prescheduled for pro-
      cessing.
   B. Tube: Blue-top.

C. Do not use plasma collected in the
   presence of fluoride, EDTA, or heparin.
D. Specimens without lipidemia or hemolysis are preferred.
E. Specimens MAY be drawn during hemodialysis.

3. Procedure:
   A. Draw and discard a 2-ml blood sample
      and discard the syringe, leaving the
      needle in place. Perform venipuncture
      and withdraw 2 ml of blood into a sy-
      ringe or vacuum tube. Remove the sy-
      ringe or tube, leaving the needle in
      place. Attach a second syringe, and
      draw a sample quantity of 2.4 ml for a
      2.7-ml tube and 4.0 ml for a 4.5-ml
      tube. Immediately place the specimens
      in a container of ice.

4. Postprocedure care:
   A. Write the collection time on the labo-
      ratory requisition.
   B. Send the specimens to the laboratory
      and refrigerate them if not processed
      within 8 hours.

5. Client and family teaching:
   A. If results are elevated, the client may
      need to change from oral contracep-
      tives to other forms of birth control.

6. Factors that affect results:
   A. Reject hemolyzed or clotted speci-
      mens.

7. Other data:
   A. Clients with decreased plasminogen
      concentration may be prone to devel-
      oping recurrent thromboses.
   B. Plasminogen concentrations are de-
      creased with acquired or secondary hy-
      pofibrinogenemia and remain normal
      when congenital causes exist.

Bibliography:

Redlitz A, Plow EF: Receptors for plasminogen and
t-PA: an update. Baillieres Clin Haem *8*(2):313–
327, 1995.

Wang H, Lottenberg R, Boyle MD: Analysis of the interaction of group A streptococci with fibrinogen,
streptokinase and plasminogen. Microbial Pathogenesis *18*(3):153–166, 1995.

PLATELET ADHESION TEST, DIAGNOSTIC

Norm: Glass bead retention: 50–95%
(most commonly, 90–95%).

Increased: Aging, atherosclerosis,
burns, carcinoma, diabetes mellitus,
exertion, homocystinuria, hypercoagulability, hyperlipemia, infection
(acute), multiple sclerosis, pregnancy,
surgery, thrombosis, and trauma.
Drugs include oral contraceptives.

Decreased: Afibrinogenemia, anemia (severe), azotemia, Bernard-
Soulier syndrome, Chediak-Higashi
syndrome, congenital heart disease,

Glanzmann's thrombasthenia, glycogen storage disease, macroglobulinemia, multiple myeloma, myeloid metaplasia, myeloproliferative disorders, plasma cell dyscrasia, platelet release defect, storage pool disease, thrombasthenia, thrombocytopathy, uremia, and von Willebrand's disease. Drugs include vitamin E and dietary fish oil supplementation.

Description: This test evaluates the ability of platelets to adhere to foreign bodies during blood clotting by running blood through a collection of glass beads and counting the number of platelets adhering to the beads.

Professional Considerations:

1. Consent form NOT required.
2. Preparation:
   A. Preschedule this test with the laboratory.
   B. Tube: Red-top, red/gray-top, or gold-top.
   C. Specimens MAY be drawn during hemodialysis.
   D. *See Client and family teaching.*
3. Procedure:
   A. Draw a 10-ml blood specimen.
4. Postprocedure care:
   A. None.
5. Client and family teaching:
   A. Do not take drugs that inhibit platelet adhesion within 10 days prior to the test.
   B. Do not take drugs that decrease platelet levels within 10 days prior to the test *(see Platelet Count, Blood).*
   C. Fast for 8 hours before this test.
   D. If results are elevated, the client may need to change from oral contraceptives to other forms of birth control.
6. Factors that affect results:
   A. Reject clotted specimens or specimens with an extremely low platelet count.
   B. Platelet adhesiveness is increased during the spring season.
   C. Platelet adhesiveness is highest during the afternoon hours.
7. Other data:
   A. This test is difficult to standardize.

Bibliography:

Gartner TK, Amrani DL, Derrick JM: Characterization of adhesion of non-exogenously stimulated and resting platelets in normal plasma to fibrinogen and its fragments. Blood Coag Fibrin 5(5): 747–754, 1994.

Hantgan RR, Endenburg SC, Sixma JJ, et al.: Evidence that fibrin alpha-chain RGDX sequences are not required for platelet adhesion in flowing whole blood. Blood 86(3):1001–1009, 1995.

Ross JM, McIntire LV, Moake JL, et al.: Platelet adhesion and aggregation on human type VI collagen surfaces under physiological flow conditions. Blood 85(7):1826–1835, 1995.

PLATELET AGGREGATION, BLOOD, PLATELET AGGREGATION, HYPERCOAGULABLE STATE, BLOOD

Norm: 60–100% or according to specific laboratory.

Hypercoagulable State: Normal values are reported in descriptive terms of rate of spontaneous platelet aggregation of samples as compared to rate of platelet aggregation of control, evaluation of a second wave of aggregation with adenosine diphosphate (ADP) reagent, and platelet response to serial dilutions of epinephrine.

Increased: Atheromatosis, diabetes mellitus, hypercoagulability, hyperlipemia, and polycythemia vera.

Decreased: Afibrinogenemia, anemia (sideroblastic), Bernard-Soulier syndrome (ristocetin test), beta-thalassemia major, Chediak-Higashi syndrome, cirrhosis, Glanzmann's thrombasthenia (ADP, epinephrine, and collagen test), gray platelet syndrome (ADP, epinephrine, thrombin, collagen tests), Hermansky-Pudlak syndrome, homocystinuria, idiopathic thrombocytopenic purpura (ADP, collagen, epinephrine), macroglobulinemia, myeloid metaplasia, plasma cell dyscrasia, platelet release defects (ADP, second phase; epinephrine, second phase; and collagen tests), preleukemia, scurvy, storage pool disease (ADP, second phase; epinephrine, second phase; and collagen tests), thrombasthenia (ADP, epinephrine, collagen), thrombocythemia (hemorrhagic), uremia, von Gierke's disease, von Willebrand's disease (ristocetin test), and Wiskott-Aldrich syndrome. Drugs include alphaprodine, antibiotics, anticoagulants, antihistamines, aspirin, azlocillin, carbenicillin indanyl sodium, cephalothin sodium, chlordiazepoxide, chloroquine hydrochloride, chloroquine phosphate, clofibrate, cocaine hydrochloride, corticosteroids, cyproheptadine hydrochloride, dextran, dextropropoxyphene, diazepam, diphenhydramine hydrochloride, dipyridamole, flufenamic acid, furosemide, gentamicin sulfate, guaifenesin, heparin calcium, heparin sodium, ibufenac, ibuprofen, imipramine, indomethacin, marijuana, mefenamic acid, naproxen sodium, nitrofurantoin, nortriptyline hydrochloride, oxyphenbutazone, penicillin G benzathine, penicillin G potassium, penicillin G procaine, phenothiazines, phenylbutazone, promethazine hydrochloride, propranolol, pyrimidine compounds, sulfinpyrazone, theophylline, ticlopidine hydrochloride, tricyclic antidepressants, vitamin E, volatile general anesthetics (methoxyflurane, halothane, nitrous oxide), and zomepirac.

Description: The platelet aggregation test assesses the ability of platelets to adhere to each other by mixing the client's platelets in solution with substances that induce aggregation and measuring the amount of light that passes through the solution after clumping has occurred. Substances that induce aggregation include ADP, epinephrine, ristocetin, collagen, arachidonic acid, and thrombin. The platelet aggregation test for a hypercoagulable state is a modification on the standard platelet aggregation test. This test assesses the ability of platelets to adhere to each other in the following ways. First, the rate and amount of spontaneous platelet aggregation of the sample is compared to a known normal control sample. Second, the platelet aggregating reagent, ADP, is added to the client's sample, which is then observed for evidence of a second wave of aggregation. Third, serial dilutions of epinephrine, another platelet aggregating reagent, are added to the sample and it is studied for an enhanced platelet response.

Professional Considerations:

1. Consent form NOT required.
2. Preparation:
   A. Preschedule this test with the laboratory.
   B. Tube: Blue-top.
   C. Do NOT draw specimens during hemodialysis.
   D. *See Client and family teaching.*
3. Procedure:
   A. Draw a 10-ml blood sample.
   B. Traumatic venipuncture may cause contamination, thereby increasing aggregation.
4. Postprocedure care:
   A. Write the specimen collection time on the laboratory requisition.
   B. Deliver the specimen to the laboratory immediately. Do not refrigerate it. Testing should be performed within 2 hours after collection. Keep the speci-

men stable at room temperature for 1–3 hours.
5. Client and family teaching:
   A. Do not take drugs that inhibit platelet aggregation within the prior 10 days unless the test is being used to evaluate the drug effect on platelet function.
   B. Do not eat or drink caffeine-containing products within 12 hours.
6. Factors that affect results:
   A. Reject hemolyzed or clotted specimens or specimens received more than 2 hours after collection.
   B. Platelet count <100,000/mm³ causes inaccurate results.
   C. A delay in testing may cause a loss of platelet ability to aggregate.
   D. Lipemia may interfere with accurate measurement.
7. Other data:
   A. Von Willebrand's disease may be ruled out by a normal response to ristocetin aggregating agent. Platelet aggregation inhibition due to ingestion of aspirin may be ruled out by an inhibited response to arachidonic acid aggregating agent. Gray platelet syndrome may be ruled out when aggregation occurs with ristocetin but not with other aggregating agents.

Bibliography:

Caple JF, Kottke-Marchant K, Miller ML: The effect of a heparin removal filter on platelet aggregation studies in heparin-induced thrombocytopenia. Am J Clin Pathol 103(6):745–747, 1995.

Chang BH, Burgess J, Ismail F: The clinical usefulness of the platelet aggregation test for the diagnosis of heparin-induced thrombocytopenia. Thromb Haemost 69(4):344–350, 1993.

PLATELET ANTIBODY, BLOOD

Norm: Negative or <1000 molecules IgG/platelet.

Positive: Thrombocytopenia due to platelet autoantibodies causing idiopathic thrombocytopenic purpura (ITP), post-transfusion purpura, platelet refractoriness, isoimmune purpura, drug-induced (quinidine, quinine, furosemide, sulfonamides), or due to platelet isoantibodies after receipt of multiple transfusions.

Description: The platelet antibody test is performed to detect the presence of platelet autoantibodies and platelet isoantibodies (alloantibodies). Platelet autoantibodies are IgG immunoglobulins of autoimmune origin and are present in all cases of ITP. A quantitative antiglobulin consumption test or other methods may be used to detect platelet autoantibodies. Platelet isoantibodies develop in clients when they become sensitized to platelet antigens of transfused blood. This results in destruction of both donor and native platelets and shortened survival time of platelets in the transfusion recipient. A complement fixation test (or other methods) may be used to detect platelet isoantibodies.

Professional Considerations:

1. Consent form NOT required.
2. Preparation:
   A. Preschedule this test with the laboratory.
   B. Tubes: Two (2) blue-top.
   C. Do NOT draw during hemodialysis.
3. Procedure:
   A. Completely fill two sodium citrate-anticoagulated, blue-top tubes with a blood sample.
   B. If testing will be delayed, collect the sample into tubes containing acid citrate dextrose obtained from the laboratory.
4. Postprocedure care:
   A. Send the specimens to the laboratory. Plasma should be separated from the red cells and frozen in a plastic tube at −25°C.
   B. For specimens collected into acid citrate dextrose, store the sample as collected at 4°C.

C. Specimens may be frozen up to 3 years.
5. Client and family teaching:
   A. If thrombocytopenia is present, avoid rough physical activity and bumping into furniture. Use a stool softener and avoid straining to have a bowel movement. Use a soft toothbrush and watch for and report signs of bleeding: bruising, petechiae, blood in the stool/urine/sputum, bleeding from invasive lines, bleeding gums, abnormal/excessive vaginal bleeding.
6. Factors that affect results:
   A. Reject hemolyzed or clotted specimens.
7. Other data:
   A. Samples with mean fluorescence greater than two standard deviations above the mean of the negative control sample are considered positive.

Bibliography:

Christie DJ, Sauro SC, Fairbanks KD, et al.: Detection of clonal platelet antibodies in immunologically-mediated thrombocytopenias: association with circulating clonal/oligoclonal B cells. Brit J Haem 85(2):277–284, 1993.

Rule SA, Erber WN, Lown JA, et al.: Cross-matched platelets in bone marrow transplantation. Pathology 26(3):288–290, 1994.

Smith JW, Hayward CP, Warkentin TE, et al.: Investigation of human platelet alloantigens and glycoproteins using non-radioactive immunoprecipitation. J Immunol Methods 158(1):77–84, 1993.

PLATELET (THROMBOCYTE) COUNT, BLOOD

Norm:

Platelets (PLT)		SI Units
Adults	150,000–400,000/µl	150–400 × 10⁹/L
Critical low	<30,000/µl	<30 × 10⁹/L
Critical high	>1,000,000/µl	>1000 × 10⁹/L
Children		
Cord	100,000–290,000/µl	100–290 × 10⁹/L
Premature	100,000–300,000/µl	100–300 × 10⁹/L
Newborn	100,000–300,000/µl	100–300 × 10⁹/L
Neonate	150,000–390,000/µl	100–390 × 10⁹/L
3 months	260,000/µl	260 × 10⁹/L
Infant	200,000–473,000/µl	200–473 × 10⁹/L
1–10 years	150,000–450,000/µl	150–450 × 10⁹/L
Critical low	<20,000/µl	<20 × 10⁹/L
Critical high	>1,000,000/µl	>1000 × 10⁹/L

Increased: Anemia (hemolytic, iron-deficiency, postmenorrhagic, sickle cell), asphyxia, asplenism, carcinoma, cirrhosis, collagen disease, cryoglobulinemia, exercise, fractures, heart disease, hemorrhage (acute), idiopathic thrombocythemia, infection (acute), inflammation, leukemia (chronic granulocytic, chronic myelogenous), malignancy, multiple myeloma, myelofibrosis, myeloproliferative disease, pancreatitis (chronic), polycythemia vera, postoperatively, postpartum, postsplenectomy, pregnancy, pseudothrombocytosis, reticulocytosis, rheumatoid arthritis, surgery, and tuberculosis. Drugs include epinephrine, epinephrine bitartrate, epinephrine borate, epinephrine hydrochloride, and oral contraceptives.

Decreased: Anemia (aplastic, megaloblastic, pernicious), aplastic or hypoplastic bone marrow, autoimmune disorders, Bernard-Soulier syndrome, blood transfusion (incompatible, large amounts), burns (severe), carcinoma (metastatic), cirrhosis, clostridial infection, collagen diseases, defibrination syndrome, diphtheria, disseminated intravascular coagulation, extracorporeal circulation, Gaucher's disease, hemorrhage, hemolytic disease of the newborn, heparin therapy, histoplasmosis, hypersplenism, idiopathic thrombocytopenic purpura, lymphoproliferative disease, infections (acute), irradiation, leukemia (acute granulocytic, acute lymphocytic, monocytic), malaria, May-Hegglin anomaly, megakaryocytic hypoplasia, menstruation, multiple myeloma, myelofibrosis, postsplenectomy (2 months), radiation, septicemia, typhoid fever, uremia, and Wiskott-Aldrich syndrome. Drugs include acetazolamide, acetohexamide, amidopyrine, aminosalicylic acid, amphotericin B, ampicillin, antimony, antimony potassium tartrate, antineoplastics, arsenicals, aspirin, aurothioglucose, barbiturates, brompheniramine maleate, carbamazepine, chloramphenicol, chlorpropamide, chloroquine hydrochloride, chloroquine phosphate, chlorothiazide, colchicine, diazoxide, digitoxin, ethacrynate sodium, ethacrynic acid, ethoxzolamide, furosemide, gold sodium thiomalate, hydroxychloroquine sulfate, indomethacin, iothiouracil, isoniazid, mefenamic acid, meprobamate, methazolamide, methimazole, methyldopa, methyldopate hydrochloride, oral hypoglycemics, organic insecticides (some), oxyphenbutazone, oxytetracycline, oxytetracycline calcium, oxytetracycline hydrochloride, penicillamine, penicillins, phenylbutazone, phenytoin, phenytoin sodium, pyrimethamine, quinidine gluconate, quinidine polygalacturonate, quinidine sulfate, quinine sulfate, rifampin, salicylates, streptomycin sulfate, sulfonamides, thiazides, tolbutamide, tricyclic antidepressants, and vaccines.

Description: Platelets are non-nucleated, disk-shaped cells that function in hemostatic plug formation, clot retraction, and coagulation factor activation. They are produced by the bone marrow from megakaryocytes released into the bloodstream to function in hemostasis.

Professional Considerations:

1. Consent form NOT required.
2. Preparation:
   A. Tube: Lavender-top.
   B. Do NOT draw specimens during hemodialysis.
3. Procedure:
   A. Leave a tourniquet in place less than 1 minute.
   B. Draw a 5-ml blood sample.
   C. Gently invert the tube two or three times.
4. Postprocedure care:
   A. Send the specimen to the laboratory within 1 hour.
   B. Closely monitor the site for bleeding with clients with known thrombocytopenia.
5. Client and family teaching:
   A. If thrombocytopenia is present, avoid rough physical activity and bumping into furniture. Use a stool softener and avoid straining to have a bowel movement. Use a soft toothbrush and watch for and report signs of bleeding: bruising, petechiae, blood in the stool/urine/sputum, bleeding from invasive lines, bleeding gums, abnormal/excessive vaginal bleeding.
6. Factors that affect results:
   A. Reject hemolyzed specimens or specimens received more than 1 hour after collection.
   B. High altitudes, chronic cold weather, and exercise increase platelet counts.
7. Other data:
   A. The serum sample is stable at room temperature for 10 hours, may be refrigerated for up to 18 hours, and should not be frozen.

Bibliography:

Evenson DA, Stroncek DF, Pulkrabek S, et al.: Posttransfusion purpura following bone marrow transplantation. Transfusion *35*(8):688–693, 1995.

Kain ZN, Mayes LC, Pakes J, et al.: Thrombocytopenia in pregnant women who use cocaine. Am J Obstet Gynecol *173*(3, Pt 1):885–890, 1995.

Mughal TI: Primary thrombocytopenia: a current perspective. Stem Cells *13*(4):355–359, 1995.

PLP

(see Pyridoxal 5' Phosphate, Plasma)

P-METHOXYAMPHETAMINE

(see Amphetamines, Blood)

PNEUMOCYSTIS IFA, SERUM

Norm: Antibodies <1:16. No organisms observed.

Usage: Diagnosis of pneumocystis pneumonia associated with acquired immune deficiency syndrome (AIDS), immunosuppressed cancers, and organ transplants.

Description: *Pneumocystis carinii* are protozoan bacteria that produce an inflammatory infection within the lungs known as pneumocystis pneumonia. This type of pneumonia does not generally develop in humans unless they are immunocompromised by steroid therapy or cell-mediated immunodeficiencies. The alveolar exudate produced by pneumocystis is a proteinous material marked by cysts and trophozoites. The antigens present in the bacterial cell walls produce antibodies that circulate in the blood. These antibodies can be examined under a microscope when stained with immunofluorescent dyes and examined under ultraviolet light.

Professional Considerations:

1. Consent form NOT required.
2. Preparation:
   A. Tube: Red-top or pink-top or Corvac tube.
   B. Specimens MAY be drawn during hemodialysis.
3. Procedure:
   A. Draw a 10-ml blood sample.
4. Postprocedure care:
   A. Handle the specimen with caution because of potential cross-infection.
5. Client and family teaching:
   A. Results are normally available within 24 hours.
6. Factors that affect results:
   A. Immunofluorescent antibody titers are elevated in only about 30% of clients with pneumocystis.
   B. Serum antibody or antigen detection is not reliable for definitive diagnosis of *Pneumocystis carinii.*
7. Other data:
   A. A diagnostic bronchoscopy for tissue brushings should be performed if the serum specimen is positive for *P carinii.*

Bibliography:

Leigh TR, Millet MJ, Jameson B, et al.: *Pneumocystis carinii* antibody in health care workers caring for patients with AIDS. Thorax *48*(6):619–621, 1993.

POLIOMYELITIS 1, 2, 3 TITER, BLOOD

Norm: <1.8 is normal. A fourfold increase in the antibody titer between the acute and convalescent blood specimens is diagnostic for poliomyelitis. Presence of a high IgM titer may also indicate recent infection.

Usage: Identification and diagnosis of the enterovirus, polio, and differentiation of the serotype (1 = Grumhilde, 2 = Lansing, 3 = Leon).

Description: Poliomyelitis is an extremely contagious systemic infection resulting in necrotic and inflammatory lesions of the motor and autonomic neurons of the brain and spinal cord. Poliomyelitis usually presents as a systemic viremia with headache, fever, vomiting, and back and neck pain progressing in severity to a prominent paralysis and, possibly, death. The virus is transmitted by ingestion of contaminated water or food. The virus incubates and replicates in the lymphoid tissue of the tonsils, Peyer's patches, pharynx, and alimentary tract. Enteroviruses (polio) are excreted in the feces and can remain active outside of the human cells for months. The incubation period for poliomyelitis is 5–35 days, with acute symptoms occurring 7–12 days after exposure. Both acute and convalescent blood samples are tested to detect a rise in titer levels. Antigen-neutralization tests quantitate titers and serotype the virus from centrifuged serum. Type I, Brumhilde poliovirus, is associated with paralysis, chronic cardiomyopathy, diabetes, fetal malformation, myocarditis, and pericarditis. Oral vaccines available since the 1950s have decreased the incidence of this disease worldwide.

Professional Considerations:

1. Consent form NOT required.
2. Preparation:
   A. Tube: Red-top, red/gray-top, or gold-top.
   B. Specimens MAY be drawn during hemodialysis.

3. Procedure:
   A. Draw an 8- to 10-ml (adults) or a 3- to 4-ml (pediatric) blood sample.
4. Postprocedure care:
   A. None.
5. Client and family teaching:
   A. Strict isolation precautions may be instituted if serum titers indicate infection secondary to the extreme contagiousness.
6. Factors that affect results:
   A. In 50% of people with poliomyelitis, the serum titers have already peaked before testing.

7. Other data:
   A. Use extreme caution when handling or transporting samples and wash hands well after handling a sample.
   B. Polio virus is human-specific.

Bibliography:

Cohen-Abbo A, Culley BS, Sannella EC, et al.: Diagnostic test for poliovirus infections: a comparison of neutralization and immunofluorescence for the identification and typing of stool isolates. J Virol Methods *52*(1–2):35–39, 1995.

PORPHYRINS, QUANTITATIVE, BLOOD

Norm:

		SI Units
Total erythrocyte		
Porphyrins	<31 µg/dl	
ALA	<1 mg/dl	
Coproporphyrin	0.5–2.3 mg/dl	
Protoporphyrin	4–52 mg/dl	0.07–0.93 µmol/L
Uroporphyrin	Negative to trace	Negative to trace

Increased ALA: Chemical toxicity, cirrhosis (alcoholic), lead poisoning, and porphyrias.

Increased Coproporphyrin: Anemia (hemolytic, pernicious, sideroblastic), cirrhosis (alcoholic), coproporphyria (erythropoietic), erythroid hyperplasia, exercise (extreme), fever, hemochromatosis, Hodgkin's disease, lead poisoning, leukemia, myocardial infarction (acute), poliomyelitis (acute), porphyria (congenital erythropoietic), protoporphyria (erythropoietic), thyrotoxicosis, and vitamin deficiencies.

Increased Protoporphyrin: Anemia (hemolytic, sideroblastic), carbon tetrachloride and benzene toxicity, erythropoiesis, infection, iron deficiency, lead poisoning, protoporphyria (erythropoietic), and thalassemia.

Increased Uroporphyrin: Cirrhosis, lead poisoning, and porphyria (acute, intermittent, congenital erythropoietic).

Decreased ALA: Not applicable.

Decreased Coproporphyrin: Not applicable.

Decreased Protoporphyrin: Anemia (megaloblastic).

Decreased Uroporphyrin: Not applicable.

Description: Porphyrins are compounds necessary for heme synthesis in hemoglobin metabolism. ALA (delta-aminovulinic acid) is the basic building block of porphyrins and is involved in the synthesis of coproporphyrin and protoporphyrin. Coproporphyrin is the main porphyrin found in urine, while protoporphyrin is the main porphyrin found in erythrocytes. When iron is added to protoporphyrin, the final heme molecule is formed. As the hemoglobin is eventually broken down, these products used for heme synthesis again appear in the blood, urine, and stool as hemoglobin breakdown products. Clients with one of the congenital or acquired diseases classified as the "porphyrias" secrete and excrete increased amounts of these compounds. The diseases are characterized by neurologic abnormalities, acute abdominal pain, photosensitivity, or psychiatric disturbances. This test is used most frequently in conjunction with the measurement of urine porphyrin levels to differentiate the etiology and type of porphyria occurring.

Professional Considerations:

1. Consent form NOT required.
2. Preparation:
   A. Tube: Green-top, lavender-top, or black-top.
   B. Do NOT draw during hemodialysis.
   C. *See Client and family teaching.*
3. Procedure:
   A. Draw a 3-ml blood sample without hemolysis.
4. Postprocedure care:
   A. None.
5. Client and family teaching:
   A. Do not drink alcohol for 24 hours before testing.
   B. Clients with positive test results should avoid ethanol, barbiturates, and anticonvulsants that might cause an acute attack of neurologic/psychotic porphyria (elevated ALA).
   C. Clients with positive test results should avoid sunlight.
   D. Genetic counseling may be necessary for the inherited form of porphyria.
6. Factors that affect results:
   A. Hemolysis of the specimen invalidates the results.
   B. Increased levels may occur during menstruation or pregnancy.
7. Other data:
   A. *See also Protophorphyrin, Free Erythrocyte, Blood; and Coproporphyrin, Urine.*

Bibliography:

Leung FY, Bradley C, Pellar TG: Reference intervals for blood lead and evaluation of zinc protoporphyrin as a screening tool for lead toxicity. Clin Biochem *26*(6):491–496, 1993.

Long C, Smyth SJ, Woolf, J, et al.: Detection of latent variegate porphyria by fluorescence emission spectroscopy of plasma. Brit J Dermatol *129*(1): 9–13, 1993.

POSITRON EMISSION TOMOGRAPHY (PET), DIAGNOSTIC

Norm: Requires interpretation according to the type of study being performed.

Usage: Enables noninvasive regional tissue physiology study of metabolic changes in body tissues. Comparison of cerebral blood flow and energy metabolism; evaluation for leakage of the blood-brain barrier; study of brain pharmacology; evaluation of brain hemodynamics in cerebrovascular disease; localization of seizure foci in clients with focal seizures; evaluation of regional myocardial blood flow and metabolism; study of the distribution of pulmonary edema; and study of solid tumor proliferation, blood flow, glucose, and oxygen utilization.

Description: Positron emission tomography (PET) is a noninvasive radiographic method for studying blood flow and metabolic changes occurring in specific organs or regions of the body tissues. It involves the injection or inhalation of gamma ray-emitting, biologically compatible radioisotopes and the creation of images of radioisotope distribution in the body. As the radioisotopes disintegrate, they emit positrons, which are positively charged particles similar to electrons. As the positrons are captured by electrons, both are destroyed, resulting in the emission of two photons, which travel outward in opposite directions. The photons are detected simultaneously by the PET camera, an event known as a "coincidence." The summation of these coincidences allows for the creation of a continuous map of the metabolic activity of the body. A computer then creates pictures of cross-sections of the body area studied, which show brighter areas according to the amount of radioisotope present.

Some examples of radioisotopes include oxygen-15, nitrogen-13, carbon-11, and fluorine-18, which are labeled onto substances such as water, carbon dioxide, or glucose. Because the radioisotopes are biologically compatible, they take the place of the body's chemical elements (e.g., oxygen, nitrogen or fluorine), and the resulting scan gives a true representation of the physiologic function of the body processes. The choice of radioisotope and material to be labeled is based on the body function to be studied. For example, blood flow is studied using O-15-labeled HO, glucose metabolism is studied using F-18-labeled glucose, tissue perfusion is studied using N-13-labeled NH, and anaerobic metabolism is studied using C-11-labeled acetate. Some conditions in which the use of PET has been studied include Alzheimer's disease, asthma, brain tumors, cerebral atrophy, cerebrovascular disorders, chronic obstructive pulmonary disease, coronary artery disease, epilepsy, head trauma, Huntington's disease, myocardial infarction, obsessive compulsive disorder, pulmonary edema, schizophrenia, and unstable angina.

Professional Considerations:
1. Consent form MAY be required.

Risks:
Hematoma, infection.

Contraindications:
During pregnancy and breast-feeding.

2. Preparation:
   A. A premedication may be prescribed to be given prior to transport to the nuclear medicine department.
   B. Diuretics should be withheld prior to the study unless an indwelling urinary catheter is present or will be inserted.
   C. If pelvic imaging will be performed, an indwelling urinary catheter should be inserted.
   D. The client should have a meal prior to the procedure. Diabetics should be given their morning insulin prior to the procedure.
   E. If abdominal imaging is indicated, a bowel preparation may be prescribed.
   F. *See Client and family teaching.*
3. Procedure:
   A. The client is placed in a supine position on the scanning table, with an arm supported in extension.
   B. Intravenous access is established.
   C. A heparin flush solution is slowly infused.
   D. An arterial line may be inserted for some procedures.
   E. For brain scans, a polyform molded face mask is placed over the temporal level of the face and secured to the headrest to immobilize the client's head. The mask is marked with a reference point to ensure exact repeat positioning for any necessary future PET studies.
   F. The scanning table is moved into position within the lumen of the positron emission scanner.
   G. Once the client is positioned, he or she must remain motionless throughout the study.
   H. Some studies are conducted by having the client inhale the radioisotope. Others use intravenous injection.
   I. An example of the steps involved in one type of scan follows.
   J. *Cardiac PET:*
      i. O-15-labeled HO is injected intravenously and a 15-minute test scan is conducted to verify proper positioning.
      ii. A 30-minute transmission scan is then performed to correct for the attenuation of the chest and lungs.
      iii. N-13-labeled NH is injected intravenously and allowed to equilibrate for 3 minutes. Then a PET study is performed for approximately 30 minutes to study cardiac tissue perfusion.
      iv. Finally, glucose metabolism of the heart is studied. If the client is a diabetic, with a glucose level >150 mg/dl, insulin may be given before this step. If the client has a low blood glucose, either oral glucose or intravenous 50% dextrose in water will be given. Fluorodeoxyglucose (FDG) is injected intravenously to study glucose metabolism of the heart. After waiting 30 minutes for the FDG to circulate, a 30-minute PET study is performed.
4. Postprocedure care:
   A. The arterial line, if inserted for the PET study, is discontinued, and the site should be monitored for the development of hematoma.
5. Client and family teaching:
   A. The client must remain motionless in an enclosed space for 1–3 hours.
   B. Wear comfortable clothing to the test.
   C. The client may bring a cassette tape to listen to during the study.
   D. Do not drink large quantities of fluid or caffeine-containing beverages within 2 hours prior to the study unless you have been informed that an indwelling catheter will be inserted.
   E. Have a meal prior to the procedure.
   F. The client may need a bowel preparation if abdominal imaging is indicated.
6. Factors that affect results:
   A. Hypoglycemia may alter the results of PET of glucose metabolism.
   B. Movement more than about 1 cm may blur the resulting pictures. The ability of the client to remain motionless in an enclosed space affects whether or not an accurate study can be obtained.
   C. Insulin-dependent diabetics must have insulin administered the day of the study if glucose metabolism will be a focus of PET.
7. Other data:
   A. PET takes 1–3 hours. The half-life of the specific radioisotope used affects the length of the study.
   B. Claustrophobia may occur during the procedure.

Bibliography:

Marchal G, Serrati C, Rox P, et al.: PET imaging of cerebral perfusion and oxygen consumption in acute ischemic stroke: relation to outcome. Lancet *341*:925–927, 1993.

POTASSIUM HYDROXIDE PREPARATION (KOH WET MOUNT PREPARATION), DIAGNOSTIC

Norm: Negative; no fungus elements identified.

Usage: Identification and diagnosis of fungal dermatitis and infections.

Description: Fungi are slow-growing, eukaryotic organisms that can grow on living and nonliving organic materials, and are subdivided into yeasts and molds. Only a few fungi species infect humans. Normal host defense mechanisms limit the damage they cause superficially. The KOH preparation allows for direct microscopic examination of skin, nail, hair, sputum, abscess exudate, or biopsy tissue for the presence of fungal fragments. A 10–20% KOH solution mixed with the specimen clears away debris, making visualization of mycelial filaments, hyphae, spores, spherules, and budding yeast cells possible under a low-power microscope.

Professional Considerations:

1. Consent form NOT required.
2. Preparation:
   A. Obtain KOH preparation, methylene blue, a clear glass slide, a glass coverslip, a teasing needle, and a heat source.
3. Procedure:
   A. Place one drop of 10–20% KOH preparation and, if indicated, methylene blue on a clear glass slide.
   B. Using a needle or scalpel, gently scrape the skin, nails, tissue, or wound, or gather several strands of hair for a specimen and place them on a glass slide.
   C. Using a teasing needle, separate the specimen to make a thin preparation on the slide.
   D. Cover the specimen with a coverslip and pass the slide over a low flame two

or three times. Gently press on the coverslip several times with a teasing needle until the specimen lies flat on the slide.
   E. Allow the slide to cool.
4. Postprocedure care:
   A. Write the specimen source on the laboratory requisition.
   B. Send the specimen to the microbiology laboratory.
5. Client and family teaching:
   A. Antifungal medication may be prescribed if results are positive.
   B. Deep coughs are necessary to produce sputum, rather than saliva. To produce the proper specimen, take several breaths in, without fully exhaling each, then expel sputum with a "cascade cough."
6. Factors that affect results:
   A. False-positive results may occur if the specimen is contaminated with cotton fibers, cellulose fibers, or cholesterol deposits, which may be mistaken for hyphae.
7. Other data:
   A. Handle the specimen with care to prevent self-contamination.
   B. Dimethyl sulfoxide (DMSO) should be added to the slide if the specimen to be examined is nail.
   C. Adding glycerol to the KOH will enable preservation of the slide for a few days if it cannot be examined promptly.

Bibliography:

Abbot J: Clinical and microscopic diagnosis of vaginal yeast infection: a prospective analysis. Ann Em Med 25(5):587–592, 1995.

De Kick CA, Samplers GO, Knottnerus JA: Diagnosis and management of cases of suspected dermatomycosis in The Netherlands: influence of general practice based potassium hydroxide testing. Brit J Gen Prac 45(396):349–351, 1995.

POTASSIUM, SERUM

Norm:

		SI Units
Adult	3.5–5.3 mEq/L	3.5–5.3 mmol/L
Premature infant		
Cord blood	5.0–10.2 mEq/L	5.0–10.2 mmol/L
2 days	3.0–6.0 mEq/L	3.0–6.0 mmol/L
Full-term newborn		
Cord blood	5.6–12.0 mEq/L	5.6–12.0 mmol/L
Newborn	3.7–5.0 mEq/L	3.7–5.0 mmol/L
Infant	4.1–5.3 mEq/L	4.1–5.3 mmol/L
Child	3.4–4.7 mEq/L	3.4–4.7 mmol/L
Panic values		
Adult	<2.5 mEq/L	<2.5 mmol/L
	or >6.6 mEq/L	or >6.6 mmol/L
Newborn	<2.5 mEq/L	<2.5 mmol/L
	or >8.1 mEq/L	or >8.1 mmol/L

Panic Level Symptoms and Treatment:

Hyperkalemia Symptoms: Irritability, diarrhea, cramps, oliguria, difficulty speaking, cardiac dysrhythmias including peaked T-waves and ventricular fibrillation/tachycardia.

Hyperkalemia Treatment:
> Provide continuous ECG monitoring.
> Administer sodium polystyrene sulfonate.
> Administer intravenous insulin/dextrose.
> Administer sodium bicarbonate.
> Administer calcium chloride or gluconate.
> Both hemodialysis and peritoneal dialysis WILL remove potassium.

Hypokalemia Symptoms: Malaise, thirst, polyurea, anorexia, weak pulse, low blood pressure, vomiting, decreased reflexes, ECG changes, including depressed T-waves and ventricular ectopy.

Hypokalemia Treatment: Potassium replacement.

Increased: Acidosis, Addison's disease, adrenocortical insufficiency, anemia (hemolytic), anxiety, asthma, burns, dialysis (hemodialysis or peritoneal), diet (excessive potassium intake), dysrhythmia, hemolysis, hypoventilation, increased osmolality, infection (acute), ketoacidosis, leukocytosis, malignant hyperthermia (early), massive rapid red blood cell transfusion, metabolic acidosis, muscle necrosis, near-drowning, obstruction (intestinal), ostomies, pneumonia, pseudohypoaldosteronism, renal failure, renal hypertension, sepsis, shock, status epilepticus, syndrome of inappropriate antidiuretic hormone secretion (SIADHS), thrombocytosis, tissue trauma, uremia, and Waterhouse-Friderichsen syndrome. Drugs include aldosterone antagonists, captopril, cyclophosphamide, digoxin, ephedrine, ephedrine sulfate, epinephrine, estrogens, heparin calcium, heparin sodium, histamine, ibuprofen, indomethacin, lithium, mannitol, methicillin, methicillin sodium, nonsteroidal anti-inflammatory agents, potassium bicarbonate, potassium chloride, potassium citrate, potassium gluconate, propranolol, spironolactone, succinylcholine, tetracyclines, timolol maleate, and triamterene.

Decreased: Acute tubular necrosis (diuretic phase), alcoholism, aldosteronism (primary), alkalosis, anorexia, barium intoxication, Bartter's syndrome, bradycardia, cancer (colon), cerebral palsy, cholera, cirrhosis (chronic), congestive heart failure, Crohn's disease, Cushing's disease, dehydration, diabetes insipidus, diabetes mellitus, diarrhea, dumping syndrome, dysrhythmias, Fanconi's syndrome, fever, fistulas, folic acid deficiency, hyperaldosteronism, hyperalimentation, hypercorticoadrenalism, hypertension, hypomagnesemia, hypothermia, hypovolemia, hysterectomy, kwashiorkor, ketoacidosis, laxative abuse, lymphoma, malabsorption, malignant hyperthermia (late-stage), metabolic alkalosis, nephritis, organic brain syndrome, ostomies, pancreatitis (acute), paralytic ileus, postsigmoidoscopy, pseudoaldosteronism, pyelonephritis (chronic), pyloric obstruction, renal tubular acidosis, salicylate intoxication, salt-losing nephropathy, sweating, suction (gastric), surgery (postoperatively), starvation, stress, toxic shock syndrome, ureterosigmoidostomy, villous adenoma, vipoma, vomiting, and Zollinger-Ellison syndrome (with diarrhea). Drugs include acetazolamide, albuterol, ammonium chloride, amphotericin, aspirin, bisacodyl, bronchodilators, carbenicillin, chlorthalidone, corticosteroids, corticotropin, EDTA, ethacrynic acid, furosemide, gentamicin sulfate, glucose, insulin, licorice, mercurial diuretics, penicillin G, piperacillin, salicylates, sodium bicarbonate, sodium chloride, succinylcholine chloride (in children), thiazides, thiopental, ticarcillin, and trimethaphan camsylate.

Description: Potassium (K^+) is the major intracellular cation. The body obtains potassium through dietary ingestion, and the kidneys either preserve or excrete it depending upon cellular need. Potassium is responsible for the regulation of cellular water balance, electrical conduction in muscle cells, and acid-based homeostasis. Although the majority of potassium is stored and used within tissue cells, serum potassium analysis can be helpful in evaluating electrolyte balance. Serum potassium levels are used in the evaluation of clients with cardiac dysrhythmias, renal dysfunction, mental confusion, gastrointestinal distress, and intravenous replacement therapy.

Professional Considerations:

1. Consent form NOT required.
2. Preparation:
   A. Tube: Red-top, red/gray-top, or gold-top or green-top.
   B. Do NOT draw specimens during hemodialysis.
3. Procedure:
   A. Draw the specimen without using a tourniquet.
   B. Using a 20-gauge or larger needle, draw a 1-ml blood sample.
   C. Do not aspirate strongly or push the plunger into the vacuum tube too forcefully.
   D. Avoid hemolysis.
4. Postprocedure care:
   A. Write the collection time on the laboratory requisition.
   B. Note on the laboratory requisition if the client is receiving potassium by pill, liquid, or intravenously.
   C. Send the specimen to the chemistry laboratory for spinning within 1 hour of collection.
   D. Serum and plasma must be separated from the red cells or elevated results may occur.
5. Client and family teaching:
   A. The client must follow the prescribed dosage of potassium.
   B. Foods high in potassium are apricots, bananas, meats, potatoes, prunes, and tomatoes.
6. Factors that affect results:
   A. Reject hemolyzed specimens or specimens received more than 1 hour after collection.
   B. Use of a tourniquet and pumping the hand prior to obtaining a venous sample can increase the laboratory value by up to 20%.
   C. Do NOT draw the specimen from a site where an intravenous infusion exists.
   D. Clients with elevated white blood counts and platelet counts may have falsely elevated serum potassium levels.
   E. Incomplete separation of the serum from the clot may cause falsely elevated results.
   F. Acidemia causes potassium to move from cells into the extracellular fluid in exchange for hydrogen ions moving intracellularly.
   G. Values are 0.2–0.4 mEq/L higher in samples collected in the afternoon and early evening.
7. Other data:
   A. For elevated potassium levels, an arterial blood gas should be evaluated for acidemia.

Bibliography:

Vanek VW, Seballos RM, Chong D, et al.: Serum potassium concentrations in trauma patients. South Med J 87(1):41–46, 1994.

POTASSIUM, URINE

Norm:

		SI Units
Adult	25–123 mEq/24 hours (intake-dependent)	25–123 mmol/day
Child	17–57 mEq/24 hours	17–57 mmol/day

Increased: Alkalosis, Cushing's disease, dehydration, diabetic ketoacidosis, diet (excessive potassium intake), fever, head trauma, hyperaldosteronism, hypokalemia, renal tubular acidosis, renal failure (chronic), salicylate intoxication, and starvation. Drugs include acetazolamide, ammonium chloride, amphotericin, fosinopril, glucocorticoids, loop diuretics, mercurial diuretics, penicillin, potassium, and thiazide diuretics.

Decreased: Addison's disease, diarrhea, hyperkalemia, hypomagnesemia, malabsorption syndrome, nephrotic syndrome, potassium deficiency, renal failure (acute), and syndrome of inappropriate antidiuretic hormone secretion (SIADHS). Drugs include laxatives, epinephrine, levarterenol, and general anesthetic agents.

Description: Potassium (K^+) is the major intracellular cation. The body obtains potassium through dietary ingestion, and the kidneys either preserve or excrete it, depending on cellular need. Potassium is responsible for the regulation of cellular water balance, electrical conduction in muscle cells, and acid-based homeostasis. A 24-hour urine collection is obtained to determine excreted potassium levels. Urine potassium levels are helpful in the assessment of endocrine abnormalities and renal tubular function.

Professional Considerations:

1. Consent form NOT required.
2. Preparation:
   A. Obtain a 3-L container without preservatives, or a pediatric urine collection device/bag and tape.
   B. Write the beginning time of the collection on the laboratory requisition.
   C. Note diuretic or glucocorticoid therapy on the laboratory requisition.
3. Procedure:
   A. Discard the first morning-urine specimen.
   B. Save all urine voided for 24 hours in a refrigerated, clean, 3-L container without preservatives. Document the quantity of urine output during the specimen collection period. Include urine voided at the end of the 24-hour period. For catheterized clients, keep the drainage bag on ice and empty urine into the collection container hourly.
   C. *Pediatric/infant specimen collection:*
      i. Place the child in a supine position with the knees flexed and the hips externally rotated and abducted.
      ii. Cleanse, rinse, and thoroughly dry the perineal area.
      iii. To prevent the child from removing the collection device/bag, a diaper may be placed over the genital area.
      iv. *Females:* Tape the pediatric collection device/bag to the perineum. Starting at the area between the anus and vagina, apply the device/bag in an anterior direction.
      v. *Males:* Place the pediatric collection device/bag over the penis and scrotum and tape it to the perineal area.
4. Postprocedure care:
   A. Compare the urine quantity in the specimen container with the urinary output record for the test. If the specimen contains less urine than was recorded as output, some of the sample may have been discarded, invalidating the test.
   B. Document the quantity of urine and the collection ending time on the laboratory requisition.
   C. Send the specimen to the laboratory and refrigerate it.
5. Client and family teaching:
   A. Save all the urine voided in the 24-hour period and urinate before defecating to avoid loss of urine. If any urine is accidentally discarded, discard the entire specimen and restart the collection the next day.
6. Factors that affect results:
   A. All urine voided for the 24-hour period must be included to avoid a falsely low result.

7. Other data:
   A. Urine potassium levels exhibit a diurnal variation, with higher levels occurring at night.

Bibliography:

Cochran, L: What you need to know about potassium imbalances. Nursing 95:32H–32J, February 1995.

PPD
(see Mantoux Skin Test, Diagnostic)

PPLP
(see Pyridoxal 5′ Phosphate, Plasma)

PRA, PLASMA
(see Renin, Plasma)

PRAZEPAM
(see Benzodiazepines, Plasma and Urine)

PREALBUMIN
(see Transthyretin, Serum)

PRECIPITIN TEST AGAINST HUMAN SPERM AND BLOOD, VAGINAL SWAB

Norm: Negative.

Usage: Used to identify the presence of semen or blood of human origin from vaginal secretions following sexual assault or rape.

Description: Human semen contains specific antibodies that are unique to the species. When vaginal secretions containing semen or blood are mixed with antisera solution, an antigen-antibody reaction or linkage will occur if the source is human sperm. The reaction is the result of the antigen binding to the antibody and forming an insoluble precipitate. This test can be performed by mixing the vaginal aspirate with antisera solution in a test tube or capillary tube. If an antigen-antibody reaction occurs, the cells will clump and fall to the bottom of the test tube, indicating that semen or blood present in the sample is from a human source. The result of the semen precipitation test is recorded as permanent evidence that coital relations occurred. Vaginal aspirations can also be tested for hemagglutination of ABO blood typing.

Professional Considerations:

1. Consent form NOT required.
2. Preparation:
   A. Obtain a rape examination tray.
   B. Use a speculum rinsed with 0.9% saline for examination and specimen collection.
3. Procedure:
   A. The collection of specimens is governed by the laws of each state.
   B. Follow the directions in the "Sex Evidence Kit" according to the requirements of the state.
4. Postprocedure care:
   A. Follow directions in the "Sex Evidence Kit" for the proper chain of command of evidence.
   B. The specimen is generally given to the police and forwarded to the proper authorities for evidence testing.
5. Client and family teaching:
   A. Vaginal douching or bathing decreases the likelihood of obtaining positive results.
   B. Survivors of sexual assault should be referred to appropriate crisis counseling agencies as well as for gynecologic follow-up.
   C. Referral for HIV testing should be reviewed and offered to all sexual assault victims.
   D. Preventive treatment for *Chlamydia*, gonorrhea, and syphilis should be provided to all survivors of sexual assault.
   E. The option of postcoital contraceptive should be reviewed with all survivors of sexual assault.
6. Factors that affect results:
   A. The laboratory must receive vaginal washing immediately, or else the specimen should be frozen.
7. Other data:
   A. No universal threshold exists for evidence of intercourse or rape. A decrease in acid phosphatase after intercourse varies from hours to 4 days.

Bibliography:

Nichols DH, Sweeney PJ: Ambulatory Gynecology. Philadelphia, JB Lippincott, pp 215–221, 1995.

PREGNANCY TEST (HCG, UCG), ROUTINE, SERUM

Norm:

HCG		SI Units
Males	<5.0 mIU/ml	<5.0 IU/L
Females		
Nonpregnant	<5.0 mIU/ml	<5.0 IU/L
≤1 week gestation	5–50 mIU/ml	5–50 IU/L
2 weeks gestation	50–500 mIU/ml	50–500 IU/L
3 weeks gestation	100–10,000 mIU/ml	100–10,000 IU/L
4 weeks gestation	1000–30,000 mIU/ml	1000–30,000 IU/L
5 weeks gestation	3500–115,000 mIU/ml	3500–115,000 IU/L
6–8 weeks gestation	12,000–270,000 mIU/ml	12,000–270,000 IU/L
12 weeks gestation	15,000–220,000 mIU/ml	15,000–220,000 IU/L

Increased: Breast cancer, bronchogenic carcinoma, choriocarcinoma, embryonal carcinoma, gastric carcinoma, hepatocarcinoma, hydatidiform mole, malignant melanoma, multiple myeloma, pancreatic cancer, pregnancy, seminoma, teratoma, and trophoblastic tumor.

Decreased: Abortion (threatened, actual) and ectopic pregnancy.

Description: Human chorionic gonadotropin (HCG) is a hormone uniquely secreted by the placenta of a fertilized ovum implanted in the uterine wall. HCG production begins 8–10 days after conception or during day 21–23 of the cycle. It reaches peak concentration at 8–12 weeks' gestation and then gradually decreases until returning to normal within 3–4 days after normal full-term delivery. This test can be most accurately performed 2 days after missed menses up to 3 weeks.

Testing is performed by incubating serum with antihuman chorionic gonadotropin (anti-HCG). If HCG is present in the sample, it combines with the anti-HCG antibodies and inactivates them. When these inactivated antibodies are exposed to the indicator, red or latex cells coated with HCG, clumping of the cells does not occur, resulting in a positive pregnancy test. If clumping does occur, the test is negative.

Professional Considerations:

1. Consent form NOT required.
2. Preparation:
   A. Tube: Red-top, red/gray-top, or gold-top.
   B. Specimens MAY be drawn during hemodialysis.
   C. *See Client and family teaching.*
3. Procedure:
   A. Draw a 1-ml blood sample.
4. Postprocedure care:
   A. None.
5. Client and family teaching:
   A. May help differentiate actual pregnancy from an ectopic pregnancy in conduction with an ultrasound.
   B. Avoid medications such as anticonvulsants, antiparkinsonian agents, hypnotics, and tranquilizers, which may cause a false-positive result.
6. Factors that affect results:
   A. False-positive results may be due to incorrect performance or handling of the test, excessive production of luteinizing hormone (LH) of the pituitary gland, absence of gonadal hormones in menopausal women, or HCG-producing tumors.
   B. False-negative results may be due to the test being performed too early in pregnancy.
7. Other data:
   A. Although not usually present in healthy males or nonpregnant females, elevated levels of HCG may be detected in these clients with certain malignant tumors.
   B. *See also Human Chorionic Gonadotropin, Beta Subunit, Serum.*

Bibliography:

Smikle CB, Sorem KA, Wians FH Jr, et al.: Measuring quantitative serum human chorionic gonadotropin. Variations in levels between kits. J Reprod Health *40*(6):439–445, 1995.

Tyrey L: Human chorionic gonadotropin: properties and assay methods. Sem Oncol *22*(2):121–129, 1995.

Wyte CD: Diagnostic modalities in the pregnant patient. Emerg Med Clin North Am *12*(1):9–43, 1994.

PREGNANETRIOL, URINE

Norm:

		SI Units
Adult female	0.5–2.0 mg/24 hours	1.5–5.9 mmol/day
Adult male	0.4–2.4 mg/24 hours	1.2–7.1 mmol/day
Child		
≤6 years	<0.2 mg/24 hours	<0.6 mmol/day
7–16 years	0.3–1.1 mg/24 hours	0.9–3.3 mmol/day

Increased: Adrenogenital syndrome, congenital adrenocortical hyperplasia, hirsutism, Stein-Leventhal syndrome, 21-hydroxylase deficiency, tumor (ovarian, adrenal cortex), and virilization.

Description: Pregnanetriol, a metabolite of 17-hydroxyprogesterone, is involved in the synthesis of adrenal corticoids and is normally excreted in the urine in only small amounts. Increased urinary excretion is caused by a deficiency in the enzyme that converts 17-hydroxyprogesterone to cortisol. The decreased cortisol production results in increased adrenocorticotropic hormone (ACTH), which leads to increased serum hydroxyprogesterone. This in turn, stimulates the release of adrenal androgens. As the increased amounts of hydroxyprogesterone are metabolized, urine pregnanetriol levels increase. This test is most commonly abnormal in adrenogenital syndrome, which results in symptoms of hypertension, craving for salt, premature physical development of sexual characteristics in males, failure to thrive in infants, and pseudohermaphrodism (females with male genitalia).

Professional Considerations:

1. Consent form NOT required.
2. Preparation:
   A. Obtain a clean, 3-L container without preservative or to which acetic acid preservative has been added.
   B. For pediatric/infant specimens, obtain a pediatric urine collection device/bag and tape.
   C. *See Client and family teaching.*
3. Procedure:
   A. Discard the first morning-urine specimen.
   B. Save all the urine voided for 24 hours in a refrigerated, clean, 3-L container without preservative or to which acetic acid preservative has been added. Doc-

ument the quantity of urine output during the specimen collection period. Include urine voided at the end of the 24-hour period. For catheterized clients, keep the drainage bag on ice and empty the urine into the collection container hourly.

C. *Pediatric/infant specimen collection:*
  i. Place the child in a supine position with the knees flexed and the hips externally rotated and abducted.
  ii. Cleanse, rinse, and thoroughly dry the perineal area.
  iii. To prevent the child from removing the collection device/bag, a diaper may be placed over the genital area.
  iv. *Females:* Tape the pediatric collection device/bag to the perineum. Starting at the area between the anus and vagina, apply the device/bag in an anterior direction.
  v. *Males:* Place the pediatric collection device/bag over the penis and scrotum and tape it to the perineal area.

4. Postprocedure care:
A. Compare the urine quantity in the specimen container with the urinary output record for the test. If the specimen contains less urine than was recorded as output, some of the sample may have been discarded, invalidating the test.
B. Document the urine quantity on the laboratory requisition.

5. Client and family teaching:
A. Save all the urine voided in the 24-hour period and urinate before defecating to avoid loss of urine. If any urine is accidentally discarded, discard the entire specimen and restart the collection the next day.
B. Avoid muscular exercise before or during the specimen collection period.

6. Factors that affect results:
A. All the urine voided for the 24-hour period must be included to avoid a falsely low result.
B. Results are invalid if the specimen was not refrigerated throughout the collection period.
C. Exercise during the collection period causes increased androgen release.

7. Other data:
A. In 21-hydroxylase deficiency, there is also an increase in serum 17-hydroxyprogesterone and urinary 17-ketosteroids.

Bibliography:

Lim YJ, Yong AB, Warne GL, et al.: Urinary 17 alpha-hydroxyprogesterone in management of 21-hydroxylase deficiency. J Pediatr Child Health *31*(1): 47–50, 1995.

PREKALLIKREIN, PLASMA
(see Factor, Fletcher, Plasma)

PRENATAL SCREEN, DIAGNOSTIC
(see ABO Group and Rh Type, Blood; and Coombs', Indirect, Serum)

PRIMIDONE (MYSOLINE), SERUM

Norm: Negative.

		SI Units
Therapeutic levels		
Adults	5–12 µg/ml	23–55 µmol/L
Children <5 years	7–10 µg/ml	32–46 µmol/L
Panic level	>24 µg/ml	>110 µmol/L

Panic Level Symptoms and Treatment:

Symptoms: Decreased level of consciousness, ataxia, anemia.

Treatment:
Discontinue primidone.
Protect airway.
Support hemodynamics.
Hemodialysis WILL remove primidone.
Treat anemia with folic acid or vitamin B_{12}.

Drugs that may speed the conversion of primidone to its metabolite phenobarbital include phenytoin and phenytoin sodium.

Usage: Monitoring the effectiveness of primidone therapy and prevention of primidone toxicity.

Increased: Drugs include carbamazepine, isoniazid, monoamine oxidase (MAO) inhibitors, phenobarbital, and sodium valproate.

Decreased: Subtherapeutic treatment. Drugs include acetazolamide.

Description: Primidone is an anticonvulsant used in the treatment of temporal lobe epilepsy and other grand mal seizures that are resistant to other anticonvulsants. When metabolized by the liver, it breaks down into phenobarbital and phenylethylmalonamide. These two metabolites have a synergistic ability to raise the seizure threshold. The metabolites of primidone are excreted by the kidneys. Half-life is 4–12 hours in adults and 4–6 hours in children. Peak time varies from 0.5–0.9 hours. Steady-state levels are reached after 16–60 hours in adults and after 20–30 hours in children.

Professional Considerations:

1. Consent form NOT required.
2. Preparation:
   A. Tube: Red-top or green-top.
   B. Do NOT draw during hemodialysis.
3. Procedure:
   A. Draw a 5-ml blood sample just prior to administration of primidone (trough level).
4. Postprocedure care:
   A. Monitor for panic level symptoms (see above).
   B. Monitor for convulsions if the drug is discontinued.

5. Client and family teaching:
   A. Take medication as prescribed and report any adverse side effects such as sedation, dizziness, nausea, vomiting, nystagmus, and loss of libido.
   B. For accidental overdose, teach the client and family early warning symptoms of overdose (see above).
   C. For intentional overdose, refer the client and family for crisis intervention.
6. Factors that affect results:
   A. Reject hemolyzed or lipemic specimens to avoid falsely elevated results.
   B. Peak levels occur 2–4 hours after the oral dose.
7. Other data:
   A. Data suggest there is no evidence of good seizure control with levels above 10 μg/ml.

Bibliography:

Miller CA, Gaylor M, Lorch V, et al.: The use of primidone in neonates with theophylline-resistant apnea. Am J Dis Child *147*(2):183–186, 1993.

Romanyshyn LA, Wichmann JK, Kucharczyk, et al.: Simultaneous determination of felbamate, primidone, phenobarbital, carbamazepine, two carbamazepine metabolites, phenytoin, and one phenytoin metabolite in human plasma by high-performance liquid chromatography. Ther Drug Monit *16*(1):90–99, 1994.

PROACCELERIN, BLOOD
(see Factor V, Blood)

PROCAINAMIDE, SERUM

Norm: Negative.

		SI Units
Procainamide	4.9–12 μg/ml	20.7–50.8 μmol/L
Toxic level	16–20 μg/ml	67.7–84.6 μmol/L
Panic level	>20 μg/ml	>84.6 μmol/L
Procainamide + NAPA	<30 μg/ml	<126.7 μmol/L
Toxic level	>30 μg/ml	>126.7 μmol/L

Toxic Level Symptoms and Treatment:

Symptoms: Torsades de Pointes, nausea, vomiting, hepatic disturbances, agranulocytosis.

Treatment:
Protect airway.
Support hemodynamic stability.
Force emesis.
Do gastric lavage.
Administer infusion of a molar sodium lactate solution.

Hemodialysis WILL, but peritoneal dialysis will NOT, remove procainamide.

Increased Procainamide: Hepatic dysfunction. Drugs include amiodarone.

Increased Procainamide and NAPA: Renal dysfunction.

Decreased NAPA: Hepatic dysfunction.

Description: Procainamide is an antidysrhythmic used in the treatment of atrial and ventricular dysrhythmias. It is most commonly administered as an oral or intravenous drug and metabolized by the liver. 25% of procainamide is metabolized to NAPA by the liver; 60% of the dose is excreted via the kidneys, with a half-life of 3–4 hours. Procainamide's primary metabolite is *N*-acetylprocainamide (NAPA), which has similar antidysrhythmic properties and a half-life of approximately 6 hours but is not metabolized by the liver. The differences in the half-lives result in slightly high NAPA levels until both reach stabilization approximately 18 hours after initiation of therapy. At this time, a 1:1 ratio exists between procainamide and NAPA. An increase or decrease in the ratio between them can alter the therapeutic effectiveness or result in toxicity. Therefore, when procainamide is assayed, NAPA levels should be monitored simultaneously. Steady-state levels of procainamide are reached after 11–20 hours. Steady-state levels of NAPA are reached after 22–40 hours.

Professional Considerations:
1. Consent form NOT required.
2. Preparation:
   A. Tube: Red-top, red/gray-top, or gold-top.
   B. Do NOT draw specimens during hemodialysis.
3. Procedure:
   A. Draw a 1-ml blood sample.
4. Postprocedure care:
   A. Monitor for panic level symptoms (see above).
5. Factors that affect results:
   A. Reject hemolyzed or lipemic specimens.
6. Client and family teaching:
   A. Take medication as prescribed.
   B. Report side effects such as anorexia, nausea, and vomiting.
7. Other data:
   A. For the initial evaluation, draw a trough level just prior to the next dose of procainamide and draw a peak level 75–90 minutes after oral administration or immediately after the loading dose and at 2, 6, 12, and 24 hours for intravenous administration.
   B. For continuous therapeutic drug monitoring, three normal-range levels within one dosing interval are required initially. Then only trough levels are required unless toxicity is suspected.

Bibliography:
Adams LE, Balakrishnan K, Roberts SM, et al.: Genetic, immunologic and biotransformation studies of patients on procainamide. Lupus *2*(2): 89–98, 1993.

Ellenbogen KA, Wood MA, Stambler BS: Procainamide: a perspective on its value and danger. Heart Dis Stroke *2*(6):473–476, 1993.

Landrum EM, Siegert EA, Hanlon JT, et al.: Prolonged thrombocytopenia associated with procainamide in an elderly patient. Ann Pharmacother *28*(10): 1172–1176, 1994.

PROCHLORPERAZINE
(see Phenothiazines, Blood)

PROCONVERTIN, BLOOD
(see Factor VII, Blood)

PROCTOSCOPY, DIAGNOSTIC

Norm: The rectal lining is continuous, reddish, and free of lesions, abscesses, inflammation, ulcerations, and polyps. The anal lining appears grayish-tan and smooth.

Usage: Melena or bleeding from the anorectal area, persistent diarrhea, changes in bowel habits, passage of pus and mucus, suspected chronic inflammatory bowel disease, bacteriologic/histologic surveillance, surveillance of known rectal disease or following rectal surgery, rectal pain, screening for suspected polyps or tumors, foreign body removal, or adjunct to barium enema.

Description: A proctoscopy is the endoscopic, direct visual examination of the lining of the rectum and anal canal using a rigid, lighted proctoscope. Specimens for biopsy, cytology, or culture may be taken during the procedure. Proctoscopy is usually performed in conjunction with a flexible sigmoidoscopy for clients demonstrating unexplained anemia, unexplained diarrhea, or the presence of blood in the stool.

Professional Considerations:
1. Consent form IS required.

Risks:
Bowel perforation, hemorrhage, peritonitis.

Contraindications:
Severe necrotizing enterocolitis, toxic megacolon, painful anal lesions or severe cardiac dysrhythmias.

2. Preparation:
   A. A tap-water, hypertonic phosphate, or saline enema may be prescribed. Clients with ulcerative colitis or acute diarrhea can be examined without an enema.
   B. Obtain drapes, gloves, 1–2% lidocaine (Xylocaine), a proctoscope with an obturator, and a light source. If a biopsy will be performed, obtain a specimen container of 10% formalin. If cytology slides will be prepared, obtain cytology slides and a Coplin jar of 95% ethyl alcohol. If cultures will be performed, obtain sterile swabs with culture tube.
   C. *See Client and family teaching.*
3. Procedure:
   A. The client is placed in a left-lateral or knee-to-chest position and draped for comfort and privacy.
   B. The physician inserts a lubricated finger through the anus to assess for patency and the presence of obstruction.
   C. After patency is determined, the lubricated proctoscope with obturator is inserted fully into the rectum through the anus and the obturator is removed.
   D. After a light is inserted, the physician carefully inspects the interior lining of the rectum and anal canal as the proctoscope is slowly withdrawn.
   E. If biopsies are taken, the site may be anesthetized first with 1–2% Xylocaine or another local anesthetic.
   F. Any liquid drainage is removed with suction during the procedure.

4. Postprocedure care:
   A. Send the specimens to the laboratory immediately.
   B. The client should lie flat for 10–15 minutes before leaving.
   C. Monitor for signs of fatigue, abdominal pain or distention, fever, hypotension, or rectal bleeding.
   D. Bloody stools are normal for 1–2 days after a rectal biopsy.
   E. No enemas or barium studies for 1 week post-rectal biopsy secondary to the increased risk of perforation.
5. Client and family teaching:
   A. Client may be asked to follow a clear liquid diet for 2 days or fast for 8 hours.
   B. Try to defecate prior to the procedure.
   C. An urge to defecate may be felt during the procedure, and slow, controlled deep breathing may help to diminish this feeling.
6. Factors that affect results:
   A. Residual barium from prior testing will impair visualization.
   B. The presence of stool in the rectum impairs visualization.
7. Other data:
   A. Complications of proctoscopy include rectal perforation, minimal bleeding from lacerations, transient abdominal discomfort, and cardiac dysrhythmias.

Bibliography:

Society of Gastroenterology Nurses and Associates: Gastroenterology Nursing Core Curriculum. St Louis, MO, Mosby Year Book, 1993, pp 24–25.

PROGESTERONE RECEPTOR ASSAY, BLOOD

Norm: Negative.

		SI Units
Negative	<5 fmol/mg protein	<5 nmol/kg protein
Positive	>10 fmol/mg protein	>10 nmol/kg protein

Usage: Determination of the likelihood of carcinoma to respond to hormone or antihormone therapy, monitoring the responsiveness of tumors to hormonal or antihormonal therapy, and determination of the need for oophorectomy.

Positive: Breast cancer, hormonal therapy, meningioma, and metastasis.

Negative: Normal finding. Normal results may be obtained in the presence of a benign and nonresponsive tumor.

Description: Progesterone receptors are located primarily in mammary gland tissue, but are also present in the corpus luteum, prostate, uterus, vaginal epithelium, and placenta. Progesterone receptors transfer and bind steroid molecules into cell nuclei to exert hormonal function. This test is usually performed in conjunction with an estrogen receptor assay and involves testing an excised or biopsied tumor for the degree of responsiveness (positivity) of the progesterone receptors in the tissue. In some clients with carcinoma, the degree of progesterone receptor positivity correlates to the amount of cellular subtype differentiation and is a measure of potential tumor responsiveness to hormonal or antihormonal therapy. Clients with positive tests are more likely to respond to these types of therapy than those with negative results. In monitoring tumor response to therapy, the best prognosis can be expected in clients whose progesterone receptor assay results remain positive. In clients who have negative tests after positive initial tests, the prognosis is poor. Clients who remain negative have the poorest outcome.

Professional Considerations:

1. Consent form NOT required for this test, but IS required for the procedure used to obtain the specimen tested. See individual procedure for risks and contraindications.
2. Preparation:
   A. The client is prepared for a surgical biopsy or resection.
   B. Arrange for a person to be standing by to transport the iced specimen to the pathology laboratory immediately after excision.
   C. Obtain a waxed cardboard specimen container without preservatives. Do not place it in formalin.
3. Procedure:
   A. A fresh tissue specimen of at least 150 mg and preferably 1 g (1 ml) is obtained via needle biopsy or resection and placed into a container free of formalin.
   B. The specimen is transported to the pathology laboratory immediately.
4. Postprocedure care:
   A. Apply a dry, sterile dressing to the biopsy or operative site.

B. Specimens must be stored at temperatures lower than –70°C. Specimens transported to another institution must be packed in dry ice.
5. Client and family teaching:
   A. Results of the test may dictate the type of anticipated therapy.
6. Factors that affect results:
   A. Reject specimens not stored at temperatures lower than –70°C or those contaminated with formalin.
   B. Reject specimens not transported to the pathology laboratory immediately, as a delay of even 15 minutes results in degradation of receptor sites.
   C. The presence of massive tumor necrosis or tumors with low cellular composition lowers the assay result.
7. Other data:
   A. The estrogen receptor assay should also be performed on all specimens.
   B. Progesterone receptors are found in up to 75% of estrogen receptor-positive mammary cancers.
   C. Estrogen and progesterone positive tumors have a 75% response rate to endocrine therapy, whereas estrogen and progesterone negative tumors have a 5–10% response rate.

Bibliography:

Horwitz KB: How do breast cancers become hormone resistant? J Steroid Biochem Molecular Biol 49(4–6):295–302.
Masood S: Prognostic and diagnostic implications of estrogen and progesterone receptor assays in cytology. Diag Cytopathol 10(3):263–267, 1994.
Wong K, Henderson IC: Management of metastatic breast cancer. World J Surg 18(1):98–111, 1994.

PROGESTERONE, SERUM

Norm:

		SI Units
Female		
Follicular phase	0.2–0.6 ng/ml	<2 nmol/L
Luteal phase	6–30 ng/ml	19–95 nmol/L
Midluteal phase	5.7–28.1 ng/ml	18–89 nmol/L
Oral contraceptives	0.1–0.3 ng/ml	<2 nmol/L
Postmenopause	0–0.2 ng/ml	<2 nmol/L
Pregnancy		
1–12 weeks	9–47 ng/ml	28–149 nmol/L
13–24 weeks	16.8–146 ng/ml	53–464 nmol/L
25 weeks–term	55–255 ng/ml	175–811 nmol/L
Male	0.1–0.3 ng/ml	<2 nmol/L
Child (prepubertal)	7–52 ng/ml	0.2–1.7 nmol/L

Usage: Assessment of corpus luteum formation and placental function, and assists in determining the day of ovulation.

Increased: Adrenal hyperplasia (congenital, males), corpus luteum cyst, lipid ovarian tumors, molar pregnancy, ovarian chorionepithelioma, ovarian neoplasms, placental tissue (retained postparturition), precocious puberty and theca lutein cyst. Drugs include adrenocortical hormones, estrogens, and progesterones.

Decreased: Adrenogenital syndrome, amenorrhea, anovular menstruation, fetal abnormality or death, luteal deficiency, menstrual abnormalities, ovarian failure, panhypopituitarism, placental failure or insufficiency, preeclampsia, Stein-Leventhal syndrome, threatened abortion, toxemia of pregnancy, Turner's syndrome, and primary/secondary hypogonadism. Drugs include ampicillin, ethinyl estradiol.

Description: Progesterone is a steroid sex hormone secreted by the corpus luteum during the latter half of the menstrual cycle in nonpregnant women, by the placenta in large amounts of pregnant women, and by the adrenal cortex in men. Progesterone causes secretory changes in the mucosa of the fallopian tubes and assists in nourishing the fertilized ovum as it travels through the tubes to the uterus. It prepares the endometrium for implantation of the fertilized ovum, stimulates growth of the breasts and proliferation of the vaginal epithelium, and decreases myometrial excitability and uterine contractions.

Professional Considerations:
1. Consent form NOT required.
2. Preparation:
   A. Tube: Red-top or green-top.
   B. Specimens MAY be drawn during hemodialysis.
3. Procedure:
   A. Draw a 7-ml blood sample.
4. Postprocedure care:
   A. Record the first day of the last menstrual cycle or the week of gestation on the laboratory requisition.
5. Client and family teaching:
   A. Results are normally available within 24 hours.
6. Factors that affect results:
   A. The sample may be refrigerated for 4 days, frozen up to 1 year, and is stable at room temperature for 7 days.
7. Other data:
   A. Serial testing is recommended.
   B. For diagnosis of a short luteal phase, correlation with endometrial biopsy is recommended.
   C. Levels are higher with twin pregnancies than with single pregnancies.

Bibliography:
Minassian SS, Wu CH: Free and protein bound progesterone during normal and luteal phase defective cycles. Int J Gynecol Obstet *43*(2):163–168, 1993.

PROLACTIN (HUMAN PROLACTIN, HPRL), SERUM

Norm: Prolactin levels do not differ between males and females prior to the onset of puberty.

		SI Units
Adult female, nonlactating	<23 ng/ml	<23 ng/dl
Follicular phase	<28 ng/ml	<28 ng/dl
Luteal phase	5–40 ng/ml	5–40 ng/dl
Postmenopause	<12 ng/ml	<12 ng/dl
Pregnancy		
Trimester 1	<80 ng/ml	<80 ng/dl
Trimester 2	<160 ng/ml	<160 ng/dl
Trimester 3	<400 ng/ml	<400 ng/dl
Adult male	<20 ng/ml	<20 ng/dl
Pituitary tumor	>100 ng/ml	>100 ng/dl
Newborn	>10 times adult levels	

Increased: Acromegaly, Addison's disease, amenorrhea, anorexia nervosa, breast stimulation, bronchogenic carcinoma, Chiari-Frommel syndrome, coitus, del Castillo's syndrome, ectopic tumors, endometriosis, exercise, Forbes-Albright syndrome, galactorrhea, hyperestrogen states, hyperpituitarism, hypothalamic disorders, hypothyroidism (primary), hysterectomy, idiopathic causes (e.g., early microadenoma that are undetectable by radiology), impotence, lactation, Nelson's syndrome, neurogenic causes, pituitary tumors, polycystic ovaries, pregnancy, renal failure (chronic), sleep, and stress. Drugs include amitriptyline, amoxapine, amphetamines, benzamides, chlorprothixene, desipramine, doxepin, droperidol, estrogens, haloperidol, imipramine, isoniazid, maprotiline, meprobamate, methyldopa, metoclopramide, nortriptyline, opiates, oral contraceptives, phenothiazines, procainamide hydrochloride, protriptyline, reserpine, thioridazine, thiothixene, thyrotropin, triavil, and trimipramine maleate.

Decreased: Gynecomastia, hirsutism, osteoporosis, and pituitary necrosis or infarction. Drugs include apomorphine hydrochloride, clonidine, bromocriptine mesylate, dihydroergotamine mesylate, dopamine, ergonovine maleate, ergotamine tartrate, ergoloid mesylate, Lergotrile, levodopa, and lisuride hydrogen maleate.

Description: Prolactin is a peptide hormone produced by the anterior pituitary gland that promotes growth of breast tissue and is essential for the initiation and maintenance of milk production. Also called the lactogenic hormone, luteotropic hormone, LTH, and mammotropin. It is identical to luteotropin.

Professional Considerations:

1. Consent form NOT required.
2. Preparation:
   A. Tube: Red-top, red/gray-top, or gold-top.
   B. Specimens MAY be drawn during hemodialysis.
   C. *See Client and family teaching.*

3. Procedure:
   A. Draw a 5-ml blood sample without trauma.
   B. Samples should be drawn in the morning.
4. Postprocedure care:
   A. None.
5. Client and family teaching:
   A. Fast for 12 hours before testing.
6. Factors that affect results:
   A. Hemolysis of the specimen invalidates the results.
7. Other data:
   A. Samples remain stable for 4 days at room temperature, and then must be frozen if analysis is delayed.
   B. Serum level >300 ng/ml is assumed to be pathognomic of a pituitary tumor.
   C. Differentiation between a pituitary tumor and other prolactin disorders can be done using thyrotropin-releasing hormone (TRH). Prolactin levels in clients with pituitary tumors do not increase.
   D. Men with elevated prolactin levels generally have low serum testosterone. Symptoms will not reverse unless prolactin is reduced.

Bibliography:

Keening KL, Tenuously P, Burning PF, et al.: Reliability of serum prolactin measurements in women. Cancer Epidemiol, Biomarkers Prevention 2(5): 411–414, 1993.

Malkowicz DE, Legido A, Jackel RA, et al.: Prolactin secretion following repetitive seizures. Neurology 45(3, Pt 1):448–452, 1995.

Reber PM: Prolactin and immunodilution. Am J Med 95(6):637–644, 1993.

PROLIFERATION MARKER MIB 1–3

(see Ki-67 Proliferation Marker, Specimen)

PROPOXYPHENE, BLOOD

Norm: Negative.

Propoxyphene Therapy Norms		SI Units
Therapeutic levels	0.1–0.4 µg/ml	0.3–1.2 µmol/L
Panic level	>0.5 µg/ml	>1.5 µmol/L

Usage: Suspected drug abuse, drug overdose, or suicide.

Panic Level Symptoms and Treatment:

Symptoms: Coma; respiratory depression; circulatory collapse; pulmonary edema; dysrhythmias, including heart block, trigeminy and prolongation of the QRS complex; and nephrogenic diabetes insipidus. Overdosage may be fatal in as little as 1 hour after ingestion.

Treatment: Supportive therapy, including maintenance of airway and hemodynamic stability; opiate antagonists; gastric lavage; forced emesis; and charcoal slurry. Hemodialysis and peritoneal dialysis will NOT remove propoxyphene.

Description: Propoxyphene is a schedule-IV, non-narcotic analgesic structurally related to methadone. It is one-half to two-thirds as potent as codeine. Propoxyphene is metabolized in the liver and excreted in the urine, with a half-life of 30–36 hours.

Professional Considerations:

1. Consent form NOT required.
2. Preparation:
   A. Tube: Red-top, red/gray-top, or gold-top or black-top.
   B. Specimens MAY be drawn during hemodialysis.
3. Procedure:
   A. Broad-spectrum drug screening: Draw a 20-ml blood sample.
4. Postprocedure care:
   A. None.
5. Client and family teaching:
   A. Take medication as prescribed to avoid an overdose.
   B. Report any adverse side effects to the physician.
   C. If activated charcoal was given for elevated levels, the client should drink 4–6 glasses of water each day for 2 days to prevent constipation. The activated charcoal will cause stools to be black for a few days.
6. Factors that affect results:
   A. Peak serum levels occur in 2–5 hours for propoxyphene hydrochloride and in 3–4 hours for propoxyphene napsylate.
   B. Metabolism and excretion are delayed with hepatic and renal dysfunction.
7. Other data:
   A. A 100-ml urine sample, collected without preservatives, should be obtained at the time of the serum sample.

Bibliography:

Stork CM, Redd JT, Fine K, et al.: Propoxyphene-induced wide QRS complex dysrhythmia responsive to sodium bicarbonate—a case report. J Toxicol Clin Toxicol 33(2):179–183, 1995.

PROPRANOLOL, BLOOD

Norm: Negative.

Propranolol Therapy Norms		SI Units
Therapeutic level	50–100 ng/ml	193–386 nmol/L
Panic level	>500 ng/ml	>1930 nmol/L

Panic Level Symptoms and Treatment:

Symptoms: Bradycardia, profound hypotension, loss of consciousness, seizures, cardiac failure, and bronchospasm.

Treatment:

Supportive therapy, including maintenance of airway and hemodynamic stability.
Perform forced emesis and gastric lavage.
Provide prophylactic transcutaneous pacemaker.
Administer atropine, isoproterenol.
Administer cardiac glycoside.
Administer diuretics.
Administer Glucagon.
Hemodialysis and peritoneal dialysis will NOT remove propranolol.

Increased: Propranolol overdosage. Drugs include flecainide, methimazole, and propylthiouracil.

Description: Propranolol hydrochloride is a beta- and beta-adrenergic blocking drug classified as a type II cardiac antidysrhythmic. It competes with epinephrine and norepinephrine for adrenoreceptors, resulting in inhibition of myocardial beta-adrenergic stimulation. Cardiac effects include reduced irritability and heart rate, as the automaticity of the SA node, AV node, and intraventricular conduction velocity is depressed. Large doses depress cardiac function. Propranolol may also cause hypoglycemia without warning in diabetics. Propranolol is bound to plasma proteins, metabolized in the liver, and excreted in the urine, with a half-life of 2–6 hours. Steady-state levels are reached after 10–30 hours.

Professional Considerations:

1. Consent form NOT required.
2. Preparation:
   A. Tube: Red-top, red/gray-top, or gold-top.
   B. Specimens MAY be drawn during hemodialysis.
3. Procedure:
   A. Draw a 7-ml blood sample in a syringe.
   B. After removing the stopper, inject the specimen promptly into the tube

(plasma propranolol binding is reduced when blood passes through the stopper of a vacuum tube).

C. Replace the stopper.

D. Collect the specimen prior to the next dose (trough) if drawing to evaluate therapeutic value.

4. Postprocedure care:

A. Monitor the client for evidence of increasing congestive heart failure.

5. Client and family teaching:

A. Take medication as prescribed to prevent overdose.

B. Report any side effects to the physician.

C. Take your pulse daily and notify the physician if it falls below the level your physician specifies.

6. Factors that affect results:

A. Smoking decreases plasma concentration of propranolol.

B. Peak propranolol levels occur 1–2 hours after oral administration.

C. Propranolol metabolism and excretion are delayed with hepatic and renal dysfunction.

7. Other data:

A. When obtaining serial levels, the same time interval between drug dosing and specimen collection should be maintained.

Bibliography:

Merk S: Adverse effects of epinephrine when given to patients taking propranolol. J Emerg Nurs *21*(1): 27–32, 1995.

Sowinski KM, Burlew BS, Johnson JA: Racial differences in sensitivity to the negative chronotropic effects of propranolol in healthy men. Clin Pharmacol Ther *57*(6):678–683, 1995.

PROSTATE SONOGRAM (PROSTATE ECHOGRAM, PROSTATE ULTRASOUND), DIAGNOSTIC

Norm: The prostate gland is round and about 3 cm in diameter. Prostatic tissue is homogeneous, and causes only a slight bladder wall indentation.

Usage: Adjunct to digital examination of the prostate, diagnosis and staging of and screening for prostate cancer, evaluation of the size and shape of the prostate gland, monitoring response to treatment in prostate disease, and provides guidance for transrectal biopsy of the prostate gland.

Description: Evaluation of the prostate gland via the creation of an oscilloscopic picture from the echoes of high-frequency sound waves passing through the anterior rectal wall or through the urethra over the pelvic area (acoustic imaging, endosonogra-

phy). The time required for the ultrasonic beam to be reflected back to the transducer from differing densities of tissue is converted by a computer to an electrical impulse displayed on an oscilloscopic screen to create a three-dimensional picture of the pelvic contents. Because of the risk of sepsis and trauma from transurethral sonography, the transrectal route is preferred. For staging prostate cancer, transrectal sonography costs less than magnetic resonance imaging, with comparable or superior accuracy. This technique may help detect prostate lesions before they become large enough to palpate.

Professional Considerations:

1. Consent form IS required.

Risks:

Transurethral route: sepsis and trauma. Transrectal route: infection.

Contraindications:

Nonprostate disease. Transurethral route: bleeding disorders, thrombocytopenia.

2. Preparation:

A. This test should be performed before intestinal barium tests, or after the barium is cleared from the system.

B. Obtain ultrasonic gel or paste.

C. For transrectal sonography, a hypertonic enema of sodium phosphate or a bisacodyl suppository may be prescribed.

D. The client must disrobe below the waist or wear a gown.

E. *See Client and family teaching.*

3. Procedure:

A. The client is positioned supine, and a short transabdominal sonogram may be performed to evaluate for kidney distention.

B. A suprapubic examination of the prostate is performed, and the rectum is examined digitally for obstruction.

C. The client is assisted to a knee-elbow, lateral decubitus, or sitting position.

D. The probe is covered with an air-free, sterile transparent cover or condom. The condom is then coated with sterile lubricant, and the probe is slowly inserted into the rectum.

E. After the probe is inserted into the rectum, the condom may be inflated with 20–60 ml of deaerated water, depending on the practitioner's preference.

F. The probe is angled anteriorly, and

sonography of the prostate is performed.

G. Photographs of the oscilloscopic display are taken.

4. Postprocedure care:
   A. Remove the gel from the skin.
   B. Sterilize the endosonography probes by soaking them in glutaraldehyde solution for 10 minutes.

5. Client and family teaching:
   A. An enema may be prescribed prior to the procedure.
   B. Drink normal amounts of fluids for 24 hours before the procedure.

6. Factors that affect results:
   A. Dehydration interferes with adequate contrast between organs and body fluids.

B. Lower intestinal barium obscures results by preventing proper transmission and deflection of the high-frequency sound waves.

7. Other data:
   A. A biopsy of the prostate lesions may be taken during ultrasound.
   B. Doppler sonography may be used to further define abnormalities in vascular supply and differentiate vascular differences in the prostate tissue.

Bibliography:

Lui PD, Terris MK, McNeal JE, et al.: Indications for ultrasound guided transition zone biopsies in the detection of prostate cancer. J Urol *153*(3, Pt 2): 1000–1003, 1995.

PROSTATE-SPECIFIC ANTIGEN (PSA), SERUM

Norm:

Immunoassay Method	
Female	<0.5 µg/L
Male	
0–39 years	<2.0 µg/L
≥40 years	<2.8 µg/L

Usage: Assists in the identification, differentiation, classification, staging, and localization of tumor; monitoring preoperatively, postoperatively, and for recurrent tumor; assists in the selection of therapeutic interventions or cytotoxic drug therapy; and assists in assessment of tumor response to treatment protocols.

Increased: Benign prostatic hypertrophy, cirrhosis, impotence, osteoporosis, prostate cancer or infarct, prostatic needle biopsy, prostatitis, pulmonary embolism, renal osteopathy, transurethral resection (TUR), urethral instrumentation, and urinary retention.

Description: Prostate-specific antigen (PSA) is a glycoprotein exclusive to the prostate epithelium. It is smaller than the prostatic acid phosphatase molecule, more stable, and does not demonstrate diurnal variations. Tumor catabolic activity and accelerated metabolic rate in prostate carcinoma elevate the serum value of PSA. PSA is, therefore, a reliable immunocytochemical marker used in the detection of prostate cancer.

Professional Considerations:

1. Consent form NOT required.

2. Preparation:
   A. Tube: Red-top, red/gray-top, or gold-top.
   B. Specimens MAY be drawn during hemodialysis.
   C. *See Client and family teaching.*

3. Procedure:
   A. Draw a 1-ml blood sample.

4. Postprocedure care:
   A. The sample is stable at room temperature for 24 hours and may be refrigerated.

5. Client and family teaching:
   A. Fast for 8 hours.
   B. Do not have the test drawn less than 24 hours after a rectal or prostate examination.

6. Factors that affect results:
   A. Falsely elevated results may be associated with blood drawn 1 to 24 hours after a rectal examination.
   B. A routine PSA in conjunction with an annual rectal exam is recommended for men older than 50.
   C. Approximately 25% of men with benign prostatic hypertrophy have an elevated PSA.

7. Other data:
   A. While this test aids in the diagnosis of malignant states, some benign diseases can also demonstrate antigen marker abnormalities.
   B. Adult levels are reached at approximately 15 years.
   C. Some recent research shows the PSA is influenced by the age of the client.

Bibliography:

Oesterling JE, Cooner WH, Jacobsen SJ, et al.: Influence of patient age on the serum PSA concentration. An important clinical observation. Urol Clin North Am 20(4):671–680, 1993.

Richie JP, Catalona WJ, Ahmann FR, et al.: Effect of patient age on early detection of prostate cancer with serum prostate-specific antigen and digital rectal examination. Urology 42(4):356–374, 1993.

Vessella RL, Lange PH: Issues in the assessment of PSA immunoassays. Urol Clin of North Am 20(4): 607–619, 1993.

PROSTATIC ACID PHOSPHATASE (PAP), BLOOD

Norm: Values are dependent upon laboratory method.

		SI Units
Fishman-Lerner	0–0.7 U/dl	
Bessey, Lowry, and Brock (BLB)		
Female	0.02–0.55 U at 37°C	0.3–9.2 U/L
Male	0.15–0.65 U at 37°C	2.5–10.8 U/L
Bodansky	0–3 U/dl	0–16.1 U/L
King-Armstrong	0–3 U/dl	0–5.3 U/L
RIA	2.5–3.7 ng/ml	

Increased: Bone cancer (metastatic), hyperparathyroidism, metastatic prostatic carcinoma, multiple myeloma, osteogenesis imperfecta, Paget's disease, prostatic carcinoma (10–25%), and prostatic infarct.

Decreased: Down syndrome. Drugs include estrogen therapy for prostatic carcinoma, and ethanol.

Description: Prostatic acid phosphatase, an isoenzyme of acid phosphatase, is a lysosomal enzyme that hydrolyzes phosphate esters. It is found mainly in the prostate, but is also present in erythrocytes and the kidneys, liver, and spleen. Prostatic tissue has a concentration of acid phosphatase 100 times greater than other tissues. Serum activity of the prostatic isoenzyme is greatly increased in metastatic cancer of the prostate in which the tumor has extended beyond the capsule surrounding the prostate gland. Therefore, this test is used as both a marker for and a monitor of the disease course.

Professional Considerations:

1. Consent form NOT required.
2. Preparation:
   A. Tube: Red-top, red/gray-top, or gold-top or lavender-top.
   B. Specimens MAY be drawn during hemodialysis.
3. Procedure:
   A. Draw an early-morning, 5-ml blood sample.
4. Postprocedure care:
   A. Transport the specimen to the laboratory immediately. Serum specimens deteriorate rapidly at room temperature.
5. Client and family teaching:
   A. Wait at least 24 hours after prostatic massage, extensive prostate palpation, or a transurethral resection before the blood test.
   B. This test may be drawn in conjunction with the prostate-specific antigen test.
6. Factors that affect results:
   A. Recent administration of clofibrate invalidates the results.
   B. Falsely elevated results may be associated with blood drawn 1 to 24 hours after a rectal examination.
   C. False-positive results have been reported in hemolyzed serum samples.
   D. False-negative results have been reported in serum specimens contaminated with fluoride, oxalate, or phosphate.
7. Other data:
   A. Refrigerated specimens or specimens frozen with 0.01 ml of 20% acetic acid per milliliter of serum can remain stable for up to 1 week.
   B. Prostatic acid phosphatase is elevated in 75–80% of those with metastatic bone lesions, 50–75% with metastatic lesions of the prostate, and in 10–25% of those with nonmetastatic prostate lesions.
   C. PAP levels exhibit a diurnal variation, with the highest levels occurring during the early morning.
   D. With the increased reliability of prostate-specific antigen (PSA), screening serum PAP testing may become more limited in value for prostate carcinoma.

Bibliography:

Huang CL, Brassil D, Rozzell M, et al.: Comparison of prostate secretory protein with prostate specific antigen and prostatic acid phosphatase as a serum biomarker for diagnosis and monitoring patients with prostate carcinoma. Prostate 20(4): 581–588, 1993.

Lowe FC, Trauzzi, SJ: Prostatic acid phosphatase in 1993. Its limited clinical utility. Urol Clin North Am *20*(4):588–595, 1993.

PROTEIN, CEREBROSPINAL FLUID, SPECIMEN

(see Cerebrospinal Fluid, Myelin Basic Protein, Oligoclonal Bands, Protein, and Protein Electrophoresis, Specimen)

PROTEIN, ELECTROPHORESIS, CEREBROSPINAL FLUID, SPECIMEN

(see Cerebrospinal Fluid, Myelin Basic Protein, Oligoclonal Bands, Protein, and Protein Electrophoresis, Specimen)

PROTEIN, ELECTROPHORESIS, SERUM

Norm: Norms are dependent on laboratory procedure. Percentage values represent the percentage of total protein for the Agarose method:

		SI Units
Adult		
Total protein	100%	5.90–8.00
Albumin	58–74%	0.58–0.74
Alpha$_1$ globulin	2.0–3.5%	0.02–0.04
Alpha$_2$ globulin	5.4–10.6%	0.05–0.11
Beta globulin	7.0–14.0%	0.07–0.14
Gamma globulin	8.0–18.0%	0.08–0.18
Adult		
Total protein	6.0–8.0 g/dl	60–80 g/L
Albumin	3.3–5.0 g/dl	35–50 g/L
Alpha$_1$ globulin	0.1–0.4 g/dl	1–4 g/L
Alpha$_2$ globulin	0.5–1 g/dl	5–10 g/L
Beta globulin	0.7–1.2 g/dl	7–12 g/L
Gamma globulin	0.8–1.6 g/dl	8–16 g/L
Premature infant		
Total protein	4.4–6.3 g/dl	44–63 g/L
Albumin	3.0–4.2 g/dl	30–42 g/L
Alpha$_1$ globulin	0.11–0.5 g/dl	1.1–5 g/L
Alpha$_2$ globulin	0.3–0.7 g/dl	3–7 g/L
Beta globulin	0.3–1.2 g/dl	3–12 g/L
Gamma globulin	0.3–1.4 g/dl	3–14 g/L
Newborn		
Total protein	4.6–7.4 g/dl	46–74 g/L
Albumin	3.5–5.4 g/dl	35–54 g/L
Alpha$_1$ globulin	0.1–0.3 g/dl	1–3 g/L
Alpha$_2$ globulin	0.3–0.5 g/dl	3–5 g/L
Beta globulin	0.2–0.6 g/dl	2–6 g/L
Gamma globulin	0.2–1.2 g/dl	2–12 g/L
Infant		
Total protein	6.0–6.7 g/dl	60–67 g/L
Albumin	4.4–5.4 g/dl	44–54 g/L
Alpha$_1$ globulin	0.2–0.4 g/dl	2–4 g/L
Alpha$_2$ globulin	0.5–0.8 g/dl	5–8 g/L
Beta globulin	0.5–0.9 g/dl	5–9 g/L
Gamma globulin	0.3–0.8 g/dl	3–8 g/L
Child		
Total protein	6.2–8.0 g/dl	62–80 g/L
Albumin	4.0–5.8 g/dl	40–58 g/L
Alpha$_1$ globulin	0.1–0.4 g/dl	1–4 g/L

		SI Units
Child *(continued)*		
Alpha$_2$ globulin	0.4–1.0 g/dl	4–10 g/L
Beta globulin	0.5–1.0 g/dl	5–10 g/L
Gamma globulin	0.3–1.0 g/dl	3–10 g/L

Usage: Assists in the diagnosis of blood dyscrasias, dysproteinemias, gastrointestinal disorders, hepatic disease, hypergammaglobulinemias, hypogammaglobulinemias, inflammatory states, neoplasms, and renal disease.

Increased Total Protein: Macroglobulinemia, multiple myeloma, and sarcoidosis.

Increased Prealbumin Zone Intensity: Alcoholism.

Increased Albumin Zone Mobility: Acute pancreatitis. Drugs include aspirin and penicillins.

Increased Albumin-Alpha$_1$ Interzone Intensity: Alcoholism (chronic), females during puberty, and pregnancy.

Increased Alpha Globulin Zone Intensity: Acute-phase response in inflammation (alpha, alpha haptoglobin), acute rheumatic fever (alpha), aged (alpha), analbuminemia (alpha), chronic glomerulonephritis (alpha), cirrhosis (increased alpha with normal or only slightly elevated alpha), diabetes mellitus (alpha), dysproteinemia (familial idiopathic), glomerular protein loss (alpha-macroglobulin), hepatic damage, hepatic metastasis (increased alpha with normal alpha), Hodgkin's disease (alpha, alpha), hypoalbuminemia, infancy (alpha zone dominated by macroglobulin), infection (acute), meningitis (alpha), metastatic carcinomatosis (alpha, alpha), myocardial infarction, myxedema, nephrosis (alpha), nephrotic syndrome (alpha), osteomyelitis (alpha), peptic ulcer disease (alpha, alpha), pneumonia (alpha), polyarteritis nodose (alpha), pregnancy (increased alpha, with normal alpha), protein-losing enteropathy (alpha, alpha), rheumatoid arthritis (alpha), sarcoidosis (alpha), stress (alpha, alpha), systemic lupus erythematosus (alpha), and ulcerative colitis (alpha, alpha). Drugs that increase alpha with little change in alpha include estrogens.

Increased Alpha$_2$-Beta$_1$ Interzone Intensity: Hypercholesterolemia (type II), nephrotic syndrome, and pregnancy.

Increased Beta Globulin Zone Intensity: Acute-phase response (beta), analbuminemia, diabetes mellitus (poorly controlled), dysproteinemia (familial idiopathic), glomerular protein loss, hepatitis (viral), hypercholesterolemia, hyperlipemia, iron-deficiency anemia (beta) jaundice (obstructive), macroglobulinemia, nephrotic syndrome, pregnancy (beta), rheumatoid arthritis, and sarcoidosis. Drugs that increase beta include estrogens and oral contraceptives.

Increased Gamma Globulin Zone Intensity: Acute viral hepatitis (sometimes), amyloidosis, analbuminemia, carcinoma (advanced), chronic aggressive hepatitis (appearance of oligoclonal bands), chronic hepatic disease (IgM), chronic lymphatic leukemia (IgM paraprotein), chronic viral infections (appearance of oligoclonal bands), cirrhosis (IgA), cryoglobulinemia, cystic fibrosis (IgG, IgA), Hashimoto's disease, hepatic disease, Hodgkin's disease, hypergammaglobulinemia, hypersensitivity reaction, infection (severe), juvenile rheumatoid arthritis (IgG, IgA, IgM), Laennec's cirrhosis, leukemia (myelogenous, monocytic), lymphosarcoma (IgM paraprotein), macroglobulinemia, multiple myeloma, respiratory infection (IgA), rheumatoid arthritis (IgA, IgM), sarcoidosis, scleroderma (sometimes), skin disease (IgA), Sjögren's syndrome (IgG), systemic lupus erythematosus (active) (IgM), and Waldenström's macroglobulinemia (IgM paraprotein).

Decreased Total Protein: Analbuminemia, cholecystitis (acute), chronic glomerulonephritis, Hodgkin's disease, hypertension (essential with congestive heart failure), hypogammaglobulinemia, leukemia (myelogenous, monocytic), nephrosis, peptic ulcer disease, and ulcerative colitis.

Decreased Prealbumin Zone Intensity: Acute-phase response (day 1) and cirrhosis.

Decreased Albumin Zone Intensity: Acute rheumatic fever, analbuminemia, carcinomatosis (metastatic), cholecystitis (acute), diabetes mellitus, gastrointestinal protein loss (inflammatory or neoplastic disease), glomerular protein loss, glomerulonephritis (chronic), hepatic disease, hepatitis (acute viral), Hodgkin's disease, hyperthyroidism, hypertension (essential with congestive heart failure), Laennec's cirrhosis, leukemia (lymphatic, myelogenous, monocytic), lymphoma, macroglobulinemia, malnutrition, meningitis, multiple myeloma, nephrosis, nephrotic syndrome, osteomyelitis, peptic ulcer disease, pneumonia, polyarteritis nodose, protein-losing enteropathy, pyrexia, rheumatoid arthritis, sarcoidosis, stress, systemic lupus erythematosus, and ulcerative colitis. Drugs include corticosteroids.

Decreased Albumin-Alpha$_1$ Interzone Intensity: Cirrhosis, hepatitis (acute), and inflammation (severe).

Decreased Alpha Globulin Zone Intensity: Acute viral hepatitis (alpha, alpha), congenital hypohaptoglobinemia (alpha haptoglobin), hepatic disease, intravascular hemolysis (hemolytic anemia, hepatic metastases, cirrhosis, and splenomegaly cause decreased alpha haptoglobin), malabsorption, pulmonary emphysema (alpha), scleroderma, starvation, and steatorrhea.

Decreased Alpha$_2$-Beta$_1$ Interzone Intensity: Diabetes mellitus, inflammation, and pancreatitis.

Decreased Beta Globulin Zone Intensity: Autoimmune disease, carcinomatosis (metastatic), hepatic disease (beta) immune complex disease (beta), leukemia (lymphatic, monocytic, myelogenous), lymphoma, malabsorption, malnutrition (beta), nephrosis, scleroderma, starvation, steatorrhea, systemic lupus erythematosus, and ulcerative colitis.

Decreased Gamma Globulin Zone Intensity: Acute viral hepatitis (sometimes), agammaglobulinemia, glomerular protein loss, hypogammaglobulinemia, leukemia (lymphatic), lymphoma, nephrosis, nephrotic syndrome, malabsorption, protein-losing enteropathy, scleroderma (sometimes), starvation, steatorrhea, and ulcerative colitis.

Description: Protein electrophoresis is the most frequent measurement of the primary blood proteins, albumin, and globulins (alpha, alpha, beta, and gamma). Under the influence of an electrical field, at a pH of 8.6, the proteins separate by electrical charge, molecular size, and shape. Plotted on treated paper, the serum proteins form five homogeneous bands of the relative protein values in percentages. These percentages, when multiplied by the total protein concentration, reflect the absolute value of each protein. High-resolution electrophoresis allows the detection of additional bands or zones. Immunoelectrophoresis may be performed to identify the nature of suspicious bands. The most rapid form of unknown band identification combines high-resolution electrophoresis with immunoprecipitation. Certain protein electrophoresis band patterns are characteristic of specific disease states.

Professional Considerations:

1. Consent form NOT required.
2. Preparation:
   A. Tube: Red-top, red/gray-top, or gold-top.
   B. Specimens MAY be drawn during hemodialysis.
3. Procedure:
   A. Draw a 1-ml blood sample, without trauma.
4. Postprocedure care:
   A. None.
5. Client and family teaching:
   A. Immunoelectrophoresis may take up to 3 days for results.
   B. Medications that interfere with serum protein levels may be prescribed to be withheld.
6. Factors that affect results:
   A. Falsely elevated total protein levels may occur with the use of contrast dyes.
   B. Hemolysis of the specimen invalidates the results.
   C. Electrophoresis may be performed on serum or plasma. The alpha-beta interzone is absent in heparinized plasma.
   D. At least a 30% drop in albumin is required before changes can be detected via electrophoresis.
   E. Aged serum samples may cause decreased beta and increased beta density.
   F. Protein electrophoresis is unreliable for diagnosis of IgA deficiency.

G. Recent dialysis distorts protein values.
7. Other data:
A. None.

Bibliography:

Astion ML, Rank J, Wener MH: Electrophoresis-tutor: an image-based personal computer program that teaches clinical interpretation of protein electrophoresis patterns of serum, urine and cerebrospinal fluid. Clin Chem 41(9):1328–1332, 1995.

Tormey WP, O'Brien PA: Clinical associations of an increased transthyretin band in routine serum and urine protein electrophoresis. Ann Clin Biochem 30(Pt 6):550–554, 1993.

PROTEIN, ELECTROPHORESIS, URINE

Norm: Interpretation of urine electrophoretic patterns is required. Normal urine electrophoretograms show individual variance and consist of a globulin pattern that is generally diffuse. Distinct bands may not be identifiable. The dominant protein, albumin, rapidly migrates to the anode, producing a spike in the pattern. Normally, there is only a trace amount of $alpha_1$ globulin and $alpha_2$ globulin. The beta globulin and gamma globulins are negligible to absent. In contrast to serum electrophoresis, urine electrophoresis does not contain beta-lipoproteins and beta globulin.

	Total Protein	SI Units
Albumin	37.9%	0.379
Alpha$_1$ globulin	27.3%	0.273
Alpha$_2$ globulin	19.5%	0.195
Beta globulin	8.8%	0.088
Gamma globulin	3.3%	0.033

Usage: Detection of albumin, Bence Jones proteins, hemoglobin, myoclonal gammopathies, myoglobin, renal disease, and systemic lupus erythematosus.

Interpretation of Abnormals:

Proteinuria associated with increased glomerular permeability exhibits an electrophoretic pattern that is dominated by albumin, with moderate beta globulin, some alpha globulin, trace alpha globulin, and trace gamma globulin. Basement membrane glomerular capillary damage occurs with amyloidosis, congestive heart failure, glomerulosclerosis (diabetic), inflammation, increased venous pressure, nonrenal infectious disease, or renal vein thrombosis. Glomerular dysfunction may occur with idiopathic nephrotic syndrome, membranous glomerulonephritis, immune complex disorders such as poststreptococcal glomerulonephritis, and systemic lupus erythematosus. These conditions produce proteinuria. Proteinuria can result from chyluria, increased circulating proteins, increased glomerular permeability, or renal tubular dysfunction.

Prerenal conditions include hemoglobinuria, inflammatory syndrome, monocytic leukemia, myoglobinuria, and paraproteinemias. Prerenal electrophoretic patterns vary, based on the specific low molecular weight excess protein present in serum. These circulating proteins may be normal or abnormal. Their excess results in the excretion of proteins in the presence of normal glomerular function.

Hemoglobinuria or intravascular hemolysis produces an electrophoretic pattern that is dominated by beta globulin, with some albumin, trace alpha globulin, trace alpha globulin, and negligible to absent gamma globulin.

Inflammatory syndromes include acute infection, burns, cancer, collagen diseases, hyperthyroidism, and pregnancy. This electrophoretic pattern consists of moderate alpha globulin, some albumin, some alpha globulin, and negligible to absent beta globulin and gamma globulin.

Monocytic and monomyelocytic leukemia result in a cationic peak or dominant migration to the cathode, moderate albumin, trace alpha globulin, trace alpha globulin, and negligible to absent beta globulin and gamma globulin.

Myoglobinuria associated with crushing injuries or electrocution demonstrates a pattern of dominant to absent gamma globulin, some albumin, trace alpha globulin, trace alpha globulin, and negligible to absent beta globulin.

Paraproteinemias such as multiple myeloma with Bence Jones proteinuria produce moderate to absent beta globulin and gamma globulin, with some albumin, trace alpha globulin, and alpha globulin.

Inflammatory conditions (such as chronic osteomyelitis), increased glomerular permeability, and tubular dysfunction (such as chronic renal failure) produce a pattern that is dominated by albumin, with moderate alpha globulin elevation, some alpha globulin, trace beta globulin, and negligible to absent gamma globulin.

Renal tubular disorders include acute renal tubular failure, Balkan neuropathy, cadmium poisoning (chronic), cystinosis, Fanconi's syndrome, galactosemia, hypokalemia (chronic, severe), intoxication (phenacetin or vitamin D), medullary cystic disease, monoclonal gammopathy, oculocerebral renal syndrome, polycystic kidney disease, pyelonephritis (chronic), renal transplantation, renal tubular acidosis, sarcoidosis, and Wilson's disease. The electrophoretic pattern is dominated by beta globulin, with some alpha globulin, some gamma globulin, trace albumin, trace alpha globulin, and a trace cationic migration or peak.

Retroperitoneal lymphatic injury from inflammation, obstruction, or trauma can result in aberrant communication of the retroperitoneal lymph vessels, chyle ducts of the intestine, and urinary tract. This condition causes chyluria. The electrophoretic pattern noted in chyluria is one dominated by albumin, with moderate gamma globulin, some alpha globulin, some beta globulins, and trace alpha globulin.

Upright or orthostatic position-dependent proteinuria is characterized by dominant albumin, moderate beta globulin, some alpha globulin, trace alpha globulin, and trace gamma globulin. The recumbent position reflects a normal electrophoretic pattern. Activity-related proteinuria demonstrates a pattern that is more accentuated than normal, but not as elevated as orthostatic proteinuria. An exercise pattern produces moderate albumin, some alpha globulin and alpha globulin, trace beta globulin, and trace gamma globulin.

Description: Normally, the urine is free of protein or contains only trace amounts of albumin and globulin, as the glomeruli prevent the passage of proteins from the plasma to the glomerular filtrate. Protein electrophoresis is a quantitative measurement of proteins, which under the influence of an electrical field, at a pH of 8.6, separate by charge, size, and shape. The separation produces homogeneous bands that are plotted on treated paper. Protein electrophoresis detects the presence of free light chains and other proteins associated with myoclonal gammopathies. The normally round and broad curves form a "church spire," or sharp peak. The immunoelectrophoretic technique is able to demonstrate a large number of components that are identical to the serum electrophoretic patterns. It is used to identify light chain, Bence Jones, kappa, lambda, and heavy chain proteins. The test helps detect specific abnormalities by identifying patterns of protein characteristic of different disease states. The meaning of the results of urine electrophoresis is best interpreted when the test is run simultaneously with a serum sample for electrophoresis.

Professional Considerations:

1. Consent form NOT required.
2. Preparation:
   A. Obtain a clean 50-ml container for a random urine collection or a 3-L container without preservatives or to which toluene or acetic acid has been added. For pediatric/infant specimen collection, also obtain a pediatric urine collection device/bag and tape.
   B. Write the beginning time of the 24-hour collection on the laboratory requisition.
   C. *See Client and family teaching.*
3. Procedure:
   A. *Random sample:* Obtain a 25-ml fresh, first morning-voided urine sample in a clean container. A fresh specimen may be taken from a urinary drainage bag.
   B. *24-hour sample:* Discard the first morning-urine specimen. Save all urine voided for 24 hours in a refrigerated, clean 3-L container without preservatives or to which toluene or acetic acid preservative has been added. Document the quantity of urine output during the specimen collection

period. Include the urine voided at the end of the 24-hour period. For catheterized clients, keep the drainage bag on ice and empty the urine into the collection container hourly.

C. *Pediatric/infant specimen collection:* Empty the urine into the refrigerated collection container after each void.

   i. The child is placed in a supine position with the knees flexed and the hips externally rotated and abducted.

   ii. Cleanse, rinse, and thoroughly dry the perineal area.

   iii. To prevent the child from removing the collection device/bag, a diaper may be placed over the genital area.

   iv. *Females:* Tape the pediatric collection device/bag to the perineum. Starting at the area between the anus and vagina, apply the device/bag in an anterior direction.

   v. *Males:* Place the pediatric collection device/bag over the penis and scrotum and tape it to the perineal area.

4. Postprocedure care:

   A. Compare the urine quantity in the specimen container with the urinary output record for the test. If the specimen contains less urine than was recorded as output, some of the sample may have been discarded, invalidating the test.

   B. Document the urine quantity on the laboratory requisition.

5. Client and family teaching:

   A. For 24-hour urine collection for home collection: Save all urine voided in the 24-hour period and urinate before defecating to avoid loss of urine. If any urine is accidentally discarded, discard the entire specimen and restart the collection the next day.

   B. Avoid drugs that may cause protein-

uria (listed below) for specific lengths of time before the test, as specified by the physician.

6. Factors that affect results:

   A. Contamination of the specimen with stool invalidates the results. The test must be repeated or restarted.

   B. Drugs that cause proteinuria include amikacin sulfate, amphotericin B, aurothioglucose, bacitracin, gentamicin sulfate, gold sodium thyiomalate, kanamycin, neomycin sulfate, netilmycin sulfate, penicillins, phenylbutazone, polymyxin B, streptomycin sulfate, sulfonamides, tobramycin sulfate, and trimethadione.

7. Other data:

   A. Urine protein electrophoresis results should be evaluated with consideration given to serum protein electrophoresis patterns.

Bibliography:

Astion ML, Rank J, Wener MH: Electrophoresis-tutor: an image-based personal computer program that teaches clinical interpretation of protein electrophoresis patterns of serum, urine and cerebrospinal fluid. Clin Chem *41*(9):1328–1332, 1995.

Bueler MR, Wiederkehr F, Vonderschmitt DJ: Electrophoresis, chromatographic and immunological studies of human urinary proteins. Electrophoresis *16*(1):124–134, 1995.

Tormey WP, O'Brien PA: Clinical associations of an increased transthyretin band in routine serum and urine protein electrophoresis. Ann Clin Biochem *30*(Pt 6):550–554, 1993.

PROTEIN, QUANTITATIVE, URINE
(see Protein, Urine)

PROTEIN, SEMIQUANTITATIVE, URINE
(see Protein, Urine)

PROTEIN, TOTAL, SERUM

Norm:

		SI Units
Adults	6.0–8.0 g/dl	60–80 g/L
Children		
Premature	4.3–7.6 g/dl	43–76 g/L
Newborn	4.6–7.4 g/dl	46–74 g/L
Infant	6.0–6.7 g/dl	60–67 g/L
Child	6.2–8.0 g/dl	62–80 g/L

Increased: Amyloidosis, Addison's disease, autoimmune collagen disorders, chronic infection, Crohn's disease, dehydration (relative increase), diarrhea, Franklin's disease, hemolysis, liver disease, macroglobulinemia, multiple myeloma, protozoal diseases (kala-azar), renal disease, sarcoidosis, vomiting, and wound drainage. Drugs include Bromsulphalein, clofibrate, corticosteroids, corticotropin, dextran, heparin calcium, heparin sodium, insulin, levothyroxine sodium/T, radiographic contrast dye, somatotropin, sonatrem, thyrotropin, and tolbutamide.

Decreased: Acute cholecystitis, analbuminemia, burns, chronic glomerulonephritis, cirrhosis, congestive heart failure, Crohn's disease, diarrhea, edema, essential hypertension, exfoliative dermatitis, frequent plasma donation, hemorrhage, hepatic disease (severe), Hodgkin's disease, hyperalimentation, hyperthyroidism, hypoalbuminemia, hypogammaglobulinemia, infectious hepatitis, kwashiorkor, leukemia (monocytic, myelogenous), malabsorption, malnutrition, nephrosis, nephrotic syndrome, peptic ulcer, pregnancy, protein-losing enteropathies, sprue, ulcerative colitis, and water intoxication. Drugs include ammonium ion, dextran, excessive intravenous fluids containing glucose, oral contraceptives, pyrazinamide, and salicylates.

Description: Total serum protein reflects the total amount of albumin and globulins in the serum. The serum proteins that are synthesized in the liver and reticuloendothelial system constitute over 100 different substances and are grouped as albumin and globulins. Serum proteins are essential to the regulation of colloid osmotic pressure, and comprise coagulation factors for hemostasis, enzymes, hormones, tissue growth and repair, and pH buffers. They produce antibodies, transport blood components (bilirubin, calcium, lipids, metals, oxygen, steroids, thyroid hormones, and vitamins) and are the preservers of chromosomes.

Professional Considerations:

1. Consent form NOT required.
2. Preparation:
   A. Tube: Red-top, red/gray-top, or gold-top.
   B. Medications that interfere with serum protein levels may be withheld.
   C. Do NOT draw specimens during hemodialysis.
   D. *See Client and family teaching.*
3. Procedure:
   A. Draw a 1-ml blood sample, without trauma.
   B. Avoid prolonged application of a tourniquet, which can cause an increase in protein concentrations.
   C. Obtain the sample away from IV solution, which can lower protein levels through local dilution.
4. Postprocedure care:
   A. Samples may be refrigerated for up to 1 week.
5. Client and family teaching:
   A. Do not ingest a high-fat diet for 8 hours before the test.
   B. Medications that interfere with serum protein levels may be prescribed to be withheld prior to the test.
6. Factors that affect results:
   A. Reject hemolyzed or lipemic specimens.
   B. Falsely elevated total protein levels occur for up to 48 hours after the use of sulfobromophthalein contrast dye.
   C. Recent dialysis distorts protein values.
   D. Hyperglycemia may cause total protein concentration to appear to be greater than actual.
   E. Serum total protein for bedridden clients is lower by approximately 0.3 g/dl than expected for the same age.
7. Other data:
   A. *See also Protein Electrophoresis, Blood.*
   B. The significance of the total protein is difficult to interpret without knowledge of the level of the individual fractions (albumin/globulin) obtained through electrophoresis.

Bibliography:

Jones DK, Dunn MI: "Vampire Syndrome": serum protein and lipid abnormalities related to frequent sale of plasma. J Fam Pract *40*(3):288–290, 1995.

PROTEIN, URINE

Norm: Negative; no detectable protein.

		SI Units
Semiquantitative Norms		
Normal	<20 mg/%	<0.2 g/L
Reagent strip/stick		
Negative	0–5 mg/dl	0–0.05 g/L

		SI Units

Semiquantitative Norms (continued)

Trace	5–20 mg/dl	0.05–0.2 g/L
1+	30 mg/dl	0.3 g/L
2+	100 mg/dl	1.0 g/L
3+	300 mg/dl	3.0 g/L
4+	1000 mg/dl	10.0 g/L

Quantitative Norms

Adults	30–150 mg/24 hours	0.03–0.15 g/day
Children <age 10	<100 mg/24 hours	<0.10 g/day

Newborn: Increased protein in urine for 3 days following delivery.

Increased or Positive:

Nonrenal Disease: Abdominal tumor, aging, anemia (severe), ascites, bacterial toxins (acute streptococcal, diphtheria, pneumonia, scarlet and typhoid fever), cardiac disease, central nervous system lesion, convulsive disorders, fever, hepatic disease (jaundice), hypersensitivity reaction, hyperthyroidism, infection (acute), ingestion of or overexposure to certain substances (arsenic, carbon tetrachloride, ether, lead, mercury, mustard, opiates, phenol, propylene glycol, sulfosalicylic acid, turpentine), intestinal obstruction, leukemia (chronic lymphocytic), subacute bacterial endocarditis, toxemia, and trauma.

Transient Proteinuria: Dehydration, diet (excessive protein), emotional stress, exposure to cold, exercise (strenuous), fever, orthostatic proteinuria, posthemorrhage, and sodium depletion. Drugs include epinephrine bitartrate, epinephrine borate, epinephrine hydrochloride, and levarterenol bitartrate.

Prerenal Disease: Amyloidosis, Bence Jones proteinuria associated with myeloma, congestive heart failure, convulsions, exercise, leukemia (myelocytic), orthostatic proteinuria, stroke, and Waldenström's macroglobulinemia.

Renal Disease: Collagen diseases, cryoglobulinemia, Henoch-Schönlein purpura, hypertension (malignant, renovascular), and thrombotic thrombocytopenic purpura.

Glomerular Disease: Amyloidosis, diabetic glomerulosclerosis and nephropathy, glomerulonephritis and lesion, Goodpasture's syndrome, high molec-ular weight proteinuria, membranous nephropathy, polycystic disease, pyelonephritis (chronic), renal vein thrombosis, and systemic lupus erythematosus.

Interstitial Disease: Bacterial pyelonephritis, deposition of calcium, uric acid, or urate, and idiosyncratic pharmacologic reactions to the following drugs: methicillin sodium, phenytoin, phenytoin sodium, phenindione, and sulfonamides.

Tubular Disease: Acute tubular necrosis, Bartter's syndrome, beta-microglobulinemia, Bright's disease, Butler-Albright syndrome, Fanconi's syndrome, galactosemia, heavy metal poisoning (cadmium, lead, mercury), Kimmelsteil-Wilson disease, nephrotic syndrome, and renal tubular acidosis.

Postrenal Disease: Cystitis (severe), tumor metastasis of the bone, and tumor (urinary bladder, renal pelvis). *Drugs that cause proteinuria include* amikacin sulfate, amphotericin B, aurothioglucose, bacitracin, gentamicin sulfate, gold sodium thiomalate, netilmicin sulfate, neomycin sulfate, penicillins, phenylbutazone, polymyxin B, streptomycin sulfate, sulfonamides, and trimethadione.

Decreased: Not applicable.

Description: The semiquantitative urine test is a random screening test for urinary protein and is part of the routine urinalysis. The reagent strip color indicators and use of sulfosalicylic acid in the laboratory are two methods used to confirm the presence of urinary protein. A small amount of protein in the urine is regarded as normal and consists of albumin and low molecular weight plasma proteins (beta-microglobulin, globulins, haptoglobulin, light chains, and Tamm-Horsfall glycoprotein). Protein in the urine is a key indicator of renal pathology.

Quantitation of urinary protein is indicated when a random urine sample is positive for more than a trace of protein. Normally, only low molecular weight proteins are small enough to pass through the glomerular membrane into the glomerular filtrate, and most of these are reabsorbed by the renal tubules. Proteinuria is a key indicator of renal pathology and can result from glomerular leakage, tubular impairment, breakdown of renal tissue, or from excessive concentrations of low molecular weight proteins. Transient proteinuria may result from nonpathologic states such as physical or emotional stress and body position. Protein substances are excreted at different rates and at varying times in a 24-hour period; thus, the 24-hour timed quantitative urine test for protein provides the most accurate reflection of kidney function.

Professional Considerations:

1. Consent form NOT required.
2. Preparation:
   A. *Semiquantitative test:*
      i. Obtain a clean, dry plastic container or a pediatric urine-collection device and a container of reagent strips.
   B. *Quantitative test:*
      i. Obtain a clean, 3-L container that is free of preservative. For pediatric/infant collections, also obtain tape and a pediatric urine-collection device/bag.
      ii. Write the beginning time of the 24-hour collection on the laboratory requisition.
3. Procedure:
   A. *Semiquantitative test:*
      i. An early-morning specimen or the first voided specimen of the day after the client stands upright is preferred.
      ii. Instruct the client to void into a clean, dry container. The specimen may be transferred to a plastic container.
      iii. Specimens may be tested immediately or sent to the laboratory for testing.
      iv. To test the sample immediately, dip the reagent strip into the urine and remove any excess urine by gently tapping the strip on the side of the collection container. The strip

should then be held at a horizontal plane to prevent mixing of any other chemicals on the strip. Immediately and carefully compare the color of the test pad on the reagent strip to the color chart provided on the container from which it was taken. Record the result according to the negative to 4+ range of approximate mg/dl of protein.
   B. *Quantitative test:*
      i. Early morning is the preferred time to begin a 24-hour collection.
      ii. Discard the first morning-urine specimen.
      iii. Save all the urine voided for 24 hours in a refrigerated, clean, 3-L container that is free of preservatives. Document the quantity of urine output during the specimen collection period. Include the urine voided at the end of the 24-hour period. For catheterized clients, keep the drainage bag on ice and empty the urine into the refrigerated collection container hourly.
      iv. Pediatric/infant specimen collection:
         a. Empty the collection bag into the refrigerated collection container after each void.
         b. The child is placed in a supine position with the knees flexed and the hips externally rotated and abducted.
         c. Cleanse, rinse, and thoroughly dry the perineal area.
         d. To prevent the child from removing the collection device/bag, a diaper may be placed over the genital area.
         e. *Females:* Tape the pediatric collection device/bag to the perineum. Starting at the area between the anus and vagina, apply the device/bag in an anterior direction.
         f. *Males:* Place the pediatric collection device/bag over the penis and scrotum and tape it to the perineal area.
4. Postprocedure care:
   A. *Semiquantitative test:*
      i. To be most accurate, specimens sent to the laboratory must be transported within 2 hours of the collection of the sulfosalicylic acid precipitation of the protein. Specimens must be refrigerated.
   B. *Quantitative test:*
      i. Compare the urine quantity in the specimen container with the urinary output record for the test. If the specimen contains less urine than was recorded as output, some of the sample may have been discarded, thus invalidating the test.

ii. Document the urine quantity and ending time on the laboratory requisition.

5. Client and family teaching.
   A. Save all the urine voided in a 24-hour period; urinate before defecating to avoid loss of urine; and avoid contamination of the specimen with stool, toilet tissue, or prostatic or vaginal secretions. If any urine is accidentally discarded, discard the entire specimen and restart the collection the next day.
   B. Parents may be taught a pediatric collection technique for specimens collected on infants at home.

6. Factors that affect results:
   A. Drugs that may cause false-positive semiquantitative results include acetazolamide, aminosalicyclic acid, cephaloridine, chlorpromazine, penicillins, phenazopyridine, promazine hydrochloride, radiographic contrast media, sodium bicarbonate, sulfisoxazole, sulfonamides, thymol, and Tolbutamide.
   B. Drugs that may cause falsely elevated quantitative results include acetazolamide, aminosalicyclic acid, aspirin, barbiturates, cephalosporins, corticosteroids, iodine, iodine contrast medium, mercurial diuretics, penicillins, sodium bicarbonate, sulfonamides, tolbutamide, and tolmetin sodium.
   C. First-voided urine samples are the most accurate for semiquantitative measurement, as they are more uniformly concentrated, with a more acidic pH, and they are more likely to exhibit abnormalities.
   D. False-positive semiquantitative results can occur with incorrect matching of the reagent strip to the color chart and with prolonged exposure of the strip/stick to the urine.
   E. False-positives have been reported with gross hematuria.
   F. Reject specimens contaminated with blood, heavy mucus, purulent drainage, stool, prostatic or vaginal secretions, or toilet tissue.

G. The presence of many white blood cells can alter the results.
H. False-negative results have been reported with very dilute urine, highly buffered alkaline urine, urine high in sodium, and urea-splitting infectious organisms of the urinary tract.
I. Reject quantitative specimens in which the last void prior to the testing period was not discarded.
J. All urine voided for the 24-hour period must be included to avoid a falsely low quantitative result.

7. Other data:
   A. The creatinine clearance test is often prescribed in conjunction with the quantitative urine protein test.
   B. The reagent strip is most sensitive to albumin and less sensitive to globulins.
   C. The reagent strip method will not detect Bence Jones protein, globulins, mucoproteins, or myeloma protein.
   D. Bence Jones protein may be present if the reagent strip method is negative and the sulfosalicylic acid test is positive. An electrophoresis and immunoelectrophoresis for light chains is indicated, as Bence Jones proteins are associated with amyloidosis, chronic lymphocytic leukemia, hyperparathyroidism, macroglobulinemia, malignant lymphoma, metastatic bone tumor, multiple myeloma, and osteomalacia.
   E. Semiquantitative testing with a regent strip will show a trace positive reaction at a protein concentration of 100–200 mg/L.
   F. Increased protein concentrations are found during the daytime and after exercise.
   G. *See also Protein Electrophoresis, Urine.*

Bibliography:

Gibble RK, Fee SC, Berg RL: The value of routine urine dipstick screening for protein at each prenatal visit. Am J Obstet Gynecol *173*(1):214–217, 1995.

Wilson DM, Anderson RL: Protein-osmolality ratio for the quantitative assessment of proteinuria from a random urinalysis sample. Am J Clin Pathol *100*(4):419–424, 1993.

PROTHROMBIN TIME (PT) AND INTERNATIONAL NORMALIZED RATIO (INR), SERUM

Norm: Each laboratory establishes a normal value, or control, based on the method and reagents used to perform the test. A value within ±2 seconds of the control set by each laboratory is considered within a normal range.

	Prothrombin Time
Adult	10–15 seconds
Newborn	<17 seconds
Child	11–14 seconds
Panic value	>40 seconds
Nonanticoagulated condition	>20 seconds
Anticoagulated condition	>3 times the control

International Normalized Ratio (INR)

Coumadin Therapy: There are, in general, two therapeutic ranges for clients on warfarin (Coumadin):

Standard therapy: 2.0–3.0 INR: Appropriate for management of acute myocardial infarction, atrial fibrillation, deep vein thrombosis, prevention of systemic embolism.

High-dose therapy: 3.0–4.5 INR: Appropriate for management of mechanical heart valves and recurrent systemic embolism; for prevention of systemic embolism; and prophylaxis in high-risk surgery.

Panic Level Symptoms and Treatment:

Symptoms: Bleeding from venipuncture/arterial/intravenous catheter sites, ecchymoses, hematoma, hematuria, blood in stool, ecchymosis, or hallmark signs of intracerebral, gastrointestinal, or retroperitoneal bleed.

Treatment:

Discontinue or reduce rate of IV anticoagulant.
Maintain patent airway.
Apply pressure × 10 minutes or more to bleeding line or venipuncture sites.
Observe and intervene for hemodynamic stability.
Administer vitamin K.

Increased PT: Afibrinogenemia, alcoholism, biliary obstruction, cancer, celiac disease, circulating anticoagulants, cirrhosis, colitis, collagen disease, congestive heart failure, diarrhea (chronic), disseminated intravascular coagulation (DIC), dysfibrinogenemia, factor deficiency (I, II, V, VII, X), fever, fibrinogen degradation products (FDP), fistula, hemorrhagic disease of the newborn, hepatic disease (abscess, biopsy, failure, jaundice, infectious hepatitis), hypernephroma of kidney, hyperthyroidism, hypervitaminosis A, hypofibrinogenemia (<100 mg/dl), idiopathic familial hypoprothrombinemia, idiopathic myelofibrosis, increased fibrinolytic activity, jaundice (hemolytic, he-patocellular, obstructive), leukemia (acute), malabsorption, malnutrition, obstetric complications, pancreatic carcinoma, pancreatitis (chronic), polycythemia vera, premature infants, prolonged hot weather, prothrombin deficiency, Reye's syndrome, snakebite, sprue, steatorrhea, toxic shock syndrome, vitamin K deficiency, and vomiting. Drugs include alcohol, allopurinol, aminosalicylic acid, amiodarone hydrochloride, anabolic steroids, antibiotics, bromelains, chenodiol, chloral hydrate, chlorpropamide, chymotrypsin, cimetidine, clofibrate, dextran, dextrothyroxine, diazoxide, diflunisal, disulfiram, diuretics, ethacrynic acid, fenoprofen, fluoroquinolone antibiotics, glucagon, hepatotoxic drugs, ibuprofen, indomethacin, influenza virus vaccine, mefenamic acid, methyldopa, methylphenidate, metronidazole, miconazole, monoamine oxidase inhibitors, nalidixic acid, naproxen, narcotics (prolonged), pentoxifylline, phenylbutazone, phenytoin sodium, propafenone, pyrazolones, quinidine, quinine, ranitidine, salicylates, sulfinpyrazone, sulfonamides (long-acting), sulindac, tamoxifen, thyroid drugs, tolbutamide, trimethoprim/sulfamethoxazole and warfarin sodium (underdosage).

Increased INR: Excess oral anticoagulant. INR is also increased by conditions that increase PT.

Decreased PT: Arterial occlusion, deep vein thrombosis, edema, hereditary coumarin resistance, hyperlipemia, hyperthyroidism, hypothyroidism, multiple myeloma, myocardial infarction, peripheral vascular disease, pulmonary embolism, spinal cord injury, thromboembolism (acute), and transplant rejection. Drugs include adrenocortical steroids, alcohol, aminoglutethimide, antacids, antihistamines, barbiturates, carbamazepine, chloral hydrate, chlordiazepoxide, cholestyramine, diuretics, ethchlorvynol, glutethimide, griseofulvin, haloperidol, meprobamate, nafcillin, oral contraceptives, paraldehyde, primidone, ranitidine, rifampin, sucralfate, trazodone, vitamin C, and warfarin sodium (underdosage).

Decreased INR: Insufficient oral anticoagulant. INR is also decreased by conditions and drugs that decrease PT.

Description: Prothrombin is a vitamin K-dependent glycoprotein produced by the liver that is necessary for firm fibrin clot formation. It converts to thrombin in the clotting cascade process and should not appear in the serum after clot formation. Prothrombin time PT measures the amount of time taken for clot formation after reagent tissue thromboplastin (brain tissue extract) and calcium are added to citrated plasma. PT is used to monitor response to warfarin therapy or to screen for dysfunction involving the extrinsic system resulting from liver disease, vitamin K deficiency, factor deficiency, or DIC. The most accurate PT values are reported as the number of seconds taken for the client's plasma to form a clot, along with the number of seconds taken for a laboratory control sample to clot. Very small PT fluctuations can have profound physiologic effects.

The INR improves usability of the PT test in monitoring response to anticoagulation therapy. Individual responses to same-dose warfarin anticoagulant therapy varies. Therefore, the efficacy and safety of management are dependent upon maintaining the anticoagulant effect within a defined therapeutic range. The INR standardizes the PT ratio by allowing all thromboplastin reagents to be compared to an international standard thromboplastin provided by the World Health Organization. An International Sensitivity Index (ISI) is assigned to each thromboplastin reagent that is used in mathematically calculating the INR to correct for varying thromboplastin sensitivities: The INR is calculated by raising the observed PT ratio to the power of the ISI specific to the particular thromboplastin reagent used, or:

$$INR = \frac{Client's\ PT\ in\ seconds^{ISI}}{Mean\ normal\ PT\ in\ seconds}$$

Professional Considerations:

1. Consent form NOT required.
2. Preparation:
   A. Baseline PT should be drawn before starting anticoagulant therapy.
   B. Tube: 2.7-ml or 4.5-ml blue-top tube and a control tube and a waste tube or syringe.
   C. Do NOT draw specimens during hemodialysis.
   D. *See Client and family teaching.*

3. Procedure:
   A. Perform venipuncture and withdraw 2 ml of blood into a syringe or vacuum tube. Remove the syringe or tube, leaving the needle in place.
   B. Attach a second syringe and completely fill a blue-top tube with a blood sample collected without trauma. The sample quantity should be 2.4 ml for a 2.7-ml tube and 4.0 ml for a 4.5-ml tube.
   C. A 9:1 ratio of blood to citrate is critical.
   D. Gently tilt the tube several times to thoroughly mix the specimen.

4. Postprocedure care:
   A. Write the specimen collection time on the laboratory requisition.
   B. Send the specimen to the laboratory immediately.
   C. The specimen should be refrigerated until testing.
   D. In the presence of a coagulation defect, the venipuncture site should have digital direct pressure to the site for 3–5 minutes after the needle is removed. The venipuncture site should be observed for bleeding or excessive ecchymosis.

5. Client and family teaching:
   A. Abstain from coffee and alcohol for 24 hours before the test, as they cause lipemia, which can cause falsely decreased levels.
   B. Follow normal dietary patterns for vitamin-K-containing foods during the 24 hours prior to the test.
   C. Oral anticoagulant medication should be taken at the same time daily. Regular PT checks may be required for clients on long-term anticoagulant medication.
   D. Report any unusual bleeding.
   E. Women of childbearing age should be advised to avoid pregnancy during oral anticoagulation, as warfarin is teratogenic and can cause fetal death. Heparin, which does not cross the placenta, should be used if pregnancy is desired.
   F. Warfarin enters breast milk. Women should not breast-feed when taking warfarin.

6. Factors that affect results:
   A. Reject hemolyzed or lipemic specimens or specimens received more than 3 hours after collection.
   B. Reject specimens in which collection tubes are incompletely filled, because the volume of the sample is not enough to thoroughly mix with the premeasured amount of anticoagulant.
   C. Reject specimens not promptly transported to the laboratory or refrigerated.
   D. Concurrent therapy with heparin can lengthen PT for up to 5 hours after dosing. To minimize this influence,

blood for PT determinations should be drawn 5 hours after IV heparin and 24 hours after SQ heparin injection.

E. The problem of loss of accuracy/precision of the INR system can be resolved by using sensitive thromboplastins with ISI values close to 1.0 (WHO reagent ISI = 1.0). However, even without this sensitivity, the INR system is more accurate than reporting the results as a PT ratio.

F. The use of automated clot detectors requires the use of sensitive thromboplastins or calibration of each new batch of thromboplastins with lyophilized plasmas with certified INR values obtained by the manual method to obtain valid and reliable results. ("True" INR values were obtained by the manual method.)

G. It is recommended that reagents insensitive to heparin be used to avoid obtaining falsely elevated INRs when on heparin and Coumadin concurrently. Innovin and Thromboplastin C Plus meet this criterion.

H. Antibiotic therapy, mineral oil, and clofibrate can affect the PT.

I. Diets excessively high in green leafy vegetables can increase the absorption of vitamin K, which shortens the PT.

J. A minimum of 100 g/dl of fibrinogen must be present for the PT to be accurate.

K. The PT is affected by many pharmacologic agents, including those that alter protein-binding patterns, those that inhibit the formation of intestinal microorganisms, and those that are precursors of enzyme production.

L. Contamination of the specimen with tissue thromboplastin may alter the results. This is the reason for the double-draw technique.

M. The PT is usually not prolonged until factors (II, V, VII, X) are decreased or less than 50% of normal or the fibrinogen is decreased to less than 80–100 mg/dl.

7. Other data:

A. PT/INR should be measured frequently: daily × 5 when treatment is initiated, twice a week the following 1–2 weeks, once a week for the next 1–2 months, and every 2–4 weeks thereafter. Also, PT/INR should be performed whenever a drug that interacts with warfarin is added to or deleted from the regimen *(see Prothrombin Time, Serum)*.

B. The INR system is invalid in clients with liver disease (different reagents do not give the same INR for the same sample) but is no less valid than the PT in this client population.

C. The PT should be evaluated daily and used as a basis for dose adjustments during initial anticoagulation therapy.

D. A time interval of 16–48 hours may occur before warfarin affects the PT value.

E. A PT >30 seconds places the client at risk for hemorrhage.

F. Oral anticoagulation therapy usually maintains the prothrombin time at 1.5–2 times the laboratory control value. Clients with cardiac disease may be maintained at 2–2.5 times the laboratory control value.

Bibliography:

Anonymous: ASHP therapeutic position statement on the use of the international normalized ratio system to monitor oral anticoagulation therapy. Am J Health-System Pharmacy 52(5):529–531, 1995.

Hirsh J, Poller L: The International Normalized Ratio: A guide to understanding and correcting its problems. Arch Intern Med 154(3):282–288, 1994.

Katz SS, White RH, Hill J, et al.: Accuracy of laboratory and portable monitor international normalized ratio determinations. Comparison with a criterion standard. Arch Intern Med 155(17):1861–1867, 1995.

Kovacs MJ, Wong A, MacKinnon K, et al.: Assessment of the validity of the INR system for patients with liver impairment. Thromb Haemost 71(6):727–730.

Lehne RA, et al.: Pharmacology for Nursing Care, 2nd ed. Philadelphia, WB Saunders, 1994, pp 583–584.

Morse EE, Panek S, Pisciotto P, et al.: Reemergence of the International Normalized Ratio for the standardization of prothrombin time. Ann Clin Lab Sci 23(3):184–188, 1993.

Nichols WL, Bowie EJ: Standardization of the prothrombin time for monitoring orally administered anticoagulant therapy with the use of the International Normalized Ratio system. Mayo Clin Proc 68(11):897–898, 1993.

Solomon HM, Randall JR, Simmons VL: Heparin-induced Increase in the International Normalized Ratio: Responses of 10 commercial thromboplastin reagents. Am J Clin Pathol 103:735–739, 1995.

PROTOPORPHYRIN, FREE ERYTHROCYTE, BLOOD

Norm:

		SI Units
Piomelli method		
Adult female	19–52 mg/dl	0.34–0.92 μmol/L
Adult male	11–45 mg/dl	0.20–0.80 μmol/L

		SI Units
Hematofluorometer		
Adult female	<40 mg/dl	0.71 µmol/L
Adult male	<30 mg/dl	0.53 µmol/L
Panic level	>190 mg/dl	>3.38 µmol/L
Erythrocyte precursors		
Protoporphyrin	4–52 mg/dl	0.07–0.92 µmol/L

Increased: Erythropoiesis, erythropoietic protoporphyria (>2200 mg/dl), hemolytic anemia (>50 mg/dl), infection (>50 mg/dl), iron deficiency (>200 mg/dl), lead poisoning (>200 mg/dl), protoporphyria, sideroachrestic anemia (acquired) (>50 mg/dl), and thalassemia.

Decreased: Megaloblastic anemia (<30 mg/dl).

Description: Protoporphyrin is a derivative of porphin that combines with iron to form the heme portion of hemoglobin and comprise the predominant porphyrin in red blood cells (RBCs). After hemoglobin breakdown, protoporphyrin is converted into bilirubin, combines with albumin, and remains unconjugated in the circulation. In conditions interfering with heme synthesis, increased amounts of protoporphyrin can be detected in erythrocytes, urine, and stool. Protoporphyria is an autosomal dominant disorder in which increased amounts of protoporphyrin are secreted and excreted. It is thought to be caused by an enzyme deficiency and is detected by the identification of increased concentrations of protoporphyrin in RBCs. Protoporphyria causes photosensitivity and may lead to cirrhosis and cholelithiasis due to protoporphyrin deposition. The free erythrocyte protoporphyrin (FEP) test measures the concentration of protoporphyrin in RBCs.

Professional Considerations:

1. Consent form NOT required.
2. Preparation:
   A. Write the current hematocrit value on the laboratory requisition.
   B. If this test is being used for evaluation of lead intoxication, a blood sample for lead measurement should also be obtained.
   C. Tube: Green-top, lavender-top, or black-top.
   D. Do NOT draw specimens during hemodialysis.
3. Procedure:
   A. Draw a 3-ml blood sample, without hemolysis.
   B. Capillary tube samples from pediatric heelsticks are acceptable. (See notation regarding infant testing in item 6 below).
4. Postprocedure care:
   A. Protect specimens from light.
5. Client and family teaching:
   A. Because protoporphyria is a hereditary disease, genetic counseling may be advised.
   B. Inform the client of lead poisoning detection and prevention.
6. Factors that affect results:
   A. Hemolysis of the specimen invalidates the results.
   B. This test is considered to be unreliable in infants under 6 months of age.
7. Other data:
   A. This test can be used to screen for elevated lead in children after iron deficiency is ruled out.
   B. See also Porphyrins, Quantitative, Blood; and Coproporphyrin, Urine.

Bibliography:

Fishbane S, Lynn RI: The utility of zinc protoporphyrin for predicting the need for intravenous iron therapy in hemodialysis patients. Am J Kidney Dis 25(3):426–432, 1995.

Mercurio MG, Prince G, Weber FL Jr, et al.: Terminal hepatic failure in erythropoietic protoporphyria. J Am Acad Dermatol 29(5, Pt 2):829–833, 1993.

Siegel RM, LaGrone DH: The use of zinc protoporphyrin in screening young children for iron deficiency. Clin Pediatr 33(8):473–479, 1994.

PROTRIPTYLINE
(see Tricyclic Antidepressants, Plasma or Serum)

PSA, SERUM
(see Prostate-Specific Antigen, Serum)

PSEUDOCHOLINESTERASE (CHOLINESTERASE, CHOLINESTERASE II, CHS, PCHE), PLASMA

Norm: Norms vary, depending on the laboratory substrate test method.

		SI Units
RID method	0.5–1.5 mg/dl	5–15 mg/L
DuPont ACA method	7–19 U/ml	7–19 kU/L
Other methods	3.0–8.0 U/ml	
	8–18 IU/L	
	0.5–1.3 pH U/h	
Female	204–500 IU/dl	
Male	274–532 IU/dl	
Dibucaine inhibition	81–87%	0.81–0.87
Fluoride inhibition	44–54%	0.44–0.54

Increased: Diabetes mellitus, hyperthyroidism, insecticide exposure of organic phosphates, and nephrotic syndrome.

Decreased: Anemia (severe pernicious, aplastic), carcinomatosis, cirrhosis, congenital deficiency, congestive heart failure (causing liver disease), dermatomyositis, hepatic carcinoma (metastatic), hepatitis (infectious), hypoproteinemia, infections (acute), infectious mononucleosis, insecticide exposure (carbamate, organophosphate), jaundice (obstructive), malnutrition, metastasis, muscular dystrophy, myocardial infarction, organophosphate insecticide poisoning (DFP, parathion, sarin, triocresyl phosphate), parenchymatous liver disease, recent plasmapheresis, shock, skin diseases, succinylcholine hypersensitivity, tuberculosis, and uremia. Drugs include estrogens, morphine sulfate, neostigmine bromide, neostigmine methylsulfate, oral contraceptives, physostigmine sulfate, physostigmine salicylate, pyridostigmine bromide, and phospholine iodine.

Description: Pseudocholinesterase (PCHE) is a nonspecific cholinesterase that hydrolyzes noncholine esters as well as acetylcholine. It exists in several forms and serves to inactivate acetylcholine. PCHE is synthesized by the liver and found in plasma and is well distributed throughout the body. This enzyme's activity is inhibited reversibly by carbamate insecticides and irreversibly by organophosphate insecticides. Clients with an inherited PCHE deficiency exhibit an increased sensitivity to the effects of succinylcholine, which is normally inactivated by PCHE. Inherited deficiencies can be detected by the identification of abnormal genotypes of PCHE through dibucaine and fluoride inhibition tests. While normal forms of PCHE are inhibited by these substances, the abnormal forms are not.

Professional Considerations:

1. Consent form NOT required.
2. Preparation:
   A. Tube: Red-top or green-top.
   B. Specimens MAY be drawn during hemodialysis.
   C. *See Client and family teaching.*
3. Procedure:
   A. Draw a 5-ml blood sample, without trauma.
4. Postprocedure care:
   A. If the test purpose is to screen for organophosphate insecticide poisoning, the sample should be transported to the laboratory for immediate spinning and refrigeration. For other purposes, serum samples remain stable at room temperature for up to 1 week, refrigerated for 2 weeks, and frozen for up to 3 months.
5. Client and family teaching:
   A. Ten percent of the population may carry the gene for an uncommon form of PCHE.
   B. Elevated results may indicate exposure to organophosphates and the source would need to be identified.
   C. If the test is to be using dibucaine/fluoride inhibition, the client should not have taken muscle relaxants or anticholinergic drugs within 24 hours.
6. Factors that affect results:
   A. Hemolysis of the specimen causes falsely elevated results.
   B. Pregnancy decreases values by 30%.
   C. Exposure of the sample to chemicals such as fluoride, citrate, and borate will cause falsely decreased results.

7. Other data:
   A. A 20% drop in PCHE activity between baseline and subsequent samples indicates overexposure to organophosphate insecticides.
   B. PCHE (pseudocholinesterase) is not to be confused with acetylcholinesterase (true cholinesterase, cholinesterase I, AcCHS).
   C. PCHE levels are an earlier indicator of organophosphate exposure than are acetylcholinesterase levels.

Bibliography:

Kutty KM, Payne RH: Serum pseudocholinesterase and very low density lipoprotein metabolism. J Clin Lab Anal *8*(4):247–250, 1994.

PSITTACOSIS TITER, BLOOD

Norm: *Chlamydia* antibody IgG test. Titer ≤1:640. Low titers may be found in psittacosis. A fourfold elevation indicates recent infection.

Usage: Screening for antibodies indicating infection with *Chlamydia psittaci.*

Description: Psittacosis (parrot fever, ornithosis) is a viral infectious disease caused by *C. psittaci. Chlamydia* transmission to humans is thought to be through inhalation of the aerosols of dried droppings and exudates from parrots, birds, and domestic fowl. Person-to-client transmission is rare. Symptoms of psittacosis include mild respiratory symptoms along with fever, headache, muscle aches, and chills. Because laboratory recovery of *C. psittaci* is often difficult, diagnosis is made after a significant rise in the titer of antibodies directed at the psittacosis-*lymphogranuloma* group of *Chlamydia* is detected.

Professional Considerations:

1. Consent form NOT required.
2. Preparation:
   A. Tube: Red-top, red/gray-top, or gold-top.
   B. Specimens MAY be drawn during hemodialysis.
3. Procedure:
   A. Draw a 10-ml blood sample, without hemolysis.
   B. Paired samples, an acute-phase specimen, and a convalescent-phase specimen, 2–3 weeks apart, should be obtained.
4. Postprocedure care:
   A. None.
5. Client and family teaching:
   A. The disease is transmitted through inhalation near bird feces.
   B. If a cough is present in the acute stage, psittacosis is communicable. The client must be placed on respiratory isolation, with close contacts wearing masks for protection. All bodily discharges must be disinfected.
6. Factors that affect results:
   A. Other infections such as brucellosis and Q fever can cause false-positive results.
7. Other data:
   A. Titer levels collected in the latter course of the infection provide more conclusive evidence of the disease.
   B. Albuminuria is common, while sputum culture and smear show normal flora. Cold agglutination is negative.
   C. In many countries, psittacosis is a reportable disease.
   D. Tetracyclines are used for the treatment of psittacosis.
   E. For diagnosis of psittacosis, prior contact with sick birds or employment in poultry business/pet shop should be documented.

Bibliography:

Kirchner JT, Boyarsky SA: *Chlamydia psittaci:* An uncommon cause of community-acquired pneumonia. Arch Fam Med *2*(9):997–1001, 1993.
Schlossberg D, Delgado J, Moore MM, et al.: An epidemic of avian and human psittacosis. Arch Intern Med *153*(22):2594–2596, 1993.
Wong KH, Skelton SK, Daugharty H: Utility of complement fixation and microimmunofluorescence assays for detecting serologic responses in patients with clinically diagnosed psittacosis. J Clin Microbiol *32*(10):2417–2421, 1994.

PTH
(see Parathyroid Hormone, Blood)

PTT
(see Partial Thromboplastin Time, Serum)

PULMONARY ANGIOGRAM (PULMONARY ANGIOGRAPHY, PULMONARY ARTERIOGRAPHY), DIAGNOSTIC

Norm: Radiopaque iodine contrast material should circulate symmetrically and without interruption through the pulmonary circulatory system.

Usage: Visualization of the size and shape of the pulmonary artery, its branches, and the pulmonary vascular bed; measurements of pressures within these structures, cardiac output, and pulmonary vascular resistance determinations; assessment of pulmonary vascular perfusion defects, including aneurysms, blood vessel displacement, stenosis, thrombi, and vascular filling defects; definitive diagnostic test for pulmonary thromboembolism, in the symptomatic client and in clients at risk on anticoagulation therapy and when lung scans are normal or inconclusive; and evaluation of the pulmonary circulatory system preoperatively in clients with congenital heart disease.

Description: Pulmonary angiography is an invasive roentgenographic, fluoroscopic procedure following injection of iodine radiopaque contrast material through a catheter inserted through an antecubital or femoral vein into the pulmonary artery or one of its branches.

Professional Considerations:

1. Consent form IS required.

Risks:
Arterial occlusion, dysrhythmias, embolism, hemorrhage, infection, allergic reaction to dye (itching, hives, rash, tight feeling in the throat, shortness of breath, bronchospasm, anaphylaxis, death), perforation of pulmonary artery or myocardium, renal toxicity from contrast medium.

Contraindications:
Previous allergy to iodine, radiographic dye, or shellfish; pregnancy; renal insufficiency. Sedatives are contraindicated in clients with central nervous system depression.

2. Preparation:
   A. Recent coagulation times, platelet count, and renal function should be noted.
   B. A mild sedative may be prescribed.
   C. Establish intravenous access for use in the event of a hypersensitivity or dysrhythmic complication.
   D. Obtain electrocardiographic patches, surgical scrub solution, povidone-iodine solution, sterile drapes, 1–2% lidocaine (Xylocaine), radiopaque contrast material, a pulmonary artery catheter, and a pulmonary angiogra-

phy tray. The amount of contrast dye used is based on the client's body weight.
   E. Have an emergency cart readily available.
   F. *See Client and family teaching.*
3. Procedure:
   A. The client is placed in the supine position. Electrodes are connected to a cardiac monitor.
   B. The femoral or antecubital vein site is cleansed with surgical scrub solution, followed by povidone-iodine solution, and covered with sterile drapes.
   C. After a local anesthetic is injected over the site, a needle puncture is made into the vein, a guidewire is placed through the needle, and a long catheter is introduced over the wire through the antecubital or femoral vein and advanced into the pulmonary vasculature. Pressures are measured as the catheter passes through the right atrium, right ventricle, and into the pulmonary artery.
   D. As the contrast material is injected, rapid, serial roentgenographic images or films record the circulation of the dye through the pulmonary vasculature.
   E. Monitor the client throughout the procedure for cardiac dysrhythmias or a hypersensitivity reaction to the contrast material.
   F. The catheter is removed and a pressure dressing is applied over the insertion site.
4. Postprocedure care:
   A. Monitor the catheter insertion site for bleeding, inflammation, or hematoma formation.
   B. Assess vital signs according to institutional protocol (usually every 15 minutes × 4, then every 4 hours × 4).
   C. Although hypersensitivity reactions usually occur during the first 30 minutes after injection of radiopaque iodine, a delayed reaction is possible.
   D. Resume previous diet.
   E. No blood pressures should be taken from the extremity used for injection for 24 hours.
5. Client and family teaching:
   A. Fast for 8 hours before the procedure.
   B. For 5 minutes after the injection of the contrast material, an urge to cough, flushing, nausea, or salty taste may occur.
   C. The client must lie motionless during the procedure.
6. Factors that affect results:
   A. The client must be able to lie motionless during the procedure.
7. Other data:
   A. Small peripheral emboli may not be visible with angiography, but these rarely produce symptoms or result in the usual outcomes of embolism.

B. Potential complications of angiography include venous occlusion, ventricular dysrhythmias, hypersensitivity reactions, myocardial perforation or rupture, acute pulmonary hypertension, and acute renal failure (related to the presence of contrast material).

Bibliography:

Greenspan RH: Pulmonary angiography and the diagnosis of pulmonary embolism. Progr Cardiovasc Dis 37(2):93–105, 1994.

Matsumoto AH, Tegtmeyer CJ: Contemporary diagnostic approaches to acute pulmonary emboli. Radiat Clin North Am 33(1):167–183, 1995.

PULMONARY ARTERIOGRAPHY, DIAGNOSTIC

(see Pulmonary Angiogram, Diagnostic)

PULMONARY ARTERY CATHETERIZATION, DIAGNOSTIC

Norm:

Adult Pressures	
Right atrial (RA) pressure	3–11 mmHg
Central venous pressure (CVP)	2–6 mmHg
	(2.7–12 cm H_2O)
Right ventricular systolic pressure	20–30 mmHg
Right ventricular end-diastolic pressure	<5 mmHg
Pulmonary artery systolic (PAS) pressure	20–30 mmHg
Pulmonary artery end-diastolic pressure (PAEDP)	8–15 mmHg
Pulmonary artery mean (PAM) pressure	<20 mmHg
Pulmonary artery wedge pressure (PAWP) or pulmonary capillary wedge pressure (PCWP)	4–12 mmHg
Cardiac output (CO)	5–8 L/minute
Cardiac index	2.5–3.5 L/minute/m²
Pulmonary vascular resistance	80–240 dyne/second/cm⁻⁵
Systemic vascular resistance	800–1300 dyne/second/cm⁻⁵

Usage: Assessment, diagnosis, and evaluation of the effects of therapy on right and left ventricular function; measurement of cardiac output and cardiac and pulmonary pressures; access to central venous blood and mixed venous blood samples; monitoring of mixed venous oxygen saturation (SVO_2); temporary atrial, ventricular, or A-V sequential pacing via a thermodilution pulmonary arterial pacing catheter; and preoperative, intraoperative, and postoperative uses, including monitoring of high-risk clients (those with a history of angina, cardiopulmonary disease, or potential fluid shifts during surgery), elderly clients, and high or low cardiac output states, and in situations when hypotensive anesthesia is used. Indications for pulmonary artery catheterization include acute myocardial infarction, angina (severe), burns (severe), cardiomyopathy, congestive heart failure, cardiac tamponade, intraoperative cardiac collapse, failure to respond to appropriate resuscitative measures, fluid-related hypotension and hypovolemia, intravascular control problems, noncardiogenic pulmonary edema, pulmonary congestive states, pulmonary edema, pulmonary failure, pulmonary hypertension, renal disease, right and left ventricular failure, shock states (cardiogenic, hypovolemic, septic, traumatic with concomitant heart failure), tissue perfusion (altered), and titration of chronotropic, inotropic, or vasoactive pharmacologic agents.

Description: Pulmonary artery (PA) catheterization is an invasive procedure using a radiopaque polyvinyl-chloride, flow-directed, balloon-tipped catheter containing fluid-filled proximal, distal, and thermistor lumens and a balloon inflation lumen with a valve. Proper placement of the catheter in the PA, in the lower one third of the lung (zone 3), where venous pressures are greater than alveolar pressure, allows for measurement of CVP, PAS, PAEDP, PAM, and PAWP pressures. Intermittent occlusion of the PA branch by inflation of the balloon tip with air or carbon dioxide (never fluid) temporarily impedes blood flow from the right side of the heart to the lungs. The mitral valve opens during diastole, permitting the distal part of the catheter to record pressure that is reflected backward through the left atrium and pulmonary capillary bed. Identical pressures in the left ventricle, left atrium, and pulmonary vasculature momentarily occur during diastole and are captured as the PAWP when the balloon is inflated.

Professional Considerations:

1. Consent form MAY be required.

Risks:

Air embolism, arterial occlusion, dysrhythmias, hemothorax, infection, perforation of the pulmonary artery or myocardium, pneumothorax, ventricular tachycardia, cardiac valvular damage, complete heart block in clients with pre-existing left bundle branch block.

Contraindications:

History of latex allergy (for catheters containing latex or latex balloons).

2. Preparation:
   A. Cardiac assessment for history of complete left bundle branch block is indicated before insertion of a PA catheter, as there is slight risk for developing a right bundle branch block during catheter insertion, resulting in complete heart block. Standby external transcutaneous pacemaker, insertion of temporary pacemaker, or use of a pacing thermodilution PA catheter can be used for those at risk for this complication.
   B. Assemble and prepare monitoring equipment according to institutional protocol. This includes the following:
      i. Program the monitor for PA pressure display.
      ii. Prepare a transducer with high-pressure tubing for hemodynamic monitoring and a pressure bag of normal saline or heparin flush so-

lution according to institutional protocol.
      iii. Balance the transducer at the phlebostatic axis (the level of the client's right atrium, the fourth intercostal space at the midaxillary line).
   C. Have an emergency cart on standby. Have lidocaine (100 mg) for intravenous use at the bedside in the event of sustained ventricular tachycardia due to catheter irritation of the right ventricle.
   D. Obtain povidone-iodine solution, sterile drapes, 1–2% lidocaine (Xylocaine), introducer (cordis) trays, a pulmonary artery catheter tray, and 0.9% saline or heparin flush solution.
   E. The physician(s) performing the procedure should wear the following: a sterile gown, a sterile mask, a cap, and sterile gloves.
   F. The procedure may be performed at the bedside or under fluoroscopy.

3. Procedure:
   A. The PA catheter may be inserted percutaneously into the external or internal jugular veins, femoral or subclavian veins, and the antecubital fossa veins via venous cutdown.
   B. The client is placed in the supine position. For subclavian or internal jugular insertions, the head of the bed is lowered slightly into a shallow Trendelenburg position. The flat supine position is preferred; however, if not tolerated by the client, a low semi-Fowler's position is acceptable, provided that the same position is maintained throughout the procedure.
   C. Electrocardiographic monitoring is performed throughout the procedure.
   D. After the site is cleansed with povidone-iodine solution and allowed to dry, it is covered with sterile drapes.
   E. A protective sleeve is placed over the PA catheter and the catheter is flushed with sterile 0.9% saline or heparin flush solution (heparin 100 U/ml 0.9% saline). The balloon at the distal end of the PA catheter is tested for proper inflation and integrity by injecting 1–1.5 ml of air into the PA distal injection port.
   F. The PA distal port is connected to the transducer tubing and a paper printout of the PA tracing is started and run continuously throughout the catheter insertion.
   G. The site is anesthetized with 1–2% Xylocaine. For subclavian or internal jugular (IJ) insertions, the Seldinger technique is used as follows. The vessel is cannulated with a 22- or 25-gauge needle (IJ insertions only; subclavian insertions omit this step). A large-bore needle is inserted over the small nee-

dle and the small needle is removed. A guidewire is inserted through the large-bore needle and the needle is removed. The introducer (cordis) is then inserted over the guidewire and the guidewire is removed. The introducer is then secured into place.

H. The PA catheter is inserted through the introducer (cordis) and directed into the right atrium and through the tricuspid valve into the right ventricle. As the catheter traverses the right ventricle, the balloon at the distal portion of the catheter is inflated to permit normal cardiac blood flow to carry (float) the catheter through the pulmonic valve into the PA. Inflation of the balloon and flow-direction minimize the potential of catheter-induced ventricular dysrhythmias and irritability. However, the risk for ventricular tachycardia is greatest while the PA catheter tip is passing through the right ventricle. If ventricular tachycardia occurs, the catheter should be either advanced through the pulmonary valve or withdrawn into the right atrium. Xylocaine and emergency measures are seldom needed, as the removal of the catheter as a ventricular irritant is usually sufficient to stop the tachycardia.

I. As the catheter is slowly inserted, placement and progress are assessed by observing the monitor for the waveform and pressure changes characteristic of the different chambers and vessels of the cardiac and pulmonary anatomy. When the waveform changes from a PA waveform to a PAWP waveform, the balloon is allowed to deflate and the catheter is secured into this position. The syringes of flush solution are removed and the ports are either connected to a continuous flush solution or capped, according to the policy of the institution.

4. Postprocedure care:
   A. Apply an occlusive sterile dressing to the PA catheter insertion site.
   B. Obtain a chest x-ray for verification of the catheter placement if fluoroscopy has not been used.
   C. PA pressures should be monitored continuously. The waveform should be frequently observed for progression of the catheter tip into a wedge position.

5. Client and family teaching:
   A. If the access is subclavian or jugular, the head will be covered with a sterile drape during the procedure.
   B. Activity may be limited during the time a PA catheter is in place.

6. Factors that affect results:
   A. The mechanical factors that invalidate pressure measurements include the following:

i. *Air bubbles* in pressure tubing system or transducer cause dampening of the waveform.

ii. *Kinking of pressure tubing* causes dampening of the waveform.

iii. *Improper tubing length:* Tubing should not exceed 48 inches in length from the client to the transducer.

iv. *Loose connections* interfere with the high pressure pathway along the tubing and may cause waveform artifact and false readings.

v. *Stopcocks* between the transducer and the PA distal port distort PA pressures slightly, but effects increase with an increased number of stopcocks. For this reason, use no more than one stopcock for ports through which pressures are monitored.

vi. *Blood return* in the transducer tubing. The continual flush counteracting pressure should be maintained at 300 mmHg.

vii. *Catheter artifact* (catheter whip, catheter fling) results from excessive catheter movement during cardiac contraction when the distal tip of the catheter is too close to the pulmonary valve.

viii. *Catheter displacement* may result from backward recoil into the right ventricle, as evidenced by large RV waveforms. It may also result from forward migration into a wedged position.

ix. *Migration of the catheter against the vessel wall* may cause a dampened waveform and affect pressure readings. Repositioning the client or asking the client to cough may help to return the tip to a floating position. The catheter should never be flushed if a spontaneous wedge position is suspected.

x. *A flush solution rate* affects pressure readings. Clot formation near the distal port due to too slow a flush rate dampens the waveform and causes falsely low readings. Falsely high readings may result from a flush rate >3–6 ml/hour.

xi. *Incorrect transducer position* below the phlebostatic axis causes falsely low pressure readings. A transducer higher than the phlebostatic axis causes falsely high pressure readings. Each 1 cm difference alters the reading by 1 mmHg.

xii. *Malfunction of equipment,* which may include the amplifier, the oscilloscope, the recording devices, or the transducer.

xiii. *Positive pressure mechanical ventilation* (PEEP) elevates pressures ·

slightly. Formulas are available to compensate for this effect. PEEP should never be discontinued to obtain pressure readings, as the discontinuation has been shown to be deleterious to the client's condition.

xiv. *Overinflation of the balloon* results in inflation larger than is necessary for the vessel size, recognized by a drifting up or down of the PAWP waveform. Overinflation may cause rupture of the pulmonary capillary. Air should be injected into the balloon very slowly while continuously watching for a waveform change to a wedge position. Proper placement of the PA catheter is indicated when a PAWP waveform is obtained with 0.8–1.2 cc of air. At no time should more than 1.5 cc of air be injected into the balloon. Assessment and/or adjustment of PA catheter placement by a physician is indicated if a PAWP waveform cannot be obtained with ≤1.5 cc of air.

xv. *A ruptured balloon* is indicated when no resistance is felt to air injection into the balloon port, along with an absence of a PAWP waveform or by the presence of blood in the PA distal (balloon) port. Balloon rupture may result from a manufacturing defect, or from balloon weakening after many inflations. Manual deflation may accelerate balloon weakening. If a ruptured balloon is suspected, no more air should be injected and a physician should immediately assess the client.

xvi. *Respiratory variation* due to inspiration and expiration cannot be accounted for by digital averaging. The most accurate readings of pressures are calculated manually from paper recordings of the waveforms at end-expiration.

xvii. *Retrograde injection* during cardiac output measurement is indicated when a backflow of blood or fluid is detected in the introducer or protective sleeve of the catheter. This is an indication that the catheter injectate opening is located within the lumen of the introducer (cordis), rather than in the right atrium. Retrograde injection results in inadequate thermodilution and falsely high cardiac output values.

B. Physiologic conditions that alter pressure measurements of the different chambers and vessels include the following:

i. *RA/CVP:* Cardiac tamponade, fluid overload, pulmonary disease, pulmonary hypertension, right heart failure, tricuspid regurgitation, and tricuspid stenosis.

ii. *RV:* Chronic congestive heart failure, constrictive pericarditis, pericardial effusion, pulmonary hypertension, pulmonary valvular stenosis, right ventricular failure, and ventricular septal defects.

iii. *PAS/PAD:* Chronic obstructive pulmonary disease, increased pulmonary blood flow, left-to-right shunts secondary to atrial or ventricular septal defects, mitral stenosis, pulmonary edema, pulmonary embolus, and pulmonary hypertension.

iv. *PAWP/PCWP:* Cardiac insufficiency, cardiac tamponade, left ventricular failure, mitral regurgitation, and mitral stenosis.

7. Other data:

A. Transducers should be balanced every 2–4 hours with position and ventilator changes and prior to each measurement of PA catheter parameters.

B. PA catheter balloons should never be manually deflated. The air should be allowed to flow back into the syringe spontaneously.

C. Potential complications of PA catheterization include perforation of the heart or pulmonary vasculature, pulmonary embolus or thrombus, and cardiac dysrhythmias.

D. The flexible PA catheter includes two-lumen, three-lumen, four-lumen thermodilutional, and five-lumen catheters of varying lengths. Sizes include 5-, 6-, 7-, and 7.5 Fr, with markings at 10-cm increments along the outer surface.

E. Later generations of catheter development include the capability for atrial, ventricular, or AV sequential pacing; continuous mixed venous oxygen saturation (SVO_2); continuous cardiac output; using fiber optic oximetry; and additional lumens/ports for fluid infusions.

Bibliography:

Johnson MK, Schumann L: Comparison of three methods of measurement of pulmonary artery catheter readings in critically ill patients. Am J Crit Care 4(4):300–307, 1995.

Kearney TJ, Shabot MM: Pulmonary artery rupture associated with the Swan-Ganz catheter. Chest 108(5):1349–1352, 1995.

Quaal SJ: Quality assurance in hemodynamic monitoring. AACN Clin Issues Crit Care Nurs 4(1): 197–206, 1993.

PULMONARY FUNCTION TEST (PFT), DIAGNOSTIC

Norm: The observed values are reported as percentages of normal using prediction equations calculated according to age, height, sex and weight. Results are considered abnormal if they are less than predicted 80% of the calculated values. Average results for adults:

Tidal volume (V_T)	500 cc
Expiratory reserve volume (ERV)	1500 cc
Residual volume (RV)	1500 cc
Inspiratory reserve volume (IRV)	2000 cc

Note:
IRV + V_T = Inspiratory Capacity (IC).
ERV + RV = Functional Residual Capacity (FRC).
IRV + V_T + ERV = Vital Capacity (VC).
V_T + ERV + RV + IRV = Total Lung Capacity (TLC).

Usage: Diagnosis and progress of pulmonary dysfunction; evaluation of the effectiveness of medications (bronchodilators); determination of whether a functional abnormality is obstructive or restrictive; identification of clients at high risk for postoperative pulmonary complications; and evaluation of the risk of pulmonary resection.

Description: Pulmonary function tests (PFTs) are a number of different tests used to evaluate lung mechanics, gas exchange, and acid-base disturbance through spirometric measurements, lung volumes, and arterial blood gases. These tests include measuring the amount of air that can be maximally exhaled after a maximum inspiration and the time required for that expiration, and determining the ability of the alveolar capillary membrane to transport oxygen into the blood and carbon dioxide from the blood into the expired air. PFTs include the following:

1. Total lung capacity (TLC), the total volume of the lungs when maximally inflated, is divided into four volumes: tidal volume (V_T), inspiratory reserve volume (IRV), expiratory reserve volume (ERV), and residual volume (RV). Increased TLC indicates over distention of the lungs associated with obstructive disease. Decreased TLC indicates restrictive disease.

   V_T is the volume of air inhaled and exhaled in normal quiet breathing. Decreased V_T may indicate fatigue, restrictive parenchymal lung disease, atelectasis, cancer, edema, pulmonary congestion, pneumothorax, or thoracic tumor, and necessitates further testing. Increased V_T may indicate bronchiolar obstruction with hyperinflation or emphysema.

   IRV is the maximum volume that can be inhaled following a normal quiet inhalation. Decreased IRV is an isolated value that does not indicate disease.

   ERV is the maximum volume that can be exhaled following a normal quiet exhalation. Decreased ERV may occur with obesity, pregnancy, or thoracoplasty.

   RV is the volume remaining in the lungs following maximal exhalation. Increased RV above 35% of the TLC indicates obstructive disease. It is also increased with aging.

2. Forced expiratory volume (FEV) is the volume expired during specified time intervals (0.5, and 1 seconds). Decreased FEV_1 after the administration of beta-blockers may indicate the presence of bronchospasm and contraindicate the continued use of the specific pharmacologic therapy involved. Decreased FEV_1 indicates restrictive disease. Decreased FEV_1 with as percent of the vital capacity ($FEV1/FVC$) indicates obstructive disease.

3. Functional residual capacity (FRC) is the amount of volume in the lungs after normal exhalation. Increased FRC indicates overdisten-

tion of the lungs and is associated with chronic obstructive pulmonary diseases. Decreased FRC can be seen in acute respiratory distress syndrome (ARDS).

4. Inspiratory capacity (IC) is the maximum volume that can be inhaled following a normal quiet exhalation. IC provides a very useful parameter in evaluating timeliness of weaning from mechanical ventilation. Decreased IC indicates restrictive disease.

5. Vital capacity (VC) is the total volume that can be exhaled after maximum inspiration. Increased or normal VC with decreased flow rates indicates an obstructive defect (airway diseases). Decreased VC with normal or increased flow rates indicates restrictive defect (diaphragmatic impairment, drug overdose, head injury, limited thoracic expansion, and neuromuscular disease).

6. Forced vital capacity (FVC) is the total volume exhaled forcefully and rapidly after maximum inhalation. Interpretation in changes are similar to vital capacity.

7. Minute volume (MV) is the total amount of gas breathed during 1 minute.

8. Thoracic gas volume (TGV) is the total volume of the lungs including nonventilated and ventilated airways. Increased TGV indicates air trapping caused by obstructive disease and requires special equipment to monitor.

Professional Considerations:

1. Consent form NOT required.
2. Preparation:
   A. Assess medication record for recent analgesic that may depress respiratory function.
   B. Bronchodilators and intermittent positive-pressure breathing therapy may be withheld prior to the tests.
   C. The client should void and then loosen any restrictive clothing.
   D. Record the client's age, sex, weight, and height on the test requisition.
   E. *See Client and family teaching.*
3. Procedure:
   A. A nose clip is applied.
   B. The client is instructed to breathe through a mouthpiece.
   C. The procedure takes 20 minutes.
4. Postprocedure care:
   A. Resume normal diet and any bronchodilators or intermittent positive-pressure breathing therapy.

B. Results are normally available within 30 minutes. Consideration of client's clinical condition may be necessary when interpreting results.

5. Client and family teaching:
   A. Refrain from smoking or eating a heavy meal for 4–6 hours.
   B. Dentures should not be removed.
6. Factors that affect results:
   A. The client's ability to voluntarily and actively participate is essential to complete the indicated tests.
   B. An inadequate seal around the mouthpiece invalidates the results.
   C. Gastric distention, hypoxia, metabolic disturbances, narcotic analgesia, pregnancy, and sedatives may alter the results.
   D. Bronchodilators administered prior to the tests may obscure true pulmonary function.
   E. Values are based on age, sex, and height.
7. Other data:
   A. Pulmonary function tests are normally performed in a pulmonary laboratory.
   B. *See also Lung Scan, Perfusion; and Ventilation, Diagnostic.*

Bibliography:

Neale AV, Demers RY: Significance of the inability to reproduce pulmonary function test results. J Occup Med *36*(6):660–666, 1994.

Sahebjami H, Doers JT, Render ML, et al.: Anthropometric and pulmonary function test profiles of outpatients with stable chronic obstructive pulmonary disease. Am J Med *94*(5):469–474, 1993.

Zeiher BG, Gros TJ, Kern JA, et al.: Predicting postoperative pulmonary function in patients undergoing lung resection. Chest *108*(1):68–72, 1995.

PULMONARY SCINTOPHOTOGRAPHY

(see Lung Scan, Perfusion and Ventilation, Diagnostic)

PULSE OXIMETRY

(see Oximetry, Diagnostic)

PULSE VOLUME RECORDER TESTING OF PERIPHERAL VASCULATURE, DIAGNOSTIC

Norm: The waveform recording demonstrates rapid upstroke or an anacrotic limb, a sharp peak, a brisk decline or catacrotic limb, and a clearly discernible visual diastolic wave. Bilateral consistent augmentation of the pulse amplitude from proximal to distal measurement sites is present throughout the waveform recordings.

Usage: Assists in the diagnosis, location, and monitoring of the progression of arterial vascular lesions and arterial narrowing; preoperative, intraoperative, and postoperative evaluations; aids in the determination of the need for arterial angiography; differentiation of aortoiliac and superficial femoral artery occlusion and neuropathies; and assists in the evaluation of the severity of arterial occlusions and the detection of arterial pressure changes in distal extremity vessels that cannot be measured by a Doppler probe.

Description: Pulse volume recording measures pressure changes of arterial vessels and displays the pressure changes as waveforms. Pressure changes are recorded via a transducer during blood pressure cuff inflation and deflation. A segmental air plethysmography records the pulse waveform tracings onto graph paper. These pressure recordings supplement segmental limb pressure studies and are a sensitive indicator of arterial vascular occlusive disease of the distal vessels of the feet and toes. Recordings may be taken before or after segmental limb pressure measurements. Arterial narrowing distal to a vascular lesion produces a loss of the diastolic wave, a prolonged catacrotic limb (prolonged downstroke tracing), rounding of the normally sharp peak, and a decrease in the slope of the anacrotic limb (vertical ascending limb). Progression of arterial occlusive disease results in a broadened, flattened, lengthened, and dampened waveform with depression in the amplitude of the diastolic wave.

Professional Considerations:

1. Consent form NOT required.
2. Preparation:
   A. Remove clothing from each extremity.
3. Procedure:
   A. The client is placed in the prone position.
   B. Blood pressure cuffs that have a length of 80% of the limb circumference, a width of 40% of the limb circumference, and a pneumatic inflatable bladder that is 20% wider than the limb diameter are selected.
   C. The pressure cuffs are placed bilaterally 2.5 cm above the antecubital crease of the arm, just above the wrist, as high as possible on the thigh, just below the knee, and just above the malleolus of the ankle.

D. Transmetatarsal and penile pressure recordings may be obtained.
E. Pulse volume recordings are measured at brachial, radial, ulnar, femoral, popliteal, dorsalis pedis, and posterior tibial levels of each resting extremity.
F. Pressure changes are recorded by a transducer during cuff inflation and deflation.
G. Cuff inflation is measured by standard mercury-gravity or aneroid manometer.
H. Cuff deflation is measured via stethoscope, plethysmography, or by the Doppler velocity detector, which is the most convenient and sensitive measurement device.
I. A segmental air plethysmography records the pulse waveform tracings onto graph paper.
J. The same procedure is used for pediatrics.
4. Postprocedure care:
   A. Remove cuffs.
5. Client and family teaching:
   A. The procedure takes 30 minutes.
   B. Results are available immediately.
6. Factors that affect results:
   A. Improper size, inflation, or loose cuff application causes inaccurate results.
   B. False-negatives have been reported in clients with a short segmental occlusion of the superficial femoral artery in which they have developed large femoral collateral circulation. The pulse volume recording produced a very depressed thigh tracing without discernible augmentation over the occluded site, while circulation to the extremity was maintained.
7. Other data:
   A. Pulse volume recording of peripheral vascular pulses reports 97% accuracy for detecting superficial femoral artery occlusion.

Bibliography:

Gertler JP, Headley A, L'Italien G, et al.: Claudication in the setting of plethysmographic criteria for resting ischemia: is surgery justified? Ann Vasc Surg 7(3):249–253, 1993.

PURE TONE AUDIOMETRY, DIAGNOSTIC
(see Audiometry Test, Diagnostic)

PYELOGRAPHY, ANTEGRADE, DIAGNOSTIC
(see Antegrade Pyelography, Diagnostic)

PYELOGRAPHY, RETROGRADE, DIAGNOSTIC
(see Retrograde Pyelography, Diagnostic)

PYP SCAN
(see Heart Scan, Diagnostic)

PYRIDOXAL
(see Vitamin B_6, Plasma)

PYRIDOXAL 5′ PHOSPHATE (PLP, PPLP), PLASMA

Norm: 5–30 ng/ml (20–121 nmol/L SI units).

Deficiency: <5 ng/ml (<20 nmol/L SI units).

Increased: Occurs only in high-dietary vitamin B_6 replacement. Levels are normally higher in infancy.

Decreased: Asthma, carpal tunnel syndrome, chronic alcoholism, malnutrition, malabsorption problems, neonatal seizures, pellagra, preeclamptic edema, renal dialysis, uremia. May also occur with industrial exposure to hydrazine compounds. Normally lower in pregnancy and during lactation, especially with gestational diabetes. Drugs that cause lower levels of plasma pyridoxal 5′ phosphate are Amiodarone, anticonvulsants, cyclocerins, disulferan, hydralazine, isoniazid, levodopa, oral contraceptives, penicillamine, prozinoic acid, and theophylline.

Description: Plasma pyridoxal 5′-phosphate levels assess the vitamin B_6 status of clients.

Professional Considerations:
1. Consent form NOT required.
2. Preparation:
   A. Fasting specimens are required.
   B. Tube: Lavender-top.
3. Procedure:
   A. Draw a 3–5-ml blood sample.
4. Postprocedure care:
   A. Send the specimen to the laboratory immediately. The specimen needs to be frozen.
5. Client and family teaching:
   A. Fast from food and fluids from midnight until the night before the blood sample is drawn.
   B. Results are normally available within 72 hours.
6. Factors that affect results:
   A. Ingestion of foods that contain vitamin B_6.
7. Other data:
   A. Hip fracture clients may be deficient in vitamin B_6.

Bibliography:

Reynolds RD: Importance of deproteinized serum samples for pyridoxal 5′-phosphate determination. Am J Clin Nutr *60*(1):148, 1994.

Reynolds TM, Marshall PD, Brain AM: Hip fracture patients may be vitamin B6 deficient. Acta Orthop Scand *63*(6):635–638, 1992.

PYRIDOXAMINE
(see Vitamin B_6, Plasma)

4-PYRIDOXIC ACID, URINE (VITAMIN B_6)

Norm:

	SI Units
0.5–1.3 mg/dl	2.7–7.1 µmol/d

Increased: Pyridoxine megavitaminosis due to excessive dietary supplementation.

Decreased: Anemia, asthma, carpal tunnel syndrome, chronic alcoholism, gestational diabetes, industrial exposure to hydrazine compounds, lactation, malnutrition, pellagra, peripheral neuritis, peritoneal dialysis and vitamin B_6 deficiency. Drugs include amiodarone, anticonvulsants, cyclosporin, disulfuram, ethanol, hydralazine, isoniazid, oral contraceptives, penicillamine, pyrazinoac acid, and tricyclic antidepressants.

Description: Urinary 4-pyridoxic acid is a major metabolite of vitamin B_6 and can be used to evaluate vitamin B_6 deficiency. As a coenzyme, vitamin B_6 aids in the synthesis and breakdown of amino acids; aids in the synthesis of unsaturated fatty acids from essential fatty acids; essential for conversion of tryptophan to niacin; involved in formation of the precursor to porphyrin compound.

Professional Considerations:
1. Consent form NOT required.
2. Preparation:
   A. Obtain a clean, 3-L container that is

free of preservative. For pediatric/infant collections, also obtain tape and a pediatric urine collection device/bag.

B. Write the beginning time of the 24-hour collection on the laboratory requisition.

3. Procedure:

A. Early morning is the preferred time to begin a 24-hour collection.

B. Discard the first morning urine specimen.

C. Save all the urine voided for 24 hours in a refrigerated, clean, 3-L container that is free of preservatives. Document the quantity of urine output during the specimen collection period. Include the urine voided at the end of the 24-hour period. For catheterized clients, keep the drainage bag on ice and empty the urine into the refrigerated collection container hourly.

D. Pediatric/infant specimen collection:

i. Empty the collection bag into the refrigerated collection container after each void.

ii. The child is placed in a supine position with the knees flexed and the hips externally rotated and abducted.

iii. Cleanse, rinse, and thoroughly dry the perineal area.

iv. To prevent the child from removing the collection device/bag, a diaper may be placed over the genital area.

v. *Females:* Tape the pediatric collection device/bag to the perineum. Starting at the area between the anus and vagina, apply the device/bag in an anterior direction.

vi. *Males:* Place the pediatric collection device/bag over the penis and scrotum and tape it to the perineal area.

4. Postprocedure care:

A. Compare the urine quantity in the specimen container with the urinary output record for the test. If the speci-

men contains less urine than was recorded as output, some of the sample may have been discarded, thus invalidating the test.

B. Document the urine quantity and ending time on the laboratory requisition.

C. Isoniazid (INH) is a pyridoxal antagonist. Note if the client is on the drug.

5. Client and family teaching:

A. Save all the urine voided in a 24-hour period, urinate before defecating to avoid loss of urine, and avoid contamination of the specimen with stool, toilet tissue, or prostatic or vaginal secretions. If any urine is accidentally discarded, discard the entire specimen and restart the collection the next day.

B. Inform the client of the possible need for a vitamin B_6 supplement during pregnancy and lactation or with the use of oral contraceptives.

6. Factors that affect results:

A. None.

7. Other data:

A. Recommended daily requirements of vitamin B_6 are complicated by differences in protein intake and the use of alcohol and oral contraceptives.

B. Daily allowances for vitamin B_6 generally are 1.6–2.0 mg.

C. Foods rich in vitamin B_6 include yeast, wheat germ, pork, glandular meats, whole grain cereal, legumes, potatoes, bananas, and oatmeal.

D. Urinary testing of 4-pyridoxic acid is not widely used and is of limited value. Plasma values are preferred.

Bibliography:

Tietz NW: Tietz Textbook of Clinical Chemistry. Philadelphia, WB Saunders, 1994, pp 1300–1304.

PYRIDOXINE

(see Vitamin B_6, Plasma)

QUINIDINE, SERUM

Norm:

		SI Units
Therapeutic	2–6 µg/ml	8.1–18.4 µmol/L
Panic level	>10 µg/ml	>30.6 µmol/L

Panic Level Symptoms and Treatment:

Symptoms: Ataxia, respiratory depression, vomiting, diarrhea, severe hypotension, syncope, anuria, cardiac dysrhythmia (heart block, widening of QRS and QT interval), asystole, hallucinations, paresthesia, irritability.

Treatment:

Maintain airway and hemodynamic stability.

Provide transcutaneous or transvenous temporary pacemaker.

Acidify urine.
Do gastric lavage.
Implement forced emesis.
Give activated charcoal.
Administer infusion of a sodium
    molar lactate.
Both hemodialysis and peritoneal
    dialysis WILL remove quinidine
    in small amounts.

Increased: Impaired hepatic function, impaired renal function, and urine alkalinity. Drugs include acetazolamide, amiodarone, antacids, carbonic anhydrase inhibitors, cimetidine, magnesium hydroxide, sodium bicarbonate, and thiazide diuretics.

Decreased: Urine acidity. Drugs include ascorbic acid, barbiturates, nifedipine, phenobarbital, phenytoin, phenytoin sodium, primidone, and rifampin.

Description: Quinidine is class 1A antidysrhythmic that exerts a depressant effect on myocardial excitability, conduction velocity, and contractility. It causes decreased sodium, potassium, and calcium influx across the cell membrane, resulting in a prolongation of the myocardial refractory period. In larger doses, the ventricular response rate is increased through anticholinergic inhibition of vagal stimulation of the AV node. Quinidine is metabolized by the liver and excreted unchanged in the urine, with a half-life of 4–10 hours. Steady-state levels are reached after 20–35 hours. Toxicity may result in prolongation of the QRS complex >25% from baseline, hypotension, and cardiac standstill.

Professional Considerations:
1. Consent form NOT required.
2. Preparation:
   A. Tube: Red-top, red/gray-top, or gold-top or green-top.
   B. Do NOT draw specimens during hemodialysis.
3. Procedure:
   A. Draw a 1-ml blood sample.
4. Postprocedure care:
   A. None.
5. Client and family teaching:
   A. Take medication as prescribed.
   B. Report any side effects, such as nausea, vomiting, and dizziness.
   C. Check pulse every day when taking quinidine. The client should notify the physician when panic level symptoms (see above) are noted.
   D. If activated charcoal was given for elevated levels, the client should drink 4–6 glasses of water each day for 2 days to prevent constipation. The activated charcoal will also cause stools to be black for a few days.
6. Factors that affect results:
   A. When obtaining serial samples, the same time interval between drug dosing and sample collection should be observed.
   B. Peak quinidine levels occur 1.5–2 hours after oral administration.
   C. Acidification of the urine increases excretion of quinidine. Alkalinization of the urine decreases excretion of this drug.
7. Other data:
   A. None.

Bibliography:

Allen NM: Relationship between quinidine concentration and quinidine dosage. Pharmacotherapy *12*(3):189–194, 1992.

RABIES, BLOOD
(see Animals and Rabies, Serum)

RADIOACTIVE IODINE (RAI) UPTAKE TEST, DIAGNOSTIC

Norm: Norms vary by different laboratories. Thyroid gland absorption of radioactive test dose: 2 hours, 1–13%; 6 hours, 2–25%; 24 hours, 15–45%.

Increased: Cirrhosis, decreased iodine intake (iodine deficiency, sodium restriction), hyperthyroidism, increased iodine excretion (chronic diarrhea, nephrotic syndrome), rebound withdrawal of thyroid hormones, thyroiditis (early Hashimoto's disease, thyroiditis in the recovery phase of a subacute clinical case), and thyroid-stimulating hormone (TSH) excess (neoplasm, overmedication, synthesis defects). Drugs include barbiturates, diuretics during testing period, estrogens (occasionally), lithium carbonate, phenothiazines, and thyrotropin.

Decreased: Excess intake (cabbage, iodized foods, iodized salt), hypothyroidism (late primary, secondary, tertiary), thyroiditis (late Hashimoto's, active stage of subacute thyroiditis), and intravenous radiographic dyes within the past 12 months. Drugs include adrenal corticoids (within the past 7 days), adrenocorticotropic hormone (within the past 7 days), aminosalicylic acid (within the past 2 weeks), amphenone, ansindione, antihistamines (within the past week), chlorpromazine, cobalt, corticotropin, dicumarol, iodinated vaginal suppositories (within the prior 4 weeks), iodothiouracil (within the past 8 days), isoniazid, levothyroxine sodium/T_4 (within the prior 2 weeks), L-triiodothyronine, Lugol's solution (within the past 3 weeks), methimazole (within the past 8 days), nitrates, orinase (within the past week), ornade (within the past 3 weeks), penicillins, pentothal (within the past week), perchlorate, phenylbutazone, phenprocoumon, potassium iodide (within the past 3 weeks), propylthiouracil (within the past 8 days), salicylates (large doses), saturated solution of potassium iodide (SSKI) (within the past 3 weeks), sodium iodide, sulfonamides (within the past week), thyroid extract (within the past 2 weeks), thiocyanate (within the past 8 days), tolbutamide, warfarin sodium, and vitamins that contain minerals.

Description: A nuclear medicine test performed to determine direct thyroid function and to detect hyperthyroidism, hyperthyroidism associated with low radioactive iodine uptake, factitious hyperthyroidism, struma ovarii or subacute thyroiditis, hypothyroidism, goiter, pituitary failure, and to evaluate post-thyroid therapy. The thyroid gland uses iodine from the diet to synthesize thyroid hormone. The rate at which the thyroid gland is able to accumulate, incorporate, and release iodine determines the ability of the thyroid gland to concentrate iodine from blood plasma. Oral or intravenous radioactive iodine (I-131 or I-123) is administered, and measurement of iodine concentration in the thyroid gland at specific timed intervals of 2 and 4 hours are obtained. A 24-hour measurement may also be done. This test has been largely re-placed by radioimmunoassay for the thyroid hormones thyroxine (T_4) and triiodothyronine (T_3).

Professional Considerations:
1. Consent form MAY be required.

Risks:
Allergic reaction to contrast material (itching, hives, rash, tight feeling in the throat, shortness of breath, bronchospasm, anaphylaxis, death); renal toxicity from contrast medium.

Contraindications:
Previous allergy to iodine, shellfish, or radiographic dye is a relative contraindication: Even in the presence of an iodine allergy, this test may be acceptable due to the small amount of iodine administered. Also contraindicated in infants, children, and during pregnancy or breast-feeding.

---

2. Preparation:
   A. List all medications taken by the client during the prior 3 weeks.
   B. Notify the nuclear medicine physician if the client has received intravenous radiographic contrast medium within the past year.
   C. *See Client and family teaching.*
3. Procedure:
   A. Radioactive isotope of iodine (I-131 or I-123) is administered via capsule, lipid oral preparation, or intravenously prior to the thyroid scan.
   B. After administration of radioactive iodine, serial thyroid scans at 2-, 4-, and 24-hour intervals are obtained. The timing of the scans is critical for accurate determinations of thyroid function.
4. Postprocedure care:
   A. Observe the client carefully for up to 60 minutes after the study for a possible (anaphylactic) reaction to the radionuclide.
   B. When urine is being discarded, rubber gloves should be worn for 24 hours after the procedure. Wash the gloved hands with soap and water before removing the gloves. Wash the ungloved hands after gloves are removed.
5. Client and family teaching:
   A. Follow a low-iodine diet for 7 days before the procedure.
   B. Fast for 1 hour after the radionuclide administration.
   C. The client must meticulously wash the hands with soap and water after each

void until 24 hours after the procedure.

6. Factors that affect results:
   A. Past administration of radiographic contrast medium may cause decreased results for extended periods as follows:
      i. *Cholecystography:* Cholografin within the prior 3 months; Telepaque within the prior 2 months; Oragrafin within the prior 2 months.
      ii. Diodrast within the prior 3 months.
      iii. *Bronchography:* Dionosil within the prior 5 months; Lipiodol within the prior 3 years.
      iv. *Myelography:* Pantopaque within the prior year.
      v. *Intravenous pyelography:* Hypaque within the prior 2 weeks; Renografin within the prior 2 weeks.
      vi. *Uterosalpingography:* Salpix within the prior month.
7. Other data:
   A. Health care professionals working in a nuclear medicine area must follow federal standards set by the Nuclear Regulatory Commission. These standards include precautions for handling the radioactive material and monitoring of potential radiation exposure.
   B. Iodine-131 half-life is 8 days. Iodine-123 half-life is 13.3 hours.

Bibliography:

Hennessey JV, Berg LA, Ibrahim MA, et al.: Evaluation of early (5 to 6 hours) iodine 123 uptake for diagnosis and treatment planning in Graves disease. Arch Intern Med 155(6):621–624, 1995.

Price DC: Radioisotopic evaluation of the thyroid and the parathyroids. Radiologic Clin North Am 31(5):991–1015, 1993.

RADIOALLERGOSORBENT TEST, SERUM

(see Allergin-Specific IgE Antibody, Serum)

RAJI CELL ASSAY, BLOOD

Norm:

Normal	<13 µg AHG Eq/ml
Borderline	13–25 µg AHG Eq/ml
Abnormal	≥26 µg AHG Eq/ml

Usage: Detection of immune complexes in the following: autoimmune disorders; celiac disease; cirrhosis; Crohn's disease; cryoglobulinemia; dermatitis herpetiformis; disseminated malignancy; drug reactions; microbial, parasitic, and viral infections; and sickle cell anemia.

Description: Complement receptors for IgG are found on the Raji cells, which are lymphoblastoid cells that contain receptors for complement, particularly C3b. Raji cells are derived from Burkitt's lymphoma and are used to recognize and bind protein-bound immune complexes that contain C3b. Results are reported in the quantity of precipitated immune complexes. Detection of circulating immune complexes is used to help determine the mechanisms of autoimmune diseases.

Professional Considerations:

1. Consent form NOT required.
2. Preparation:
   A. Preschedule this test with the laboratory.
   B. Tube: Chilled green-top.
   C. Specimens MAY be drawn during hemodialysis.
3. Procedure:
   A. Draw a 5-ml blood sample.
   B. Heelstick is acceptable, collected in a microtainer.
   C. Place the tube in a container of ice and water.
4. Postprocedure care:
   A. Transport the specimen to the laboratory immediately.
5. Client and family teaching:
   A. The test is used to help diagnose autoimmune diseases.
6. Factors that affect results:
   A. Results may be unreliable if the client has undergone a recent scan involving the injection of radioactive dye.
7. Other data:
   A. AHG measurement stands for aggregated human gamma globulin equivalents.
   B. *See also Immune Complex Assay, Blood.*

Bibliography:

Bouvier G, Hergenhahn M, Polack A, Bornkamm GW, Bartsch H: Validation of two test systems for detecting tumor promoters and EBV inducers: comparative responses of several agents in DR-CAT Raji cells and in human granulocytes. Carcinogenesis 14(8):1573–1578, 1993.

Polack A, Laux G, Hergenhahn M, Kloz U, Roeser H, Bornkamm GW: Short-term assays for detection of conditional cancerogens. I. Construction of DR-CAT Raji cells and some of their characteristics as tester cells. Int J Cancer 50(4):611–616, 1992.

RAPID PLASMA REAGIN (RPR) TEST, BLOOD

Norm: Negative, nonreactive sample.

Positive: Borderline, reactive, and weakly reactive are considered positive results for the syphilis antibody. A reactive result suggests contraction of syphilis, but diagnosis must be confirmed by medical examination and history.

Negative: RPR nonreactive results may be reported in clients who are treated before the appearance of the primary chancre (in the primary phase), those treated after the appearance of the primary chancre but before the appearance of the reagin, and in clients treated in the secondary phase of the disease. This test can be substituted for the venereal disease research laboratory (VDRL) test. Seronegative results occur with alcohol ingestion prior to the test and during inactive or latent-phase syphilis.

Description: Syphilis is a complex sexually transmitted disease characterized by a wide range of symptoms that imitate other diseases. It is caused by the organism *Treponema pallidum*. The RPR test is a macroscopic agglutination screening test for the presence of reagin, the antibody specific for the treponemal spirochete. In this test, an antigen (cardiolipin phospholipid derived from beef heart) to reagin is used to detect an agglutination reaction, indicating a positive test. The RPR test is most useful during the secondary stage of syphilis, at the peak of reagin antibody presence in the blood. This test is inexpensive and widely used for mass testing for syphilis. However, its sensitivity in primary syphilis is fairly poor and many biologic false-positives are possible.

Professional Considerations:

1. Consent form NOT required.
2. Preparation:
   A. Tube: Red-top, red/gray-top, or gold-top.
   B. *See Client and family teaching.*
   C. Specimens MAY be drawn during hemodialysis.
3. Procedure:
   A. Draw a 7-ml blood sample.
   B. Heelstick is acceptable, collected in a microtainer.
4. Postprocedure care:
   A. State law may require completion of a confidential Department of Health form when a specimen is reported as reactive.
5. Client and family teaching:
   A. Do not drink alcohol for 24 hours prior to the test.
   B. Assess the client's understanding of safe sexual practices.
   C. If testing is positive and a syphilis diagnosis is confirmed:

   i. Notify all sexual contacts from the last 90 days (if early stage) to be tested for syphilis.
   ii. Syphilis can be cured with antibiotics. These may worsen the symptoms for the first 24 hours.
   iii. Do not have sex for 2 months and until after repeat testing has confirmed that the syphilis is cured. Use condoms after that for 2 years. Return for repeat testing every 3–4 months for the next 2 years to make sure the disease is cured.
   iv. Do not become pregnant for 2 years, because syphilis can be transmitted to the fetus.
   v. If left untreated, syphilis can damage many body organs, including the brain, over several years' time.
6. Factors that affect results:
   A. Alcohol ingestion within the prior 24 hours produces transient nonreactive results.
   B. Hemolysis of the specimen invalidates the results.
   C. Serum samples should be drawn before meals, as chyme alters the reaction.
   D. Refrigeration destroys *Treponema* spirochetes in 72 hours.
   E. Conditions that may cause false-positive results include active immunization in children, antinuclear antibodies, blood loss (with multiple transfusions), chancroid, chickenpox, cirrhosis, the common cold, diabetes mellitus, fever (relapsing), hepatitis (infectious), HIV, hypergammaglobulinemia, leprosy, leptospirosis (Weil's disease), Lyme disease, lymphogranuloma venereum, lymphoma, infection (chronic), malaria, measles, mononucleosis (infectious), *Mycoplasma* pneumonia, nonsyphilitic treponemal diseases (bejel, pinta, yaws), periarteritis nodosa, pneumococcal pneumonia, pneumonia, pregnancy, rat-bite fever, rheumatic fever, rheumatic heart disease, rheumatoid arthritis, scarlet fever, scleroderma, senescence, subacute bacterial endocarditis, systemic lupus erythematosus, tuberculosis (advanced pulmonary), treponematosus, trypanosomiasis, tuberculosis, typhus fever, and vaccinia.
7. Other data:
   A. Results may be nonreactive while infectious organisms are present in the bloodstream, as immunologic response is not detectable for 14–21 days after contraction of the spirochetes.
   B. The greatest risk for transmission of syphilis occurs in freshly drawn blood products that must be administered immediately (platelets) or those not refrigerated for 72 hours prior to infusion.
   C. Negative results in the presence of definite clinical signs of syphilis or sus-

pected biologic false-positive tests necessitate the *Fluorescent Treponemal Antibody Absorption test.*

Bibliography:

Rusnak JM, Butzin C, McGlasson D, Blatt SP: False-positive rapid plasma reagin tests in human immunodeficiency virus infection and relationship to anti-cardiolipin antibody and serum immunoglobulin levels. J Infect Dis *169*(6):1356–1359, 1994.

Van Dyck E, Bogaerts J, Piot P: Rapid plasma reagin card test: evaluation of a hand-rotation procedure and stability of RPR antigen. Bull WHO *72*(5): 741–743, 1994.

RAST TEST, SERUM
(see Allergin-Specific IgE, Serum)

RAYNAUD'S COLD STIMULATION TEST, DIAGNOSTIC

Norm: Within 15 minutes, digital temperature returns to prebath temperature. Recovery time >20 minutes indicates Raynaud's syndrome.

Usage: Detection of Raynaud's syndrome after ruling out occlusive disease of the peripheral arteries.

Description: This test records digital temperature changes after submersion of the digits in an ice-water bath. Raynaud's syndrome is an idiopathic, vasospastic disorder of small cutaneous arteries and arterioles of the extremities characterized by intense paroxysmal bilateral pallor and cyanosis of the fingers or toes, with or without local gangrene. The attacks may occur in response to exposure of the affected extremities to cold temperature. Idiopathic or primary occurrence of this syndrome is referred to as Raynaud's disease. Raynaud's phenomenon is accompanied by paresthesia and caused by underlying disease processes such as connective tissue disorders.

Professional Considerations:

1. Consent form NOT required.

Risks:
Increased infection in open wounds on fingers.

Contraindications:
Gangrenous digits, or open or infected wounds on the hands.

2. Preparation:
   A. All jewelry should be removed from the fingers and wrists.
3. Procedure:
   A. Digital temperatures are measured via thermistors attached to each digit.
   B. The hands are then submerged in an ice-water bath for 20 seconds.
   C. Serial temperature recordings are taken beginning immediately after the hands are removed from the bath and continue every 5 minutes for 20 minutes.
4. Postprocedure care:
   A. None.
5. Client and family teaching:
   A. Avoid exposing the hands to extreme cold.
   B. Smoking greatly increases difficulties in clients with peripheral circulatory problems.
6. Factors that affect results:
   A. Excessively cold or warm ambient temperature can alter the physiologic response.
7. Other data:
   A. If the arteriospastic disorder is primary, it is called Raynaud's disease. If the disorder is secondary, such as from scleroderma or systemic lupus erythematosus, it is called Raynaud's phenomenon.

Bibliography:

The Merck Manual, 16th ed. Rahway, NJ, Merck and Company, 1992, p 584.

Strandness DE, Van Breda A: Vascular Diseases: Surgical and Interventional Therapy. New York, Churchill Livingstone, 1994, p 529.

Wyngaarden JB, Smith LH, Bennett JC: Cecil Textbook of Medicine, 19th ed. Philadelphia, WB Saunders, 1992, pp 356–358.

RBC, BLOOD
(see Red Blood Cell, Blood)

RECOMBIGEN LATEX AGGLUTINATION ASSAY
(see Acquired Immune Deficiency Syndrome Evaluation Battery, Diagnostic)

RECTAL BIOPSY, DIAGNOSTIC

Norm: Negative.

Usage: Assists in the diagnosis of aganglionosis (anal achalasia), amebic ulceration, cancer of the rectosigmoid, Crohn's disease, chronic inflammation, infection, Hirschsprung's disease, rectosigmoid polyps, schistosomiasis (in the absence of visible lesions), secondary amyloidosis, ulcerative colitis, and villous adenoma; evaluation of myenteric plexus ganglia; and differentiation and staging of Crohn's disease and ulcerative colitis.

Description: Rectal biopsy is the excision of a small piece of living tissue for gross microscopic and histologic examination and may include mucosal and muscle layers. Biopsies from multiple sites may be obtained during proctosigmoidoscopy or proctoscopy using fiberoptic endoscopic instruments. Excisional biopsy is the excision of an entire lesion as well as the surrounding tissue margin and is the most ideal for determinations of benign or borderline histology. Incisional biopsy includes the tissue below and surrounding the lesion and is obtained after either local or general anesthesia. Alligator forceps may be used when a specific lesion is not present and is the preferred technique for anorectal lesions. Needle biopsy is useful for tissue diagnosis and may be used for prostatic lesions. The urinary bladder and peritoneum should be avoided, and the risks with needle biopsy of large tumors leave this biopsy approach as the least preferred for the anorectal structures.

Professional Considerations:

1. Consent form IS required.

Risks:

Hematoma, bleeding, and infection with needle biopsy of large tumors.

Contraindications:

Anticoagulant therapy, bleeding disorder, hypertensive crisis, thrombocytopenia.

2. Preparation:
   A. The client should disrobe below the waist.
   B. Obtain equipment for proctologic examination, proctoscopy, or sigmoidoscopy.
   C. Obtain a rectal biopsy tray, gloves, a water-soluble lubricant, fixative, and a specimen slide or container.
3. Procedure:
   A. *Adults:*
      i. The client is draped in the left lateral position with the knees and hips flexed.
      ii. An analgesic is given as prescribed.
      iii. A physician performs the proctologic examination.
      iv. The biopsy is obtained using straight or curved alligator forceps.
      v. The first valve of Houston is an easy and common site for rectal biopsy when a lesion is not present.
      vi. A posterior mucosa site, below the peritoneal reflection within 7–10 cm of the anal verge, decreases the incidence of peritoneal invasion.
   B. *Children and infants:*
      i. A rectal biopsy in the child or infant is obtained, using a Parks' retractor for visualization, from the upper anal canal 1 cm from the mucocutaneous junction.
   C. *Newborn:*
      i. The rectal biopsy is obtained starting 1 cm above the anal canal.
4. Postprocedure care:
   A. Transfer the tissue biopsy to a slide or sterile specimen container and fix with phosphate-buffered 1% formalin solution or other fixative specified by the laboratory in an amount 5–20 times the size of the tissue specimen.
   B. Label the specimen and record the specimen source and site on the laboratory requisition and the label.
   C. Transport the specimen to the pathology laboratory immediately.
   D. Cleanse the anal area.
5. Client and family teaching:
   A. A small amount of spotting of blood may occur initially. Contact the physician immediately if continued or increased bleeding is observed.
6. Factors that affect results:
   A. Bacterial cultures, electron microscopy, estrogen or progesterone receptor assay, or frozen section examination cannot be performed on specimens fixed in formalin.
   B. Reject specimens that have dried from prolonged exposure to air.
7. Other data:
   A. Biopsies in which lymphoproliferative disease is suspected must be fresh and should be transported immediately to the pathologist on a moist sponge. Immersion in a fixative or saline prior to examination with the use of Wright's stain obscures cytologic detail.

Bibliography:

Cusick EL, Buick RG: Injury to the common iliac artery during suction rectal biopsy. J Pediatr Surg *30*(1):111–112, 1995.

Idoate MA, Vazquez JJ, Civeira P: Rectal biopsy as a diagnostic procedure of chronic visceral leishmaniasis. Histopathology *22*(6):589–590, 1993.

Lessells AM, Beck JS, Burnett RA, Howatson SR, Lee FD, McLaren KM, Moss SM, Robertson AJ, Simpson JG, Smith GD, et al.: Observer variability in the histopathological reporting of abnormal rectal biopsy specimens. J Clin Pathol *47*(1):48–52, 1994.

RECTAL CULTURE, SWAB, DIAGNOSTIC

Norm: Negative for pathogenic organisms.

Usage: Screening for causes of bacterial diarrhea such as *Campylobacter, Chlamydia, Neisseria gonorrhoeae, Salmonella,* and *Shigella;* and detection of aerobic and anaerobic intestinal flora.

Description: The rectal swab culture is a screening test for pathogenic organisms of the rectum.

Professional Considerations:

1. Consent form NOT required.
2. Preparation:
   A. Obtain a sterile culture swab, a closed sterile container, and drapes.
   B. The client should disrobe below the waist.
3. Procedure:
   A. Drape the client in the left lateral position with the knees and hips flexed.
   B. Gently insert a sterile, cotton-tipped swab at least 2.5–3 cm into the rectum. Rotate the swab from side to side and leave it in place for a few seconds to allow absorption of rectal flora.
   C. If the swab is being obtained for *N. gonorrhoeae* culture, the swab must be discarded and the procedure repeated if fecal material contaminates the swab.
   D. Place the swab in a sterile container and cover it tightly. If a Culturette is used, insert the swab into the medium compartment of the culture tube and crush the distal end to release the ampule of medium.
4. Postprocedure care:
   A. Label the specimen with the site and collection time.
5. Client and family teaching:
   A. The test is used to determine the potential bacterial cause of diarrhea.
6. Factors that affect results:
   A. Swabs should be sent to the laboratory immediately.
   B. Refrigerate specimens not tested immediately.
7. Other data:
   A. The rectal culture is not used to determine carrier state.

Bibliography:

Rabello AL: Parasitological diagnosis of schistosomiasis mansoni: fecal examination and rectal biopsy. Memorias do Instituto Oswaldo Cruz. 87(Suppl 4):325–331, 1992.

Rabello AL, Rocha RS, de Oliveira JP, Katz N, Lambertucci JR: Stool examination and rectal biopsy in the diagnosis and evaluation of therapy of schistosomiasis mansoni. Revista do Instituto de Medicina Tropical de São Paulo, 34(8):601–608, 1992.

Tay YK, Goh CL, Chan R, Ali K, Nadarajah M, Sng J: Evaluation of enzyme immunoassay for the detection of anogenital infections caused by *Chlamydia trachomatis.* Singapore Med J *36*(2):173–175, 1995.

RECTAL EXAMINATION FOR MUCUS AND BLOOD, DIAGNOSTIC

Norm: Guaiac negative for blood. Rectal mucus should be a clear, viscid fluidlike substance.

Usage: Screening for colorectal disease. Detection of friability of the mucosa or punctate bleeding. Assists in the diagnosis of anal fissures; asymptomatic carcinoma; hemorrhoids; perianal, sphincteric, and ampullary lesions; peritoneal metastasis (Blumer's shelf); perirectal tissue deformities; prostatic and uterine abnormalities; tumefaction; rectal masses; and rectal prolapse (mucosal).

Description: This procedure consists of a digital exploration of the rectum and testing of rectal mucus for occult blood. All rectal bleeding should be investigated because bleeding is the most apparent sign of colonic disease.

Professional Considerations:

1. Consent form NOT required.
2. Preparation:
   A. *See Client and family teaching.*
   B. The client should disrobe below the waist.
   C. Obtain disposable gloves, lubricant, and a slide or a guaiac-impregnated card for occult blood.
3. Procedure:
   A. *Adults:*
      i. The client is placed in the left lateral position with the knees and hips flexed and draped.
      ii. When the rectal examination is performed after a vaginal examination, the lithotomy position may be used.
      iii. The index finger of the examiner should be covered with a glove or finger cot and well lubricated with a water-soluble lubricant.
      iv. The buttocks are separated, the anal area is inspected, and the client is asked to bear down.
      v. As the sphincter relaxes, the examiner's finger, while fully extended, is inserted slowly and in the direction of the umbilicus.
      vi. The examiner's finger is withdrawn and the material on the glove should be immediately smeared

onto a guaiac-impregnated card for occult blood.

B. *Children and infants:*

 i. With feet held together, flex the knees and hips onto the abdomen.

 ii. Because of the increased tactile sensitivity of the index finger, this digit is used even with the infant.

 iii. Slight bleeding and protrusion of the rectal mucosa upon withdrawal is expected, independent of the size of the examiner's index finger.

4. Postprocedure care:

 A. Cleanse the anal area.

 B. Send the guaiac card to the laboratory.

5. Client and family teaching:

 A. Follow a meat-free, high-residue diet for 24–48 hours prior to the procedure. The diet should also be free of vegetables with high peroxidase activity (including turnips, broccoli, beets, horseradish, cauliflower, cantaloupe, and parsnips).

 B. Once home, alert the physician of further rectal bleeding.

6. Factors that affect results:

 A. Specimens will be positive if contaminated by menstrual blood, hemorrhoidal blood, or povidone-iodine.

7. Other data:

 A. Over 50% of rectal carcinomas lie within reach of the index finger.

 B. Abnormalities of the right colon produce dark red to black blood. Abnormalities of the left colon produce bright red blood. Hemorrhoids produce very bright red blood.

Bibliography:

Chelmowski MK: Checking for fecal occult blood with digital rectal examinations [letter, comment]. Arch Intern Med *152*(9):1929, 1992.

RECTAL MANOMETRY, DIAGNOSTIC

(see Rectal Motility Test, Diagnostic)

RECTAL MOTILITY TEST (RECTAL MANOMETRY), DIAGNOSTIC

Norm: Adult: 40–120 mmHg. Distention of the rectum produces relaxation of the internal sphincter and contraction of the external sphincter.

Usage: Assists in the diagnosis of colonic dilation, constipation, diarrhea, external sphincter disorders (hypothyroidism, myasthenia gravis, myotonic dystrophy, polymyositis), Hirschsprung's disease, incontinence, and internal sphincter disorders (scleroderma); detection of anal achalasia; and evaluation of intrinsic ganglionic innervation of the internal sphincter of the rectum.

Description: This test measures the pressures within the rectum and evaluates the strength and function of the internal and external anal sphincters. Rectal distention produces relaxation of the internal sphincter and contraction of the external sphincter. The anal canal length is 5 cm, with a functional length of 3–5 cm. Functional length is determined by the extent of pressure generated by the involuntary internal and voluntary external anal sphincter muscles within the anal canal. This test is a more sensitive indicator of short segments of anal achalasia than barium enema. A small, thin, flexible balloon catheter with four sensing ports is introduced into the proximal rectum. The catheter is connected to three pressure transducers. Pressure readings of the rectum and sphincter are measured and recorded onto a graph or computer.

Professional Considerations:

1. Consent form NOT required.

2. Preparation:

 A. The client should disrobe below the waist.

 B. If a large amount of stool is present, a Fleet's enema is given and the examination is performed 1 hour after rectal evacuation.

3. Procedure:

 A. *Adults:*

 i. The client is placed in the left lateral position.

 ii. A small, thin, flexible balloon catheter with four sensing ports is introduced into the proximal rectum.

 iii. The catheter is inserted 8–10 cm above the mucocutaneous level, with the balloon portion in the proximal rectum and the sensing ports in the anal canal.

 iv. The catheter is connected to three pressure transducers.

 v. The rectum is distended with an inflated balloon for 7–12 seconds until resistance to balloon distention is demonstrated by passive movement of a syringe. Usually, 30–50 cc of air is required and is dependent on the client's age, the balloon size, and rectal dilation capacity.

 vi. The amount of air required for the client to feel resistance is recorded as the internal anal sphincter response.

vii. Air is withdrawn in 5–10-cc amounts until distention is no longer felt. This smallest volume reflects the threshold of rectal sensation. Most people have relaxation of the internal sphincter with a distention volume of 15 cc.

viii. The client is asked to squeeze the external sphincter tightly for 2 seconds and then relax.

ix. Anal canal pressures are measured at eight points, in 0.5- to 1.0-cm increments, with the highest resting and voluntary squeeze pressures recorded at each point.

x. Pressure readings of the rectum and sphincters are recorded onto graph paper, or images are configured on a computer.

xi. The catheter is removed.

B. *Children:*
   i. The procedure as above is consistent with the following changes: The catheter is inserted 5 cm above the mucocutaneous level, and the child may be sedated to prevent unnecessary movements and crying.

C. *Infants:*
   i. A cleansing enema is not given.

4. Postprocedure care:
   A. Cleanse the anal area.
5. Client and family teaching:
   A. Once home, alert the physician if rectal bleeding or discharge occurs.
6. Factors that affect results:
   A. Rectal stool decreases pressure readings.
   B. Insufficient rectal distention results in decreased pressure readings.
   C. Improper placement of the anal balloon or equipment malfunction.
7. Other data:
   A. Rectal manometry has not been demonstrated to be reliable in the newborn.

Bibliography:

Bassoti G, Betti C, Pelli MA, Morelli A: Prolonged (24-hour) manometric recording of rectal contractile activity in patients with slow transient constipation. Digestion *49*(2):72–77, 1991.

Nagashima M, Iwai N, Yanagihara J, Shimotake T: Motility and sensation of the rectosigmoid and the rectum in patients with anorectal malformations. J Pediatr Surg *27*(10):1273–1277, 1992.

RECTOSPHINCTERIC MANOMETRY, DIAGNOSTIC
(see Rectal Motility Test, Diagnostic)

RED BLOOD CELL (RBC), BLOOD

Norm:

		SI Units
Adult female	4–5.5 million/µl	4–5.5×10^{12}/L
Pregnant	3–5.0 million/µl	3–5.0×10^{12}/L
Adult male	4.5–6.2 million/µl	4.5–6.2×10^{12}/L
Infant	3.8–6.1 million/µl	3.8–6.1×10^{12}/L
1–2 years	3.6–5.5 million/µl	3.6–5.5×10^{12}/L
6–15 years	4.7–4.8 million/µl	4.7–4.8×10^{12}/L

Increased: Anoxia, burns (severe), cardiovascular disease, cerebellar hemangioblastoma, Cushing's disease, dehydration (severe), diarrhea, erythema, erythropoietin production increase, hemorrhage, hemoconcentration (exercise, fright, stress), hepatic carcinoma, hereditary spherocytosis, high-oxygen-affinity hemoglobinopathy, hypernephroma, poisoning, polycythemia vera, pulmonary disease and fibrosis, renal cyst, shock, sickle cell disease, surgery, thalassemia, and trauma. Drugs include gentamicin sulfate, methyldopa, and methyldopate hydrochloride.

Decreased: Addison's disease, anemias (aplastic, hemolytic, hemorrhagic, iron deficiency, pernicious, pure red cell), bone marrow suppression, cirrhosis, fatty liver, fluid overload, Gaucher's disease, hemorrhage, hemodilution, hemolysis, Hodgkin's disease, hydremia in pregnancy, hypothyroidism, idiopathic steatorrhea, infection (chronic), leukemia (chronic myelogenous), malaria, multiple myeloma, myxoma of left atrium of the heart, rheumatic fever, systemic lupus erythematosus, subacute bacterial endocarditis, and vitamin deficiency (B_6, B_{12}, folic acid). Drugs include acetaminophen, aminosalicylic acid, ampicillin, antineoplastics, carbamazepine, chloramphenicol, chloroquine hydrochloride or phosphate, haloperidol, hydralazine hydrochloride, hydroxychloroquine sulfate, indomethacin, isoniazid, mefenamic acid, methsuximide, methyldopa, methyldopate hydrochloride, nitrofurantoin, novobiocin sodium, penicillamine, phenobarbital, phenylbutazone, phenytoin, phytonadione, rifampin, spectinomycin hydrochloride, tetracyclines, thiazide diuretics, thiocyanates, tolbutamide, tripelennamine hydrochloride, valproic acid, and vitamin A.

Description: Red blood cells constitute the majority of peripheral blood cells. They are formed by red bone marrow, have a lifespan of about 120 days, and are removed from the blood by the liver, spleen, and bone marrow. Red blood cells function in hemoglobin transport, which results in delivery of oxygen to the body tissues. Red blood cell development is characterized by passage through several characteristic stages, beginning with erythroblasts, which are immature, nucleated red blood cells.

Professional Considerations:

1. Consent form NOT required.
2. Preparation:
   A. Tube: Lavender-top.
   B. Draw the sample from an extremity that does not have intravenous fluids infusing.
   C. Do NOT draw specimens during hemodialysis.
3. Procedure:
   A. Draw a 4-ml blood sample.
   B. Heelstick is acceptable, collected in a microtainer.
4. Postprocedure care:
   A. Invert the tube 10 times to mix the contents.
   B. The sample is stable at room temperature for 10 hours and refrigerated for 18 hours.
5. Client and family teaching.
   A. This test evaluates the body's ability to produce red blood cells in sufficient numbers.
6. Factors that affect results:
   A. False low values occur in the presence of cold agglutinins.
   B. Traumatic venipuncture and hemolysis invalidate the results.
7. Other data:
   A. Red blood cell indices are useful in further differentiating conditions.

Bibliography:

Davis BH, Bigelow NC: Reticulocyte analysis and reticulocyte maturity index. Methods Cell Biol *42*(Pt B):263–274, 1994.

Souweine B, Serre AF, Philippe P, Conio N, Aumaitre O, Marcheix JC: Serum erythropoietin and reticulocyte counts in inflammatory process. Ann Med Intern *146*(1):8–12, 1995.

RED BLOOD CELL ENZYME DEFICIENCY, SCREEN, BLOOD

Norm: Red blood cell enzyme is present.

Usage: Assists in the differential diagnosis of chronic nonspherocytic hemolytic anemias.

Description: Erythrocytes contain many enzymes that are involved in numerous metabolic activities. Any of the red blood cell enzymes may be congenitally deficient or become deficient due to acquired abnormalities. Either type of deficiency falls under the category of nonspherocytic anemia. The red blood cell enzyme deficiency screen is a battery of tests that assists in the differential diagnosis of chronic nonspherocytic hemolytic anemias.

Glucose-6-phosphate dehydrogenase (G6PD) is an enzyme present in red blood cells that plays an important role in the hexose monophosphate shunt. The majority of those affected by G6PD deficiency remain asymptomatic, and few exhibit chronic hemolytic anemia. After exposure to certain drugs, deficiency of this enzyme may result in hemolytic anemia. This trait is carried on the $\times$ chromosome, is expressed in the hemizygous male and the homozygous female, and is one of the most common red blood cell deficiencies, with over 50 variants of this sex-linked disorder.

Glutathione reductase (GR) is a red blood cell enzyme that is a catalyst in the reduction of NADPH to glutathione in the hexose monophosphate shunt. Exposure to certain drugs may cause a deficiency of this enzyme, resulting in hemolytic anemia.

Pyruvate kinase (PK) is a red blood cell glycolytic enzyme, of the Embden-Meyerhof pathway, and when deficient, is the second most frequent cause (after G6PD deficiency) of congenital, homozygous, nonspherocytic hemolytic anemia.

2,3-Diphosphoglycerate (2,3-DPG) is the most abundant intracellular organic phosphate in red blood cells. It is a byproduct of the glycolytic pathway in the Rapoport-Luebering shunt. 2,3-DPG controls oxygen transport to the tissues and binds to specific amino acid sites on proteins. In the presence of decreased levels of hemoglobin (anemia),

2,3-DPG acts on the beta chains of the deoxyhemoglobin to decrease oxygen affinity or release oxygen to the tissues. Increased production of 2,3-DPG causes the oxyhemoglobin dissociation curve to "shift to the right." Conversely, deficiency of this enzyme or conditions that increase oxygen affinity results in defects in the unloading of oxygen to the tissues.

Professional Considerations:

1. Consent form NOT required.
2. Preparation:
   A. Tube: Lavender-top, red-top, red/gray-top, or gold-top; or capillary tube.
   B. Specimens MAY be drawn during hemodialysis.
3. Procedure:
   A. Draw a 7-ml blood sample, without trauma.
   B. Fingerstick samples should be collected into seven microhematocrit tubes, three-fourths full and gently rotated 7 times to ensure complete mixing of the sample and anticoagulant.
   C. For 2,3-DPG, draw a 3-ml blood sample.
4. Postprocedure care:
   A. None.
5. Client and family teaching:
   A. This test evaluates and helps differentiate the different anemias.
6. Factors that affect results:
   A. Reject hemolyzed or clotted specimens.
   B. High altitudes increase 2,3-DPG results.
   C. Banked/stored blood decreases 2,3-DPG results.
   D. False-normal G6PD results may occur in black clients if the sample is collected during a hemolytic episode.
7. Other data:
   A. Phenotyping of RBC enzymes has been applied to paternity testing.

Bibliography:

Isselbacher KJ, et al.: Harrison's Principles of Internal Medicine, 13th ed. New York, McGraw-Hill, 1994, pp 1746–1748.

The Merck Manual, 16th ed. Rahway, NJ, Merck and Company, 1992, pp 1168–1169.

RED BLOOD CELL MORPHOLOGY, BLOOD

Norm: Microscopic interpretation is required.

Color	Uniformly normochromic
Size	6–8 μ, only slight size variation
Shape	Round, biconcave disk
Stained appearance	Mature erythrocytes stain uniformly and contain a normal concentration of hemoglobin with an area of central pallor.
Nucleus	Absent
Nuclear remnants	Absent
Cellular inclusions	Absent
Acanthocytes	Absent
Crescent bodies	Absent
Drepanocytes	Absent
Echinocytes	Absent
Leptocytes	Absent
Poikilocytes	Absent
Schizocytes	Absent
Spherocytes	Absent
Stomatocytes	Absent
Cabot rings	Absent
Heinz bodies	Absent
Siderocytes	Absent

CLASSIFICATION OF VARIATION FROM NORMAL

Abnormal RBCs/HPF	Score	Interpretation
3–6	1+	Slight
7–10	2+	Moderate
11–20	3+	Marked
>20	4+	Very marked

Usage: Detection of blood dyscrasias; and differentiation of anemias, leukemia, and thalassemia.

Description of Abnormalities of RBC Color	Possible Causes of Abnormal RBC Color
Anisochromia is demonstrated by variable staining intensities indicating unequal hemoglobin content due to multiple populations of red blood cells (RBCs).	*Anisochromatism:* Iron-deficiency anemia treated with transfused blood
Hyperchromia is demonstrated by the presence of cells having a smaller than normal area of central pallor, causing the cells to take on excessive staining and demonstrate higher than normal pigmentation. Increased amounts of these cells are called hyperchromatism.	*Hyperchromatism:* Dehydration, increased bone marrow iron stores, inflammation (chronic), and in the presence of spherocytes that have increased cell wall thickness
Hypochromia is demonstrated by the presence of cells having a larger than normal area of central pallor, causing the cells to stain weakly and appear to have less than normal pigmentation. Increased amounts of these cells are called hypochromatism.	*Hypochromatism:* Anemia (iron deficiency) and decreased hemoglobin concentration
Polychromatophils are cells that are stainable with many types of stains, such as stains with both an acid and base component. They are demonstrated by a bluish-pink tinge caused by the presence of both hemoglobin stained by acid and cytoplasmic ribonucleic acid (RNA) stained by the basic component. Both the larger-than-normal cell size and the presence of cytoplasmic RNA indicate that polychromatophils are reticulocytes (newly made red blood cells). Increased amounts of polychromatophils are called polychromatosis and occur in accelerated RBC production.	*Polychromatosis:* Hemorrhage, hemolysis, reticulocytosis, and therapy for iron deficiency anemia or pernicious anemia

Description of Abnormalities of RBC Shape	Possible Causes of Abnormal RBC Shape
Acanthocytes are cells with irregular, thorny, spiculated membrane surface projections containing bulbous, rounded ends. They result from an irreversible defect in the lipid content of the RBC membrane. The presence of acanthocytes is called acanthocytosis.	*Acanthocytosis:* Abetalipoproteinemia (most common cause), alcoholic cirrhosis, hemolytic anemia (induced by pyruvate kinase deficiency), hepatic disease, postsplenectomy, and retinitis pigmentosa. Drugs include heparin calcium and heparin sodium.

Description of Abnormalities of RBC Shape *(continued)*	Possible Causes of Abnormal RBC Shape *(continued)*
Crescent bodies (achromocytes) are cells with a faint quarter-moon shape caused by RBC rupture.	*Achromocytosis:* Any condition that increases the fragility of red blood cells (i.e., sickle cell anemia, reduced oxygen supply)
Drepanocytes/sickle cells are cells formed in the shape of a sickle with a point at one end. The presence of these cells is called drepanocytosis.	*Drepanocytosis:* Anemia (hemolytic, sickle cell) and hemoglobin SC disease
Echinocytes/burr cells/crenated RBCs have a cell surface with 10–30 uniformly distributed, blunt spicules. Echinocytes may be commonly due to pH changes due to faulty drying during smear preparation, but certain physiologic conditions, including a reversible defect in the lipid content of the RBC membrane, have been associated with their presence. The presence of these cells is called echinocytosis.	*Echinocytosis:* Bile acid abnormalities, blood loss (acute), burns (extensive), carcinoma of the stomach, disseminated intravascular coagulation (DIC), gastric ulcers (bleeding), increased free fatty acids, microangiopathic hemolytic anemia, pyruvate kinase deficiency, renal failure, thrombotic thrombocytopenic purpura, and uremia. Drugs include barbiturates, heparin calcium, heparin sodium, and salicylates.
Elliptocytes/ovalocytes have a cigar shape, which distinguishes them from the more oval shape of the ovalocytes. They are normal constituents of mature RBCs. Higher than normal amounts of these cells are called elliptocytosis.	*Elliptocytosis:* Anemias (iron deficiency, pernicious, sickle cell), hereditary elliptocytosis, leukemia, megaloblastic hematopoiesis, and thalassemia
Leptocytes/target cells have an increased ratio of surface to volume, often due to a shape that looks like a cup, bell, or hat. They have a colorless center and are thinner and lighter staining than normal RBCs due to abnormally low amounts of hemoglobin. When stained, the depth of the "cup" collapses, causing a bulls-eye appearance. The presence of leptocytes is termed leptocytosis.	*Leptocytosis:* Anemia (iron deficiency, sickle cell), cellular dehydration, cirrhosis, hemoglobin C disease, hemoglobin SC disease, hepatitis, jaundice (obstructive), postsplenectomy, and thalassemia
Poikilocytes occur in varying shapes, ranging from slightly irregular to dumbbell-like, pear-shaped, or teardrop-shaped. Defective bone marrow production causes poikilocytosis, a general term used to describe the presence of cells demonstrating variation from the normal shape of the RBC.	*Poikilocytosis:* Anemia (iron deficiency, hemolytic, megaloblastic, pernicious), myelofibrosis, myeloid metaplasia, and thalassemia

Description of Abnormalities of RBC Shape (continued)	Possible Causes of Abnormal RBC Shape (continued)
Schizocytes/schistocytes are RBCs with adhesions of spiral and triangular red blood cell fragments due to hemolysis, hemoglobinopathies, or erythrocytic mechanical damage from fibrin strands. The presence of these cells is called schizocytosis.	*Schizocytosis or Schistocytosis:* Anemia (acute hemolytic, microangiopathic hemolytic), burns (severe), disseminated intravascular coagulation (DIC), prosthetic heart valves, pyruvate kinase deficiency, renal graft rejection, uremic-hemolytic syndrome, valve prosthesis, and valvular stenosis
Spherocytes are cells that are globe-like rather than biconcave, with an abnormally small dimple. They are thicker than normal, with many fine-needle-like projections. Spherocytes lack an area of central pallor (due to an increased mean corpuscular hemoglobin concentration) and have a smaller surface area relative to their size. Spherocytes are caused by mechanical fibrin strand damage to circulating RBCs. The presence of spherocytes is called spherocytosis.	*Spherocytosis:* ABO hemolytic disease of the newborn, accelerated reticuloendothelial red blood cell destruction, anemia (hemolytic), following blood transfusion, hereditary spherocytosis, and thermal injury of the cell membrane
Stomatocytes are cup-shaped RBCs with an abnormal area of central pallor that may be oval or rectangular, elongated, or slitlike. These cells are produced by antibodies or hydrocytosis. The presence of these cells is called stomatocytosis.	*Stomatocytosis:* Alcoholism, cirrhosis, erythrocyte sodium pump defect, hepatic disease (obstructive), hereditary spherocytosis, hereditary stomatocytosis, and Rh null cells

Description of Abnormalities of RBC Size	Possible Causes of Abnormalities of RBC Size
Anisocytosis is a general term that describes any variation in the size of the RBC.	*Anisocytosis:* Anemias (iron deficiency, pernicious), folic acid deficiency, following blood transfusion of normal cells into an abnormal red blood cell population, leukemia, newborns, and reticulocytosis
Macrocytes are large erythrocytes having a diameter >8 μ, a mean corpuscular volume <95 μ, and higher than normal hemoglobin content. They are usually increased due to stress erythropoiesis. Increased amounts of macrocytes are called macrocytosis.	*Macrocytosis:* Anemia (hemolytic, pernicious), folic acid deficiency, following hemorrhagic states, hepatic disease, hyperthyroidism, idiopathic steatorrhea, newborns, reticulocytosis, and thalassemia

Description of Abnormalities of RBC Size *(continued)*	Possible Causes of Abnormalities of RBC Size *(continued)*
Microcytes have a RBC diameter <6 μ, a mean corpuscular volume <80 μ, and mean corpuscular hemoglobin concentration <27%. Increased amounts of microcytes are called microcytosis.	*Microcytosis:* Anemia (from chronic hemorrhage, iron deficiency), hemoglobinopathies, hereditary spherocytosis, and thalassemia

Description of Abnormalities of RBC Content or Structure	Possible Causes of Abnormal RBC Structure or Content
Agglutination: Clumping together of RBCs is an immune mechanism caused by antibody formation.	*Agglutination:* Invading antigen(s)
Basophilic stippling is demonstrated by the presence of minute basophilic granules that cause a bluish/purple color when reticulocytes are stained. They are caused by ribosomal aggregation that occurs as smears are prepared. Small amounts of basophilic stippling normally occur as the smears are dried. Increased amounts occur in conditions in which RNA has aggregated in the cells.	*Increased basophilic stippling:* Alcoholism, anemia (megaloblastic, sickle cell), heavy metal intoxication (bismuth, lead, mercury, and silver), hemorrhage (gastrointestinal), leukemia, and thalassemia
Cabot's rings are cells containing mitotic spindle remnants appearing as fine, threadlike filaments of bluish purple color in the shape of a single ring or a double ring (figure-eight shape).	*Presence of Cabot's rings:* Anemia (severe, pernicious), lead poisoning, myelofibrosis, and myeloid metaplasia
Heinz bodies are denatured particles of hemoglobin attached to the RBC membrane that appear when stained with cresyl blue or new methylene blue. Heinz bodies usually indicate abnormal erythrocyte stability due to hemolytic conditions or hemoglobinopathies.	*Presence of Heinz bodies:* Alpha-thalassemia, anemia (hemolytic), glucose-6-phosphate dehydrogenase deficiency, hemoglobinopathies, methemoglobinemia, and post-splenectomy. Drugs include analgesics, antipyretics, chlorates, phenacetin, phenothiazines, phenylacetamide, phenylhydrazine, phenylamine, primaquine phosphate, resorcinol, and sulfapyridine
Howell-Jolly bodies are nuclear fragments contained in red cells that stain purple or violet. They are normally present in immature RBCs and in mature erythrocytes before they pass through the splenic circulation. In conditions causing increased RBC production, erythrocytes contain higher than normal amounts of these bodies.	*Presence of Howell-Jolly bodies:* Anemia (hemolytic, megaloblastic), leukemia, splenic absence (congenital or surgical removal), and splenic atrophy

Description of Abnormalities of RBC Content or Structure *(continued)*	Possible Causes of Abnormal RBC Structure or Content *(continued)*
Platelets on red blood cells appear as a halo that resists staining and can be easily confused with RBC inclusion bodies.	*n/a*
Rouleaux formation is demonstrated by a cellular configuration in stacks or rolls. Increased rouleaux formation may be caused by increased fibrinogen or globulins in the blood. Rouleaux formation is decreased by the presence of abnormally shaped RBCs, which inhibits adherence of the cells in a stacked shape. Rouleaux formation may also result from a delay in slide preparation.	*Increased rouleaux formation:* Hyperfibrinogenemia, macroglobulinemia, and multiple myeloma *Decreased rouleaux formation:* Hereditary spherocytosis
Siderocytes/Pappenheimer bodies are cells with mitochondrial concentrations of ferritin (nonhemoglobin iron) deposits. These cells stain as purple-bluish granules only in the presence of iron stains such as Prussian-blue reactions. Pappenheimer bodies are noniron basophilic granules contained in the iron-protein matrix and stain positive for iron in the presence of noniron stains. Ferritin is normally absent in RBCs. During hemoglobin formation in the premature infant and newborn, siderocyte free-iron granules commonly occur in developing normoblasts and reticulocytes. The presence of siderocytes is called siderocytosis.	*Siderocytosis/Pappenheimer bodies:* Anemia (chronic hemolytic, congenital spherocytic, dyserythropoietic, megaloblastic, pernicious, refractory, sideroblastic), burns (severe), hemochromatosis, infection, lead poisoning, postsplenectomy, and thalassemia

Description: Red blood cells (RBCs) constitute the majority of peripheral blood cells and function in hemoglobin transport, which results in delivery of oxygen to the body tissues. RBC development is characterized by passage through several characteristic stages, beginning with erythroblasts, which are immature, nucleated RBCs. RBC morphology is the examination of red cells under a microscope, comparing the actual appearance with calculated values for each indice of color, size, shape, developmental stage, and structure or content.

Professional Considerations:
1. Consent form NOT required.
2. Preparation:
   A. Tube: Lavender-top.
   B. Specimens MAY be drawn during hemodialysis.
3. Procedure:
   A. Draw a 7-ml blood sample.
   B. Heelstick is acceptable, collected in a microtainer.
4. Postprocedure care:
   A. None.
5. Client and family teaching:
   A. This test evaluates the structure of the RBCs.
6. Factors that affect results:
   A. Automated methods of counting and

sizing of the RBCs should not be used in the presence of red cell agglutination. Instead, hand counts must be performed.

7. Other data:
   A. RBC morphology stained smear is usually carried out at the same time as the differential white blood cell count.

Bibliography:

Brugnara C, Hipp MJ, Irving PJ, Lathrop H, Lee PA, Minchello EM, Winkelman J: Automated reticulocyte counting and measurement of reticulocyte cellular indices. Evaluation of the Miles H*3 blood analyzer. Am J Clin Pathol *102*(5):623–632, 1994.

Davis BH, Bigelow NC: Automated reticulocyte analysis. Clinical practice and associated new parameters [review]. Hematol Oncol Clin North Am *8*(4): 617–630, 1994.

Lee GR, et al.: Wintrobe's Clinical Hematology, 9th ed, Vol 1. Philadelphia, Lea and Febiger, 1993, pp 724–726.

The Merck Manual, 16th ed. Rahway, NJ, Merck and Company, 1992, pp 1138–1139.

RED BLOOD CELL SURVIVAL, BLOOD

(see Cr-51 [Chromium] Red Cell Survival, Blood)

RED CELL COUNT, SERUM

(see Red Blood Cell, Blood)

RED CELL MASS, BLOOD

Norm:

Female	24.24 ± 2.59 ml/kg (standard deviation)
Male	28.27 ± 4.11 ml/kg (standard deviation)

Increased: Addison's disease, burns, carboxyhemoglobinemia, cerebellar hemangioblastoma, Cushing's disease, dehydration, emphysema, hepatoma, high altitude, increased erythropoietin production, left-to-right shunt (due to cardiovascular disease), lung disease (producing hypoxia), methemoglobinemia, myeloproliferative syndrome, pickwickian syndrome, polycythemia vera, renal cell adenocarcinoma, renal cyst, secondary polycythemia, smokers, stress states, and uterine myoma.

Decreased: Addison's disease, anemias, blood loss (acute), carcinoma, edema (severe), hemorrhage, infection (chronic), inflammation (chronic), myxedema, panhypopituitarism, radiation, renal failure (chronic), and starvation.

Description: Red cell mass is a direct measurement of the total number of red blood cells in the systemic circulation and is expressed in relation to body weight as ml/kg. Red cell mass reflects the equilibrium between the rate that the bone marrow produces and releases erythrocytes and the rate of peripheral erythrocyte destruction. This test assists in differential diagnosis of absolute and relative polycythemia, anemia, erythrocytosis, and Gaisbock's syndrome.

Professional Considerations:

1. Consent form NOT required.

Risks:
Hematoma, infection.

Contraindications:
During pregnancy or breast-feeding.

2. Preparation:
   A. Tube: Two (2) green-top.
3. Procedure:
   A. Draw an 8-ml blood sample.
   B. The sample is mixed with a radioactive isotope (Cr-51, I-131-labeled albumin, or I-125-tagged albumin) and is reinjected into the client after 15 minutes.
   C. Draw an 8-ml blood sample 15 minutes after reinjection.
4. Postprocedure care:
   A. Observe the client carefully for up to 60 minutes after the study for a possible (anaphylactic) reaction to the radionuclide.
   B. When urine is being discarded, rubber gloves should be worn for 24 hours after the procedure. Wash the gloved hands with soap and water before removing the gloves. Wash the ungloved hands after gloves are removed.
5. Client and family teaching:
   A. This test is a measurement of the body's ability to produce RBCs.
   B. Instruct the client to meticulously wash the hands with soap and water after each void × 24 hours.
6. Factors that affect results:
   A. Active bleeding, edematous extremities, or intravenous infusions during measurement may alter the results.
   B. Recent scans involving the administra-

tion of radioactive isotopes will obscure the results.

7. Other data:
   A. Total blood volume and plasma volume are obtained at the time of this test.
   B. Health care professionals working in a nuclear medicine area must follow federal standards set by the Nuclear Regulatory Commission. These standards include precautions for handling the radioactive material and monitoring of potential radiation exposure.
   C. Iodine-131 half-life is 8 days. Iodine-125 half-life is 60 days. Chromium-51 half-life is 27.8 days.

Bibliography:

Korbet SM: Comparison of hemodialysis and peritoneal dialysis in the management of anemia related to chronic renal disease. Semin Nephrol *9*(1, Suppl 1):9–15, 1989.

Levin N: Management of blood pressure changes during recombinant human erythropoietin therapy. Semin Nephrol *9*(1, Suppl 2):16–20, 1989.

Wyngaarden JB, Smith LH, Bennett JC: Cecil Textbook of Medicine, 19th ed. Philadelphia, WB Saunders, 1992, p 491, 921.

5. Client and family teaching:
   A. This test will evaluate iron intake and utilization in the body.
6. Factors that affect results:
   A. RDW is obtained by electronic evaluation (anisocytosis).
   B. *See Reticulocyte Count, Blood; and Hematocrit, Blood.*
7. Other data:
   A. *See Reticulocyte Count, Blood; and Hematocrit, Blood.*

Bibliography:

Baqar MS, Khurshid M, Molla A: Does red blood cell distribution width (RDW) improve evaluation of microcytic anemias? J Pakistan Med Assoc *43*(8):149–151, 1993.

Fernandes J: Automated hematology: the value of the red blood cell distribution width (RDW). JAOA *91*(3):260–264, 1991.

Lee GR, et al.: Wintrobe's Clinical Hematology, 9th ed, Vols 1 and 2. Philadelphia, Lea and Febiger, 1993, pp 15, 793–794, 797–798, 826.

The Merck Manual, 16th ed. Rahway, NJ, Merck and Company, 1992, pp 1142, 1149.

RED CELL SIZE DISTRIBUTION WIDTH (RDW), BLOOD

Normal: 13.4–14.6%. Microscopic electronic interpretation is required.

Increased: Iron deficiency. *See Red Blood Cell (RBC), Blood. See Red Blood Cell Morphology, Blood.*

Decreased: Defects in iron reutilization. *See Red Blood Cell (RBC), Blood. See Red Blood Cell Morphology, Blood.*

Description: Red cell volume distribution width, or RDW, is a coefficient of variation (CV) in red cell volume. This is derived from anisocytosis. RDW becomes abnormal earlier in iron deficiency than any other blood cell parameters. RDW may be a useful tool in differential diagnosis of microcytic anemia. It should be remembered that RDW is a CV, and it should be correlated with other erythrocytic indices for most accurate diagnoses. *(See Red Blood Cell Morphology, Blood.)*

Professional Considerations:

1. Consent form NOT required.
2. Preparation:
   A. Tube: Lavender-top.
   B. Specimens MAY be drawn during hemodialysis.
3. Procedure:
   A. Draw a 5-ml blood sample.
4. Postprocedure care:
   A. None.

REDUCING SUBSTANCES, STOOL

Norm:

Normal	<2 mg/g stool
Borderline	2–5 mg/g stool
Abnormal	>5 mg/g stool

Increased: Dissacharidase deficiencies, intestinal mucosal defects, and metabolic disorders.

Decreased: Beta-lipoprotein deficiency, blind loop syndrome, celiac disease, cystic fibrosis of the pancreas, *Giardia* infestation, and malnutrition (severe). Drugs include colchicine, neomycin sulfate, and oral contraceptives.

Description: The presence of reducing substances in the stool demonstrates the inability of intestinal border enzymes to absorb disaccharides, especially sucrase and lactase. These unabsorbed sugars are reduced by metal ions, such as copper contained in the frequently used Clinitest reduction tablet.

Professional Considerations:

1. Consent form NOT required.
2. Preparation:
   A. Obtain a clean, dry plastic specimen container.
3. Procedure:
   A. Collect at least 1 g of stool in a clean, dry plastic specimen container with a lid.

4. Postprocedure care:
   A. Send the specimen to the laboratory immediately.
   B. Freeze the specimen if not tested immediately.
5. Client and family teaching:
   A. This test measures the digestive tract's ability to absorb disaccharides.
   B. Urinate before defecating to avoid contaminating the stool sample with urine.
6. Factors that affect results:
   A. False-low results due to bacterial fermentation may occur when analysis is delayed in nonfrozen specimens.

B. Reject specimens that have been placed on an absorbent surface (diaper, cardboard).
7. Other data:
   A. The weight and pH of the specimen are usually obtained and included in the results.

Bibliography:

Aneen VZ, Powell GK, Jones LA: Quantitation of fecal carbohydrate excretion in clients with short bowel syndrome. Gastroenterology 92(2):493–500, 1987.

Krom EA, Frank CG: Clinitesting neonatal stools. Neonat Network 8(2):37–40, 1989.

REFRACTION VISION TEST, DIAGNOSTIC

Norm: Emmetropia or no refractive error.

Refractive Power of the Human Eye, Without Accommodation:	58 diopters
Refractive Power of the Structures of the Eye:	
Cornea	44 diopters
Aqueous humor	44 diopters
Lens	10–14 diopters

Note: The vitreous humor has little refractive power and primarily transmits light.

Usage: Assists in the evaluation of visual acuity; diagnosis of ametropias (refractive errors), including astigmatism, hyperopia (farsightedness), and myopia (nearsightedness); and determination of the need for the prescription of corrective lenses.

Description: Refraction is the process by which light rays entering the eye bend or pass obliquely over the curved surfaces of the eye (cornea, aqueous humor, lens, and vitreous humor), which have differing densities. Clear images are produced as a point of light is focused directly on the retina.

Professional Considerations:

1. Consent form NOT required.

Risks:

Allergic reaction to eye drops (itching, hives, rash, tight feeling in the throat, shortness of breath, bronchospasm, anaphylaxis, death).

Contraindications:

Previous allergy to mydriatic drops; narrow-angle glaucoma.

2. Preparation:
   A. Eye drops may be placed in both eyes to dilate the pupils and to prevent lens accommodation during the examination.
3. Procedure:
   A. The examiner locates the pupillary opening with a retinoscope, then assesses for stasis of the red/orange retinal reflection of the retinoscope light.
   B. Brightness, clarity, shape, size, vascularity, and uniformity of the retina are observed.
   C. A variety of lenses with varying lens powers are inserted into the client's test glasses.
   D. This process continues until the lens power that best neutralizes retinal reflex motion, produces the most clarity and brightness, and produces the most consistently correct reading of a visual chart is determined.
4. Postprocedure care:
   A. *See Client and family teaching.*
5. Client and family teaching:
   A. This is a simple eye test to determine if you do or do not need corrective lenses.
   B. Bring sunglasses to wear after the procedure.
   C. Do not drive or operate any machinery until distant vision returns.
6. Factors that affect results:
   A. Inadequate pupil dilation, excessive lens accommodation, or incomplete cooperation of the client prevents accurate results.
7. Other data:
   A. Most clients show some degree of ametropia or refractive error.

Bibliography:

Isselbacher KJ, et al.: Harrison's Principles of Internal Medicine, 13th ed. New York, McGraw-Hill, 1994, p 99.

Lavery JR, Gibson JM, Shaw DE, Rosenthal AR: Vision and visual acuity in an elderly population. Ophthalmic Physiol Opt *8*(4):390–393, 1988.

RENAL ANGIOGRAM (RENAL ARTERIOGRAM), DIAGNOSTIC

Norm: Radiopaque iodine contrast material should circulate symmetrically and without interruption through the renal parenchyma and renal vasculature.

Usage: Visualization of the renal parenchyma and renal vasculature; assists in differentiation of renal masses; identification of renovascular abnormalities such as abscesses, aneurysms, arteriovenous fistula, hypervascularity, hypovascularity, emboli, fibrosis, infarction, intrarenal hematoma, parenchymal laceration, renal artery dysplasia, stenosis, thrombolic occlusions, and traumatic injury; and evaluation of chronic renal disease, renal failure, and transplant donors and recipients, as well as post-transplant evaluation of vascular flow and rejection of the donor organ.

Description: Renal angiogram is an invasive roentgenographic procedure involving injection of iodine radiopaque contrast material through a catheter inserted into the aorta near the bifurcation of the renal arteries or directly into the renal arteries.

Professional Considerations:

1. Consent form IS required.

Risks:

Embolus, hematoma, hemorrhage, infection, allergic reaction to contrast material (itching, hives, rash, tight feeling in the throat, shortness of breath, bronchospasm, anaphylaxis, death), renal toxicity from contrast medium.

Contraindications:

Previous allergy to iodine, shellfish, or radiographic dye; renal insufficiency. The procedure may be contraindicated during pregnancy.

Caution should be taken with clients who have bleeding tendencies and those with renal failure due to end-stage renal disease. Sedatives are contraindicated in clients with central nervous system depression.

2. Preparation:
   A. Establish intravenous access.
   B. A narcotic or sedative may be prescribed.
   C. The client should void and remove all jewelry and metal objects.
   D. Have an emergency cart readily available.
   E. Obtain local anesthetic, povidone-iodine solution, intravenous fluid, contrast material, guidewire, vascular and renal catheters, and sterile gloves.
   F. *See Client and family teaching.*
3. Procedure:
   A. The client is positioned supine.
   B. A peripheral intravenous infusion is started.
   C. The arterial site is cleansed and anesthetized.
   D. A catheter is introduced via the Seldinger technique into the femoral artery or into the transaxillary, transbrachial, or translumbar vessels, and advanced under fluoroscopy to the aorta. Test aortograms with a small amount of contrast material are completed.
   E. The catheter is then replaced with a renal catheter and larger amounts of radiopaque contrast material are injected through the catheter directly into the aorta near the bifurcation of the renal arteries or directly into the renal arteries.
   F. Rapid, serial roentgenographic films are then taken to record circulation of the contrast material through the renal parenchyma and vasculature.
   G. The catheter is removed and a pressure dressing is applied over the insertion site.
4. Postprocedure care:
   A. If sedation was used, continue assessment of respiratory status. If deep sedation was used, follow institutional protocol for postsedation monitoring. Typical monitoring includes continuous ECG monitoring and pulse oximetry, with continual assessments (q 5–15 minutes) of airway, vital signs, and neurologic status until the client is lying quietly awake, is breathing independently, and responds to commands spoken in a normal tone.
   B. Monitor the catheter insertion site for bleeding, inflammation, and/or hematoma formation.
5. Client and family teaching:
   A. This test determines the adequacy of blood flow through both renal arteries.
   B. Fast for 8 hours before the procedure.

C. For 5 minutes after injection of the contrast material, an urge to cough, a flushed sensation, nausea, or a salty taste may occur.

D. It is important to lie motionless throughout the procedure. Sedation may be used to help you relax.

6. Factors that affect results:

A. Interpretation of the results may be impaired by the presence of gas, feces, or contrast material such as barium in the gastrointestinal tract.

B. Movement of the client during the procedure obscures the radiography.

7. Other data:

A. None.

Bibliography:

Kushner FG, Helm MJ: Successful directional atherectomy of eccentric renal artery stenosis using the Simpson directional coronary atherocath as a primary therapy. Cathet Cardiovasc Diagn *29*(2): 128–130, 1993.

Sonpal GM, Sharma A, Killer A: Primary antiphospholipid antibody syndrome, renal infarction and hypertension. J Rheumatol *20*(7):1221–1223, 1993.

RENAL ARTERIOGRAM, DIAGNOSTIC

(see Renal Angiogram, Diagnostic)

RENAL ECHOGRAM

(see Kidney Sonogram, Diagnostic)

RENAL FUNCTION TEST, DIAGNOSTIC

(see Concentration Test, Urine; Creatinine Clearance, Serum, Urine; Inulin Clearance Test, Diagnostic; and Phenolsulfonphthalein Test, Diagnostic)

Description: The renal function test may consist of up to four tests: the urine concentration test, the phenolsulfonphthalein (PSP) test, and the creatinine clearance or inulin clearance tests. These four indices reflect glomerular filtration, tubular reabsorption, renal blood flow, and tubular secretion. Measurement of these separate kidney functions assists in the determination of the origin and degree of renal dysfunction and renal tissue destruction. These tests are limited in their scope to detect early or mild renal disorders. *(See individual test listings for more information.)*

RENAL SCAN, DIAGNOSTIC

(see Renocystogram, Diagnostic)

RENAL ULTRASOUND, DIAGNOSTIC

(see Kidney Sonogram, Diagnostic)

RENIN (PLASMA RENIN ACTIVITY, PRA), PLASMA

Norm: Norms are age-, diet-, position-, and vein-site-dependent:

		SI Units
Normal-Sodium Diet, Upright and from the Peripheral Vein		
Age 20–39	0.6–4.3 ng/ml/h	0.6–4.3 µg/L/h
Mean	1.9 ng/ml/h	1.9 µg/L/h
Age ≥40	0.6–3.0 ng/ml/h	0.6–3.0 µg/L/h
Mean	1.0 ng/ml/h	1.0 µg/L/h
Low-Sodium Diet, Upright and from the Peripheral Vein		
Age 20–39	2.9–24.0 ng/ml/h	2.9–24.0 µg/L/h
Mean	10.8 ng/ml/h	10.8 µg/L/h
Age ≥40	2.9–10.8 ng/ml/h	2.9–10.8 µg/L/h
Mean	5.9 ng/ml/h	5.9 µg/L/h

Note: Samples obtained during renal vein catheterization are compared with levels obtained in the inferior vena cava to obtain the renal venous renin ratio. Renal venous renin ratio: <1.5:1.

Increased: Addison's disease, aldosteronism (secondary), ambulatory clients (compared to clients on bedrest), Bartter's syndrome, chronic renal failure, cirrhosis, erect posture for 4 hours (twofold increase), essential hypertension (rare), hypokalemia, hypovolemia (hemorrhage-induced), last half of menstrual cycle (twofold increase), low-sodium diet, nephropathy (sodium-losing), normal pregnancy, pheochromocytoma, renal hypertension, renin-producing renal tumors, and transplant rejection. Drugs include antihypertensives, diazoxide, estrogens, furosemide, guanethidine sulfate, hydralazine hydrochloride, minoxidil, nitroprusside sodium, saralasin, spironolactone, and thiazides.

Decreased: Adrenocortical hypertension, advancing age, Cushing's syndrome, essential hypertension, high-sodium diet, licorice-ingestion syndrome, and primary aldosteronism. Drugs include clonidine hydrochloride, desmopressin acetate, lypressin, methyldopa, propranolol, reserpine, steroids (sodium-retaining), and vasopressin.

Description: Renin is a proteolytic enzyme that is synthesized, stored, and secreted by the juxtaglomerular cells of the kidney. Renin is the primary catalyst that regulates the body's blood pressure, potassium, and fluid volume balance. Hydrolytic activity of the renin-angiotensin-aldosterone cycle results in the production of angiotensin II, a potent vasoconstrictor that stimulates the production of aldosterone in the adrenal cortex. Decreased renal blood flow stimulates renin secretion and an increased secretion of aldosterone. Blood loss and sodium depletion stimulate the release of renin. Hypertensive states with low plasma renin activity are suggestive of body fluid expansion imbalance. High plasma renin activity suggests hypertension from the vasoconstrictive effects of angiotensin.

Professional Considerations:

1. Consent form NOT required.
2. Preparation:
   A. Preparation and cooperation of the client are critical for accurate results.
   B. The client must be assessed for medications that affect the results (estrogens can affect results for up to 6 months), and certain medications may be withheld for 2–4 weeks prior to the test.
   C. *See Client and family teaching.*
   D. Preschedule this test with the laboratory.
   E. Tube: Lavender-top, ice cold.
   F. A local anesthetic may be administered prior to renal vein catheterization.
3. Procedure:
   A. Completely fill an ice-cold lavender-top tube with blood.

B. Tilt the tube several times to mix the sample.
   C. The same procedure is used in handling blood samples obtained during renal vein catheterization.
4. Postprocedure care:
   A. Place the specimen immediately on ice.
   B. Send the specimen to the laboratory immediately.
   C. Monitor vital signs, the catheterization site, and distal pulses q 15 minutes × 2, then q 30 minutes × 2.
5. Client and family teaching:
   A. This test measures one of the fluid balance mechanisms within the body.
   B. Follow a 3 g/day sodium diet for 3–14 days prior to the test. Do not eat licorice prior to the test.
   C. If the sodium depletion renin level will be measured, follow a low-sodium diet for 3 days prior to the test. Diuretics may also be prescribed prior to the test.
   D. Fast for 8 hours prior to the test.
   E. The recumbent position test requires that the client remain supine for at least 1 hour. The upright position test requires that the client stand or sit upright for 2 hours.
6. Factors that affect results:
   A. Improper position of the client, diet, sodium intake, or medication regulation prior to the test invalidates the results.
   B. Results are invalidated if the collection tube was not chilled prior to venipuncture and if the specimen was not placed on ice after collection.
   C. Reject tubes incompletely filled or specimens not well mixed.
7. Other data:
   A. Renin is very unstable and samples must be handled properly.
   B. The 24-hour urine sample for sodium should be indexed against renin levels.
   C. A second nonfasting blood sample, with exercise, may also be prescribed.

Bibliography:

Kasuga A, Takei I, Tasaka S, Shibata H, Maruyama H, Saruta T, Kataoka K: A case of aldosterone producing adenoma associated with high PRA after long-term angiotensin converting enzyme inhibitor treatment. Endocr J *40*(1):47–52, 1993.

Sonpal GM, Sharma A, Miller A: Primary antiphospholipid antibody syndrome, renal infarction and hypertension. J Rheumatol *20*(7):1221–1223, 1993.

Van Vliet AA, Kroger R, Dubbelman R, Ten Bokkel-Huinink WW: Treatment of patients with IVCS and gross oedema and ascites with diuretic combination and ACE-inhibitors: relation to baseline PRA and PAC. Neth J Med *46*(2):62–72, 1995.

RENOCYSTOGRAM (RENOGRAM SCAN, RENAL SCAN), DIAGNOSTIC

Norm: Radionuclide contrast material should circulate bilaterally, symmetrically, and without interruption through the renal parenchyma, ureters, and urinary bladder; 50% of radionuclide should be excreted within the first 10 minutes. The initial uptake or vascular phase occurs within 30–45 seconds after administration of the radionuclide. The transit or tubular phase follows over the next 2–5 minutes, and drainage of the radionuclide from the kidneys occurs during the excretory phase.

Usage: Azotemia, excretory defects, nephroureteral dilation, renal ischemia (acute tubular necrosis), renal obstruction or mass, renal parenchymal disease, renovascular hypertension, unilateral kidney disease, and upper urinary obstruction; assessment of renal perfusion, pretransplantation, and post-transplantation; and evaluation of hydroureteronephrosis and urinary tract patency, also used for clients hypersensitive to iodine-based contrast material used with intravenous pyelography or those in whom urethral catheterization is contraindicated.

Description: The renocystogram is a dynamic nuclear medicine study of the kidneys and ureters in which the dispersion, clearance, and excretion of a radionuclide is recorded via a gamma radiographic scan. Radionuclide uptake, transit, and excretion times are computed, and renogram curves are plotted on a graph for each kidney and ureter. Quantitative evaluation of renal function occurs as the external radiation detectors record vascular, tubular filtration, and excretory phases. A renogram curve is produced as the radionuclide dispersion is plotted on a graph or computed. Comparison of the right and left kidney, curve shape, and relative function is calculated. Curve shapes are characteristic of certain disorders.

Professional Considerations:

1. Consent form IS required.

Risks:
Allergic reaction, bleeding, infection, urinary tract obstruction.

Contraindications:
During pregnancy, this test is performed only when imperative. It is contraindicated during breast-feeding, with congenital renal abnormality, and with previous allergic reaction to the same radionuclide.

2. Preparation:
   A. Obtain the client's current weight.
   B. Unless contraindicated, the client should be well hydrated with 10 ml of water per kilogram of body weight.
   C. Establish intravenous access.
3. Procedure:
   A. The client is positioned upright.
   B. Following placement of external posterior radiation detectors over both kidneys, an intravenous injection of radionuclide technetium-99m DTPA (technetium with the chelating agent diethylenetriaminepentacetic acid) or I-131 orthoiodohippurate (radioiodine hippuran) is administered. Detectors record the uptake and excretion radiation counts as gamma scanning of both kidneys is completed.
4. Postprocedure care:
   A. Urine or serum blood samples may be obtained.
   B. Observe the client carefully for up to 60 minutes after the study for a possible (anaphylactic) reaction to the radionuclide.
   C. When urine is being discarded, rubber gloves should be worn for 24 hours after the procedure. Wash the gloved hands with soap and water before removing the gloves. Wash the ungloved hands after gloves are removed.
5. Client and family teaching:
   A. This is a screening test for suspected renal blood flow insufficiency.
   B. Immediately flush the toilet after each voiding following the procedure, and meticulously wash your hands with soap and water after each void for 24 hours after the procedure.
6. Factors that affect results:
   A. The presence of contrast material from prior diagnostic testing interferes with accuracy.
   B. Abnormalities may be accentuated in the presence of dehydration or masked in the presence of overhydration.
   C. Injection of radiographic contrast material within 24 hours prior to the test invalidates the results.
7. Other data:
   A. This study records the activity of the entire kidney, but does not distinguish between specific areas of disease within the kidneys.
   B. Health care professionals working in a nuclear medicine area must follow the federal standards set by the Nuclear Regulatory Commission. These standards include precautions for handling the radioactive material and monitoring of potential radiation exposure.
   C. Technetium half-life is 6 hours.

Bibliography:

Kushner FG, Helm MJ: Successful directional atherectomy of eccentric renal artery stenosis using the Simpson directional coronary atherocath as a primary therapy. Cathet Cardiovascul Diagn *29*(2): 128–130, 1993.

Pelsang RE, Rezai K: Abnormal captopril renogram in a patient without renovascular hypertension. Clin Nucl Med *17*(4):303–305, 1992.

RENOGRAM SCAN, DIAGNOSTIC

(see Renocystogram, Diagnostic)

REPTILASE TIME, SERUM

Norm: 18–20 seconds.

Increased: Congenital afibrinogenemia and dysfibrinogenemia.

Decreased: Not clinically significant.

Description: Reptilase is an enzyme from Russell's viper venom used to determine blood coagulation time. It is a variation of the thrombin time used to detect the presence of adequate fibrinogen levels without interference from heparin, fibrin-fibrinogen degradation products, or increased concentrations of plasmin. Prolonged thrombin time in the presence of a normal reptilase time is confirmation that heparin, rather than low fibrinogen levels, is the cause of the coagulation defect.

Professional Considerations:

1. Consent form NOT required.
2. Preparation:
   A. Tube: 2.7-ml or 4.5-ml blue-top.
   B. Specimens MAY be drawn during hemodialysis.
3. Procedure:
   A. Draw a 3-ml blood sample and discard, leaving the needle in place.
   B. Withdraw 2-ml of blood into a syringe or vacuum tube. Remove the syringe or tube, leaving the needle in place. Attach a second syringe, and draw a blood sample quantity of 2.4 ml for a 2.7-ml tube and 4.0 ml for a 4.5-ml tube.
4. Postprocedure care:
   A. None.
5. Client and family teaching:
   A. The test will measure your blood's ability to clot properly.
   B. Results are normally available within 24 hours.
6. Factors that affect results:
   A. Send specimens to the laboratory immediately.
   B. Contamination of the sample with tissue thromboplastin causes falsely elevated results. This is the reason for the double-draw technique.

7. Other data:
   A. The reptilase time may be used in place of the thrombin time in fibrinogen evaluation in clients anticoagulated with heparin.

Bibliography:

Carr ME Jr, Qureshi GD: The impact of delayed fibrinopeptide-A release on fibrin structure. Studies of an abnormal fibrinogen. J Biol Chem *262*(32): 15568–15574, 1987.

Lee GR, et al.: Wintrobe's Clinical Hematology, 9th ed, Vols 1 and 2. Philadelphia, Lea and Febiger, 1993, pp 569, 1313.

Levy J, Pettei MJ, Weitz SI: Dysfibrinogenemia in obstructive liver disease. J Pediatr Gastroenterol Nutr *6*(6):967–970, 1987.

RESERPINE, SERUM

Norm: Negative. Serum therapeutic level: 20 ng/ml.

Overdose Symptoms and Treatment:

Symptoms: Lethargy, drowsiness, respiratory depression.

Treatment:
   Protect airway.
   Support blood pressure with vasopressors.
   Monitor neurologic checks q 1 hour.
   Hemodialysis and peritoneal dialysis will NOT remove reserpine.

Increased: Parkinson's disease.

Description: Reserpine, an alkaloid of the *Rauwolfia serpentina* plant, is used primarily as an antihypertensive, sedative, or tranquilizer. It acts at adrenergic receptor sites, primarily of the central and peripheral nervous systems and heart, by interfering with the binding of serotonin. Reserpine is metabolized in the liver and excreted as an inactive metabolite in small amounts in the urine and stool. Reserpine has a very slow onset of peak action (2–3 weeks), with a prolonged effect (4–6 weeks); thus, alterations in dosage occur in small increments and at 7- to 14-day intervals. Half-life is 4.5 hours, with a duration of 45–168 hours.

Professional Considerations:

1. Consent form NOT required.
2. Preparation:
   A. Tube: Lavender-top.
   B. Specimens MAY be drawn during hemodialysis.

3. Procedure:
   A. Draw a 7-ml blood sample.
   B. Heelstick is acceptable, collected in a microtainer.
4. Postprocedure care:
   A. None.
5. Client and family teaching:
   A. This test measures the level of reserpine in your body.
   B. Results are normally available within 24 hours.
   C. Know and understand the side effects of this drug, and recognize the signs of overdose (see above).

6. Factors that affect results:
   A. Specimens collected in heparin invalidate results.
7. Other data:
   A. *Rauwolfia* alkaloids lower seizure threshold. Clients with convulsive disorders should be observed closely.

Bibliography:

Cieri UR: Determination of reserpine in tablets by liquid chromatography with fluorescence detection: revised procedure. J AOAC Int 77(3):758–760, 1994.

RETICULOCYTE COUNT, BLOOD

Norm: Comprises 1–2% of the total RBC count:

		SI Units
Adult females	0.5–2.5%	$0.005–0.025 \times 10^{-3}$
Adult males	0.5–1.5%	$0.005–0.015 \times 10^{-3}$
Cord blood	3.0–7.0%	$0.030–0.070 \times 10^{-3}$
Newborn	1.1–4.5%	$0.011–0.045 \times 10^{-3}$
Neonates	0.1–1.5%	$0.010–0.015 \times 10^{-3}$
Infants	0.5–3.1%	$0.005–0.031 \times 10^{-3}$
Children >6 months	0.5–4.0%	$0.005–0.040 \times 10^{-3}$

Increased: Acquired autoimmune hemolytic anemia, DiGuglielmo disease, erythremic myelosis (chronic), erythroblastosis fetalis, hemolytic anemias, hemoglobin C disease, hemorrhage (chronic), hereditary spherocytosis, infants, leukemia, malaria, metastatic carcinoma, myxoma of left heart atrium, paroxysmal nocturnal hemoglobinuria, polycythemia, posthemorrhagic anemia (acute), pregnancy, sickle cell disease, thalassemia major, thrombotic thrombocytopenic purpura, transfusion therapy, treatment of iron-deficiency anemia, and vitamin B_{12} deficiency or folic acid deficiency.

Decreased: Alcoholism, anemia (aplastic, iron deficiency, megaloblastic, pernicious, pure red cell), aregenerative crisis, aplastic crisis of hemolytic anemia, chronic infection, iron-deficiency anemias, myxedema, and radiation therapy. Drugs include carbamazepine and chloramphenicol.

Description: A reticulocyte is a nonnucleated red blood cell containing a basophilic network of granules or filaments characteristic of an immature cell of the erythrocyte class. Formed in the bone marrow, reticulocytes reach maturity after 1 day in the circulating blood and are an index of bone marrow function. The reticulocyte count is the number of reticulocytes per 1000 erythrocytes and is significant only when reported as a percentage of the total number of erythrocytes. This test assists in the diagnosis and differentiation of bone marrow depression from anemias, hemorrhage, hemolysis, or radiation, and evaluates bone marrow activity and response to therapeutic interventions.

Professional Considerations:

1. Consent form NOT required.
2. Preparation:
   A. Obtain venipuncture supplies and a lavender-top tube or white blood cell pipette and supravital dye (such as brilliant cresyl blue or new methylene blue).
   B. Do NOT draw specimens during hemodialysis.
3. Procedure:
   A. *Adult:*
      i. Leaving the tourniquet on no more than 1 minute, draw a 4-ml blood sample without trauma.
      ii. Gently tilt or roll the specimen six to eight times to mix the anticoagulant and the blood.
   B. *Infant:*
      i. Draw a fresh drop of capillary blood into a white blood cell

pipette and mix with an equal volume of a supravital dye.

4. Postprocedure care:
   A. None.
5. Client and family teaching:
   A. This test measures your body's ability to make adequate numbers of red blood cells.
   B. Results are normally available within 4 hours.
6. Factors that affect results:
   A. Reject hemolyzed specimens or specimens not thoroughly mixed with EDTA anticoagulant.
   B. Hemodilution of the sample may occur if the specimen is drawn from an extremity that is being infused with intravenous solution.
   C. False-positive results have been reported with laboratory handling of the specimen that included drying of the coverslip preparation; incorrect concentration of sodium metabisulfite; and mixture with fibrinogen, gelatin, or thrombin on the slide.
   D. After transfusion with blood containing sickle cell trait, cells with the sickle cell trait are present for 4 months.
   E. False low results may occur when the sample is drawn soon after a blood transfusion.
   F. Drugs that may cause false-positive results include antipyretics, chloroquine hydrochloride, chloroquine phosphate, corticotropin, furazolidone (in infants), hydroxychloroquine sulfate, levodopa, primaquine phosphate, pyrimethamine, quinacrine hydrochloride, quinine sulfate, and sulfonamides.
   G. Drugs that may cause false-negative results include azathioprine, chloramphenicol, dactinomycin, methotrexate sodium, and sulfonamides.
7. Other data:
   A. Reticulocyte count corrected for abnormal hematocrit only = reticulocyte % × (Hct/45).

Bibliography:

Barbone AG, Aparicio B, Anderson DW, Natarajan J, Ritchie DM: Reticulocyte measurements as a bioassay for erythropoietin. J Pharmaceutical Biomed Anal *12*(4):515–522, 1994.

Davis BH, Bigelow NC: Reticulocyte analysis and reticulocyte maturity index. Methods Cell Biology *42*(Pt B):263–274, 1994.

Newman TB, Easterling MJ: Yield of reticulocyte counts and blood smears in term infants. Clin Pediatr *33*(2):71–76, 1994.

RETICULOCYTE PRODUCTION INDEX (RPI), DIAGNOSTIC

Norm: Index of 1.

Increased: Accelerated red blood cell production.

Decreased: Alcoholism, anemia (aplastic, iron deficiency, megaloblastic, pernicious, pure red cell), aregenerative crisis, aplastic crisis of hemolytic anemia, chronic infection, iron-deficiency anemias, myxedema, and radiation therapy.

Description: The reticulocyte production index (RPI) is a calculated measurement of the number of circulating reticulocytes in relation to packed cell volume of hematocrit. The raw reticulocyte count is expressed as a percentage of erythrocytes. In anemia, a 1–2% reticulocyte count is not really normal, because it is based on a lower than normal amount of erythrocytes. Also, the normal lifespan of reticulocytes is 2 days, but in the presence of accelerated red blood cell production, reticulocytes are released prematurely and circulate for up to 4 days. The RPI normalizes the reticulocyte count by multiplying it by the hematocrit divided by 45 and by correcting for the increased lifespan of reticulocytes (based on the degree of anemia) to give a more accurate portrayal of the rate of reticulocyte production. This index is used to calculate the degree of increased erythropoietic activity associated with the premature release of reticulocytes (shift) from the bone marrow in anemia.

Professional Considerations:

1. Consent form NOT required.
2. Preparation:
   A. *See Reticulocyte Count, Blood; and Hematocrit, Blood.*
   B. Do NOT draw specimens during hemodialysis.
3. Procedure:
   A. Obtain samples for reticulocyte count and for VPRC (volume of packed red cells, hematocrit). *See Reticulocyte Count, Blood; and Hematocrit, Blood.*
   B. Calculation: Reticulocyte maturation time in the circulating blood changes as follows:

Hematocrit	Reticulocyte Maturation Time
35	1.5 days
30	1.75 days
25	2.0 days
20	2.25 days
15	2.5 days

The RPI is calculated as:

$$RPI = \frac{Reticulocyte\ percentage,}{Reticulocyte\ maturation\ time\ (days)}$$
$$\times \frac{Client's\ VPRC\ (1/1)}{0.45}$$

4. Postprocedure care:
   A. *See Reticulocyte Count, Blood; and Hematocrit, Blood.*
5. Client and family teaching:
   A. This test measures the number of immature red blood cells in your bloodstream.
   B. Results are normally available within 24 hours.

6. Factors that affect results:
   A. *See Reticulocyte Count, Blood; and Hematocrit, Blood.*
7. Other data:
   A. *See Reticulocyte Count, Blood; and Hematocrit, Blood.*

Bibliography:

Barbone AG, Aparicio B, Anderson DW, Natarajan J, Ritchie DM: Reticulocyte measurements as a bioassay for erythropoietin. J Pharmaceut Biomed Anal *12*(4):515–522, 1994.

Davis BH, Bigelow NC: Reticulocyte analysis and reticulocyte maturity index. Methods Cell Biology *42*(Pt B):263–274, 1994.

Newman TB, Easterling MJ: Yield of reticulocyte counts and blood smears in term infants. Clin Pediatr *33*(2):71–76, 1994.

RETINOBLASTOMA CHROMOSOME ABNORMALITIES, DIAGNOSTIC

Norm:

Female	44 autosomes + 2X chromosomes
Karyotype	46,XX
Male	44 autosomes + 1X and 1Y chromosome
Karyotype	46,XY
Retinoblastoma chromosomal defect is identified as:	Female 46,XX,13q–; Male 46,XY,13q–

Usage: Screening for retinoblastoma, identification of numerical chromosomal defects, and genetic counseling.

Description: Retinoblastoma is the most frequently occurring congenital ocular tumor in children, occurring in 1 in 20,000 births. Tumor occurrence is usually bilateral, nonmetastatic, and may occur up to several years later in the second eye. Clinical symptoms include strabismus, impaired vision, and the appearance of white to yellow reflex from the pupil, referred to as "cat's eye." Left untreated, this tumor is fatal, because optic nerve, subarachnoid space, and cerebral tissue invasion occurs. Heredity accounts for 40% of the incidence of retinoblastoma through autosomal dominant transmission, from an unaffected gene carrier parent or from germinal mutation in a normal parent. The retinoblastoma gene is located on the long arm of chromosome 13, q band 14. Deletion in the q band occurs in 50% of clients with retinoblastoma. Leukocyte screening of peripheral blood is the most common technique for chromosomal abnormality detection and analysis. Tissue cultures are cultivated from the blood sample, fixed, and stained. The chromosomes are then counted, photographed, and the karyotype is arranged according to the Denver nomenclature from cut photographs. Diagnosis is confirmed by computed tomography and/or magnetic resonance imaging, and radiotherapy is a common approach to treatment. Prognosis is dependent on location, size, and the amount of ocular and extraocular involvement.

Professional Considerations:

1. Consent form NOT required.
2. Preparation:
   A. *See Client and family teaching.*
   B. Tube: Green-top.
   C. Specimens MAY be drawn during hemodialysis.
3. Procedure:
   A. A morning sample is preferred. Draw a 10-ml blood sample.
4. Postprocedure care:
   A. None.
5. Client and family teaching:
   A. This test is a genetic screen.
   B. Fast for 3 hours before the blood is drawn.
6. Factors that affect results:
   A. Insufficient number of cells in sample.

7. Other data:
  A. Retinoblastoma is also associated with elevated plasma somatostatin levels.

Bibliography:

Pratt CB, Raimondi SC, Kaste SC, Heaton DM, Mounce KG, Mandrell B, Crom D, Meyer D: Outcome for patients with constitutional 13q chromosomal abnormalities and retinoblastoma. Pediatr Hematol Oncol *11*(5):541–547, 1994.

RETROGRADE PYELOGRAPHY, DIAGNOSTIC

Norm: Bilateral, symmetrical, and uniform opacification of ureters, renal calyces, and renal pelves. Normal size and architecture of these structures. Superimposed films on inspiration and expiration normally show two outlines of the renal pelvis 2 cm apart.

Usage: Assessment of displacement, drainage, enlargement, or fixation of the structures of the renal collecting system; and detection of complete or partial obstruction due to blood clot, calculus, perinephric abscess, inflammation, stricture, or tumor formation. This examination is used in clients with severe renal insufficiency, those with hypersensitivity to iodine-based contrast material, and when visualization of the renal collecting system with excretory urography is inadequate.

Description: Retrograde pyelography is an invasive radiographic (fluoroscopic) examination of the kidneys from a distal direction via the ureters. During cystoscopy, catheters are passed into the ureters and radiopaque contrast material is injected. The mucous membrane absorbs minimal amounts of the iodine radiopaque contrast material. Thus, the complications of hypersensitivity reactions or delayed excretion of the dye in renal impairment that are associated with intravenous dye injections are avoided.

Professional Considerations:

1. Consent form IS required.

Risks:

Bladder perforation, hemorrhage, nausea, vomiting, urinary tract infection, vasovagal response.

Contraindications:

Severe dehydration. Sedatives are contraindicated in clients with central nervous system depression.

2. Preparation:
  A. *See Client and family teaching.*
  B. The client should disrobe below the waist.
3. Procedure:
  A. If deep sedation or anesthesia is used, monitor respiratory status and ECG continuously throughout the procedure.
  B. The client is placed in a dorsal lithotomy position and a cystoscopic examination is performed. *(See Cystoscopy, Diagnostic.)*
  C. A catheter is then advanced through the ureter(s) into the renal pelvis. After drainage of the renal pelvis, iodine radiopaque contrast material is injected through the catheter(s) into the kidney(s) and anterior, posterior, lateral, and oblique radiographic films are obtained. A small amount of contrast material may be injected into the ureters as the catheter is removed, and radiography of the ureters may then be taken.
  D. The procedure may also be performed without cystoscopy by injecting the radiopaque contrast material into the lower ureter after wedging a bulb catheter at the distal end of the ureter.
4. Postprocedure care:
  A. A ureteral and/or Foley catheter may be left in place after the examination.
  B. Continue assessment of respiratory status. If deep sedation or anesthesia was used, follow institutional protocol for postsedation monitoring. Typical monitoring includes continuous ECG monitoring and pulse oximetry, with continual assessments (q 5–15 minutes) of airway, vital signs, and neurologic status until the client is lying quietly awake, is breathing independently, and responds to commands spoken in a normal tone.
  C. Monitor vital signs at the end of the procedure, then every 4 hours × 24 hours.
  D. Observe for signs of allergic reaction to the dye × 24 hours.
  E. Encourage the oral intake of fluids when not contraindicated. Monitor urinary output for quantity and hematuria × 24 hours. Notify physician for bladder distention, anuria, oliguria, or hematuria. Gross hematuria or persistent hematuria, after the third voiding, is abnormal.
  F. Notify the physician if there are symptoms of infection (fever, tachycardia, hypotension, chills, dysuria, flank pain).

G. Resume previous diet.

H. Administer analgesic as prescribed.

5. Client and family teaching:

A. This test evaluates kidney structure.

B. Fast for 8 hours before the procedure if general anesthesia will be administered.

C. A laxative may be prescribed the evening prior to the procedure. A cleansing enema may be prescribed to be given the morning of the procedure.

D. A sedative may be prescribed to be given just prior to the procedure.

E. After the procedure is over, save all the urine voided and report chills or pain with urination. Notify the physician if there are symptoms of infection (see above, section 4F).

6. Factors that affect results:

A. Views are obscured by the presence of feces, gas, or barium in the bowel.

7. Other data:

A. Impaired renal function does not affect test results.

B. If the renal pelves are not visualized by this exam, ureteral obstruction may be present and may be localized via antegrade pyelography (*see separate test listing*).

Bibliography:

Rushton HG, Salem Y, Belman AB, Majd M: Pediatric pyelography: is routine retrograde pyelography necessary? J Urol *15*(2, Pt 2):604–606, 1994.

Weese DL, Greenberg HM, Zimmern PE: Contrast media reactions during voiding cystourethrography or retrograde pyelography. Urology *41*(1): 81–84, 1993.

RETROSYNCYNTIAL VIRUS (RSV), CULTURE

Normal: Negative for retrosyncyntial virus (RSV).

Usage: Detection of the presence of RSV in obtained medium.

Description: RSV is an important cause of lower respiratory infections in infants. It typically afflicts children 1–3 years of age, and can be very severe and even fatal in the immunocompromised. In adults, RSV manifests itself as an upper respiratory infection. The elderly and others with pulmonary disease can be quite susceptible.

Professional Considerations:

1. Consent form NOT required.

2. Preparation:

A. Obtain a chilled viral transport medium and a sterile wire swab in a pack.

B. Open the transport medium, and place it in ice.

C. Obtain assistance for restraint of the client if necessary.

3. Procedure:

A. Explain the procedure to the client, and offer reassurance.

B. Bend the wire swab; open the pack.

C. Restrain the client if necessary, pass the wire through one nare and into the nasopharynx, and rotate the swab quickly.

D. Remove the swab, place it in the medium, and close.

E. Transport to the laboratory immediately.

4. Postprocedure care:

A. None.

5. Client and family teaching:

A. This test is performed to try to isolate the pathogen causing the illness.

B. Results are normally available within 48–72 hours.

6. Factors that affect results:

A. Specimens must remain cold.

B. Inaccurate swabbing or swabbing of the wrong location.

7. Other data:

A. Specimens do not tolerate freezing and thawing well.

B. Serologic isolation should also be considered.

Bibliography:

Becker S, Soukup J, Yankaskas JR: Respiratory syncytial virus infection of human primary nasal and bronchial epithelial cell cultures and bronchoalveolar macrophages. Am J Respir Cell Mol Biol *6*(4):369–374, 1992.

Isselbacher KJ, et al.: Harrison's Principles of Internal Medicine, 13th ed. New York, McGraw-Hill, 1994, pp 805–806.

Mendoza J, Rojas A, Navarro JM, de la Rosa M: Evaluation of three rapid enzyme immunoassays and cell culture for detection of respiratory syncytial virus. Eur J Clin Microbiol Infect Dis *11*(5):452–454, 1992.

The Merck Manual, 16th ed. Rahway, NJ, Merck and Company, 1992, pp 2177–2178.

Wyngaarden JB, Smith LH, Bennett JC: Cecil Textbook of Medicine, 19th ed. Philadelphia, WB Saunders, 1992, pp 1845–1851.

REVERSE GIEMSA, DIAGNOSTIC

(*see Banding in Genetic Disorders, Diagnostic*)

REVIEW OF PERIPHERAL BLOOD SMEAR: RED BLOOD CELL MORPHOLOGY

(*see Red Blood Cell Morphology, Blood*)

Rh TYPE, BLOOD

(*see ABO Group and Rh Type, Blood*)

RHEUMATOID FACTOR (RF), BLOOD

Norm:

Qualitative	Negative
Quantitative	
Normal	<1:20
Chronic inflammatory disease	<1:40
Diagnostic for rheumatoid arthritis	1:40–1:60
Advanced rheumatoid arthritis	>1:60

Increased: Allografts (skin, renal), ankylosing rheumatoid spondylitis, cancer, cirrhosis, dermatomyositis, diabetes mellitus, diseases (of the kidney, liver, or lung), endocarditis, healthy clients over age 60, hepatic neoplasms, hepatitis, hypertension, infectious mononucleosis, juvenile rheumatoid arthritis, kala-azar, leishmaniasis, leprosy, lymphomas, macroglobulinemia, malaria, mixed connective tissue disease, neuropathy, osteoarthritis, paraproteinemia, polyarteritis nodosa, pulmonary interstitial fibrosis, sarcoidosis, schistosomiasis, scleroderma, Sjögren's syndrome, splenomegaly, subacute bacterial endocarditis, syphilis, systemic lupus erythematosus, transfusions (multiple), tuberculosis, vaccinations (multiple), vasculitis, viral infections, and yaws.

Decreased after Previous Elevations: Gold salt therapy.

Description: Rheumatoid factor is an immunoglobulin present in the serum of 50–95% of adults with rheumatoid arthritis. It appears in the serum and synovial fluid several months after the onset of rheumatoid arthritis and is present for up to years after therapy. The macroglobulin-type antibody produced in the synovium appears in the presence of autoimmunity, chronic infections, or connective tissue defects. This factor, though not specific for rheumatoid arthritis, is very helpful in diagnosis, because high titers correlate with severe disease as compared to titers with other diseases. Analgesia and anti-inflammatory pharmacologic preparations do not affect the presence of rheumatoid factor.

Professional Considerations:

1. Consent form NOT required.
2. Preparation:
   A. Tube: Red-top, red/gray-top, or gold-top.

B. Specimens MAY be drawn during hemodialysis.
3. Procedure:
   A. Draw a 2-ml blood sample.
4. Postprocedure care:
   A. None.
5. Client and family teaching:
   A. This is a screening test for many different disorders.
   B. Results are normally available within 24 hours.
6. Factors that affect results:
   A. Anticoagulant in the specimen tube invalidates the results.
7. Other data:
   A. Clients who have rheumatoid factor demonstrated early in the course of rheumatoid arthritis have a greater risk of developing articular destruction.

Bibliography:

Saraux A, Valls I, Voisin V, Koreichi A, Baron D, Youinou P, Le Goff P: How useful are tests for rheumatoid factors, antiperinuclear factors, antikeratin antibody, and the HLA DR4 antigen for the diagnosis of rheumatoid arthritis? Rev Rhuma, English ed 62(1):16–20, 1995.

Schmitz JL, Folds JD: Evaluation of the Rheuma-Lex latex agglutination test for the detection of rheumatoid factor. J Clin Lab Immunol 40(4): 187–193, 1993.

RINNE TEST, DIAGNOSTIC
(see Tuning Fork Test of Weber, Rinne, and Schwabach Tests, Diagnostic)

ROCHALIMAEA HENSELAE ANTIBODY, SERUM

Norm: Titer <1:64.

Increased: Titer >1:64 or a fourfold rise in titer between acute and convalescent sera: cat scratch disease.

Description: A serologic test to identify antibodies to *Rochalimaea henselae* (Bartonella species), an organism thought to be causative of cat scratch disease in humans who have been bitten or scratched by an infected cat. The disease is characterized by unexplained regional lymphadenopathy, fever, malaise, and skin lesion at the site of injury. Although the etiology of cat scratch disease is not firmly established, *R. henselae* has been found in significantly higher levels in cats owned by clients infected with the disease and recently wounded by the cat. *R. henselae* is thought to be transmitted through the saliva or other body fluids of the sick cat when biting or scratching a human. In this indirect fluorescent antibody test, a sample of the client's serum with the *R. henselae* antigen and titers of antibodies to the antigen are measured. This test is more sensitive and specific than the skin test for Bartonella species.

Professional Considerations:

1. Consent form NOT required.
2. Preparation:
   A. Tube: Red-top, red/gray-top, or gold-top.
   B. Specimens MAY be drawn during hemodialysis.
3. Procedure:
   A. Draw a 2-ml blood sample.
4. Postprocedure care:
   A. None.
5. Client and family teaching:
   A. Avoid traumatic contact, such as rough playing, with kittens and cats because this disease may be transmitted through bites and scratches from the animals.
   B. Results are normally available within 24 hours.
6. Factors that affect results:
   A. None found.
7. Other data:
   A. Zangwill et al. (1993) found an 84% sensitivity and 96% specificity for this serologic test.
   B. Fleas have also been suspected as transmission sources for this disease.
   C. Many antibiotics are not effective against *R. henselae* infections. Musso et al. (1995) found aminoglycosides to be bactericidal against the organism.

Bibliography:

Bergmans AM, Groothedde JW, Schellekens JF, van Embden JD, Ossewaarde JM, Schouls LM: Etiology of cat scratch disease: comparison of polymerase chain reaction detection of Bartonella (formerly Rochalimaea) and Afipia felis DNA with serology and skin tests. J Infect Dis *171*(4):916–923, 1995.

Musso D, Drancourt M, Raoult D: Lack of bactericidal effect of antibiotics except aminoglycosides on Bartonella (Rochalimaea) henselae. J Antimicrob Chemother *36*(1):101–108, 1995.

Zangwill KM, Hamilton DH, Perkins BA, Regnery RL, Plikaytis BD, Hadler JL, Cartter ML, Wenger JD: Cat scratch disease in Connecticut: epidemiology, risk factors, and evaluation of a new diagnostic test. N Engl J Med *329*(1):8–13.

ROCKY MOUNTAIN SPOTTED FEVER (RMSF) SEROLOGY, SERUM

Norm: Negative.

Indirect fluorescent antibody assay (most sensitive): diagnostically significant: titer >128 in a single specimen, or fourfold rise in paired serum titers, or any positive titer for IgM.

Latex agglutination test: Active Rocky Mountain spotted fever: titer >128.

Complement fixation for rickettsial infection: >1:160 or fourfold increase in paired samples within 7 days.

Weil-Felix agglutination reaction for rickettsial disease (least sensitive test): Strong agglutination response to *Proteus* Ox-19 ++++ suggests rickettsial disease.

Positive: High titers occur with continuous exposure to bacterial, *Proteus,* or rickettsial infection and recent vaccinations.

Negative: Normal finding. Low titers occur with antibiotic therapy (early in the disease course), and in symptomatic clients who are unable to produce antibodies during active infection (immunodeficiency disorders).

Description: Rocky Mountain spotted fever (RMSF) is an infectious disease caused by the parasite *Rickettsia rickettsii* transmitted to man by the bite of an infected tick (usually the wood tick, *Dermacentor andersoni;* the dog tick, *Dermacentor variabilis;* and occasionally by the lone star tick, *Amblyomma americanum*). Although thought to exist in the Western Hemisphere, this disease can occur anywhere that the vector is present. Symptoms include the sudden onset of fever lasting 2–3 weeks, and the appearance of a rash spreading from the palms of the hands and soles of the feet to the entire body. Death may occur if RMSF is left untreated.

Professional Considerations:

1. Consent form NOT required.
2. Preparation:
   A. Tube: Red-top, red/gray-top, or gold-top.
   B. Specimens MAY be drawn during hemodialysis.
3. Procedure:
   A. Draw a 5-ml blood sample, without trauma.

B. An acute sample should be drawn with the onset of symptoms.

C. Draw a convalescent sample 7 days later.

4. Postprocedure care:

A. Send specimens to the laboratory immediately.

5. Client and family teaching:

A. This is a screening test to determine exposure to certain bacteria, including *Rickettsia.*

B. Return in 1 week to have a convalescent sample drawn. This will help determine if the disease is responding to treatment.

6. Factors that affect results:

A. Weil-Felix false-positive reactions have been reported in *Borrelia* infection, *Proteus* infection, endemic typhus, leptospirosis, liver disease (severe), and in clients who have been recently vaccinated.

B. Weil-Felix false-negative reactions have been reported when antibiotic therapy is started before the first specimen is drawn.

C. The latex agglutination test is useful only during active infection.

7. Other data:

A. The Weil-Felix test is able to establish titers, but does not use the causal agent as the reactive antigen. It is useful in screening for rickettsial infections, but is unable to distinguish murine typhus from spotted fever. Indirect fluorescent antibody testing can be used for specific identification of RMSF.

B. If the Weil-Felix agglutination test is positive, the possibility of a *Proteus* urinary tract infection should be considered.

Bibliography:

Sexton DJ, Kanj SS, Wilson K, Corey GR, Hegarty BC, Levy MG, Breitschwerdt EB: The use of a polymerase chain reaction as a diagnostic test for Rocky Mountain spotted fever. Am J Tropical Med Hyg *50*(1):59–63, 1994.

ROSE BENGAL SCAN
(see Liver I-131 Scan, Diagnostic)

ROTAVIRUS ANTIGEN, BLOOD

Norm: Negative antigen screen.

Positive: Presence of rotavirus antibodies and postviral lactase deficiency.

Negative: Normal finding. Also, disaccharidase deficiencies.

Description: Rotavirus is a sporadic, acute, infectious, diarrheal disease of the reoviridae viral class, in which five serographs have been identified. It replicates exclusively in the epithelial cells of the small intestine and is pathogenic primarily in infants and children during the winter or cooler months. This virus is the major cause of sporadic acute enteritis in infants and epidemic acute gastroenteritis in small children. Rotavirus is presumed to be transmitted via the fecal-oral route and is detectable only during the first 7–8 days of illness. Radioimmunoassay and complement-fixing antibody titers are used for rotavirus detection.

Professional Considerations:

1. Consent form NOT required.

2. Preparation:

A. Tube: Red-top, red/gray-top, or gold-top.

B. Specimens MAY be drawn during hemodialysis.

3. Procedure:

A. Draw a 5-ml blood sample without trauma.

B. Heelstick is acceptable, collected in a microtainer.

4. Postprocedure care:

A. None.

5. Client and family teaching:

A. These clients are most often children; therefore, emotional support and comfort measures should be offered during blood draws.

B. Results are normally available within 24 hours.

C. Parents should maintain enteric precautions during the client's diarrheal symptoms.

6. Factors that affect results:

A. Hemolysis of the specimen invalidates the results.

7. Other data:

A. Clients with the rotavirus may be free of symptomatic illness.

B. There is no specific treatment for rotavirus. Fluid and electrolyte balance should be supported to prevent severe dehydration.

C. Rectal swabs and stool samples should be examined for the presence of rotavirus antigen. (*See Rotavirus Antigen, Stool.*)

Bibliography:

Dar VS, Ghosh S, Broor S: Rapid detection of rotavirus by using colloidal gold particles labeled with monoclonal antibody. J Virol Methods *47*(1–2): 51–58, 1994.

Saavedra JM, Bauman NA, Oung I, Perman JA, Yolken RH: Feeding Bifidobacterium and Streptococcus thermophilus to infants in hospital for prevention of diarrhoea and shedding of rotavirus. Lancet *344*(8929):1046–1049, 1994.

Tsunemitsu H, Jiang B, Saif LJ: Detection of group C rotavirus antigens and antibodies in animals and humans by enzyme-linked immunosorbent assays. J Clin Microbiol *30*(8):2129–2134, 1992.

ROTAVIRUS ANTIGEN, STOOL

Norm: Negative. The presence of rotavirus in neonates under 2 weeks of age is inconclusive.

Usage: Directly detects the rotavirus antigen that is shed in large amounts in the stool.

Description: Diarrheal disease of the reoviridae viral class, in which five serogroups have been identified. It replicates exclusively in the epithelial cells of the small intestine and is pathogenic primarily in infants and children during the winter or cooler months. This virus is the major cause of sporadic acute enteritis in infants and epidemic acute gastroenteritis in small children. Rotavirus is presumed to be transmitted via the fecal-oral route. Rotavirus antigen in the stool is detected by direct visualization with electron microscopy or by the more common enzyme-linked immunosorbent assay (ELISA) screen. Rotavirus is an acute, infectious disease.

Professional Considerations:

1. Consent form NOT required.
2. Preparation:
   A. Obtain a clean, dry, preservative-free, covered cardboard specimen container or a tube with a screw-top cap, and a larger container of ice; or obtain a sterile culture swab and a closed, sterile container.
   B. The client should disrobe below the waist for rectal swab collection.
3. Procedure:
   A. *Stool collection:*
      i. Obtain 5 ml or 5 g of liquid stool in a closed container or soiled diaper as soon as possible after evacuation from the bowel.
   B. *Rectal swab collection:*
      i. Place the client in the left lateral position with knees and hips flexed and draped.
      ii. Gently insert a sterile cotton-tipped swab at least 2.5–3.0 cm into the rectum. Rotate the swab from side to side and leave it in place for a few seconds to allow absorption of rectal flora.
      iii. Place the swab into a sterile container without preservatives and cover tightly.
4. Postprocedure care:
   A. The stool container should be placed on ice and transported promptly to the laboratory.
   B. The rectal swab container should be labeled with the site and time of collection, packed in ice, and sent promptly to the laboratory.
5. Client and family teaching:
   A. These clients are most often children; therefore, supportive measures should be offered if collection occurs via rectal swabbing.
   B. Results are normally available within 24 hours.
   C. Parents should maintain enteric precautions during the client's diarrheal symptoms.
6. Factors that affect results:
   A. Reject specimens placed in preservatives or those not placed on ice.
7. Other data:
   A. Clients with the rotavirus may be free of symptomatic illness.

Bibliography:

Albrecht H, Stellbrink HJ, Fenske S, Ermer M, Raedler A, Greten H: Rotavirus antigen detection in patients with HIV infection and diarrhea. Scand J Gastroenterol *28*(4):307–310, 1993.

RPR, DIAGNOSTIC
(see Rapid Plasma Reagin Test, Diagnostic)

RUBELLA SEROLOGY, SERUM

Norm: Negative. A fourfold rise in titer of paired titer or a sample positive for rubella-specific IgM is diagnostic of exposure to rubella.

Hemagglutination Inhibition Test

Susceptibility to rubella infection	<1:8
Immunity uncertain	1:8
Immunity from prior infection or vaccination	>1:8
Resistance to rubella infection	>1:64

Fluorescent Antibody Test

Susceptibility to rubella infection	<1+
Positive for rubella antibodies	>1+

Usage: Determination of rubella immune status. Differentiation of rubella, measles, scarlet fever, erythema infectiosum, and exanthem subitum during pregnancy.

Description: Rubella, also known as German measles, is an acute viral communicable disease of children and young adults. This infection is caused by the togavirus and produces a discrete red or pink macular rash that desquamates and vanishes in 2–3 days. It is transmitted client to client via direct contact with the discharges of infected clients or droplet spray inhalation. This test is useful when a pregnant woman is exposed to the rubella virus or an illness similar to rubella. Apparent or nonapparent transplacental fetal infection during the first trimester of pregnancy can result in spontaneous abortion or fetal congenital defects such as cataracts, cardiac lesions, congenital heart defects, deafness, encephalitis, hepatitis, growth and mental retardation, microcephaly, ocular lesions, pulmonary stenosis, radiolucencies of long bones, or retinopathy.

Professional Considerations:

1. Consent form NOT required.
2. Preparation:
   A. Tube: Red-top, red/gray-top, or gold-top.
   B. Specimens MAY be drawn during hemodialysis.
3. Procedure:
   A. Draw a 3-ml blood or umbilical cord blood sample.
   B. Heelstick is acceptable, collected in a microtainer.
   C. An acute sample should be drawn as soon as possible after symptoms appear.
   D. The convalescent sample should be drawn at least 7–14 days after the acute sample and preferably 14–21 days after the onset of symptoms.
4. Postprocedure care:
   A. None.
5. Client and family teaching:
   A. This test will reveal exposure to togavirus, the causative virus of rubella.
   B. If pregnant, avoid anyone known to have rubella.
   C. Return in 7–14 days for repeat testing.
   D. A negative test result in the mother rules out infection in the fetus.
   E. Rubella is highly communicable from adults for a week before and 4 days after the appearance of rash. Infants may transmit the virus in feces for up to 6 months.

6. Factors that affect results:
   A. Rubella antibodies remain present and static for many years.
7. Other data:
   A. Confirmation of congenital infection requires that samples be drawn from the mother and the infant.

Bibliography:

Deshmukh CT, Nadkarni UB, Nair K, Gharpure VP, Jain MK, Shah MD: Hydranencephaly/multicystic encephalomalacia: association with congenital rubella infection. Indian J Pediatr *30*(2):253–257, 1993.

Granberg C, Meurman O: Performance of two new immunoassays for the detection of IgM and IgG antibodies to rubella. Eur J Clin Microbiol Infect Dis *13*(6):512–515, 1994.

Schoub BD, Johnson S, McAnerney JM, Blackburn NK, Guidozzi F, Ballot D, Rothberg A: Is antenatal screening for rubella and cytomegalovirus justified? South Afr Med J *83*(2):108–110, 1993.

RUBEOLA SEROLOGY, SERUM

Norm: Negative. The presence of antibodies 1 week after the onset of symptoms is indicative of susceptibility to rubeola infection. Recent exposure to the virus shows a fourfold or greater increase in antibody titers in two consecutive samples (acute and convalescent) drawn 1–4 weeks apart, using hemagglutination inhibition or complement fixation methods.

Usage: Diagnosis of measles.

Description: Rubeola is an acute, contagious, viral, communicable disease caused by the measles virus of the paramyxovirus family. It is transmitted by direct contact with or inhalation of the infected oral or nasal secretions of infected clients. Rubeola is characterized by the appearance of a blotchy red facial rash appearing 3 days after a fever, with progression to a generalized rash lasting about 1 week. Other symptoms include Koplick's spots in the mouth, rose-colored maculopapular skin eruptions, photosensitivity, and catarrhal symptoms. Uncomplicated cases are usually self-limiting, but death may occur from complications and in undernourished children.

Professional Considerations:

1. Consent form NOT required.
2. Preparation:
   A. Tube: Red-top, red/gray-top, or gold-top.
   B. Specimens MAY be drawn during hemodialysis.

3. Procedure:
   A. Draw a 2-ml blood sample.
   B. Heelstick is acceptable, collected in a microtainer.
4. Postprocedure care:
   A. None.
5. Client and family teaching:
   A. This test can reveal exposure to the paramyxovirus family, which includes measles.
   B. Results are normally available within 24 hours.
6. Factors that affect results:
   A. Hemolysis or contamination alters the results.
7. Other data:
   A. ELISA assay is 20 times more sensitive than the complement fixation test and the hemagglutination inhibition test and is the assay of choice.

Bibliography:

Jenkerson SA, Beller M, Middaugh JP, Erdman DD: False positive rubeola IgM tests [letter]. N Engl J Med.*332*(16):1103–1104, 1995.

Swift JD, Barruga MC, Perkin RM, Van Stralen D: Respiratory failure complicating rubeola. Chest *104*(6):1786–1787, 1993.

RUBIN'S TEST (UTEROTUBAL INSUFFLATION), DIAGNOSTIC

Norm: Bilaterally patent fallopian tubes.

Normal patency: Pressure rises to 80–100 mmHg, then decreases as carbon dioxide passes through the fallopian tubes.

Partial patency: Pressure rises to between 120 and 130 mmHg.

Occlusion of tubes: Pressure rises above 200 mmHg.

Usage: Diagnosis of obstruction, stenosis, or stricture of the fallopian tubes; and detection of spasm of the uterine end of the fallopian tubes.

Description: Rubin's test involves transuterine fallopian tube insufflation with carbon dioxide. A flow meter and pressure gauge are attached to the source of the carbon dioxide. Changes in pressure are recorded on a kymograph. Displacement of adhesions and removal of debris from the tubes may occur during the procedure.

Professional Considerations:

1. Consent form NOT required.

Risks:

Air embolism, hemorrhage, infection, and referred shoulder pain.

Contraindications:

Infections of the cervix, fallopian tubes, or vagina; in suspected pregnancy; and with uterine bleeding.

2. Preparation:
   A. *See Client and family teaching.*
   B. An analgesic may be given 1 hour prior to the procedure to minimize tubal spasm from anxiety or discomfort.
   C. Obtain povidone-iodine, a vaginal speculum, cervical swabs, and a cervical cannula.
   D. The client should void.
3. Procedure:
   A. The client is placed in the dorsal lithotomy position and the perineal area is cleansed with 1% povidone-iodine solution.
   B. The physician introduces a vaginal speculum and exposes the cervix.
   C. The cervix is swabbed.
   D. A sterile cannula with a rubber tip is inserted into the cervical canal.
   E. The cannula tip is pressed tightly against the cervical os to seal the opening and is secured with a tenaculum.
   F. A rest period of approximately 2 minutes permits relaxation of the fallopian tubes.
   G. 60 cc/minute of carbon dioxide (never air, due to risk of embolism) is administered into the uterus and pressures are recorded using a kymograph.
   H. During insufflation, a swishing sound may be heard with a stethoscope as the carbon dioxide passes through the tubes.
   I. Shoulder pain due to gas-induced subphrenic pneuperitoneum is an indication of patency of at least one fallopian tube.
4. Postprocedure care:
   A. Nausea, vomiting, cramping, dizziness, and pain associated with carbon dioxide gas absorption may be reduced by having the client rest for 2–3 hours with the pelvis elevated.
5. Client and family teaching:
   A. This test will determine the patency of the fallopian tubes.
   B. Rubin's test takes approximately 30 minutes and is performed on an ambulatory care basis.
   C. You may be prescribed a laxative to take the night before the examination or may be given a suppository or enema prior to the procedure.
   D. Shoulder-top pain may be felt with insufflation.

E. You may rest with the pelvis elevated for several hours to reduce discomfort secondary to gas absorption.

6. Factors that affect results:
   A. Anxiety can cause fallopian tube spasm.
7. Other data:
   A. This test is performed 4–5 days after the last day of menstruation.
   B. Because Rubin's test can only ensure that at least one fallopian tube is patent, it is of limited value.
   C. *See also Hysterosalpingography, Diagnostic.*

Bibliography:

Confino E, Tur-Kaspa I, DeCherney A, et al.: Transcervical balloon tuboplasty. A multicenter study. JAMA *264*(16):2079–2082, 1990.

Corbett JV: Laboratory Tests and Diagnostic Procedures with Nursing Diagnosis, 2nd ed. Norwalk, CT, Appleton and Lange, 1987, pp 631–632.

Pagana, KD, Pagana TJ: Diagnostic Tests and Nursing Implications. St Louis, MO, CV Mosby, 1982.

Thurmond AS, Rosch J: Nonsurgical fallopian tube recanalization for treatment of infertility. Radiology *114*(2):371–374, 1990.

RUMPEL-LEEDE TOURNIQUET TEST, DIAGNOSTIC
(see Capillary Fragility Test, Diagnostic)

SAECG, DIAGNOSTIC
(see Signal-Averaged Electrocardiography, Diagnostic)

SALICYLATE (ASPIRIN, ACETYLSALICYLIC ACID), BLOOD

Norm: Negative.

		SI Units
Analgesia therapeutic level	<100 µg/ml	0.72 mmol/L
Anti-inflammatory therapeutic level	100–200 µg/ml	1.09–1.45 mmol/L
Panic level	>50 µg/dl	3.62 mmol/L

Overdose Symptoms and Treatment:

Symptoms: Acidemia, alkalosis, convulsions, dizziness, hyperactivity, hyperglycemia, hyperpnea, hyperthermia, ketosis, nausea, respiratory arrest, tinnitus, vomiting.

Treatment:

1. Early emptying of the stomach is important; use ipecac syrup if the client is conscious.
2. Monitor salicylate levels with serial serum draws.
3. Oral activated charcoal should be given as vomiting ceases.
4. Urine alkalinization to pH>7.5 with bicarbonate and fluids. Measure urine pH q 1 hour.
5. Fluid resuscitation may be necessary. This may be orally in mild cases, IV in severe cases.
6. A single dose of vitamin K may be given for the rare case of hypoprothrombinemia.
7. In the case of renal failure, dialysis is indicated. Both hemodialysis and peritoneal dialysis WILL remove acetylsalicylic acid.

Usage: Monitoring for salicylate toxicity during salicylate therapy or when overdose is suspected.

Description: Salicylates are a group of non-narcotic drugs with analgesic, antipyretic, anti-inflammatory, and platelet aggregation-inhibiting (aspirin only) effects. Salicylates are absorbed in the gastrointestinal tract, metabolized in the liver, and excreted in the urine, with a half-life of 2–3 hours in short-term use, and 15–30 hours in chronic use.

Professional Considerations:

1. Consent form NOT required.
2. Preparation:
   A. Optimal sampling time for blood is 2–6 hours after salicylate ingestion.
   B. Tube: Red-top, red/gray-top, or gold-top.
   C. Do NOT draw specimens during hemodialysis.
3. Procedure:
   A. Draw a 1-ml blood sample.
   B. Heelstick is acceptable, collected in a microtainer.
4. Postprocedure care:
   A. Assess for tinnitus and dizziness, signs of mild salicylate toxicity.

5. Client and family teaching:
   A. Watch for and seek medical attention for signs of toxicity, such as tinnitus and dizziness.
   B. If activated charcoal was given for elevated levels, the client should drink 4–6 glasses of water each day for 2 days to prevent constipation. The activated charcoal will cause stools to be black for a few days.
6. Factors that affect results:
   A. Negative result found in ketoacidosis.
   B. Bilirubin of 5–20 mg/dl depresses results by 1–5 mg/dl.
   C. Sodium azide increases results.
   D. Urine alkalinization (e.g., by antacids) speeds renal excretion.
7. Other data:
   A. Salicylate poisoning may include alkalemia, followed by acidemia, ketosis, and hyperglycemia.
   B. Salicylate hepatitis can occur at blood concentrations of 20–25 mg/dl.

Bibliography:

Chan TY, Chan AY, Ho CS, Critchley JA: The clinical value of screening in acute poisoning. Vet Human Toxicol 37(1):37–38, 1995.

The Merck Manual, 16th ed. Rahway, NJ, Merck and Company, 1992, pp 2123–2124.

SALIVARY SCAN
(see Parotid Scan, Diagnostic)

SALMONELLA TITER, BLOOD

Norm: Less than a fourfold rise in titer between acute and convalescent specimens.

Positive: Fever of undetermined origin, and salmonellosis.

Description: *Salmonella* is a complex genus of gram-negative, non-spore-forming rods that are facultatively anaerobic. There are four subgenera of *Salmonella* (*S. typhi, S. choleraesuis, S. enteritidis,* and *S. arizonae*), as well as 1500 serotypes. *Salmonella* causes salmonellosis; typhoid fever; paratyphoid fever; septicemia; and, sometimes, inflammations of the joints and/or organs. The mode of transmission is through the fecal-oral route, most commonly by ingestion of food contaminated with the feces of infected clients or animals. This test uses cellular (O) antigens and flagellar (H) antigens to detect the presence of *Salmonella* antibodies in a sample of serum.

Professional Considerations:
1. Consent form NOT required.
2. Preparation:
   A. Specify for *Salmonella* antigens of groups A, B, C, or D on the laboratory requisition.
   B. Tube: Red-top, red/gray-top, or gold-top.
   C. Specimens MAY be drawn during hemodialysis.
3. Procedure:
   A. Draw a 7-ml blood sample. Label the specimen as the acute sample.
   B. Repeat the test in 3–5 days and label the tube as the convalescent sample.
   C. Heelstick is acceptable, collected in a microtainer.
4. Postprocedure care:
   A. None.
5. Client and family teaching:
   A. Thoroughly cook food, and avoid ingesting raw eggs or foods that have been sitting at room temperature for more than 2 hours.
   B. In addition to universal precautions, practice enteric precautions with the clothing and linen of infected clients.
6. Factors that affect results:
   A. Hemolysis or insufficient volume invalidates the results.
   B. Titers on a single specimen are not diagnostically significant.
   C. False-positives may occur due to cross-reacting bacterial antibodies.
   D. Antibiotic treatment may cause false-negative results.
7. Other data:
   A. Stool culture is the definitive technique for diagnosing bacterial diarrhea.

Bibliography:

Keller LH, Benson CE, Garcia V, Nocks E, Battenfelder P, Eckroade RJ: Monoclonal antibody-based detection system for Salmonella enteritidis. Avian Dis 37(2):501–507, 1993.

Konrad H, Smith BP, Dilling GW, House JK: Production of Salmonella serogroup D (09)-specific enzyme-linked imunosorbent assay antigen. Am J Vet Res 55(12):1647–1651, 1994.

SAO₂, BLOOD
(see Blood Gases, Arterial, Blood)

SCHICK TEST FOR DIPHTHERIA, DIAGNOSTIC

Norm: Negative test.

Usage: Measurement of immunity to diphtheria. To eliminate the carrier state of strains during epidemics.

Description: The Schick test is an intracutaneous skin test to determine the immunity strain for diphtheria by detecting the presence of antitoxins in the blood to this respiratory disease. The test is performed by injecting 1/50th of the minimum lethal dose of diphtheria toxin, then observing the site for a reaction, which would indicate lack of diphtheria immunity. A negative response indicates the presence of diphtheria antitoxin in the client's bloodstream.

Professional Considerations:

1. Consent form NOT required.
2. Preparation:
   A. Obtain two intradermal needles with syringes, and two alcohol pads.
3. Procedure:
   A. Cleanse the forearm sites for injection with alcohol pads and allow the areas to dry.
   B. Inject intracutaneously 0.1 ml of purified diphtheria toxin into one forearm and 0.1 ml of inactivated diphtheria toxoid into the other forearm.
   C. Observe the sites for reaction 24–48 hours (no longer than 120 hours) later. Absence of erythema, induration, and necrosis at the site is indicative of immunity to diphtheria.
4. Postprocedure care:
   A. Leave the injection sites open to air.
   B. For positive responses, inject 1/13 U of diphtheria antitoxin to neutralize the toxin.
5. Client and family teaching:
   A. This test will indicate whether or not you are immune to diphtheria.
   B. The recommended schedule for active immunization of children is 2 months, 4 months, 6 months, 18 months, and 4–6 years of age.
6. Factors that affect results:
   A. Expired toxin will cause false-negative results.
7. Other data:
   A. If a client has been actively immunized but the Schick test is positive, then the client is unable to produce antibodies.

Bibliography:

Durbaca S, Stoean C: Investigations concerning the possibility to replace the Schick test by the passive hemagglutination reaction for evaluating the diphtheria immunity level in population. Roumanian Arch Microbiol Immunol *51*(3):141–146, 1992.

SCHILLING TEST, DIAGNOSTIC

Norm: Over 10% absorption of vitamin B_{12} or $\geq 7\%$ of a 1-mg dose excreted within the first 24 hours. Clients lacking intrinsic factor will excrete <2% of the administered dose in the first 24 hours. Clients with intestinal malabsorption will excrete 3–5% of the administered dose in the first 24 hours.

Usage: Alcoholism, Crohn's disease in terminal ileum, differential diagnosis of macrocytic anemias, enteric steatorrhea, folic acid anemia, gastritis, malabsorption, megaloblastic anemia, pernicious anemia, and small intestine malabsorption.

Description: The Schilling test is a vitamin B_{12} absorption test that indicates if a client lacks intrinsic factor by measuring excretion of orally administered, radiolabeled cyanocobalamin (vitamin B_{12}) in a 24-hour urine sample. Vitamin B_{12} normally combines with intrinsic factor from the stomach and is absorbed in the terminal ileum. The test is based on the fact that, in normal clients, absorbed vitamin B_{12} in excess of the body's needs is excreted in the urine. Because parenteral nonradiolabeled cyanocobalamin is also administered to saturate the vitamin B_{12} binding sites, all of the radiolabeled cyanocobalamin should eventually be excreted in the urine.

Professional Considerations:

1. Consent form NOT required.

Risks:
Increased renal dysfunction.

Contraindications:
Pregnancy, breast-feeding.

2. Preparation:
   A. Assess kidney function by serum urea nitrogen and creatinine levels.
   B. *See Client and family teaching.*
   C. Obtain a 3-L urine container without a preservative.
3. Procedure:
   A. 0.5 mCi of cyanocobalamin CO-57 is administered in capsule form, followed 2 hours later by an intramuscular injection of vitamin B_{12}.
   B. Collect all urine over the next 24 hours in a clean container without preservatives.
   C. If excretion is low (<7%) in 24 hours, the procedure should be repeated using hog intrinsic factor given orally along with radioactive cyanocobalamin. If this excretion is normal, then the original values were due to intrin-

sic factor deficiency. However, if this second test remains abnormal, then malabsorption is due to an intestinal disease. A normal test after antibiotic treatment would indicate malabsorption of vitamin B_{12} due to bacterial infection.

4. Postprocedure care:
   A. Food and drink are permitted after the intramuscular dose of vitamin B_{12}.
   B. Observe the client carefully for up to 60 minutes after injection for a possible (anaphylactic) reaction to the radionuclide.
   C. When urine is being handled, rubber gloves should be worn for 24 hours after the procedure. Wash the gloved hands with soap and water before removing the gloves. Wash the ungloved hands after gloves are removed.
   D. Send the entire specimen to the laboratory. The test is performed on an aliquot of the 24-hour specimen.
5. Client and family teaching:
   A. This test will indicate whether or not you lack intrinsic factor, which helps your body absorb vitamin B_{12}.
   B. The client should fast for 8–12 hours before the test.
   C. Do not take B vitamins for at least 3 days or laxatives for at least 24 hours before the test.
   D. Save all the urine voided, urinate before defecating, and avoid contaminating the urine with stool or toilet tissue. If any urine is accidentally discarded, discard the entire specimen and restart the collection the next day.
   E. Instruct the client to meticulously wash the hands with soap and water after each void × 24 hours.
6. Factors that affect results:
   A. Incomplete urine collection or stool mixed with urine invalidates the results.
   B. A radioactive scan within 7 days prior to the test invalidates the results.
   C. Diabetes mellitus, hypothyroidism, intestinal bacterial overgrowth by decreasing intestinal vitamin B_{12} absorption, kidney disease, liver disease, myxedema, pancreatic insufficiency.
   D. Partial gastrectomy will cause no detection of vitamin B_{12}, due to lack of the intrinsic factor that enables vitamin B_{12} absorption.
7. Other data:
   A. At least 5 days should pass between Schilling tests.
   B. Bone marrow procedures should be performed prior to the Schilling test.
   C. Half-life of CO-57 is 270 days.

Bibliography:

Krynyckyi BR, Zuckier LS: Accuracy in using dual-isotope Schilling test to measure urine samples: a multicenter study [see comments]. J Nucl Med 36(9):1659–1665, 1995.

SCHIRMER TEARING EYE TEST, DIAGNOSTIC

Norm: ≥10 mm of moisture from each eye after 5 minutes.

Usage: Aging that results in tearing, leukemia, lymphoma, Sjögren's syndrome, and rheumatoid arthritis.

Description: The simultaneous testing of both eyes to assess the function of the lacrimal glands by assessing the amount of moisture accumulating on filter paper held against the conjunctival sac. Filter paper that remains dry for 15 minutes indicates insufficient tear formation.

Professional Considerations:

1. Consent form NOT required.
2. Preparation:
   A. Two sterile strips of filter paper ruled in millimeters.
   B. Topical anesthetic such as proparacaine.
3. Procedure:
   A. To measure the function of accessory lacrimal glands, instill one drop of topical anesthetic into each conjunctival sac before inserting the strips.
   B. Position the client sitting upright with the head tilted back against a headrest.
   C. Instruct the client to look upward and gently lower the inferior lids. Hook the folded ends of the filter paper strips over the inferior eyelids.
   D. After 5 minutes, remove the strips and measure the length of the moistened area in millimeters, starting from the folded ends of the strips.
   E. If the paper remains dry, repeat the test for up to 15 minutes.
4. Postprocedure care:
   A. Assess for corneal abrasion caused by rubbing the eyes before the topical anesthetic has worn off.
5. Client and family teaching:
   A. This test assesses the tearing ability of the eyes.
   B. After the test, do rub your eyes until the topical anesthetic has worn off (usually about 30 minutes). Rubbing the eyes before this time can cause a corneal abrasion, which is painful and takes several days to heal.
6. Factors that affect results:
   A. Rubbing or squeezing the eyes increases tearing.
7. Other data:
   A. None.

Bibliography:

Cho P, Yap M: Schirmer test. I. A review [review]. Optom Vis Sci 70(2):152–156, 1993.

Cho P, Yap M: Schirmer test. II. A clinical study of its repeatability. Optom Vis Sci 70(2):157–159, 1993.

Sherman MD, Whitcher JP, Daniels TE: Retrospective use of frozen Schirmer strips for the measurement of tear lysozyme. Adv Exp Med Biol *350*: 367–370, 1994.

SCHLICHTER TEST (SBT, INHIBITION LEVEL, ANTIBIOTIC), SPECIMEN

Norm: Bactericidal activity >1:8 dilution.

Usage: Endocarditis and osteomyelitis.

Description: Determination of the maximal dilution necessary to be bactericidal for 99.9% of clients with an infecting organism.

Professional Considerations:

1. Consent form NOT required.
2. Preparation:
   A. Obtain venipuncture supplies and a red-top, red/gray-top, or gold-top tube, or a sterile tube and sterile aspiration set for body fluid testing.
   B. List any recent antibiotic therapy on the laboratory requisition.
   C. Specimens MAY be drawn during hemodialysis.
3. Procedure:
   A. Draw a 5-ml blood sample in the blood tube or a 2-ml body fluid sample via sterile aspiration.
4. Postprocedure care:
   A. None.
5. Client and family teaching:
   A. This test evaluates the success of antibiotic treatment.
6. Factors that affect results:
   A. Specimens over 4 hours old invalidate the results.
7. Other data:
   A. It is preferred that two specimens be obtained: one prior to antibiotic treatment and the other 30–45 minutes after an antibiotic dose.
   B. Results take 2–3 days.

Bibliography:

Korzeniowski OM, Kaye D: Infective endocarditis. *In* Braunwald E (ed): Heart Disease: A Textbook of Cardiovascular Medicine, 4th ed. Philadelphia, WB Saunders, 1992, p 1090.

Wyngaarden JB, Smith LH, Bennett JC: Cecil Textbook of Medicine, 19th ed. Philadelphia, WB Saunders, 1992, p 1644.

SCLERODERMA ANTIBODY, BLOOD

Norm: Negative.

Positive: CREST (calcinosis, Raynaud's, esophageal dysfunction, scle-rodactyly, telangiectasia) syndrome, and scleroderma.

Description: Scleroderma antibody (Scl-70), is found in the blood of clients with progressive systemic sclerosis.

Professional Considerations:

1. Consent form NOT required.
2. Preparation:
   A. Tube: Red-top, red/gray-top, or gold-top.
   B. Specimens MAY be drawn during hemodialysis.
3. Procedure:
   A. Draw a 5-ml blood sample.
4. Postprocedure care:
   A. Refrigerate separated serum.
5. Client and family teaching:
   A. This test evaluates you for possible systemic sclerosis.
   B. Results are normally available within 24 hours.
6. Factors that affect results:
   A. False-positives may be created by aminosalicylic acid, diphenylhydantoin, ethosuximide, isoniazid, methyldopa, penicillin, propylthiouracil, streptomycin sulfate, tetracycline, and trimethadione.
7. Other data:
   A. Absence of scleroderma antibody does not exclude diagnosis.

Bibliography:

Bunce TD, Black CM, Bruckdorfer KR: Systemic sclerosis, plasma antioxidants and lipids. Biochem Soc Trans *23*(2):274S, 1995.

Csipo I, Czirjak L, Szanto S, Szerafin L, Sipka S, Szegedi G: Decreased serum trytophan neopterin levels in systemic sclerosis. Clin Exp Rheumatol *13*(2):269–270, 1995.

Kadono T, Kikuchi K, Sato S, Soma Y, Tamaki K, Takehara K: Elevated plasma endothelin levels in systemic sclerosis. Arch Dermatol Res *287*(5):439–442, 1995.

SCOUT FILM, DIAGNOSTIC

(see Flat Plate X-Ray of Abdomen, Diagnostic)

SECRETIN PROVOCATION TEST

(see Secretin Stimulation for ZE Syndrome, Diagnostic)

SECRETIN STIMULATION FOR ZE SYNDROME (SECRETION PROVOCATION TEST), DIAGNOSTIC

Norm: Serum gastrin: ≤200 pg/ml with no increase in production.

Increased: Gastrinoma (gastrin levels increase <100 pg/ml), and Zollinger-Ellison (ZE) syndrome (gastrin levels increase ≥110 pg/ml within 10 minutes).

Decreased: Duodenal ulcer, G-cell hyperplasia (antral), and pancreatic dysfunction.

Description: A stimulation test to assess for gastrinomas that can be correlated with chemical findings for diagnostic purposes. Secretin is a polypeptide secreted by the duodenal mucosa and the upper jejunum in response to gastric acidity. It acts to stimulate gastric pepsinogen, hepatic duct bicarbonate and water, pancreatic juice, bile and intestinal fluid secretion, and to inhibit gastric acid and gastrin secretion and intestinal smooth muscle contraction. ZE syndrome is a gastrointestinal disease in which elevated gastrin is formed, and pancreatic gastrinomas are present. In clients with ZE syndrome, the intravenous administration of secretin produces a paradoxical increase in serum gastrin levels. This test aids diagnosis of ZE syndrome for clients with baseline gastrin levels of 100–500 pg/ml (equivocal levels).

Professional Considerations:

1. Consent form NOT required.

Risks:

Allergic reaction to secretin.

Contraindications:

Positive reaction to secretin skin testing.

2. Preparation:
   A. *See Client and family teaching.*
   B. Establish intravenous access.

C. Obtain secretin for intravenous administration, a tourniquet, and seven each of: alcohol wipes, needles, syringes, and red-top tubes. Number the tubes sequentially.
D. Perform secretin skin testing to assess for allergy to the foreign protein. Inject 0.1 ml intradermally and observe 30 minutes for development of a wheal at the injection site.

3. Procedure:
   A. Draw a 5-ml blood sample for the gastrin level.
   B. Inject intravenously 2–3 U/kg body weight of secretin over 30 seconds. Repeat step 3A every 5 minutes × 6 for a total of 30 minutes postinjection, using the tubes in sequential order.
   C. An alternate procedure is to infuse secretin 9 U/kg body weight over 1 hour and draw blood specimens every 15 minutes. In ZE syndrome, gastrin levels peak after 45–90 minutes.

4. Postprocedure care:
   A. Label all the tubes and laboratory requisitions with the time the specimens were collected.

5. Client and family teaching:
   A. This test helps diagnose ZE syndrome.
   B. Fast from food and fluids from midnight prior to the test.

6. Factors that affect results:
   A. Amino acids, calcium, catecholamines, coffee, and insulin increase results.
   B. Atropine decreases results.

7. Other data:
   A. Gastrin secretion may increase by 100–200 pg/ml (ng/L) every 5 minutes after secretin injection when gastrinoma is present.
   B. Calcium provocation tests are also sometimes performed to aid in the diagnosis of ZE syndrome.

Bibliography:

Brady CE III: Secretin provocation test in the diagnosis of Zollinger-Ellison syndrome. Am J Gastroenterol 86(2):129–134, 1991.

Imamura M, Takahashi K: Use of selective arterial injection test to guide surgery in patients with Zollinger-Ellison syndrome. World J Surg 17(4): 433–438, 1993.

SECRETIN TEST FOR PANCREATIC FUNCTION, DIAGNOSTIC

Norm:

		SI Units
Duodenal Fluid		
Volume	95–235 ml/h	
Bicarbonate	74–121 mEq/L	74–121 mmol/L
Amylase	87,000–267,000 mg	
Lipase	<1.5 U/ml	<415 IU/L

Usage: Assessment of exocrine secretory ability of the pancreas for carcinoma, ductal obstruction, or chronic pancreatitis.

Description: Secretin is a polypeptide secreted by the duodenal mucosa and the upper jejunum in response to gastric acidity. Some of its actions are to stimulate pancreatic enzyme secretion and bicarbonate pancreatic juice production. This test allows an assessment of pancreatic endocrine function by assessing duodenal contents for volume, bicarbonate, amylase, lipase, and trypsin before and after pancreatic stimulation by secretin. In chronic pancreatitis and cystic fibrosis, all values are low, due to pancreatic tissue destruction. In early stages of obstructive pancreatic cancer, volume may be low, with other values normal. In pancreatic pseudocyst, bicarbonate may be decreased, with other values normal.

Professional Considerations:

1. Consent form IS required.

Risks:

Allergic reaction to secretin. Complications of nasogastric tube insertion include bleeding, dysrhythmias, esophageal perforation, laryngospasm, and decreased mean PO_2.

Contraindications:

Positive reaction to secretin skin testing.

2. Preparation:
   A. Obtain a double-lumen orogastric tube, pH paper, secretin, and two aspiration syringes or mechanical suction.
   B. Perform secretin skin testing to assess for allergy to the foreign protein. Inject 0.1 ml intradermally and observe 30 minutes for development of a wheal at the injection site.
   C. Establish intravenous access.
   D. *See Client and family teaching.*
3. Procedure:
   A. An orogastric tube is passed into the duodenum to the ligament of Treitz. Placement is assessed by analyzing the pH of secretions. Gastric pH is acidic, while duodenal secretions are alkaline.

B. The gastric (proximal) lumen is continuously aspirated to prevent acidic gastric secretions from contaminating duodenal contents.
C. All the duodenal fluid is aspirated from the distal lumen and placed in a sterile container. The container is labeled with the date, time, and specimen source and sent to the laboratory for baseline volume, bicarbonate, and amylase measurement.
D. Secretin, 1–2 U/kg of body weight, is administered intravenously.
E. All fluid is aspirated from the distal lumen every 20 minutes and analyzed for volume, bicarbonate, amylase, and lipase levels, as for the baseline sample.
4. Postprocedure care:
   A. Remove the orogastric tube.
5. Client and family teaching:
   A. This test is one of several used to screen for pancreatic cancer or pancreatitis.
   B. A nasogastric tube will be inserted through your nose into your stomach. Insertion may be uncomfortable and cause a pressurelike feeling or cause you to gag and cough. You will be asked to take sips of water and swallow to make tube insertion easier.
6. Factors that affect results:
   A. Failure to insert the tube fully into the duodenum causes unreliable results.
7. Other data:
   A. There is a 5.1% chance of false-positive and a 5.2% chance of false-negative results.
   B. This test is somewhat in disfavor because duodenal intubation is unpopular, and pancreatic disease is usually far advanced before exocrine function is appreciably reduced.
   C. This test is of little help in distinguishing chronic pancreatitis from advanced pancreatic cancer.
   D. Pancreozymin may be used in place of secretin for pancreatic stimulation but is more expensive.

Bibliography:

Brady CE III: Secretin provocation test in the diagnosis of Zollinger-Ellison syndrome. Am J Gastroenterol 86(2):129–134, 1991.

Glaser J, Mann O, Pausch J: Diagnosis of chronic pancreatitis by means of a sonographic test. Int J Pancreatol 15(3):195–200, 1994.

Ikeda M, Sato T, Ochiai M, Morozumi A, Nakamura T, Fukino MA: Morphological changes of small pancreatic cysts in response to secretin stimulation. Observation by endoscopic ultrasonography. Dig Dis Sci 38(4):648–652, 1993.

Laugier R: Dynamic endoscopic manometry of the response to secretin in patients with chronic pancreatitis. Endoscopy 26(2):222–227, 1994.

SEDIMENTATION RATE, ERYTHROCYTE (ESR, ZETA SEDIMENTATION RATE), BLOOD

Norm:

Westergren and Modified Westergren Methods

Adult females	
<Age 50	20 mm/hour
Age 50–85	30 mm/hour
>Age 85	42 mm/hour
Adult males	
<Age 50	15 mm/hour
Age 50–85	20 mm/hour
>Age 85	30 mm/hour
Children	0–10 mm/hour

Wintrobe Method

Females	0.36–0.45
Males	0.41–0.51

Zeta Sedimentation Ratio   41–54% (41–54 arbitrary units, SI units)

Increased: Anemia, ankylosis spondylitis, arteritis (temporal), arthritis (rheumatoid), cat scratch disease, cholesterol, coccidioidomycosis, colon cancer, Crohn's disease, dermatomyositis, endocarditis, fever of undetermined origin, fibrinogen elevation, hemolytic anemia, hyperfibrinogenemias, industrial-related diseases, infection, inflammation, macroglobulinemia, malignancy, multiple myeloma, obstructive hepatic disease, osteomyelitis, pain (acute, chronic, abdominal, pelvic), paraproteinemia, pelvic inflammatory disease, pericarditis, peritonitis, polyclonal hyperglobulinemias, polymyalgia rheumatica, pregnancy, pulmonary embolism, sickle cell disease, sinusitis, Sjögren's syndrome, subacute bacterial endocarditis, systemic lupus erythematosus, and tissue destruction. Drugs include dextran, fat emulsion, oral contraceptives, and vitamin A.

Decreased: Congestive heart failure and poikilocytosis. Drugs include albumin, corticotropin, cortisone, and lecithin.

Description: When a tube of well-mixed venous blood is positioned vertically, the red blood cells will tend to fall to the bottom. The rate at which they fall is the erythrocyte sedimentation rate (ESR). The ESR is a reflection of acute-phase reaction in inflammation and infection. A limitation of this test is that it is nonspecific for disease process. Various methods are used to measure the ESR. The Westergren method is used most often, due to the simplicity of the procedure. The Wintrobe method is more accurate for borderline elevations in the ESR. The zeta sedimentation ratio is a sedimentation rate calculation that provides more accurate data than the ESR in clients with anemia, requires the smallest amount of blood for testing, and provides the fastest results.

Professional Considerations:

1. Consent form NOT required.
2. Preparation:
   A. Specimens MAY be drawn during hemodialysis.
   B. *Westergren method:*
      i. Obtain venipuncture supplies and a blue-top tube, a 30-cm-long pipette with a 2.5-mm internal diameter and calibrated 0–200 mm, and a Westergren rack.
      ii. For the modified Westergren method, substitute a lavender-top tube for the blue-top tube.
   C. *Wintrobe method:*
      i. Obtain venipuncture supplies, a lavender-top tube, and a Wintrobe hematocrit tube.
   D. *Zeta sedimentation ratio:*
      i. Obtain venipuncture supplies, a lavender-top tube, and a capillary tube.

3. Procedure:
   A. *Westergren method:*
      i. Draw a 4-ml blood sample in a blue-top tube. Gently roll the tube to mix the sample.
      ii. Fill a pipette to the 0 mark with the blood sample.
      iii. Place the filled pipette vertically in the Westergren rack at room temperature.
      iv. After exactly 60 seconds, measure and record the distance to the top of the column of cells.
   B. *Modified Westergren method:*
      i. Draw a 2-ml blood sample in a lavender-top tube.
      ii. Add 0.5 ml of 3.8% sodium citrate or 0.85% sodium chloride to the sample, and follow the steps as for the Westergren method above.
   C. *Wintrobe method:*
      i. Draw a 7-ml blood sample in a lavender-top tube.
      ii. Fill a 7-cm-long Wintrobe capillary hematocrit tube with the blood sample, then place the cap on the tube.
      iii. Spin the tube for 5 minutes.
   D. *Zeta sedimentation ratio:*
      i. Draw a 7-ml blood sample. Gently roll the tube to mix the sample.
      ii. Heelstick is acceptable, collected in a microtainer.
      iii. Fill a capillary tube with 100 ml of the blood sample.
      iv. Place the capillary tube vertically in a centrifuge.
      v. Spin for 45-second cycles.
      vi. Read the capillary tube like a standard hematocrit tube. The results are called the "zetacrit."
      vii. Divide the true hematocrit by the zetacrit and express the result as a percentage.
4. Postprocedure care:
   A. Perform the Westergren method within 2 hours, the modified Westergren method within 12 hours, the Wintrobe method within 4 hours, and the zeta method within 4 hours of collection.
5. Client and family teaching:
   A. This test is used in situations in which acute infection or inflammation is suspected. It is a screening test only.

B. Results are normally available within 4 hours.
6. Factors that affect results:
   A. *All methods:*
      i. Conditions that counteract accelerated ESR in the conditions listed in the above *Increased* category include hypofibrinogenemia, polycythemia vera, sickle cell anemia, and spherocytosis.
      ii. Hemolysis or clotting invalidates the results.
   B. *Westergren or modified Westergren method:*
      i. Heparin falsely increases the results.
      ii. Bubbles in the pipette decrease the results.
      iii. Tilting the pipette more than 3 degrees from vertical can increase the results by as much as 30%.
   C. *Wintrobe method:*
      i. Inadequate duration or speed of the centrifuge, or specimens overdiluted with EDTA, causes unreliable results.
7. Other data:
   A. ESR is often normal in clients with connective tissue disease or neoplasms.

Bibliography:

Miettinen AK, Heinonen PK, Laippala P, Paavonen J: Test performance of erythrocyte sedimentation rate and C-reactive protein in assessing the severity of acute pelvic inflammatory disease. Am J Obstet Gynecol 169(5):1143–1149, 1993.

Thomas RD, Westengard JC, Hay KL, Bull BS: Calibration and validation for erythrocyte sedimentation test. Role of the International Committee on Standardization in Hematology reference procedure. Arch Pathol Lab Med 117(7):719–723, 1993.

Zlonis M: The mystique of the erythrocyte sedimentation rate. A reappraisal of one of the oldest laboratory tests still in use. Clin Lab Med 13(4):787–800, 1993.

SEGMENTED NEUTROPHILS, BLOOD
(see Differential Leukocyte Count, Peripheral Blood)

SENSITIVE TSH ASSAY
(see Thyroid-Stimulating Hormone, Sensitive Assay, Blood)

SEMEN ANALYSIS, SPECIMEN

Norm:

pH	>7, with average being 7.7
Appearance	Highly viscid, opaque, white, or gray-white
Odor	Musty or acrid odor
Sperm density	$>20 \times 10^6/L$
Spermatazoa total number	$>80 \times 10^6/$ejaculate
Sperm motility	>60% or progressive motility score of 3–4

Volume	1.5–5.0 ml (0.0015–0.005 L, SI units)
Normal spermatazoa	≥60
Defective heads	<35
Defective midpieces	≤20
Defective tails	≤20
Immature	<4

Increased: Not applicable.

Decreased: Cryptorchidism, hyperpyrexia, infertility, and Klinefelter's syndrome.

Description: Semen consists of spermatozoa in seminal plasma, which provides a nutritive medium for conveying the sperm to the endocervical mucus. The components of semen are obtained from the testes, seminal vesicles, prostate, epididymis, vas deferens, bulbourethral glands, and urethral glands.

Professional Considerations:

1. Consent form NOT required.
2. Preparation:
   A. Obtain a clean glass container.
   B. *See Client and family teaching.*
3. Procedure:
   A. Collect a fresh specimen in a clean glass jar. The client may obtain the specimen at home if he is unable to masturbate or uncomfortable with masturbation.
4. Postprocedure care:
   A. Specimens must be received within 1 hour and examined within 3 hours.
5. Client and family teaching:
   A. This test is used to estimate the number of sperm and evaluate fertility.
   B. Do not have intercourse or masturbate for 48 hours before specimen collection.
   C. Collect a fresh semen specimen in a plastic cup. The specimen may be collected by masturbation at the institution or at home, but it must be collected by masturbation. Do not use a condom or a lubricant, other than saliva.
   D. Keep track of the time the semen was collected.
   E. *For home collection:* After collecting the specimen, keep the container of

semen warm by putting it in a pocket next to the body.
   F. If the specimen is collected at home, it must be delivered to the laboratory within 1 hour.
6. Factors that affect results:
   A. Temperature extremes decrease the sperm count.
   B. Drugs that may decrease the sperm count include chemotherapeutics, cimetidine, and ketoconazole.
   C. Testicular irradiation decreases the sperm count.
   D. Reject semen specimens more than 1 hour old.
   E. Heavy tobacco smoking and heavy coffee consumption may decrease the number of motile spermatozoa.
7. Other data:
   A. Repeat testing may be necessary, because results vary with samples.
   B. Males with infertility tend to have increased semen volume, which is associated with diminished sperm count.
   C. Motility is graded as 0 = none, 1 = poor, 2 = moderate, 3 = good, and 4 = excellent.
   D. *See also Infertility Screen, Specimen.*

Bibliography:

Drudy L, Lewis SE, Barry-Kinsella C, Harrison RF, Thompson W: The influence of peritoneal fluid from patients with minimal stage or treated endometriosis on sperm motility parameters using computer-assisted semen analysis. Hum Reprod 9(12):2418–2423, 1994.

Irvine DS, Aitken RJ: Seminal fluid analysis and sperm function testing [review]. Endocrinol Metab Clin North Am 23(4):725–748, 1994.

Mandat KM, Wieczorkiewicz B, Bubala-Kacala M, Sypniewski J, Bujok G: Semen analysis of patients who had orchidopexy in childhood. Eur J Pediatr Surg 4(2):94–97, 1994.

Matson PL: External quality assessment for semen analysis and sperm antibody detection: results of a pilot scheme. Hum Reprod 10(3):620–625, 1995.

SEROTONIN (5-HYDROXYTRYPTAMINE), PLASMA

Norm:

	SI Units
10–30 µg/dl	570–1700 nmol/L
0.1–0.3 µg/ml	
50–200 ng/ml	0.28–1.14 µmol/L

Increased: Carcinoid syndrome, cystic fibrosis, dumping syndrome, endocarditis, metastasis, myocardial infarction, nontropical sprue, oat cell carcinoma of the lung (causing ectopic production), pain (chronic), pancreatic islet cell tumor (causing ectopic production), primary pulmonary hypertension, and thyroid medullary carcinoma (causing ectopic production). Drugs include imipramine, methyldopa, monoamine oxidase (MAO) inhibitors, reserpine, and tramodol (decreases serotonin reuptake).

Decreased: Depression, Down syndrome, Parkinson's disease, phenylketonuria, renal insufficiency, and teratomas (benign cystic).

Description: Serotonin is an indole amine synthesized by the argentaffin cells of the intestinal mucosa. Serotonin is stored in and transported by platelets, but it is also found in many body tissues, including the central nervous system. Serotonin acts as a vasoconstrictor, neurotransmitter, and stimulant of smooth muscle contraction, prolactin release, and growth hormone release, and functions in hemocoagulation. This test is used to confirm the diagnosis of carcinoid tumors, in which the highest increases in levels are found.

Professional Considerations:

1. Consent form NOT required.
2. Preparation:
   A. Preschedule this test with the laboratory. Clarify whether the client must follow a low-indole diet for a period of time prior to testing.
   B. MAO inhibitor drugs should be discontinued 1 week prior to the test.
   C. Avoid radionuclide scans for 7 days prior to the test.
   D. Tube: Chilled lavender-top, and a container of ice.
   E. Specimens MAY be drawn during hemodialysis.
3. Procedure:
   A. Draw a 7-ml blood sample. Place the specimen on ice.
   B. Heelstick is acceptable, collected in a microtainer.
4. Postprocedure care:
   A. Send specimens to the laboratory promptly. Specimens must be transferred to a plastic container of 10 mg EDTA and 75 mg ascorbic acid and frozen within 4 hours of collection.

5. Client and family teaching:
   A. This test is used to screen for carcinoid tumors.
   B. Results are normally available within 48 hours.
6. Factors that affect results:
   A. Lithium either increases or decreases the level of serotonin in the brain.
   B. A radioactive scan within 7 days prior to this test invalidates the results of the radioimmunoassay method.
7. Other data:
   A. Because blood serotonin samples are unstable, urine measurements of 5-hydroxyindoleacetic acid are more commonly measured.

Bibliography:

Cubeddu LX, O'Connor DT, Parmer RJ: Plasma chromogrannin A: a marker of serotonin release and emesis associated with cisplatin chemotherapy. J Clin Oncol *13*(3):681–687, 1995.

Herve P, Launay JM, Scrobohaci ML, Brenot F, Simonneau G, Petitpretz P, Poubeau P, Cerrina J, Duroux P, Drouet L: Increased plasma serotonin in primary pulmonary hypertension. Am J Med *99*(3):249–254, 1995.

Matuchansky C, Launay JM: Serotonin, catecholamines, and spontaneous midgut flush: plasma studies from flushing and nonflushing sites. Gastroenterology *108*(3):743–751, 1995.

SERUM GLUTAMIC OXALOACETIC TRANSAMINASE (SGOT), SERUM

(see Aspartate Aminotransferase, Serum)

SERUM GLUTAMIC PYRUVIC TRANSAMINASE (SGPT), SERUM

(see Alanine Aminotransferase, Serum)

SESTAMIBI-DIPYRIDAMOLE STRESS TEST AND SCAN

(see Heart Scan, Diagnostic)

SESTAMIBI EXERCISE TESTING AND SCAN

(see Heart Scan, Diagnostic)

SGOT, SERUM

(see Aspartate Aminotransferase, Serum)

SGPT, SERUM

(see Alanine Aminotransferase, Serum)

SICKLE CELL TEST, BLOOD

Norm: Sickling test: negative, no sickled red blood cells seen, 0% hemoglobin S; solubility test: negative.

Positive: Pain (chronic) and sickle cell anemia.

Negative: Drugs include phenothiazines at concentrations >128 mg/ml.

Description: A screening test used to demonstrate hemoglobin S, which causes red blood cells to assume a sickle shape or crescent shape under reduced oxygen supply. Sickling test is positive in sickle cell anemia or trait, or in combinations of other hemoglobin S abnormalities.

Professional Considerations:
1. Consent form NOT required.
2. Preparation:
   A. Tube: Lavender-top, green-top, or black-top.
   B. Note whether the client received a blood transfusion within the prior 4 months, as this may produce false-negative results.
   C. Specimens MAY be drawn during hemodialysis.
3. Procedure:
   A. Draw a 3-ml blood sample. Gently roll the tube to mix the specimen.
4. Postprocedure care:
   A. Observe for signs of sickle cell disease: fatigue, dyspnea, bone pain, joint swelling, and chest pain.
5. Client and family teaching:
   A. This test is used in screening for sickle cell disease.
   B. Clients with sickle cell disease should avoid hypoxic situations such as high altitudes, strenuous activity, extreme cold, and traveling in an unpressurized aircraft.
   C. Refer clients with sickle cell disease for genetic counseling.
6. Factors that affect results:
   A. If hemoglobin S concentration is <25%, erythrocytes will not sickle.
   B. False-positive results may be caused by polycythemia, hemoglobin abnormalities, or high blood protein levels (e.g., systemic lupus erythematosus, multiple myeloma).
   C. Collection of more than 7 ml of blood may cause false-positive results.
   D. False-negative results may be caused by anemia in combination with less than 7 ml of blood drawn, blood transfusion of normal hemoglobin within the prior 4 months, phenothiazine drug therapy, concurrent iron deficiency or thalassemia, elevated hemoglobin F, and in infants under 6 months of age.

E. Hemolysis, clotting, or lipemia of the specimen invalidates the results.
7. Other data:
   A. This test cannot reliably differentiate the homozygous sickle cell state from the heterozygous trait.
   B. The Sickledex Test is a trade name for the sickle cell test.

Bibliography:
Brugnara C: Membrane transport of Na and K and cell dehydration in sickle erythrocyte. Experientia *49*(2):100–109, 1993.

Croizat H: Early circulating erythroid progenitors (BFU-E) in sickle cell anemia. Experientia *49*(2): 118–125, 1993.

Ferrone FA: The polymerization of sickle hemoglobin in solutions and cells. Experientia *49*(2):110–117, 1993.

Robins EB, Khan AJ, Atrak T, Torrijos E: Erythrocyte sedimentation rate. A valuable test in infants and children with sickle cell disease. Clin Pediatr *32* (11):681–683, 1993.

SICKLEDEX TEST, DIAGNOSTIC
(see Sickle Cell Test, Blood)

SIDEROCYTE STAIN, DIAGNOSTIC
(see Hemosiderin Stain, Diagnostic)

SIGMOIDOSCOPY, DIAGNOSTIC

Norm: Negative.

Usage: Bowel obstruction, carcinoma of sigmoid colon, celiac sprue, colitis, Crohn's disease, diverticulitis, diverticulosis, and malabsorption.

Description: Sigmoidoscopy is the endoscopic visualization of the sigmoid colon, using a sigmoidoscope. A sigmoidoscope is a 50-cm fiberoptic tube with a lighted mirror lens system that illuminates the sigmoid colon for visualization.

Professional Considerations:
1. Consent form IS required.

Risks:
Bowel perforation, peritonitis, hemorrhage.

Contraindications:
Anorectal fistula, diverticulitis, paralytic ileus, third-trimester pregnancy. Sedatives are contraindicated in clients with central nervous system depression.

2. Preparation:
    A. *See Client and family teaching.*
    B. Obtain sterile specimen containers if a biopsy is planned.
    C. The client should disrobe below the waist or wear a gown.
3. Procedure:
    A. The client is placed in the left lateral position.
    B. Monitor blood pressure, heart rate, and oxygen saturation rate by pulse oximeter prior to analgesic and sedative being given and then every 5 minutes during the procedure.
    C. An analgesic or sedative may be administered. Monitor respiratory status continually after sedation.
    D. The sigmoidoscope is lubricated and inserted into the anus and rectum, then slowly advanced into the sigmoid colon.
    E. During the procedure, biopsies may be taken and suction used to remove excess secretions.
4. Postprocedure care:
    A. Assess for side effects of the sedative: hypotension, depressed respirations, and bradycardia.
    B. Continue the assessment of the respiratory status. If deep sedation was used, follow institutional protocol for postsedation monitoring. Typical monitoring includes continuous ECG monitoring and pulse oximetry, with continual assessments (q 5–15 minutes) of airway, vital signs, and neurologic status until the client is lying quietly awake, is breathing independently, and responds to commands spoken in a normal tone.
5. Client and family teaching:
    A. This test is performed to evaluate the colon for several different disorders.
    B. Consume a full liquid diet the evening before the test.
    C. Laxatives may be prescribed to be administered the night before the test and/or an enema/suppository 1 hour before the test, except in pregnant women.
    D. The urge to defecate as the sigmoidoscope is inserted into the rectum is normal.
    E. The procedure takes approximately 30 minutes.
    F. Resume normal activities and diet as soon as you feel ready.
    G. Call a physician if your temperature is higher than 101°F (38.3°C), or if you have trouble breathing or experience stomach pain, nausea, or bright red rectal bleeding.
6. Factors that affect results:
    A. Retained barium from previous studies makes visualization impossible.
    B. Fixation of bowel from previous radiation therapy or surgery may inhibit the passage of the sigmoidoscope.
7. Other data:
    A. Perforation of the intestinal wall is a rare complication.

Bibliography:

Jensen J, Kewenter J, Swedenborg J: The correlation of symptoms, occult blood test, and neoplasms in patients referred for double-contrast barium enema [review]. Scand J Gastroenterol 28(10): 911–914, 1993.

McGahan TP, Gilinsky NH: Colonic tumors [review]. Endoscopy 26(1):70–87, 1994.

Moran JA: Flexible fiberoptic sigmoidoscopy. Safe and effective for family practice [see comments] [review]. Can Fam Phys 39:1927–1934, 1994.

SIGNAL-AVERAGED ELECTROCARDIOGRAPHY (SIGNAL-AVERAGED ECG, SAECG), DIAGNOSTIC

Norm: No late potentials detected.

Usage: Determination of the risk for developing life-threatening dysrhythmias for the following high-risk conditions: myocardial infarction, clients with a history of reentrant dysrhythmias, survivors of sudden cardiac death, and syncope. Aids decision making about the need for further evaluation and treatment, including electrophysiologic study, drug treatment, antitachycardia pacemaker, or coronary artery bypass grafting.

Description: Signal-averaged electrocardiography (SAECG) is an inexpensive, noninvasive method for detection of late ventricular potentials (late potentials). Late potentials are low-amplitude electrical activity occurring in diastole during a normally isoelectric phase. Their presence signals slowed conduction velocity and is usually associated with disease, ischemia, or scarring of the heart muscle. The existence of late potentials is thought to indicate a potential for the development of reentrant dysrhythmias, which may lead to sudden cardiac death. Traditional electrocardiography is not sensitive enough to detect the very low-amplitude electrical activity of late potentials. Signal averaging is an electrocardiographic method that amplifies and averages up to 10,000 samples of electrical activity per second from the electrocardiographic signals of 100–1000 cardiac cycles in order to reduce the effect of random noise and artifact, thus allowing the detection of late potentials. The procedure may take up to 20 minutes, depending on the number of cardiac cycles averaged and the amount of electrical interference present. The presence of late potentials in the SAECG is determined by examination of the duration of the QRS complex, the root mean square voltage of the last 40 ms of the QRS complex, and the duration of the terminal QRS complex that measures under 40 mV.

Professional Considerations:

1. Consent form NOT required.
2. Preparation:
   A. Provide a private, comfortable, calm, warm environment to help the client relax skeletal muscles and avoid shivering.
   B. To minimize artifact caused by electrical interference, turn off all nonessential electrical equipment in the area. For example, run IV pumps on battery, and turn off the hypothermia machine, television, and radio. Plug the SAECG machine into an outlet different from that of essential equipment such as a ventilator or monitor.
   C. Obtain electrodes, conduction gel, and an SAECG machine.
3. Procedure:
   A. Position the client supine or with the head of the bed slightly elevated.
   B. For electrode placement, clip hair from the sites, then cleanse the sites with an alcohol wipe and scrape them lightly with the edge of an electrode.
   C. Lead placement varies by institutional protocol and SAECG machine manufacturer recommendations, but generally involves the placement of bipolar lead sets on the anterior and posterior torso. Apply leads according to institutional protocol.
   D. Follow the manufacturer's recommendations for obtaining the SAECG. This generally involves activating the SAECG machine, which runs an electrocardiographic template of the client's common cardiac cycle and then compares it to the template, amplifies it, and averages the electrical signals from a set number of subsequent cardiac cycles.
4. Postprocedure care:
   A. Remove the electrodes and cleanse the skin of conductive gel.
5. Client and family teaching:
   A. This test is performed to determine the risk of developing life-threatening dyshythmias in high-risk conditions. This is a special kind of electrocardiogram that takes longer than a normal electrocardiogram.
   B. It is important to lie motionless and try to relax the muscles as much as possible throughout the procedure.
6. Factors that affect results:
   A. Because a specific number of cardiac cycles will be averaged, the procedure will take longer than normal for brady-

cardia and less time than normal for tachycardia.
   B. Ectopic beats are not included in the averaging. Thus, the procedure time increases for clients demonstrating a great deal of ectopy.
   C. Artifact is not included in the averaging. Thus, movement or shivering of the client as well as electrical interference by nearby equipment will increase the procedure time.
7. Other data:
   A. SAECG has not been found useful for atrial dysrhythmias, continuously irregular rhythms, or rhythms with wide QRS complexes.

Bibliography:

Denes P, el-Sherif N, Katz R, Capone R, Carlson M, Mitchell LB, Ledingham R: Prognostic significance of signal-averaged electrocardiogram after thrombolytic therapy and/or angioplasty during acute myocardial infarction (CAST substudy). Cardiac Arrhythmia Suppression Trial (CAST) SAECG Substudy Investigators. Am J Cardiol 74 (3):216–220, 1994.

el-Sherif N, Denes P, Katz R, Capone R, Mitchell LB, Carlson M, Reynolds-Haertle R: Definition of the best prediction criteria of the time domain signal-averaged electrocardiogram for serious arrhythmic events in the postinfarction period. The Cardiac Arrhythmia Suppression Trial/Signal-Averaged Electrocardiogram (CAST/SAECG) Substudy Investigators. J Am Coll Cardiol 25(4):908–914, 1995.

Merva J: A closer look at the heart SAECG [published erratum]. RN 56(5):50–54, 1993.

SIMS-HUHNER TEST, DIAGNOSTIC

Norm: Mucus tenacity: stretches ≥10 cm. Number of motile sperm: ≥6–20/HPF.

Usage: Infertility testing; rape trauma.

Description: Examination of the postcoital endocervical mucus to detect its quality and the ability of the spermatozoa to penetrate the mucus. This test is included in infertility work-ups when prior semen analysis results are normal.

Professional Considerations:

1. Consent form NOT required, unless the specimen is being collected for medico-legal purposes.
2. Preparation:
   A. The test should be timed to coincide with midovulation. The male should abstain from ejaculation for 3 days prior to this test. Intercourse should be performed without using a lubricant. The woman should lie recumbent for 15–30 minutes after intercourse in which male ejaculation has occurred, then arrive for testing within 1–5 hours.

B. Obtain a glass cannula with a rubber tube, a syringe, a Petri dish, slides, and a ruler.

C. The client should disrobe below the waist or wear a gown.

D. Obtain a speculum and a glass slide.

3. Procedure:

A. Specimen collection must be witnessed if used for medicolegal purposes.

B. The client is placed in the dorsal lithotomy position and draped for privacy and comfort.

C. The external cervical os is wiped clear of mucus.

D. An endocervical mucus sample is obtained by aspiration in a glass cannula attached by a rubber tube to a syringe.

4. Postprocedure care:

A. For medicolegal specimens, place the specimen in a sealed plastic bag and label it as legal evidence. All persons handling the specimen must sign a record with the date and time received.

B. Deliver the specimen in a syringe to the laboratory, where the following occurs:

i. After the mucus volume is measured, the specimen is placed in a Petri dish, and color and viscosity are noted.

ii. The tenacity of the mucus is measured (spinnbarkeit) by grasping a portion of the mucus and noting the distance it can be drawn before it breaks.

iii. Next, a drop of mucus is placed on a microscope slide and covered with a coverslip, and the number of motile sperm are counted.

5. Client and family teaching:

A. This test is performed to evaluate endocervical mucus as part of a fertility work-up when sperm counts have been normal.

6. Factors that affect results:

A. Specimens collected more than 6 hours after coitus yield unreliable results.

7. Other data:

A. Mucus can also be microscopically examined for leukocytes, erythrocytes, and trichomonads.

Bibliography:

Gerhard I, Lenhard K, Eggert-Kruse W, Runnebaum B: Clinical data which influence semen parameters in infertile men. Hum Reprod 7(6):830–837, 1992.

SINGLE PHOTON EMISSION COMPUTED TOMOGRAPHY (SPECT SCAN), BRAIN, DIAGNOSTIC

Norm: Normal brain and structures.

Usage: Evaluate AIDS, Alzheimer's disease, anoxia, cerebrovascular accident, head trauma, transient ischemic attack; helps differentiate type of dementia (Alzheimer's, focal, multi-infarct, diffuse) by identifying pattern of cerebral ischemia; identifies the focus of seizure activity.

Description: SPECT scan is a nuclear medicine procedure in which the radiopharmaceutical technetium-99m hexamethyl propylenamine oxime is injected intravenously. This substance crosses the blood-brain-barrier, decomposes, and remains for several hours in the brain tissue, where it can be detected with the SPECT camera. The camera sends images to a computer that can reproduce visual images or "slices" of the brain along several planes. Advantages of SPECT imaging over older nuclear medicine scans are that it can identify patterns of dementia earlier in the process and allow for early intervention for potentially reversible types of dementia.

Professional Considerations:

1. Consent form IS required.

Risks:

Allergic reaction to the radiopharmaceutical (itching, hives, rash, tight feeling in the throat, shortness of breath, anaphylaxis, death).

Contraindications:

Inability to lie motionless during the scan; during pregnancy or breast-feeding. Previous allergic reaction to the radiopharmaceutical.

2. Preparation:

A. Remove all metal objects from the client's clothes, hair, and body.

B. *See Client and family teaching.*

3. Procedure:

A. The client is transported to the nuclear medicine department, positioned supine on the scanning table, and left to rest quietly for approximately 10 minutes to allow the brain to reach a basal activity level.

B. A radiopharmaceutical is injected intravenously and allowed to circulate and cross the blood-brain barrier.

C. The SPECT scan is then taken while the client lies motionless, with open eyes.

4. Postprocedure care:

A. *See Client and family teaching.*

5. Client and family teaching:
    A. Do not drink caffeine-containing beverages for 24 hours before the scan.
    B. It is important to lie motionless during this scan. If the client is confused, a family member familiar to the client may remain in the room to reassure the client during the scan.
    C. The scan takes about 30 minutes.
    D. For about 24 hours after the scan, meticulously wash your hands after urination to remove any radioactivity from contaminated urine.
6. Factors that affect results:
    A. The presence of metal objects, such as metal eyeglasses, over the scanning area may block some views.
    B. Movement of the client during imaging obscures the clarity of the images.
7. Other data:
    A. The radiopharmaceutical half-life is about 6 hours.

Bibliography:

Fleming KC, Adams AC, Petersen RC: Dementia: diagnosis and evaluation. Mayo Clin Proc *70*(11): 1093–1107, 1995.

Souder E: A comparison of neuroimaging modalities for diagnosing dementia. Nurse Pract *20*(1): 66–74, 1995.

Talbot PR, Testa HJ: The value of SPECT imaging in dementia. Nucl Med Commun *16*(6):425–437, 1995.

SINUS X-RAYS, DIAGNOSTIC

Norm: Negative.

Usage: Cysts, postoperative nasal/ sinus surgery, rhinitis, and sinusitis.

Description: Sinus x-rays (roentgen rays) are short electromagnetic waves that penetrate the soft sinus tissues to produce an image that is recorded on radiographic film. The sinuses are usually radiolucent due to the air content. Any deviation from total radiolucence indicates tumor or infection.

Professional Considerations:

1. Consent form NOT required.
2. Preparation:
    A. Shield the pregnant uterus during x-ray exposure.
    B. Remove earrings, glasses, hairpins, or other radiopaque objects from the head area.
3. Procedure:
    A. The head is placed in a fixed position.
    B. Radiographs of sinuses are taken from several angles.
    C. The exam takes 10–15 minutes.
4. Postprocedure care:
    A. Remove the lead apron.
5. Client and family teaching:
    A. This test is performed to evaluate sinus cavities for signs of infection or growth.

6. Factors that affect results:
    A. Movement during radiography distorts the images.
7. Other data:
    A. Anaerobic organisms are the predominant pathogens of chronic sinusitis.
    B. *See also Tomography Paranasal Sinuses, Diagnostic)*

Bibliography:

Friedman WH, Katsantonis GP: Staging systems for chronic sinus disease. Ear Nose Throat J *73*(7): 480–484, 1994.

Garcia DP, Corbett ML, Eberly SM, Joyce MR, Le HT, Pence HL, Nguyen KL: Radiographic imaging studies in pediatric chronic sinusitis. J Allergy Clin Immunol *94*(3, Pt 1):523–530, 1994.

Libanore M, Pastore A, Frasconi PC, Rossi MR, Bedetti A, Sighinolfi L, Ghinelli F: Invasive multiple sinusitis by Aspergillus fumigatus in a patient with AIDS. Int J STD AIDS *5*(4):293–295, 1994.

Rossi OV, Pirila T, Laitman J, Huhti E: Sinus aspirates and radiographic abnormalities in severe attacks of asthma. Int Arch Allergy Immunol *103*(2):209–213, 1994.

SJÖGREN'S ANTIBODIES (SS-A [RO] AND SS-B [LA]), BLOOD

(see Anti-La/SS-B Test, Diagnostic; and Anti-Ro/SS-A Test, Diagnostic)

SKELETAL MUSCLE ANTIBODY, SPECIMEN

(see Striational Antibody, Specimen)

SKIN CULTURE

(see Culture, Skin, Specimen)

SKIN FUNGUS, CULTURE

Norm: Negative.

Usage: Dermatitis and fungal infections.

Description: Culture of skin scrapings, nails, scalp, hair, or debris under the nails is taken to isolate and identify fungi. A single negative culture does not rule out a fungal infection.

Professional Considerations:

1. Consent form NOT required.
2. Preparation:
    A. Obtain a sterile scraper and a dermatophyte test medium or a sterile container.
3. Procedure:
    A. Place the skin or scalp scrapings, nail clippings, hair stubs, or nail debris scrapings into a dermatophyte medium or sterile container.
4. Postprocedure care:
    A. Store the specimens at room temperature.

5. Client and family teaching:
   A. Culture results for *Candida* are usually available within 1 week and for dermatophytes within 2 weeks.
   B. All negative cultures are final after 4 weeks.
6. Factors that affect results:
   A. Cotton-plugged tubes should not be used, because they may cause the specimen to become trapped in the cotton and lost.
   B. Closed rubber stopper tubes should not be used, because they keep the specimen moist and aid in bacterial growth.
7. Other data:
   A. None.

Bibliography:

Shrum JP, Millikan LE, Bataineh O: Superficial fungal infections in the tropics. Dermatol Clin *12*(4): 687–693, 1994.

SKIN MYCOBACTERIA, CULTURE

Norm: No growth.

Usage: Abscess, AIDS, amyloidosis, buruli ulcers, granulomatous cutaneous lesions, and osteomyelitis.

Description: Isolation of mycobacteria on the skin as the cause of infection. Some of the common mycobacteria are *M. tuberculosis* and the non-tubercular *M. avium-intracellular, genavense* and *marinum* found in clients with acquired immune deficiency syndrome (AIDS) or immunosuppression.

Professional Considerations:

1. Consent form NOT required.
2. Preparation:
   A. Obtain a sterile scraper and a mycobacterial culture medium.
3. Procedure:
   A. Scrape the skin or lesion (do not use a swab) and place the specimen in the mycobacterial culture medium.
4. Postprocedure care:
   A. Transport the specimen directly to the laboratory.
5. Client and family teaching:
   A. Negative cultures are reported after 9 weeks.
6. Factors that affect results:
   A. Specimens not incubated at 30°C may not grow.
7. Other data:
   A. The yield on cultures is proportional to the amount of specimen submitted.

Bibliography:

Kirschner P, Vogel U, Hein R, Bottger E: Bias of culture technique for diagnosing mixed *Mycobacterium genavense* and *Mycobacterium avium* infection in AIDS. J Clin Microbiol *32*(3):828–831, 1994.

Street ML, Umbert-Millet IJ, Roberts GD, Su WPD: Nontuberculous mycobacterial infections of the skin. J Amer Acad Dermatol *24*(2):208–215, 1991.

SKIN TEST FOR HYPERSENSITIVITY, DIAGNOSTIC

Norm: Negative.

Positive: There is no agreement on a threshold value for a positive skin test result.

Usage: Allergies and cat scratch disease.

Description: An intradermal test using allergen extracts to determine sensitivity to various drugs, materials, and pollens that a client may react to in an allergic manner, such reaction possibly resulting in anaphylaxis. The result is based on an immediate hypersensitivity reaction.

Professional Considerations:

1. Consent form NOT required.
2. Preparation:
   A. Obtain an alcohol wipe, 0.1 ml of the test substance in question, and an intradermal 26- or 27-gauge needle.
   B. Have emergency equipment and medications on hand for possible anaphylaxis.
   C. *See Client and family teaching.*
3. Procedure:
   A. Wipe the skin with an alcohol wipe and let it air-dry.
   B. Intradermally inject 0.1 ml of the test substance in question in the underpart of the forearm.
4. Postprocedure care:
   A. Observe for redness and swelling (a wheal) at the site of the injection.
   B. Results are read 15 minutes after injection. Assess the wheal size of the skin reaction by measuring the mean wheal diameter (MWD) or the mean of the largest wheal diameter and that perpendicular to it. MWDs of skin tests may be expressed in absolute values (millimeters) or they may be related to the size of a control. An MWD >7 mm has a higher diagnostic value for symptomatic allergies. An MWD greater than or equal to a histamine control also has a greater diagnostic value.
   C. Assess for anaphylaxis symptoms for ½ hour.
5. Client and family teaching:
   A. Withhold allergy medications and antihistamines for 48 hours prior to the test.
   B. Report drowsiness, skin rash or itching, difficulty breathing, and palpitations immediately.

6. Factors that affect results:
   A. A subcutaneous rather than an intra-dermal injection will produce a false-negative result.
7. Other data:
   A. Most skin tests are available in prepack-aged sterile kits.

Bibliography:

Brand PLP, Kerstjens HAM, Jansen HM, et al.: Interpre-tation of skin tests to house dust mite and relation-ship to other allergy parameters in patients with asthma and chronic obstructive pulmonary disease. J Allergy Clin Immunol 91(2):560–569, 1993.

Merget R, Stollfuss J, Wiewrodt R, et al.: Respiratory pathophysiologic responses: Diagnostic tests in en-zyme allergy. J Allergy Clin Immunol 91(2):264–277, 1993.

Silviu-Dan F, McPhillips S, Warrington, RJ: Clinical as-pects of allergic disease: the frequency of skin test reactions to side-chain penicillin determinants. J Allergy Clin Immunol 91(3), 1993.

SLIT-LAMP VISION TEST, DIAGNOSTIC

Norm: Normal.

Usage: Detection of conjunctivitis, corneal abrasions, iritis, and opacities.

Description: The slit lamp is a special microscopic instrument with a lighting system that allows detailed visualiza-tion of the anterior segment of the eye. Slit-lamp vision testing involves visual-ization of the anterior chamber, con-junctiva, cornea, crystalline lens, eye-lashes, eyelids, iris, sclera, tear film, and vitreous face, and evaluation of oc-ular fluid and tissue size and shape by using a slit-lamp light source.

Professional Considerations:
1. Consent form NOT required.

Risks:
Allergic reaction to eye drops (itching, hives, rash, tight feeling in the throat, shortness of breath, anaphylaxis).

Contraindications:
Allergy to mydriatic eye drops; narrow-angle glaucoma.

---

2. Preparation:
   A. Remove contact lenses and glasses.
3. Procedure:
   A. The client is positioned sitting upright with the chin resting on a chin rest and the forehead touching the fore-head bar of the slit-lamp instrument.
   B. The client is instructed to gaze into the eye of the microscope as the exam-iner examines the eye from the other side of the microscope.
   C. Pupillary dilation drops may be needed, such as in iritis.
4. Postprocedure care:
   A. See Client and family teaching.
5. Client and family teaching:
   A. If dilatory drops are used, vision will be blurred for up to 2 hours. The client should bring sunglasses to wear after the test. The client should not drive or operate machinery during this time period.
   B. The test takes 10 minutes and is pain-less.
6. Factors that affect results:
   A. Inability of the client to remain still during the examination prevents proper examination.
7. Other data:
   A. Three other slit-lamp procedures may be used: fluorescein staining to detect scratches on the cornea or conjunc-tiva; Hruby lens to better visualize the posterior vitreous and retina; and go-nioscopy, where special contact lens eliminates the corneal curve so glau-coma testing can be performed.

Bibliography:

Cohen JS, Tilton T: Technique for slit lamp compari-son of anterior chamber depth. Ophthalmic Surg 19(1):58–59, 1988.

Duran JA, Labella F: Keratoscopy through the slit lamp. Ophthalmic Surg 21(11):810–811, 1990.

Javitt JC: A modified slit lamp for examination of wheelchair-bound patients [see comments]. Arch Ophthalmol 107(3):453–454, 1989.

SMA-6, -7, -12, -20 (CHEM-6, -7, -12, 20), BLOOD

Norms: See individual test listings.

Increased or Decreased: See indi-vidual test listings.

Description: SMA is an acronym for the sequential multiple analyzer (SMA) automated system that analyzes multiple blood values from one tube of blood.

For the blood values of an SMA-6 see Carbon dioxide, Total Content, Blood; Chloride, Serum; Creatinine, Serum; Potassium, Serum; Sodium, Plasma or Serum; and Urea Nitrogen, Plasma or Serum.

For the blood values of an SMA-7 see Carbon dioxide, Total Content, Blood; Chloride, Serum; Creatinine, Serum; Glucose, Blood; Potassium, Serum; Sodium, Plasma or Serum; and Urea Nitrogen, Plasma or Serum.

For the blood values of an SMA-12

see *Albumin, Serum; Alkaline phosphatase, Serum; Aspartate Aminotransferase, Serum; Bilirubin, Serum; Calcium, Serum; Cholesterol, Blood; Glucose, Blood; Lactate Dehydrogenase, Blood; Phosphorus, Serum; Protein, Total, Serum; Urea Nitrogen, Plasma or Serum; and Uric Acid, Serum.*

For the blood values of an SMA-20 see *Alanine Aminotransferase, Serum; Alkaline phosphatase, Serum; Aspartate Aminotransferase, Serum; Bilirubin, Serum; Calcium, Serum; Carbon dioxide, Total Content, Blood; Chloride, Serum; Cholesterol, Blood; Creatine Kinase, Serum; Creatinine, Serum; Gamma-Glutamyl Transpeptidase, Blood; Glucose, Blood; Lactate Dehydrogenase, Blood; Phosphorus, Serum; Potassium, Serum; Protein, Total, Serum; Sodium, Plasma or Serum; Triglycerides, Blood; Urea Nitrogen, Plasma or Serum; and Uric Acid, Serum.* For further information, see individual test listings.

Professional Considerations:
1. Consent form NOT required.
2. Preparation:
   A. Tube: Red-top, red/gray-top, or gold-top.
   B. Do NOT specimens draw during hemodialysis.
3. Procedure:
   A. Draw a 5-ml blood sample.
4. Postprocedure care:
   A. None.
5. Client and family teaching:
   A. *See individual test listings.*
6. Factors that affect results:
   A. *See individual test listings.*
7. Other data:
   A. *See individual test listings.*

Bibliography:
Kulpmann WR, Maibaum P, Sonntag O: Analyses with the KODAK-Ektachem. Accuracy control using reference method values and the influence of protein concentration. Part II. Substrates. J Clin Chem Clin Biochem 28(11):835–843, 1990.

Schotters SB, McBride JH, Rodgerson DO, et al.: Clinical assessment of the Hitachi 736–730 chemistry analyzer. J Clin Lab Anal 4(2):157–160, 1990.

van Suijlen JD, Blijenberg BG, Boerma GJ, et al.: Calibration of Technicon Chem 1 multitest analyzers. Eur J Clin Chem Clin Biochem 29(3):205–208, 1991.

SMALL BOWEL SERIES, DIAGNOSTIC

Norm: No abnormalities in the small bowel contour, position, or motility.

Usage: Cancer, Crohn's Disease, diarrhea, enteritis, hematemesis, Hodgkin's disease, lymphosarcoma, malabsorption syndrome, melena, polyps, ulcers, and weight loss.

Description: Fluoroscopic examination of the small intestine after ingestion of barium sulfate. The barium enters the stomach and empties into the duodenal bulb. Circular folds appear as barium enters the duodenal loop. These folds deepen in the jejunum and then lessen in the ileum. The procedure takes 2–6 hours depending on barium transit time through the small bowel.

Professional Considerations:
1. Consent form NOT required.

Risks:
Aspiration of contrast material, bowel obstruction, constipation.

Contraindications:
In obstruction or perforation of the small intestine, as the barium may intensify the obstruction or cause seeping of the barium into the abdominal cavity.

2. Preparation:
   A. *See Client and family teaching.*
3. Procedure:
   A. Preliminary radiographs are taken in supine, erect, and lateral side positions.
   B. The client is given 500 ml flavored but chalky-tasting barium orally.
   C. Radiographs are taken at 30- to 60-minute intervals with the client in supine, erect, and lateral side positions for 2–6 hours to track the barium passage through the small intestine.
3. Postprocedure care:
   A. Encourage fluids (4–6 glasses of water per day × 2 days, when not contraindicated) to promote the passage of the barium through the intestines.
   B. A cathartic may be prescribed to prevent barium impaction.
5. Client and family teaching:
   A. Fast from food and fluids and refrain from smoking from midnight prior to the test.
   B. A cathartic may be prescribed to be administered the evening before the test.
   C. Bring reading material or other diversion to the test, as the procedure is lengthy.
   D. Stool will be barium-colored for up to 72 hours.

6. Factors that affect results:
   A. Chronic narcotic use can cause delayed motility.
7. Other data:
   A. Barium enema, oral cholecystography, and routine radiography should precede a small bowel series, since retained barium clouds details on the radiographs.

Bibliography:

Herlinger H: Guide to imaging of the small bowel. Gastroenterol Clin North Am 24(2):309–329, 1995.

Sampson MA, deLacey G, Twomey B, et al.: The small bowel follow-through: Time to sit up. Clinical Radiology 49:478–480, 1994.

SMOOTH MUSCLE ANTIBODY, BLOOD

(see Anti-Smooth Muscle Antibody, Serum)

S MUCOPOLYSACCHARIDE TURNOVER, DIAGNOSTIC

Norm: Normal turnover.

Usage: Glucuronidase deficiency, Hurler's syndrome, Maroteaux-Lamy syndrome, mucopolysaccharidoses I–VII (except Morquio syndrome), Sanfilippo's syndrome type A or B, and Scheie syndrome.

Description: The mucopolysaccharidoses are a group of inherited disorders caused by the deficiency of enzymes required for the lysosomal degradation of glycosaminoglycans. Evaluation of the rate of turnover of S-35 labeled mucopolysaccharidoses in cultures of the skin assists in their diagnosis. Skin containing fibroblasts that lack an enzyme necessary for the breakdown of mucopolysaccharides will accumulate polysaccharides.

Professional Considerations:

1. Consent form NOT required.
2. Preparation:
   A. Obtain a 4-mm punch biopsy instrument, sterile gauze, tape, and a sterile plastic container.
3. Procedure:
   A. Obtain a skin biopsy using a 4-mm punch biopsy instrument.
   B. Place the specimen in the sterile plastic container.
4. Postprocedure care:
   A. Transport the specimen to the laboratory immediately.
5. Client and family teaching:
   A. Genetic counseling is necessary for clients and families undergoing genetic testing.
6. Factors that affect results:
   A. An inadequate amount of biopsy tissue can cause false-negative results.
7. Other data:
   A. The mucopolysaccharidoses, besides involving diseases of connective and vascular tissues, also secrete substantial amounts of chondroitin—6-sulfate heparin sulfate, and keratin sulfate.

Bibliography:

Scott HS, Litjens T, Nelson PV, et al.: Identification of mutations in the alpha-l-iduronidase gene (IDUA) that cause Hurler and Scheie syndromes. Am J Hum Genet 53:973–986, 1993.

SO₂, BLOOD

(see Blood Gases, Arterial, Blood)

SODIUM, PLASMA, SERUM OR URINE

Norm:

		SI Units
Plasma or Serum		
Adult	136–145 mEq/L	136–145 mmol/L
Umbilical cord	116–166 mEq/L	116–166 mmol/L
Infant	139–146 mEq/L	139–146 mmol/L
Child	138–145 mEq/L	138–145 mmol/L
Panic level	≤110 mEq/L	≤110 mmol/L
Urine		
Adults	75–200 mEq/24 hours	75–200 mmol/day
Children		
Newborn	14–40 mEq/24 hours	14–40 mmol/day
6–10 years		
Female	20–69 mEq/24 hours	20–69 mmol/day
Male	41–115 mEq/24 hours	41–115 mmol/day

	SI Units

Urine (continued)

Children (continued)

10–14 years

Female	48–168 mEq/24 hours	48–168 mmol/day
Male	63–177 mEq/24 hours	63–177 mmol/day

Panic Level Symptoms and Treatment:

Symptoms (low sodium): Impaired cognition, depressed level of consciousness, convulsions.

Treatment (sodium <110 mEq/L, 110 mmol/L SI units):

Measure serum osmolality via blood test or by calculated means to determine if relative or true hyponatremia. Measure urine specific gravity.

Maintain a patent airway.

Monitor for convulsions due to brain cell edema.

Monitor hourly neurologic checks.

The use of hypertonic saline is controversial due to its association with osmotic demyelinating syndrome. The literature demonstrates uncertainty over the cause of osmotic demyelinating syndrome, with the possible causes being rapid infusions of hypertonic saline, cerebral ischemia that occurs in severely hyponatremic clients, or some other unknown cause. However, most sources agree that slow infusions are indicated when levels reach the panic (low) level above. Give hypertonic saline (3–5%) slowly and with extreme caution. Change to a less hypertonic infusion as soon as possible. Sodium should be replaced at about the amount of time over which the loss occurred.

Increased (Hypernatremia): Congestive heart failure, Cushing's disease, dehydration, diabetes insipidus, diaphoresis, diarrhea, hyperaldosteronism, hypertension, hypovolemia, insensible water loss, ostomies, salicylate toxicity, toxemia, vomiting, and Zollinger-Ellison syndrome with diarrhea. Drugs include ACTH, androgens, carbenicillin, clonidine, corticosteroids, estrogens, lactulose, licorice, mannitol, methyldopa, oral contraceptives, oxyphenbutazone, phenylbutazone, rauwolfia alkaloids, reserpine, and sodium bicarbonate. Urinary sodium concentration is decreased if hypernatremia is caused by volume depletion. Urinary sodium concentration is increased if hypernatremia is caused by renal losses due to osmotic diuresis.

Urinary Sodium Concentration (Increased): If hyponatremia is due to renal salt losses or to renal failure with water retention, urinary sodium concentration is increased. Also: dehydration, fever, head trauma, hypernatremia, hyponatremia, kidney stone, nephrotic syndrome, salicylate toxicity, starvation and syndrome of inappropriate antidiuretic hormone secretion (SIADHS). Drugs include caffeine, calcitonin, cisplatin, diuretics, dopamine, heparin, lithium, niacin, sulfates, tetracycline, and vincristine.

Decreased (Hyponatremia): Addison's disease, adrenal insufficiency, aminoglycoside toxicity, ascites in cardiac failure, bowel obstruction, burns, cerebral palsy, chronic renal failure, cirrhosis, congenital adrenal hyperplasia, diabetes mellitus, emphysema, glomerulonephritis, hyperglycemia, hyperosmolality, hyperthermia, hypophosphatemia, hypotension, hypothyroidism, hysterectomy, malabsorption, malnutrition, meningitis, metabolic acidosis, myxedema, nephrotic syndrome, ostomies, overhydration, pain (abdominal), paracentesis, paralytic ileus, psychogenic polydipsia, pyelonephritis (chronic), renal hypertension, sigmoidoscopy, sprue, syndrome of inappropriate antidiuretic hormone secretion syndrome (SIADHS), toxemia, toxic shock syndrome, and vomiting. Drugs include aminoglutethimide, ammonium chloride, amphotericin B, carbamazepine, chlorpropamide, cisplatin, clofibrate, cyclophosphamide, diuretics (oral and mercurial), fosinopril, heparin, miconazole, nonsteroidal anti-inflammatory agents (NSAIDs), spironolactone, tolbutamide, tricyclic antidepressants, vasopressin, and vincristine.

Urinary Sodium Concentration (Decreased): If hyponatremia is associated with edema or with volume depletion from extrarenal causes, urinary sodium concentration is decreased. Also: acute renal failure, diarrhea, emphysema, fluid retention, malabsorption, pyloric obstruction and sprue. Drugs include corticosteroids, diazoxide, epinephrine, levarterenol, and propranolol.

Description: Sodium is the major cation of extracellular fluid. Its primary function is to maintain osmotic pressures and acid-base balance, and to transmit nerve impulses. It is absorbed from the small intestine and excreted in the urine in amounts dependent on dietary intake. In normal clients, the sodium content of the body remains fairly constant despite wide variations in sodium intake.

Professional Considerations (Serum or Plasma):

1. Consent form NOT required.
2. Preparation:
   A. *Serum or plasma:*
      i. Tube: Red-top, red/gray-top, or gold-top.
      ii. Do NOT draw specimens during hemodialysis.
   B. *Urine:*
      i. Obtain a clean, 3-L container without preservatives.
      ii. Write the beginning time of collection on the laboratory requisition.
3. Procedure:
   A. *Serum:* Draw a 1-ml blood sample.
   B. *Urine:*
      i. Discard the first morning urine specimen.
      ii. Save all the urine voided for 24 hours in a refrigerated, clean 3-L container without preservatives. Document the quantity of urine output during the collection period. Include the urine voided at the end of the 24-hour period. For catheterized clients, keep the drainage bag on ice and empty the urine into the collection container hourly.
4. Postprocedure care:
   A. Compare the urine quantity in the specimen container with the urinary output record for the test. If the specimen contains less urine than was recorded as output, some of the sample may have been discarded, thus invalidating the test.

B. Document the quantity of urine output and the ending time for the collection period on the laboratory requisition.
C. Send the entire 24-hour urine specimen to the laboratory for testing.
5. Client and family teaching:
   A. Save all the urine voided in the 24-hour period and urinate before defecating to avoid loss of urine. If any urine is accidentally discarded, discard the entire specimen and restart the collection the next day.
   B. Routine blood results are normally available within 2 hours.
6. Factors that affect results:
   A. Drawing blood samples proximal to intravenous infusion of sodium chloride will falsely elevate the results.
7. Other data:
   A. An average dietary intake of 90–250 mEq/day will maintain sodium balance in adults.
   B. Minimum daily requirement is 15 mEq.
   C. The rate of sodium excretion during the night is one-fifth the peak rate during the day.
   D. Urinary excretion of sodium is highly dependent on dietary intake, state of hydration, and renal function.
   E. Signs of hypernatremia include dry and sticky mucous membranes, fever, thirst, and rubbery skin turgor.
   F. Signs of hyponatremia include abdominal cramping, apprehension, oliguria, and rapid weak pulse.

Bibliography:

Rutecki GW, Whittier FC: Cause of hypotonicity directs management. Consultant 35(5):705–707, 711–712, 1994.
Rutecki GW, Whittier FC: Physiologic clues to a state of disordered tonicity. Consultant 35(5):688–690, 700–702, 1994.

SOMATOMEDIN-C, BLOOD
(see Insulin-like Growth Factor-I, Blood)

SOMATOSENSORY EVOKED POTENTIAL, DIAGNOSTIC

Norm: Results of the somatosensory evoked potential (SEP) are interpreted by a physician trained in neurophysiology.

Usage: Aids in the diagnosis of demyelinating diseases, including multiple sclerosis; neurodegenerative diseases, including adrenoleukodystrophy, adrenomyeloneuropathy, and Friedreich's ataxia; and spinal cord lesions. May help predict recovery prognosis in coma, especially nontraumatic coma.

Description: SEP testing utilizes peripheral electrical nerve stimulation to examine the conduction velocity of impulses through the somatosensory pathway along peripheral nerves to the cortex of the brain in a fashion similar to that of the electroencephalogram (EEG). The test uses sophisticated signal averaging to filter out the effect of other brain activity during testing. Of significance are conduction time for the SEP to occur after stimulation (latency), and the amplitude of the SEP waveform.

Professional Considerations:

1. Consent form NOT required.
2. Preparation:
   A. Obtain EEG electrodes, an EEG machine, and electroconductive gel.
   B. Remove jewelry and metal objects from the client's head and limbs.
3. Procedure:
   A. Scalp electrodes are placed over the sensory cortex of the scalp on the side opposite that to be stimulated.
   B. Small painless electrical stimuli are administered to large sensory fibers in the median or posterior tibial nerves.
   C. The afferent volley is recorded as well as waves that reflect peripheral nerve trunk activity.
4. Postprocedure care:
   A. Remove electrodes from the scalp and cleanse it of electroconductive gel.
5. Client and family teaching:
   A. The hair should be clean, dry, and free of hair spray or other hair fixatives.
   B. Small painless electrical stimuli are administered to peripheral nerves. The brain's response is recorded via scalp electrodes.
6. Factors that affect results:
   A. The client must be able to lie motionless during the test.
   B. Results must be compared with the norms of the laboratory performing the test, as different variations of the test will be performed, depending on the client's history and the purpose of the test.
   C. Complete lesion of the spinal cord results in no SEP recording when nerves distal to the lesion are stimulated.
   D. Lesions between the stimulated nerve and the thalamus increase the latency of the SEP.
   E. Lesions of the somatosensory cortex reduce the amplitude of the SEP wave.
   F. SEPs are a useful diagnostic tool for infants and children; however, growth and maturation of the nervous system complicate the technical application and interpretation of the results.
   G. SEP examines a restricted anatomic pathway and does not reflect general brainstem or cerebral function.
7. Other data:
   A. This test is unaffected by general anesthesia, medications, and metabolic abnormalities.

Bibliography:

Gilmore R: Somatosensory evoked potential testing in infants. J Clin Neurophysiol 9(3):324–341, 1992.
Jordan KG: Continuous EEG and evoked potential monitoring in the neuroscience intensive care unit. J Clin Neurophysiol 10(4):445–475, 1993.

SOMATOTROPIN, BLOOD
(see Growth Hormone, Blood)

SPECIFIC GRAVITY, URINE

Norm:

		SI Units
Adults	1.016–1.022	1.016–1.022
No fluids for 12 hours	1.007–1.030	1.007–1.030
No fluids for 24 hours	≥1.026 indicates normal renal concentrating ability	
Stress conditions	1.001–1.040	1.001–1.040
Newborn	1.012	1.012
Infants	1.002–1.006	1.002–1.006

Increased: Adrenal insufficiency, bactiuria, congestive heart failure, diabetes mellitus, diarrhea, fever, fluid volume deficit, glomerulonephritis, obstruction uropathy, proteinuria, syndrome of inappropriate antidiuretic hormone secretion (SIADHS), toxemia of pregnancy, and vomiting. Drugs include dextran, radiographic contrast media, and sucrose.

Decreased: Chronic renal insufficiency, diabetes insipidus, fluid volume excess, hypothermia, intracranial pressure increase, and malignant hypertension. Drugs include aminoglycosides, carbenoxolone, lithium, and methoxyflurane.

Description: Specific gravity is the ratio of the density of urine compared to the density of an equal volume of water, which has a density of 1.000. Specific gravity is dependent on the number, size and weight of urine solutes (chloride, creatinine, glucose, phosphates, protein, sodium, sulfates, urea, uric acid) dissolved in solvent. Specific gravity evaluates the kidneys' ability to regulate fluid balance, as well as the hydration status of the body.

Professional Considerations:

1. Consent form NOT required.
2. Preparation:
   A. Obtain a calibrated hydrometer (urinometer) or a temperature-compensated refractometer and a random urine specimen.
3. Procedure:
   A. Urinometer procedure:
      i. The urinometer should be clean and dry prior to use.
      ii. Place the urinometer on a level surface and fill it with 15 ml of urine.
      iii. Insert a glass cylinder into the urinometer, using a spinning motion.
      iv. When the spinning stops, read the base meniscus, avoiding surface bubbles.
      v. Subtract 0.001 from the reading for every 3°C room temperature below 20°C to determine the specific gravity. Alternatively, add 0.001 to the reading for every 3°C room temperature above 20°C to determine the specific gravity.
      vi. For every 1 g/dl proteinuria, subtract 0.003 from the specific gravity.
      vii. For every 1 g/dl glucosuria, subtract 0.004 from the specific gravity.
   B. Refractometer procedure:
      i. Clean the cover and prism with a drop of distilled water and allow them to dry.
      ii. Close the cover.
      iii. Hold the instrument horizontally.
      iv. Apply a drop of urine at the notched bottom of the cover so that the drop flows over the prism surface.
      v. Point the instrument toward a light.
      vi. Rotate the eyepiece until the scale is in focus.
      vii. Read the specific gravity between the sharp dividing line of the dark and light contrast.

4. Postprocedure care:
   A. Cleanse the urinometer.
5. Client and family teaching:
   A. Give instructions about obtaining a urine specimen.
6. Factors that affect results:
   A. The reading is invalid if the glass cylinder touches the sides or bottom of the urinometer while the meniscus is being read.
   B. The urine specimen must be at room temperature.
7. Other data:
   A. The urinometer needs to be calibrated in order to produce accurate readings.

Bibliography:

Gibbs TD: Health assessment of the adult urology patient. *In* Karlowicz KA (ed) Urological Nursing: Principles and Practice. Philadelphia, WB Saunders, 1994.

Gouyon JB, Houchan N: Assessment of urine specific gravity by reagent strip test in newborn infants. Ped Nephrol 7(1):77–78, 1993.

SPECT SCAN, BRAIN
(see Single Photon Emission Computed Tomography, Brain, Diagnostic)

SPEECH AUDIOMETRY
(see Audiometry Test, Diagnostic)

SPERM COUNT, SPECIMEN
(see Infertility Screen, Specimen and Semen Analysis, Specimen)

SPHINGOMYELINASE, DIAGNOSTIC

Norm: 1.53–7.18 U/g.

Increased: Not clinically significant.

Decreased: Niemann-Pick disease, Types A and B.

Description: Sphingomyelinase is an enzyme that acts as a catalyst in the metabolism of sphingomyelin. Sphingomyelin is a phospholipid ubiquitously distributed in all membranes of mammalian cells and in serum lipoproteins. Niemann-Pick disease is an autosomal recessive lysosome storage disease caused by sphingomyelinase deficiency. Massive tissue accumulation of sphingomyelin results. Two types of Niemann-Pick disease have been identified: Type A—a severe, neurodegenerative infantile form leading to death by age 4; and Type B—a chronic, non-neurono-pathic form. A subacute form, similar to Type B but with mild neuronal involvement (retinal storage, peripheral neuropathy, mild neurologic changes, or psychiatric disorders) has also been identified. In this test, a skin biopsy is used to perform fibroblast tissue culture and fibroblast assay for sphingomyelinase activity.

Professional Considerations:

1. Consent form NOT required.
2. Preparation:
    A. Obtain a skin punch biopsy setup and a sterile plastic cup.
3. Procedure:
    A. Cleanse the biopsy site with alcohol and allow it to air-dry.
    B. Obtain a skin punch biopsy with a 4-mm punch.
4. Postprocedure care:
    A. Place the biopsy specimen in a sterile cup.
5. Client and family teaching:
    A. A mild analgesic may be used for site tenderness.
    B. Contact the physician for redness, swelling, increasing tenderness, purulent drainage, or slow healing noted at the site.
    C. Genetic counseling must be provided for individuals and families undergoing genetic testing.
6. Factors that affect results:
    A. Inadequate punch biopsy specimen may cause false-negative results.
7. Other data:
    A. Timeliness of results depends on laboratory availability.

Bibliography:

Ferlinz K, Hurwitz R, Weiler M, et al.: Molecular analysis of the acid sphingomyelinase deficiency in a family with an intermediate form of Niemann-Pick disease. Am J Hum Genet 56:1343–1349, 1995.

Spence MW: Sphingomyelinases. Adv Lipid Res 26:3–23, 1993.

Taki T, Chatterjee S: An improved method for the measurement and detection of sphingomyelinase activity. Anal Biochem 224:490–493, 1995.

SPINAL PUNCTURE
(see Lumbar Puncture, Diagnostic)

SPIROMETRY, DIAGNOSTIC

Norm: Forced vital capacity, forced expiratory volumes, and peak expiratory flow rates are at predicted value for age.

Usage: Asthma, bronchitis, chronic obstructive pulmonary disease (COPD), emphysema, and myasthenia gravis.

Description: A spirometer is an instrument that measures lung capacity, volume, and flow rates. The instrument consists of a bell suspended in a container of water. The bell rises and falls in response to the client's breathing. The movement of the bell is recorded on a kymograph or electrical potentiometer.

Professional Considerations:

1. Consent form NOT required.
2. Preparation:
    A. Assess baseline vital signs.
    B. Obtain a spirometer, recording paper, a mouthpiece, and a nose clip.
    C. *See Client and family teaching.*
3. Procedure:
    A. Connect the mouthpiece to the spirometer and place the mouthpiece in the client's mouth.
    B. Place the clip over the nose so that only breathing through the mouth is possible.
4. Postprocedure care:
    A. Assess vital signs q 5 minutes until they return to baseline.
    B. The client may resume bronchodilator medication if no further (same day) pulmonary testing is indicated or planned.
5. Client and family teaching:
    A. Withhold bronchodilator medication for 5 hours before the test.
    B. Take a maximal inhalation, hold it, then maximally and forcibly exhale.
    C. After a short rest period, the procedure is repeated two more times.
    D. The procedure takes 15 minutes.
6. Factors that affect results:
    A. An ineffective nose clip causes unreliable results.
    B. The client must be able to cooperate to obtain meaningful results.
7. Other data:
    A. A modified technique with an initial forced exhalation followed by a relaxed exhalation continued for as long as possible may be used.

Bibliography:

Johns DP, Abramson M, Bowes G: Evaluation of a new ambulatory spirometer for measuring forced expiratory volume in one second and peak expiratory flow rate. Am Rev Respir Dis 147:1245–1250, 1993.

Stoller JK, Basheda S, Laskowski D, et al.: Trial of standard versus modified expiration to achieve end-of-test spirometry criteria. Am Rev Respir Dis 148(2):275–280, 1993.

SPLEEN ECHOGRAM
(see Spleen Sonogram, Diagnostic)

SPLEEN SCAN, DIAGNOSTIC

Norm: Homogenous distribution of the radiolabeled erythrocytes throughout the spleen.

Usage: Evaluation of the size, shape, and location of the spleen in suspected congenital anomalies, in cancer, or following trauma.

Description: The spleen scan is a nuclear medicine examination of the left upper quadrant of the abdomen after intravenous administration of either technetium-99m-labeled or chromium-51-labeled, heat-treated, red blood cells. Because erythrocytes are sequestered by the spleen, the radiolabeled cell accumulation in the spleen can be identified with the scinticounter.

Professional Considerations:

1. Consent form IS required.

Risks:
Hematoma, infection.

Contraindications:
Inability to lie motionless during the scan; during pregnancy or breast-feeding.

2. Preparation:
   A. Establish intravenous access.
   B. Have emergency equipment available for potential anaphylaxis.
3. Procedure:
   A. A 5-ml sample of the client's blood is removed with a heparinized syringe via venipuncture. It is heat treated and labeled with the selected radionuclide in the nuclear medicine department.
   B. The labeled blood is injected via the established intravenous access into the client.
   C. After 1 hour, scintiscans are taken of the left upper quadrant of the abdomen from anterior, posterior, left lateral, and oblique views.
   D. Scanning is repeated in 24 hours.
4. Postprocedure care:
   A. Observe the individual for 1 hour after the study for possible anaphylactic reaction to the radionuclide.
   B. General body substance isolation precautions protect the health care professional from potential radiation exposure.
5. Client and family teaching:
   A. Technetium half-life is 6 hours. Chromium-51 half-life is 27.8 days.
   B. General body substance isolation pre-

cautions protect the client's family from potential radiation exposure.
6. Factors that affect results:
   A. Impaired hepatic function causes a greater than normal splenic uptake of the labeled cells.
   B. Hematoma, infarct, abscess, or tumor causes decreased uptake.
   C. Amyloidosis, sarcoidosis, or granulomas may cause many filling defects.
7. Other data:
   A. This test may be performed in conjunction with a liver scan.
   B. Health care professionals working in a nuclear medicine area must follow federal standards set by the Nuclear Regulatory Commission. These standards include precautions for handling the radioactive material and monitoring of potential radiation exposure.

Bibliography:

Bakir M, Bilgic A, Ozmen M, et al.: The value of radionuclide splenic scanning in the evaluation of asplenia in patients with heterotaxy. Pediatr Radiol 2425–2428, 1994.

SPLEEN SONOGRAM (SPLEEN ECHOGRAM, SPLEEN ULTRASOUND), DIAGNOSTIC

Norm: Proper size, shape, and position of the spleen. Negative for abscess, cyst, tumor, or splenomegaly. Spleen tissue stipples with fine, homogenous, low-level echoes. Spleen is not visualized until the transducer reaches 9–11 cm above the umbilicus.

Usage: Assessment of status following trauma; detection of and/or differentiation of splenic abnormalities such as abscess or cyst; and ongoing monitoring of the spleen during medical therapy.

Description: Evaluation of the spleen's size, shape, and position via the creation of an oscilloscopic picture from the echoes of high-frequency sound waves passing over the abdominal area (acoustic imaging). The time required for the ultrasonic beam to be reflected back to the transducer from differing densities of tissue is converted by a computer to an electrical impulse displayed on an oscilloscopic screen to create a three-dimensional picture of the spleen. The echomorphology of splenic lesions assists in the diagnosis of the lesion and can be described as isoechogenic, hyperechogenic, hypoechogenic, or complex in comparison to the normal spleen echogenicity. The differing tissue densities of specific lesions assists in the diagnosis of the lesion.

Professional Considerations:
1. Consent form NOT required.
2. Preparation:
   A. This test should be performed before intestinal barium tests, or after the barium is cleared from the system.
   B. Obtain ultrasonic gel or paste.
   C. *See Client and family teaching.*
3. Procedure:
   A. The client is positioned supine in a bed or on a procedure table.
   B. The skin overlying the spleen is covered with ultrasonic gel and a lubricated transducer is passed slowly and firmly over the left upper quadrant of the abdomen at various angles and at specific intervals 1–2 cm apart. The transducer is passed between rather than over the ribs. This may be performed with the client in several positions. The right lateral decubitus position provides the best information.
   C. Photographs are taken of the oscilloscopic display.
4. Postprocedure care:
   A. Wipe the ultrasonic gel from the skin.
5. Client and family teaching:
   A. Fast from food and fluids overnight (when possible), and abstain from smoking for several hours prior to the test.
   B. The procedure is painless and carries no risks.
   C. The procedure takes less than 30 minutes.
6. Factors that affect results:
   A. Dehydration interferes with adequate contrast between organs and body fluids.
   B. Intestinal barium, food, or gas (particularly in the supine position) obscures the results by preventing the proper transmission and deflection of the high-frequency sound waves.
7. Other data:
   A. Further testing may include tomography or magnetic resonance imaging.

Bibliography:
Gorg C, Weide R, Schwerk WB, Loppler H, et al.: Ultrasound evaluation of hepatic and splenic microabcesses in the immunocompromised patient: Sonographic patterns, differential diagnosis and follow-up. J Clin Ultrasound 22:525–529, 1994.

Kessler A, Mitchell DG, Israel HL, et al.: Hepatic and splenic sarcoidosis: ultrasound and MR imaging. Abdom Imaging 18:159–163, 1993.

Tsuda K, Nakamura H, Murakami T, et al.: Peliosis of the spleen with intraperitoneal hemorrhage. Abdom Imaging 18:283–285, 1993.

SPLEEN ULTRASOUND
(see Spleen Sonogram, Diagnostic)

SPLENOPORTOGRAPHY, DIAGNOSTIC

Norm: Splenic pulp pressure: 50–180 mm H_2O or 3.5–13.5 mmHg. Smooth flow of dye through the splenic venous system, without obstruction or diversion. Timely flow of the dye through the hepatic portal system, without evidence of collateral veins.

Usage: Cirrhosis, hepatocellular carcinoma, and portal hypertension.

Description: Splenoportography is the radiographic examination of the venous system of the spleen and portal system of the liver after injection of contrast media directly into the splenic vein. The measurement of splenic pulp pressure prior to dye injection helps detect portal hypertension.

Professional Considerations:
1. Consent form IS required.

Risks:
Allergic reaction to contrast media (itching, hives, rash, tight feeling in the throat, shortness of breath, anaphylaxis); renal toxicity from contrast medium; hemorrhage requiring blood transfusion and/or splenectomy.

Contraindications:
Previous allergy to iodine, shellfish, or radiographic contrast media; renal insufficiency; ascites, coagulation disorders, impaired hepatic or renal function, or splenic infection. Sedatives are contraindicated in clients with central nervous system depression.

---

2. Preparation:
   A. Establish intravenous access.
   B. Assess platelet count, prothrombin time (PT), partial thromboplastin time (PTT), urea nitrogen, creatinine, and liver enzymes.
   C. Administer a sedative and an analgesic, as prescribed, 30 minutes prior to the test.
   D. Obtain antiseptic, sterile drapes, 1–2% lidocaine (Xylocaine) local anesthetic, a percutaneous injection tray, a manometer, contrast medium, and material for a dry, sterile dressing.
   E. *See Client and family teaching.*

3. Procedure:
   A. The client is positioned supine with the left hand under the head.
   B. The left sides of the thorax and abdomen are washed with an antiseptic.
   C. The spleen is located via fluoroscopy.
   D. The puncture site is marked, usually the ninth or tenth intercostal space at the mid- or post-axillary line.
   E. After local anesthesia is injected around the puncture site, a sheathed needle is inserted percutaneously into the spleen. The needle is removed and the sheath is connected to a spinal manometer for splenic pulp pressure measurement.
   F. After sheath placement is verified, radiographic contrast medium is injected through the splenic parenchyma into the splenic vein and cineradiographic films are taken to record splenic venous system filling.
   G. The needle is removed, and a dry, sterile dressing is applied to the puncture site.
   H. The procedure takes less than 1 hour.
4. Postprocedure care:
   A. Assess vital signs every 15 minutes × 4, then every 30 minutes × 4, then hourly × 4, then every 4 hours until 24 hours after the procedure.
   B. Observe for bleeding and swelling at the puncture site each time vital signs are taken.
5. Client and family teaching:
   A. Fast from food and fluids from midnight prior to the test.
   B. A sensation of warmth or flushing after the dye injection is normal and will be transient.
   C. Immediately report any left upper quadrant pain.
   D. The client must assume a left-side lying position × 24 hours.
   E. The client may resume previous diet after the procedure. The oral intake of fluids, where not contraindicated, is encouraged.
6. Factors that affect results:
   A. Cirrhosis causes delayed emptying of the intrahepatic radicles.
   B. Portal hypertension causes elevated splenic pulp pressure and evidence of the development of collateral veins.
7. Other data:
   A. The newer computed tomographic percutaneous transsplenic portography (CT-PTSP) utilizes thinner needles for splenic puncture and CT rather than cineradiography. The use of thinner needles decreases the amount of pain and the risk of hemorrhage associated with the procedure. CT has a higher contrast resolution and can thus detect a lower dose of contrast dye. CT-PTSP thus decreases the length of time that the client must be monitored and on bedrest after the procedure and allows the procedure to be performed on an outpatient basis.
   B. CT during arterial portography (CTAP) is an alternative method of visualizing the portal venous system.

Bibliography:

Conn HO, Atterbury CE: Cirrhosis. *In* Schiff L, Shiff ER (eds): Diseases of the Liver, 7th ed. Philadelphia, JB Lippincott, 1993, pp 875–934.

Sawada S, Nakamura K, Tanigawa N, et al.: Computed tomographic transcutaneous transsplenic portography. Acta Radiol *34*(5):529–531, 1993.

SPONDEE THRESHOLD SPEECH TEST, DIAGNOSTIC

Norm: Spondee threshold differs 510 decibels (db) within pure tone audiometry threshold.

Usage: Evaluates the ability to hear conversational speech and provides more specific evaluation after abnormal pure tone audiometry results.

Description: Spondees are two-syllable words (i.e., baseball, airplane) presented to a client through earphones to measure the lowest level at which the client repeats 50% of the words. This test measures degree of hearing loss and is often performed following audiometric testing.

Professional Considerations:

1. Consent form NOT required.
2. Preparation:
   A. Obtain a speech audiometer, earphones, and a recorded spondee list.
3. Procedure:
   A. Explain to the client that a series of two-syllable words in decreasing loudness will be transmitted through the earphones. The client should repeat these words when he or she hears them to the best of his or her ability.
4. Postprocedure care:
   A. A client with abnormal results should be referred to an audiologist.
5. Client and family teaching:
   A. The earphones are placed over the client's ears, and testing proceeds as described above, with only one ear tested at a time.
6. Factors that affect results:
   A. Unfamiliarity with the language or words used may make the results unreliable.
   B. This test is unreliable in young children who do not yet have fully developed speech.
7. Other data:
   A. *See also Audiometry Test, Diagnostic.*

Bibliography:

Browning GG, Swan IR, Chew KK: Clinical role of informal tests of hearing. J Laryngol Otol *103*(1): 7–11, 1989.

Macpherson BJ, Elfenbein JL, Schum RL, et al.: Thresholds of discomfort in young children. Ear Hear *12*(3):184–190, 1991.

Rei G, Fu BT: Diagnostic significance of the staggered spondaic word test and 40-Hz auditory event—related potentials. Audiology *27*(1):8–16, 1988.

SPUTUM, FUNGUS, CULTURE

Norm: No growth.

Usage: AIDS, actinomyces, aspergillosis, candidiasis, coccidioidomycosis, fungal infections, histoplasmosis, neoplastic disease, and pneumonia.

Description: Fungi are slow-growing, eukaryotic organisms that can grow on living and nonliving organic materials and are subdivided into yeasts and molds. Only a few fungi species infect humans. Normal host defense mechanisms limit the damage these fungi cause superficially. When inhaled or inoculated deep into tissues, or when acquired by an immunocompromised client, fungi can cause serious infections.

Professional Considerations:

1. Consent form NOT required.
2. Preparation:
   A. A first morning specimen is preferred because it represents overnight secretions of the tracheobronchial tree.
   B. Obtain a sterile plastic container or a sputum trap.
3. Procedure:
   A. Obtain 1–3 ml of sputum in a sterile container and cover it with a lid, or obtain a specimen in a sputum trap.
4. Postprocedure care:
   A. Refrigerate the specimen or deliver it to the laboratory within 1 hour.
   B. Preliminary reports will be available in 48–72 hours and negative reports after 4 weeks.
5. Client and family teaching:
   A. Cough deeply and expectorate 5–10 ml of sputum into a sterile plastic container and then cap it tightly. Deep coughs are necessary to produce sputum, rather than saliva. To produce the proper specimen, take several breaths in, without fully exhaling each, then expel sputum with a "cascade cough."
6. Factors that affect results:
   A. A contaminated specimen cup invalidates the results.
7. Other data:
   A. Pathogenic fungi include *Alternaria*,

Aspergillus, Blastomyces dermatitis, Candida, Coccidioides immitis, Cryptococcus, Histoplasma capsulatum, Monilia, Mucor, Penicillium, Rhizopus, Scopuleriopsis, and *Sporothrix schenckii.*
   B. A single negative culture does not rule out a fungal infection.

Bibliography:

Flournoy DJ: Sputum specimen quality. Chest *106*(6): 1930, 1994.

Keating JJ, Rogers T, Petrou M, et al.: Management of pulmonary aspergillosis in AIDS: An emerging clinical problem. J Clin Pathol *47*(9):805–809, 1994.

SPUTUM, GRAM STAIN, DIAGNOSTIC
(see Gram Stain, Diagnostic)

SPUTUM, MYCOBACTERIA, CULTURE

Norm: No growth.

Usage: Acquired immune deficiency syndrome, hemoptysis, mycobacteria, splenomegaly, and tuberculosis.

Description: Mycobacteria are rod-shaped, aerobic bacteria that resist decolorizing chemicals after staining, hence "acid-fast." A number of new species of nontuberculous mycobacteria (or new components of species complexes) as well as multiple drug-resistant isolates of *M. tuberculosis* have been recognized. Mycobacteria species are capable of producing human disease characterized by destructive granulomas that can necrose, ulcerate, and cavitate. *M. tuberculosis* is transmitted via the airborne route, most commonly to the lungs, where it survives well, causes areas of granulomatous inflammation and, if not dormant, causes cough, fever, and hemoptysis. In this test, an acid-fast culture and stain of sputum are performed to detect mycobacteria.

Professional Considerations:

1. Consent form NOT required.
2. Preparation:
   A. A first morning specimen is preferred because it represents an accumulation of overnight secretions of the tracheobronchial tree.
   B. Obtain a sterile plastic cup with a lid.
3. Procedure:
   A. Sputum may be induced by inhalation of hypertonic saline aerosol.

B. Laryngeal swabs and gastric isolates may also be useful in individuals unable to produce sputum or cooperate with induction procedures.

4. Postprocedure care:
   A. Refrigerate the specimens if not delivered to the laboratory within an hour.
   B. A preliminary report is available in 72 hours, the final report in 4–6 weeks.

5. Client and family teaching:
   A. Cough deeply and expectorate 5–10 ml of sputum into a sterile plastic container and then cap it tightly. Deep coughs are necessary to produce sputum, rather than saliva. To produce the proper specimen, take several breaths in, without fully exhaling each, then expel sputum with a "cascade cough."
   B. Repeat the procedure for three consecutive mornings.

6. Factors that affect results:
   A. Contamination of the specimen invalidates the results.
   B. An insufficient sputum amount may cause false-negative results.

7. Other data:
   A. Because 5–10 ml of sputum are required, the specimen may be collected over a 2-hour period. However, a 24-hour period is unacceptable.
   B. Bronchial washings often do not contain enough sputum, as they are diluted with anesthetics and irrigating fluid.

Bibliography:

Witebsky FG, Conville PS: The laboratory diagnosis of mycobacterial diseases. Infect Dis Clin North Am 7(2):359–375, 1993.

SPUTUM, ROUTINE, CULTURE

(see Culture, Routine, Specimen)

SPUTUM ACID FAST BACTERIA (AFB), CULTURE

(see Acid Fast Bacteria, Culture and Stain)

SPUTUM CULTURE AND SENSITIVITY (C & S), SPECIMEN

(see Culture, Routine, Specimen)

SPUTUM CYTOLOGY, SPECIMEN

(see Cytologic Study of Respiratory Tract, Diagnostic)

SPUTUM FOR *HAEMOPHILUS* SPECIES, CULTURE

Norm: No *Haemophilus* species isolated.

Positive: Chronic bronchitis, epiglottitis, *Haemophilus influenzae*, meningitis, otitis media, and pneumonia.

Negative: Viral pulmonary disease.

Description: The gram-negative *Haemophilus* coccobacillus is the leading cause of pediatric otitis, meningitis, epiglottitis, and adult pneumonia.

Professional Considerations:

1. Consent form NOT required.
2. Preparation:
   A. A first morning specimen is preferred because it represents overnight secretions of the tracheobronchial tree.
   B. Obtain a sterile plastic cup with a lid.
3. Procedure:
   A. Obtain 3–5 ml of sputum in a sterile container and cover it with a lid, or obtain a specimen in a sputum trap.
4. Client and family teaching:
   A. Cough deeply and expectorate 3–5 ml of sputum into a sterile plastic container and then cap it tightly.
5. Postprocedure care:
   A. Refrigerate the specimen within 2 hours of collection.
   B. Results are normally available within 24 hours, the final report within 48 hours.
6. Factors that affect results:
   A. Specimens over 2 hours old and not refrigerated may cause false-negative results.
7. Other data:
   A. 5–15% of *Haemophilus influenzae* pathogens produce penicillinase and therefore are resistant to treatment with ampicillin.

Bibliography:

Flournoy DJ, Adkins LJ, Laughlin KJ: Value of oral hygiene before expectoration of sputum for routine bacterial culture. Chest 107(6):1923, 1994.

Minocha A, Moravec CL: Gram's stain and culture of sputum in the routine management of pulmonary infection. S Med J 86(11):1225–1228, 1993.

SPUTUM HEMOSIDERIN PREPARATION, SPECIMEN

Norm: Negative.

Usage: Blood in the alveolar space.

Description: Hemosiderin are iron-storage granules normally found in the liver cytoplasm, spleen, and bone marrow. Hemosiderin is also a byproduct of macrophage degradation of erythrocytes. This test uses Prussian blue stain on a smear of sputum to detect the presence of hemosiderin in the lungs, representing previous alveolar hemorrhage (AH). AH has a variety of etiologies, including anti-basement-membrane-mediated diseases, pulmonary infection, and vasculitis. AH can also occur in immunocompromised people with invasive fungal pneumonia and thrombocytopenia and in people who have undergone heart transplantation for chronic congestive heart failure.

Professional Considerations:

1. Consent form NOT required.
2. Preparation:
   A. Obtain a sterile plastic sputum cup, a sterile container with a lid, glass slides, and a cytologic sputum fixative.
3. Procedure:
   A. Obtain a sputum specimen in a sterile plastic container.
4. Postprocedure care:
   A. Smear sputum on a glass slide and apply cytologic fixative. Place the slide in a sterile container and cap it tightly.
5. Client and family teaching:
   A. Cough deeply and expectorate 3–5 ml of sputum into a sterile plastic container. Deep coughs are necessary to produce sputum, rather than saliva. To produce the proper specimen, take several breaths in, without fully exhaling each, then expel sputum with a "cascade cough."
6. Factors that affect results:
   A. Failure to "fix" the specimen invalidates the results.
7. Other data:
   A. Results are available within hours but require interpretation with other clinical data.

Bibliography:

Grebski E, Hess T, Hold G, et al.: Diagnostic value of hemosiderin-containing macrophages in bronchoalveolar lavage. Chest *102*(6):1794–1799, 1992.

Merrill WW: Bronchoalveolar lavage: Let's focus on clinical utility. Chest *102*(6):1641, 1992.

ST. LOUIS ENCEPHALITIS VIRUS SEROLOGY, SERUM

Norm: A less than fourfold rise in titer between acute and convalescent samples.

Usage: Hemagglutination titer <1:10. Complement fixation titer <1:8.

Description: St. Louis encephalitis virus is a group B arbovirus, a member of flavivirus, that is transmitted to humans by the bite of infected mosquitos, with the donor host being birds. This virus causes inflammation of the tissues of the central nervous system. Symptoms may range from mild headache and fever to encephalitis and death. This virus occurs in the western, central, and southern United States, and in Jamaica, Panama, Brazil, and Trinidad.

Professional Considerations:

1. Consent form NOT required.
2. Preparation:
   A. Tube: Red-top, red/gray-top, or gold-top.
   B. Specimens MAY be drawn during hemodialysis.
3. Procedure:
   A. Draw a 7-ml blood sample as soon as possible after symptoms appear, and label it as the acute sample.
   B. Repeat the test in 10–14 days, and label the tube as the convalescent sample.
4. Postprocedure care:
   A *See Client and family teaching.*
5. Client and family teaching:
   A. Return in 10–14 days to have a convalescent sample drawn, which is necessary to interpret the results of the acute sample.
6. Factors that affect results:
   A. Failure to collect a convalescent sample.
   B. False-positive results may occur in clients recently vaccinated for yellow fever.
7. Other data:
   A. 10–15% of clients with St. Louis encephalitis do not develop complement fixation antibodies.
   B. There is no specific treatment for this disease.
   C. Universal precautions and vector-control practices are adequate to prevent spread of this disease.

Bibliography:

Anonymous: Arboviral disease—United States 1994. Morbidity and Mortality Weekly Report *44*(35): 641–644, 1995.

Anonymous: Rapid assessment of vector borne diseases during the Midwest flood—United States, 1993. Morbidity and Mortality Weekly Report *43*(26):481–483, 1994.

Okhuysen PC, Crane JK, Pappas J: St. Louis encephalitis in patients with human immunodeficiency virus infection. Clin Infect Dis *17*(1):140–141, 1993.

STABLE FACTOR, BLOOD
(see Factor VII, Blood)

STEMLINE DNA ANALYSIS, SPECIMEN
(see DNA Ploidy, Specimen)

STEREOTACTIC BREAST BIOPSY, DIAGNOSTIC

Negative: Benign.

Positive: Atypical or malignant cells.

Description: Stereotactic breast biopsy is an x-ray guided method of localizing and sampling nonpalpable breast lesions discovered on mammography and considered to be suspicious for malignancy. The position of the lesion in the breast can be calculated relative to a fixed grid and a needle placed within the lesion with direct confirmation of its position on a stereotactic x-ray. The placement is accurate to within 2 mm. Stereotactic breast biopsy can be performed via fine-needle aspiration cytology or core needle histology.

Professional Considerations:

1. Consent form IS required.

Risks:

Bruising, infection at needle aspiration site.

Contraindications:

Large abnormal breast tissue area.

---

2. Preparation:
   A. This procedure is performed by a radiologist with mammographic experience.
   B. Equipment is assembled according to the type of biopsy (fine-needle aspiration or core needle) and the radiologist's preference.
   C. The client is assessed for any allergies, use of anticoagulants or antiplatelet agents, or bleeding disorders.
3. Procedure:
   A. The client is positioned prone on the x-ray table with the breasts hanging down for the mammogram films and biopsy.
   B. The skin is prepared according to the radiologist's preference and institutional policy.
   C. A local anesthetic is injected into the biopsy site.
   D. A small incision is made at the site of needle insertion.
   E. The needle is inserted into the lesion with placement confirmed by x-ray.

F. Multiple samples are taken from different positions in the lesion.
G. The specimen obtained from core needle biopsies is placed in formalin and sent immediately to the laboratory.
H. The specimen obtained from fine-needle aspiration is fixed on cytology slides and sent immediately to the laboratory.
4. Postprocedure care:
   A. Place steri-strips and a pressure dressing over the site.
5. Client and family teaching:
   A. The client may eat or drink as usual.
   B. The procedure generally takes 1 hour.
   C. Most individuals are able to return to their usual routine, including driving or work, after the procedure.
   D. The dressing may be removed the next day.
   E. There may be some tenderness, swelling, bruising, or slight bleeding at the site. An ice pack or nonaspirin pain reliever will help to relieve the above.
6. Factors that affect results:
   A. None found.
7. Other data:
   A. If inadequate tissue was obtained or if a malignancy is suspected but not confirmed, an open surgical biopsy is recommended. Open surgical biopsy is also recommended if atypical cells are identified.
   B. While complications from this procedure may include infection and hematoma, the complication rate is low.
   C. Results from either fine-needle aspiration or core needle biopsy are available within 24 hours.
   D. A one-year follow-up mammography is recommended for benign lesions.

Bibliography:

Rubin E, Dempsey PJ, Pile NS, et al.: Needle-localization biopsy of the breast: Impact of a selective core needle biopsy program on yield. Radiology *195*(3):627–631, 1995.

Schmidt RA: Stereotactic breast biopsy. CA *44*(3): 172–191, 1994.

Vazquez MF, Mitnick JS, Pressman P, et al.: Stereotactic aspiration biopsy of nonpalpable nodules of the breast. J Am Coll Surg *178*(1):17–23, 1994.

STOOL CULTURE, ROUTINE, STOOL

Norm: Negative for pathogens; no growth other than normal flora.

Usage: Coccidioidomycosis, dysentery, enteric fever, failure to thrive (fat, ova, and parasites), gastroenteritis, salmonellosis, typhoid with salmonella, and ulcerative colitis.

Description: To screen for common enteric pathogens such as *Helicobacter, Salmonella, Shigella, Campylobacter,*

Vibrio, Yersinia, or *Clostridium difficile.* This test may be indicated in clients with persistent or bloody diarrhea accompanied by fever and/or recent out-of-country travel (to third-world country), in clients with a history of recent antibiotic usage, or in clients known to be exposed to enteric pathogens.

Professional Considerations:
1. Consent form NOT required.
2. Preparation:
   A. Obtain a bedpan or a plastic toilet-seat specimen hat, a wooden tongue blade, and a sterile container with a lid.
3. Procedure:
   A. Using a wooden tongue blade, place a fresh stool sample 1 inch in diameter in a sterile container and cap it tightly.
4. Postprocedure care:
   A. Send the specimen to the laboratory immediately.
   B. If there will be a 2- or 3-hour delay before testing, place the specimen in a transport medium such as buffered saline-glycol or alkaline peptone water.
5. Client and family teaching:
   A. Defecate in a bedpan or toilet-seat specimen hat, and avoid contaminating the stool with urine, toilet tissue, soap, or water.
6. Factors that affect results:
   A. Refrigerate the specimens if they are not sent to the laboratory immediately.
   B. Barium or mineral oil inhibit bacterial growth.
   C. Keep the specimens free of toilet tissue, bismuth, soap, water, or urine, as these speed up deterioration of ova.
7. Other data:
   A. Rectal swabs can be used, but they are less likely to yield positive results.
   B. *Vibrio parahaemolyticus,* a marine bacterium, causes gastrointestinal symptoms due to improperly refrigerated crab, lobster, or shrimp.
   C. *Vibrio cholerae,* rice-watery in appearance with a fishy odor, causes both epidemic and environmental cholera.
   D. *Helicobacter pylori* has been cultured from the diarrheal stools of infected individuals in developing countries. Immigration is responsible for the development of isolated areas of high prevalence in some Western countries.
   E. The optimal specimen for the diagnosis of *C. difficile*-associated diarrhea is a watery or loose stool.
   F. Results are normally available in 48 hours.

Bibliography:
Liesenfeld O, Saeger F, Hahn H: Detection of *Clostridium difficile* toxin by enzyme immunoassay, tissue culture test and culture. Infection *22*(1): 29–31, 1994.

Peterson LR, Kelly PJ: The role of the clinical microbiology laboratory in the management of *Clostridium difficile*-associated diarrhea. Infect Dis Clin North Am *7*(2):277–290, 1993.

STOOL, FUNGUS, CULTURE

Norm: Negative for fungus; no growth.

Usage: Fungal infections and immunosuppressed clients.

Description: Fungi are slow-growing, eukaryotic organisms that can grow on living and nonliving organic materials and are subdivided into yeasts and molds. Only a few fungi species infect humans. Normal host defense mechanisms limit the damage these fungi cause superficially. This is a screening test performed on a sample of stool to determine the presence of fungi in clients at risk for fungal infection (those on antibiotic therapy, parenteral nutrition, and those who are immunocompromised).

Professional Considerations:
1. Consent form NOT required.
2. Preparation:
   A. Obtain a bedpan or a plastic toilet-seat specimen hat, a wooden tongue blade, and a sterile container with a lid.
3. Procedure:
   A. Using a wooden tongue blade, place a fresh stool sample 1 inch in diameter in a sterile container and cap it tightly.
4. Postprocedure care:
   A. Refrigerate the specimen if it is not sent to the laboratory immediately.
5. Client and family teaching:
   A. Defecate in a bedpan or toilet-seat specimen hat, and avoid contaminating the stool with urine, toilet tissue, soap, or water.
6. Factors that affect results:
   A. Dried specimens are not acceptable.
7. Other data:
   A. Negative cultures are reported after 1 week. Results may take 4 weeks if a systemic fungal infection is indicated.
   B. Fungi in stool may be *Aspergillus, Candida, Cryptococcus, Geotrichum, Histoplamosis, Rhodotorula,* or *Torulopsis* species.

Bibliography:
Friedman SL: GI manifestations of AIDS. *In* Sleisenger MH, Fordtran JS (eds): Gastrointestinal Diseases: Pathophysiology, Diagnosis, and Management, 5th ed. Philadelphia, WB Saunders, 1993, pp 239–267.

STOOL LEUKOCYTES, STOOL
(see Methylene Blue Stain, Stool)

STREPTODORNASE, SERUM

(see Antideoxyribonuclease B Titer, Serum)

STREPTOZYME, BLOOD

Norm: Titer <166 Todd units or <100 streptozyme units.

Positive: Bacterial endocarditis, glomerulonephritis, pharyngitis, reactive arthritis, recent streptococcal infection, rheumatic and connective tissue diseases, rheumatic fever, scarlet fever, and upper respiratory infections.

Negative: Hematuria.

Description: A nonspecific screening test for the detection of antibodies to multiple exoenzymes of various species of streptococci using a commercial reagent containing erythrocytes coated with streptococcal antigens (Dnase, streptokinase, streptolysin-O, and hyaluronidase). This test can determine current or recent streptococcal infection earlier than the ASO titer, but cannot determine the location or type of streptococcal infection. In a positive test, antibodies begin rising by week 3 after infection and decrease by week 10.

Professional Considerations:

1. Consent form NOT required.
2. Preparation:
   A. Tube: Red-top, red/gray-top, or gold-top.
   B. Specimens MAY be drawn during hemodialysis.
3. Procedure:
   A. Draw a 1-ml blood sample as soon as possible after symptoms appear, and label it as the acute sample.
4. Postprocedure care:
   A. Repeat testing in 10 days, and label the tube as the convalescent sample.
   B. Subsequent samples, taken biweekly for the next 4–6 weeks, are recommended.
5. Client and family teaching:
   A. Serial testing is recommended.
6. Factors that affect results:
   A. Antibiotic therapy may cause decreased results.
7. Other data:
   A. Serial testing over a period of weeks is more significant than a single determination.
   B. This test is not as sensitive in children as it is in adults.
   C. *See also Antistreptolysin O Titer, Blood.*

Bibliography:

Gray GC, Struewing JP, Hyams KC, et al.: Interpreting a single antistreptolysin O test: A comparison of the "upper limit of normal" and likelihood ratio methods. J Clin Epidemiol 46(10):1181–1185, 1993.

Valtonen JM, Koskimies S, Miettinen A, et al.: Various syndromes in adult patients associated with high antistreptolysin O titres and their differential diagnosis with rheumatic fever. Ann Rheum Dis 52:527–530, 1993.

STRESS/EXERCISE TEST, DIAGNOSTIC

Norm: Negative.

Usage: Coronary artery disease; evaluation of cardiopulmonary fitness and exercise tolerance; assessment of the efficacy of interventions such as coronary artery bypass graft, coronary angioplasty, medications and cardiac rehabilitation; dysrhythmias; and valvular competence.

Description: Stress testing measures the efficiency of the heart during a period of physical stress on a treadmill or on a stationary bicycle. The effects of exercise on cardiac output and myocardial oxygen consumption are evaluated by concurrently monitoring electrocardiograms, blood pressure, and oxygen consumption. An advantage of exercise testing is that it can identify (in a safe environment) individuals prone to cardiac ischemia during activity, when resting electrocardiograms are normal.

Professional Considerations:

1. Consent form IS required.

Risks:

Cardiac ischemia, including myocardial infarction, dysrhythmias, hypotension, hypertension, dizziness.

Contraindications:

Active unstable angina, recent significant changes in ECG, alcohol intoxication, uncontrolled dysrhythmias, chest pain, acute infection, cardiac inflammation (myocarditis, pericarditis), acute congestive heart failure, coronary insufficiency syndrome, digitalis toxicity, heart blocks (2°, 3°), thrombophlebitis, recent pulmonary embolism, inability to walk on a treadmill or pedal a bicycle.

2. Preparation:
   A. Have emergency equipment readily available.
   B. *See Client and family teaching.*
3. Procedure:
   A. The stress test is performed by specially trained (i.e., ACLS certified) nurses, exercise physiologists, and physical therapists. The American Association of Cardiovascular and Pulmonary Rehabilitation has recommended direct physician supervision of all initial stress tests and tests for individuals considered at high risk for complications.
   B. Attach electrocardiogram leads and a blood pressure cuff.
   C. While the client is on a treadmill, stationary bicycle, or stair stepper, computerized electrocardiographic recordings and blood pressure readings are obtained. Oxygen consumption may be measured by having the client breathe through a special mouthpiece during exercise.
   D. The client is stressed in stages by increases in miles per hour and the percentage grade of elevation of the treadmill.
   E. The test is terminated when any of the following occurs:
      i. Signs of ischemia are present (ST segment depression of ≥1–2 mm for a duration >0.06 second, or ST segment elevation).
      ii. Maximum effort has been achieved.
      iii. A predetermined target has been achieved.
      iv. Dyspnea, hypertension >250 mmHg systolic blood pressure.
      v. Tachycardia >200 minus the client's age.
      vi. New dysrhythmias, new conduction disturbances (i.e., heart block), or increasing ectopy.
      vii. Chest pain with or without ECG changes.
      viii. Faintness, weakness, dizziness, or confusion.
      ix. Blood pressure fails to rise as body exercise stress increases.
      x. Extreme fatigue, or request by the client that the test be stopped.
4. Postprocedure care:
   A. The client should be monitored at rest until the heart rate, blood pressure, and electrocardiogram are at baseline.
   B. Remove the electrodes and the blood pressure cuff.
5. Client and family teaching:
   A. Wear flat walking or tennis shoes and comfortable attire.
   B. According to physician preference and instructions, gradually discontinue beta-blocker drugs prior to the test.
   C. Fast from food and fluids, and refrain from smoking and caffeine usage, for 4 hours prior to the test.
   D. Clients may take all of their medications as usual.
   E. During the test, immediately report any chest pain, dizziness, lightheadedness, nausea, or discomfort you experience to the technician.
   F. After the test, rest for a few hours at home.
6. Factors that affect results:
   A. False-positive electrocardiogram responses are caused by anemia, baseline ECG abnormalities, digitalis, diuretics, estrogen, hypertension, hypoxia, left bundle branch block, left ventricular hypertrophy, Lown-Ganong-Levine syndrome, syndrome X in women, or valvular heart disease.
   B. False-positive results occur more frequently in women than in men.
   C. False-negative tests occur when individuals with known significant CAD fail to demonstrate exercise-induced ST segment depression.
   D. Conditions that may affect performance include lung disease, muscle pain, and electrolyte imbalances.
7. Other data:
   A. Ischemic ST segment displacement >0.1 mm of 80 ms duration during exercise but not found at rest means a five times greater risk of coronary heart disease in males.
   B. Exertional hypotension may indicate left coronary artery disease, myocardial ischemia, or left ventricular dysfunction.
   C. The exercise stress test may also be performed with radionuclide (thallium) or radiopharmaceutical (sestamibi) perfusion studies. See *Heart Scan, Diagnostic.*
   D. *See also Stress Test, Pharmacologic, Diagnostic.*

Bibliography:

Franklin BA: Diagnostic and functional exercise testing: Test selection and interpretation. J Cardiovasc Nurs *10*(1):8–29, 1995.

Ryan PT: Physiologic responses to forward and retrograde simulated stair stepping. Arch Phys Med Rehabil *75*(7):798–802, 1994.

STRESS TEST, PHARMACOLOGIC, DIAGNOSTIC

Norm: Negative.

Usage: Coronary artery disease; detection of ischemia and assessment of myocardial viability; evaluation of left ventricular function; preoperative cardiac risk stratification; and valvular competence.

Description: Pharmacologic stress testing is used to evaluate individuals with suspected or proven coronary artery disease who are unable to perform satisfactory levels of exercise. A pharmacologic agent is used to elevate heart rate and blood pressure. The dobutamine echocardiographic stress test induces pharmacologic cardiac stress. Cardiac response is examined through an imaging technique. Dobutamine is a synthetic amine that increases myocardial contractility by directly stimulating cardiac α_1- and β_1-adrenergic receptors thereby increasing oxygen demand. When this occurs in the presence of an impaired oxygen supply, echocardiography can directly visualize myocardial wall motion abnormalities in individuals with fixed coronary artery stenosis.

Professional Considerations:

1. Consent form IS required.

Risks:

Cardiac ischemia, including myocardial infarction, dysrhythmias, hypotension, hypertension, dizziness.

Contraindications:

Active unstable angina, recent significant changes in ECG, uncontrolled dysrhythmias, severe aortic stenosis, uncontrolled hypertension, poor left ventricular function, chest pain, congestive heart failure.

2. Preparation:
   A. Have emergency equipment readily available.
   B. Establish intravenous access.
   C. *See Client and family teaching.*
3. Procedure:
   A. The stress test is performed by specially trained (i.e., ACLS certified) nurses and echocardiographers. The American Association of Cardiovascular and Pulmonary Rehabilitation has recommended direct physician supervision of all initial stress tests and tests for individuals considered at high risk for complications.
   B. Attach electrocardiogram leads and a blood pressure cuff.
   C. Obtain a baseline 12-lead ECG and blood pressure.
   D. The individual is placed in the best position to obtain echocardiographic images (usually left lateral decubitus), and baseline images are obtained.

E. Dobutamine is diluted according to institutional policy and procedure and administered via an infusion pump at an initial rate of 5 µg/kg/minute.
F. The infusion rate is increased every 3 minutes to 10, 20, and a maximum of 40 µg/kg/minute unless end points develop.
G. Heart rate and ECG rhythm strip are monitored continuously, and blood pressure and 12-lead ECG are recorded at each stage of drug infusion.
H. Continuous echocardiography is also performed. Direct recordings of images are made at rest, at midinfusion, at peak infusion, and at 1–2 minutes postinfusion.
I. The test is terminated when any of the following occurs:
   i. Signs of ischemia are present (ST segment depression of ≥1–2 mm for a duration >0.06 second, or ST segment elevation).
   ii. Heart rate >75–85% of predicted maximum for age.
   iii. Development of new wall motion abnormality.
   iv. Hypertension >210–260 mmHg systolic blood pressure or diastolic blood pressure >100 mmHg.
   v. New dysrhythmias.
   vi. Chest pain with or without ECG changes.
   vii. Symptomatic hypotension or blood pressure decrease more than 20 mmHg.
   viii. Heart rate decrease more than 20 beats per minute.
   ix. Prespecified dosage of dobutamine has been reached or target heart rate has been reached.
   x. The client requests to terminate test.
4. Postprocedure care:
   A. The client should be monitored until the heart rate, blood pressure, and electrocardiogram are at baseline.
   B. Remove the electrodes and the blood pressure cuff.
5. Client and family teaching:
   A. The entire procedure lasts approximately 60 minutes.
   B. According to physician preference and instructions, gradually discontinue beta-blocker drugs prior to the test. Antianginal agents may also be discontinued 24–48 hours before testing to maximize test sensitivity.
   C. Fast from food and fluids, and refrain from smoking and caffeine usage, for 4 hours prior to the test.
   D. Clients may take all of their medications as usual.
   E. The administration of dobutamine is associated with mild side effects such as chest tightness, dyspnea, flushing, nausea, headache, paresthesias, chills,

anxiety, or palpitations. Individuals are instructed to immediately report any side effects they experience to the technician. Side effects generally subside quickly after the dobutamine is discontinued.

6. Factors that affect results:
   A. Chest wall deformities, emphysema, and severe obesity limit visualization of the heart with transthoracic probes.

7. Other data:
   A. The half-life of dobutamine is 2 minutes.
   B. Side effects may be treated with intravenous beta-blockers.
   C. Abnormalities of ventricular contraction detected by echocardiography precede ECG signs or symptoms of ischemia.
   D. The adenosine or dipyridamole stress tests also induce pharmacologic cardiac stress that is examined through radionuclide (thallium, sestamibi) imaging. *See also Heart Scan, Diagnostic.*
   E. *See also Stress/Exercise Test, Diagnostic.*

Bibliography:

Daoud EG, Pitt A, Armstrong WF: Electrocardiographic response during dobutamine stress echocardiography. Am Heart J *129*(4):673–677, 1995.

Johns JP, Abraham SA, Eagle KA: Dipyridamole-thallium versus dobutamine echocardiographic stress testing: a clinician's viewpoint. Am Heart J *130*(2):373–385, 1995.

Latcham AP, Orsinelli DA, Pearson AC: Recognition of the segmental tendency of false-positive dobutamine stress echocardiograms and its effects on test sensitivity and specificity. Am Heart J *129*(5):1047–1050, 1995.

STRIATIONAL ANTIBODY, SPECIMEN

Norm: Negative, titer <60.

Positive: Autoimmune liver disorders, Lambert Eaton myasthenic syndrome, myasthenia gravis, myopathic disorders, and small cell lung carcinoma. Recipients of D-penicillamine and bone marrow allografts may have positive titers.

Description: Striational antibodies are immunoglobulins that react to contractile elements of skeletal muscle. They are detected by enzyme-linked immunoassay or immunofluorescence microscopy. Striational antibodies are a valuable marker of myasthenia gravis in the adult and are associated with thymoma. Their prevalence increases with the age of onset of myasthenia gravis. They are rarely positive at ages under 20.

Professional Considerations:

1. Consent form NOT required.
2. Preparation:
   A. Tube: Red-top, red/gray-top, or gold-top.
   B. Specimens MAY be drawn during hemodialysis.
3. Procedure:
   A. Draw a 7-ml blood sample.
4. Postprocedure care:
   A. None.
5. Client and family teaching:
   A. Results are normally available in 1 week.
6. Factors that affect results:
   A. None found.
7. Other data:
   A. Titer rarely positive in adolescence.

Bibliography:

Lanska DJ: Diagnosis of thymoma in myasthenics using anti-striational muscle antibodies: predictive value and gain in diagnostic certainty. Neurology *42*:520–524, 1991.

Lennon VA: Serological diagnosis of myasthenia gravis and the Lambert Eaton Syndrome. *In* Lisak RP (ed): Handbook of Myasthenia Gravis and Myasthenic Syndromes. New York, Marcel Dekker, 1994.

STUART-PROWER FACTOR, BLOOD
(see Factor X, Blood)

SUCROSE HEMOLYSIS TEST, DIAGNOSTIC

Norm: <5% hemolysis, or negative.

Usage: Screening for paroxysmal nocturnal hemoglobinuria (PNH).

Description: Paroxysmal nocturnal hemoglobinuria is an acquired anemia characterized by the production of abnormal hemopoietic cells, red blood cells with an abnormal sensitivity to complement, and erythrocyte hemolysis. Symptoms include leukopenia and/or thrombocytopenia, as well as nocturnal hemoglobinuria, chronic anemia, and thrombosis. Symptom severity is related to the degree of red blood cell sensitivity to complement and varies from client to client. In this test, sucrose provides a medium of low ionic strength that promotes the binding of complement to red cells. Blood from clients with PNH demonstrates the results of excessive lysis.

Professional Considerations:

1. Consent form NOT required.
2. Preparation:
   A. Tube: Blue-top.
   B. Specimens should NOT be drawn during hemodialysis.

3. Procedure:
   A. Draw a 5-ml blood sample.
   B. Mix the washed red blood cells with ABO-compatible normal serum and 10% isotonic sucrose.
   C. Incubate the tube 30 minutes at room temperature.
   D. Centrifuge the tube.
   E. Read the percentage of hemolysis that results.
4. Postprocedure care:
   A. None.
5. Client and family teaching:
   A. Results are normally available within 2 hours of the test.
6. Factors that affect results:
   A. Hemolysis or clotting of the specimen invalidates the results.
   B. False-positive results occur with megaloblastic anemia, autoimmune hemolytic anemias, dyserythropoietic anemia, lymphoma, adenocarcinoma of the colon, eosinophilia, renal failure, or bronchogenic carcinoma.
   C. False-negative results may occur in clients who have received recent blood transfusions, or if the specimen has been collected in a lavender-top tube containing EDTA or a green-top tube containing heparin.
7. Other data:
   A. Recent advances in the diagnosis of PNH include direct identification of affected cells by flow cytometry, detection of impaired synthesis of GPI anchor, and cytogenic analysis of the abnormal expression of the PIG-A gene.

Bibliography:

Iwamoto N, Kawaguchi T, Takatsuki K, et al.: Positivity of the sugar-water test in the screening for paroxysmal nocturnal hemoglobinuria. Blood 84(4): 1349, 1994.

Miyata T, Yamada N, Iida Y, et al.: Abnormalities of PIG-A transcripts in granulocytes from patients with paroxysmal nocturnal hemoglobinuria. N Eng J Med 330(4):249–255, 1994.

SUDAN BLACK B STAIN, DIAGNOSTIC

Norm: Lymphocytes do not stain; granulocytes do stain.

Usage: Differentiation of acute leukemias and lipid and phospholipid staining.

Description: The microscopic examination of a sample of bone marrow or blood stained with Sudan black stain, a fat-soluble dye. This stain differentiates acute granulocytic leukemia (which accepts the stain) from acute lymphocytic leukemia (which does not accept the stain).

Professional Considerations:

1. Consent form NOT required.
2. Preparation:
   A. Obtain a bone marrow biopsy tray or a red-top tube.
   B. Blood samples MAY be drawn during hemodialysis.
3. Procedure:
   A. After a bone marrow biopsy or venipuncture, place the aspirate/blood on a slide.
   B. Place the Sudan black stain on the slide and examine it under a microscope.
4. Postprocedure care:
   A. Apply a pressure bandage to the bone marrow aspiration site.
5. Client and family teaching:
   A. Bone marrow aspiration is painful, but only briefly. The client may receive premedication and an analgesic to ease the pain.
   B. The bone marrow aspiration site may be sore and bruised for several days after the biopsy.
6. Factors that affect results:
   A. Inadequate specimen amounts may produce inaccurate results.
7. Other data:
   A. Lymphocytes, plasma cells, and lymphoblasts, because they do not hold the Sudan black stain, are called sudanophilic cells.
   B. Myeloblasts, although they do not stain with Wright's stain, may stain with Sudan black stain.

Bibliography:

Cuneo A, Demuynck H, Ferrant A, et al.: Minor myeloid component in pH chromosome-positive acute lymphoblastic leukemia: Correlation with cytogenic pattern and implication for poor response to therapy. Br J Haematol 87(3):515–522, 1994.

SUDS

(see Acquired Immune Deficiency Syndrome Evaluation Battery, Diagnostic)

SUGAR WATER TEST SCREEN, DIAGNOSTIC
(see Sucrose Hemolysis Test, Diagnostic)

SUPREME BG, DIAGNOSTIC
(see Glucose Monitoring Machines, Diagnostic)

SWAN-GANZ CATHETER PULMONARY WEDGE PRESSURE, DIAGNOSTIC
(see Pulmonary Artery Catheterization, Diagnostic)

SWEAT TEST, DIAGNOSTIC
(see Chloride, Sweat, Specimen)

SYNOVIAL FLUID ANALYSIS, SPECIMEN
(see Body Fluid Analysis, Specimen)

SYNOVIAL FLUID MUCIN TEST, DIAGNOSTIC
(see Mucin Clot Test, Specimen)

SYPHILIS, SERUM
(see Microhemagglutination Treponema Pallidum (MHA-TP) Test, Serum)

T AND B LYMPHOCYTE SUBSET ASSAY (LYMPHOCYTE [T & B] ASSAY, LYMPHOCYTE SUBSET TYPING, LYMPHOCYTE MARKER STUDIES), BLOOD

Norm:

T-cells	60–80%
B-cells	5–15%

Usage: AIDS, autoimmune diseases, DiGeorge syndrome, Graves' disease, Hodgkin's disease, humoral immune deficiency, leukemia, lymphoma, multiple myeloma, systemic lupus erythematosus, Waldenström's macroglobulinemia, and X-linked agammaglobulinemia.

Description: Quantification of T and B cells as a percentage of total peripheral blood lymphocytes in order to determine immunodeficiency states. Lymphocyte stem cells are produced in the bone marrow and released into the peripheral circulation. The tissue that traps the lymphocyte stem cells determine whether they mature into a T or B lymphocyte. T lymphocytes mature in the thymus gland or the precortical areas of lymph nodes and are responsible for cell mediated immunity. B lymphocytes mature in the tonsils, spleen, germinating centers of the lymph nodes and nodules of the intestinal tract and are responsible for antibody-mediated immunity.

Professional Considerations:

1. Consent form NOT required.
2. Preparation:
   A. Tube: Two lavender-top.
   B. Do NOT draw specimens during hemodialysis.
3. Procedure:
   A. Draw two 7-ml blood samples.
4. Postprocedure care:
   A. Keep the specimens at room temperature and process them within 3 hours.
5. Client and family teaching:
   A. Explain the rationale for the test and explain the results, which should be available the same day.
6. Factors that affect results:
   A. Drugs that may increase lymphocytes include steroids and immunosuppressives.
   B. Refrigerating or freezing blood decreases lymphocyte counts.
7. Other data:
   A. Fresh tissue, bone marrow, and suspensions of lymph node or spleen can also be used for analysis.
   B. This test is also useful for monitoring clients on chemotherapy or immunosuppressive agents.
   C. *See also Acquired Immune Deficiency Syndrome Evaluation Battery, Diagnostic,* when applicable.

Bibliography:

Minguela A, Alvarez-Lopez MR, Sanchez-Bueno F, et al.: Presence of different T and B-peripheral blood lymphocyte subsets in liver transplantation after cyclosporine or OKT3 immunosuppressive treatment. Transplant Proc *27*(4):2317–2318, 1995.

Workman ML: The immune system: Your defensive partner and offensive foe. AACN Clin Issues *4*(3): 453–470, 1993.

T₃ OR T₄ THYROID TEST, BLOOD
(see Thyroid Test: Thyroxine, Blood or Thyroid Test: Triiodothyronine, Blood)

T₃ RESIN UPTAKE TEST, DIAGNOSTIC
(see Thyroid Test: Thyroid Hormone Binding Ratio, Blood)

TANGENT SCREEN TEST, DIAGNOSTIC

Norm: Normal, no loss of visual field.

Usage: Detection and monitoring of central visual field loss.

Description: A screening test that measures central vision. It is often used in the diagnosis of optic neuritis. The test involves having the client indicate when an object moving across a visual field of concentric circles can be seen.

Professional Considerations:

1. Consent form NOT required.
2. Preparation:
   A. The client should wear corrective lenses during the test.
3. Procedure:
   A. Have the client sit 1 m from the target screen.
   B. Occlude one eye and perform the tangent screen test.
   C. Repeat the procedure with the other eye occluded.
4. Postprocedure care:
   A. If the test is positive, the client should be referred to a neuro-ophthalmologist.
5. Client and family teaching:
   A. The client should fixate on a central target.
   B. The examiner will move an object into the client's visual field at 30-degree intervals while he or she remains fixated on a central target.
   C. The client will signal when he or she sees the object come into view.
6. Factors that affect results:
   A. The client must be able to cooperate with signaling when the object enters his or her visual field.
   B. Central visual boundaries vary with object size, brightness, contrast background, pupil size, and the client's age.
7. Other data:
   A. Abnormal results warrant further examination with a perimeter to measure peripheral visual fields.

Bibliography:

Dowen PA: Tangent screen examination. *In* Hamilton HK, Cahill M (eds): Diagnostics, 2nd ed. Springhouse, PA, Springhouse Corporation, 1986, pp 552–554.

Glaser JS, Goodwin JA: Neuro-ophthalmologic examination: The visual sensory system. *In* Glaser JS (ed): Neuro-ophthalmology, 2nd ed. Philadelphia, JB Lippincott, 1990, pp 9–36.

Scheie HG, Albert DM: Textbook of Ophthalmology, 9th ed. Philadelphia, WB Saunders, 1977.

TARTRATE RESISTANT ACID PHOSPHATASE (TRAP), BLOOD

Norm: Negative.

Positive: Hairy cell leukemia, lymphoma, mononucleosis, and prolymphocytic leukemia.

Description: Hairy cell leukemia (leukemic reticuloendotheliosis) is a chronic form of leukemia characterized by distinctive cells called "hairy cells," which have many fine, cytoplasmic projections that look like hair. Most leukocytes have an acid phosphatase reaction inhibited by L-tartrate. Hairy cells, however, are thought to contain an isoenzyme of acid phosphatase that is tartrate resistant (isoenzyme 5). Thus, this test is used to help diagnose hairy cell leukemia and assess response to treatment. In a positive test, leukocytes are not inhibited by L-tartrate.

Professional Considerations:

1. Consent form NOT required.
2. Preparation:
   A. Obtain four glass microslides for smears and fixative (glutaraldehyde-acetone).
   B. Specimens MAY be drawn during hemodialysis.
3. Procedure:
   A. Draw a 2-ml blood sample in a heparinized syringe.
   B. Place two drops of blood on each of the four slides.
4. Postprocedure care:
   A. Spray fixative on the slides immediately.
5. Client and family teaching:
   A. Results are normally available in 1–2 days.
6. Factors that affect results:
   A. Rare false-negatives occur.
7. Other data:
   A. Serum levels of acid phosphatase isoenzyme 5 may also be elevated in hairy cell leukemia.

Bibliography:

Janckila AJ, Cardwell EM, Yam LT, et al.: Hairy cell identification by immunohistochemistry of tartrate-resistant acid phosphatase. Blood 85(10): 2839–2844, 1995.

Robbins BA, Ellison DJ, Spinosa JC, et al.: Diagnostic application of two-color flow cytometry in 161 cases of hairy cell leukemia. Blood 82(4):1277–1287, 1993.

TB TEST, DIAGNOSTIC
(see Mantoux Skin Test, Diagnostic)

TECHNETIUM-PENTAACETIC ACID (Tc-99m-DTPA), CLEARANCE, DIAGNOSTIC

Norm: Glomerular filtration rate varies widely and is affected by numerous factors, including age, gender, body size, physiologic variables, and disease. The GFR of children and adults is frequently "normalized" to an average adult surface area of 1.73 m². The mean value in men is 131 ml/minute/1.73 m² with a standard deviation of 18 percent. The mean value in women is 120 ml/minute/1.73 m² with a standard deviation of 14 percent.

Increased: Amino acid infusions, burns, high-protein diet, overhydration, pregnancy.

Decreased: Acute or chronic renal failure, dehydration, exercise, renal insufficiency, severe exertion.

Description: The GFR is used as a clinical assessment of renal function. This test measures the GFR by external scintigraphy over the kidneys after injection of the radionuclide, technetium-99m-diethylenetriamine pentaacetic acid (Tc-99m-DTPA). Tc-99m-DTPA is freely filtered by the glomerulus and not reabsorbed and thus is used to calculate GFR. This test is also used to measure renal function and flow, to determine the contribution of each kidney to overall renal function, to evaluate renal transplants, to detect obstruction or trauma, and to evaluate renovascular disease.

Professional Considerations:

1. Consent form IS required:

Risks:
Infection or hematoma at the injection site.

Contraindications:
Inability to lie motionless during the scan; during pregnancy or breast-feeding.

2. Preparation:
    A. Establish intravenous access.
    B. The client should void before beginning the study.
    C. Have emergency equipment available for potential anaphylaxis.
3. Procedure:
    A. The radionuclide is injected via the established intravenous access.
    B. Scintiscans of the kidneys are taken at 1-, 3-, 5-, 10-, 15-, and 20-minute intervals.
    C. GFR is calculated based on the net in-

jected dose, the determined kidney depth, and the uptake of the injected dose in each kidney.
4. Postprocedure care:
    A. The client should void after the procedure to significantly reduce gonadal radiation dose.
    B. Observe the client for 1 hour after the study for possible anaphylactic reaction to the radionuclide.
    C. General body substance isolation precautions protect the health care professional from potential radiation exposure.
5. Client and family teaching:
    A. The entire procedure takes 45 minutes.
    B. No special precautions must be taken following this test, and there is no radiation hazard.
6. Factors that affect results:
    A. This test is valid for adults with normal cardiac output and normal vascular volume.
    B. A normal diurnal variation in GFR does occur, with the highest values occurring in the afternoon and the lowest values in the middle of the night. This is thought to be related to variations in protein intake during the day.
    C. GFR changes predictably with age. In the first 2 weeks of life, the GFR is 50 percent of the value achieved at age 1. After age 1, the GFR remains constant until the fourth decade of life, when it gradually declines. By the eighth decade, the GFR is only 30 percent of that observed in young adults.
7. Other data:
    A. Health care professionals working in a nuclear medicine area must follow the federal standards set by the Nuclear Regulatory Commission. These standards include precautions for handling the radioactive material and monitoring of potential radiation exposure.
    B. Technetium half-life is 6 hours.

Bibliography:

Carlson JA, Harrington JT: Laboratory evaluation of renal function. *In* Schrier RW, Gottschalk CW (eds): Diseases of the Kidney, 5th ed. Boston, Little, Brown, 1993, pp 361–405.

Danovitch GM, Wilkinson AH: Evaluation of renal function. *In* Massry SG, Glassock RJ (eds): Textbook of Nephrology, 2nd ed. Baltimore, Williams and Wilkins, 1989, pp 1619–1627.

Levey AS, Madaio MP, Perrone RD: Laboratory assessment of renal disease: Clearance, urinalysis and renal biopsy. *In* Brenner BM, Rector FC (eds): The Kidney, 4th ed. Philadelphia, WB Saunders, 1991, pp 919–968.

TEE
(see Transesophageal Sonogram, Diagnostic)

TEICHOIC ACID ANTIBODY, BLOOD

Norm: Titer ≤1:2 or less than a four-fold rise in titer between acute and convalescent samples.

Increased: Endocarditis, infections caused by *Staphylococcus aureus*, osteomyelitis, and subacute bacterial endocarditis.

Description: Teichoic acid is a macromolecule present on the cell wall of gram-positive bacteria. Antibodies to teichoic acid can be seen in some infections. Monitoring teichoic acid antibody levels may be helpful in assessing response to therapy in clients with gram-positive infections.

Professional Considerations:
1. Consent form NOT required.
2. Preparation:
   A. Tube: Red-top, red/gray-top, or gold-top.
   B. Specimens MAY be drawn during hemodialysis.
3. Procedure:
   A. Draw a 5-ml sample as soon as possible after symptoms appear or diagnosis is suspected, and label the tube as the acute sample.
   B. Repeat the test in 14 days and label the tube as the convalescent sample.
   C. Serial testing may also be performed.
4. Postprocedure care:
   A. *See Client and family teaching.*
5. Client and family teaching:
   A. The client must return in 2 weeks for convalescent sample testing.
6. Factors that affect results:
   A. Technical variability.
7. Other data:
   A. The clinical significance of this test has not been fully established.

Bibliography:

Arizono T, Umeda A, Amako K: Distribution of capsular materials on the cell wall surface of strain smith diffuse of *Staphylococcus aureus*. J Bacteriol *173*(14):4333–4340, 1991.

Wise KA, Tosolini FA: Detection of teichoic acid antibodies in *Staphylococcus aureus* infections. Pathology *24*(2):102–108, 1992.

TEMAZEPAM

(see Benzodiazepines, Plasma and Urine)

TENSILON TEST, DIAGNOSTIC

Positive: Unequivocal improvement in a single weakened muscle.

Negative: Equivocal or no improvement in a weakened muscle. False negative tests are fairly common and repeated tests are of use.

Usage: Diagnosis of myasthenia gravis.

Description: Myasthenia gravis is an autoimmune neuromuscular disease characterized by fatigue of the limb, facial, bulbar, and ocular muscles with repetitive activity and by improvement with rest. Respiratory muscle fatigue can also occur. It is caused by circulating antibodies directed toward the skeletal muscle acetylcholine receptor. The factors that trigger the autoimmune response are unknown. In the Tensilon (edrophonium chloride) test, a short-acting anticholinesterase is administered intravenously, and muscle response is observed. The test is most useful if improvement in ptosis or the strength of an extraocular muscle is demonstrated because of the objective nature of this response. Following intravenous administration of Tensilon, muscle strength will improve quickly in clients with myasthenia gravis.

Professional Considerations:
1. Consent form NOT required.
2. Preparation:
   A. Assess for use of medications that affect muscle function, allergies, and respiratory disease.
   B. Establish intravenous access with a butterfly needle or an infusion of 5% dextrose in water or 0.9% saline.
   C. Obtain baseline vital signs.
   D. Have emergency respiratory support equipment and atropine available for use in the event of complications.
3. Procedure:
   A. Determine the muscle to observe for response.
   B. An initial test dose is administered because some people may be sensitive to Tensilon and may experience bradycardia or bronchospasm. These individuals should not receive additional Tensilon.
   C. Administer an initial dose of Tensilon intravenously as follows:
      i. Adults: 2 mg.
      ii. Children weighing >75 pounds: 2 mg.
      iii. Children weighing <75 pounds: 1 mg.
      iv. Infants: 0.5 mg.
   D. Muscle strength may improve within 45 seconds. If no improvement is noted, additional Tensilon should be infused as follows:

i. Adults: up to 8 mg over 30 seconds.
ii. Children weighing >75 pounds: up to 8 mg at a rate of 1 mg/30–45 seconds.
iii. Children weighing <75 pounds: up to 5 mg at a rate of 1 mg/30–45 seconds.
iv. Infants: Do not administer further Tensilon.
E. Flush the IV access line between doses to ensure that the medication has infused.
F. Be prepared for possible respiratory distress because Tensilon may stimulate a cholinergic crisis that causes extreme muscle weakness. If this occurs, up to 1 mg of intravenous atropine should be administered promptly.
G. Atropine may be administered during the test to clients with respiratory diseases, such as asthma, to minimize the side effects of Tensilon.
H. Once an unequivocal response is noted, the test is complete, and Tensilon administration should be stopped.
4. Postprocedure care:
A. Monitor vital signs every 5 minutes × 4.
5. Client and family teaching:
A. Instruct the client on the procedure and on the potential side effects of Tensilon.
6. Factors that affect results:
A. Prednisone delays the effect of Tensilon.
B. Quinidine and anticholinergics inhibit the action of Tensilon.
C. Skeletal muscle relaxants may mask the effect of Tensilon.
7. Other data:
A. The side effects of Tensilon include abdominal cramps, bradycardia, diaphoresis, diarrhea, hypotension, incontinence, pupillary constriction, respiratory distress, and salivation.

Bibliography:

Hopkins LC: Clinical features of myasthenia gravis. Neurol Clin North Am *12*(2):243–261, 1994.
Kernich CA, Kaminski HJ: Myasthenia gravis: Pathophysiology, diagnosis and collaborative care. J Neurosci Nurs *27*(4):207–218, 1995.

TERMINAL DEOXYNUCLEOTIDYL TRANSFERASE (TDT), BLOOD

Norm:

Adult		0–4 TdT U/10 cells or 0–0.67 pU/cell
Child		0–3.5 TdT U/10 cells or 0–0.58 pU/cell

Usage: Acute lymphoblastic leukemia, blast crisis, Hodgkin's disease, lymphoma, and myelogenous leukemia.

Description: Terminal deoxynucleotidyl transferase (TdT) is an intracellular protein that is a biochemical marker that aids in the diagnosis and classification of acute leukemias. It acts as a catalyst in the synthesis of deoxynucleotide triphosphates in the absence of a template. Approximately 1–5% of normal mononuclear cells express TdT in normal peripheral blood and bone marrow, respectively.

Professional Considerations:

1. Consent form NOT required.
2. Preparation:
   A. Contact the laboratory to determine if the test must be prescheduled.
   B. Tube: Lavender-top.
   C. Specimens should NOT be drawn during hemodialysis.
3. Procedure:
   A. Draw a 10-ml blood sample.
4. Postprocedure care:
   A. None.
5. Client and family teaching:
   A. Results are normally available in 1–2 days.
6. Factors that affect results:
   A. Heparin in the blood tube may decrease the results.
7. Other data:
   A. Some children with acute lymphoblastic leukemia have low TdT activity.

Bibliography:

Orazi A, Cotton J, Cattoretti G, et al.: Terminal deoxynucleotidyl transferase staining in acute leukemia and normal bone marrow in routinely processed paraffin sections. Am J Clin Pathol *102*(5):640–644.
Paietta E, Meenan B, Heavey C, Thomas D: Detection of terminal transferase in acute myeloid leukemia by flow cytometry. Cytometry *16*:256–261, 1994.
Sasaki R: Detection of terminal deoxynucleotidyl transferase (TdT) in nonlymphocytic leukemia by immunofluorescent (IF) assay. Leukemia *9*(3):520–521, 1995.

TERMINAL DEOXYNUCLEOTIDYL TRANSFERASE (TDT), BONE MARROW, DIAGNOSTIC

Norm:

Adult		0–5.7 TdT U/10 cells or 0–0.95 pU/cell
Child		2.9–8.9 TdT U/10 cells or 0.48–1.49 pU/cell

Usage: Acute lymphoblastic leukemia, blast crisis, Hodgkin's disease, lymphoma, and myelogenous leukemia.

Description: Terminal deoxynucleotidyl transferase (TdT) is an intracellular protein that is a biochemical marker that aids in the diagnosis and classification of acute leukemia. It catalyzes the polymerization of deoxynucleotide triphosphates in the absence of a template. In this test, a smear of bone marrow is tested for the presence of TdT. Approximately 1–5% of mononuclear cells express TdT in normal adult peripheral blood and bone marrow, respectively.

Professional Considerations:

1. Consent form IS required for bone marrow aspiration. See *Bone Marrow Aspiration Analysis, Specimen* for procedural risks and contraindications.
2. Preparation:
   A. Obtain a bone marrow biopsy tray, sterile gloves, 1–2% lidocaine (Xylocaine), and a sterile bone marrow specimen cup with formalin.
3. Procedure:
   A. Position the client so he or she is lying on the side, with the knees flexed.
   B. Scrub antiseptic over the potential biopsy site.
   C. Anesthetize the area with 1–2% Xylocaine.
   D. Perform the bone marrow biopsy.
   E. Place the specimen in a formalin cup and secure the lid.

4. Postprocedure care:
   A. Place a small sterile dressing on the biopsy site.
   B. Assess for bleeding from the biopsy site for 24 hours, especially in thrombocytopenic clients.
5. Client and family teaching:
   A. A bone marrow biopsy is painful, but only briefly. A preanalgesic may be given to lessen discomfort.
   B. The bone marrow biopsy site may be bruised and sore for several days after the procedure.
6. Factors that affect results:
   A. Insufficient bone marrow sample.
7. Other data:
   A. TdT-positive leukemics that relapse can show a change in phenotype and can then be TdT-negative.

Bibliography:

Orazi A, Cotton J, Cattoretti G, et al: Terminal deoxynucleotidyl transferase staining in acute leukemia and normal bone marrow in routinely processed paraffin sections. Am J Clin Pathol *102* (5):640–644, 1995.

Paietta E, Meenan B, Heavey C, Thomas D: Detection of terminal transferase in acute myeloid leukemia by flow cytometry. Cytometry *16*:256–261, 1994.

Sasaki R: Detection of terminal deoxynucleotidyl transferase (TdT) in nonlymphocytic leukemia by immunofluorescent (IF) assay. Leukemia *9*(3): 520–521, 1995.

TESTOSTERONE, FREE, BLOOD

Norm:

	pg/ml	SI Units pmol/L	Percentage of Total Testosterone
Male Values			
Adults	50–210	174–729	1.0–2.7
Children			
Cord blood	5–22	17.4–76.3	2.0–4.4
Newborn	1.5–31.0	5.2–107.5	0.9–1.7
4 weeks–3 months	3.3–8.0	11.5–62.5	0.4–0.8
3–5 months	0.7–14.0	2.4–48.6	0.4–1.1
5–7 months	0.4–4.8	1.4–16.6	0.4–1.0
6–9 years	0.1–3.2	0.3–11.1	0.9–1.7
10–11 years	0.6–5.7	2.1–19.8	1.0–1.9
12–14 years	1.4–156	4.9–541	1.3–3.0
15–17 years	80–159	278–552	1.8–2.7
Female Values			
Adults	1.0–8.5	3.5–29.5	0.5–1.8
Children			
Cord blood	4.0–16.0	13.9–55.5	2.0–3.9
Newborn	0.5–2.5	1.7–8.7	0.8–1.5
4 weeks–3 months	0.1–1.3	0.3–4.5	0.4–1.1

	pg/ml	SI Units pmol/L	Percentage of Total Testosterone
Female Values (continued)			
Children (continued)			
3–5 months	0.3–1.1	1.0–3.8	0.5–1.0
5–7 months	0.2–0.6	0.7–2.1	0.5–0.8
6–9 years	0.1–0.9	0.3–3.1	0.9–1.4
10–11 years	1.0–5.2	3.5–18.0	1.0–1.9
12–14 years	1.0–5.2	3.5–18.0	1.0–1.9
15–17 years	1.0–5.2	3.5–18.0	1.0–1.9

Increased: Androgen resistance, hirsutism, polycystic ovary syndrome, tumor (virilizing). *See also Testosterone, Total, Blood.*

Decreased: Hypogonadism, P-450$_{C17}$ enzyme deficiency. *See also Testosterone, Total, Blood.*

Description: Free testosterone is that portion of circulating testosterone that is not bound to the sex hormone-binding globulin (SHBG) plasma protein. This test is used to differentiate true abnormal testosterone levels from those caused by abnormally low or high amounts of circulating SHBG. *(See also Testosterone, Total, Blood.)*

Professional considerations:

1. Consent form NOT required.
2. Preparation:
   A. Tube: Green-top or red-top, red/gray-top, or gold-top (serum) or green-top (plasma).
   B. Specimens MAY be drawn during hemodialysis.
3. Procedure:
   A. Draw a 3-ml blood sample.
4. Postprocedure care:
   A. None.
5. Client and family teaching:
   A. Discuss the test results and the implications thereof with the physician.
   B. Results may not be available for several days.
6. Factors that affect results:
   A. In adult men, serum testosterone levels peak in the early morning and after exercise and decrease after glucose loading and immobilization. Due to this diurnal rhythm of circulating testosterone levels, the blood is generally drawn in the morning.
   B. Results are invalidated if the client has undergone a radioactive scan within the past 7 days.
7. Other data:
   A. None.

Bibliography:

Lucky AW: Hormonal correlates of acne and hirsutism. Am J Med *98*(Suppl 1A):89–94, 1995.
Redmond GP: Androgenic disorders of women: Diagnostic and therapeutic decision making. Amer J Med *98*(Suppl 1A):120–129, 1995.
Winters SJ: Endocrine evaluation of testicular function. Endocrinol Metab Clin North Am *23*(4): 709–721, 1994.

TESTOSTERONE, TOTAL, BLOOD

Norm:

	Male		Female	
	ng/dl	SI Units nmol/L	ng/dl	SI Units nmol/L
Adult	300–1200	10.4–41.6	30–95	1.0–3.3
Prepubertal values				
Cord blood	13–55	0.45–1.91	5–45	0.17–1.56
Premature infant	37–198	1.28–6.87	5–22	0.17–0.76
Newborn	75–400	2.6–13.9	20–64	0.69–2.22
1–5 months	1–177	0.03–6.14	1–5	0.03–0.17
6–11 months	2–7	0.07–0.24	2–5	0.07–0.17

| | Male | | Female | |
	ng/dl	SI Units nmol/L	ng/dl	SI Units nmol/L
Prepubertal values *(continued)*				
12 months–5 years	2–25	0.07–0.87	2–10	0.07–0.35
6–9 years	3–30	0.10–1.04	2–20	0.07–0.69
Pubertal values				
Tanner stage				
1	2–23	0.07–0.80	2–10	0.07–0.35
2	5–70	0.17–2.43	5–30	0.17–1.04
3	15–280	0.52–9.72	10–30	0.35–1.04
4	105–545	3.64–18.91	15–40	0.52–1.39
5	265–800	9.19–27.76	10–40	0.35–1.39

Increased: Adrenal hyperplasia, adrenal tumor, arrhenoblastoma, central nervous system lesions, hirsutism (idiopathic), hyperthyroidism, ovarian tumor (virilizing), testicular feminization, testicular tumor, virilizing luteoma, and virilization. In women, idiopathic hirsutism, cystic acne, polycystic ovary syndrome, adrenogenic alopecia, abnormal menstruation, anovulation, adrenogenital syndrome with virilization, ovarian tumor, and Stein-Leventhal syndrome with virilization. Drugs include anticonvulsants, barbiturates, cimetidine, clomiphene, estrogens, gonadotropin (males), and oral contraceptives.

Decreased: Anemia, cirrhosis, cryptorchidism, Down syndrome, gynecomastia, hypogonadism (male), hypopituitarism, impotence, Klinefelter's syndrome, male climacteric, obesity, and orchidectomy. Drugs include androgens, cyproterone, dexamethasone, diethylstilbestrol, digoxin (males), digitalis, estrogens (males), ethanol, glucose, glucocorticoids, gonadotropin-releasing hormone analogs, halothane, ketoconazole, metoprolol, metyrapone, phenothiazines, spironolactone, and tetracycline.

Description: Testosterone is the dominant androgen found in the adrenal glands, brain, ovary, pituitary, skin, kidney, and testes. It circulates both freely, and bound to plasma proteins (sex hormone-binding globulin [SHBG]). Testosterone promotes the growth and development of the male sexual organs, and increases body mass and hair replacement. This test measures total testosterone levels in clients with normal SHBG levels.

Professional Considerations:
1. Consent form NOT required.
2. Preparation:
   A. Tube: Green-top (plasma) or red-top, red/gray-top, or gold-top (serum).
   B. Specimens MAY be drawn during hemodialysis.
3. Procedure:
   A. Draw a 1.5-ml blood sample.
4. Postprocedure care:
   A. None.
5. Client and family teaching:
   A. Discuss the test results and the implications thereof with the physician.
   B. Results may not be available for several days.
6. Factors that affect results:
   A. In adult men, serum testosterone levels peak in the early morning and after exercise and decrease after glucose loading and immobilization. Due to this diurnal rhythm of circulating testosterone levels, the blood is generally drawn in the morning.
   B. Results are invalidated if the client has undergone a radioactive scan within the past 7 days.
7. Other data:
   A. Free testosterone should be measured, instead of total testosterone, if the client has a condition that increases or decreases the level of SHBG. Some conditions that increase SHBG are hyperthyroidism and low estrogen production states (pregnancy, taking oral contraceptives or anticonvulsant drugs). Some conditions that decrease SHBG include excess androgen states, hypothyroidism, and obesity.

Bibliography:
Lucky AW: Hormonal correlates of acne and hirsutism. Amer J Med *98*(Suppl 1A):89–94, 1995.
Redmond GP: Androgenic disorders of women: Diagnostic and therapeutic decision making. Amer J Med *98*(Suppl 1A):120–129, 1995.
Winters SJ: Endocrine evaluation of testicular function. Endocrinol Metab Clin North Am *23*(4): 709–721, 1994.

THALLIUM, SERUM OR 24-HOUR URINE

Norm:

		SI Units
Serum	<0.5 µg/dl	<24.5 nmol/L
Panic level	10–800 µg/dl	0.5–39 nmol/L
Urine		
Adult	<2 µg/L	<9.8 µmol/L
	or <10 µg/24 h	
Panic level	1–20 µg/L	4.9–97.8 µmol/L

Panic Level Symptoms and Treatment:

Symptoms: Abdominal pain, alopecia, ataxia, constipation, coma, delirium, diaphoresis, hypertension, intractable insomnia, optic neuritis, pulmonary edema, rash, tachycardia, and vomiting.

Treatment: Give syrup of ipecac followed by 50 g of activated charcoal placed into the stomach by a nasogastric tube. Prussian blue (ferric ferrocyanide) is then given, because it binds to thallium and prevents absorption in the gastrointestinal tract. The dose is 125 mg/kg in 50 ml of 15% mannitol twice daily via nasogastric tube. Continue this until excretion of thallium is <0.5 mg/day. Neither chelating agents nor hemodialysis seems beneficial. Hemoperfusion may be helpful.

Increased: Metal poisoning.

Description: Thallium is an extremely toxic heavy metal used in manufacturing and found in chlorinated chemicals, cosmetics, dyes, fireworks, jewelry, medications, pesticides, photoelectric cells, rat poison, and semiconductors. Thallium accumulates in the bone, kidney, liver, and muscle tissue. Thallium poisoning may cause blindness, liver damage, paralysis, paresthesia, peripheral neuropathy, and/or renal damage. This test helps identify clients who have acquired abnormal body amounts of thallium through ingestion or inhalation or through skin absorption.

Professional Considerations:

1. Consent form NOT required.
2. Preparation:
   A. *Serum:*
      i. Tube: Metal-free green-top.
      ii. Specimens MAY be drawn during hemodialysis.
   B. *Urine:*
      i. Obtain a 3-L, metal-free urine collection container.
      ii. Provide a plastic, metal-free urinal or bedpan for specimen collection.
3. Procedure:
   A. *Serum:* Draw a 5-ml blood sample in a metal-free, green-top tube.
   B. *Urine:*
      i. Collect all the urine voided in a 24-hour period in a plastic, metal-free bedpan or urinal.
      ii. The urine is mixed with 0.4% sodium bismuth in 20% nitric acid and 10% sodium iodine. If thallium is present, a red precipitate forms.
4. Postprocedure care:
   A. Observe the client for symptoms of thallium poisoning.
5. Client and family teaching:
   A. For urine collection, urinate before defecating and avoid contaminating the specimen with stool or toilet tissue. If any urine is accidentally discarded, discard the entire specimen and restart the collection the next day.
   B. Blood and urine thallium levels tend to decrease rapidly following exposure.
   C. If activated charcoal was given for elevated levels, the client should drink 4–6 glasses of water each day for 2 days to prevent constipation. The activated charcoal will cause stools to be black for a few days.
6. Factors that affect results:
   A. Urine or blood allowed to come into contact with metal will falsely elevate results.
7. Other data:
   A. Poisoning occurs 1–10 days after exposure. A lethal dose is 1 g or 8–12 mg/kg.
   B. The urine of a client with thallium poisoning will also show proteinuria, increased red cells, casts, eosinophils,

lymphocytes, or polymorphonuclear leukocytes.

Bibliography:

Herrero F, Fernandez E, Gomez J, et al.: Thallium poisoning presenting with abdominal colic, paresthesia, and irritability. Clin Toxicol *33*(3):261–264, 1995.

Mauras Y, Premel-Cabic A, Berre S, Allain P: Simultaneous determination of lead, bismuth and thallium in plasma and urine by inductively coupled plasma mass spectrometry. Clin Chem Acta *218*: 201–205, 1993.

THALLIUM-DIPYRIDAMOLE STRESS TEST AND SCAN
(see Heart Scan, Diagnostic)

THALLIUM EXERCISE SCINTIGRAPHY, DIAGNOSTIC
(see Heart Scan, Diagnostic)

THALLIUM IMAGING, DIAGNOSTIC
(see Heart Scan, Diagnostic)

THEOPHYLLINE (AMINOPHYLLINE), BLOOD

Norm:

		SI Units
Therapeutic	10–20 µg/ml	44–111 µmol/L
Toxic level	>20 µg/ml	>111 µmol/L
Panic level	>30 µg/ml	>160 µmol/L

Panic Level Symptoms and Treatment:

Symptoms: Dysrhythmias, gastrointestinal bleeding, headache, hypotension, nausea, restlessness, seizures, syncope, tachycardia, and vomiting.

Treatment:

Maintain a patent airway.
Withhold theophylline.
Do gastric lavage if it can be done within 6 hours of ingestion.
Induce vomiting with syrup of ipecac.
Give activated charcoal.
Provide hydration.
Give diazepam for convulsions.
Provide continuous ECG monitoring for dysrhythmias.
Monitor theophylline levels q 2 hours.
Monitor and treat electrolyte imbalance.
Administer charcoal hemoperfusion for severe overdose.
40% of theophylline may be removed by hemodialysis. Peritoneal dialysis will NOT remove theophylline.

Increased: CHF, COPD, liver dysfunction, and overdose. Drugs that may cause increased levels include allopurinol, cimetidine, ciprofloxin, clindamycin, erythromycin, lin-comycin, oral contraceptives, and probenecid.

Decreased: Smoking. Drugs that may cause decreased levels include barbiturates, carbamazepine, furosemide, isoniazid, nortriptyline, phenytoin, and rifampin.

Description: Theophylline is a methylxanthine drug that decreases breakdown of intracellular cyclic adenosine monophosphate (cAMP) that, in turn, stimulates dilation of the smooth muscles of the bronchial airways and relaxation of the pulmonary blood vessels. It is 60% plasma protein bound, with a half-life of 6–10 hours in adults and 2–5 hours in children (half-life is reduced 40% in cigarette smokers); 90% of theophylline is metabolized in the liver. Steady-state levels occur in 15–20 hours in adults and in 5–40 hours in children.

Professional Considerations:

1. Consent form NOT required.
2. Preparation:
   A. Tube: Red-top, red/gray-top, or gold-top.
   B. The client should not ingest substances that contain xanthene for 12 hours prior to the test. The substances to avoid include chocolate, cocoa, coffee, cola, and tea.
   C. Do NOT draw specimens during hemodialysis.

3. Procedure:
   A. Draw a 3-ml blood sample.
4. Postprocedure care:
   A. Refrigerate the specimen. Do not freeze it.
5. Client and family teaching:
   A. Explain the significance of therapeutic drug levels and the periodic monitoring thereof.
   B. If activated charcoal was given for elevated levels, the client should drink 4–6 glasses of water each day for 2 days to prevent constipation. The activated charcoal will cause stools to be black for a few days.
6. Factors that affect results:
   A. Peak levels with oral dosing occur 1–3 hours after uncoated or liquid preparations and 4–7 hours after enteric coated or extended release preparations.
   B. Ingestion of xanthines within 12 hours prior to the test may elevate levels.
7. Other data:
   A. A minor metabolite of theophylline is caffeine.

Bibliography:

Hassan E: Clinical significance of theophylline drug interactions. J Cardiopulm Rehab *14*(2):102–103, 1994.

Perry AG: Aminophylline use in the critically ill: An old ally or new foe? AACN Clin Issues *6*(2):297–306, 1995.

THERMOGRAPHY, DIAGNOSTIC

Norm: Normal temperature pattern.

Usage: May aid in the diagnosis of chronic pain, distinguishing between psychosomatic pain and disorders such as dystrophy and nerve root irritation/compression. May be used to study vascular diseases. No longer recommended for breast tumor mass evaluation.

Description: Thermography is the measurement of the skin heat patterns, based on heat radiation from the skin surfaces. The test involves scanning the tissue with an infrared camera, which then displays on a screen, an image with shades varying according to areas of differing heat radiation.

Professional Considerations:

1. Consent form NOT required.
2. Preparation:
   A. Reassure the client that there is no pain or discomfort associated with this test.
3. Procedure:
   A. The client should disrobe the area to be studied and then wait in a cool room for 10 minutes to promote heat emission.
   B. The thermoscope takes pictures from the sides and front of the area.
4. Postprocedure care:
   A. Results are normally available within 2 days.
5. Client and family teaching:
   A. The test takes 10 minutes.
   B. The test is painless and safe.
6. Factors that affect results:
   A. Fluctuations in room temperature will cause faulty results.
   B. Inflammation and abscesses may generate enough heat to produce hot spots.
7. Other data:
   A. Due to the high incidence of false-negative and false-positive results, thermography is seldom used.
   B. The American Medical Association's Council on Scientific Affairs and the American College of Radiology recommend against the use of thermography for diagnostic purposes.

Bibliography:

Cotton P: AMA's council on scientific affairs takes a fresh look at thermography. JAMA *267*(14):1885–1887, 1992.

Harper CM Jr, Low PA, Fealey RD, et al.: Utility of thermography in the diagnosis of lumbosacral radiculopathy. Neurology *41*(7):1010–1014, 1991.

Lolly J: Thermography: A prototype of failed technology. Del Med J *65*(12):789–790, 1993.

Stern EE, Zee B: Thermography as a predictor of prognosis in cancer of the breast. Cancer *67*(6):1678–1680, 1991.

THIAMINE, SERUM
(see Vitamin B₁, Serum)

THIOCYANATE, BLOOD OR URINE

Norm: Negative for blood or urine.

Therapeutic Levels:

		SI Units
Serum		
Nonsmokers	1–4 µg/ml	0.02–0.07 mmol/L
Smokers	3–12 µg/ml	0.05–0.21 mmol/L
Pediatric	≤0.1 µg/ml	

Therapeutic Levels (continued)

		SI Units
Urine		
Nonsmokers	1–4 mg/24 hours	
Smokers	7–17 mg/24 hours	
Panic levels		
Serum	>35 µg/ml	>0.6 mmol/L
Urine	>0.2 mg/dl	

Poisoning Symptoms and Treatment:

Symptoms: Agitation, confusion, focal brain damage, hyperreflexia, hypotension, metabolic acidosis, myocardial damage, psychotic behavior, thrombophlebitis, and thyroid enlargement.

Treatment:

Do gastric lavage.
Administer intravenous fluids at 3 L/day (if normal renal function is present) to maintain adequate output.
Monitor amyl nitrate inhalation.
Give sodium nitrite and sodium thiosulfate infusions.
Both hemodialysis and peritoneal dialysis WILL remove thiocyanate.

Increased: Poisoning from nitroprusside; smoking.

Description: Thiocyanate is a major metabolite of the drug nitroprusside, and is the important gauge of nitroprusside-induced toxicity during prolonged administration or with unusually high rates of infusion (*see also Cyanide, Blood,* which has a more important role in early toxicity of nitroprusside.) Both sodium and potassium thiocyanate depress the metabolic activities of all cells, but mostly those of the brain and heart. Half-life is 7 days. Formerly, this drug was used to treat hypertension by producing peripheral vasodilation. More recently this measure has been studied for detection of smoking deceivers in smoking cessation programs.

Professional Considerations:

1. Consent form NOT required.

2. Preparation:
   A. Tube: Red-top, red/gray-top, or gold/top.
   B. Obtain a sterile plastic container for urine sample.
   C. Do NOT draw specimens during hemodialysis.
3. Procedure:
   A. *Blood:* Draw a 2-ml blood sample.
   B. *Urine:* Obtain a 20-ml, fresh urine sample in a sterile plastic cup.
4. Postprocedure care:
   A. Tighten the top of the plastic urine container.
5. Client and family teaching:
   A. The treatment for poisoning will take at least 1 week.
   B. Death is possible from thiocyanate poisoning.
6. Factors that affect results:
   A. Eating cabbage or smoking cigarettes can falsely increase blood and urine results.
7. Other data:
   A. It takes 1 week to reduce thiocyanate by 50% if normal kidney function is present.
   B. Some clients show a temporary improvement for several days, only to relapse and die as long as 2 weeks later.

Bibliography:

Chen Y, Pederson LL, Lefcoe NM: Exposure to environmental tobacco smoke (ETS) and serum thiocyanate level in infants. Arch Environ Health 45(3):163–167, 1990.

Jacobs N, Lamaire L, Bellini M: Measurement of urinary tobacco markers in a smoking-cessation program. Clin Chem 37(9):1655–1656, 1991.

Linhakis J, Lacouture P, Woolf A: Cyanide and thiocyanate concentrations during infusion of sodium nitroprusside in children. Pediatr Cardiol 12(4):214–218, 1991.

Woodward M, Tunstall-Pedoe H: An iterative technique for identifying smoking deceivers with application to the Scottish heart study. Prev Med 21(1):88–97, 1992.

THIORIDAZINE

(see Phenothiazines, Blood)

THORACENTESIS, DIAGNOSTIC

Norm:

Amount	<20 ml
Color	Clear

Specific gravity	<1.016
pH	Equal to serum level
Protein	<3 g/dl
Fibrinogen	None
Cells	Few lymphocytes, few red blood cells
Lactate dehydrogenase	Equal to serum level
Glucose	Equal to serum level
Amylase	Equal to serum level

Usage:

Therapeutic: relieves dyspnea due to pleural effusion.

Diagnostic: evaluates underlying cause of pleural effusion. Abnormal accumulation of fluid in the pleural space may be classified as either transudate or exudate.

	Transudate	Exudate
Amount	>20 ml	None
Color	Clear	Cloudy, turbid
Specific gravity	<1.016	>1.016
pH	Equal to serum level	<7.3
Protein	<3 g/dl	>3 g/dl
Fibrinogen	None or may be present	
Cells	Few lymphocytes	Many; may be a few red blood cells or purulent
Lactate	Equal to serum level	May be >lactate dehydrogenase, serum
Glucose	Equal to serum level	May be <serum
Amylase	Equal to serum level	May be >serum

Description: Thoracentesis is the removal of fluid or air from the pleural space via transthoracic aspiration. It is performed to determine the nature or cause of an effusion, to relieve dyspnea caused by an effusion, or to obtain fluid for testing.

Professional Considerations:

1. Consent form IS required.

Risks:

The risk of pneumothorax as a complication is small if the needle is withdrawn immediately. Also: air embolism, bradycardia, hypertension, pulmonary edema.

Contraindications:

Bleeding disorders or anticoagulated state, uncontrolled coughing.

2. Preparation:
   A. The procedure may be preceded by ultrasound or chest x-ray.
   B. Identify the upper border of the effusion by the loss of fremitus and the presence of flat percussion. The thoracentesis will be performed in the interspace below this level and 5–10 cm lateral to the spine.
   C. Obtain sterile gloves, injectable lidocaine, a thoracentesis tray, collection bottles with heparin, sterile 4 × 4 gauze pads, tape, and povidone-iodine.
   D. Obtain baseline vital signs.
   E. List any recent antibiotic therapy on the laboratory requisition.
3. Procedure:
   A. The client is positioned sitting upright, often in the orthopneic position, with arms and head supported by a table at the bedside. Clients who cannot sit up are placed in the lateral decubitus position, lying on the side of the effusion, near the edge of the bed. This procedure can be performed on those who are ventilator dependent.
   B. The skin is cleansed with povidone-iodine.
   C. The underlying tissue at the previously identified effusion site is anesthetized.
   D. A 20-gauge or larger needle is placed immediately above the superior aspect of the lower rib and advanced until the parietal membrane is penetrated and no more than 1 L of fluid is aspirated.
   E. At least 50 ml of fluid is needed for diagnostic studies.
4. Postprocedure care:
   A. Apply a pressure dressing and assess the puncture site for bleeding and crepitus every 5 minutes × 6.

B. Assess vital signs every 30 minutes × 4.

C. A follow-up chest x-ray should be taken within several hours of the procedure, or immediately if respiratory distress is exhibited.

5. Client and family teaching:

A. Describe the procedure and the usual sensations the client may expect related to the test.

B. Do not cough, breathe deeply, or move during the procedure.

6. Factors that affect results:

A. Complications that affect results include an air embolism, a hemothorax, a pneumothorax, and a pulmonary edema.

B. Transudate in the pleural space may be caused by ascites, cirrhosis (hepatic), congestive heart failure, hypertension (pulmonary, systemic), nephritis, and nephrosis.

C. Exudate in the pleural space may be caused by blocked lymphatic drainage, empyema, esophageal rupture, infarction (pulmonary), infection, neoplasm, pancreatitis, rheumatoid arthritis, systemic lupus erythematosus, thoracic duct disruption, traumatic injury, and tuberculosis.

D. Allowing fluid to stand for a prolonged period before processing may cause deterioration and artifacts.

7. Other data:

A. If the thoracentesis is performed below the tenth intercostal space, be careful not to lacerate the spleen or liver or penetrate the diaphragm (ipsilateral shoulder pain is a sign of diaphragmatic penetration).

B. Malignant cells cannot be recovered from all fluids for clients with malignancies.

C. Increased amylase levels in the effusion are associated with pancreatitis, lung cancer, and esophageal perforation.

D. The most common pathogens found in pleural effusions are *M. tuberculosis, S. aureus, S. pneumoniae,* and *H. influenzae.*

Bibliography:

Duvall CP: Complications associated with thoracentesis [letter; comment]. Arch Intern Med *151*(1): 201, 1991.

Qureshi N, Zahir M, Brandstetter R: Thoracentesis in clinical practice. Heart Lung *23*(5):376–383, 1994.

Weber A, Philipson E: Fetal pleural effusion. Obstet Gynecol *79*(2):281–286, 1992.

THROAT CULTURE FOR *CANDIDA ALBICANS,* CULTURE

Norm: Negative, no growth.

Usage: Immunosuppressive diseases, stomatitis, and thrush.

Description: *Candida albicans* is an opportunistic fungus that occurs in the aged, debilitated, newborns, and clients with acquired immune deficiency syndrome (AIDS) or cancer who are immunosuppressed. Steroid use is also a causative factor. This fungus occurs mostly on the buccal mucosa, tongue, palate, and mucous membranes. It appears as patches or plaques that are white to gray in color.

Professional Considerations:

1. Consent form NOT required.

2. Preparation:

A. Obtain a sterile cotton swab, a sterile container, and a tongue blade.

3. Procedure:

A. Swab suspicious lesions and place the swab in a sterile container.

4. Postprocedure care:

A. List the specific site of the specimen on the laboratory requisition.

B. Deliver the swab to the laboratory immediately or refrigerate the sample immediately.

5. Client and family teaching:

A. The turnaround time for results is normally 3–7 days.

6. Factors that affect results:

A. Dry swab or insufficient specimen volume.

7. Other data:

A. A Gram stain or potassium hydroxide (KOH) preparation may be prescribed to obtain a more rapid diagnosis.

B. Other *Candida* species (*C. tropicalis, C. glabrata, C. Kruei*) are being reported in individuals following lengthy imidazol or triazole antifungal therapy. These species are less susceptible to treatment.

Bibliography:

Coleman D, Bennett D, Sullivan D, et al.: Oral *Candida* in HIV infection and AIDS: New perspectives/new approaches. Crit Rev Microbiol *19*(2): 61–82, 1993.

Tang C, Cohen J: Diagnosing fungal infections in immuno-compromised hosts. J Clin Pathol *45*(1): 1–5, 1992.

THROAT CULTURE FOR *CORYNEBACTERIUM DIPHTHERIAE,* CULTURE
(see Culture, Throat for Corynebacterium, Specimen)

THROAT CULTURE FOR GROUP A-BETA-HEMOLYTIC STREPTOCOCCI, CULTURE

Norm: Negative, no growth.

Usage: Glomerulonephritis, pharyngitis, scarlet fever, strep throat, and tonsillitis.

Description: Group A beta-hemolytic streptococci is a bacteria usually introduced into the respiratory tract whose incubation period is 3–5 days. The onset of streptococcal sore throat is sudden, with frank chills, headache, malaise, fever, throat soreness, and exudative gray-white patches on the tonsils or pharynx.

Professional Considerations:

1. Consent form NOT required.
2. Preparation:
   A. Obtain a sterile cotton swab or Culturette, and a tongue blade.
   B. Obtain the specimen before initiating antibiotic therapy.
3. Procedure:
   A. Depress the tongue and take a swab of the throat and pharynx (both tonsils). Avoid swabbing the tongue, saliva, buccal mucosa, or the lips.
   B. Place the swab in a sterile container, or return the swab to the Culturette tube and crush the distal end to release the ampule of medium.
4. Postprocedure care:
   A. Send the specimen to the laboratory within 2 hours or refrigerate the specimen.
5. Client and family teaching:
   A. It is important to obtain the specimen prior to beginning antibiotics. Strep throat remains contagious until 24 hours after starting antibiotic therapy.
   B. If there is no improvement within 2 days, return to the health professional for further examination.
   C. Place a cool mist humidifier in the bedroom to relieve any tight, dry feeling in the throat. A sore throat may be relieved with salt water gargle (1 cup warm water + 1 teaspoon salt).
   D. For a schoolchild with positive culture, wait 24 hours after antibiotics have been started before letting the child return to school.
   E. Call the physician if developing a rash or coughing up green, yellow, or bloody sputum.
6. Factors that affect results:
   A. Technical proficiency is required to avoid false-positive and false-negative results.
   B. Previous antibiotic therapy may cause false-negative results. Up to 10% of clients who deny the use of antibiotics have been shown to have taken unprescribed antibiotics prior to contact with the health professional.
   C. The use of antibacterial gargles may cause false-negative results.
7. Other data:
   A. For a faster diagnosis, the swab can be incubated for 2 hours and then examined for fluorescent organisms; a rapid strep test for direct antigen detection can obtain results in 7–20 minutes, (the highest sensitivity with high colony counts); however, results should be confirmed with a throat culture.
   B. Penicillin is the treatment of choice, but erythromycin and clindamycin are also effective.

Bibliography:

Feldman W: Pharyngitis in children. Postgrad Med *93*(3):141–145, 1993.

Pichichero M, Disney F, Green J, et al.: Comparative reliability of clinical, culture, and antigen detection methods for the diagnosis of group A betahemolytic streptococcal tonsillopharyngitis. Pediatr Ann *21*(12):798–805, 1992.

Vukmir R: Adult and pediatric pharyngitis: a review. J Emerg Med *10*(5):607–616, 1992.

THROAT CULTURE FOR *NEISSERIA GONORRHOEAE,* CULTURE

Norm: Negative; no *Neisseria gonorrhoeae* isolated.

Usage: Gonococcal infection of pharynx, gonorrhea, and pharyngitis.

Description: *N. gonorrhoeae* is a pyogenic, gram-negative, oxidase-positive cocci that is an obligate parasite of humans. It is the causative organism of the sexually transmitted infection gonorrhea. *N. gonorrhoeae* inhabits the mucous membranes of the genital tract and may also be found in the oral mucosa of clients who engage in oral sex (gonococcal pharyngitis). Left untreated, gonorrhea leads to skin lesions, arthritis, meningitis, and reproductive problems.

Professional Considerations:

1. Consent form NOT required.
2. Preparation:
   A. Obtain a Thayer-Martin culture medium, sterile cotton swabs, and a tongue blade.
3. Procedure:
   A. Depress the tongue and swab from the tonsilar regions and the posterior pharynx.
   B. Place the specimen immediately onto the Thayer-Martin medium and incubate it in a carbon dioxide environment.
4. Postprocedure care:
   A. Transport the specimen to the laboratory within 2 hours.
5. Client and family teaching:
   A. Gonorrhea infection is treatable with antibiotics.
   B. Evaluate the client's knowledge of safe sex practices and review appropriate measures.
   C. If the results are positive, provide the

client with the appropriate information on sexually transmitted diseases.

   i. Notify all sexual partners from the last 90 days to be tested for gonorrhea infection.

   ii. Do not have sexual relations until the physician confirms that the infection is gone.

6. Factors that affect results:

   A. Refrigerating the specimen invalidates the culture.

7. Other data:

   A. Preliminary reports are available within 24 hours and the final report within 48 hours.

   B. For a faster diagnosis, the swab can be incubated for 2 hours and then examined for fluorescent organisms.

   C. Penicillin is the treatment of choice (plus probenecid), but erythromycin and clindamycin are also effective.

   D. For positive results, the client should also be serologically tested for syphilis. Consider also testing for AIDS.

   E. Positive results must usually be reported to the local health department.

Bibliography:

Roochvarg L, Lovechik J: Screening for pharyngeal gonorrhea in adolescents. J Adolesc Health *12*(3): 269–272, 1991.

Vlaspolder F, Mutsaers J, Blog F, et al.: Value of a DNA probe assay (Gen-Probe) compared with that of culture for diagnosis of gonococcal infection. J Clin Microbiol *31*(1):107–110, 1993.

THROAT CULTURE, ROUTINE, CULTURE

(see Culture, Routine, Specimen)

THROAT CULTURE, SWAB, DIAGNOSTIC

(see Culture, Routine, Specimen)

THROMBIN TIME, SERUM

Norm: Within 2 seconds of 9- to 13-second control value. Within 5 seconds of 15- to 20-second control value; <1.5 times control value.

Increased: Acute leukemia, afibrinogenemia, amyloidosis, cirrhosis, disseminated intravascular coagulation (DIC), dysfibrinogenemia, epistaxis, factor deficiency, fibrinopenia, lymphoma, obstetric complications, polycythemia vera, shock, and stress. Drugs include asparaginase, fibrin degradation products, heparin, streptokinase, tissue plasminogen activator (TPA), uremia, and urokinase.

Decreased: Thrombocytosis.

Description: Thrombin is an enzyme that functions in the release of fibrin from fibrinogen in the final stage of the clotting cascade. This test measures the clotting time of a sample of plasma to which thrombin has been added. Thrombin time is longer than normal when abnormalities in the conversion of fibrinogen into fibrin are present.

Professional Considerations:

1. Consent form NOT required.

2. Preparation:

   A. Tube: 2.7-ml blue-top or 4.5-ml blue-top and a control tube, and a waste tube or syringe.

3. Procedure:

   A. Withdraw 2 ml of blood into a syringe or vacuum tube. Remove the syringe or tube, leaving the needle in place. (From a heparinized line, discard an amount equal to the volume of the tubing prime.) Attach a second syringe, and draw a blood sample volume of 2.4 ml for a 2.7-ml tube and 4.0 ml for a 4.5-ml tube.

   B. Gently tilt the tube five or six times to mix the sample.

4. Postprocedure care:

   A. Send the sample to the laboratory within 2 hours.

   B. Refrigerate the sample. The plasma should be frozen if it is not tested promptly.

5. Client and family teaching:

   A. Results can be available within an hour.

6. Factors that affect results:

   A. Hemolyzed specimens invalidate the results.

   B. Failure to discard the first 1–2 ml of blood may result in specimen contamination with tissue thromboplastin.

   C. Heparin therapy within 2 days prior to the test increases the results. Collecting a sample from a heparinized line without discarding the first blood withdrawn can falsely prolong results.

   D. A recent blood or plasma transfusion will invalidate the results.

7. Other data:

   A. The test is used as a rapid screening device to detect profound fibrinogen deficiency.

   B. This test is not reliable to monitor heparin therapy in clients with DIC.

   C. This test will NOT differentiate primary fibrinolysis from DIC.

Bibliography:

Gastineau DA, Gertz MA, Daniels TM, et al.: Inhibitor of the thrombin time in systemic amyloidosis: A common coagulation abnormality. Blood *77*(12): 2637–2640, 1991.

Wang J, Lin C, Karp R: Comparison of high-dose thrombin time with activated clotting time for monitoring of anticoagulant effects of heparin in cardiac surgical patients. Anesthesia Analgesia 79(1):9–13, 1994.

THROMBOPLASTIN TIME, ACTIVATED PARTIAL, DIAGNOSTIC
(see Partial Thromboplastin Time, Plasma)

THYROCALCITONIN, SERUM
(see Calcitonin, Plasma or Serum)

THYROID ANTIMICROSOMAL ANTIBODY, BLOOD

Norm: Negative (hemagglutination, IFA methods); titer <1:100 (complement fixation method); titer ≤25 U/ml (≤25 kU/L, SI units) (radioimmunoassay method).

Positive or Increased: Anemia (pernicious), goiter (nontoxic nodular), granulomatous thyroiditis, Grave's disease, Hashimoto's (chronic) thyroiditis, hyperthyroidism, lupus erythematosus, myasthenia gravis, myxedema, primary hypothyroidism, rheumatoid arthritis, Sjögren's syndrome, and thyroid cancer. Drugs include hypersensitivity reactions to anticonvulsants and sulfonamides.

Description: Thyroid antimicrosomal antibody is an autoantibody (primarily IgG) directed against the lipoprotein microsomal antigen present in the epithelium of the thyroid gland. This antibody (which is neither sensitive nor specific) may be present in inflammation of the thyroid gland, or may be the cause of hypothyroidism secondary to thyroid tissue destruction. The test is also helpful in identifying thyroid autoimmunity in clients who have other autoimmune diseases.

Professional Considerations:
1. Consent form NOT required.
2. Preparation:
   A. Tube: Red-top, red/gray-top, or gold-top.
3. Procedure:
   A. Draw a 7-ml blood sample.
4. Postprocedure care:
   A. Separate and freeze the serum if it is not to be tested within 24 hours after collection.

5. Client and family teaching:
   A. Results are normally available within 72 hours.
6. Factors that affect results:
   A. Antibody may be present in up to 15% of clients with no disease symptoms and in up to 20% age 70 and over.
   B. Positive titers may decrease during pregnancy. They may also briefly increase after giving birth.
   C. The radioimmunoassay method should not be used if the client received radioactive therapy within 30 days prior to the test.
7. Other data:
   A. The thyroid antithyroglobulin antibody test should also be performed to eliminate other causes of thyroiditis.

Bibliography:
Intenzo C, Park C, Kim S, et al.: Clinical laboratory and scintographic manifestation of subacute and chronic thyroiditis. Clin Nucl Med 18(4):302–306, 1993.

Kawai K, Tamai H, Mori T, et al.: Thyroid histology of hyper thyroid Graves's disease with undetectable thyrotropin receptor antibodies. J Clin Endorinol Metab 27(3):716–719, 1993.

Poropatich C, Marcus D, Oertel Y: Hashimoto's thyroiditis: fine-needle aspiration of 50 asymptomatic cases. Diagn Cytopathol 11(2):141–145, 1994.

Wallach, J (ed): Interpretation of Diagnostic Tests, 5th ed. Boston, Little, Brown, 1992, p 751.

THYROID ANTITHYROGLOBULIN ANTIBODY, SERUM

Norm: Negative, or titer <1:100.

Positive or Increased: Anemia (autoimmune hemolytic, pernicious), goiter (nontoxic nodular), granulomatous thyroiditis, Grave's disease, Hashimoto's (chronic) thyroiditis, hyperthyroidism, hypothyroidism, myxedema, rheumatoid arthritis, Sjögren's syndrome, systemic lupus erythematosus, thyroid cancer, and thyrotoxicosis.

Description: Thyroid antiglobulin antibody is an autoantibody directed against the antigen thyroglobulin, a thyroid glycoprotein that functions in the synthesis of triiodothyronine (T_3) and thyroxine (T_4). This antibody may be present in inflammation of the thyroid gland, or may be the cause of hypothyroidism secondary to thyroid tissue destruction. The test is also helpful in identifying thyroid autoimmunity in clients who have other autoimmune diseases.

Professional Considerations:

1. Consent form NOT required.
2. Preparation:
   A. Tube: Red-top, red/gray-top, or gold-top.
3. Procedure:
   A. Draw a 7-ml blood sample.
4. Postprocedure care:
   A. None.
5. Client and family teaching:
   A. Results are normally available within a few days.
6. Factors that affect results:
   A. Antibody may be present in a small number of clients with no disease symptoms.
7. Other data:
   A. The thyroid antimicrosomal antibody test should also be performed to eliminate other causes of thyroiditis.

Bibliography:

Chow F, Wang P, Sheen-Chen S: The presence of higher levels of thyroglobin, but not thyroid autoantibodies in the thyroid vein in Graves' disease. J Endo Invst *17*(1):41–44, 1994.

Shechner C, Kraiem Z, Luckerman E, et al.: Toxic Graves' disease with thyroid hemangenisis: Diagnosis using thyroid stimulating immunoglobulin measurements. Thyroid *2*(2):133–135, 1992.

Wallach, J (ed): Interpretation of Diagnostic Tests, 5th ed. Boston, Little, Brown, 1992, p 571.

THYROID ECHOGRAM
(see Thyroid Sonogram, Diagnostic)

THYROID FUNCTION TESTS, BLOOD

Norm:

		SI Units
Free Thyroxine Index		**Mean**
Puberty through adulthood	4.2–13.0	8.0
Children and infants:		
Cord blood	6.0–13.2	9.8
First 72 hours	9.9–17.5	13.9
7 days	7.5–15.1	11.2
4–52 weeks	5.0–13.0	8.4
1–3 years	5.4–12.5	8.1
3–10 years	5.7–12.8	8.2
Thyroxine (T_4) Radioimmunoassay		
Adults	5.0–12.0 µg/dl	65–155 nmol/L
Pregnant >14 weeks	9.1–14.0 µg/dl	117–181 nmol/L
Elderly (>age 60):		
Female	5.5–10.5 µg/dl	71–135 nmol/L
Male	5.0–10.0 µg/dl	65–129 nmol/L
Children		
Cord blood	7.4–13.0 µg/dl	95–168 nmol/L
First 72 hours	11.8–22.6 µg/dl	152–292 nmol/L
7–14 days	9.8–16.6 µg/dl	126–214 nmol/L
4–16 weeks	7.2–14.4 µg/dl	93–186 nmol/L
4–12 months	7.8–16.5 µg/dl	101–213 nmol/L
12 months–5 years	7.3–15.0 µg/dl	94–194 nmol/L
5–10 years	6.4–13.3 µg/dl	83–172 nmol/L
10–15 years	5.6–11.7 µg/dl	72–151 nmol/L
Triiodothyronine (T_3) Radioimmunoassay		
Adults	80–230 ng/dl	1.2–3.5 nmol/L
Children		
Cord blood	15–75 ng/dl	0.23–1.16 nmol/L
First 72 hours	32–216 ng/dl	0.49–3.33 nmol/L
7–14 days	Average 250 ng/dl	Average 3.85 nmol/L
2–4 weeks	160–240 ng/dl	2.46–3.70 nmol/L
4–16 weeks	117–209 ng/dl	1.80–3.22 nmol/L
16–52 weeks	110–280 ng/dl	1.70–4.31 nmol/L

		SI Units
Triiodothyronine (T₃) Radioimmunoassay *(continued)*		**Mean**
Children *(continued)*		
1–5 years	105–269 ng/dl	1.62–4.14 nmol/L
5–10 years	94–241 ng/dl	1.45–3.71 nmol/L
10–15 years	83–213 ng/dl	1.28–3.28 nmol/L
Thyroid-Stimulating Hormone (TSH)		
Adults	<10 μU/ml	3.0–20 mU/L
Adults >age 60		
Female	2.0–16.8 μU/ml	2.0–16.8 mU/L
Male	2.0–7.3 μU/ml	2.0–7.3 mU/L
Newborn (days 1–3)	3.0–20.0 μU/ml	3.0–20.0 mU/L

Usage: Work-up of suspected thyroid disorder; and differentiation of primary thyroid disease from secondary causes and from abnormalities in thyroxin-binding globulin levels.

Description: Thyroid function testing involves performing several measurements on one sample of blood. These tests have largely been replaced by the thyroid-stimulating hormone assay. Tests included are as follows: *Thyroid Test: Free Thyroxine Index, Serum; Thyroid Test: Thyroid-Stimulating Hormone, Blood and Sensitive Assay, Blood; Thyroid Test: Thyroxine, Blood; and Thyroid Test: Triiodothyronine, Blood.* See individual test listings for further description.

Professional Considerations:
1. Consent form NOT required.
2. Preparation:
   A. Tube: Red-top, red/gray-top, or gold-top.
3. Procedure:
   A. Completely fill the tube with venous blood.
4. Postprocedure care:
   A. None.
5. Client and family teaching:
   A. Results are normally available within a few days.
6. Factors that affect results:
   A. Results are invalidated if the client has undergone a radionuclide scan within 7 days prior to the test.
7. Other data:
   A. See individual test listings.

Bibliography:

Martinez M, Derksen D, Kapner P: Making sense of hypothyroidism. Postgrad Med *93*(6):135–138, 141–145, 1993.

Price DE, O'Malley BP, Northover B, Rosenthal FD: Changes in circulating thyroid hormone levels and systolic time intervals in acute hypothyroidism. Clin Endocrinol *35*(1):67–69, 1991.

Radunovic N, Dumez Y, Nastic D, et al.: Thyroid function in fetus and mother during the second half of normal pregnancy. Biol Neonate *59*(3):139–148, 1991.

THYROID HORMONE BINDING RATIO, BLOOD

Norm:

		SI Units
T₃Uptake		
Adult	24–34%	24–34 arb. units
Elderly (>age 60)		
Female	22–32%	22–32 arb. units
Male	24–32%	24–32 arb. units
Neonates	25–37%	25–37 arb. units
Thyroid Hormone Binding Ratio		
Adults (≤age 50)	0.85–1.14	0.85–1.14 arb. units
Adults (>age 50)		
Female	0.80–1.04	0.80–1.04 arb. units
Male	0.87–1.11	0.87–1.11 arb. units

		SI Units

Thyroid Hormone Binding Ratio (*continued*)

Children

Cord blood	0.75–1.05	0.75–1.05 arb. units
First 72 hours	0.90–1.40	0.90–1.40 arb. units
7–14 days	0.82–1.15	0.82–1.15 arb. units
4–16 weeks	0.75–1.05	0.75–1.05 arb. units
1–15 years	0.88–1.12	0.88–1.12 arb. units

Free Thyroxine Index		**Mean**
Puberty through adulthood	4.2–13.0	8.0
Infants and children		
Cord blood	6.0–13.2	9.8
First 72 hours	9.9–17.5	13.9
7 days	7.5–15.1	11.2
4–52 weeks	5.0–13.0	8.4
1–3 years	5.4–12.5	8.1
3–10 years	5.7–12.8	8.2

Increased T_3 Uptake and THBR: Decreased TBG (genetic deficiency or due to other causes), hyperandrogenic state, hyperthyroidism, hypoproteinemia, liver disease (severe), malnutrition, metastasis, nephrosis, nephrotic syndrome, protein loss, and thyrotoxicosis factitia. Drugs include adrenocorticotropic hormone, androgens, barbiturates, corticosteroids, glucocorticoids, furosemide, penicillin (large doses), phenylbutazone, phenytoins, salicylates (high doses), thyroid extract, and thyroxine.

Decreased T_3 Uptake and THBR: Cretinism, endocrine-secreting tumors, hepatitis (acute), hypothyroidism, increased TBG (congenital excess or due to other causes), and pregnancy. Drugs include chlorpromazine, estrogens, heroin, lithium carbonate, methadone, oral contraceptives, perphenazine (long-term use), and propylthiouracil.

Description: This test measures the amount of unbound thyroid hormone binding sites on thyroxine-binding globulin (TBG), a major protein carrier of thyroid hormones. The measurement is obtained by measuring the amount of radiolabeled T_3 bound by a T_3-binding resin (T_3 uptake) after all TBG binding sites in a client's blood sample are saturated. The number of sites available is dependent upon the amount of thyroxine (T_4) present, as it is present in greater quantities than triiodothyronine (T_3) and has a greater

affinity for TBG than does T_3. The greater the number of TBG binding sites available, the lower will be the T_3 uptake by the resin. The greater the amount of T_4 present, the smaller will be the proportion of unbound TBG binding sites, and the greater will be the T_3 uptake by the resin. T_3 uptake is used to calculate the thyroid hormone binding ratio (THBR) as follows:

$$\frac{\% \ T_3 \ \text{Uptake}}{\text{Mean} \ \% \ T_3 \ \text{uptake of reference serum}}$$

THBR compared to T_4 level is useful in determining whether thyroid hormone changes are due to thyroid disease or to abnormalities in TBG. If the values show parallel changes, a problem in thyroid function is indicated. However, if the results show opposite changes, an abnormality in the amount of TBG is more likely. Use of these results in a further calculation provides an indirect measurement of free T_4 in the bloodstream by multiplying the T_3 uptake by the client's T_4 level to obtain the free thyroxine index (FTI).

Professional Considerations:

1. Consent form NOT required.
2. Preparation:
   A. Tube: Red-top, red/gray-top, or gold-top.
3. Procedure:
   A. Draw a 7-ml blood sample.
4. Postprocedure care:
   A. Refrigerate specimens until tested. Freeze specimens at –20°C if the test is not performed within 1 week after collection.

5. Client and family teaching:
   A. Results are normally available within 72 hours.
6. Factors that affect results:
   A. THBR results may be falsely increased in acidosis (severe) and atrial fibrillation.
   B. Drugs that cause falsely elevated results include dicumarol, heparin, phenytoin, and salicylates.
7. Other data:
   A. "THBR" replaces nomenclature of "T$_3$ uptake."
   B. *See also Thyroid Test: Thyroxine, Blood; and Thyroid Test: Triiodothyronine, Blood.*

Bibliography:

Faix J, Rosen H, Velazquez F: Indirect estimate of thyroid-binding protein to calculate free thyroxine index: Comparison of nonisotopic methods that use labeled thyroxine ("T-uptake"). Clin Chem *41*(1):41–47, 1995.

Pakarinen A, Hakkinen K, Alen M: Serum thyroid hormones, thyrotropin and thyroxine binding globulin in elite athletes during very intense strength training of one week. J Sports Med Phys Fitness *31*(2):142–146, 1991.

THYROID PROFILE, BLOOD
(see Thyroid Function Tests, Blood)

THYROID SCAN, DIAGNOSTIC

Norm: Homogeneous uptake of radioactive tracer; and normal size, shape, and position of the thyroid gland.

Usage: Differentiation of hyperfunctioning nodule and of thyroid tissue hyperplasia; of help in diagnosing thyroid cancer; evaluation of thyroid in client with history of irradiated head and neck; and monitoring of the thyroid gland during therapy.

Description: A thyroid scan is a nuclear medicine scan of the thyroid after injection of a radioactive tracer (I-123, I-125, I-131, or Tc-99m) for the purpose of detecting areas of increased or decreased tracer uptake by thyroid and area tissue. Hyperfunctioning thyroid nodules (usually nonmalignant) cause areas of increased uptake labeled as "hot nodules." "Cold nodules" are nodules that do not take up the tracer (i.e., tissue is not functioning as normal thyroid tissue) and are more likely to be malignant.

Professional Considerations:

1. Consent form NOT required.

Risks:
Allergic reaction to tracer (itching, hives, rash, tight feeling in the throat, shortness of breath, anaphylaxis).

Contraindications:
Previous allergy to iodine, shellfish, or radioactive tracer; pregnancy; breast-feeding.

2. Preparation:
   A. *See Client and family teaching.*
   B. Have emergency equipment readily available.
   C. Jewelry and metal objects near the head or neck area should be removed prior to scanning.
3. Procedure:
   A. Oral radioactive tracer is administered 6 hours prior to scanning. Intravenous radioactive tracer is administered ½ hour prior to scanning.
   B. The client is positioned supine, with a pillow, rolled towel, or sponge beneath the shoulder blades, and the neck hyperextended.
   C. The thyroid gland is scanned with a gamma camera that moves over one or more sections of the thyroid gland.
   D. Scan takes ½ hour.
4. Postprocedure care:
   A. Resume previous diet 2 hours after oral radioactive tracer administration.
   B. Observe the client carefully for up to 60 minutes after the study for a possible (anaphylactic) reaction to the radionuclide.
   C. Rubber gloves should be worn by health care providers when discarding urine for 24 hours after the procedure. Wash the gloved hands with soap and water before removing the gloves. Wash the ungloved hands after the gloves are removed. An incontinent client requires special handling of any soiled linen or disposable pads. These should be placed in special storage for a few weeks before cleaning or discarding. Consult with your radiation safety officer for details.
5. Client and family teaching:
   A. Drugs that may be discontinued up to 21 days prior to the scan include anticoagulants, antihistamines, corticosteroids, cough syrup, radiopaque dyes (28–42 days), phenothiazines, salicylates, thyroxine (10 days), triiodothyronine (3 days), iodides, vitamins, and antithyroid medications such as propylthiouracil or Tapazole (3 days).
   B. Foods that should not be ingested for 14–21 days prior to the test include shellfish and salt or salt substitutes containing iodine.

C. Fast from food and fluids for 4 hours before and 1 hour after, if radioactive tracer will be administered orally.

D. There is no discomfort with this test.

E. Describe the procedure and expected sensations.

F. Meticulously wash your hands with soap and water after each void × 24 hours. The toilet should be flushed 2–3 times after each voiding.

6. Factors that affect results:

A. If a radioactive iodine tracer is used, uptake may be increased in clients on a diet with subnormal iodine levels, or those on phenothiazine therapy.

B. Ingestion of drugs listed under "Client and family teaching" within 2–3 weeks prior to the test may cause decreased tracer uptake.

C. Gastroenteritis may interfere with absorption of orally administered radioactive tracer.

D. Receipt by the client of intrathecal or intravenous contrast material within 21 days prior to the scan invalidates the results.

7. Other data:

A. Health care professionals working in a nuclear medicine area must follow federal standards set by the Nuclear Regulatory Commission. These standards include precautions for handling the radioactive material and monitoring of potential radiation exposure.

B. Technetium half-life is 6 hours. Iodine-131 half-life is 8 days. Iodine-123 half-life is 13.3 hours.

Bibliography:

Foldes I, Levay A, Stotz G: Comparative scanning of thyroid nodules with technetium-99m pertecnetate and technetium-99 methoxyisobutylisonitrile. Eur J Nucl Med *20*(4):330–333, 1993.

Gordon K, Wagner R, Dillehay G, et al.: The effect of fine-needle aspiration biopsy on the thyroid scan. Clin Nucl Med *18*(6):495–497, 1993.

Kasagi K, Hatabu H, Miyamoto S, et al.: Scintigraphic findings of the thyroid in hypothyroid patients with blocking type TSH-receptor antibodies. Eur J Nucl Med *21*(9):962–967, 1994.

Kasagi K, Hidaka A, Misaki T, et al.: Scintigraphic findings of the thyroid in Euthyroid ophthalmic Graves' disease. J Nucl Med *35*(5):811–817, 1994.

Persuhn, PG: Nuclear medicine: What exactly is it? Images *15*(1): 11–14, 1996.

THYROID SONOGRAM (THYROID ECHOGRAM, THYROID ULTRASOUND), DIAGNOSTIC

Norm: Proper size, shape, and position of the thyroid gland. Negative for cyst or tumor. Thyroid tissue demonstrates an even mixture of medium-level echoes.

Usage: Differentiation between cyst and tumor not distinguishable by other studies, guidance for aspiration of thyroid cyst, monitoring of thyroid nodules during pregnancy, and ongoing monitoring of size of thyroid during radioactive therapy.

Description: Evaluation of the thyroid gland size, shape, and position via the creation of an oscilloscopic picture from the echoes of high-frequency sound waves passing over the neck area (acoustic imaging). The time required for the ultrasonic beam to be reflected back to the transducer from differing densities of tissue is converted by a computer to an electrical impulse displayed on an oscilloscopic screen to create a three-dimensional picture of the thyroid gland. The differing tissue densities of cysts and tumors enable the sonogram to be helpful in determining which is present. Cysts are clearly demarcated by smooth borders and do not demonstrate internal echoes. Adenoma appearance varies, but usually demonstrates a halo. Multinodular goiter may also demonstrate a halo. In thyroiditis, the gland appears enlarged, with a greater than normal amount of low-level echoes. Thyroid cancer is usually poorly defined, with low-level echoes, and without a halo. Advantages of this test are that it is safe for use during pregnancy, it can detect smaller nodules (2 mm) than can nuclear medicine scanning, and it can differentiate cysts from solid nodules (which nuclear medicine scans cannot).

Professional Considerations:

1. Consent form NOT required.

2. Preparation.

A. Remove any metallic objects or jewelry from the head and neck area.

B. Obtain ultrasonic gel.

3. Procedure:

A. The client is positioned supine, with a towel roll, pillow, or sponge beneath the shoulder blades, and the neck hyperextended, with the head turned away from the side of the thyroid gland being scanned. This permits better transducer access to the area by moving the mandible out of the scanning area.

B. The neck area is covered with ultrasonic gel, and a lubricated transducer is passed slowly and firmly over the thyroid gland and neck at specific intervals. Each lobe of the thyroid gland is examined separately and completely, beginning with transverse scanning followed by longitudinal scanning. Finally, the isthmus is scanned transversely.

C. Photographs are taken of the oscilloscopic display.

D. The procedure takes less than 20 minutes.

4. Postprocedure care:
   A. Remove ultrasonic gel from the skin.
   B. If thyroid cyst aspiration is performed under sonogram guidance, see separate test listing, *Needle Aspiration, Diagnostic.*

5. Client and family teaching:
   A. The procedure is painless.

6. Factors that affect results:
   A. None found.

7. Other data:
   A. Ultrasound alone should not be relied upon for diagnosis of malignant thyroid nodules. Aspiration biopsy cytology is necessary to confirm or add to the diagnosis.

Bibliography:

Freitas J: Thyroid and parathyroid imaging. Sem Nuc Med *24*(3):234–245, 1994.

Jarlov A: Observer variation in ultrasound assessment of the thyroid gland. Brit J Rad *66*(787):625–627, 1993.

Reading C, Gorman C: Thyroid imaging techniques. Clin Lab Med *13*(3):711–724, 1993.

THYROID-STIMULATING HORMONE (TSH, THYROTROPIN), BLOOD

Norm:

		SI Units
Adults	<10 µU/ml	3.0–20 mU/L
Adults (>age 60)		
Female	2.0–16.8 µU/ml	2.0–16.8 mU/L
Male	2.0–7.3 µU/ml	2.0–7.3 mU/L
Newborn (days 1–3)	3.0–20.0 µU/ml	3.0–20.0 mU/L

Increased: Addison's disease (primary), anti-TSH antibodies, euthyroid goiter (with enzyme defect), fasting state, goiter (iodine-deficiency type), hyperpituitarism, hypothyroidism (primary), hypothermia, pituitary adenoma (that secretes thyrotropin), postoperatively (subtotal thyroidectomy), psychiatric illness (acute), status following therapy with radioactive iodine, and thyroiditis. Drugs include amiodarone, benserazide, clomiphene, iopanoic acid, ipodate, lithium, methimazole, metoclopramide, morphine, propylthiouracil, radiographic dye, SSKI, and thyroid-releasing hormone.

Decreased: Hashimoto's thyroiditis, hyperthyroidism, hypothyroidism (secondary, tertiary) (sometimes), and organic brain syndrome. Drugs include ASA, corticosteroids, heparin, ketoconazole, T_3, and TSH.

Description: Thyroid-stimulating hormone (TSH) is produced as a glycoprotein by the anterior lobe of the pituitary gland in response to low blood levels of thyroid hormone and to stimulation of thyrotropin-releasing hormone from the hypothalamus. After release, TSH stimulates production and release of triiodothyronine (T_3) and thyroxine (T_4), thyroid uptake of iodine, iodination of tyrosine, and an increased rate of body metabolism. This test is helpful in differentiating primary hypothyroidism (in which TSH is elevated, indicating normal pituitary and hypothalamic function) from other causes. *See also Thyroid Test: Thyroid-Stimulating Hormone Assay, Blood and Filter Paper.*

Professional Considerations:

1. Consent form NOT required.
2. Preparation:
   A. Tube: Red-top, red/gray-top, or gold-top.
3. Procedure:
   A. Draw a 7-ml blood sample.
   B. Handle the sample gently to prevent hemolysis.
4. Postprocedure care:
   A. None.
5. Client and family teaching:
   A. Results are normally available within 48 hours.
6. Factors that affect results:
   A. Results are invalid if the client received a radioactive isotope within the prior 7 days.
   B. TSH is released in a diurnal, pulsatile

pattern, with the highest levels occurring in the late evening and the lowest levels occurring in the midmorning. High levels may be three times greater than low levels. Preferred collection time is early morning.

C. Results are unreliable in clients receiving dopamine or glucocorticoids, or in those who are seriously ill.

D. Cross-reactions are possible with the alpha-subunit of human chorionic gonadotropin when it is extremely elevated.

7. Other data:

A. Conventional TSH tests have been made obsolete by the TSH ultrasensitive assays.

B. Some of the older literature recommends confirmatory thyrotropin-stimulation testing for elevated TSH levels; however, TSH stimulation testing is almost never needed.

C. The dose of levothyroxine needed for replacement with primary hypothyroidism diminishes with age.

Bibliography:

Klee G, Hay I: Role of thyrotropin measurements in the diagnosis and management of thyroid disease. Clin Lab Med *13*(3)673–682, 1993.

Martinez M, Derksen D, Kapner P: Making sense of hypothyroidism. Postgrad Med *93*(6):135–138, 141–145, 1993.

Polk D: Diagnosis and Management of altered fetal thyroid status. Clin Perinatol *21*(3):647–663, 1994.

Shigemasa C, Tetsuo K, Yoshihiko U: Evaluation of thyroid function in patients with isolated adrenocorticotropin deficiency. Am J Med Sci *304*(5): 279–284, 1992.

THYROID-STIMULATING HORMONE, FILTER PAPER, BLOOD

Norm:

		SI Units
Newborn		
At birth, peak occurs of up to	30 µU/ml	30 mU/L
3 days old	<20 µU/ml	<20 mU/L
10 days old	<10 µU/ml	<10 mU/L

Usage: Newborn screening for congenital hypothyroidism. May also be used to follow children known to have congenital hypothyroidism. Must be interpreted in light of T_4 levels.

Description: *See also Thyroid Test: Thyroid-stimulating Hormone (TSH), Blood.* Thyroid screening is recommended for all newborns from birth to up to 4 weeks. With congenital hypothyroidism, TSH will be elevated. Test kits developed in the late 1980s are considered specific enough to use for screening purposes. Early detection of congenital hypothyroidism enables treatment and prevents complications, which include mental retardation and subnormal growth patterns.

Professional Considerations:

1. Consent form NOT required.
2. Preparation:
   A. Obtain alcohol wipe, lancet, and TSH filter paper card.
   B. Prewarming the heel is not necessary.
3. Procedure:
   A. Cleanse the lateral curvature of the infant's heel with alcohol and allow it to dry.
   B. Puncture the lateral heel curvature with a lancet.
   C. Saturate a spot on the TSH filter paper card with heelstick blood.
   D. Allow the blood spot to dry before sending the sample to the lab.
4. Postprocedure care:
   A. Apply pressure to the puncture site until the bleeding stops. Let the site air-dry.
5. Client and family teaching:
   A. Results are normally available immediately.
6. Factors that affect results:
   A. The test must be repeated if the blood amount is not enough to completely saturate a spot on the card.
   B. Touching the filter paper or exposure to extremes of heat and light can cause errors in the results.
7. Other data:
   A. None.

Bibliography:

Bourdoux PP, Van Thi HV, Courtois PA, et al.: Superiority of thyrotropin to thyroxine as a tool in the screening for congenital hypothyroidism by the filter paper spot technique. Clin Chem Acta *195*(3):97–105, 1991.

Eldar D, Gelernter L, Sack J: Blood-spotted filter paper measurements of thyroxine and thyroid-stimulating hormone in the follow-up of children with congenital hypothyroidism. Horm Res *34*(5–6): 219–223, 1990.

Grant DB: Monitoring TSH concentrations during treatment for congenital hypothyroidism. Arch Dis Child *66*(6):669–670, 1991.

THYROID-STIMULATING HORMONE, SENSITIVE ASSAY (SENSITIVE TSH ASSAY, SENSITIVE THYROTROPIN ASSAY), BLOOD

Norm:

Adults	0.5–5.0 µU/ml*
Adults (>age 80)	up to 10 µU/ml
Newborn (by day 3)	<20 µU/ml
Diagnostic values	
1° hypothyroidism	<0.3µU/ml
2–3° hypothyroidism	<0.1µU/ml
Hyperthyroidism	>20 µU/ml
Desired level when receiving thyroxine therapy	0.5–3.5 µU/ml

*The middle 95% of adults have values in the range of 0.5–3.5 µU/ml. The upper reference limit is set at 5.0 µU/ml to prevent inappropriate treatment with thyroxine.

Increased: Addison's disease (primary), anti-TSH antibodies, euthyroid goiter (with enzyme defect), fasting state, goiter (iodine-deficiency type), hyperpituitarism, hypothyroidism (primary), hypothermia, pituitary adenoma (that secretes thyrotropin), postoperatively (subtotal thyroidectomy), psychiatric illness (acute), status following therapy with radioactive iodine, and thyroiditis. Drugs include amiodarone, benserazide, clomiphene, iopanoic acid, ipodate, lithium, methimazole, metoclopramide, morphine, propylthiouracil, radiographic dye, SSKI, and thyroid-releasing hormone.

Decreased: Hashimoto's thyroiditis, hyperthyroidism, hypothyroidism (secondary, tertiary) (sometimes), and organic brain syndrome. Drugs include ASA, corticosteroids, dopamine, heparin, ketoconazole, T_3, and TSH.

Description: Serum TSH assay is an ultrasensitive indicator that has largely replaced all of the other tests used to diagnose hypothyroidism and monitor treatment, although some controversy with this practice exists. If the assay is normal, further testing is not indicated. If the assay is abnormal, a T_4 assay should be prescribed. *See also Thyroid Test: Thyroid-Stimulating Hormone (TSH, Thyrotropin), Blood.*

Professional Considerations:

1. Consent form NOT required.
2. Preparation:
   A. Tube: Red-top, red/gray-top, or gold/top.
3. Procedure:
   A. Draw a 1-ml blood sample.
4. Postprocedure care:
   A. None.
5. Client and family teaching:
   A. Results are normally available within 24 hours.
6. Factors that affect results:
   A. Levels are elevated temporarily when recovering from illness, but return to normal after recovery.
7. Other data:
   A. None.

Bibliography:

Feldcamp C, McKenna M: Contemporary approach to thyroid disease emphasizing use of high-sensitivity thyrotropin assays. Henry Ford Hosp Med J *39*(1):25–29, 1991.

Klee G, Hay I: Role of thyrotropin measurements in the diagnosis and management of thyroid disease. Clin Lab Med *13*(3):673–682, 1993.

Spencer C, Schwarzbein D, Guttler R, et al.: Thyrotropin (TSH)-releasing hormone stimulating test responses employing third and fourth generation TSH assays. J Clin Endocrinol *76*(2):494–498, 1993.

Spencer C, Takeuchi M, Kazarosyan M: Interlaboratory-intermethod differences in functional sensitivity of immunometric assays of thyrotropin (TSH) and impact on reliability of measurement of subnormal concentration of TSH. Clin Chem *41*(3):367–374, 1995.

THYROID-STIMULATING HORMONE STIMULATION TEST (THYROTROPIN-STIMULATION TEST), DIAGNOSTIC

Norm: Uptake (or increased uptake) of radioactive iodine occurs after administration of exogenous thyrotropin.

Usage: Differentiation of primary hypothyroidism from hypothyroidism secondary to pituitary deficiency.

Description: Thyroid-stimulating hormone (TSH) is produced as a glycoprotein by the anterior lobe of the pituitary gland both in response to low blood levels of thyroid hormone, and stimulation of thyrotropin-releasing hormone from the hypothalamus. One action of TSH is to stimulate thyroid uptake of iodine. In this 5-day test, thyroid uptake of radioactive iodine after exogenous administration of TSH is evaluated. The test is performed to confirm a suspected diagnosis of primary hypothyroidism, in which baseline TSH levels are elevated. In clients with normal thyroid glands, exogenous TSH stimulates uptake of the radioactive iodine, which is identified by nuclear medicine scanning. In clients with primary hypothyroidism, the thyroid gland does not respond to the exogenous TSH.

Professional Considerations:

1. Consent form NOT required.

Risks:

Allergic reaction to dye (itching, hives, rash, tight feeling in the throat, shortness of breath, anaphylaxis).

Contraindications:

Previous allergy to iodine, shellfish, or radiographic dye. The client may develop antibodies to the exogenous TSH.

2. Preparation:
    A. Have emergency equipment readily available.
    B. Baseline levels of radioactive iodine and thyroxine (T_4) should be known.
    C. Tube: Red-top, red/gray-top, or gold-top for each T_4 level.
3. Procedure:
    A. First day:
        i. 2–15 µCi of I-131 is administered orally.
    B. Second day:
        i. 24 hours after the I-131 dose, nuclear medicine scanning of the thyroid gland is performed to measure radioactive iodine uptake.
        ii. T_4 levels are drawn (1-ml blood sample).
        iii. Thyrotropin, 10 U (adults) or 5 U (children), is administered intramuscularly.
    C. Third day:
        i. Thyrotropin, 10 U (adults) or 5 U

(children), is administered intramuscularly.
    D. Fourth day:
        i. Thyrotropin, 10 U (adults) or 5 U (children), is administered intramuscularly.
    E. Fifth day:
        i. Nuclear medicine scanning of the thyroid gland is performed to measure radioactive iodine uptake.
        ii. T_4 levels are drawn (1-ml blood sample).
4. Postprocedure care:
    A. Observe the client carefully for up to 60 minutes after each I-131 study for a possible (anaphylactic) reaction to the radionuclide.
    B. When urine is being discarded, rubber gloves should be worn for 24 hours after each injection. Wash the gloved hands with soap and water before removing the gloves. Wash the ungloved hands after the gloves have been removed.
5. Client and family teaching:
    A. Meticulously wash your hands with soap and water after each void × 24 hours.
6. Factors that affect results:
    A. The test may be normal with secondary hypothyroidism.
7. Other data:
    A. A normal response is an increase of ≥10% in radioactive iodine uptake, and 1.5 mg/dl of T_4.
    B. The half-life of I-131 is 8 days.
    C. This test is seldom used, due both to the risks and to the improved specificity of TSH testing kits, which are often considered adequate to diagnose primary hypothyroidism.

Bibliography:

Chazenbalk GD, Nagayama Y, Kaufman KD, Rapoport B: The functional expression of recombinant human thyrotropin receptors in nonthyroidal eukaryotic cells provides evidence that homologous desensitization to thyrotropin stimulation requires a cell-specific factor. Endocrinology *127*(3): 1240–1244, 1990.

Surks MI: Thyroid-stimulating hormone: reference range validity. JAMA *266*(11):1573, 1991.

THYROID-STIMULATING IMMUNOGLOBULINS, BLOOD

Norm: Negative.

Usage: Helps diagnose hyperthyroidism and Graves' disease.

Description: Thyroid-stimulating immunoglobulin, also called thyrotropin-receptor antibody, is an autoimmune antibody that binds to or near the TSH receptor on thyroid cells. It also stimulates cyclic adenosine monophosphate production, which in turn causes thyroxine (T_4) and triiodothyronine (T_3) release and subsequent symptoms of hyperthyroidism. This IgG immunoglobulin is present in the majority of clients with Graves' disease.

Professional Considerations:

1. Consent form NOT required.
2. Preparation:
   A. Tube: Red-top, red/gray-top, or gold-top.
3. Procedure:
   A. Draw a 7-ml blood sample.
4. Postprocedure care:
   A. Separate and freeze the serum.

5. Client and family teaching:
   A. Results are normally available within days.
6. Factors that affect results:
   A. Up to 4% of results may be false-positive.
   B. Levels may be elevated in autoimmune thyroiditis or nonspecific goiter.
   C. Administration of radioactive iodine within 48 hours of this test may increase autoimmune antibodies.
7. Other data:
   A. None.

Bibliography:

Gupta M: Thyrotropin receptor antibodies: Advances and importance of detection techniques in thyroid disease. Clin Biochem 25(3):193–199, 1992.

THYROID TEST: FREE THYROXINE INDEX (FT_4I, T_7), SERUM

Norm:

		Mean
Puberty through adulthood	4.2–13.0	8.0
Infants and children		
Cord blood	6.0–13.2	9.8
First 72 hours	9.9–17.5	13.9
7 days	7.5–15.1	11.2
4–52 weeks	5.0–13.0	8.4
1–3 years	5.4–12.5	8.1
3–10 years	5.7–12.8	8.2

Increased: Dysalbuminemic, hyperthyroxinemia, hyperthyroidism and psychiatric illness (acute). Drugs include amiodarone, propranolol, radiographic dyes, and thyroxine.

Decreased: Anorexia nervosa, heparin, hypothyroidism, and illness (severe).

Description: Thyroxine (T_4) is a hormone produced in the thyroid gland from iodide and thyroglobulin in a multistep process. Less than 0.05% of thyroxine circulates freely and is thus biologically active. Biologically active T_4 stimulates the basal metabolic rate, including usage of carbohydrates and lipids, protein synthesis, bone calcium release, and vitamin metabolism. In infants, T_4 plays an important role in central nervous system growth and development. Circulating T_4 levels affect the release of thyroid-stimulating hormone (TSH) and hypothalamic thyroid-releasing hormone (TRH) through a negative feedback mechanism. Due to the tiny quantity of free T_4 normally present, direct measurement is difficult and expensive. An alternative, the free thyroxine index (FT_4I), is derived from a calculation and provides an indirect measurement of free T_4 levels, based on total T_4 levels and thyroid uptake (TU) expressed as the percentage of hormone unbound to the thyroid binding protein. The calculation is as follows:

$$FT_4I = T_4 \times \frac{TU\%}{Mean\ TU\%}$$

This calculation takes into account both the quantity of total T_4 and the availability of thyroxin-binding globulin binding sites.

Professional Considerations:

1. Consent form NOT required.
2. Preparation:
   A. Tube: Red-top, red/gray-top, or gold-top.
3. Procedure:
   A. Draw a 5-ml blood sample.

4. Postprocedure care:
   A. None.
5. Client and family teaching:
   A. Results are normally available in 72 hours.
6. Factors that affect results:
   A. Results are invalidated if the client has undergone a radionuclide scan within 7 days prior to the test. Schedule any needed scans after the thyroid profile tests.
   B. During pregnancy, both T_4 and THBR are elevated, but the FT_4I is normal.
   C. The value may be normal in hypothy-

roid clients receiving phenytoin or salicylate therapy.
7. Other data:
   A. *See also Thyroid Test: Thyroxine, Blood; and Thyroid Test: Thyroid Hormone Binding Ratio, Blood.*
   B. Older methods calculated the FT_4I by multiplying total T_4 and T_3 uptake.

Bibliography:

Baer D: Tips on technology: Free thyroxine index. MLO (6):14, 1995.

Deam D, Goodwin M, Ratnaike S: Comparison of four methods for free thyroxin. Clin Chem 37(4):569–572, 1991.

THYROID TEST: THYROXINE (T₄), BLOOD

Norm:

Radioimmunoassay		SI Units
Adults	5.0–12.0 µg/dl	65–155 nmol/L
Pregnant >14 weeks	9.1–14.0 µg/dl	117–181 nmol/L
Elderly (>age 60)		
Female	5.5–10.5 µg/dl	71–135 nmol/L
Male	5.0–10.0 µg/dl	65–129 nmol/L
Children		
Cord blood	7.4–13.0 µg/dl	95–168 nmol/L
First 72 hours	11.8–22.6 µg/dl	152–292 nmol/L
7–14 days	9.8–16.6 µg/dl	126–214 nmol/L
4–16 weeks	7.2–14.4 µg/dl	93–186 nmol/L
4–12 months	7.8–16.5 µg/dl	101–213 nmol/L
12 months–5 years	7.3–15.0 µg/dl	94–194 nmol/L
5–10 years	6.4–13.3 µg/dl	83–172 nmol/L
10–15 years	5.6–11.7 µg/dl	72–151 nmol/L

Whole Blood Newborn Screening (Filter Paper Method):

Infants		
First 5 days	>7.5 µg/dl	>97 nmol/L
6 days	>6.5 µg/dl	>84 nmol/L
Panic levels		
Thyroid storm possible	>20 µg/dl	>257 nmol/L
Myxedema possible	<2.0 µg/dl	<26 nmol/L

Panic Level Symptoms and Treatment:

Thyroid Storm Symptoms: Hyperthermia, diaphoresis, vomiting, dehydration, and shock.

Thyroid Storm Treatment:
   Supportive treatment for shock.
   Fluid and electrolyte replacement for dehydration.
   Antithyroid drugs (propylthiouricil and Lugol's solution).

Myxedema Symptoms: Hypothermia, hypotension, bradycardia, hypoventilation, CO_2 narcosis, lethargy, and coma.

Myxedema Treatment:
   Support airway and blood pressure.
   Monitor neurologic checks q 1 hour.
   Administer thyroid hormone (levothyroxine) intravenously.

Increased: Acute intermittent porphyria, cirrhosis (primary biliary), congenital excess of thyroxine-binding globulin, excess dietary iodine intake, familial dysalbuminemic hyperthyroxinemia, goiter (toxic multinodular, uninodular), Graves' disease, hyperemesis gravidarum, hyperthyroidism, liver disease (early stage), lymphoma, newborn infants, obesity, pregnancy, psychiatric disorder (acute), subacute thyroiditis (first stage), and thyrotoxicosis. Drugs include amiodarone (within the prior 4 months), amphetamines, Betadine, clofibrate, dextrothyroxine, dinoprost tromethamine, estrogens (within the past 4 weeks), floraquin, 5-fluorouracil, halothane, heparin, heroin, iodinated vaginal suppositories (within the prior 4 weeks), iodothiouracil (within the past several weeks), iopanoic acid, ipodate, levarterenol, levodopa, methadone, metrecal, oral contraceptives, perphenazine (long-term use, occasional increase), progesterone, beta-blockers, thyroid extract (within the prior 6 weeks), thyroid-releasing hormone, thyrotropin, thyroxine (within the prior 4 weeks), and Vioform.

Decreased: Acromegaly, cirrhosis, cretinism, exercise (strenuous), genetic deficiency of thyroxine-binding globulin, goiter (some), Hashimoto's thyroiditis (chronic thyroiditis), hypoproteinemia, hypothyroidism (primary, secondary), iodide deficiency (severe), liver disease (chronic), malnutrition, myxedema, nephrosis, nephrotic syndrome, pancreatic malabsorption, panhypopituitarism, postoperatively (due to stress), radioactive iodine therapy, Sheehan's syndrome, Simmonds' disease, subacute thyroiditis (third stage), thyroidectomy, thyroid gland agenesis, and tumor (pituitary). Drugs include adrenal corticoids (within the past 2 weeks), adrenocorticotropic hormone (within the past 2 weeks), amiodarone (rare), androgens (within the past 3 weeks), anabolic steroids, antithyroid drugs, asparaginase, barbiturates, carbamazepine, chlorpromazine, corticotropin, cortisone (long-term use), danazol, diphenylhydantoin, ethinonamide, furosemide (high doses), gold salts (within the past several weeks), iodides, isoniazid (long-term use), isotretinoin, lithium carbonate, L-triiodothyronine (within the past 4

weeks), methimazole (within the past 7 days), oxyphenbutazone, penicillin, phenylbutazone (within the past 2 weeks), phenytoin (within the past 10 days), prednisone, propranolol, propylthiouracil (within the past 7 days), reserpine, salicylates, somatotropin, SSKI (early in therapy), sulfonamides, and thiocyanate (within the past 3 weeks).

Description: Thyroxine (T₄) is a hormone produced in the thyroid gland from iodide and thyroglobulin in a multistep process. Production occurs in response to the effects of pituitary thyroid-stimulating hormone (TSH) on the thyroid gland. T₄ is the major hormone synthesized by the gland and the hormone from which triiodothyronine (T₃) is derived. When released from the thyroid gland, almost all (99.96%) of T₄ is bound to protein (thyroxine-binding globulin thyroxine-binding prealbumin, and albumin). The remainder of T₄ (0.04%) is called "free thyroxine" and is the only portion of this hormone that is biologically active. Biologically active T₄ stimulates the basal metabolic rate, including usage of carbohydrates and lipids, protein synthesis, bone calcium release, and vitamin metabolism. In infants, T₄ plays an important role in central nervous system growth and development. Circulating T₄ levels affect the release of TSH and hypothalamic thyroid-releasing hormone (TRH) through a negative feedback mechanism. This test measures total T₄ (protein-bound and free).

Professional Considerations:

1. Consent form NOT required.
2. Preparation:
   A. Tube: Red-top; or for whole blood newborn screening, obtain an alcohol wipe, a lancet, and filter paper for T₄ testing.
   B. The most accurate picture of T₄ levels is obtained when the client has been free of thyroid medications for 1 month.
   C. Newborn screening for hypothyroidism should be performed at least 72 hours after birth, and after newborn has been taking feedings containing protein for at least 24 hours.
3. Procedure:
   A. Draw a 1-ml blood sample.
   B. Whole-blood newborn screening:
      i. Prewarming the heel is not necessary.
      ii. Cleanse the lateral curvature of the

heel with an alcohol wipe, and allow the area to dry.

   iii. Puncture the lateral curvature of the heel with a lancet until free flow of blood is obtained.

   iv. Completely saturate all test circles on the filter paper with heelstick blood. The circles should be completely filled.

   v. Place the filter paper in a light-protected container for delivery to the laboratory.

   vi. Cord blood may also be used.

4. Postprocedure care:
   A. Let the heelstick site air-dry.
   B. Indicate pregnancy status on the laboratory requisition.
5. Client and family teaching:
   A. Results are normally available within 72 hours.
6. Factors that affect results:
   A. Results are invalidated if the client has undergone a radionuclide scan within 7 days prior to the test.
   B. Results are invalidated in hemolyzed or lipemic specimens.
   C. With the double-antibody testing method, results may be increased in the presence of antithyroxine antibodies.
   D. With the single-antibody testing method, results may be decreased in the presence of antithyroxine antibodies.
   E. Cord blood levels are lower in premature infants than in full-term infants.
   F. The following iodine contrast media may increase test results:
      i. *Cholecystography:* Telepaque within the prior 6 weeks; Orografin.
7. Other data:
   A. Test results are usually evaluated in conjunction with free T$_4$ and TSH levels.

Bibliography:

McConell R: Abnormal thyroid function test results in patients taking salsalate. JAMA *267*(9):1242–1443, 1992.

Price DE, O'Malley BP, Northover B, et al.: Changes in circulating thyroid hormone levels and systolic time intervals in acute hypothyroidism. Clin Endocrinol *35*(1):67–69, 1991.

THYROID TEST: THYROXINE (T$_4$) BY RIA, BLOOD

(see Thyroid Test: Thyroxine, Blood)

THYROID TEST: THYROXINE (T$_4$) FREE, SERUM

Norm: Radioimmunoassay, 0.7–1.8 ng/dl (9–23 pmol/L, SI Units). Norms vary among newer test kits, and should be compared with those from the manufacturer.

Increased: Hyperthyroidism and psychiatric illness (acute). Drugs include amiodarone, heparin, propranolol, radiographic dyes, and thyroxine.

Decreased: Anorexia nervosa, hypothyroidism, illness (severe), and pregnancy. Drugs include carbamazepine and heparin.

Description: Thyroxine (T$_4$) is a hormone produced in the thyroid gland from iodide and thyroglobulin in a multistep process. Less than 0.05% of thyroxine circulates freely and is thus biologically active. Biologically active T$_4$ stimulates the basal metabolic rate, including usage of carbohydrates and lipids, protein synthesis, bone calcium release, and vitamin metabolism. In infants, T$_4$ plays an important role in central nervous system growth and development. Circulating T$_4$ levels affect the release of thyroid-stimulating hormone (TSH) and hypothalamic thyroid-releasing hormone (TRH) through a negative feedback mechanism. Due to the tiny quantity of free T$_4$ normally present, direct measurement is difficult and expensive. Equilibrium dialysis is the "Gold Standard" for measuring free T$_4$, but is seldom used, due to cost. Radioimmunoassay is often used but is subject to the influence of the serum albumin and lipid levels. Newer testing kits are being developed to improve the accuracy and ease of direct measurement of free T$_4$.

Professional Considerations:

1. Consent form NOT required.
2. Preparation:
   A. Tube: Red-top, red/gray-top, or gold-top.
3. Procedure:
   A. Draw a 1-ml blood sample.
4. Postprocedure care:
   A. The serum should be separated within 48 hours after collection.
5. Client and family teaching:
   A. Results are normally available within 72 hours.
6. Factors that affect results:
   A. RIA results are invalidated if the client has undergone a radionuclide scan within 7 days prior to the test.
   B. Value may be normal in hypothyroid clients receiving phenytoin or salicylate therapy.
7. Other data:
   A. *See also Thyroid Test: Thyroxine, Blood; and Thyroid Test: Thyroid Hormone Binding Ratio, Blood.*

Bibliography:

Elkins R: Analytical measurements of free thyroxine. Clin Lab Med *13*(3):599–630, 1993.

Kaptein E: Clinical application of free thyroxine determinations. Clin Lab Med *13*(3):653–671, 1993.

O'Leary P, Boyne P, Atkinson G, et al.: Longitudinal study of serum thyroid hormone levels during normal pregnancy. Int J Gynecol Obstet *38*(3): 171–179, 1992.

Rosen H, Greenspan S, Landsberg L, et al.: Distinguishing hypothyroxinemia due to euthyroid sick syndrome from pituitary insufficiency. Isr J Med Sci *30*(30):746–750, 1994.

THYROID TEST: TRIIODOTHYRONINE (T$_3$), BLOOD

Norm:

		SI Units
Adults	80–230 ng/dl	1.2–3.5 nmol/L
Children		
Cord blood	15–75 ng/dl	0.23–1.16 nmol/L
First 72 hours	32–216 ng/dl	0.49–3.33 nmol/L
7–14 days	Avg. 250 ng/dl	Avg. 3.85 nmol/L
2–4 weeks	160–240 ng/dl	2.46–3.70 nmol/L
4–16 weeks	117–209 ng/dl	1.80–3.22 nmol/L
16–52 weeks	110–280 ng/dl	1.70–4.31 nmol/L
1–5 years	105–269 ng/dl	1.62–4.14 nmol/L
5–10 years	94–241 ng/dl	1.45–3.71 nmol/L
10–15 years	83–213 ng/dl	1.28–3.28 nmol/L

Increased: Congenital excess of thyroxine-binding globulin, Familial dysalbuminemic hyperthyroxinemia, fasting state, Graves' disease, high altitudes, hyperthyroidism, pregnancy, psychiatric illness (acute), and T$_3$ thyrotoxicosis. Drugs include amiodarone (rarely), antithyroid medications, dextrothyroxine, dinoprost tromethamine, estrogens, heroin, L-triiodothyronine, methadone, oral contraceptives, terbutaline, and thyroxine.

Decreased: Anorexia nervosa, elderly, genetic deficiency of thyroxine-binding globulin, goiter (due to iodine deficiency), hepatic cirrhosis, iodine deficiency (severe), myxedema, obesity, postoperatively (due to stress), radioactive iodine therapy, renal failure, starvation, and thyroidectomy. Drugs include amiodarone, androgens, antithyroid drugs, asparaginase, cimetidine, dexamethasone, iopanoic acid, ipodate, isotretinoin, lithium, phenytoin, propranolol, propylthiouracil, radiographic dyes, salicylates, and valproic acid.

Description: Triiodothyronine (T$_3$) is a hormone produced primarily in peripheral tissues from conversion of thyroxine (T$_4$), but also is produced in small amounts by the thyroid gland; 99.96% of T$_3$ is bound to protein (thyroxine-binding globulin, thyroxine-binding prealbumin, and albumin), and the remainder is the biologically active form. About four times as much T$_3$ as T$_4$ circulates freely, partly due to its lower affinity for serum proteins. Additionally, T$_3$ has a shorter half-life than T$_4$. Biologically active T$_3$ stimulates the basal metabolic rate, including usage of carbohydrates and lipids, protein synthesis, bone calcium release, and vitamin metabolism. In infants, T$_3$ plays an important role in central nervous system growth and development. Circulating T$_3$ levels affect the release of thyroid-stimulating hormone (TSH) and hypothalamic thyroid-releasing hormone (TRH) through a negative feedback mechanism. T$_3$ levels are used to confirm a diagnosis of hyperthyroidism when T$_4$ levels are borderline high, and to diagnose T$_3$ thyrotoxicosis. This test is a radioimmunoassay measurement of total T$_3$ levels.

Professional Considerations:

1. Consent form NOT required.
2. Preparation:
   A. Tube: Red-top, red/gray-top, or gold-top.
   B. List the dose and administration time of any thyroid drugs on the laboratory requisition.

3. Procedure:
   A. Draw a 1-ml blood sample. Cord blood may be used.
4. Postprocedure care:
   A. Indicate pregnancy status on the laboratory requisition.
5. Client and family teaching:
   A. Results are normally available within 72 hours.
6. Factors that affect results:
   A. Results are invalidated if the client has undergone a radionuclide scan within 7 days prior to the test.
   B. Results are invalidated in hemolyzed or lipemic specimens.
   C. With the double-antibody testing method, results may be increased in the presence of antithyroxine antibodies.
   D. With the single-antibody testing method, results may be decreased in the presence of antithyroxine antibodies.
7. Other data:
   A. Results are normally evaluated in conjunction with T_4 and TSH levels.

Bibliography:

Celani MF, Corradini MC, Rota C, et al.: A rise in haemoglobin levels may enhance serum triiodothyronine (T_3) concentrations in prepubertal patients with beta-thalassemia major. Exp Clin Endocrinol *96*(2):169–176, 1990.

Sapin R, Gasser F, Chambron J: Different sensitivity to anti-triiodothyronine autoantibodies of two direct radioimmunoassays of free triiodothyronine. Clin Chem *36*(12):2141–2142, 1990.

Verma N, Haidukewych D: Differential but infrequent alterations of hepatic enzyme levels and thyroid hormone levels by anticonvulsant drugs. Arch Neurol *51*(4):381–384, 1994.

THYROID TEST: TRIIODOTHYRONINE (T_3) BY RIA, BLOOD
(see Thyroid Test: Triiodothyronine, Blood)

THYROID TEST: TRIIODOTHYRONINE (T_3) UPTAKE, BLOOD
(see Thyroid Hormone Binding Ratio, Blood)

THYROID ULTRASOUND
(see Thyroid Sonogram, Diagnostic)

THYROTROPIN-STIMULATING HORMONE, SENSITIVE ASSAY, BLOOD
(see Thyroid-Stimulating Hormone, Sensitive Assay, Blood)

THYROTROPIN STIMULATION TEST, DIAGNOSTIC
(see Thyroid-Stimulating Hormone Stimulation Test, Diagnostic)

THYROXINE, BLOOD
(see Thyroid Test: Thyroxine, Blood)

TILT TABLE TEST (HEAD UP TILT TABLE TEST), DIAGNOSTIC

Norm: Negative or absence of hypotension and/or bradycardia with position changes.

Usage: Evaluation of recurrent idiopathic syncope once cardiac causes have been ruled out. Vasovagal syncope (also known as vasodepressor, neurodepressor, dysautonomia, or neurogenic syncope) is a sudden, short-term loss of consciousness due to malfunction in the regulatory mechanisms between the nervous and cardiac systems.

Description: The head-upright table, by sudden assumption of an upright position, can produce passive orthostatic stress, which induces syncope in individuals affected by vasovagal syncope. Administration of an intravenous isoproterenol (Isuprel) infusion increases sensitivity of the tilt table test for those susceptible to vasovagal syncope by producing the elevation of circulating catecholamines associated with this type of an event.

Professional Considerations:

1. Consent form IS required.

Risks:
Dizziness, dysrhythmias, hypotension, tachycardia.

Contraindications:
Gradual loss of more than 500 ml of blood, hypertension, hypotension.

2. Preparation:
   A. *See Client and family teaching.*
   B. Start an IV at KO rate for administration of isoproterenol or emergency medication.
3. Procedure:
   A. The test can be run while the client is medicated or unmedicated.
   B. Baseline monitoring of heart rate (HR),

rhythm (ECG), blood pressure (BP), with the client in a supine resting state q 5 minutes for 15–30 minutes.

C. The table is then tilted up to 80 degrees for usually 5–7 minutes (up to 20 minutes).

D. BP and HR are monitored/documented q 1 minute for 25–45 minutes by automatic cuff or arterial line and ECG.

E. The test is terminated and the client returned to the supine position when presyncopal hypotension and bradycardia or full syncope develop.

F. Isoproterenol provocation may be added if no symptoms are produced during the unmedicated test.

  i. Return the client to the supine position for 5 to 10 minutes for the recovery period.

  ii. Isoproterenol may then be added as a single stage (1 µg/minute for 5 minutes) or as a multistage protocol (repeated 3 times with progressively increasing doses of 1 µg, 2 µg, and 3 µg/minute).

  iii. The table is tilted 60–80 degrees after each stage, and the test proceeds as previously described.

4. Postprocedure care:

A. Monitor the vital signs for 15 minutes.

B. Full return to consciousness and baseline BP and HR is usually rapid when the client is placed in the supine position.

C. Normal intake and activity can be resumed immediately after the test.

D. Occasionally temporary residual pallor, weakness, headache, and bradycardia (rarely) last up to 30 minutes.

5. Client and family teaching:

A. Any medication known to cause postural hypotension or bradycardia should be stopped at least 3 days prior to the test. Your physician will tell you which drugs to stop.

B. Fast from food and fluids for 4–8 hours prior to the test.

C. Describe the procedure and the usual sensations the client can expect related to the tilt table test (see above, under "Procedure"). With the medicated test,

mild stomach cramping, salty taste in the mouth, and minor vision changes are not unusual. Increased heart rate and lightheadedness are common.

D. An IV will be inserted before the test.

E. The goal of the test is to reproduce syncope or near syncope in a carefully controlled environment in which the client will not fall.

F. Usual testing time takes 1–2 hours.

G. Normal diet and activity may be resumed after the test is complete.

H. If you develop chest pain after the procedure, call 911. Do not drive yourself to the hospital.

I. Call the doctor if you experience shortness of breath, a fainting spell, a severe headache or dizziness, or pain in your back.

6. Factors that affect results:

A. The positive effect of the isoproterenol-tilt table declines with age.

7. Other data:

A. Abrupt infusion of 5 g of isoproterenol may cause intolerable changes in HR and BP.

B. This test is up to 75% effective in reproducing vasovagal syncope.

Bibliography:

Campbell B: Vasovagal syncope and head upright tilt table testing. Crit Care Nurs Q *17*(3):27–34, 1994.

Futterman L, Lemberg L: Unexplained syncope: Diagnostic value of tilt-table testing. Am J Crit Care *3*(4):322–325, 1994.

Sheldon R: Evaluation of a single-stage isoproterenol-tilt table test in patients with syncope. J Am Coll Cardiol *22*(1):114–118, 1993.

Tonnessen G, Haft J, Fulton J, et al.: The value of tilt table testing with isoproterenol in determining therapy in adults with syncope and presyncope of unexplained origin. Arch Intern Med *154*(14): 1613–1617, 1994.

TISSUE PATHOLOGY
(see Histopathology, Specimen)

TISSUE TYPING, BLOOD
(see Human Leukocyte Antigen Typing, Blood)

T-LYMPHOCYTES, BLOOD

Norm:

	SI Units
500–2400/mm³ or /µl	500–2400 cells × 10⁶/L
45–85% of total lymphocytes	0.45–0.85 fraction of total lymphocytes
75–80% of circulating lymphocytes	

Increased: Autoimmune disease, delayed hypersensitivity reactions, and Graves' disease.

Decreased: Agammaglobulinemia (sex-linked, Swiss-type), AIDS, antibody to human T-cell lymphotropic virus, ataxia telangiectasia, chronic mucocutaneous candidiasis, Hodgkin's disease, immunosuppression, leukemia (chronic lymphocytic), lepromatous leprosy, lymphoma, Nezelof syndrome, systemic lupus erythematosus, thymic hypoplasia, transplant rejection, and Wiskott-Aldrich syndrome. Drugs include immunosuppressives and steroids.

Description: T lymphocytes are white blood cells with a long lifespan that are produced by, and receive an antigenic imprint in, the thymus gland. T lymphocytes are responsible for a cell-mediated type of immunity and control of the immune system response. Subsets of T lymphocytes secrete lymphokines such as interferon, chemotaxin, and macrophage migration inhibition factor that function in cell-mediated immune response to varying antigens. Three of the T lymphocyte subsets are "helper T cells" (OKT-4 cells), which help B cells produce certain antibodies; "suppressor T cells" (OKT-8 cells), which prevent unnecessary formation of antibodies; and "cytotoxic killer T cells," which have the ability to cause lysis of specific targeted cells such as those containing viral antigens. Overall, T lymphocytes function in delayed hypersensitivity reactions, autoimmune responses, rejection of transplanted tissue, and resistance to tumors, as well as the immune response to bacterial and viral antigens.

This test is used to type and classify lymphocytic leukemias and lymphomas, as well as define immunodeficient states such as AIDS. Identification of T lymphocytes is accomplished by the "rosette technique" in which sheep erythrocytes gather around T cells to form a rosette pattern.

Professional Considerations:

1. Consent form NOT required.
2. Preparation:
   A. Tube: Heparinized green-top tube.
   B. Do NOT draw specimens during hemodialysis.
3. Procedure:
   A. Draw a 5-ml blood sample.
4. Postprocedure care:
   A. Send specimens to the laboratory for processing within 2 hours.
5. Client and family teaching:
   A. Results are normally available within 24 hours.
6. Factors that affect results:
   A. Prolonged refrigeration decreases levels of helper T cells (OKT-4 cells).
7. Other data:
   A. *See also Acquired Immune Deficiency Syndrome Evaluation Battery, Diagnostic; and T- and B-Lymphocyte Subset Assay, Blood.*

Bibliography:

Cohen J: Programmed cell death and apoptosis in lymphocyte development and function. Chest *103*(2, Suppl):996–1015, 1993.

Sneller M, Strober W, Eisentein, et al.: NIH conference: New insights into common variable immunodeficiency. Ann Intern Med *118*(9):720–730, 1993.

Voss S, Hong R, Sondel P: Severe combined immunodeficiency interleukins (IL-2), and the IL-2 receptor. Blood *83*(3):626–635, 1994.

TOBRAMYCIN, SERUM

Norm: Negative.

		SI Units
Therapeutic levels		
Peak	4–10 µg/ml	8 µmol/L
Trough	1–2 µg/ml	2–4 µmol/L
Panic levels		
Peak	>12 µg/ml	>25 µmol/L
Trough	>2 µg/ml	>4 µmol/L

Overdose Symptoms and Treatment:

Symptoms: Weight gain, edema, oliguria, hearing loss, dizziness, nystagmus, ataxia, and respiratory paralysis (when administered with anesthetics).

Treatment:
Intravenous fluids at 3 L/day (if normal renal function is present) to maintain adequate output. Both hemodialysis and peritoneal dialysis WILL remove tobramycin.

Usage: Monitoring for therapeutic and safe levels during tobramycin therapy.

Description: Tobramycin is an aminoglycoside antibiotic used to treat infections caused by certain gram-negative bacilli that are resistant to gentamicin. It causes misreading of the genetic code to prevent protein synthesis by the bacterial ribosome. Tobramycin is minimally metabolized, with most of the dose excreted in the urine, with a half-life of 2 hours and peak levels reached within 30 minutes after intravenous infusion and within 3 hours after intramuscular administration. Nephrotoxicity (probably reversible) and ototoxicity (probably irreversible) are possible at levels only slightly above the therapeutic peak and trough levels. Therefore, it is very important to monitor tobramycin levels during its usage. Clients with any degree of pre-existing renal failure are at higher risk for toxicity, because of impaired ability to clear the drug from the body.

Professional Considerations:

1. Consent form NOT required.
2. Preparation:
   A. Tube: Red-top, red/gray-top, or gold-top.
   B. Do NOT draw specimens during hemodialysis.
3. Procedure:
   A. Draw trough levels just prior to the dose. Draw peak levels 30 minutes after the last intravenous dose or 30 minutes to 3 hours after the last intramuscular dose.
   B. Draw a 1-ml blood sample. Label the specimen as "trough" or "peak."
4. Postprocedure care:
   A. Record the collection time on the laboratory requisition.
5. Client and family teaching:
   A. In origin, the need for this test is for monitoring. The information is needed to make sure the safe and effective dose of tobramycin is being given.
   B. Results are normally available within 4 hours.
6. Factors that affect results:
   A. In clients with normal renal function, 24–36 hours are required before steady-state levels are reached.
7. Other data:
   A. Renal function (creatinine, beta$_2$-microglobulin, muramidase, albumin) and hearing should be monitored throughout therapy with tobramycin.
   B. A once-daily dosing regimen has been shown to be safe and effective for mother and fetus during pregnancy.

C. An every-6-hour dosing regimen with a larger daily dosage administered has been shown in one study to provide better pulmonary function and longer time of wellness in clients with cystic fibrosis than an every-8-hour dosing regimen.
D. Usual methods of continuous peritoneal dialysis (CAPD) result in relatively low drug clearance during any specific dialysate exchange, but cumulative drug removal may necessitate dosage supplementation with increased flow rates. Tobramycin added to the peritoneal dialysate absorbs into the bloodstream.
E. Aminoglycosides are inactivated when used concomitantly with antipsuedomonal penicillins in the treatment of gram-negative infections in the client with renal failure.

Bibliography:

Bourget P, Fernandez H, Delouis C, et al.: Pharmacokinetics of tobramycin in pregnant women. J Clin Pharm Ther *16*(3):167–176, 1991.

Gilbert D: Once-daily aminoglycoside therapy. Antimicrob Agents Chemother *35*(3):399–405, 1991.

Uber W, Brundage R, White R, et al.: In vivo inactivation of tobramycin by piperacillin. DICP: Ann Pharmacother *25*(4):357–359, 1991.

Winnie GB, Cooper JA, Witson J, et al.: Comparison of 6 and 8 hourly tobramycin dosing intervals in treatment of pulmonary exacerbations in cystic fibrosis patients. Pediatr Infect Dis J *10*(5):381–386, 1991.

Ylitalo P, Morsky P, Parviainen MT, et al.: Nephrotoxicity of tobramycin. Value of examining various protein and enzyme markers. Methods Find Exp Clin Pharmacol *13*(4):281–287, 1991.

TOMOGRAPHY PARANASAL SINUSES, DIAGNOSTIC

Norm: Negative for foreign body, fracture, or tumor.

Usage: Adjunct to conventional radiography for clients with suspected fracture (status post-trauma), delineation of inflammatory sinus disease, bony tumor invasion of the paranasal sinus area, or foreign body introduction into the paranasal sinus area. Improves planning and safety of paranasal sinus surgery.

Description: Computed tomography (CT) of the paranasal sinuses is a radiographic scan that reconstructs an image of the paranasal sinus area based on differing densities and composition of the tissues. A detector records the intensity of the x-rays from multiple angles as they are transmitted through the paranasal sinus area. A computer then reconstructs the differing intensities into pixels, which appear in differing shades for differing tissues and represent "slices" across the plane of the area. This test may provide additional information that standard radiography cannot, because it can portray boundaries between tissues that are normally indistinguishable by traditional radiography. In particular, CT provides a sensitive display of the deep air passages and posterior ethmoid and sphenoid sinuses that are difficult to reach via nasal endoscopy.

Professional Considerations:

1.   Consent form NOT required.

Risks:

None.

Contraindications:

Clients who are unable to lie motionless.

2.   Preparation:
  A.   Remove radiopaque objects such as jewelry, eyeglasses, or hairpins from the head area.
3.   Procedure:
  A.   The client is positioned supine, with the head secured in a hyperextended position on a headrest (coronal imaging) or prone, resting on chin with head hyperextended (axial imaging) on a motorized handling table.
  B.   The client must lie motionless as the table slowly advances through the circular opening of the scanner. The CT scanner sends a narrow beam of x-rays across the area to be imaged in a linear fashion.
  C.   Imaging in both axial and coronal planes is recommended.
4.   Postprocedure care:
  A.   Replace radiopaque objects that were removed prior to the scan.
5.   Client and family teaching
  A.   It is necessary to lie motionless during the scan. Because this can be a frightening test, it should be carefully described before the client enters the CT room.
6.   Factors that affect results:
  A.   Radiopaque objects left in place obscure visualization.
7.   Other data:
  A.   Further testing may include magnetic resonance imaging (MRI), which is more sensitive than CT for identification of neoplasm. MRI is replacing CT of the paranasal sinuses as the study of choice for oropharyngeal and paranasal sinus lesions.

Bibliography:

Babbel R, Harnsberger HR, Nelson B, et al.: Optimization of techniques in screening CT of the sinuses. Am J Neuroradiol 12(5):849–854, 1991.

Duvoisin B, et al.: Low-dose CT and inflammatory diseases of the paranasal sinuses. Neuroradiology 33(5):403–406, 1991.

Farrell V, Emby D: Meningitis following fractures of the paranasal sinuses: Accurate non-invasive localization of the dural defect by direct coronal computed tomography. Surg Neurol 40(5):378–382, 1993.

White PS, Cowan IA, Robertson MS: Limited CT scanning techniques of the paranasal sinuses. J Laryngol Otolaryngol 105(1):20–23, 1991.

TONOMETRY TEST FOR GLAUCOMA, DIAGNOSTIC

Norm: 12–20 mmHg.

Warning: 22–28 mmHg. More testing required.
Major concern: >38 mmHg.
Panic levels: There is lack of definitive IOP cutoff level for glaucoma.

Usage: Screening for glaucoma. Ongoing monitoring for clients with glaucoma.

Description: Tonometry testing involves measuring intraocular pressure using a tonometer, an instrument that is pressed directly against the anesthetized eye. In glaucoma, intraocular pressure increases either due to blocked drainage or excessive production of aqueous humor. The tonometer makes an indentation in the eye with a specific amount of weight and records the amount of resistance to the indentation, which is then converted to an intraocular pressure. The Schiotz' tonometer, which comes into direct contact with the eye, has been the most widely used device in the primary care setting. Noncontact tonometry is also available; this has been found to improve compliance with testing in children and there has been improvement in the accuracy of the handheld units.

Professional Considerations:

1.   Consent form NOT required.

Risks:

Corneal abrasion or infection.

Contraindications:

Corneal infection, unless absolutely necessary. It is also contraindicated in clients who may be unable to hold very still during the test (i.e., those with persistent coughing or sneezing).

2. Preparation:
   A. Remove contact lenses and loosen any jewelry or clothing (tie, tight collar, necklace) around the neck area.
   B. Obtain anesthetic eye drops and sterile tonofilms for the contact tonometer.
3. Procedure:
   A. The client is positioned supine.
   B. Anesthetic eye drops are instilled bilaterally.
   C. One eye is tested at a time. After the tonometer is zeroed, the eyelids are held open as the tonometer is placed against the eyeball. The tonometer is pressed against the eye with a specific amount of weight, and the tonometer scale reflects a number that is converted to mmHg for an intraocular pressure (IOP) reading.
4. Postprocedure care:
   A. Eyeglasses may be worn in place of contact lenses.
   B. *See Client and family teaching.*
5. Client and family teaching:
   A. Provide a thorough explanation of the procedure, emphasizing that the client must cooperate by keeping the eyes open during testing.
   B. Contact lenses must be removed. Bring eyeglasses to wear, if needed, after the test.
   C. Avoid rubbing the eyes or replacing contact lenses until the local anesthesia has worn off (about 2 hours). Rubbing the eyes before this time can cause corneal abrasion, which is painful and takes several days to heal.
6. Factors that affect results:
   A. It may be necessary to adjust the weight placed against the eyeball to obtain a consistent pressure reading.
7. Other data:
   A. IOP evaluation in the detection of glaucoma has approximately 50% specificity.
   B. Applanation tonometry performed by an ophthalmologist/optometrist with an applanation tonometer is another method of measuring IOP.
   C. Pneumotonometry is another specialized method of measuring IOP and is used in cases of irregular corneas or after keratoplasty when the applanation tonometer can not be used.
   D. For abnormal findings, the client should have a full ophthalmological examination, including cup to disc ratio and field studies.

Bibliography:

Brencher H, Kohl P, Reinke A, et al.: Clinical comparison of air-puff and Goldman tonometers. J Am Optom Assoc 62(5):395–402, 1991.
Buscemi M, Capoferri C, Garavaglia A, et al.: Noncontact tonometry in children. Optom Vis Sci 68(6):461–464, 1991.
Goldberg I: Glaucoma—diagnostic hints. Aust Fam Physician 20(2):150–151, 1991.
Pearce C, Kohl P, Yolton R, et al.: Clinical evaluation of the Keeler PULSAIR 2000 tonometer. J Am Optom 63(2):106–110, 1992.
Ralston M, Choplin N, Hollenbach K, et al.: Glaucoma screening in primary care: The role of non-contact tonometry. J Fam Pract 34(1):73–76, 1992.

TORCH, BLOOD
(see Toxoplasmosis, Other, Rubella, Cytomegalovirus, Herpes Virus Serology, Blood)

TOTAL BODY SCAN, DIAGNOSTIC
(see Bone Scan, Diagnostic)

TOTAL IRON-BINDING CAPACITY (TIBC), SERUM
(see Iron and Total Iron-Binding Capacity/Transferrin, Serum)

TOURNIQUET TEST, DIAGNOSTIC
(see Capillary Fragility Test, Diagnostic)

TOXICOLOGY, DRUG SCREEN, BLOOD OR URINE

Norm: Negative.

Treatment of Overdose: Prepare for activated charcoal orally in the awake client or for gastric lavage in the client not awake who has ingested drugs within the last 4 hours or who has ingested aspirin within the last 8 hours. Hemodialysis and peritoneal dialysis WILL remove morphine. *(See also individual test listings.)*

Usage: Monitor toxic, overdose, or newly comatose situations, or screen for drug abuse. Determine causes for agranulocytosis, impotence, and pruritus.

Description: Common drugs included in this test are acetaminophen, alcohol, amphetamines, barbiturates, benzodiazepines, cannabinoids, cocaine metabolite, hypnotics, methadone, methaqualone, narcotics, opiates, organic bases, phencyclidine, phenothiazines, phenytoins, propoxyphene, salicylates, and tricyclics antidepressants. *(See also Toxicology: Volatiles Group by GLC, Blood or Urine; and many are also in individual test listings.)*

Professional Considerations:

1. Consent form NOT required unless results may be used for legal purposes.
2. Preparation:
   A. Tube: Red-top, red/gray-top, or gold-top or lavender-top.
   B. *Urine:* Obtain a clean container with a tight-fitting lid.
3. Procedure:
   A. If the specimen may be used as legal evidence, have the specimen collection witnessed.
   B. *Blood:* Draw a 2-ml blood sample in a red-top, red-gray-top, or gold top tube, or draw a 5-ml blood sample in a lavender-top tube.
   C. *Urine:* Obtain a 50-ml random urine specimen in a clean container. Tightly cap the container.
4. Postprocedure care:
   A. Specify suspected drug(s) on the requisition.
   B. If the specimen may be used for legal purposes, write the client's name, date, exact time of collection, and specimen source on the laboratory requisition. Sign and have the witness sign the laboratory requisition. Transport the specimen to the laboratory immediately in a sealed plastic bag marked as legal evidence. All clients handling the specimen should sign and mark the time of receipt on the laboratory requisition.
   C. Assess for possible signs of drug withdrawal.
5. Client and family teaching:
   A. Results are normally not available for days.
   B. If activated charcoal was given for elevated levels, the client should drink 4–6 glasses of water each day for 2 days to prevent constipation. The activated charcoal will also cause stools to be black for a few days.
6. Factors that affect results:
   A. Failure to maintain a clear chain of custody may invalidate results for legal purposes.
   B. Failure to tightly cap the specimen container may cause falsely decreased results for volatiles.
7. Other data:
   A. The test provides only qualitative detection of drugs. Any drug identified in a screening should be confirmed by a test specific to that drug.
   B. The blood drug screening is usually performed in conjunction with urine drug screening.
   C. *See also individual listings of specific drugs or classes of drugs for therapeutic ranges and panic levels.*

Bibliography:

Caprino L: Evaluation of drug safety by toxicological test procedures as provided by regulatory laws: An overview. Pharmacol Res *22*(3):253–262, 1990.

Halbach J, Guder W: Mechanized toxicological serum tests in screening hospitalized patients. Eur J Clin Chem Biochem *29*(9):537–547, 1991.

Henderson A, Wright M, Pond S: Experience with 732 acute overdose patients admitted to an intensive care unit over six years. Med J Aust *158*(4):28–30, 1993.

Schwartz JG, Zollars PR, Okorodudu AO, et al.: Accuracy of common drug screen test. Am J Emerg Med *9*(2):166–170, 1991.

Wiley JF II: Difficult diagnoses in toxicology. Poisons not detected by the comprehensive drug screen. Pediatr Clin North Am *38*(3):725–737, 1991.

TOXICOLOGY, VOLATILES GROUP BY GLC, BLOOD OR URINE

Norm: Negative for acetone, ethanol, isopropanol, and methanol.

Positive: Ingestion of substances.

		SI Units
Blood panic levels		
Acetone	>20 mg/dl	>3.44 mmol/L
Ethanol	>100 mg/dl	>21.7 mmol/L
Isopropanol	>400 mg/L	>6.64 mmol/L
Methanol	>200 mg/L	>6.24 mmol/L
Urine panic levels		
Acetone	>27 mg/dl	>4.65 mmol/L
Ethanol	>100 mg/dl	>21.7 mmol/L
Isopropanol	>500 µg/ml	>8.32 mmol/L
Methanol	>50 mg/L	>1.56 mmol/L

Overdose Symptoms and Treatment:

Acetone Panic Level Symptoms:
Coma, hypotension, respiratory depression.

Acetone Panic Level Treatment:
Support airway, breathing, and circulation.

Monitor hourly neurologic checks.

Administer blood glucose, serum and urine acetone levels, and provide arterial pH monitoring.

Hemodialysis WILL remove acetone. Hemoperfusion will NOT remove acetone.

Ethanol Poisoning Symptoms:

<50 mg/dl	Muscular incoordination
50–100 mg/dl	Worsening incoordination of movement
100–150 mg/dl	Mood and behavior changes
150–200 mg/dl	Delayed reactions
200–300 mg/dl	Ataxia, double vision, nausea, vomiting
300–400 mg/dl	Amnesia, dysarthria, hypothermia
400–700 mg/dl	Respiratory failure, coma, death possible

Ethanol Poisoning Treatment:
Administer tap water or 3% sodium bicarbonate lavage.

Support oxygenation and breathing.

Hemodialysis WILL remove ethanol but is seldom necessary unless levels rise >300 mg/dl. During hemodialysis, levels drop an average of 62 mg%/hour.

Isopropanol Panic Level Symptoms:
Coma, hypotension, respiratory depression.

Isopropanol Panic Level Treatment:
Give activated charcoal (use is controversial, effect is not proven).

Do gastric lavage with tap water.

Support airway with oxygen and mechanical ventilation as needed.

Administer vasopressors for hypotension.

Hemodialysis will NOT remove isopropanol, but WILL remove its acetone metabolite. Hemodialysis is usually indicated when levels exceed 400 mg/dl.

Give a normal saline infusion intravenously.

Monitor closely for central nervous system depression.

Methanol Poisoning Symptoms:
Eight to thirty-six hours after ingestion: headache, weakness, abdominal and back pain, nausea and vomiting, dizziness, hallucinations and confusion, metabolic acidosis possible blindness, respiratory depression, and coma; death is possible.

Methanol Poisoning Treatment:
Within 2 hours of ingestion:
Administer gastric lavage with 5% NaHCO$_3$, leaving a portion of solution to dwell.

Reverse acidosis.

Administer ethanol to block breakdown of methanol into its toxic metabolites.

Support airway, breathing, and circulation.

Keep environment dark to reduce stress on vision.

Description: The toxicology volatiles screen tests for the presence of acetone, ethanol, isopropanol, and methanol in a blood sample. Acetone level helps identify isopropanol alcohol (rubbing alcohol) ingestion or toxicity because when ingested, isopropanol is converted to acetone. Isopropanol is also an ingredient of perfumes, aftershaves, and antifreeze. Ethanol, also known as grain alcohol, is a substance, often abused, that depresses the central nervous system and may lead to coma progressing to death at levels above the panic level listed above. Methanol and isopropanol may be ingested by alcoholics accustomed to taking ethanol when ethanol is unavailable. Methanol, also known as wood alcohol, is an ingredient in antifreeze and moonshine. Both blood and urine levels of these substances are important. While blood levels reflect the most recently ingested substance(s), urine levels may reflect substances ingested over a longer time period. This test is frequently routine for clients who are newly unconscious, with unknown cause.

Professional Considerations:
1. Consent form NOT required unless results may be used as legal evidence.
2. Preparation:
   A. Tube: Gray-top (contains glycolytic inhibitor) for the blood sample.
   B. Obtain a clean container with a tight-

fitting lid, and a container of ice for the urine sample.

C. Do NOT draw specimens during hemodialysis.

3. Procedure:
   A. Specimen collection should be witnessed if it may be used as legal evidence.
   B. *Blood sample:* Do NOT use alcohol for venipuncture. Instead, cleanse the site with a povidone-iodine wipe and allow the area to dry. Draw a 5-ml blood sample. Tightly cap the tube.
   C. *Urine sample:* Obtain a 50-ml random urine specimen in a clean container. Tightly cap the container. Transport it on ice.

4. Postprocedure care:
   A. Place the urine specimen on ice.
   B. Write the client's name, the date, the contents of the tube, and the exact time of specimen collection, along with your signature and the signature of the witness, on the tube label and laboratory requisition if the specimen may be used as legal evidence. Transport the specimen on ice to the laboratory in a sealed plastic bag labeled as legal evidence.

5. Client and family teaching:
   A. Results may be available within hours.

6. Factors that affect results:
   A. Failure to tightly cap the specimen container may cause false low results.
   B. Failure to maintain a clear chain of custody may invalidate the results for legal purposes.

7. Other data:
   A. In the event of an overdose, be prepared to provide respiratory and circulatory support.

Bibliography:

Burkhart KK, Kulig KW: The other alcohols. Methanol, ethylene glycol, and isopropanol. Emerg Med Clin North Am *8*(4):913–928, 1990.

TOXOPLASMOSIS, OTHER, RUBELLA, CYTOMEGALO-VIRUS, HERPES VIRUS SEROLOGY (TORCH), BLOOD

Norm: Negative for all diseases.

Usage: Maternal and infant screening.

Description: This serologic test is performed to detect the congenitally acquired diseases of toxoplasmosis, rubella, cytomegalovirus, herpes virus, and others such as syphilis, varicella, and group B beta-hemolytic streptococcal infections in infants who manifest symptoms of viral or other infections during the first year of life. The test may also be performed on the mother during pregnancy to screen for diseases that are likely to cause birth defects. The literature discounts the value of *routine* TORCH screening and discusses the value of various methods of testing. One study recommends enzyme immunoassay to document past infection. IgM enzyme-linked immunosorbent assay (ELISA) is recommended to detect recent toxoplasmosis or rubella infection. Finally, several studies relate that culture is required to confirm herpes or cytomegalovirus infection.

Professional Considerations:

1. Consent form NOT required.
2. Preparation:
   A. Tube: Red-top, red/gray-top, or gold-top.
3. Procedure:
   A. Draw a 3-ml blood sample.
4. Postprocedure care:
   A. Any individual positive test or higher than normal titer should be repeated in 7–10 days to observe for changing titer.
5. Client and family teaching:
   A. Return in 7–10 days for repeat testing if the results are positive.
6. Factors that affect results:
   A. See individual test listings.
7. Other data:
   A. For positive tests, genetic counseling may be indicated.
   B. See individual test listings for full descriptions.
   C. TORCH test sera should be held in the laboratory for a year in the event repeat testing is necessary.

Bibliography:

Stamos J: Timely diagnosis of congenital infections. Pediatr Clin North Am *41*(5):1017–1033, 1994.

TOXOPLASMOSIS SEROLOGY, SERUM

Norm:

Immunofluorescence	
Adults	IgM titer <1:64
	IgG titer <1:1024
Neonates	IgM undetectable

Indirect hemagglutination
  No previous infection   Titer <1:4
  Probable past infection   Titers >1:4 and <1:256
  Suggestive of recent infection   Titer >1:256

Increased: Current or past infection with *Toxoplasma gondii.*

Decreased: Not applicable.

Description: Toxoplasmosis is a systemic, parasitic disease caused by the protozoa *Toxoplasma gondii.* It is transmitted to humans by ingestion of the undercooked meat of infected animals, or often by the ingestion of oocysts acquired from handling cat litter containing contaminated cat feces. It may also be transmitted to a fetus through the placenta of an infected mother. After ingestion, this parasite travels to various body tissues and is found grouped together in oocysts. Acquired toxoplasmosis often causes no symptoms in clients with intact immune systems. In immunosuppression, it may cause hyperpyrexia, lymphadenopathy, lymphocytosis, and in some cases, encephalitis, pneumonitis, myocarditis, myositis, and possible death. Fetal congenital toxoplasmosis can cause severe birth defects, including blindness, hydrocephalus, and mental retardation, and may lead to fetal or postnatal death. Serologic testing for *T. gondii* antibody titer is recommended for all pregnant females. If antibody titer is low-positive, indicating past infection, there is no risk to the fetus. However, the fetus is at risk for birth defects if the disease is acquired during pregnancy. Thus, if antibody titer is initially high (indicating current active infection) or initially negative, the test should be repeated at each prenatal checkup throughout the first 5 months of pregnancy, and just prior to delivery. Toxoplasmosis occurs in advanced AIDS.

Professional Considerations:

1. Consent form NOT required.
2. Preparation:
   A. Assess whether the woman has handled cat feces during pregnancy.
   B. Assess whether the client has eaten any raw or undercooked meat.
   C. Tube: Red-top, red/gray-top, or gold-top.
3. Procedure:
   A. Draw a 3-ml blood sample as soon as pregnancy is known or as soon as possible after symptoms appear. Label the specimen as the acute sample. Repeat the test in 7–14 days to detect rising antibody titer and label the tube as the convalescent sample. For pregnancy, repeat the test as described under "Description," above.
4. Postprocedure care:
   A. None.
5. Client and family teaching
   A. Cat owners who are pregnant or who have AIDS must feed the cat commercially prepared and/or well-cooked food and prevent the cat from roaming and scavenging. Avoid handling the cat litter, if possible. Cat litter should be handled (preferably by another household member) with gloved hands and discarded every day, with daily disinfection of the litter container by rinsing it with boiling water. If you must handle the cat litter or litter box, avoid touching anything else afterward, until you have performed meticulous handwashing. Also avoid handling other cats and avoid gardening (where you may come in contact with contaminated cat feces).
   B. Thoroughly cook any meat to be ingested.
6. Factors that affect results:
   A. None found.
7. Other data:
   A. Except for placental-fetal transfer, toxoplasmosis is not communicable between clients.
   B. When toxoplasmosis is acquired early in pregnancy, abortion may be recommended.
   C. Pyrimethamine and sulfonamides are used to treat toxoplasmosis.

Bibliography:

Takahashi E, Rossi C: Use of three immunological techniques for the detection of Toxoplasmosis spIgA antibodies in acute toxoplasmosis. J Clin Pathol *47*(5):1101–1104, 1994.

TOXOPLASMOSIS SKIN TEST, DIAGNOSTIC

Norm: Negative.

Positive: Current or past infection with *Toxoplasma gondii.*

Description: Toxoplasmosis is a systemic, parasitic disease caused by the protozoa *T. gondii.* It is transmitted to humans by ingestion of the undercooked meat of infected animals, or often by the ingestion of oocysts acquired from handling cat litter containing contaminated cat feces. It may also be transmitted to a fetus through the placenta of an infected mother. After ingestion, this parasite travels to various body tissues and is found grouped together in oocysts. Acquired toxoplasmosis often causes no symptoms in clients with intact immune systems. In immunosuppression, it may cause hyperpyrexia, lymphadenopathy, lymphocytosis, and in some cases, encephalitis, pneumonitis, myocarditis, myositis, and possible death. Fetal congenital toxoplasmosis can cause severe birth defects, including blindness, hydrocephalus, and mental retardation, and may lead to fetal or postnatal death.

Professional Considerations:

1. Consent form NOT required.
2. Preparation:
   A. Assess whether a pregnant woman has handled cat feces during her pregnancy.
   B. Assess whether the client has eaten any raw or undercooked meat.
   C. Obtain an alcohol wipe, a 1-ml syringe, an intradermal needle, *Toxoplasma* antigen, and a control.
3. Procedure:
   A. Cleanse the forearm injection site with an alcohol wipe, and allow the area to dry.
   B. Inject *Toxoplasma* antigen intradermally and record the site of injection. Inject the control in the other arm, and record the site of injection.
   C. Read the skin test in 24–48 hours. A positive test is indicated by redness and induration >10 mm in diameter.
4. Postprocedure care:
   A. *See Toxoplasmosis Serology, Serum* for pregnancy precautions and precautions for persons with AIDS.
5. Client and family teaching:
   A. After the injection, return in 24–48 hours for a skin test reading.
6. Factors that affect results:
   A. None found.
7. Other data:
   A. Many clients may be infected with *T. gondii* but are free of symptoms. Therefore, any pregnant woman should be tested for the presence of antibodies to *T. gondii*. See *Toxoplasmosis Serology, Serum.*

Bibliography:

Ambroise-Thomas P, Rougier D: New prospects in immunology of toxoplasmas: Skin tests for control of immunity and immuno-assays and agglutination tests for the detection of specific IgM antibodies. Parasitologia 28(2-3):85–93, 1986.

Rougier D, Ambroise-Thomas P: Detection of toxoplasmic immunity by multipuncture skin test with excretory-secretory antigen. Lancet 2(8447):121–123, 1985.

TRACER, DIAGNOSTIC
(see Glucose Monitoring Machines, Diagnostic)

TRANSESOPHAGEAL ECHOCARDIOGRAM
(see Transesophageal Sonogram, Diagnostic)

TRANSESOPHAGEAL SONOGRAM (TRANSESOPHAGEAL ECHOCARDIOGRAM, TEE), DIAGNOSTIC

Norm: Negative or normal structure/function and absence of pathology.

Usage: Transesophageal echocardiogram (TEE) is especially indicated for examination of prosthetic heart valves, detection of mitral valve regurgitation, aortic dissection (site and extent), congenital heart disease of the adult, cardiac tumors and masses, embolic/thrombotic disorders (particularly of the left atrium), vegetative endocarditis, intraoperative guide to left ventricular function, and for clients with conditions making standard transthoracic echocardiograms unreliable: obesity, chest deformities, chronic lung disease, or intubation.

Description: Ultrasound uses high frequency sound waves to induce vibrations that echo or reflect from the solid structures within the body. These echoes create images from which chamber/valve size, function, and pericardial effusion can be determined. A specially adapted flexible gastroscope is fitted with a high-frequency transducer to send, receive, and translate the reflected vibrations. This tube, when swallowed or advanced into the esophagus, is positioned behind the heart and related structures. It can be rotated anteriorly, laterally, or posteriorly to allow an unimpeded route for sound wave reflection off of the heart chambers, walls, and valves. Abnormalities can be displayed that are missed by standard diagnostic techniques. Only the upper aortic view is limited by the interference of the left mainstem bronchus.

Professional Considerations:

1. Consent form IS required.

Risks:

Vasovagal bradycardia and drug-induced tachycardia are likely dysrhythmias; esophageal perforation; transient hypoxemia.

Contraindications:

Esophageal obstructions, stenosis, fistula or dysphagia; history of radiation therapy to the esophagus or surrounding area (mediastinum); acute penetrating chest injuries. Neonates and young children are not candidates due to the unavailability of sized TEE scopes. Sedatives are contraindicated in clients with central nervous system depression.

2. Preparation:
   A. *See Client and family teaching.*
   B. Obtain a chest x-ray, ECG, and laboratory work, including CBC, electrolytes, PT, and PTT.
   C. Start an IV at KO rate for administration of sedation or emergency medications.
   D. Remove dentures and glasses. Have the client void prior to the procedure.
   E. A drying agent is typically given to reduce secretions (i.e., glycopyrrolate 0.1 to 0.2 mg IV). Some clients require a small IV dose of an antianxiety agent (i.e., midazolam or diazepam). Prophylactic antibiotics are usually given if the client has a prosthetic valve.
3. Procedure:
   A. The client is monitored continuously: heart rate and rhythm via cardiac monitor, blood pressure via noninvasive monitor, and O_2 via pulse oximetry.
   B. Position the client in the left lateral decubitus position.
   C. Topical anesthesia per physician preference is used to numb the throat and suppress the gag reflex. This may be repeated several times during the procedure.
   D. The client should be awake enough to follow commands, but drowsy. This procedure may also be performed on a fully anesthetized or intubated client.
   E. The client is asked to open the mouth and flex the neck forward in a chin-to-chest position.
   F. The xylocaine-lubricated probe is inserted and the client asked to swallow.
   G. Over the next 5–20 minutes the probe is gently withdrawn and cardiac images are viewed/recorded at different levels.
   H. The nurse remains with the client to monitor respiratory status, vital signs, and cardiac rhythm, and assess the need for further sedation or suctioning.
4. Postprocedure care:
   A. Continue assessment of respiratory status. If deep sedation was used, follow institutional protocol for postsedation monitoring. Typical monitoring includes continuous ECG monitoring and pulse oximetry, with continual assessments (q 5–15 minutes) of airway, vital signs, and neurologic status until client reaches level 3, 2, or 1 on the Ramsay Sedation Scale.
   B. Once the gag reflex has returned, the client can resume fluids. Full diet is not recommended until 3 hours postprocedure.
5. Client and family teaching:
   A. Fast for 6–8 hours prior to the test. Medications may be taken with a small amount of water, as directed by the physician. You will have to remove your dentures and eyeglasses, but you should keep your hearing aid on so that you can hear the physician's instructions.
   B. You will be given a sedative for the procedure. You should arrange for someone to drive you home, because you may be drowsy after the procedure and will not be permitted to drive.
   C. Do not eat or drink for 4–6 hours before the procedure. Take any prescription medications with a small sip of water.
   D. This procedure lets the physician look at your heart and its major blood vessels from the back, without the lungs blocking the view. A flexible tube about the thickness of a pen is inserted into the mouth and moved down into the esophagus. The tip of the tube produces sound waves that bounce off the heart and are changed into pictures on a video screen.
   E. Breathe through the nose and swallow during introduction of the probe, and breathe through the mouth for the remainder of the procedure, which takes about 30 minutes.
   F. The tongue and throat may feel swollen after the topical anesthetic; the mouth and lips will feel sticky and dry if a drying agent is used. Do not eat or drink after the procedure until the numbness is gone.
   G. The doctor must review the videotape of the procedure before discussing the test results.
   H. Homegoing instructions: Promptly report persistent sore throat, dysphagia, stiff neck, and epigastric, and substernal or abdominal pain that worsens with breathing or movement.

6. Factors that affect results:
   A. See the description of the test.
7. Other data:
   A. None.

Bibliography:

Brown L, Brown A: Transesophageal echocardiography: Implications for the critical care nurse. Crit Care Nurs *14*(3):55–59, 1994.

Cheney AM, Maquindang ML: Patient teaching for x-ray and other diagnostics. RN 4:54–56, 1993 (April).

Smith M, Cassidy J, Souther S, et al.: Transesophageal echocardiography in the diagnosis of traumatic rupture of the aorta. New Engl J Med *332*(6):356–362, 1995.

Thompson E: Transesophageal echocardiography: a new window on the heart and great vessels. Crit Care Nurs *13*(5):55–66, 1993.

TRANSFERRIN, SERUM

Norm:

		SI Units
Adult	200–400 mg/dl	2–4.0 g/L
Maternal (term)	305 mg/dl	3.0 g/L
Fetal	190 mg/dl	1.9 g/L
Newborn	130–275 mg/dl	1.3–2.8 g/L

Increased: Iron deficiency states with normal protein levels and pregnancy. Drugs include oral contraceptives.

Decreased: Congenital absence of transferrin (hereditary atransferrinemia), hemolytic states, hepatic disease (acquired), inflammation (chronic), iron overload, low iron states combined with protein malnutrition, neoplasm, proteinuria (severe) and other protein-losing states, and renal disease.

Description: Transferrin is a beta globulin and glycoprotein with a short (7-day) half-life. Formed in the liver, transferrin transports dietary iron from the intestinal mucosa to iron storage sites and hemoglobin synthesis sites in the body (bone, muscle, erythrocytes, lymphocytes). Transferrin enables iron storage by binding to transferrin receptors at the iron storage sites. Transferrin is capable of binding more than its own weight in iron. That is, 1 g of transferrin can carry 1.43 g of iron. Normally, iron saturation of transferrin (transferrin saturation) is between 20% and 45%. Because of its short half-life, values will decrease more quickly in protein malnutrition states than will albumin. Thus, transferrin is sometimes used to evaluate nutritional status. Transferrin also has growth-stimulating properties that are separate from its iron transport properties.

Professional Considerations:

1. Consent form NOT required.
2. Preparation:
   A. *See Client and family teaching.*
   B. Tube: Red-top, red/gray-top, or gold-top.
3. Procedure:
   A. Draw the specimen during the morning hours if it will be used to evaluate transferrin saturation, as a diurnal pattern with an A.M. peak exists.
   B. Draw a 1-ml blood sample.
4. Postprocedure care:
   A. None.
5. Client and family teaching:
   A. Fast from food and fluids (except water) for 12 hours before the test.
   B. Results are normally available within 24 hours.
6. Factors that affect results:
   A. None found.
7. Other data:
   A. Transferrin is also called siderophilin and iron-binding protein.
   B. *See also Iron and Total Iron Binding Capacity/Transferrin, Serum.*

Bibliography:

Bali PK, Zak O, Aisen P: A new role for the transferrin receptor in the release of iron from transferrin. Biochemistry *30*(2):324–328, 1991.

Hamill R, Woods J, Cook B: Congenital atransferrinemia. Clin Chem *96*(2):215–218, 1991.

Hayashi A, Wada Y, Suzuki T, et al.: Studies in familial hypotransferrinemia: unique clinical course and molecular pathology. Am J Hum Gen *53*(1):201–213, 1993.

TRANSFUSION REACTION WORK-UP, DIAGNOSTIC

Norm: Not applicable.

Transfusion Reaction Symptoms and Treatment:

Mild Febrile Reaction:

Symptoms
- Slight, nonsustained temperature rise <1°C
- Urticaria, rash, or hives
- Headache
- Malaise
- Mild chills

Treatment
- Slow the transfusion rate. Verify that the information on the client's blood band, hospital bracelet, blood bag, and blood transfusion requisition all correspond properly and notify the physician.

If all information matches properly, possible courses of action available to the physician include:
- Continue the transfusion while monitoring the recipient closely for further development of hemolytic or nonhemolytic reaction.
- Add a microaggregate filter to filter the blood, if not already being used.
- Administer antipyretic and antihistamine and continue the transfusion, while monitoring the client closely for further development of hemolytic or nonhemolytic reaction.
- Stop the transfusion, and return the blood to the blood bank.
- Stop the transfusion, and complete transfusion-reaction blood work and urine tests as described below.

Hemolytic Reaction:

Symptoms
Early signs:
- Sustained rise in temperature >1°C
- Nausea and/or vomiting
- Pronounced chills and shivering
- Palpitations
- Pain in the chest or back
- Apprehension
- Infusion site tenderness and warmth

Progressive signs:
- Shock
- Oliguria
- Hemoglobinuria
- Bleeding tendencies (disseminated intravascular coagulation)
- Acute renal failure
- Anaphylaxis

Treatment
- Stop the transfusion immediately, and leave a normal saline infusion at a keep-open rate. Notify the physician immediately.
- Monitor vital signs every 5–15 minutes.
- Completely fill a red-top tube and a lavender-top tube with a blood sample.
- Obtain a 50-ml random, fresh urine sample in a clean container.
- Document pretransfusion and post-transfusion vital signs on the blood bank requisition.
- Return the blood bank requisition, laboratory requisition for the transfusion reaction work-up, the bag of blood, the urine specimen, and the red-top and lavender-top tubes to the blood bank promptly.
- If DIC is suspected, additional testing should include fibrinogen level, fibrin split products, platelet count, PT/PTT, and thrombin time.

Acute Nonimmune Febrile Reaction:

Symptoms
- Sustained rise in temperature >1°C
- Hematemesis
- Diarrhea
- Hypotension
- Tachycardia
- Shock
- Sepsis

Treatment
In addition to following the procedures above for a hemolytic reaction:
- Draw blood for aerobic and anaerobic culture and Gram stain.

Anaphylactic Reaction:

Symptoms

- Tachycardia
- Dyspnea, wheezing (bronchospasm and upper airway edema)
- Apprehension
- Flushing
- Urticaria, hives
- Angioedema
- Shock
- Circulatory collapse
- Bowel spasm, with diarrhea

Treatment

In addition to following procedures above for a hemolytic reaction:

- Have an emergency cart readily available.
- Maintain a patent airway and blood pressure.
- Administer epinephrine intravenously as follows:
  a. Bolus with epinephrine 0.2–0.5 mg of 1:1000 dilution mixed in 10-ml 0.9% saline over 5–10 minutes.
  b. Follow the bolus with a continuous infusion of epinephrine at 1–4 mg/minute.
- Other drugs used to treat anaphylaxis may include aminophylline, atropine (for bradycardia), cimetidine, diphenhydramine, and hydrocortisone.
- Use IgA-deficient blood or plasma-deficient blood for future transfusions.

Usage: Helps determine the cause of transfusion reaction.

Description: An acute transfusion reaction work-up is indicated whenever an unexpected reaction to transfusion of blood products is noted. Symptoms are most likely to occur within the first 15–30 minutes of transfusion, and may be stimulated by as little as 10 ml of incompatible blood. Recombinant erythropoietin should be considered as an alternative to transfusion for anemic clients with nonmyeloid cancers.

Mild febrile reactions and urticaria may occur in clients who have been immunized to blood protein constituents through past receipt of donor blood or past pregnancies. A microaggregate filter used with transfusion can minimize the transfusion of such blood constituents.

Hemolytic transfusion reaction: With correctly administered blood, a hemolytic transfusion reaction may be due to recipient antibodies reacting to donor antigens not identified during type and crossmatch or type and screen procedures. Reactions are more likely to occur in clients who have had recent transfusions of blood, as new antibodies to past donor blood may have developed since the last type and crossmatch was performed. In blood administered incorrectly (i.e., to the wrong recipient), a transfusion reaction is most likely caused by ABO incompatibility or antigen-antibody reactions. An incompatible or contaminated transfusion may cause fatal hemolytic reactions and disseminated intravascular coagulation. Thus, it is important to observe recipients closely for early signs of reaction, so that the transfusion may be promptly stopped, and complications minimized.

Acute nonimmune febrile reactions may be caused by bacterial contamination of the donor blood. This type of reaction may cause fever and erythrocyte hemolysis and may progress to shock and sepsis.

Anaphylactic transfusion reactions may occur in clients with subnormal immunoglobulin A (IgA) who have a history of recurrent infections. The receipt of IgA in donor blood stimulates an antibody response to IgA that causes anaphylaxis.

Delayed transfusion reactions include delayed hemolytic reactions, graft-versus-host disease, purpura, and hemosiderosis. Delayed hemolytic reactions usually are caused by recipient anti-Rh antibodies, anti-Duffy antibodies, and anti-Kidd antibodies that were not detected during type and crossmatch procedures. A transfusion of blood containing these antigens causes delayed hemolysis and continued anemia. Graft-versus-host disease is usually fatal and occurs in immunosuppressed clients whose immune systems are unable to provide resistance against donor lymphocytes. Purpura with thrombocytopenia may develop about 7 days following transfusion in clients deficient in and who have developed antibodies to platelet antigen PLA-1. Hemosiderosis (iron overload) may occur in clients receiving multiple transfusions over a short period of time.

Laboratory procedures for an acute transfusion reaction work-up include direct Coombs' testing; repeated type and crossmatch on original recipient and donor samples; type and crossmatch on postreaction recipient sample with donor sample; hemoglobin and hematocrit level; serum haptoglobin; urea nitrogen, plasma or serum; recipient and donor blood culture and Gram stain; and urine measurement of bilirubin, hemoglobin, urobilinogen, and hemosiderin.

Professional Considerations:

1. Consent form NOT required.
2. Preparation:
   A. Assess the client during the transfusion for signs of a transfusion reaction listed above.
3. Procedure:
   A. Follow procedures described above under *Treatment.*
4. Postprocedure care:
   A. Continue monitoring vital signs every 5–15 minutes until they are stable.
5. Client and family teaching:
   A. Complete results may take several days.
   B. *See "Other data,"* and provide infor-

mation appropriate to the type of reaction that occurred.
6. Factors that affect results:
   A. See individual test listings.
7. Other data:
   A. For delayed transfusion reactions, the following should be performed if future transfusions are needed:
      i. *Delayed hemolytic reactions:* The client should be advised to carry the information in writing that any blood transfusions received must be negative for Rh (c and E), Duffy, and Kidd antigens.
      ii. *Graft-versus-host disease:* If the client survives this complication, future donor blood should be irradiated prior to transfusion.
      iii. *Purpura:* The client should be advised to carry the information in writing that any blood transfusions received must be PLA-1-negative.
      iv. *Hemosiderosis:* Hemosiderosis may be fatal. The risk for developing this complication may be minimized in clients who need multiple transfusions by performing lead chelation therapy.
   B. Card or slide hemagglutination or dipstick methods are available for use in ABO blood grouping at the bedside just prior to transfusion.

Bibliography:

Jeter E, Spivey MA: Noninfectious complications of blood transfusion in transfusion medicine II. Hematol Clin North Am 9(1):187–202, 1995.

Mohandas K, Aledort L: Transfusion requirements, risks, costs for patients with malignancy. Transfusion 35(5):427–430, 1995.

Williams A (ed): Transfusion medicine II (anthology). Hematol Clin North Am 9(1):115–118, 1995.

TRANSTHYRETIN (TTR, PREALBUMIN, PA, TRYPTOPHAN-RICH PREALBUMIN), SERUM

Norm:

		SI Units
Adult	10–40 mg/dl	100–400 mg/L
Male	(mean) 21.5 mg/dl	(mean) 215 mg/L
Female	(mean) 18.2 mg/dl	(mean) 182 mg/L
Maternal	17–18.6 mg/dl	170–186 mg/L
Children		
Cord blood	(mean) 13 mg/dl	(mean) 130 mg/L
Newborn	10.4–11.4 mg/dl	104–114 mg/L
12 months	(mean) 10 mg/dl	(mean) 100 mg/L
24–36 months	16–28.1 mg/dl	160–281 mg/L

Increased: Adrenal hyperfunction, Hodgkin's disease, shigellosis. Drugs include corticosteroids (high-dose) and NSAIDs (high-dose).

Decreased: Abdominal peritoneal dialysis, cirrhosis, chronic illness (with concomitant subnormal nutritional status), cystic fibrosis, diabetes mellitus, disseminated malignant disease, epithelial ovarian carcinoma, hereditary amyloidosis, protein/calorie malnutrition. Drugs include amiodarone, estrogens, and oral contraceptives (containing estrogen).

Description: Transthyretin is a transport protein, synthesized in the liver, that carries thyroid hormone and retinol in the body. Transthyretin is a precursor of albumin and its half-life of 2–4 days makes it a much more sensitive marker for nutritional status and for liver dysfunction than albumin, which has a half-life of 22 days. Because transthyretin reflects changes in nutritional status more quickly than albumin, it is frequently used to evaluate nutritional needs in postoperative and critically ill clients.

Professional Considerations:
1. Consent form NOT required.
2. Preparation:
   A. Tube: Red-top, red/gray-top, or gold-top.
   B. Do NOT draw specimens during hemodialysis.
3. Procedure:
   A. Draw a 1-ml blood sample without hemolysis.
4. Postprocedure care:
   A. None.
5. Client and family teaching:
   A. Results are normally available within 24 hours.
6. Factors that affect results:
   A. Hemolyzed or lipemic specimens interfere with the nephelometric testing method.
7. Other data:
   A. Avram et al. (1994) found prealbumin levels of less than 30 mg/dl to be a predictor of mortality in a sample of 33 continuous ambulatory peritoneal dialysis clients.

Bibliography:

Avram MM, Goldwasser P, Erroa M, Fein PA: Predictors of survival in continuous ambulatory peritoneal dialysis patients: the importance of prealbumin and other nutritional and metabolic markers. Am J Kidney Dis 23(1):91–98, 1994.

Ingenbleek Y, Young V: Transthyretin (prealbumin) in health and disease: nutritional implications. Ann Rev Nutr 14:495–533, 1994.

Jain SK, Sah M, Ransonet L, Wise R, Bocchini JA: Maternal and neonatal plasma prealbumin (prealbumin) concentrations and birth weight of newborn infants. Biol Neonate 68(1):10–14, 1995.

Khan WA, Salam MA, Bennish ML: C reactive protein and prealbumin as markers of disease activity in shigellosis. Gut 37(3):402–405, 1995.

Mahlck CG, Grankvist K: Plasma prealbumin in women with epithelial ovarian carcinoma. Gynecol Obstet Invest 37(2):135–140, 1994.

Measurement of visceral protein status in assessing protein and energy malnutrition: Standard of care. Prealbumin in Nutritional Care Consensus Group. Nutrition 11(2):169–171, 1995.

TRANYLCYPROMINE
(see Amphetamines, Blood)

TRAP
(see Tartrate-Resistant Acid Phosphatase, Blood)

TRAZODONE
(see Tricyclic Antidepressants, Plasma or Serum)

TRIAZOLAM
(see Benzodiazepines, Plasma and Urine)

TRICHINOSIS SEROLOGY, SERUM

Norm: Negative or titer <1:16. Possible current or past infection: titer >1:5.

Positive: A fourfold rise in titer is diagnostic for trichinosis.

Description: Trichinosis is a parasitic disease caused by the larva of *Trichinella spiralis*, a roundworm acquired in humans by ingestion of raw or poorly cooked pork or other animals it inhabits (cats, dogs, swine, and some wild animals such as walrus and bear). The ingested worm larvae mature and reproduce in the intestinal tract, then migrate through the lymphatic system and bloodstream to other sites in the body. Those reaching muscle tissue become encapsulated as cysts, causing inflammation and necrosis. The symptoms of trichinosis are progressive. Soon after ingestion, hyperpyrexia, gastrointestinal upset, eosinophilia, and muscle edema occur. These symptoms are followed by muscle soreness and may progress to neurotoxicity and myocarditis. Clients with chronic trichinosis may experience myalgia, eye burning, headache, and easy fatigability. This test detects the presence of *T. spiralis* antibodies by mixing serial dilutions of the client's serum with *T. spiralis* antigen and observing for antigen-antibody reactions. Titers may be negative soon after symptoms appear, but begin rising about 21 days after infection. Levels peak about 60 days after infection, then slowly return to higher than baseline levels until about 2 years later.

Professional Considerations:

1. Consent form NOT required.
2. Preparation:
   A. Tube: Red-top, red/gray-top, or gold-top.
   B. Assess for history of recent ingestion of raw pork or poorly cooked pork or other susceptible animals.
   C. The test may need to be prescheduled with the laboratory.
   D. Specimens MAY be drawn during hemodialysis.
3. Procedure:
   A. Draw a 5-ml blood sample. Repeat the test every 3–5 days to detect rising titer.
4. Postprocedure care:
   A. None.
5. Client and family teaching:
   A. Before eating it, thoroughly cook pork or meat from other susceptible animals until it turns gray.
   B. Serial testing is necessary to confirm *T. spiralis* infection.
6. Factors that affect results:
   A. Titers may be negative in the presence of infection if drawn during the first 3 weeks after exposure.
7. Other data:
   A. Other tests used to diagnose trichinosis include skin testing, muscle biopsy, or examination of cerebrospinal fluid for *T. spiralis*.
   B. Trichinosis has been treated with thiabendazole (intestinal phase), mebendazole (muscular stage), and corticosteroids.

Bibliography:

Dzbenski T, Bitkowska E, Wojciech P: Detection of circulating parasitic antigen in acute infection with trichinella spiralis. Diagnostic significance of findings. Int J Microbiol Vir Parasitol Infect Dis *281*(4):519–525, 1994.
Morse J, Ridenour R, Unterseher P: Trichinosis: Infrequent or frequent misdiagnosis. Ann Emerg Med *24*(5):969–971, 1994.

TRICHINOSIS SKIN TEST, DIAGNOSTIC

Norm: Negative.

Positive: Current or past infection with *T. spiralis*.

Description: Trichinosis is a parasitic disease caused by the larva of *Trichinella spiralis*, a roundworm acquired in humans by ingestion of raw or poorly cooked pork or other animals it inhabits (cats, dogs, swine, and some wild animals such as walrus and bear). The ingested worm larvae mature and reproduce in the intestinal tract, then migrate through the lymphatic system and bloodstream to other sites in the body. Those reaching muscle tissue become encapsulated as cysts, causing inflammation and necrosis. The symptoms of trichinosis are progressive. Soon after ingestion, hyperpyrexia, gastrointestinal upset, eosinophilia, and muscle edema occur. These symptoms are followed by muscle soreness and may progress to neurotoxicity and myocarditis. This test is based on an immediate hypersensitivity reaction. The presence of *T. spiralis* antibodies is indicated when intradermal injection of the killed larvae of *T. spiralis* produces signs of an antigen-antibody reaction.

Professional Considerations:

1. Consent form NOT required.
2. Preparation:
   A. Obtain an alcohol wipe, a 1-ml syringe with an intradermal needle, *T. spiralis* antigen, and a control.
   B. Assess for history of recent ingestion of raw pork or poorly cooked pork or other susceptible animals.
   C. Specimens MAY be drawn during hemodialysis.
3. Procedure:
   A. Cleanse the forearm site for injection with an alcohol wipe and allow the area to dry.
   B. Inject *T. spiralis* antigen intradermally. Inject the control into the site in the opposite forearm. Record the sites of injection.
   C. 20 minutes later, observe the injection site for a blanched wheal with surrounding erythema, a symptom of a positive reaction.
4. Postprocedure care:
   A. None.
5. Client and family teaching:
   A. Before eating it, thoroughly cook pork or meat from other susceptible animals until it turns gray.
   B. In positive tests, the wheal and redness should disappear within a few hours.
6. Factors that affect results:
   A. Positive results may also indicate past trichinosis infection.
7. Other data:
   A. Injected corticosteroids may help mediate an excessive reaction to the skin test.
   B. *See also Trichinosis Serology, Serum.*

Bibliography:

Woodcock RW, Wahl JM: Trichinosis: Recent case reports and current intervention. J Emerg Nurs *13*(1):42–46, 1987.

TRICHOMONAS PREPARATION, SPECIMEN

Norm: Negative. No *Trichomonas* identified.

Positive: Trichomoniasis.

Description: Trichomoniasis is a sexually transmitted protozoan infection of the genitourinary tract. This infection causes considerable foamy, yellow drainage as well as petechiae and vaginal burning and itching in females, and a persistent, white urethral discharge or frequently no symptoms in males. The causative organism, *Trichomonas vaginalis,* is transmitted by direct contact with the vaginal and urethral fluids of infected individuals. Diagnosis of trichomoniasis is made via direct microscopic examination of a wet mount of the secretions of infected individuals.

Professional Considerations:

1. Consent form NOT required.
2. Preparation:
   A. Obtain a speculum, a pipette, a sterile tube to which 1 ml of sterile nonbacteriostatic 0.9% saline has been added, and a sterile swab approved for microbiologic use.
   B. *See Client and family teaching.*
   C. The client should disrobe below the waist for the collection of a vaginal, cervical, or urethral swab.
3. Procedure:
   A. *Female: Vaginal, cervical, or urethral specimen:*
      i. Place the client in the dorsal lithotomy position and drape her for comfort and privacy.
      ii. For the vaginal specimen, collect it by pipette aspiration from the vaginal pool, or by swabbing the circumference of the vagina with a sterile swab. Express the secretions into the sterile tube of saline and cover the tube.
      iii. For the cervical swab, place the speculum over the cervical os and gently express secretions onto the sterile swab. Alternatively, aspirate endocervical secretions through a pipette. Transfer the secretions to the sterile tube of saline and cover the tube.
   B. *Male or female: urethral specimen:*
      i. Insert the cotton-tipped end of sterile swab into the urethral meatus. Rotate the swab and hold it in place for 10 seconds to allow absorption of secretions. Transfer the secretions to the sterile tube of saline and cover the tube.

C. *Male: prostatic specimen:*
   i. Provide privacy for the client.
   ii. Instruct the client to stimulate ejaculation by masturbation. The semen should be collected into a clean container. If the client is uncomfortable with masturbation or unable to collect the specimen, it may be collected into a plastic condom at home and brought in within 1 hour. The client should be instructed to empty the condom into a clean container and cover it tightly to prevent the specimen from drying out.
D. *Urine collection for examination of sediment:*
   i. Instruct the client to cleanse the area surrounding the urethral meatus with four soapy sponges and then to rinse and dry the area.
   ii. While holding the labia open or the foreskin back, the client should void about 20 ml of urine into a clean container, and then stop the stream and cap the container.
4. Postprocedure care:
   A. Write the specimen source and the collection time on the laboratory requisition.
   B. Send the specimen to the laboratory immediately.
   C. Do not refrigerate the specimen.
5. Client and family teaching:
   A. For vaginal or cervical specimens, avoid douching for 72 hours.
   B. If results are positive, notify any sexual contacts to be tested. Do not have sexual relations until your physician confirms that follow-up testing is negative.
   C. Assess the client's knowledge of and teach safe sex practices.
6. Factors that affect results:
   A. Results are invalidated if the specimen dries before microscopic examination.
   B. The test is less sensitive for asymptomatic females. Wet mounts are negative in 30–50% of females positive for trichomonas. Unfortunately, negative microscopy results give false reassurance.
7. Other data:
   A. Trichomoniasis may be treated with metronidazole.
   B. Consider testing for *Chlamydia* and *Neisseria gonorrhoeae* with positive results.

Bibliography:

Andrews H, Acheson N, Huengsberg M, et al.: The role of microscopy in the diagnosis of sexually transmitted infections in women. Genitourin Med 70(2):118–120, 1994.

Beal C, Goldsmith R, Kotby M, et al.: The plastic envelope method, a simplified technique for culture diagnosis of trichomoniasis. J Clin Microbiol 30(9): 2265–2268, 1992.

Hart G: Factors associated with trichomoniasis, candidiasis and bacterial vaginitis. Int J STD AIDS 4(1):21–25, 1993.

Krieger J, Verdon M, Siegel N, et al.: Natural history of urogenital trichomoniasis in men. J Urol 149(6): 1455–1458, 1993.

TRICYCLIC ANTIDEPRESSANTS, PLASMA OR SERUM

Norm: Negative.

		SI Units
Therapeutic Levels		
Amitriptyline	100–250 ng/ml	360–900 nmol/L
Panic level	>400 ng/ml	>1275 nmol/L
Amoxapine	20–100 ng/ml	64–319 nmol/L
Panic level	>500 ng/ml	>1594 nmol/L
Desipramine	150–300 ng/ml	563–1126 nmol/L
Panic level	>400 ng/ml	>1500 nmol/L
Doxepin	100–200 ng/ml	360–720 nmol/L
Panic level	>400 ng/ml	>1440 nmol/L
Imipramine	75–250 ng/ml	279–890 nmol/L
Panic level	>400 ng/ml	>1440 nmol/L
Maprotiline	150–400 ng/ml	541–1442 nmol/L
Nortriptyline	50–150 ng/ml	190–570 nmol/L
Panic level	>500 ng/ml	>1900 nmol/L
Protriptyline	50–150 ng/ml	190–570 nmol/L
Panic level	>200 ng/ml	>760 nmol/L
Trazodone	300–2500 ng/ml	1000–6000 nmol/L
Panic level	>4000 ng/ml	>9600 nmol/L

Note: Life-threatening cardiac toxicity or seizures are seen if concentrations are over 1000 ng/ml.

Overdose Symptoms and Treatment:

Symptoms: Confusion, agitation, hallucinations, seizures, coma, dysrhythmias, hyperthermia, flushing, and dilation of the pupils; death may occur.

Treatment:

1. Administer activated charcoal or induce emesis (if soon after ingestion).
2. Do gastric lavage with 0.9% saline × 24 hours.
3. Give physostigmine (IV) to counteract anticholinergic actions and side effects of coma, hypertension, respiratory depression, or uncontrollable convulsions.
4. Give bicarbonate 1–2 mmol/kg IV for delayed cardiac conduction or ventricular dysrhythmias. Adjust the dose according to arterial pH and correction of symptoms.
5. Control dysrhythmia with propranolol, lidocaine, or phenytoin.
6. Monitor cardiac pattern for QRS elongation, dysrhythmias, and conduction abnormalities for 72 hours (adults) or 96 hours (children).
7. Hemodialysis and peritoneal dialysis will NOT remove amitriptyline, desipramine, doxepin, imipramine, nortriptyline, or protryptiline. No information is available on the effectiveness of dialysis in removing amoxapine, maptroline, and trazodone.
8. Hemoperfusion will remove amitriptyline.
9. Provide supportive intervention for lethargy, confusion, hallucinations, urinary retention, hypotension, hypertension, hyperpyrexia, and respiratory depression progressing to convulsions, coma, and death.

Usage: Monitoring for therapeutic or toxic levels during tricyclic antidepressant therapy, or for toxic levels in attempted suicide.

Description: "Tricyclic antidepressants" is a term describing a group of drugs with similar cyclic chemical structures, frequently used to treat depression on a long-term basis. These drugs act by blocking norepinephrine and serotonin reuptake in the central nervous system and have anticholinergic properties. They are metabolized in the liver, with a variable half-life and peak levels occurring 4–8 hours after an oral dose. Because certain drugs of this group are metabolized to others in the group, the levels of all of them should be measured and considered when evaluating clinical symptoms. Therapeutic blood monitoring is important, both because the drugs have a narrow window of therapeutic effectiveness, and because levels have been shown to correlate poorly with clinical effectiveness. Thus, toxicity is a risk when doses are increased to improve clinical symptoms.

Professional Considerations:

1. Consent form NOT required.
2. Preparation:
   A. Tube: Tube: Red-top, red/gray-top, or gold-top (for serum); green-top (for plasma).
   B. Samples for amitriptyline, desipramine, doxepin, imipramine, nortriptyline, or protryptiline levels MAY be drawn during hemodialysis. Do NOT draw samples for amoxapine, maptroline, or trazodone during hemodialysis.
   C. Write the name of the drug ingested (if known) on the laboratory requisition.
3. Procedure:
   A. Draw blood 12 hours after the last dose.
   B. Draw a 7-ml blood sample in a syringe. Remove the stopper from either a red-top, red/gray-top, or gold-top tube (for serum), or from a green-top tube (for plasma), and eject the blood into the tube. Replace the stopper. For a plasma specimen, gently roll the tube several times to mix the blood with the anticoagulant.
4. Postprocedure care:
   A. Send the specimen to the laboratory promptly. The serum should be separated within 2 hours, and the sample should be frozen or refrigerated if not tested promptly.
   B. If concurrent monoamine oxidase inhibitors have been ingested, monitor the client for hyperpyrexia and provide convulsion precautions.
5. Client and family teaching:
   A. It will take 7–21 days of therapy for a steady state to be reached.
   B. For overdose, intensive care may be required.
   C. For an intentional overdose, refer the client and family for crisis intervention and offer resource information for counseling.
   D. If activated charcoal was given for elevated levels, the client should drink 4–6 glasses of water each day for 2 days to prevent constipation. The activated charcoal will also cause stools to be black for a few days.
   E. Cardiac deaths have occurred up to 6 days after an overdose.
6. Factors that affect results:
   A. Drugs that may cause increased levels include cimetidine, corticosteroids, methylphenidate, neuroleptics, and oral contraceptives.
   B. Drugs that may cause decreased levels include barbiturates, chloral hydrate, glutethimide, nicotine (cigarette smoking), and phenobarbital.
   C. Levels for black clients may be as much as 50% higher than for white clients taking the same dosage regimen.
   D. Toxicity occurs more readily and at lower levels with advancing age, due to slowed metabolism.
7. Other data:
   A. Tricyclic antidepressants cause serum glucose to increase and glucose tolerance to decrease. Monitor diabetics for hyperglycemia when using these drugs.
   B. Neurotoxicity and cardiotoxicity are less likely to occur with trazodone than with other drugs of this group.
   C. Children are more sensitive than adults to toxic effects.

Bibliography:

Caravati EM, Bossart PJ: Demographic and electrocardiographic factors associated with severe tricyclic antidepressant toxicity. J Toxicol Clin Toxicol 29(1): 31–43, 1991.

Davis M: Hepatotoxicity of antidepressants. Int Clin Psychopharm 6(2):97–103, 1991.

Levin G, DeVane L: A review of cyclic antidepressant-induced blood dyscrasias. Annals Pharm 26(3): 378–383, 1992.

Preskorn S, Fast G: Tricyclic antidepressant induced seizures and plasma drug concentration. J Clin Psychiatry 53(5):160–162, 1992.

TRIFLUOPERAZINE
(see Phenothiazines, Blood)

TRIGLYCERIDES, BLOOD
Norm:

		SI Units
Serum Values		
Adult females		
Age 20–29	10–100 mg/dl	0.11–1.13 mmol/L
Age 30–39	10–110 mg/dl	0.11–1.24 mmol/L
Age 40–49	10–122 mg/dl	0.11–1.38 mmol/L
Age 50–59	10–134 mg/dl	0.11–1.51 mmol/L
Age >59	10–147 mg/dl	0.11–1.66 mmol/L
Adult males		
Age 20–29	10–157 mg/dl	0.11–1.77 mmol/L
Age 30–39	10–182 mg/dl	0.11–2.05 mmol/L
Age 40–49	10–193 mg/dl	0.11–2.18 mmol/L
Age 50–59	10–197 mg/dl	0.11–2.22 mmol/L
Age >59	10–199 mg/dl	0.11–2.24 mmol/L
Children		
Female, age 1–19	10–121 mg/dl	0.11–1.36 mmol/L
Male, age 1–19	10–103 mg/dl	0.11–1.16 mmol/L

Note: Plasma values are lower by about 3%.

Classification of Triglyceride Levels

Borderline high	200–400 mg/dl	2.3 mmol/L
High	400–1000 mg/dl	4.5–11.3 mmol/L
Very high	>1000 mg/dl	>11.3 mmol/L

Increased: Alcoholism, aortic aneurysm, aortitis, arteriosclerosis, diabetes mellitus, diet (recent high-carbohydrate, prolonged high-fat) familial hypertriglyceridemia, fat embolism, glycogen storage diseases, gout, hepatic cholesterol ester storage disease, hypercholesterolemia, hyperlipoproteinemia, hypothyroidism, myocardial infarction (for up to 1 year), myxedema, nephrotic syndrome, pancreatitis, pregnancy, renal insufficiency (chronic), starvation (early), Tangier disease, and von Gierke's disease. Tobacco use.

Decreased: Abetalipoproteinemia, acanthocytosis, cirrhosis (portal), hyperalimentation, malabsorption, and malnutrition. Drugs include ascorbic acid, asparaginase, clofibrate, dextrothyroxine, gemfibrozil, heparin, lovastatin, metformin, niacin, phenformin, pravastatin, and sulfonureas.

Description: Also known as "fat," triglyceride is a compound consisting of fatty acid/glycerol ester that comprises a major part (up to 70%) of very low-density lipoproteins (VLDL) and a small part (<10%) of low-density lipoproteins (LDL) in fasting serum samples. Dietary triglycerides are carried as part of chylomicrons through the lymphatic system and bloodstream to adipose tissue, where they are released for storage. Triglycerides are also synthesized in the liver from fatty acids and from protein and glucose above the body's current needs, and then stored in adipose tissue. They may be later retrieved and formed into glucose through gluconeogenesis when needed by the body. Triglyceride levels are taken into consideration with total cholesterol, high-density lipoprotein cholesterol, and chylomicron levels when categorizing a client's serum into lipoprotein phenotypes that represent genetic lipoprotein abnormalities. Treatments differ for the different phenotypes.

Professional Considerations:
1. Consent form NOT required.
2. Preparation:
   A. Tube: Red-top, red/gray-top, or gold-top; or lavender-top.

B. A fasting specimen is preferred.

C. *See Client and family teaching.*

3. Procedure:

A. Draw a 1-ml blood sample.

4. Postprocedure care:

A. None.

5. Client and family teaching:

A. Avoid variations in diet and weight for 21 days; avoid alcohol and refined carbohydrates for 3 days.

B. Fast 12 hours prior to the test. Water is permitted.

6. Factors that affect results:

A. Drugs that may cause falsely elevated results include cholestyramine, estrogens, furosemide, miconazole, and oral contraceptives.

B. Triglyceride levels for black clients have been demonstrated to be lower than those for white clients.

7. Other data:

A. Sacher reference provides good summary of triglycerides in context with other lipids, as well as lipid phenotyping.

Bibliography:

Axelsen M, Eliasson B, Joheim R, et al.: Lipid intolerance in smokers. J Intern Med 237(5):449–455, 1995.

Expert Panel on Detection, Evaluation and Treatment of High Blood Cholesterol in Adults. Summary of the second report of the national cholesterol education program (NCEP) on detection, evaluation, and treatment of high blood cholesterol in adults. JAMA 269:3015–3023, 1993.

Joly J, Sesboue H, Martin J: Serum trypsin-like activity in chronic alcoholized men: possible relationships with lipids, apoA-1 and apoB lipoproteins. Alcohol Alcohol 27(5):563–569, 1992.

Lemay A, Dodin S, Cedrin I, et al.: Phasic serum lipid excursions occur during cyclical oral conjugated estrogens but not during transdermal estradiol sequentially combined with oral medroxyprogesteroneacetate. Clin Endocrinol 42:341–351, 1995.

Mougious V, Kotzamanidis C, Koutsari C, et al.: Exercise induced changes in the concentration of individual fatty acids and triacylglycerols of human plasma. Metabolism 44(5):681–688, 1995.

TRIIODOTHYRONINE, BLOOD
(see Thyroid Test: Triiodothyronine, Blood)

TROPONIN I OR T (CTN-I OR CTN-T), SERUM

Norm:

		SI Units
Troponin I	<3.1 µg/L	<3.1 µg/L
Troponin T	<0.2 µg/L	<0.2 µg/L

Ranges vary according to the specific method and technology used.

Increased Troponin I: Acute myocardial infarction.

Increased Troponin T: Acute myocardial infarction, muscle damage, renal failure.

Description: Cardiac Troponin 1 is a contractile protein of the myofibril manufactured only in the myocardium. Troponin-T and cardiac specific Troponin-I are two isoforms that have been identified. Because of the low-to-undetectable values in the serum of healthy people and the quick elevation (detectable within 1 hour after myocardial cell injury), these ultrasensitive markers have been praised for their usefulness in the early diagnosis of acute myocardial infarction (MI), especially in detecting silent MIs, microinfarctions, and in the case of chest pain not accompanied by typical electrocardiogram changes. It will be some time before the role of these newer markers is fully realized in clinical practice.

Professional Considerations:

1. Consent form NOT required.

2. Preparation:

A. Tube: Red-top.

3. Procedure:

A. Draw a 5-ml blood sample.

4. Postprocedure care:

A. None.

5. Client and family teaching:

A. Results are normally available within 4 hours.

6. Factors that affect results:

A. Troponin T is also elevated in renal disease and with certain surgical procedures. No circumstance has been found in which Troponin I has not reflected cardiac injury.

7. Other data:

A. The only FDA-approved test has a 90-minute turnaround time, a bit slow for triaging purposes in an emergency room.

B. The Troponin I assay costs less than the Troponin T assay. Test kits are not widely available in the United States.

Bibliography:

Adams J, Sicard G, Allen B, et al.: Diagnosis of peri-operative myocardial infarction with measurement of cardiac troponin. New Engl J Med *330*(10): 670–674, 1994.

Antman E, Grudzien C, Sacks D: Evaluation of a rapid bedside assay for detection of serum cardiac troponin-T. JAMA *273*(16):1279–1282, 1995.

Apple F: Acute myocardial infarction and coronary reperfusion: Serum cardiac markers for the 1990's. Am J Clin Pathol *97*(2):217–226, 1992.

Hamm C, Ravkilde J, Gerhardt W, et al.: The prognostic value of serum troponin T in unstable angina. New Engl J Med *327*(3):146–150, 1992.

Ravkilde J: Independent prognostic value of serum creatine kinase isoenzyme MB mass, cardiac troponin T, myosin light chain levels in suspected acute myocardial infarction. J Am Coll Cardiol *25*(3):574–581, 1995.

TRYPANOSOMIASIS SEROLOGIC TEST (CHAGAS' DISEASE SEROLOGIC TEST), BLOOD

Norm: Negative titer.

Positive: American trypanosomiasis (Chagas' disease).

Description: American trypanosomiasis, also known as "Chagas' disease," is endemic in Latin America. Serologic testing is useful after the acute stage of the disease, when blood films are not very sensitive. Symptoms may include central nervous system (CNS) changes, CNS lesions in immunocompromised clients, and meningoencephalitis in children. The course of the disease may run months to years and is frequently fatal.

Professional Considerations:

1. Consent form NOT required.
2. Preparation:
   A. Tube: Red-top, red/gray-top, or gold-top.
   B. Obtain a container of ice.
   C. Specimens MAY be drawn during hemodialysis.
3. Procedure:
   A. Draw a 5-ml blood sample. Place the tube on ice.
4. Postprocedure care:
   A. Write the name of the suspected parasite and the place and date of recent travel on the laboratory requisition.
5. Client and family teaching:
   A. Results may not be available for several days because testing is performed by the Centers for Disease Control (Atlanta, GA) or sent to a parasitology laboratory.
6. Factors that affect results:
   A. Reject specimens that are not frozen.
7. Other data:
   A. Transmission of American trypanosomiasis is possible by transfusion of contaminated blood to immunocompromised clients.
   B. A complement fixation test is being tested for rapid diagnosis of American trypanosomiasis.
   C. *See also African Trypanosomiasis, Blood; and Parasite Screen, Blood.*

Bibliography:

Garcia E, Ramirez LE, Monteon V, Sotelo J: Diagnosis of American trypanosomiasis (Chagas' disease) by the new complement fixation test. J Clin Microbiol *33*(4):1034–1035, 1995.

TRYPSIN, PLASMA OR SERUM

Norm:

Behringwerke Antibody Method	
Young adult (age 18–36)	185–272 µg/L
Middle adult (age 37–66)	185–272 µg/L
Older adult (>age 66)	147–1438 µg/L
Immunoreactive (Cationic) Trypsin by RIA Method	
Adults	16.7–32.3 µg/L
RIA Double-Antibody (Geokas') Method	
Adults	22.2–44.4 µg/L
Children	
Cord	21.4–25.2 µg/L
<6 months	25.9–36.7 µg/L
6–12 months	30.2–44.0 µg/L
1–3 years	28.0–31.6 µg/L
3–5 years	25.1–31.5 µg/L
5–7 years	32.1–39.3 µg/L
7–10 years	32.7–37.1 µg/L

Sorin Antibody Method

Adults   5.0–85.0 µg/L
Children   11.1–51.3 µg/L

Increased: Beta-thalassemia, chronic renal failure, cystic fibrosis (initial years), hepatic disease, malnutrition (acute), pancreatitis (acute), pancreatic viral infection, peptic ulcer disease, and recent endoscopic retrograde cholangiopancreatography. Drugs include bombesin, cerulein, cholecystokinin, and secretin.

Decreased: Beta-thalassemia, cystic fibrosis (advanced), diabetes mellitus, malnutrition (chronic), pancreatic cancer, and pancreatitis (chronic).

Description: Trypsin is a proteolytic enzyme produced in the pancreas in the precursor form of inactive trypsinogen. Trypsinogen is converted to trypsin in the duodenum by enterokinase. Trypsin exists in several forms in the bloodstream. One form includes as trypsinogen that is bound to alpha-antitrypsin, to alpha-macroglobulin, and free trypsin. During the initial years of cystic fibrosis, serum trypsin levels are elevated as a result of pancreatic cell destruction and liberation of trypsin into the bloodstream. Over time, pancreatic insufficiency leads to abnormally low trypsin levels. Because of the possibility of overlap with normal values as pancreatic function declines, the value of this test is limited when diagnosing cystic fibrosis. Elevations reflect either pancreatic damage or impairment or organs involved in its clearance. Trypsin is thought to play a role in activating the complement cascade.

Professional Considerations:

1. Consent form NOT required.
2. Preparation:
   A. Tube: Red-top, red/gray-top, or gold-top (serum sample), or green-top (plasma sample).
   B. Specimens MAY be drawn during hemodialysis.
   C. *See Client and family teaching.*
3. Procedure:
   A. Draw a 7-ml blood sample.
4. Postprocedure care:
   A. Transport the specimen to the laboratory and refrigerate it at 4°C or freeze it at –20°C until testing.
5. Client and family teaching:
   A. Fast from food for 8 hours prior to the test.
6. Factors that affect results:
   A. Levels are elevated in nonfasting samples.
   B. Trypsin levels demonstrate a diurnal variation, with the highest levels occurring during the late evening.
   C. Due to the problem of wide variability in trypsin norms, values should be compared to the norms of the laboratory performing the test.
   D. Values are not affected by hemodialysis.
7. Other data:
   A. Sensitivity is 90%, false-negative rate approximately 7%.
   B. For elevated immunoreactive trypsin levels, refer clients for confirmatory sweat testing.

Bibliography:

Goldberg D, Durie P: Biochemical tests in the diagnosis of chronic pancreatitis and in the evaluation of pancreatic insufficiency. Clin Biochem *26*(4): 253–275, 1993.

Hassemer D, Laessig R, Hoffman G, et al.: Laboratory quality control issues related to screening newborns for cystic fibrosis using immunoreactive trypsin. Pediatr Pulmonol *7* (Suppl):76–83, 1991.

LeMoine O, Devaster JM, Deviere J, et al.: Trypsin activity: A new marker of acute alcoholic pancreatitis. Dig Dis Sci *39*(12):2634–2638, 1994.

Montalto G, Lorello D, Carroccio A, et al.: Trypsin in chronic renal failure and transplant patients. Am J Gastroenterol *87*(9):1175–1179, 1992.

Pizzilli R, Gullo L, Ricchi E, et al.: Serum pancreatic enzymes in HIV-serosensitive patients. Dig Dis Sci.*37*(2):286–288, 1992.

TRYPSIN, STOOL

Norm: Positive.

Gelatin digestion	2+ to 4+
≤Age 1	Positive at dilutions >1:80
>Age 1	Positive at dilutions >1:40
Cystic fibrosis	Negative at dilutions >1:10

Negative: Cystic fibrosis (advanced), malabsorption in children, pancreatic insufficiency, and pancreatitis (chronic).

Description: Trypsin is a proteolytic enzyme produced in the pancreas in the precursor form of inactive trypsinogen. Trypsinogen is converted to trypsin in the duodenum by enterokinase. Trypsin is present in the stool of young children, but amounts lessen in older children and adults due to intestinal bacterial destruction of trypsin. In clients with pancreatic insufficiency, stool trypsin tests are negative. This test is performed by observing the digestive activity of serial dilutions of stool or duodenal fluid on the gelatin of unexposed radiographic film after incubation. A negative result necessitates test repetition on at least two more stool samples.

Professional Considerations:
1. Consent form NOT required.
2. Preparation:
   A. Obtain a tongue blade and a clean container.
   B. *See Client and family teaching.*
3. Procedure:
   A. Obtain a dime-sized sample of stool and place it in a covered, dry clean container.
4. Postprocedure care:
   A. Send the specimen to the laboratory promptly. The specimen must be tested within 2 hours.
5. Client and family teaching:
   A. Defecate in a bedpan. For infants, the stool sample may be taken from a diaper.
   B. Avoid laxatives or barium procedures the week prior to the specimen collection.
6. Factors that affect results:
   A. The stool from constipated samples may produce false-negative results, due to the extended time allowed for intestinal bacteria to destroy trypsin.
   B. False-positive results may be caused by the presence of bacterial proteases in the sample.
7. Other data:
   A. *See also Trypsin, Serum.*

Bibliography:

Goldberg D, Durie P: Biochemical tests in the diagnosis of chronic pancreatitis and in the evaluation of pancreatic insufficiency. Clin Biochem *26*(4): 253–275, 1993.

Roxvall L, Bengtson A, Sennerby L, et al.: Activation of the complement cascade by trypsin. Biol Chem Hoppe Seyler *372*(4):273–278, 1991.

TRYPTOPHAN, PLASMA

Norm:

		SI Units
Adults	0.51–1.49 mg/dl	25–73 µmol/L
Infants (first day of life)		
Premature	0.32–0.92 mg/dl	15–45 µmol/L
Full-term	0.51–1.49 mg/dl	25–73 µmol/L

Increased: Sepsis and tryptophanuria.

Decreased: Blue diaper syndrome (tryptophan malabsorption syndrome), carcinoid syndrome, Hartnup disease, hypothermia, kwashiorkor, and postoperative abdominal surgery (first 48 hours). Drugs include alclofenac, aspirin, glucose, and indomethacin.

Description: Tryptophan is an essential amino acid that functions as a precursor for serotonin and niacin. Some tryptophan also occurs naturally in the body. Tryptophan metabolism involves action by the enzyme, tryptophan pyrrolase. Tryptophanuria is an inherited, X-linked trait in which an enzyme, tryptophan pyrrolase, is deficient. The resulting accumulation of nonmetabolized tryptophan results in elevated serum levels, as well as tryptophan excretion in the urine after renal reabsorption sites for tryptophan become saturated. Symptoms of tryptophanuria include dwarfism, photosensitivity, and ataxia. In blue diaper syndrome, an autosomal recessive trait, intestinal absorption of tryptophan is impaired. Dietary tryptophan is broken down into indoles and excreted in the stool, where they are hydrolyzed to the blue-tinged pigment, indigo blue. Other symptoms of blue diaper syndrome include hypercalcemia, growth defects, nephrocalcinosis, and frequent infections. This test aids diagnosis of these two genetic traits.

Professional Considerations:

1. Consent form NOT required.
2. Preparation:
   A. Tube: Heparinized, green-top tube.
   B. Obtain a container of ice water.
   C. Specimens MAY be drawn during hemodialysis.
   D. *See Client and family teaching.*
3. Procedure:
   A. Draw a 7-ml blood sample. Place the tube immediately in a container of ice water.
4. Postprocedure care:
   A. Send specimens to the laboratory promptly. Plasma should be separated and frozen within 60 minutes of collection.
5. Client and family teaching:
   A. Fast for 8 hours prior to the test.
6. Factors that affect results:
   A. A delay in sample separation and freezing over 1 hour invalidates the results.
7. Other data:
   A. Dietary supplementation of tryptophan is associated with an eosinophilia-myalgia syndrome, which includes myalgia, arthralgia, fatigue, rash, hair loss, edema, impaired motion of the joints, muscle cramping, and paresthesias, as well as several laboratory value abnormalities.

Bibliography:

Chen Y, Wu L, Xiong Q: The ocular abnormalities of blue diaper syndrome. Metab Pediatr Syst Ophthalmol *14*(3–4):73–75, 1991.

Criswell LA, Sack KE: Tryptophan-induced eosinophilia-myalgia syndrome. West J Med *153*(3):269–274, 1990.

Martin J, Mellor C, Fraser F: Familial hypotryptophanemia in two siblings. Clin Genet *47*(4):180–183, 1995.

TRYPTOPHAN-RICH PREALBUMIN

(see Transthyretin, Serum)

TSH ASSAY

(see Thyroid-Stimulating Hormone, Sensitive Assay, Blood)

TTR

(see Transthyretin, Serum)

T-TUBE CHOLANGIOGRAPHY, POSTOPERATIVE, DIAGNOSTIC

Norm: Even filling of the biliary ductal system. Absence of strictures, obstruction, calculi, abnormal pathways, or delays in emptying.

Usage: Evaluation of biliary ducts after gallbladder surgery or liver transplant.

Description: T-tube cholangiography is the instillation of radiographic contrast medium through a T-tube (percutaneously inserted, T-shaped, bile duct drainage tube), followed by fluoroscopic examination of the biliary ducts. Use of intraoperative cholangiography minimizes the number of biliary calculi remaining after surgery, but up to 3% of surgeries miss some calculi, and bile duct damage, resulting in strictures, can result. Because of this possibility, T-tube cholangiography is usually performed 7–10 days after exploratory gallbladder or duct surgery or cholecystectomy for the purpose of evaluating duct patency, and identifying any remaining stones or further ductal obstruction. Biliary duct obstruction or anastomotic leakage is also possible after liver transplant, thus a T-tube is also placed after this type of surgery. If retained stones are identified, the T-tube is left in place, as this is the route of choice for removal of the remaining stones. Four to six weeks are required for the sinus tract surrounding the T-tube to be well-healed prior to percutaneous removal of remaining stones.

Professional Considerations:

1. Consent form IS required.

Risks:

Allergic reaction to dye (itching, hives, rash, tight feeling in the throat, shortness of breath, anaphylaxis, death); renal toxicity from contrast medium.

Contraindications:

Previous allergy to iodine, shellfish, or radiographic dye; renal insufficiency.

2. Preparation:
   A. A cleansing enema may be prescribed.
   B. Have emergency equipment readily available.
   C. The T-tube may be clamped for 24 hours prior to the procedure.
   D. *See Client and family teaching.*
3. Procedure:
   A. The client is positioned supine.
   B. Local anesthesia may be injected

around the T-tube site if the site is inflamed and painful.

C. After the T-tube is cleansed with 70% alcohol, radiographic contrast medium is instilled through the tube via a large-caliber catheter.

D. Fluoroscopic radiographs are taken in a variety of positions to track dye progress through the biliary duct system. Upright films are taken to detect inadvertent injection of air through the T-tube.

E. The procedure is concluded with films of contrast medium emptying into the duodenum. Delays in emptying prolong the procedure, which normally takes less than ½ hour.

F. If findings are normal, the T-tube is removed, and a dry, sterile dressing is applied to the site.

4. Postprocedure care:

A. If the T-tube has been removed, assess the site for redness, edema, pain, or drainage every hour × 4, then every 4 hours until 24 hours after removal. A T-tube left in place should be reconnected to drainage.

B. Assess for allergic reaction to the dye (listed above) × 24 hours.

C. Resume previous diet.

5. Client and family teaching:

A. Fast from food and fluids for 6 hours prior to the procedure.

6. Factors that affect results:

A. Inadvertent injection of air may cause bubbles that look like biliary calculi. These may be differentiated by observing for movement when the client is positioned upright. Calculi move down with gravity, whereas air bubbles rise.

7. Other data:

A. This procedure uses a low-dilution or high-dilution iodine contrast medium. A low-dilution medium requires longer x-ray exposure than a high-dilution medium.

B. The administration of morphine sulfate 0.05 mg/kg intravenously preoperatively may result in spasm of the ampulla Vater and duodenum, resulting in improved quality of cholangiography.

C. Routine antibiotic prophylaxis postprocedure is not necessary under selected conditions.

Bibliography:

Barton P, Steininger R, Maier A, et al.: Biliary sludge after liver transplantation: 1. Imaging findings and efficiency of various imaging procedures. Am J Roentgenol *164*(4):859–864,1995.

Sheen-Chen SM, Cheng YF, Chou FF, et al.: Postoperative T-tube cholangiography: is routine antibiotic prophylaxis necessary? A prospective, controlled study. Arch Surg *130*(1):20–23, 1995.

Siddiqui MN, Jafarey AM, Ahmed M: Use of intravenous morphine to improve preoperative imaging of the biliary system. Br J Surg *82*(2):211, 1995.

TUBERCULIN SKIN TEST (TB), DIAGNOSTIC
(see Mantoux Skin Test, Diagnostic)

TUBERCULOSIS TEST
(see Mantoux Skin Test, Diagnostic)

TULAREMIA AGGLUTININS, SERUM

Norm: <1:40. Current or past tularemia infection: >1:80.

Positive: A fourfold rise in titer is considered diagnostic of *Francisella tularensis* infection.

Negative: Normal finding. May also occur the first few days after infection.

Description: Tularemia is an infectious disease caused by the organism *F. tularensis,* which inhabits wild animals such as rabbits, muskrats, beavers, and some domestic animals such as cats, as well as ticks and deerflies. The mode of transmission is through direct contact of human skin or mucous membranes with the blood, tissue, or lesions of infected animals; ingestion of poorly cooked, infected animal meat; or through the bite of infected ticks. Airborne transmission is also possible from contaminated dust. Tularemia infection causes ulceration, lymph node edema, headache, pharyngeal inflammation, and/or pneumonia in humans 2–10 days after exposure. After infection, antibody levels begin rising within 7–21 days, peak in 60–90 days, then decline over several months to higher than normal levels. Titers at peak antibody levels are as high as 1:640. This test is a febrile agglutinin test.

Professional Considerations:

1. Consent form NOT required.

2. Preparation:

A. Tube: Red-top, red/gray-top, or gold-top.

B. This test should be drawn before skin testing for tularemia.

3. Procedure:

A. Draw a 5-ml blood sample, without hemolysis. Draw the first sample about 1 week after suspected exposure, and repeat the test every 3–5 days to observe for rising titers.

4. Postprocedure care:

A. None.

5. Client and family teaching:

A. If routinely handling wild animals (e.g., skinning rabbits), wear gloves and goggles during contact, and thoroughly cook any wild animal meat to be ingested.

B. Serial testing is required in order to interpret the results.

6. Factors that affect results:

A. Hemolysis of the specimen invalidates the results.

B. False-positive results may occur in the presence of *Brucella abortus* or *Proteus vulgaris* (OX-19) with the Weil-Felix agglutination test.

C. False-negative results may occur when the specimen is drawn early in the infective process.

D. False-positive results may occur if skin testing for tularemia has been performed within the prior 7 days.

E. Microagglutination testing has been shown to be more specific and faster than traditional tube agglutination testing for tularemia serodiagnosis.

7. Other data:

A. Avoid contact with open lesions of clients suspected of having tularemia.

B. If present, lesions should be cultured for *F. tularensis*.

C. Streptomycin, tetracyclines, gentamicin, and chloramphenicol are used to treat tularemia.

Bibliography:

Burnett JW: Tularemia. Cutis *54*(2):77–78, 1994.

Cross JT Jr, Schutze GE, Jacobs RF: Treatment of tularemia with gentamicin in pediatric patients. Pediatr Infect Dis J *14*(2):151–152, 1995.

Enderlin G: Streptomycin and alternative agents for the treatment of tularemia: review of the literature. Clin Infect Dis *19*(1):42–47, 1994.

Liles WC, Burger RJ: Tularemia from domestic cats. West J Med *158*(6):619–622, 1993.

TULAREMIA SKIN TEST, DIAGNOSTIC

Norm: Negative. No redness, induration, or wheal.

Positive: Current or past infection with *Francisella tularensis.*

Negative: Normal finding. May also occur the first few days after infection.

Description: Tularemia is an infectious disease caused by the organism *F. tularensis,* which inhabits wild animals such as rabbits, muskrats, beavers, squirrels, and some domestic animals, as well as ticks and deerflies. The mode of transmission is through direct contact of human skin or mucous membranes with the blood, tissue, or lesions of infected animals; ingestion of poorly cooked, infected animal meat; or through the bite of infected ticks. Airborne transmission is also possible from contaminated dust. Tularemia infection causes ulceration, lymph node edema, headache, pharyngeal inflammation, and/or pneumonia in humans 2–10 days after exposure. After infection, antibody levels begin rising within 7–21 days, peak in 60–90 days, then decline over several months to higher than normal levels. After recovery, lifetime immunity exists. The Foshay skin test for tularemia is based on a delayed hypersensitivity reaction. Results will be positive for clients with current infection of at least 7 days, or for up to 5 years after recovery.

Professional Considerations:

1. Consent form NOT required.

2. Preparation:

A. Obtain a 1-ml syringe with an intradermal needle and purified *F. tularensis* antigen.

3. Procedure:

A. Cleanse the forearm site for injection with an alcohol wipe and allow the area to dry.

B. Inject *F. tularensis* antigen, derived from culture, intradermally.

C. Record the site of injection.

D. Inspect the injection site in 48 hours. Reaction is positive if redness and induration of >5 mm diameter are present at the site.

4. Postprocedure care:

A. Let the site air-dry.

5. Client and family teaching:

A. If routinely handling wild animals (e.g., skinning rabbits), wear gloves and goggles during contact, and thoroughly cook any wild animal meat to be ingested.

B. Return in 48 hours to have the injection site viewed and the skin test interpreted.

6. Factors that affect results:

A. False-negative results may occur during the first week after infection, due to insufficient antibody formation. If tularemia is suspected, the test should be repeated in 1 week.

7. Other data:

A. If serum testing for tularemia agglutinins is to be done, it should be performed prior to this test.

Bibliography:

Cerny Z: Skin manifestations of tularemia. Int J Dermatol *33*(7):468–470, 1994.

Craven RB, Barnes AM: Plague and tularemia. Infect Dis Clin North Am *5*(1):165–175, 1991.

Taylor JP, Istre GR, McChesney TC, et al.: Epidemiologic characteristics of human tularemia in the southwest-central states, 1981–1987. Am J Epidemiol *133*(10):1032–1038, 1991.

TUNING FORK TEST OF WEBER, RINNE, AND SCHWABACH TESTS, DIAGNOSTIC

Norms:

Weber's test: The tone is heard equally well in both ears.

Rinne's test: The tone is heard twice as long by air conduction (AC) as by bone conduction (BC).

Schwabach test: The tone is heard for the same length of time by both the client and the examiner.

Usage: Assists in the differential diagnosis of conduction and perceptive or sensorineural hearing loss, hearing disorders, and tinnitus.

Description: The Weber, Rinne, and Schwabach tests are three simple tuning-fork hearing tests.

Weber's test helps determine whether hearing loss is due to conductive or sensorineural causes. In clients with normal hearing, a vibrating tuning fork positioned midline on the skull is heard equally well by both ears. However, in conductive hearing loss, the tone seems loudest in the affected ear, and in sensorineural hearing loss, the tone seems loudest in the unaffected ear.

Rinne's test also helps differentiate conductive from sensorineural hearing loss by comparing the duration of tone perception by bone conduction to the duration of tone perception by air conduction. In a client with normal hearing, a vibrating tuning fork that can no longer be heard via bone conduction can still be heard via air conduction for twice as long. Conductive hearing loss may be secondary to blocked pathways of sound conduction in the middle or external ear, thus bone conduction will be longer than air conduction (BC > AC). Perceptive or sensorineural loss may be secondary to inner ear disease or vestibulocochlear (8th cranial nerve) disorders, thus air conduction will be longer than bone conduction (AC > BC), but not as high as the 2:1 ratio expected in normal clients.

The *Schwabach test* helps evaluate bone conduction by comparing the length of time the client hears a tuning fork placed against his or her mastoid process with the length of time it is heard by a client with normal hearing.

Professional Considerations:

1. Consent form NOT required.
2. Preparation:
   A. Obtain a low-frequency tuning fork of 256–512 Hz.
   B. The test should take place in a quiet room, free of noise and visual distractions.
3. Procedure:
   A. *Weber's test:*
      i. The tuning fork is set into light vibration by pinching the prongs between the thumb and index finger or by tapping it on the examiner's knuckles.
      ii. The tuning fork is placed on the skull at the midpoint, or on the maxillary incisors.
      iii. The client is asked to state whether the sound can be heard better in one ear than the other and, if so, to state which ear hears the tone more loudly.
   B. *Rinne's test:*
      i. The tuning fork is set into light vibration by pinching the prongs between the thumb and index finger or by tapping it on the examiner's knuckles.
      ii. The ear not being tested should be masked from detecting sound via bone conduction by providing a sound stimulus into it during step B-iii.
      iii. The vibrating fork is held by its stem on the mastoid process of the ear until vibration is no longer heard by the client.
      iv. The fork is then held close to the external auditory meatus (within 2.5 cm of the pinna). If the client still hears the vibrations, this is called a positive Rinne's test. If the fork is not heard by air conduction, the test is repeated, but air conduction is first tested until the sound is no longer heard, then the stem of the fork is placed on the mastoid process of the ear. If the sound is still heard, this is called a negative Rinne's test.
   C. *Schwabach test:*
      i. The tuning fork is set into light vibration by pinching the prongs between the thumb and index finger or by tapping it on the examiner's knuckles.
      ii. The ear not being tested should be masked from detecting sound via bone conduction by providing a sound stimulus into it during step C-iii.
      iii. The vibrating fork is held by its stem on the mastoid process of the client, who is instructed to indicate whether the tone is heard. Each time he or she hears the

tone, the tuning fork is quickly transferred to the mastoid process of the examiner, who listens for the tone. This process continues back and forth between the client and the examiner, until the tone is no longer heard by one of them, and the results are recorded. The process is then repeated in the other ear.

4. Postprocedure care:
   A. None.
5. Client and family teaching:
   A. Testing is noninvasive and can take up to 15 minutes.
   B. Thorough audiologic testing is indicated if results are abnormal.
6. Factors that affect results:
   A. The examiner should strike the tuning fork with equal intensity for each repetition of the tests.
   B. For the Schwabach test, the examiner must have normal hearing for the results to be meaningful.
7. Other data:
   A. None.

Bibliography:

Browning GG, Swan IR: Sensitivity and specificity of Rinne tuning fork test. Br Med J 297(6660):1381–1382, 1988.

Hall JW 3d, Baer JE: Current concepts in hearing assessment of children and adults. Compr Ther 19(6):272–280, 1993.

Liniger C, Albeanu A, Bloise D, et al.: The tuning fork test revisited. Diabetic Med 7(10):859–864, 1990.

TUTTLE TEST
(see Esophageal Acidity Test, Diagnostic)

TYPE-AND-CROSSMATCH, BLOOD

Norm: Recipient blood type is determined to be either type A, B, O, or AB, and either Rh-positive or Rh-negative. Antibodies present in the recipient sample and donor blood are identified. Recipient and donor samples are mixed and observed for antigen-antibody reactions.

Usage: Determination of compatibility of recipient and donor blood prior to blood product transfusion.

Description: The type-and-crossmatch technique includes a series of procedures designed to identify donor blood that may be potentially safe to transfuse into a particular recipient with the lowest possible risk of causing a hemolytic reaction. The ABO group and Rh-type of the recipient's blood

sample is first determined. Donor blood of the same ABO blood group and Rh-type is then chosen for further testing prior to transfusion. General antibody screening (indirect Coombs' testing) is then performed on both recipient and donor blood. If antibody screening is positive, more specific antibody identification is performed to determine the specific nature of irregular antibodies, that may cause a transfusion reaction. The exact antibody is identified by combining the recipient or donor serum with a panel of red blood cell samples, each containing a known antigen, and observing for antigen-antibody reactions. Finally, recipient and donor blood samples are combined (crossmatched) and observed for antigen-antibody reactions that may cause a transfusion reaction. If no such reaction occurs, the donor blood is considered to be compatible for transfusion into the recipient. Absence of antigen-antibody reaction during crossmatching decreases, but does not completely eliminate, the possibility of a hemolytic transfusion reaction.

Professional Considerations:

1. Consent form NOT required.
2. Preparation:
   A. Tube: Red-top, red/gray-top, or gold-top AND lavender-top. Also obtain a 30-ml syringe; a blood band (if required); two labels, stamped with the client's addressograph plate; and blood.
   B. Note the client's age, medications, past transfusions of blood products, and number of pregnancies on the laboratory requisition.
   C. Consult institutional protocol for any additional requirements.
   D. Do NOT draw specimens during hemodialysis.
3. Procedure: The entire procedure should be performed by the person who performs the venipuncture.
   A. Ask the client to state his or her full name and social security number. Verify that this information matches the client's wrist identification band and addressograph stamp on the blood bank requisition and labels.
   B. Some institutions use blood bands as an extra precaution to validate the proper recipient:
      i. Write the client's name, social security number, and hospital number and the date on the blood band, and place the band on the client's wrist, cutting off the distal end of the number stickers.
      ii. Write the blood band number on

both addressograph labels and place a label on each tube. Alternatively, place addressograph labels on each tube and place a number sticker from the blood band on each tube.

iii. Place a blood band number sticker on the blood bank requisition.

C. Do NOT draw specimens from an extremity into which blood or dextran is infusing. Draw a 25-ml blood sample, without hemolysis, in a 30-ml syringe. Completely fill the red-top tube and the lavender-top tube with the sample.

D. The caregiver performing this procedure should initial the following after drawing the blood: the blood band (if used), the label on each tube, and the blood bank requisition.

E. Staple the remaining blood band number stickers (if used) to the requisition.

4. Postprocedure care:
   A. Send both tubes with the requisition and blood band number stickers (if used) to the blood bank.
   B. Testing must be performed within 48 hours of specimen collection.

5. Client and family teaching:
   A. Screening for antibodies may take longer, up to several hours, if initial screening is positive.
   B. Type-and-crossmatches are good for only 72 hours due to the possibility of the recipient developing irregular antibodies in response to a recent blood transfusion.
   C. A type-and-crossmatch takes approximately 1 hour to complete.

6. Factors that affect results:
   A. Hemolysis of the specimen invalidates the results.

B. Drugs causing a false-positive Rh test include levodopa, methyldopa, and methyldopate hydrochloride.

7. Other data:
   A. A type-and-screen involves only the ABO group and Rh-type determinations and the general antibody screening. It is sometimes prescribed instead of a type-and-crossmatch if there is only a small possibility of the client needing blood, or if the blood must be transfused in an emergency. Donor blood should not be transfused if the general antibody screen is positive.
   B. Identification of cold reacting antibodies reactive at 30°C may require the use of a blood warmer during transfusion.
   C. *See also ABO Group and Rh Type, Blood; Antibody Identification, Red Cell, Blood; and Coombs', Indirect, Serum.*

Bibliography:

Duguid JK: New approaches to cross-matching. Clin Lab Haematol 16(3):281–284, 1994.

Hooker, EA: Do all trauma patients need early cross-matching for blood? J Emerg Med 12(4):447–451, 1994.

Napier JA: The crossmatch. Br J Haematol 78(1):1–4, 1991.

Shulman IA, Calderon C: Effect of delayed centrifugation or reading on the detection of ABO incompatibility by the immediate-spin crossmatch. Transfusion 31(3):197–200, 1991.

TYPHUS TITER, BLOOD
(see Bacterial Serology, Blood and Weil-Felix Agglutinins, Blood)

UBT
(see Urea Breath Test, Diagnostic)

UGI, DIAGNOSTIC
(see Upper Gastrointestinal Series, Diagnostic)

UGP, URINE
(see Urinary Gonadotropin Peptide, Urine)

ULCERATIVE LESIONS, CULTURE
(see Body Fluid, Routine, Culture; and Culture, Routine, Specimen)

ULTRA, DIAGNOSTIC
(see Glucose Monitoring Machines, Diagnostic)

ULTRAFAST COMPUTED TOMOGRAPHY (ELECTRON BEAM CT, EBCT), DIAGNOSTIC

Norm: No coronary artery stenosis, no pulmonary embolism.

Usage: Depicting central and peripheral pulmonary emboli; visualization of coronary arteries for calcific deposits, plaques, and stenosis.

Description: A noninvasive electron beam computed tomography (EBCT) of the heart or lungs is obtained while the client holds in breath and during intravenous administration of the contrast agent.

Professional Considerations:

1. Consent form NOT required.

Risks:

Allergic reaction to the contrast agent (itching, hives, rash, tight feeling in the throat, shortness of breath, anaphylaxis); renal toxicity from the contrast medium.

Contraindications:

Previous allergy to shellfish, iodine, or eggs, or previous allergic reaction to the contrast agent; renal insufficiency.

2. Preparation:
   A. Remove all jewelry and metal objects from the client's body.
   B. Assess for patent venous access and obtain the contrast medium.
   C. Have emergency equipment readily available.
   D. *See Client and family teaching.*
3. Procedure:
   A. The client is supine on a radiologic table.
   B. Contrast medium is injected.
   C. The client is asked to hold breath.
   D. Operating in the multislice scan mode, the scanner takes several pictures as the table is advanced by a 2-mm step.
4. Postprocedure care:
   A. Assess the venous access site for infiltration.
5. Client and family teaching:
   A. The client will have to hold breath for several seconds.
   B. It is important to lie still for the test.
   C. A sensation of burning may be felt from the injection of the contrast medium.
6. Factors that affect results:
   A. Body movement during the study obscures the clarity of radiographs.
7. Other data:
   A. For chest examinations the average breast dose from EBCT was comparable to that of conventional CT scanners, despite differences in dose distribution.
   B. EBCT has the potential to replace ventilation-perfusion scanning as the primary screening diagnostic test for pulmonary emboli.

Bibliography:

McCollough CH, Liu HH: Breast dose during electron-beam CT: measurement with film dosimetry. Radiology *196*(1):153–157, 1995.

Moshage WE, Achenbach S, Seese B, et al.: Coronary artery stenosis: three-dimensional imaging with electrocardiographically triggered, contrast agent-enhanced, electron-beam CT. Radiology *196*(3):707–714, 1995.

Teigen CL, Maus TP, Aheedy PF 2nd, et al.: Pulmonary embolism: diagnosis with contrast-enhanced electron-beam CT and comparison with pulmonary angiography. Radiology *194*(2):313–319, 1995.

Thomas PJ, McCollough CH, Ritman EL: An electron-beam CT approach for transvenous coronary arteriography. J Comput Assist Tomogr *19*(3):383–389, 1995.

ULTRASOUND, ABDOMINAL AORTA, DIAGNOSTIC

(see Abdominal Aorta Sonogram, Diagnostic)

ULTRASOUND, BRAIN, DIAGNOSTIC

(see Brain Sonogram, Diagnostic)

ULTRASOUND, BREAST, DIAGNOSTIC

(see Breast Sonogram, Diagnostic)

ULTRASOUND, CAROTID ARTERY, DIAGNOSTIC

(see Carotid Doppler, Diagnostic)

ULTRASOUND, CORONARY, DIAGNOSTIC

(see Coronary Intravascular Ultrasound, Diagnostic)

ULTRASOUND, EYE AND ORBIT, DIAGNOSTIC

(see Eye and Orbit Sonogram, Diagnostic)

ULTRASOUND, GALLBLADDER, DIAGNOSTIC

(see Gallbladder and Biliary System Sonogram, Diagnostic)

ULTRASOUND, GYNECOLOGIC, DIAGNOSTIC

(see Gynecologic Sonogram, Diagnostic)

ULTRASOUND, HEART, DIAGNOSTIC

(see Echocardiogram, Diagnostic)

ULTRASOUND, KIDNEY, DIAGNOSTIC
(see Kidney Sonogram, Diagnostic)

ULTRASOUND, LIVER, DIAGNOSTIC
(see Liver Sonogram, Diagnostic)

ULTRASOUND, LYMPH NODE, DIAGNOSTIC
(see Lymph Node and Retroperitoneal Sonogram, Diagnostic)

ULTRASOUND, OBSTETRIC, DIAGNOSTIC
(see Obstetric Sonogram, Diagnostic)

ULTRASOUND, PANCREAS, DIAGNOSTIC
(see Pancreas Sonogram, Diagnostic)

ULTRASOUND, PELVIC, DIAGNOSTIC
(see Gynecologic Sonogram, Diagnostic)

ULTRASOUND, PROSTATE, DIAGNOSTIC
(see Prostate Sonogram, Diagnostic)

ULTRASOUND, SPLEEN, DIAGNOSTIC
(see Spleen Sonogram, Diagnostic)

ULTRASOUND, THYROID, DIAGNOSTIC
(see Thyroid Sonogram, Diagnostic)

ULTRASOUND, URINARY BLADDER, DIAGNOSTIC
(see Urinary Bladder Sonogram, Diagnostic)

UPPER GASTROINTESTINAL (UGI) SERIES, DIAGNOSTIC

Norm: Mucosa is smooth and regular, and free of lesions, polyps, narrowing, or filling defects. Barium fills smoothly and does not leak into the abdominal cavity. The passage of barium progresses at a normal rate and there is no reflux into the esophagus (indicating hiatal hernia or incompetent cardiac sphincter). Gastric folds measure approximately 5 mm in the antrum and body of the stomach, and are slightly wider near the fundus.

Usage: Investigation of abnormal gastrointestinal symptoms. Allows fluoroscopic visualization of the esophagus, stomach, and duodenum; helps evaluate organ size, lumen size, outline, and position of the examined areas; and detection of strictures, scarring, varices, ulcers, tumors, hiatal hernia, and/or inflammation of the upper gastrointestinal tract.

Description: Upper gastrointestinal series (UGI) involves examining the upper gastrointestinal tract under fluoroscopy after the client drinks barium sulfate. Barium sulfate is a chalky substance of "milkshake" consistency that has radiopaque properties. Films of specific portions of the tract are taken as the barium passes through and outlines the structures. Barium swallow studies of the esophagus and/or a small bowel series may be performed in conjunction with this test. *(See Barium Swallow, Diagnostic; and Small Bowel Series, Diagnostic.)*

Professional Considerations:

1. Consent form NOT required.

Risks:
Aspiration of contrast material, bowel obstruction, constipation.

Contraindications:
Suspected ileus, obstruction, or gastrointestinal perforation.

2. Preparation:
   A. Notify the physician before preparation if the client is pregnant.
   B. When possible, medications that affect the motility of the gastrointestinal tract should be withheld for 24 hours prior to the study.
   C. If this test will be followed by a small bowel series, for a bowel cleansing routine, *see also Small Bowel Series, Diagnostic.*
   D. The client should disrobe and put on a gown. All jewelry and metal objects should be removed.
   E. Obtain 8 ounces of barium sulfate solution.
   F. *See Client and family teaching.*

3. Procedure:
   A. The client is positioned supine on the fluoroscopic tilt table and strapped into place. The hydraulic table is then moved into a vertical position.
   B. Baseline fluoroscopic radiographs are taken of the area to be studied.
   C. The client is then given 8 ounces of barium sulfate solution and is instructed to drink portions of it at specified intervals as the table is tilted to various angles.
   D. Initial films are taken of the esophagus as the barium travels downward.
   E. Stomach films are taken as barium mixed with air enters the stomach. The lower esophagus is examined for reflux of the barium from the stomach or for free-flowing barium between the stomach and the esophagus, both of which conditions indicate hiatal hernia.
   F. As the client finishes ingesting the barium, the filled stomach and the emptying of the barium into the duodenum are radiographed from several angles. Gastric folds are examined for thickening, indicated by a rugal pattern that is not obliterated by filling the stomach with barium sulfate.
   G. The test takes less than 1 hour.
4. Postprocedure care:
   A. Resume previous diet.
   B. *See Client and family teaching.*
5. Client and family teaching:
   A. Fast from food and fluids, and do not chew gum or smoke overnight prior to the study.
   B. A laxative or suppository may be prescribed to be taken the night before the study.
   C. If this test will be followed by a small bowel series, bring something to read, if desired, as the procedure time may increase to 4–6 hours.
   D. After swallowing a chalky barium solution, you will be asked to move to several positions and, at times, to hold your breath while the x-rays are taken.
   E. Drink 6–8 glasses of water or other fluids each day for 2 days following the test to help pass the barium through the gastrointestinal system.
   F. Observe stools for passage of barium for 1–3 days. This will make the stools look chalky white.
   G. Call the physician if unable to defecate. A mild laxative may be prescribed prophylactically, or cathartics and/or enemas may be prescribed as needed if pending impaction is suspected.
6. Factors that affect results:
   A. The client must be able to cooperate in swallowing the barium sulfate.
7. Other data:
   A. None.

Bibliography:

Douglas BR, Johnson CD, Czaja AJ, et al.: Portal hypertensive gastropathy: upper gastrointestinal X-ray appearance. Mayo Clin Proc *69*(12):195–196, 1994.

Gunderson LL, Martenson JA, Smalley SR, et al.: Upper gastrointestinal cancers: rationale, results, and techniques of treatment. Front Radiat Ther Oncol *28*:121–139, 1994.

Hammerman AM, Shady K, Fry R, et al.: Postgastrostomy tube deformity on upper GI series. Gastrointest Radiol *16*(1):13–14, 1991.

UREA BREATH TEST (UBT), DIAGNOSTIC

Norm: Negative for *Helicobacter pylori*.

Usage: Diagnosis of gastric *H. pylori* colonization.

Description: This simple, noninvasive test involves the measurement of gas released in the breath after ingestion of a radiolabeled urea isotope. The urease of *H. pylori* bacteria in the stomach generates labeled carbon dioxide (CO_2), known as 13C, within 10–30 minutes. This 13C is measured in the client's breath with a sensitivity of 95–98% and a specificity of 97% for the diagnosis of gastric *H. pylori* colonization. This test is useful in pediatrics and is a sensitive indicator of *H. pylori* eradication 6 weeks after treatment with antibiotics.

Professional Considerations:

1. Consent form NOT required.
2. Preparation:
   A. Obtain urea-labeled water for client ingestion.
   B. *See Client and family teaching.*
3. Procedure:
   A. The client drinks 75 mg of radiolabeled urea liquid that tastes like pure water.
   B. Breath samples are taken by blowing into a bag or balloon. The samples are measured every 10 minutes in the first hour, then at 1½ and 2 hours after ingestion.
4. Postprocedure care:
   A. The client may resume eating and drinking.
5. Client and family teaching:
   A. Do NOT eat or drink for at least 6 hours prior to the test.
   B. The test takes 2 hours.
   C. The radioactivity received from this test is much less than that received from a regular chest x-ray and less than what you normally receive from a natural day of radiation.
6. Factors that affect results:
   A. A fatty meal profoundly affects results by increasing values at 30-, 40-, 50-, 60-, 90-, and 120-minute intervals.

B. Taking antibiotics or Pepto Bismol for 1 month or Prilosec or Carafate for 1 week prior to the test can cause false-negative results.

7. Other data:

A. *H. pylori* infection is treated with 7 days of tetracycline, metronidazole, and bismuth subsalicylate.

B. The mini-dose 14C urea breath test has a sensitivity of 98% and a specificity of 97% using the minidose 1 – μCi or 37 kBq.

C. *See also Campylobacter-Like-Organism Test, Specimen; Helicobacter pylori Quick Office Serology, Serum; Helicobacter pylori Titer, Blood.*

Bibliography:

Atherton JC, Washington N, Blackshaw PE, et al.: Effect of a test meal on the intragastric distribution of urea in the 13C-urea breath test for *Helicobacter pylori*. Gut 36(3):337–340, 1995.

Slomianski A, Schubert T, Cutler AF: [13C] urea breath test to confirm eradication of *Helicobacter pylori*. Am J Gastroenterol 90(2):225–226, 1995.

Yamashiro Y, Oguchi S, Otsuka Y: *Helicobacter pylori* colonization is children with peptic ulcer disease. III. Diagnostic value of 13C-urea breath test to detect gastric *H. pylori* colonization. Acta Paediatr Jpn 37(1):12–16, 1995.

UREA NITROGEN, PLASMA OR SERUM

Norm:

		SI Units
Young adult <40	5–18 mg/dl	1.8–6.5 mmol/L
Adult	5–20 mg/dl	1.8–7.1 mmol/L
Elderly >60	8–21 mg/dl	2.9–7.5 mmol/L
Mild azotemia	20–50 mg/dl	7.1–17.7 mmol/L
Children		
Cord blood	21–40 mg/dl	7.5–14.3 mmol/L
Premature infant, first 7 days	3–25 mg/dl	1.1–7.9 mmol/L
Full-term newborn	4–18 mg/dl	1.4–6.4 mmol/L
Infant	5–18 mg/dl	1.8–6.4 mmol/L
Child	5–18 mg/dl	1.8–6.4 mmol/L
Panic level	>100 mg/dl	>35.7 mmol/L

Panic Level Symptoms and Treatment:

Symptoms: Acidemia, agitation, coma, confusion, fatigue, nausea, stupor, and vomiting.

Treatment:

Correct the cause.

Administer sodium bicarbonate IV for severe acidemia.

Prescribe a low-protein diet.

Hemodialysis and peritoneal dialysis WILL remove urea nitrogen.

Avoid/reduce drug usage of long-acting barbiturates, narcotics, sulfonamides, anticoagulants, and antibiotics such as vancomycin, kanamycin, and polymycin.

Increased: Addison's disease, allergic purpura, amyloidosis, analgesic abuse, blood transfusions, cachexia, cardiac failure, congenital hypoplastic kidneys, dehydration, diabetes mellitus, diabetic ketoacidosis, diet (high-protein), Fanconi's syndrome, fluid therapy (excessive), gastrointestinal bleeding, glomerulonephritis, Goodpasture's syndrome, gout, heavy-metal poisoning, hemoglobinurias, infection, intestinal obstruction, multiple myeloma, myocardial infarction (acute), nephritis, nephropathy (hypercalcemic, hypokalemic), nephrosclerosis, pancreatitis, peritonitis, pneumonia, polyarteritis nodosa, polycystic disease, postoperative state, protein intake (excessive), pyelonephritis, renal artery stenosis or thrombosis, renal cortical necrosis, renal malignancy, renal tuberculosis, renal vein thrombosis, scleroderma, sepsis, shock, sickle cell anemia, starvation, stress, subacute bacterial endocarditis, suppuration, systemic lupus erythematosus, thyrotoxicosis, tumor necrosis, uremia, and urinary tract obstruction. Drugs include acetohexamide, acetone, alkaline antacids, aminophenol, ammonium salts, amphotericin B, anabolic steroids, androgens, antimony compounds, arginine, arsenicals, ascorbic acid, asparaginase, bacitracin, calcium salts, capreomycin, captopril, carmustine, carbutamide, cephaloridine, chloral hydrate, chloramphenicol, chlorobutanol, chlorothiazide sodium, chlorthalidone, clonidine, colistimethate sodium, dextran, dextrose infusions, disopyramide phosphate, doxapram, ethacrynic acid, fluorides, fluphenazine, fosinopril, furosemide, guanethidine sulfate, gentamicin sulfate, guanachlor, guanethidine analogs, hydroxyurea, indomethacin, kanamycin, lipomul, lithium carbonate, marijuana, meclofenamate sodium, mephenesin, mercury compounds, mercurial diuretics, methicillin, methoxyflurane, methsuximide, methyldopa, methylprednisolone sodium succinate, methysergide, metolazone, metoprolol tartrate, minoxidil, mithramycin, morphine, nalidixic acid, naproxen sodium, neomycin, nitrofurantoin, paramethasone, pargyline, polymyxin B, propranolol, salicylates, spectinomycin, streptodornase, streptokinase, sulfonamides, tetracycline, thiazide diuretics, tolmetin sodium, triamterene, and vancomycin.

Decreased: Acromegaly, alcohol abuse, amyloidosis, celiac disease, cirrhosis, diet (inadequate protein), fluid intake (excessive), hemodialysis, hepatitis, infancy, liver destruction, malnutrition, nephrosis, plasma volume expansion, and pregnancy (late). Drugs include streptomycin and thymol.

Description: Commonly referred to as BUN (blood urea nitrogen), this measurement is actually performed on plasma or serum. Plasma or serum levels of urea nitrogen are about 12% higher than BUN levels, resulting from the relatively higher percentage of protein contained in erythrocytes. Urea nitrogen is the nitrogen portion of urea, a substance formed in the liver through an enzymatic protein breakdown process. Urea is normally freely filtered through the renal glomeruli, with a small amount reabsorbed in the tubules and the remainder excreted in the urine. Elevated urea nitrogen in the bloodstream is called azotemia. However, the value is nonspecific as to cause and thus may be a result of either prerenal, renal, or postrenal etiologies. Prerenal etiologies may be grouped under factors that result in inadequate renal circulation or conditions resulting in abnormally high levels of blood protein. Renal etiologies are those of impaired renal filtration and excretion of urea nitrogen. Postrenal etiologies are lower urinary tract obstructive conditions that result in diffusion of urea nitrogen in dormant urine back into the bloodstream through the tubules. Uremia is a term used to describe symptoms occurring at very high elevations of urea in the bloodstream, and may occur at urea nitrogen levels of about 200 mg/dl (>70 mmol/L). Also of significance are low urea nitrogen levels in severe hepatic disease. A damaged liver that is unable to synthesize urea from protein results in a buildup of blood ammonia (NH), causing hepatic encephalopathy.

Professional Considerations:

1. Consent form NOT required.
2. Preparation:
   A. Tube: Red-top, red/gray-top, or gold-top.
   B. Do NOT draw specimens during hemodialysis.
3. Procedure:
   A. Draw a 1-ml blood sample without hemolysis.
4. Postprocedure care:
   A. None.
5. Client and family teaching:
   A. This test result alone is of little diagnostic value but must be compared to itself over time or used in conjunction with other test results.
6. Factors that affect results:
   A. Falsely elevated results may occur in hemolyzed specimens.
   B. Values are somewhat affected by hemodilution.
7. Other data:
   A. Both creatinine levels and urea nitrogen levels should be considered when evaluating renal function.
   B. One study indicated that a BUN/creatinine ratio suggested upper, rather than lower, gastrointestinal bleeding.

Bibliography:

Jones BF: Metabolic mimicry-renal failure with normal renal function [letter]. New Engl J Med *331*(26):1778, 1994.

Lum G, Leal-Khouri S: Significance of low serum urea nitrogen concentrations. Clin Chem *35*(4):639–640, 1989.

Richards RJ, Donica MB, Grayer D: Can the blood urea nitrogen/creatinine ratio distinguish upper from lower gastrointestinal bleeding? J Clin Gastroenterol *12*(5):500–504, 1990.

Slotman GJ, Fisher CJ Jr, Bone RC, et al.: Detrimental effects of high-dose methylprednisolone sodium succinate on serum concentrations of hepatic and renal function indicators in severe sepsis and septic shock. Crit Care Med *21*(2):191–195, 1993.

URETHROGRAPHY, RETROGRADE, DIAGNOSTIC

Norm: Negative for congenital anomaly, diverticula, fistula, obstruction, or stricture. Normal size, shape, and position of the urethra.

Usage: Aids in the diagnosis of urethral abnormalities and anomalies, including diverticula, fistula, obstruction, and strictures; and evaluation of status following urethral surgery.

Description: Retrograde urethrography is a procedure in which radiographs are taken as radiopaque contrast medium is instilled into the urethra. Autourethrography, in which the client performs the instillation (injection) of the contrast medium, has been found to enhance the client's tolerance, cause less anxiety, and decrease the instance of extravasation of contrast medium outside of the urethra. In addition, the radiologist does not have to remain with the client during x-ray exposure. Retrograde urethrography is primarily performed in males.

Professional Considerations:

1. Consent form IS required.

Risks:

Bladder infection, allergic reaction to dye (itching, hives, rash, tight feeling in the throat, shortness of breath, anaphylaxis), renal toxicity from contrast medium.

Contraindications:

Pregnancy, previous allergic reaction to radiographic dye; renal insufficiency. Sedatives are contraindicated in clients with central nervous system depression.

------

2. Preparation:
   A. Have emergency equipment readily available.
   B. Obtain sterile towels, a balloon urinary catheter, 10- and 60-ml syringes, and contrast medium.
   C. An analgesic and/or sedative may be prescribed. Monitor respiratory status continually if sedation is used.
   D. Record baseline vital signs.
   E. The client should disrobe below the waist.
   F. If autourethrography is to be performed, the client must be instructed about the dye instillation technique.
3. Procedure:
   A. With the client positioned supine, baseline radiographs of the lower urinary tract structures are taken.
   B. Using a sterile technique, a catheter filled with radiopaque dye is advanced into the urethra until the balloon is just proximal to the urethral meatus. The balloon is then inflated with air.
   C. Standard or fluoroscopic radiographs are taken as dye is injected by the radiologist or the client (autourethrography) through the catheter, with the client in various positions.
   D. The balloon is deflated and the catheter removed.
   E. The client is instructed to urinate to expel the contrast medium.
4. Postprocedure care:
   A. Monitor vital signs at the end of the procedure, then in 4 hours. If deep sedation was used, follow institutional protocol for postsedation monitoring. Typical monitoring includes continuous ECG monitoring and pulse oximetry, with continual assessments (q 5–15 minutes) of airway, vital signs, and neurologic status until the client is lying quietly awake, is breathing independently, and responds to commands spoken in a normal tone.
   B. Administer analgesic as prescribed.
   C. *See Client and family teaching.*
5. Client and family teaching:
   A. Arrange for someone to drive you home. You will not be permitted to drive for 24 hours after the procedure.
   B. Expect discomfort with dye instillation, but this will be relieved when the radiographs are completed and the catheter is removed.
   C. Observe for signs of allergic reaction to the dye (listed above) × 24 hours. Call the physician in the event of itching or hives. Go to the nearest emergency room or call an ambulance for shortness of breath.
   D. Drink 6–8 glasses of water or other fluids during the next 24 hours (when not contraindicated).
   E. Save all the urine voided. Inspect the urine for quantity and hematuria (pink or red color) × 24 hours. Notify the physician for no urine in 8 hours, less than 1 ounce (30 ml) of urine per hour, or pain with urination.
   F. Notify the physician for symptoms of infection: fever, fast heart rate, hypotension (feeling faint, weak, or dizzy), chills, dysuria, flank pain.
6. Factors that affect results:
   A. Urethral obstruction will block the flow of dye through the urethra.
7. Other data:
   A. This test is often combined with voiding cystourethrography.

Bibliography:

Dardenne AN: Anaphylactoid reactions during voiding cystourethrography [letter]. Am J Roentgenol *164*(6):1551–1552, 1995.

Sandler CM: Is fluoroscopy necessary for retrograde urethrography? Am J Roentgenol *163*(5):1263, 1994.

URIC ACID, SERUM

Norm:

		SI Units
Adult females	2.4–6.0 mg/dl	143–357 µmol/L
Adult males	3.4–7.0 mg/dl	202–416 µmol/L
Children	2.5–5.5 mg/dl	119–327 µmol/L
Panic level	>12 mg/dl	>714 µmol/L

Panic Level Symptoms and Treatment:

Symptoms: Painful swelling of great toe, hypertension, arthritis.

Treatment:
Acute phase: Allopurinol, Colchicine, Indomethacin, or Phenylbutazone, orally; or Corticotropin (ACTH), intramuscularly. Also analgesics for severe pain.
Chronic phase: Allopurinol, Probenecid, or Sulfinpyrazone, orally.

Increased Uric Acid: Alcoholism, anemia (hemolytic, pernicious, sickle cell), arteriosclerosis, arthritis, berylliosis (chronic), Blackfoot Indians, body size (larger than average), calcinosis universalis and circumscripta, congestive heart failure, dehydration, diabetes mellitus, diet (high-protein, excess nucleoproteins), Down syndrome, eclampsia, exercise, fasting, Filipinos, glomerulonephritis (chronic), Graves' disease, gout, hemolysis (prolonged), hypertension, hyperuricemia, hypoparathyroidism, hypothyroidism, infections (acute), intestinal obstruction, ketoacidosis, ketosis, lead poisoning, Lesch-Nyhan syndrome, leukemia, lipoproteinemia (type III), lymphoma, maple syrup urine disease, mononucleosis (infectious), multiple myeloma, neoplasm (disseminated), nephritis, nephropathy, New Zealand Maoris, Pima Indians, pneumonia (resolving), polycystic kidneys, polycythemia vera, pregnancy (onset of labor), psoriasis, renal failure, sarcoidosis, starvation, stress, toxemia of pregnancy, uremia, urinary obstruction, and von Gierke's disease. Drugs include acetazolamide, asparaginase, busulfan, chlorothiazide sodium, chlorthalidone, corticosteroids, cyclophosphamide, dactinomycin, daunorubicin hydrochloride, dextran, diazoxide, diuretics (except spironolactone, mercurials, and ticrynafen), epinephrine, ethacrynic acid, ethambutol, ethanol, fructose, furosemide, gentamicin sulfate, glucose, hydralazine, hydrocortisone, hydroxyurea, ibufenac, levodopa, mecamylamine, mechlorethamine hydrochloride, 6-mercaptopurine, methicillin, methotrexate, methyldopa, metoprolol tartrate, niacin, nitrogen mustards, norepinephrine, phenothiazines, probenecid, propranolol, propylthiouracil, pyrazinamide, quinethazone, rifampin, salicylates (low doses), theophylline, thiazide diuretics, 6-thioguanine, triamterene, and vincristine.

Decreased Uric Acid: Acromegaly, carcinomas, celiac disease, Dalmation dog mutation, Fanconi's syndrome, Hodgkin's disease, pernicious anemia, Wilson's disease, yellow atrophy of liver, and xanthinuria. Drugs include acetohexamide, ACTH, allopurinol, anticoagulants, azlocillin, azothioprine, bacitracin, benziodaroni, chlorine, chlorpromazine hydrochloride, chlorprothixene, chlorthalidone, cincophen, corticosteroids, corticotropin, cortisone, coumarins, dicumarol, ethacrynic acid, glyceryl guaiacolate, lithium carbonate, mannitol, marijuana, oxyphenbutazone, phenothiazines, phenylbutazone, piperazine, potassium oxalate, probenecid, radiographic dyes, salicylates (long-term, large doses), saline infusions, sodium oxalate, sulfinpyrazone, thyroid hormone, and triamterene.

Description: Uric acid (lithic acid) is formed as the purines, adenine and guanine, are continuously metabolized during the formation and degradation of ribonucleic acid (RNA) and deoxyribonucleic acid (DNA), and from metabolism of dietary purines. After synthesis in the liver triggered by the action of xanthine oxidase, part of the uric acid is excreted in the urine. Elevated amounts of serum uric acid (uricemia) become deposited in joints and soft tissues and cause gout, an inflammatory reaction to the urate crystal deposition. Conditions of fast cell turnover as well as slowed renal excretion of uric acid may both cause uricemia. Elevated amounts of urinary uric acid precipitate into urate stones in the kidneys.

Professional Considerations:

1. Consent form NOT required.
2. Preparation:
   A. Tube: Red-top, red/gray-top, or gold-top.
   B. *See Client and family teaching.*
3. Procedure:
   A. Draw a 1-ml blood sample.

4. Postprocedure care:
   A. None.
5. Client and family teaching:
   A. Fast for 8 hours prior to sampling.
   B. Foods high in purines that can contribute to gout include caffeine-containing beverages, legumes, mushrooms, organ meats, spinach, gravies, and baker's and brewer's yeast.
   C. Switching from a normal diet to a low-purine diet may potentially decrease urine uric acid levels by half.
6. Factors that affect results:
   A. Drugs that may cause falsely elevated results include aminophylline, caffeine, and vitamin C.
7. Other data:
   A. Mortality rate for women with ischemic heart disease increases fivefold if their uric acid level is ≥7 mg/dl (416 μmol/L).

Bibliography:

Freeman DS, Williamson DF, Gunter EW, et al.: Relation of serum uric acid to mortality and ischemic heart disease: The NHANES 1 Epidemiologic Follow-up Study. Am J Epidem *141*(7):637–644, 1995.

Reiter L, Brown MA, Edmonds J: Familial hyperuricemic nephropathy. Am J Kid Dis *25*(2):235–241, 1995.

Sato A, Shirato T, Shinoda T, et al.: Hyperuricemia in patients with hyperthyroidism due to Graves' disease. Metabolism *44*(2):207–211, 1995.

Shimizu T, Morikawa A, Maeda S, et al.: Effect of theophylline on serum uric acid levels in children with asthma. J Asthma *31*(5):387–391, 1994.

URIC ACID, URINE

Norm:

		SI Units
Adult female	250–750 mg/24 hours	1.5–4.5 mmol/day
Adult male	250–800 mg/24 hours	1.5–4.8 mmol/day

Usage: Determines whether renal calculi may be due to hyperuricosuria.

Description: Uric acid (lithic acid) is formed as the purines, adenine and guanine, are continuously metabolized during the formation and degradation of ribonucleic acid (RNA) and deoxyribonucleic acid (DNA), and from metabolism of dietary purines. After synthesis in the liver triggered by the action of xanthine oxidase, part of the uric acid is excreted in the urine. Elevated amounts of serum uric acid (uricemia) become deposited in joints and soft tissues and cause gout, an inflammatory reaction to the urate crystal deposition. Conditions of fast cell turnover as well as slowed renal

excretion of uric acid may both cause uricemia. Elevated amounts of urinary uric acid precipitate into urate stones in the kidneys.

Professional Considerations:

1. Consent form NOT required.
2. Preparation:
   A. Obtain a 3-L container to which 10 ml of 12.5 M sodium hydroxide solution has been added.
   B. Write the beginning time of collection on the laboratory requisition.
3. Procedure:
   A. Discard the first morning voided urine.
   B. Save all the urine voided for the next 24 hours in a 3-L container to which 10 ml of 12.5 M sodium hydroxide solution has been added. For specimens

collected from an indwelling urinary catheter, empty the urine into the collection container hourly. Document the quantity of urinary output during the collection period. Do not refrigerate the specimen.

4. Postprocedure care:
   A. Write the ending time on the laboratory requisition.
   B. Compare the quantity of urine with the urinary output record for the collection. If the specimen contains less than was recorded as output, some urine may have been discarded, thus invalidating the test.

5. Client and family teaching:
   A. Save all the urine voided during the collection period, urinate before defecating, and avoid contaminating the specimen with stool or toilet tissue. If any urine is accidentally discarded, discard the entire specimen and restart the collection the next day.
   B. Foods high in purines that can contribute to gout include caffeine-containing beverages, legumes, mushrooms, organ meats, spinach, gravies, and baker's and brewer's yeast.
   C. Switching from a normal diet to a low-purine diet may potentially decrease urine uric acid levels by half.

6. Factors that affect results:
   A. Drugs that increase the rate of uric acid excretion include ascorbic acid, cytotoxics, probenecid, radiographic dyes, salicylates (long-term, large doses), and sulfinpyrazone.
   B. Drugs that slow uric acid excretion include diuretics and insulin.
   C. Trauma has been shown to increase the rate of urinary uric acid excretion.

7. Other data:
   A. None.

Bibliography:

Emmerson BT: Identification of the causes of persistent hyperuricaemia. Lancet *337*(8755):1461–1463, 1991.

Galvan AQ, Natali A, Baldi S, Frascerra S et al.: Effect of insulin on uric acid secretion in humans. A J Physiol *31*(1):E1–E5, 1995.

Wolfe F: Gout and hyperuricemia. Am Fam Physician *43*(6):2141–2150, 1991.

URINALYSIS (UA), URINE

Norm:

Albumin	Negative
Appearance	Clear to faintly hazy
Bilirubin	Negative
Color	Yellow
Glucose or reducing substances	Negative
Ketones	Negative
Nitrite	Negative
Occult blood	Negative
pH	4.5–8.0
Odor	Faint (not fruity, musty, fishy, or fetid)
Protein	Negative
Specific gravity	1.003–1.030
Urobilinogen	Negative or 0.1–1 Ehrlich U/dl
Cells	
Erythrocytes	≤3 cells/HPF
Leukocytes	≤4 cells/HPF
Urinary tract	
Epithelium	≤10 cells/HPF
Casts	Moderate clear protein casts
Crystals	Small amount
Bacteria or fungi	None or <1000/ml
Parasites	None

Increased or Decreased: For specific causes of increased or decreased values of constituents, see individual test listings as follows: *Albumin, 24-Hour, Urine; Bilirubin, Urine; Glucose, Qualitative, Semiquantitative, Urine; Ketone, Semiquantitative, Urine; Nitrite, Bacteria Screen, Urine; Occult Blood, Urine; pH, Urine; Protein, Urine; Specific Gravity, Urine; or Urobilinogen, Urine.*

Changes in Urine Color: A variety of substances may alter urine color as follows:

Color	Possible Cause
Black	Cascara, ferrous sulfate, homogentisic acid, indicans, indigo carmine dye used in renal function tests and cystoscopy, Levodopa, melanin, methemoglobin, phenols, urobilin.
Blue	Amitriptyline, some diuretics, Methylene blue, nitrofurans, pseudomonas.
Brown	Acid hematin, Addison's disease, bile pigment, furazolidone, levodopa, metronidazole, myoglobin, nitrofurantoin, porphyrinuria, renal disease, some sulfonamides.
Dark yellow to amber	Bilirubin, cascara, chlorpromazine, food (carrots), nitrofurantoin, phenacetin, quinacrine, riboflavin, urobilinogen.
Green	Bacterial infection, biliverdin, some diuretics, vitamins.
Light	Diuresis due to alcohol ingestion or diuretics, diabetes insipidus, glycosuria.
Orange	Bile pigment, chlorzoxazone, dehydration, fever, fluorescein sodium, jaundice, some oral anticoagulants, phenazopyridine, phenothiazines, pyridium, rifampin, sulfasalazine.
Red	Deferoxamine mesylate, foods (beets, rhubarb, senna), hemoglobin, malaria, myoglobin, porphobilinogen, phenolphthalein, phenolsulfonphthalein, porphyrins, renal injury, rifampin, sulfobromphthalein.

Description: A frequently performed screening test that gives a general indication of the client's overall state of health, as well as the health of the urinary tract. The dipstick reagent strip method is commonly used to measure pH, ketones, protein, sugars, and other reducing substances. Additional reagent strips are available to measure bilirubin and urobilinogen levels. The sample is also centrifuged, with the sediment then examined microscopically for determination of the presence and type of cells, casts, crystals, and organisms such as bacteria or fungi. Urine color should correlate with specific gravity. That is, dilute urine with low specific gravity should be almost colorless, and concentrated urine with high specific gravity should be dark yellow. Glucose content should also correlate positively with specific gravity. pH should correlate inversely with ketone (acetone) level. A sweet or fruity urine color indicates the presence of ketones in the sample. A fish or fetid odor indicates urinary tract infection. An odor of maple syrup may indicate maple syrup urine disease. A musty urine odor may be caused by recent ingestion of asparagus. An increase in epithelial cells may signal an inflammatory process in the kidneys. Erythrocytes present in the urine signal damage to the renal glomeruli. Elevated leukocytes indicate inflammation and/or infection in the urinary tract and indicate the need for urine culture. Both erythrocytes and leukocytes, if present, will appear trapped in casts and can be observed microscopically. Crystals may form at room temperature in voided urine before testing or may be caused by a variety of drugs. More detailed descriptions of other aspects of urine analysis may be found under individual test listings described above under "Increased or Decreased."

Professional Considerations:
1. Consent form NOT required.
2. Preparation:
   A. Obtain a soapy sponge and a clean specimen container.
   B. If bilirubin or urobilinogen results are of specific interest, the specimen con-

tainer should be wrapped in foil to protect it from light.

3. Procedure: A first morning void is preferred.

   A. *Female:* Instruct the client to wash the area surrounding the urethral meatus with soap and water. Then, while holding the labia open, position the specimen container beneath the urethral meatus and void into the container, filling it about half full (about 50 ml). *Also see Client and family teaching.*

   B. *Male:* Instruct the client to retract the foreskin, if present. Then wash the distal end of the penis surrounding the urethral meatus with soap and water. The client should then void into the specimen container, filling it about half full (about 50 ml).

4. Postprocedure care:

   A. Write the collection method, date, and time on the laboratory requisition.

   B. Send the specimen to the laboratory promptly and refrigerate it until testing. The best results are obtained if testing is performed within 2 hours.

5. Client and family teaching:

   A. Urinate before defecating and avoid contaminating the specimen with vaginal or perineal secretions or stool.

   B. Menstruating females should insert a tampon into the vagina before cleansing and voiding.

6. Factors that affect results:

   A. First morning-voided specimens provide the most accurate reflection of the presence of bacteria and formed elements such as casts and crystals.

   B. A delay in testing after collection may cause falsely decreased glucose, ketone, bilirubin, and urobilinogen values. Delayed testing with specimens left at room temperature may cause falsely elevated bacteria levels due to bacterial overgrowth. Delays also inhibit microscopic clarity due to the dissolution of urates and phosphates.

   C. For detailed listings of factors that affect results, see individual test listings described above under "Increased or Decreased."

7. Other data:

   A. Abnormal results should be confirmed by more specific, or quantitative, follow-up testing.

Bibliography:

Bailey BL: Urinalysis predictive of urine culture results. J Fam Pract 40(1):45–50, 1995.

Bergus GR: Urinalysis to diagnose UTI. J Fam Pract 40(6):601–602, 1995.

Brigden ML, Leadbeater A: Stick 'em up: Optimizing results with urinalysis dipsticks. MLO (June):32–36, 1994.

Cooper C: What color is that urine specimen? Am J Nurs 93(8):37, 1993.

Hofmann W, Regenbogen C, Edel H, et al.: Diagnostic strategies in urinalysis. Kidney Int 47(Suppl): S111–S114, 1994.

URINALYSIS, FRACTIONAL, URINE

Norm: Sugars: negative. Acetone: negative. Calculated albumin excretion rate (nephorimetric method):

		SI Units
Adult		
At rest	2–80 mg/24 hours	0.03–0.08 g/day
Ambulatory	<150 mg/24 hours	<0.15 g/day
Child <age 10	<100 mg/24 hours	<0.10 g/day

Usage: Monitoring for clients with diabetes mellitus (infrequently used). Assessment of urinary albumin excretion rate.

Description: A fractional urine involves testing up to four timed urine collections within a 24-hour period for the presence of sugars, acetone, or albumin, all of which are abnormal. Glucose results are reflective of the level of serum glucose levels, as levels above the renal threshold for glomerular glucose reabsorption into the bloodstream are excreted in the urine. Acetone levels are an indication of the state of fatty acid metabolism in diabetics. The detection of microalbuminuria in an aliquot of a fractional specimen has been demonstrated to be predictive of diabetic nephropathy at an early and potentially reversible stage. This test used to be performed more frequently for diabetics. However, as studies demonstrated that renal thresholds for glucose reabsorption vary from client to client, this test is no longer considered the most accurate reflection of insulin needs. Routine daily blood glucose monitoring has replaced fractional urine analysis for ongoing diabetic monitoring. Fractional urine testing is more often used to measure the excretion rate of albumin.

Professional Considerations:

1. Consent form NOT required.
2. Preparation:
   A. Obtain four clean 1-L specimen containers to which toluene preservative has been added (for glucose measurement) or without preservative (for albumin measurement) and reagent strips, or Clinitest and Acetest tablets.
   B. Number the containers sequentially.
3. Procedure:
   A. Specimens for albumin measurement should be refrigerated.
   B. *First collection period:*
      i. The first morning void, 1 hour before breakfast, is discarded.
      ii. The client should drink 8 ounces of water.
      iii. One-half hour later, the client should void and test the specimen for sugar and acetone, then transfer the specimen to container 1, and record the results, as well as the beginning time of the collection period.
      iv. The client should eat breakfast.
      v. All additional urine voided until 1 hour before the midday meal should be added to container 1, and the ending time of the collection period should be recorded.
   C. *Second collection period:*
      i. The client should drink 8 ounces of water 1 hour before the midday meal.
      ii. One-half hour later, the client should void and test the specimen for sugar and acetone, then transfer the specimen to container 2 and record the beginning time of the collection period.
      iii. The client should eat the midday meal and an afternoon snack.
      iv. All additional urine voided until 1 hour before the evening meal should be added to container 2, and the ending time of the collection period should be recorded.
   D. *Third collection period:*
      i. The client should drink 8 ounces of water 1 hour before the evening meal.
      ii. One-half hour later, the client should void and test the specimen for sugar and acetone, then transfer the specimen to container 3 and record the results as well as the beginning time of the collection period.

iii. The client should eat the evening meal.
iv. All additional urine voided until 1 hour before the bedtime snack should be added to container 3, and the ending time of the collection period should be recorded.
   E. *Fourth collection period:*
      i. The client should drink 8 ounces of water 1 hour before the bedtime snack.
      ii. One-half hour later, the client should void and test the specimen for sugar and acetone, then transfer the specimen to container #4 and record the results as well as the beginning time of the collection period.
      iii. The client should eat a bedtime snack.
      iv. All additional urine voided until 1 hour before breakfast the next day should be added to container 4.
      v. The client should include the void at 1 hour before breakfast in container 4, and record the time ended.
4. Postprocedure care:
   A. Send all four containers to the laboratory.
5. Client and family teaching:
   A. Collect specimens according to the procedure above.
   B. All testing should be performed on freshly voided urine with reagent strips (Keto-Diastix, Multi-Six) or Clinitest and Acetest tablets according to manufacturer's directions. Compare the results with the color chart on the container.
6. Factors that affect results:
   A. Expired reagent strips, Clinitest tablets, or Acetest tablets, or those that have had prolonged exposure to air or moisture should not be used, as the results will be invalid.
   B. Many drugs and factors affect the accuracy of the test media used. For detailed information, see the specific test listing for the method used as follows: *Acetone, Urine; Albumin, 24-Hour, Urine; or Glucose, Qualitative, Semiquantitative, Urine.*
7. Other data:
   A. A computerized system is now available to document client outcomes.

Bibliography:

Bilous R: Diabetes: should you be screening for microalbuminemia? Practitioner *239*(1550):343–345, 1995.

Brigden ML, Leadbeater A: Stick 'em up: Optimizing results with urinalysis dipsticks. MLO (June): 32–36, 1994.

Ferris NA, Stoupa RA, Mandenhall JD, et al.: A computerized diabetes education module for documenting patient outcomes. Comput Nurs *12*(6): 272–276, 1994.

URINARY BLADDER SONOGRAM (URINARY BLADDER ECHOGRAM, URINARY BLADDER ULTRASOUND), DIAGNOSTIC

Norm: Negative for tumor, cyst, overdistention, or residual urine. Proper size, shape, and position of the urinary bladder.

Usage: Assessment for residual urine in or for overdistention of the bladder; evaluation of the size, shape, and position of the urinary bladder; helps diagnose, localize, monitor, and stage bladder tumor and evaluate hemorrhagic cystitis following bone marrow transplant as well as detect urinary bladder involvement in Crohn's disease; differentiation of superficial from deep infiltrative bladder tumors (transurethral sonogram); and measurement of urinary bladder volumes (transrectal sonogram or transvaginal sonogram).

Description: Evaluation of the urinary bladder size, shape, and position via the creation of an oscilloscopic picture from the echoes of high-frequency sound waves passing over the bladder area (acoustic imaging) via the transpelvic or transurethral route. The time required for the ultrasonic beam to be reflected back to the transducer from differing densities of tissue is converted by a computer to an electrical impulse displayed on an oscilloscopic screen to create a three-dimensional picture of the urinary bladder. Additionally, transvaginal or transrectal endosonography can provide an advantage in evaluating the neck of the bladder, the bladder base, and the urethra in females.

Professional Considerations:

1. Consent form NOT required for transabdominal method. Consent form IS required for transrectal, transurethral, and transvaginal methods.

Risks:

Transabdominal procedure: none. Transvaginal procedure: vaginal infection.

Contraindications:

Transabdominal procedure: none. Transvaginal procedure: third-trimester pregnancy.

---

2. Preparation:
   A. The client should disrobe below the waist or wear a gown.
   B. Obtain ultrasonic gel or paste.
   C. For transrectal sonography, an enema may be prescribed.
   D. *See Client and family teaching.*
3. Procedure:
   A. *Transabdominal sonogram:*
      i. The client is positioned supine.
      ii. Ultrasonic gel or paste is applied to the skin overlying the bladder.
      iii. A lubricated transducer is placed firmly against the skin over the bladder area and moved slowly back and forth at intervals 1–2 cm apart. The oscilloscope displays a three-dimensional image of the full bladder.
      iv. The client is instructed to void, and the procedure is repeated to check for the presence of residual urine.
      v. Photographs are taken of the oscilloscopic display.
      vi. The procedure takes less than 30 minutes.
   B. *Transvaginal sonogram:*
      i. After uroflowmetry studies are completed, 0.9% saline solution is instilled through a urethral catheter to fill the bladder.
      ii. A transducer probe is inserted into an ultrasonic-gel-filled condom. The condom is covered with a sterile lubricant.
      iii. The probe is inserted into the vagina by the client or the examiner, and moved to touch the vesicourethral area.
      iv. The bladder and urethra are identified via sonography. Pictures are taken of the oscilloscopic display, with the client at rest, or during micturition.
   C. *Transrectal sonogram:*
      i. The client is positioned supine, and a short transabdominal sonogram is performed to evaluate for kidney distention.
      ii. The rectum is examined digitally for obstruction.
      iii. The client is assisted to a knee-elbow, lateral decubitus, or sitting position.
      iv. The probe is covered with an air-free, sterile, transparent cover or condom. The condom is then coated with a sterile lubricant, and the probe is slowly inserted into the rectum.
      v. After the probe is inserted into the rectum, the condom is inflated with 20–60 ml of deaerated water.
      vi. The probe is angled anteriorly, and sonography of the bladder is performed.
      vii. Photographs of the oscilloscopic display are taken.

D. *Transurethral sonogram:*
   i. The bladder is filled with sterile, 0.9% saline solution.
   ii. The probe is covered with an air-free, sterile, transparent cover and inserted into the bladder through a cystoscope.
   iii. The probe is rotated within the bladder as transverse sectional scans are taken.
   iv. Oscilloscopic images may be recorded on videotape or photographs.
4. Postprocedure care:
   A. Remove the gel from the skin.
   B. Sterilize the endosonography probes by soaking in glutaraldehyde solution for 10 minutes.
5. Client and family teaching:
   A. This test should be performed before intestinal barium tests, or else after the barium is cleared from the system.
   B. Drink three to four 8-ounce glasses of fluid within 2 hours prior to the test (where not contraindicated, as the purpose of the test is to evaluate the bladder when full), and refrain from voiding.
   C. The transabdominal procedure is painless and carries no risks.
6. Factors that affect results:
   A. Dehydration interferes with adequate contrast between organs and body fluids.
   B. Lower intestinal barium obscures results by preventing proper transmission and deflection of the high-frequency sound waves.
   C. The more lower abdominal fat present, the greater the attenuation (reduction in sound wave amplitude and intensity), which interferes with the clarity of the transabdominal picture.
7. Other data:
   A. Computed tomography is preferred to ultrasound for staging and measuring urinary bladder tumors.

Bibliography:

Cartoni C, Arcese W, Avvisati G, et al.: Role of ultrasonography in the diagnosis and follow-up of hemorrhagic cystitis after bone marrow transplantation. Bone Marrow Transplant *12*(5):463–467, 1993.

Haylen BT, Parys BT, West CR: Transrectal ultrasound to measure bladder volumes in men. J Urol *143*(4):687–689, 1990.

Murandali D, Gold WL, Phillips A, et al.: Can ultrasound probes and coupling gel be a source of nosocomial infection in patients undergoing sonography? Am J Roentgenol *164*(6):1521–1524, 1995.

Woo HH, O'Driscoll DM, Saalfeld J: Non-deflation of Foley catheter balloon: use of transrectal ultrasound. Aust N Z J Surg *64*(8):576–577, 1994.

Yanushpolsky EH, Brown DL, Smith BL: Localization of small ovarian Sertoli-Leydig cell tumors by transvaginal sonography with color Doppler. Ultrasound Obstet Gynecol *5*(2):133–135, 1995.

URINARY GONADOTROPIN PEPTIDE (UGP), URINE

Norm: <0.2 ng/ml or <5 fmol/mg creatinine.

Increased: Down syndrome, gynecologic cancers (cervical, endometrial, ovarian, and vulvovaginal), pregnancy, recurrence of gynecologic cancer.

Decreased: Survival rate from gynecologic cancer is increased; nonpregnant.

Description: Urinary gonadotropin peptide (UGP), also known as urinary gonadotropin fragment (UGF), is a beta-core fragment that is found in pregnancy and is also known to originate from cancer tissue itself. UGP is secreted into the circulation and rapidly cleared and is generally not detected in the serum.

Professional Considerations:

1. Consent form NOT required.
2. Preparation:
   A. Obtain a soapy sponge and a clean specimen container.
3. Procedure:
   A. Wash the area around the meatus with a soapy sponge.
   B. Hold the labia open and position the specimen container beneath the urethral meatus.
   C. Void into the container at least 10 ml of urine. A first morning specimen is preferred.
4. Postprocedure care:
   A. Write the collection date and time and the suspected diagnosis on the laboratory requisition.
   B. Send the specimen to the laboratory within 2 hours.
   C. Freeze the specimen.
5. Client and family teaching:
   A. This test shows sensitivity as a survival and prognostic indicator for cancers of the cervix, ovary, and vulvovaginal area.
6. Factors that affect results:
   A. The sensitivity of the test is increased when results are corrected for urinary concentration.
7. Other data:
   A. Use of UGP alone, or together with serum CA-125 levels, as a test for ovarian cancer, at the time of annual PAP test, or in women with benign pelvic masses, should be carefully evaluated.
   B. False-positives have been detected in 2% of healthy postmenopausal women.
   C. A past history of gynecologic malignancy does not falsely increase UGP levels.

Bibliography:

Carter PG, Iles RK, Neven P, et al.: Measurement of urinary beta core fragment of human chorionic gonadotropin in women with vulvovaginal malignancy and its prognostic significance. Br J Cancer *71*(2):350–353, 1995.

Carter PG, Iles RK, Neven P, et al.: The prognostic significance of urinary beta core fragment in premenopausal women with carcinoma of the cervix. Gynecol Oncol *55*(2):271–276, 1994.

Cole LA, Schwartz PE, Wang Y: Urinary gonadotropin fragments (UGF) in cancers of the female reproductive system. Gynecol Oncol *31*(82):90 pp, 1988.

Cuckle HS: Urinary beta-core human chorionic gonadotropin: a new approach to Down syndrome screening. Prenat Diag *14*(10):953–958, 1994.

Walker R, Crebbin V, Stern J: Urinary gonadotropin peptide (UGP) as a marker of gynecological malignancies. Anticancer Res *14*(5A):1703–1709, 1994.

URINE, ANAEROBIC CULTURE, SUPRAPUBIC PUNCTURE, CULTURE
(see Body Fluid, Routine, Culture)

URINE, CULTURE AND SENSITIVITY (C & S), URINE
(see Culture, Routine, Specimen)

URINE, FUNGUS, CULTURE
(see Body Fluid, Fungus, Culture)

URINE, MYCOBACTERIA, CULTURE
(see Body Fluid, Mycobacteria, Culture)

URINE CULTURE, ROUTINE, URINE
(see Body Fluid, Routine, Culture)

URINE CULTURE, ROUTINE, CATHETERIZED, URINE
(see Body Fluid, Routine, Culture)

URINE CULTURE, ROUTINE, CLEAN-CATCH, URINE
(see Body Fluid, Routine, Culture)

URINE CULTURE, ROUTINE, SUPRAPUBIC PUNCTURE, URINE
(see Body Fluid, Routine, Culture)

URINE CULTURE FOR *NEISSERIA GONNORHOEAE*, URINE

Norm: Negative. No *Neisseria gonorrhoeae* isolated.

Positive: Gonorrhea.

Description: Gonorrhea is a sexually transmitted disease caused by the organism *N. gonorrhoeae*. *N. gonorrhoeae* is a gonococcus, transmitted from client to client by direct contact with exudates from the mucous membranes of infected clients. This disease causes purulent urethral discharge within 7 days of infection. Other symptoms may include rectal pruritus cervicitis, endometritis, epididymitis, salpingitis, pelvic peritonitis, or vulvovaginitis. A culture is performed on the sediment of centrifuged urine.

Professional Considerations:
1. Consent form NOT required.
2. Preparation:
   A. Obtain four soapy sponges and a sterile specimen container.
3. Procedure:
   A. Instruct the client to void and discard the urine.
   B. Cleanse the penis or vulva × 4 with the soapy sponges, moving distal to proximal or front to back, discarding each sponge after one use.
   C. Collect the first 10 ml of the first morning-voided urine in a sterile container; OR collect the entire first morning void in a sterile container; OR at least 2 hours after the last void, collect the first 10 ml of urine voided in a sterile container.
4. Postprocedure care:
   A. Write the collection date and time, any recent antibiotic therapy, and the suspected diagnosis on the laboratory requisition.
   B. Send the specimen to the laboratory within 1 hour. Do not refrigerate it.
5. Client and family teaching:
   A. At least 2 days are required for results.
   B. Gonorrhea is a reportable disease in the United States.
   C. The follow-up culture should be performed 7–10 days after treatment.
   D. Gonorrhea infection is treatable with antibiotics.
   E. If results are positive, provide the client with the appropriate information on sexually transmitted diseases.
      i. Notify all sexual partners from the last 90 days to be tested for gonorrhea infection.
      ii. Do not have sexual relations until

your physician confirms that the infection is gone.

F. Do not use feminine hygiene sprays or douche during treatment.

G. Wear underpants and pantyhose that have a cotton lining in the crotch.

H. Take showers instead of tub baths until the infection is gone.

6. Factors that affect results:

A. False-negative results may occur for some strains of *N. gonorrhoeae* when Thayer-Martin or Martin-Lewis growth medium is used (due to vancomycin content of the medium).

B. Specimen contamination with other genital flora may result in overgrowth of normal flora.

7. Other data:

A. Gonorrhea is treated with aqueous procaine penicillin G (note that penicillin resistant strain has been reported) or ampicillin or spectinomycin or tetracycline or ciprofloxacin (note that ciprofloxacin resistant gonococci reported).

B. The client should also be tested for syphilis.

C. Dipstick methods are available for purposes of screening for *N. gonorrhoeae*.

Bibliography:

Duvauchelle DA, Pien FD: Gonococcal osteomyelitis: report of a penicillin-resistant strain. Orthopedics *17*(8):719–721, 1994.

Lewis DA, Forster GE, Goh BT: Ciprofloxacin resistant gonococci arriving from Thailand [letter]. Genitourin Med *70*(5):360, 1994.

Pec J Jr, Kliment J, Moravcik P, et al.: Isolation of *Neisseria gonorrhoeae* and concomitant bacterial microflora from urine obtained by suprapubic bladder puncture in women with gonococcal urethritis. Int Urol Nephrol *22*(2):167–171, 1990.

Wong KC, Ho BS, Egglestone SI, et al.: Diagnosis of urogenital gonorrhea: evaluation of an enzyme immunoassay and use of urine as a non-invasive specimen. Br J Biomed Sci *51*(4):312–315, 1994.

URINE CYTOLOGY, URINE
(see Cytologic Study of Urine, Diagnostic)

UROBILINOGEN, URINE

Norm:

		SI Units
24-hour specimen	0.5–4.0 mg or 0.5–4.0 Ehrlich units	0.9–7.2 µmol
2-hour specimen Female	0.1–1.1 mg or 0.1–1.1 Ehrlich units	0.2–1.9 µmol
Male	0.3–2.1 mg or 0.3–2.1 Ehrlich units	0.5–3.6 µmol
Random specimen (dipstick method)	Negative = yellow-green or 0.1–1 Ehrlich units/dl	

Increased: Anemia (hemolytic, pernicious), bananas eaten within 48 hours prior to the test, cholangitis, cirrhosis, congestive heart failure causing hepatic dysfunction, Dubin-Johnson syndrome, hepatic parenchymal damage, hemolytic processes, hepatitis (early), idiopathic pulmonary hemosiderosis, infectious mononucleosis, jaundice (hemolytic), lead poisoning, malaria, polycythemia vera, portal hypertension, pulmonary infarction, sickle cell disease, thalassemia major, and tissue hemorrhage. Drugs include sodium bicarbonate.

Decreased: Carcinoma of the head of the pancreas, cholelithiasis, complete common bile duct obstruction, diarrhea (severe), inflammation (severe), and renal insufficiency. Drugs include antibiotics that suppress the normal flora of the intestine such as chloramphenicol, cholestatics, and vitamin C.

Description: Urobilinogen is a reduction product formed by the action of bacteria on conjugated bilirubin in the gastrointestinal tract. The majority of urobilinogen is excreted in the stool. A small portion is reabsorbed via the enterohepatic pathway and reexcreted in bile. The remainder is excreted in the urine. A random dipstick check for urine bilinogen is normally negative due to its rapid oxidation to urobilin. An increase in urine urobilinogen indicates that some type of hemolytic process or hepatic dysfunction is occurring in the body. Urine urobilinogen levels are usually the highest in early to mid-afternoon. Thus, when reagent strips test positive, a 2-hour urine collection between 1 and 3 P.M. is indicated.

Professional Considerations:

1. Consent form NOT required.
2. Preparation:
   A. *Dipstick method:*
      i. A dipstick method should not be used for clients taking the drug phenazopyridine.
      ii. Obtain a container of Bili-Labstix, Multistix, Urobilistix, or other reagent strip for urine urobilinogen testing, and a clean container.
   B. *2-hour specimen:*
      i. Obtain a light-protected, 1- to 2-L urine collection container without preservatives, a cup for drinking, and a pitcher of water (500 ml).
   C. *24-hour specimen:*
      i. Obtain a light-protected 3-L urine collection container without preservative.
      ii. Instruct the client to save all the urine voided for the next 24 hours, to urinate before defecating, and to avoid contaminating urine with stool or toilet tissue.
      iii. Write the beginning time of collection on the container and the laboratory requisition.
      iv. Plan collection so that the test ends during laboratory open hours.
   D. *See Client and family teaching.*
3. Procedure:
   A. *Dipstick method:*
      i. Obtain a 20-ml random urine sample in a clean plastic container.
      ii. Immediately dip the reagent strip into the specimen and slide the strip along the edge of the container to remove excess urine.
      iii. Hold the strip horizontally next to the color chart on the container, and time the reading according to the manufacturer's directions (most are 45–60 seconds).
      iv. When the timing is completed, compare the color of the reagent pad for the urobilinogen measurement to the color chart, and record the measurement as follows:

   B. *2-hour specimen:*
      i. Collect the specimen during early to mid-afternoon.
      ii. Instruct the client to void and to discard the urine.
      iii. Instruct the client to drink all of the 500 ml of water in the pitcher over the next 10 minutes.
      iv. Save all the urine voided over the next 2 hours in a refrigerated, light-protected urine collection container. The urine must be transferred into the container *immediately* after each void.
   C. *24-hour specimen:*
      i. Discard the first morning void.
      ii. Save all the urine voided in a refrigerated, light-protected 3-L container without preservatives. For specimens collected from an indwelling urinary catheter, keep the foil-covered drainage bag on ice, and empty the urine into the light-protected collection container hourly. Document the quantity of urinary output during the collection period.
4. Postprocedure care:
   A. *2-hour collection:*
      i. Send the specimen to the laboratory immediately for prompt measurement.
   B. *24-hour collection:*
      i. Write the ending time of collection on the laboratory requisition.
      ii. Compare the urine quantity in the container with the urinary output record for the test. If the container has less urine than was recorded as output, some of the urine may have been discarded, thus invalidating the test. The test must be restarted.
      iii. Send valid specimens to the laboratory immediately for prompt measurement.
5. Client and family teaching:
   A. Avoid eating bananas for 2 days prior to the test.
   B. Collect specimens according to the appropriate procedure, as described above.
6. Factors that affect results:
   A. Drugs that may cause falsely increased results include acetazolamide, aminosalicylic acid, antipyrine, aspirin, Bromsulphalein, cascara, chlorpromazine, 5-hydroxyindoleacetic acid, phenazopyridine, phenothiazines, and sulfonamides.

	Ehrlich Units/DL	Color
Normal	0.1–1	Yellow to yellow-green
Positive	2–4	Yellow-orange
	8–12	Orange-brown

B. Urine alkalinization increases the excretion rate of urine urobilinogen. Urine acidification decreases the excretion rate of urine urobilinogen.
C. Dipstick methods can detect only abnormally high levels, not abnormally low levels.
D. The level may be normal in clients with incomplete common bile duct obstruction.
E. False-positive or falsely increased results may occur in porphyria.

7. Other data:
A. None.

Bibliography:

Binder L, Smith D, Kupka T, et al.: Failure of prediction of liver function test abnormalities with the urine urobilinogen and urine bilirubin assays. Arch Pathol Lab Med *113*(1):73–76, 1989.

Kotal P, Fevery J: Quantitation of urobilinogen in feces, urine, bile and serum by direct spectrophotometry of zinc complex. Clin Chem Acta *14* (202):1–9, 1991.

UROFLOWMETRY, DIAGNOSTIC

Norm: Normal uroflow curve, with normal peak and normal voiding time for quantity voided.

	Volume	Rate	
		Female	Male
Adults			
Young (<age 45)	≥200 ml	18 ml/second	21 ml/second
Middle (age 46–65)	≥200 ml	15 ml/second	12 ml/second
Older (>age 65)	≥200 ml	10 ml/second	9 ml/second
Children			
Younger (<age 8)	≥100 ml	10 ml/second	10 ml/second
Older (age 8–13)	≥100 ml	15 ml/second	12 ml/second

Usage: Part of diagnostic evaluation for voiding abnormalities.

Description: Uroflowmetry involves measuring the voiding duration, amount, and rate of urine voided into a funnel with a urine flowmeter that records the above information in a graphic format. This simple, noninvasive test is usually performed in combination with other tests such as cystometry and voiding cystourethrography.

Professional Considerations:

1. Consent form NOT required.
2. Preparation:
   A. Provide a private environment for voiding.
3. Procedure:
   A. Several types of urine flowmeters are available. The exact procedure depends on the type of flowmeter used, and should be followed according to the manufacturer's instructions and institutional protocol.
   B. In general, the flowmeter is activated just prior to the void, as described above. The volume voided and the rate, pattern, and duration of voiding are analyzed and displayed graphically by the urine flowmeter. A uroflow curve displays the changes in the urine flow rate throughout the void.
   C. Serial recordings of each void over 2–3 days may be performed to provide the most accurate evaluation of the client's urine flow patterns. This helps correct for aberrancies such as hesitancy due to nervousness, or single voided specimens of extremely small or large volume.
   D. The client's position during each void, and the amount and route of fluid intake throughout testing, should be recorded.
4. Postprocedure care:
   A. None.
5. Client and family teaching:
   A. When the urge to void is felt, assume a normal voiding position and perform a normal void, completely emptying the bladder urine into the funnel of the flowmeter. The void should be performed without straining and while holding the rest of the body as motionless as possible. Urinate before defecating, and do not allow stool or toilet tissue to enter the funnel.
6. Factors that affect results:
   A. The quantity of urine voided affects the flow rate. Optimal amounts for evaluation of bladder function are between 200 and 400 ml. Quantities over 400 ml cause deterioration of bladder extrusor muscle function.
   B. Recent urethral instrumentation may cause decreased flow rates.

7. Other data:
   A. None.

Bibliography:

Barry MJ, Girman CJ, O'Leary MP, et al.: Using repeated measures of symptom score, uroflowmetry and prostate specific antigen in the clinical management of prostate disease. J Urol *153*(1):99–103, 1995.

Griffiths D, Harrison G, Moore K, et al.: Long-term changes in urodynamic studies of voiding in the elderly. Urol Res *22*(4):235–238, 1994.

Kaplan SA, Te AE: Uroflowmetry and urodynamics. Urol Clin North Am *22*(2):309–320, 1995.

UROGRAPHY, EXCRETORY, DIAGNOSTIC

(see Intravenous Pyelography, Diagnostic)

UTEROSALPINGOGRAPHY, DIAGNOSTIC

(see Hysterosalpingography, Diagnostic)

UTEROTUBAL INSUFFLATION, DIAGNOSTIC

(see Rubin's Test, Diagnostic)

VAGINAL ASPIRATE FOR MOTILE/NONMOTILE SPERM, SPECIMEN

(see Sims-Huhner Test, Diagnostic)

VAGINAL CULTURE

(see Genital, Routine, Culture)

VAGINAL CYTOLOGY

(see Hormonal Evaluation, Cytologic, Specimen)

VALPROIC ACID, BLOOD

Norm:

		SI Units
Therapeutic level	50–100 µg/ml	350–690 µmol/L
Toxic level	>100 µg/ml	>690 µmol/L
Panic level	>200 µg/ml	>1380 µmol/L

Panic Level Symptoms and Treatment:

Symptoms: Burning feet paresthesia, numbness, tingling, weakness, mental changes.

Treatment: Activated charcoal and Naloxone. Hemodialysis and peritoneal dialysis will NOT remove valproic acid

Usage: Monitoring for therapeutic levels during valproic acid therapy.

Description: Valproic acid is an anticonvulsant effective against myoclonus and grand mal, petit mal, and complex partial seizures. It is being used experimentally for panic disorders, bipolar disorders, and migraine treatment. After oral or rectal administration, it is metabolized by the liver and excreted in the urine, with a half-life of 6–8 hours and elimination half-life of 15–20 hours.

Professional Considerations:

1. Consent form NOT required.
2. Preparation:
   A. Tube: Red-top, red/gray-top, or gold-top (for serum level), or green-top (for plasma level).
   B. Specimens MAY be drawn during hemodialysis.
3. Procedure:
   A. Draw a 1-ml blood sample. Draw the trough level immediately prior to dose administration. Draw the peak level 1–3 hours after dose administration.
4. Postprocedure care:
   A. Specimens must be kept in a tightly capped tube until testing to prevent evaporation of valproic acid from the sample.
5. Client and family teaching:
   A. Long-term use of this drug may result in hepatotoxicity.
   B. Overdose of this drug can cause neurotoxicity.

C. If activated charcoal was given for elevated levels, the client should drink 4–6 glasses of water each day for 2 days to prevent constipation. The activated charcoal will also cause stools to be black for a few days.

6. Factors that affect results:
   A. Absorption is slowed by the presence of food in the gastrointestinal tract; thus, peak levels occur later for doses given on a full stomach than for doses given on an empty stomach.
   B. Valproic acid reaches steady-state levels in about 96 hours.
   C. Drugs that may decrease valproic acid half-life include carbamazepine, phenobarbital, phenytoin, and primidone.
   D. Hepatic failure may cause elevated results.

7. Other data:
   A. Periodic liver function tests should be performed throughout valproic acid therapy.

B. Valproic acid increases serum levels of phenobarbital.
C. A case has been reported of fatal acute pancreatitis caused by valproic acid.

Bibliography:

Bowden CL, McElroy SL: History of the development of valproate for treatment of bipolar disorders. J Clin Psychiatry 56(3, Suppl):3–5, 1995.

Dupuis RE, Lichtman SN, Pollack GM: Acute valproic acid overdose. Clinical course and pharmacokinetic disposition of valproic acid and metabolites. Drug Safety 5(1):65–71, 1990.

Evans RJ, Miranda RN, Jordan J, et al.: Fatal acute pancreatitis caused by valproic acid. Am J Forensic Med Pathol 16(1):62–65, 1995.

Heller AJ, Chesterman P, Elwes RD, et al.: Phenobarbitone, phenytoin, carbamazepine, or sodium valproate for newly diagnosed adult epilepsy: a randomized comparative monotherapy trial. J Neurol Neurosurg Psychiatry 58(1):44–50, 1995.

Mathew NT, Saper JR, Silberstein SD, et al.: Migraine prophylaxis with divalproex. Arch Neurol 52(3): 281–286, 1995.

VANCOMYCIN, BLOOD

Norm:

		SI Units
In general	5–10 μg/ml	3.4–6.8 μmol/L
Panic level	>25 μg/ml	>17 μmol/L

Panic Level Symptoms and Treatment:

Symptoms: Renal failure, nausea, vomiting, hearing loss.

Treatment: Hemofiltration WILL remove vancomycin. Hemodialysis will NOT remove vancomycin.

Usage: Monitoring for therapeutic (and safe) levels during vancomycin therapy.

Description: Vancomycin is an aminoglycoside antibiotic that inhibits cell wall synthesis of gram-positive bacteria. It is frequently used in the treatment of infections caused by methicillin-resistant *Staphylococcus aureus* (MRSA), and in treatment for pseudomembranous colitis. Vancomycin is metabolized in the liver, with 80% excreted via the kidneys and a small amount in bile. Oral doses are primarily excreted in the feces. Vancomycin half-life is very dependent on renal glomerular function. Rapid infusions of this drug have been associated with histamine release causing "redman's syndrome," in which the skin becomes flushed, erythematous, and pruritic.

Professional Considerations:

1. Consent form NOT required.
2. Preparation:
   A. Tube: Red-top, red/gray-top, or gold-top.
   B. Specimens MAY be drawn during hemodialysis.
3. Procedure:
   A. Draw the trough level just prior to dose. Draw the peak level 30 minutes after intravenous administration.
   B. Draw a 1-ml blood sample.
4. Postprocedure care:
   A. Send the sample to the laboratory promptly. Serum should be separated and frozen within 4 hours.
5. Client and family teaching:
   A. Overdoses can cause renal failure and hearing loss.
   B. Slowing the rate of drug infusion can decrease feelings of the skin being flushed, red, and itchy.
6. Factors that affect results:
   A. Minimum inhibitory concentration

(MIC) of vancomycin varies for different organisms and will affect the therapeutic trough level needed. MIC should be included in sensitivity testing results. In general, an average peak vancomycin level that is two to four times higher than the MIC is considered adequate for control of the organism. *See Minimum Inhibitory Concentration, Specimen.*

B. Clients with impaired glomerular renal function will have elevated levels if dosages are not adjusted accordingly.

7. Other data:

A. Renal function and hearing should be assessed prior to and throughout vancomycin therapy. Clients that demonstrated increased nephrotoxicity in one study were those also receiving another aminoglycoside concurrently, those who received vancomycin for over 3 weeks, and those who had trough levels >10 mg/L.

B. Vancomycin administered intravenously over 2 hours, as compared to 1 hour, has been shown to reduce the occurrence of red-man's syndrome.

C. Resistance of enterococcus to Vancomycin has been documented.

Bibliography:

Clem JR: Vancomycin therapy: resistance and appropriate usage guidelines. South Dak J Med *48*(3): 94–95, 1995.

Ducharme MP, Slaughter RL, Edwards DJ: Vancomycin pharmacokinetics in a patient population: effect of age, gender, and body weight. Ther Drug Monit *16*(5):513–518, 1994.

Mulhern JG, Branden, GL, O'Shea MH, et al.: Trough serum vancomycin levels predict the relapse of gram-positive peritonitis in peritoneal dialysis patients. Am J Kid Dis *25*(4):611–615, 1995.

Rice LB, Shlaes DM: Vancomycin resistance in the enterococcus. Relevance in pediatrics. Ped Clin North Am *42*(3):601–618, 1995.

Saunders NJ: Why monitor peak vancomycin concentrations? Lancet *344*(8939–8940):1748–1750, 1994.

VANILLYLMANDELIC ACID (VMA), URINE

Norm:

		SI Units
Norms in	**g/mg creatinine**	**mmol/mol creatinine**
Adults	≤7 µg/mg	4.0 mmol/mol
Children		
Birth–11 months	<27 µg/mg	15.4 mmol/mol
12–23 months	<18 µg/mg	10.3 mmol/mol
2–4 years	<13 µg/mg	7.4 mmol/mol
5–9 years	<8.5 µg/mg	4.9 mmol/mol
10–14 years	<7 µg/mg	4.0 mmol/mol
15–18 years	<5 µg/mg	2.9 mmol/mol
Norms in	**mg/24 hours**	**mol/day**
Adults	7–9 mg/24 hours	35–45 µmol/day
Children		
≤12 months	≤1.8 mg/24 hours	≤9 µmol/day
12 months–4 years	≤3 mg/24 hours	≤15 µmol/day
4–15 years	≤4 mg/24 hours	≤20 µmol/day

Increased: Ganglioblastoma, ganglioneuroma, neuroblastoma, and pheochromocytoma. Drugs include aspirin, aminosalicylic acid, Bromsulphalein, epinephrine, glyceryl guaiacolate, levodopa, lithium carbonate, mephenesin, methocarbamol, nalidixic acid, norepinephrine, oxytetracycline, penicillin, phenazopyridine, phenosulfonphthalein, salicylates, and sulfonamides.

Decreased: Familial dysautonomia (Riley-Day syndrome). Drugs include chlorpromazine, clofibrate, clonidine, guanethidine analogs, imipramine, levodopa, methyldopa, monoamine oxidase (MAO) inhibitors, reserpine, and salicylates.

Description: Vanillylmandelic acid (VMA) occurs as an end-product of epinephrine and norepinephrine metabolism and is freely excreted in the urine. This test aids in the diagnosis and monitoring for clients with catecholamine-secreting tumors.

Professional Considerations:

1. Consent form NOT required.
2. Preparation:
   A. Withhold drugs that may cause increased or decreased results (listed above) for 72 hours prior to the test. Diuretics, antihypertensives, and sympathomimetics (including nonprescriptive cold and allergy medications) must be withheld for 5–14 days.
   B. Obtain a clean, 3-L container with hydrochloric acid (HCl) or acetic acid preservative.
   C. Write the starting time of collection on the laboratory requisition and container.
   D. *See Client and family teaching.*
3. Procedure:
   A. Discard first morning urine specimen.
   B. Save all the urine voided for a 24-hour period in a refrigerated, clean, 3-L plastic container to which HCl or acetic acid preservative has been added. For specimens collected from indwelling urinary catheters, keep the drainage bag on ice and empty urine into the collection container hourly. Add preservative as needed to maintain pH at about 3.0 (range, 2.0 to 4.0). Document the quantity of urine output throughout the collection period.
4. Postprocedure care:
   A. Compare the urine quantity in the container with the record of urine output during the collection period. If the container contains less urine than was documented as output, some may have been discarded, invalidating the test.
5. Client and family teaching:
   A. Avoid the following foods for 72 hours prior to the test: avocados, bananas, beer, cheese (aged), Chianti wines, chocolate, citrus fruits, cocoa, coffee, fava beans, grains, tea, vanilla, walnuts, and wine.
   B. Save all the urine voided for 24 hours, urinate before defecating, and avoid contaminating urine with stool or toilet tissue. If any urine is accidentally discarded, discard the entire specimen and restart the collection the next day.
   C. Avoid stress, strenuous exercise, and smoking of tobacco prior to and throughout the urine collection period.
6. Factors that affect results:
   A. Drugs that cause decreased results in normal clients may not suppress levels to below normal level in clients with catecholamine-secreting tumors.
7. Other data:
   A. Consistency in results has been demonstrated between random, 6-hour, 12-hour, and 24-hour specimens.

Bibliography:

Noyes R Jr, Woodman C, Laukes C, et al.: The association of urinary 5-hydroxyindoleacetic acid and vanillylmandelic acid in patients with generalized anxiety. Neuropsychobiology *31*(1):6–9, 1995.

Riddhimat R, Prabhant C, Sirisali K, et al.: Comparative study of vanillylmandelic acid in random and 24-hour urine collections. J Med Assoc Thai *73*(5):239–243, 1990.

VARICELLA-ZOSTER VIRUS SEROLOGY, SERUM

Norm: Less than a fourfold increase in titer between acute and convalescent samples.

Increased: Chickenpox and *Herpes zoster* (shingles).

Description: Varicella-zoster virus, also known as human herpesvirus 3, is the causative agent of chickenpox and shingles, which are time-limited viral infections that produce skin lesions or vesicles. The mode of transmission is directly from client to client, airborne spread of infected respiratory secretions or vesicle fluid, or indirectly through contact with contaminated secretions on inanimate objects. The virus multiplies in the respiratory tract, then spreads through the bloodstream to the skin and internal organs. After causing chickenpox in childhood, the latent virus may re-emerge to cause shingles in the elderly. In this test, complement fixation, indirect immunofluorescence, or agglutination methods are used to detect the antibody to the varicella-zoster virus. A varicella vaccine is available.

Professional Considerations:

1. Consent form NOT required.
2. Preparation:
   A. Tube: Red-top, red/gray-top, or gold-top.
3. Procedure:
   A. Draw a 3-ml blood sample as soon as possible after symptoms appear. Label the tube as the "acute sample." Repeat the test in 10–14 days and label the tube as the "convalescent sample."
4. Postprocedure care:
   A. None.
5. Client and family teaching:
   A. Return for convalescent sampling in 10–14 days.
6. Factors that affect results:
   A. None found.
7. Other data:
   A. Chickenpox and shingles are contagious for up to 6 days after lesions or vesicles appear. Immunocompromised

clients may be contagious for longer periods of time.

B. For clients exposed to varicella-zoster, varicella-zoster immune globulin from zoster convalescent clients or human immune globulin given within 4 days may limit or prevent symptoms.

C. Anabolic steroid use may increase severity of varicella-associated pneumonia.

Bibliography:

Amlie-Lefond C, Kleinschmidt-DeMasters BK, Mahalingam R, et al.: The vasculopathy of varicella-zoster virus encephalitis. Ann Neurol 37(6): 784–790, 1995.

CDC: Licensure of varicella virus vaccine, live. Morbidity and Mortality Weekly Report, April 7, 44(13): 264, 1995.

Johnson AS, Jones M, Morgan-Capner P: Severe chickenpox in anabolic steroid user [letter]. Lancet 345(8962):1447–1448, 1995.

Morgan M: Is Bell's palsy a reactivation of varicella zoster virus? J Infect 30(1):29–36, 1995.

Simon PH, Steele DW: Varicella: pediatric genital/rectal vesicular lesions of unclear origin. Ann Emerg Med 25(1):111–114, 1995.

Watson B, Boardman C, Laufer D, et al.: Humoral and cell-mediated immune responses in healthy children after one or two doses of varicella vaccine. Clin Infect Dis 20(2):316–319, 1995.

VASOACTIVE INTESTINAL POLYPEPTIDE (VIP), BLOOD

Norm: Adults and children: <50 pg/ml (<50 ng/ml SI Units).

Increased: Achlorhydria (WDHA) syndrome, Ectopic islet cell tumor, hypokalemia, islet cell hyperplasia, islet cell tumor, laxative abuse, pancreatic-cholera syndrome, tachycardia, Verner-Morrison syndrome, vipoma, and watery diarrhea.

Decreased: Asthma exacerbation.

Description: Vasoactive intestinal polypeptide (VIP) is a gastrointestinal hormone produced by neuroendocrine cells in the small and large intestine, pancreas, brain, and peripheral nervous system. Its actions include stimulating watery pancreatic secretions with a high pH, stimulating glycogenolysis, inhibiting stomach secretions, stimulating the release of insulin and glucagon, causing peripheral vasodilation, slowing gastric motility, stimulating intestinal chloride secretion, and inhibiting intestinal sodium absorption. Clients with vipoma neoplasms have symptoms of watery diarrhea that is high in potassium and bicarbonate.

Professional Considerations:

1. Consent form NOT required.
2. Preparation:
   A. When possible, medications should be withheld for 1–2 days.
   B. Observe clients with watery diarrhea closely for symptoms of dehydration during the 12-hour preparation fast.
   C. Preschedule this test with the laboratory and verify collection instructions with the laboratory performing the test.
   D. Obtain a chilled plastic syringe to which 1.2 mg EDTA has been added.
   E. See Client and family teaching.
3. Procedure:
   A. Draw a 7-ml blood sample.
4. Postprocedure care:
   A. Transport the specimen to the laboratory immediately.
   B. The specimen must be separated and transferred to a special VIP container, then frozen.
5. Client and family teaching:
   A. Fast from food and fluids for 12 hours prior to the test.
6. Factors that affect results:
   A. Results are invalidated if the client has undergone a radioactive scan within 1 week prior to the test.
7. Other data:
   A. None.

Bibliography:

Anderson FL, Kralios AC, Cluff N, et al.: Vagal-induced tachycardia: release of vasoactive intestinal peptide and peptide HI. Am J Physiol 267(5, Pt 2):H2019–H11024, 1994.

Cardell LO, Uddman R, Edvinsson L: Low plasma concentrations of VIP and elevated levels of other neuropeptides during exacerbations of asthma. Eur Respir J 7(12):2169–2173, 1994.

Hill MR, Wallick DW, Martin PJ, et al.: Effects of repetitive vagal stimulation on heart rate and on cardiac vasoactive intestinal polypeptide efflux. Am J Physiol 268(5, Pt 2):H1939–H1946, 1995.

VDRL, SERUM

(see Venereal Disease Research Laboratory Test, Serum)

VECTORCARDIOGRAM, DIAGNOSTIC

Norm: Requires interpretation by an expert. P, QRS, and T loops are evaluated for direction, magnitude, and inscription.

Usage: Identification and classification of myocardial infarction; evaluation of risk for myocardial infarction progression to complete heart block; and aids in the diagnosis of ventricular pre-excitation and localization of ventricular bypass tracts.

Description: A vectorcardiogram (VCG) is a spatial representation of the sequence of changes in the heart's electrical activity measured three-dimensionally along the X- (horizontal, transverse, left-to-right) axis, Y- (vertical, head-to-foot) axis, and Z- (sagittal, anterior-posterior) axis. A vector represents the heart's electrical potential with respect to specific direction and magnitude. The vectorcardiograph simultaneously records two lead axes at a time to represent the frontal plane vector (X,Y), the horizontal plane vector (X,Z), and the sagittal plane vector (Y,Z), and provides a screen display or graphic recording of P, QRS, and T vector loops that move in the same direction as the heart's electrical activity. The literature demonstrates controversy regarding the ability of VCG to better detect and classify myocardial infarction than ECG. This expensive procedure is infrequently performed in clinical settings, but is used as a teaching tool.

Professional Considerations:

1. Consent form NOT required.
2. Preparation:
   A. Obtain a vectorcardiogram machine, electrodes, and conductive gel.
3. Procedure:
   A. The client is positioned supine.
   B. Conductive electrodes are applied according to institutional protocol (usually to the anterior and posterior upper torso, left lower extremity, and the forehead or nape of the neck).
   C. The machine is activated, and the vectorcardiogram is completed in about 10 minutes.
4. Postprocedure care:
   A. Remove the electrodes. Cleanse the skin of conductive gel.
5. Client and family teaching:
   A. It is important to relax, breathe normally, and lie very still throughout the recording.
6. Factors that affect results:
   A. The client's sex, age, medications, and clinical picture must be considered when interpreting the results.
   B. One study recommends that respiratory status be identical for serial vectorcardiograms due to the effect of respiration and ventilation on the results.
7. Other data:
   A. The vectorcardiogram is most useful when evaluated in combination with an electrocardiogram.

Bibliography:

Gannedahl P, Edner ,M, Lindahl SG, et al.: Minimal influence of anaesthesia and abdominal surgery on computerized vectorcardiography recordings. Acta Anaesthesiol Scand *39*(1):71–78, 1995.

Jensen SM, Johansson G, Osterman G, et al.: On-line computerized vector cardiography monitoring of myocardial ischemia during coronary angioplasty: comparison with 12-lead electrocardiography. Coron Artery Dis *5*(6):507–514, 1994.

Lundin P, Erikson SV, Fredrikson M, et al.: Prognostic information from on-line vectorcardiography in unstable angina pectoris. Cardiology *86*(1):60–66, 1995.

VENEREAL DISEASE RESEARCH LABORATORY TEST (VDRL), SERUM

Norm: Negative. Nonreactive.

Positive: Treponemal disease: bejel, pinta, syphilis, yaws.

Description: Syphilis is a complex sexually transmitted disease characterized by a wide range of symptoms that imitate other diseases. It is caused by the organism *Treponema pallidum*. The venereal disease research laboratory test (VDRL) is a sensitive screening test for the presence of reagin, the antibody specific for the treponemal spirochete. In this test, the sample is heat inactivated, then mixed with an antigen (cardiolipin phospholipid derived from beef heart in complex with lecithin and coated on particles of cholesterol) to reagin. The mixture is then examined microscopically to detect flocculation of the cholesterol particles, indicating a positive test. The VDRL is more sensitive than the rapid plasma reagin (RPR) test for primary syphilis. The test becomes reactive during primary stage syphilis (about 14 days after a chancre is visible) and is reactive in virtually all cases of secondary stage syphilis. Results will revert to negative with treatment or by the tertiary stage. Many biologic false-positives are possible; thus, specificity is low. A newer test, the VDRL enzyme-linked immunosorbent assay (ELISA) is being studied for possible replacement of this cardiolipin test for large-scale screening for syphilis.

Professional Considerations:

1. Consent form NOT required.
2. Preparation:
   A. Tube: Red-top, red/gray-top, or gold-top.
3. Procedure:
   A. Draw a 3-ml blood sample.
4. Postprocedure care:
   A. None.

5. Client and family teaching:
   A. Syphilis is a sexually transmitted disease; information regarding sexual partners is necessary for control of the disease.
   B. If testing positive for syphilis and diagnosis is confirmed:
      i. Notify all sexual contacts from the last 90 days (if early stage) to be tested for syphilis.
      ii. Syphilis can be cured with antibiotics. These may worsen the symptoms for the first 24 hours.
      iii. Do not have sex for 2 months and until after repeat testing has confirmed that the syphilis is cured. Use condoms after that for 2 years. Return for repeat testing every 3–4 months for the next 2 years to make sure the disease is cured.
      iv. Do not become pregnant for 2 years, because syphilis can be transmitted to the fetus.
      v. If left untreated, syphilis can damage many body organs, including the brain, over several years' time.
6. Factors that affect results:
   A. Refrigeration destroys *Treponema* spirochetes in 72 hours.
   B. Conditions that may cause false-positive results include active immunization in children, antinuclear antibodies, blood loss (with multiple transfusions), brucellosis, chancroid, chickenpox, cirrhosis, the common cold, diabetes mellitus, fever (relapsing), first week of life, hepatitis (infectious), hypergammaglobulinemia, leprosy, leptospirosis (Weil's disease), lyme disease, lymphogranuloma venereum, lymphoma, infection (chronic), malaria, measles, mononucleosis (infectious), mycoplasmal pneumonia, nonsyphilitic treponemal diseases (bejel, pinta, yaws), periarteritis nodosa, pneumococcal pneumonia, pneumonia, pregnancy, rat-bite fever, rheumatic fever, rheumatic heart disease, rheumatoid arthritis, scarlet fever, scleroderma, senescence, subacute bacterial endocarditis, systemic lupus erythematosus, tuberculosis (advanced pulmonary), treponematosus, trypanosomiasis, tuberculosis, typhus fever, and vaccinia.
7. Other data:
   A. Suspected biologic false-positive tests necessitate the Fluorescent Treponemal Antibody-Absorbed Double Stain test.
   B. The greatest risk for transmission of syphilis occurs in freshly drawn blood products that must be administered immediately (platelets) or those not refrigerated for 72 hours prior to infusion.
   C. Syphilis is treated with penicillin.

Bibliography:

Larsen SA, Steiner BM, Rudolph AH: Laboratory diagnosis and interpretation of tests for syphilis. Clin Microbiol Rev *8*(1):1–21, 1995.

Phaosavasdi S, Snidvongs W, Thasanapradit P, et al.: Rapid plasma reagin test (RPR) compared to venereal disease research laboratory test (VDRL) for the diagnosis of syphilis in pregnancy. J Med Assoc Thai *72*(4):202–206, 1989.

Young H, Walker PJ, Merry D, et al.: A preliminary evaluation of a prototype western blot confirmatory test kit for syphilis. Int J STD AIDS *5*(6): 409–414, 1994.

VENEREAL DISEASE RESEARCH LABORATORY (VDRL) TEST, CEREBROSPINAL FLUID, SPECIMEN

Norm: Nonreactive.

Usage: The only test approved for cerebrospinal fluid testing for neurosyphilis.

Description: Syphilis is a complex, sexually transmitted disease characterized by a wide range of symptoms that imitate other diseases. It is caused by the organism *Treponema pallidum*. The venereal disease research laboratory test (VDRL) is a screening test for the presence of reagin, the antibody specific for the treponemal spirochete. In this test, the sample is heat inactivated, then mixed with an antigen (cardiolipin phospholipid derived from beef heart in complex with lecithin and coated on particles of cholesterol) to reagin. The mixture is then examined microscopically to detect flocculation of the cholesterol particles, indicating a positive test. Unlike serum results, cerebrospinal fluid (CSF) results may remain positive long after treatment, thus this test is not useful for monitoring response to therapy.

Professional Considerations:

1. Consent form NOT required for the test, but IS required for the procedure used to obtain the specimen. For procedural risks and contraindications, *see Lumbar Puncture, Diagnostic.*
2. Preparation:
   A. *See Lumbar Puncture, Diagnostic.*
3. Procedure:
   A. Obtain a 5-ml sample of CSF in a sterile, capped vial via lumbar puncture, or from the ventricles of the brain during special procedures *(see Lumbar Puncture, Diagnostic).*

4. Postprocedure care:
   A. *See Lumbar Puncture, Diagnostic.*
5. Client and family teaching:
   A. Syphilis is a sexually transmitted disease; information regarding sexual partners is necessary for control of the disease.
   B. *See also Venereal Disease Research Laboratory Test, Serum for additional teaching related to syphilis.*
6. Factors that affect results:
   A. False-negative results may occur in clients with tabes dorsalis.
7. Other data:
   A. Serial testing is recommended for clients with AIDS who are suspected of having syphilis but have a negative VDRL.

Bibliography:

Feraru ER, Aronow HA, Lipton RB: Neurosyphilis in AIDS patients: Initial CSF VDRL may be negative. Neurology *40*(3, Pt 1):541–543, 1990.

Friedman RF, Ganiban GJ, Liss RA, et al.: Ocular syphilis and neurosyphilis in a patient with human immunodeficiency virus infection. Md Med J *44*(4):284–288, 1995.

Russouw HG, Roberts MC, Emsley RA, et al.: The usefulness of cerebrospinal fluid tests in neurosyphilis. S Afr Med J *84*(10):682–684, 1994.

VENEZUELAN EQUINE ENCEPHALITIS VIRUS SEROLOGY, SERUM

Norm: A less than fourfold rise in titer between acute and convalescent samples.

Usage: Confirmation of diagnosis of Venezuelan equine encephalitis.

Description: Venezuelan equine encephalitis is caused by a group A arbovirus (arthropod-borne virus) that results in fever and mild, flulike symptoms (most commonly), but may progress to severe encephalitis symptoms of disorientation, convulsions, paralysis, coma, and death in children. Occurrence is primarily in South America, Central America, Mexico, and the United States. Mode of transmission to humans from horses is through the bite of an infected mosquito. Identification of the virus is performed through viral neutralization, complement fixation, hemagglutin inhibition, fluorescent antibody, and agar gel precipitation.

Professional Considerations:

1. Consent form NOT required.

2. Preparation:
   A. Tube: Red-top, red/gray-top, or gold-top.
3. Procedure:
   A. Draw a 7-ml blood sample as soon as possible after symptoms appear and label it as the acute sample. Repeat the test in 10 days and label the sample as the convalescent sample.
4. Postprocedure care:
   A. None.
5. Client and family teaching:
   A. The mode of transmission is a mosquito bite.
   B. Hypertension can be a result of this viral infection.
6. Factors that affect results:
   A. None found.
7. Other data:
   A. Testing may also be performed on cerebrospinal fluid.
   B. Venezuelan equine encephalitis is not transmitted client to client.
   C. There is no specific treatment for this illness.

Bibliography:

Agapov EV, Razumov IA, Frolov IV, et al.: Localization of four antigenic sites involved in Venezuelan equine encephalomyelitis virus protection. Arch Virol *139*(1-2):173–181, 1994.

Grieder FB, Davis NL, Aronson JF, et al.: Specific restrictions in the progression of Venezuelan equine encephalitis virus-induced disease resulting from single amino acid changes in the glycoproteins. Virology *206*(2):994–1006, 1995.

VENOGRAPHY (PHLEBOGRAPHY), DIAGNOSTIC

Norm: Negative. Absence of thrombosis. No obstructions to flow or filling defects identified.

Usage: Detection of site and presence of venous thrombosis of the lower extremities.

Description: Venography is an invasive, radiographic, or nuclear medicine procedure whereby radiopaque dye or a radionuclide is injected intravenously and the lower extremities are radiographed for the detection of venous thrombosis. Procedure time is 1–1.5 hours.

Professional Considerations:

1. Consent form IS required.

Risks:

Thrombophlebitis, venipuncture site infection/cellulitis (onset 2–12 hours, peak 12–24 hours), vasospasm, allergic reaction to dye (itching, hives, rash, tight feeling in the throat, shortness of breath, anaphylaxis); renal toxicity from contrast medium.

Contraindications:

Severe congestive heart failure, severe pulmonary hypertension, previous allergy to radiographic dye, iodine or shellfish, pregnancy, renal insufficiency.

2. Preparation:
   A. Have emergency equipment readily available.
   B. Obtain radiographic dye, heparin/ saline flush solution, and a tourniquet.
3. Procedure:
   A. The client is positioned supine on the scanning table, and the camera is positioned over the lower extremities.
   B. A tourniquet may be placed on the extremity to control the speed of blood flow.
   C. After intravenous access is established in a foot vein, radiographic dye is injected and several rapid, sequential radiographs are taken of the extremity as the dye flows in the bloodstream. Alternatively, a nuclear medicine study may be conducted, whereby a radionuclide is injected, followed by scintigraphic scanning of the extremity.
   D. The intravenous access site is flushed with heparin/saline solution, and the access is removed.
4. Postprocedure care:
   A. Assess injection site for symptoms of dye infiltration (redness, edema, warmth, tenderness).
   B. Assess vital signs; peripheral pulses; and color, motion, temperature, and sensation of lower extremities every 15 minutes × 4, then every 30 minutes × 4, then hourly × 4, then every 4 hours until 24 hours after the procedure.
5. Client and family teaching:
   A. A feeling of warmth around the neck and face is normally felt after the injection.
6. Factors that affect results:
   A. None.
7. Other data:
   A. Potential complications of venography include bacteremia, cellulitis, embolism, and thrombophlebitis.

Bibliography:

Hommeyer SC, Freeny PC, Crabo LG: Carcinoma of the head of the pancreas: evaluation of the pancreaticoduodenal veins with dynamic CT-potential for improved accuracy in staging. Radiology *196*(1):233–238, 1995.

Palmer LS, Cohen S, Reda EF, et al.: Intraoperative spermatic venography reconsidered. J Urol *154*(1):225–227, 1995.

VENTILATION/PERFUSION LUNG SCAN, DIAGNOSTIC
(see Lung Scan, Perfusion and Ventilation, Diagnostic)

VIRAL CULTURE, SPECIMEN

Norm: Negative. No virus isolated.

Positive: Acquired immune deficiency syndrome, adenovirus, chickenpox, conjunctivitis, cytomegalovirus, enteroviruses, herpes simplex, herpes zoster, keratitis, mumps virus, parainfluenza, pneumonia (viral), respiratory syncytial virus, rhinovirus, shingles, and varicella-zoster virus.

Description: Viruses are the tiniest known infectious agents and are made up of a single type of deoxyribonucleic acid (DNA) or ribonucleic acid (RNA) surrounded by an envelope of protein (proteinaceous coat). Viruses are parasites in that they reproduce with the aid of the enzymes of their living host. Thus, they will not grow on artificial (nonliving) media. Viruses must be inoculated onto special viral culture media consisting of growing cells.

Professional Considerations:

1. Consent form NOT required.
2. Preparation:
   A. Blood cultures MAY be drawn during hemodialysis.
   B. Clarify specific instructions with the laboratory performing the test.
   C. Obtain the proper supplies, as listed below, depending on the site to be cultured.
      Blood: Chilled, heparinized green-top tube.
      Biopsy: Biopsy tray and sterile container.
      Conjunctiva: Virocult or Culturette swab, or sterile spatula and viral transport medium.
      Cerebrospinal fluid: Sterile vial with cap.
      Lesion: Virocult or Culturette swab, and 1-ml syringe with intradermal needle.
      Pharynx: Virocult or Culturette swab.
      Rectal swab: Virocult or Culturette swab.
      Stool: Clean, dry container.
      Urine: Sterile specimen container.
   D. Obtain ice for packing around specimens to be cultured for influenza or cytomegalovirus.
3. Procedure:
   A. *Blood:* Draw a 5-ml blood sample as soon as possible after symptoms appear. Label the date as the acute specimen. Repeat the test in 14–28 days and label the sample as the convalescent specimen.

B. *Biopsy:* Using a sterile technique, collect an individual tissue sample into a cold, sterile container. Label it with the collection site and date.

C. *Conjunctiva:* Gently pull the lower eyelid down. Firmly swab the lower conjunctival border back and forth several times with a sterile swab. Place the swab in a chilled viral transport medium. Alternately, gently but firmly scrape the conjunctiva with a sterile spatula and smear the sample onto a chilled viral transport medium.

D. *Cerebrospinal fluid:* Obtain a 5-ml sample of cerebrospinal fluid via lumbar puncture into a chilled, sterile vial.

E. *Lesion:* Aspirate fluid from the vesicle with an intradermal needle and a 1-ml syringe. Eject the fluid into 1–2 ml of chilled viral transport medium. Firmly swab the base of the opened lesion and place the swab into a chilled viral transport medium.

F. *Pharynx:* With the client's head tilted back and the mouth open, have him or her say "Ah" to elevate the uvula. Firmly swab any visible lesions as well as the posterior surface of the nasopharyngeal area. Place the swab into a chilled viral transport medium.

G. *Rectal swab:* Insert a sterile swab into the rectum about 2–4 inches. Leave the swab in place for 10 seconds to allow absorption of fluid. Firmly rub the swab several times around the circumference of the rectum. Remove the swab and place it in a chilled viral transport medium.

H. *Stool:* Place a marble-sized stool sample in a clean, dry container.

I. *Urine:* Obtain a midstream, clean-catch urine specimen in a sterile container. *See clean-catch collection instructions in the test Body Fluid, Routine, Culture.*

4. Postprocedure care:
   A. Keep the specimen cold (not frozen) and transport it to the laboratory immediately. Specimens for influenza or cytomegalovirus culture should be transported in an ice bath.
   B. Write the client's name, age, specimen source, recent antibiotic therapy, symptoms, and suspected diagnosis on the laboratory requisition.

5. Client and family teaching:
   A. The convalescent blood sample is needed 14–28 days after the first blood sample.
   B. Results may take up to 4 weeks, but prophylactic antibiotics are normally started immediately.

6. Factors that affect results:
   A. Failure to keep the specimen cold after collection invalidates the results.

7. Other data:
   A. None.

Bibliography:

Ogburn JR, Hoffpauir JT, Cole E, et al.: Evaluation of new transport medium for detection of herpes simplex virus by culture and direct enzyme-inked immunosorbent assay. J Clin Microbiol 32(12): 3082–3084, 1994.

Printz M, Reynolds J, Mento SJ, et al.: Recombinant retroviral vector interferes with the detection of amphotropic replication competent retrovirus in standard culture assays. Gene Ther 2(2):143–150, 1995.

VISCOSITY, SERUM

Norm: 1.4–1.8 relative to water.

Increased: Arthritis (rheumatoid), dysproteinemias, hyperfibrinogenemia, myeloma (IgA), systemic lupus erythematosus, and Waldenström's macroglobulinemia.

Decreased: Not applicable.

Description: Serum viscosity is a term describing a physical property of fluid related to the resistance to flow generated by friction. Low-viscosity fluids flow freely, while high-viscosity fluids flow more slowly. In this test, the viscosity of serum is compared to that of water at room temperature. Serum is normally more viscous than water.

Professional Considerations:

1. Consent form NOT required.
2. Preparation:
   A. Tubes: Two (2) red-top, red/gray-top, or gold-top.
3. Procedure:
   A. Completely fill two tubes with blood.
4. Postprocedure care:
   A. None.
5. Client and family teaching:
   A. Clinical symptoms do not correlate well with test results.
6. Factors that affect results:
   A. None.
7. Other data:
   A. For evaluation of polycythemia vera and neonatal hyperviscosity syndrome, whole-blood viscosity should be measured. Draw the specimen in a heparinized, green-top tube.
   B. Increased viscosity may cause dilation of the retinal veins, causing fundus changes in clients.

Bibliography:

Alonso C, Pries AR, Kisslich O, et al.: Transient rheological behavior of blood in low-shear tube flow: velocity profiles and effective viscosity. Am J Physiol 268(1, Pt 2):H25–H32, 1995.

Crowley JP, Metzger J, Assaf A, et al.: Low density lipoprotein cholesterol and whole blood viscosity. Ann Clin Lab Sci 24(6):533–541, 1994.

Levine GN, O'Malley C, Balady GJ: Exercise training and blood viscosity in patients with ischemic heart disease. Am J Cardiol 76(1):80–81, 1995.

Muldoon MF, Herbert TB, Patterson SM, et al.: Effects of acute psychological stress on serum lipid levels, hemoconcentration, and blood viscosity. Arch Intern Med *155*(6):615–620, 1995.

VISUAL ACUITY TESTS, DIAGNOSTIC

Norm:

	Distance Vision
Snellen chart	
Adults	20/20 (Near vision, 14/14)
Children	
<Age 4	20/40 or better
Age 4–7	20/30 or better
>Age 7	20/20
Allen cards	
Age 3	15/30
Age 4	20/30
Infant testing for optokinetic nystagmus	Present at 2 months of age
Strabismus	Absent
Stereopsis	Present
Color vision	Present bilaterally
Peripheral vision	Intact bilaterally

Usage: Part of routine ophthalmologic examination; community health screening for vision testing.

Description: Visual acuity testing involves testing a client's ability to read a standard Snellen chart of symbols (usually letters) at a specified distance to test distance vision, and a Jaeger card to test near vision. A Snellen chart consists of numbered rows of letters that progressively decrease in size from top to bottom. A Jaeger card contains text in progressively decreasing size. For young children and infants, substitute testing in place of the Snellen chart is performed as described below. Children are tested for distance vision, nystagmus, strabismus, stereopsis, color vision, and peripheral vision. The tests may be performed with and without current corrective lenses. For unsatisfactory tests, they will be repeated with new combinations of corrective lenses, until the best possible vision correction is obtained.

Professional Considerations:

1. Consent form NOT required.
2. Preparation:
   A. Obtain charts, a handheld eye occluder wand, an eye patch for children, and glasses for testing for stereopsis.
3. Procedure:
   A. The client is positioned sitting 20 feet away from the Snellen chart.

B. Each eye is tested separately as follows:
   i. The eye not being tested is occluded.
   ii. The client is instructed to read the line closest to the bottom of the chart that he or she can read and then to attempt to read one line lower.
   iii. The fractionated visual acuity is recorded as follows: The distance in feet the client is positioned away from the chart is the numerator (i.e., 20) and the number of the lowest line read correctly is the denominator. If the client can read one symbol of a line farther down, the results are recorded as 20/number of the lowest line read perfectly + the number of symbols read correctly on the line below. For example, "20/100 + 1" means the client, at a distance of 20 feet, read the line at which a normal eye could read at 100 feet, plus 1 symbol on the line below. A passing score for a line requires that the client read the entire line with no more than one error.
C. *Near vision testing:*
   i. The client is instructed to read a Jaeger card at normal reading distance. The numerator score is the distance at which the card was read and the denominator score is the line number of the smallest sized letters read correctly.
D. *Testing in young children:*
   i. For young children, the "E" chart is substituted for the Snellen chart.

The child must indicate which direction the letter E is pointing. Pictures of familiar objects may be placed above, below, left, and right of the chart for the child to use in identification of direction. The test is performed for each eye separately.

ii. Other substitutes for young children are Allen cards, which contain pictures of objects familiar to children. The numerator score is the distance at which three of the objects can be recognized by the child, and the denominator is 30. The eyes are tested separately.

iii. *Strabismus testing:* A light is shined into the child's eyes from 16 inches away, and the bilateral reflection of the light in the eyes is observed. Strabismus causes an off-center reflection in one eye. A second test involves occluding one eye at a time as the child gazes at an object 1 foot away, and observing for inward or outward movement of the uncovered eye, which indicates strabismus.

iv. *Stereopsis testing:* Wearing stereoscopic glasses, the child is shown a stereo picture and asked if the object is on the page or in front of the page. With intact stereopsis, the child should be able to see a three-dimensional object that appears to be in front of the page. Without stereopsis, the object appears flat on the page.

v. *Color vision testing:* The child is asked to identify objects made of specifically patterned colored dots fused into gray dots.

vi. *Peripheral vision testing:* As the child gazes ahead, he or she is asked to indicate on which side of the visual field an object is appearing.

E. *Testing of infants:*

i. Infants are tested for optokinetic nystagmus by passing a bright object back and forth in front of the eyes and observing whether nystagmus occurs.

ii. The infant is also assessed for the ability to follow a lighted object moved in front of the visual field.

iii. *Peripheral vision testing:* As the child is distracted, a bright object is moved into the peripheral visual field, and the child's response to the object is noted.

4. Postprocedure care:
   A. None.
5. Client and family teaching:
   A. Young children may cooperate best if testing is practiced at home prior to this test.
   B. Eye exercises may be prescribed for very young children with strabismus. Simple exercises that can be performed at home involve using small pictures pasted on Popsicle sticks to strengthen the muscle. The child holds the stick at arm's length in front of the visual field. While focusing on the picture, he or she slowly and steadily moves the stick in toward the eyes and attempts to maintain single vision. When double vision occurs, the child restarts the exercise.
6. Factors that affect results:
   A. The client must be able to follow directions.
7. Other data:
   A. None.

Bibliography:

Holmes JM, Coates CM: Assessment of visual acuity in children with trisomy 18. Ophthalmic Gene *15* (3–4):115–120, 1994.

Jayatunga R, Sonksen PM, Bhide A, et al.: Measures of acuity in primary-school children and their ability to detect minor errors of vision. Dev Med Child Neurol *37*(6):515–527, 1995.

Schmidt PP: Visual acuity measurement in exceptional children. J Am Optom Assoc *65*(9):627–633, 1994.

VISUAL EVOKED POTENTIAL, DIAGNOSTIC

Norm: P-100 is of normal latency. Latency is equivalent bilaterally (test results require expert interpretation.)

Usage: Diagnosis and/or monitoring of demyelinating diseases, glaucoma, maculopathy, nitrous oxide toxicity (chronic), papilledema, Parkinson's disease, pressure on the optic pathway due to tumors or granulomas, pseudotumor cerebri, retinal diseases of the optic nerve, toxic optic neuropathies, and vitamin B deficiency. Also used intraoperatively during eye surgery to provide early warning of potential optic nerve damage.

Description: Visual evoked potential (VEP) is a low-amplitude, electrical waveform representation of the brain's response to a visual stimulus. Because the amplitude is too low to be noted on a traditional electroencephalogram (EEG), sophisticated computer signal-averaging techniques are used to average out the effect of other brain activity during testing. The test involves placing repetitive, patterned stimuli such as a striped, checkerboard, or dotted pattern in the visual field while recording VEP waveforms and measuring the amount of time taken for the VEP to occur. Variations of the technique include varying the pattern size, intensity, and visual field size, as well as alternating the pattern itself in an effort to selectively stimulate portions of the visual field. Results are analyzed according to an algorithm and are related to the "P-100" wave. The P-100 wave occurs at about 100 ms after each stimulus in normal clients. Of significance is the amount of time required for the VEP to occur after stimulation (latency), and a comparison of latency measurements of both eyes. Factors that affect latency include head size, electrode location, visual field position of the stimulus, and integrity of the visual nerve pathways.

Professional Considerations:

1. Consent form NOT required.
2. Preparation:
   A. *See Client and family teaching.*
   B. Obtain EEG electrodes, a machine and cap, and electroconductive gel.
   C. Remove jewelry and metal objects from the client's head.
3. Procedure:
   A. The client is positioned sitting with his or her eyes located about 1 meter away from the screen. One eye is patched.
   B. Scalp electrodes are placed in occipital, parietal, and midline locations.
   C. The client is instructed to focus the eyes on the screen.
   D. The chosen pattern(s) is (are) displayed in a rapid, flashing sequence as the client gazes at the screen and a recording of VEPs is made. A computer signal average of the brain's electrical activity at a specifically chosen time after each stimulus is displayed.
   E. The other eye is patched, and the test is repeated on the opposite eye.
4. Postprocedure care:
   A. Remove the electrodes and cleanse the scalp of electroconductive gel.
5. Client and family teaching:
   A. The client must gaze continuously at a lighted screen of flashing patterns.
   B. Hair should be shampooed the night before the exam and should be free of hair spray or other hair fixatives.
   C. The test may take more than 1 hour.
6. Factors that affect results:
   A. Results must be compared with the norms of the laboratory performing the test, as different patterns and variations of the test will be performed, depending on the client's history and the purpose of the test.
   B. Cataracts or a miotic pupil may increase the latency of the response.
   C. Female P-100 latency has been shown to be shorter than that of male latency.
   D. After age 50, latency increases by about 2 ms every 10 years.

E. The client must be able to concentrate on the test. Breaking the gaze on the screen hinders the usefulness of the results.
7. Other data:
   A. None.

Bibliography:

Clarke JM, Halgren E, Scarabin JM: Auditory and visual sensory representations in human prefrontal cortex as revealed by stimulus-evoked spike-wave complexes. Brain *118*(Pt 2):473–484, 1995.

Hartmann EE: Infant visual development: an overview of studies using visual evoked potential measures from Harter to the present. Int J Neurosci *80* (1–4):203–235, 1995.

VITAMIN A, SERUM

Norm: 30–65 µg/dl (1.05–2.27 µmol/L, SI Units) or 125–150 IU/dl.

Increased: Excessive supplementary intake.

Decreased: Celiac disease, cystic fibrosis of the pancreas, infectious hepatitis, jaundice (obstructive), low prealbumin, malabsorption, nephritis (chronic), night blindness, and protein-calorie malnutrition.

Description: Vitamin A is a fat-soluble vitamin formed in the intestines and liver from carotenes of dietary plant intake. It is absorbed from the intestines in the presence of bile and lipase, transported to the liver in the form of chylomicrons, and stored there as retinyl ester. Vitamin A is necessary for mucous membrane epithelial cell integrity, proper growth, and proper night vision.

Professional Considerations:

1. Consent form NOT required.
2. Preparation:
   A. Tube: Red-top, red/gray-top, or gold-top, and a paper bag.
   B. *See Client and family teaching.*
3. Procedure:
   A. Draw a 5-ml blood sample without hemolysis. Place the tube in the paper bag to protect it from light.
4. Postprocedure care:
   A. None.
5. Client and family teaching:
   A. Fast from food and fluids (except for water) overnight prior to the test.
   B. Do not drink alcohol for 24 hours before sampling.
6. Factors that affect results:
   A. Hemolysis or prolonged exposure of the specimen to light invalidates the results.
7. Other data:
   A. None.

Bibliography:

Carlson SE, Peeples JM, Werkman SH, et al.: Plasma retinol and retinol binding protein concentrations in premature infants fed preterm formula past hospital discharge. Eur J Clin Nutr *49*(2): 134–136, 1995.

Nesher G, Zucker J: Rheumatologic complications of Vitamin A and retinoids. Semin Arthritis Rheum *24*(4):291–296, 1995.

VITAMIN B₁ (THIAMINE), SERUM OR URINE

Norm: Serum: 5.3–7.9 µg/dl; urine: 100–200 µg/24 hours.

Increased: Excessive supplemental intake.

Decreased: Alcoholism (chronic), beriberi, diarrhea (chronic), hyperthyroidism, pregnancy, and Wernicke-Korsakoff syndrome (cerebral beriberi). Drugs include diuretics (long-term use).

Description: Vitamin B₁ is a water-soluble vitamin of particular salt compounds. It is found widely in foods, especially organ meats, yeast, and whole grains. Vitamin B₁ is absorbed in the duodenum in the presence of folic acid, and excreted via the urine. This vitamin acts as an enzyme in alpha-ketoacid decarboxylation, connects the glycolytic cycle to the Krebs cycle, and activates the guanylate cyclase/cyclic guanosine monohosphate system. Deficiency of B₁ causes three types of beriberi. "Wet" beriberi is characterized by congestive heart failure. "Dry" beriberi is characterized by peripheral neuritis, muscle paralysis and atrophy, myelin sheath degeneration, weakness, and confusion. "Cerebral" beriberi (Wernicke-Korsakoff syndrome) occurs in chronic alcoholics and is characterized by encephalopathy, ataxia, ocular disturbances, and ocular neuropathy.

Professional Considerations:

1. Consent form NOT required.
2. Preparation:
   A. Tube: Red-top, red/gray-top, or gold-top (for serum level), and a paper bag.
   B. For urine level, obtain a clean, brown, 3-L container. Write the beginning time of collection on the laboratory requisition.
   C. *See Client and family teaching.*
3. Procedure:
   A. *Serum level:*
      i. Draw a 5-ml blood sample. Place the sample immediately in a paper bag to protect it from light.

   B. *24-hour urine collection:*
      i. Discard the first morning void.
      ii. Save all the urine voided in a 24-hour period in a refrigerated, clean, light-protected, 3-L container without preservatives. For catheterized specimens, keep the drainage bag on ice and empty the urine into the collection container hourly. Document the quantity of urine output during the collection period.
4. Postprocedure care:
   A. Send the serum specimen to the laboratory immediately.
   B. For urine collections, write the ending time and total 24-hour urine output quantity on the laboratory requisition. Send the specimen to the laboratory and refrigerate it.
5. Client and family teaching:
   A. Fast overnight prior to blood draw.
   B. For the urine test, save all the urine voided, void before defecating, and avoid contaminating the specimen with stool or toilet tissue. Empty each void into the refrigerated, light-protected collection container. If any urine is accidentally discarded, discard the entire specimen and restart the collection the next day.
6. Factors that affect results:
   A. Prolonged exposure of the specimen to light invalidates the results.
   B. Clients who consume a diet high in freshwater fish, or tea made from tea leaves, may have low levels because these foods contain thiamine antagonists.
7. Other data:
   A. None.

Bibliography:

Baumgartner TG: What the practicing nurse should know about thiamine. J Intravenous Nurs *14*(2): 130–135, 1991.

Shimon I, Almog S, Vered Z, et al.: Improved left ventricular function after thiamine supplementation in patients with congestive heart failure receiving long-term furosemide therapy. Am J Med *98*(5): 485–490, 1995.

VITAMIN B₆ (PYRIDOXINE, PYRIDOXAL AND PYRIDOXAMINE), PLASMA

Norm: 25–80 ng/ml (122–389 nmol/L, SI Units); or >50 ng/ml (>243 nmol/L, SI Units). (Norms are method dependent.)

Increased: Pyridoxine megavitaminosis due to excessive dietary supplementation.

Decreased: Alcoholism (chronic), anemia (sideroblastic), diabetes (gestational), inadequate dietary intake, lactation, malabsorption, malnutrition, pregnancy, and small bowel inflammatory disease. Drugs include cycloserine, disulfiram, hydralazine, isoniazid, levodopa, oral contraceptives, penicillamine, and pyrazinoic acid.

Description: Vitamin B_6 is a term that collectively refers to three water-soluble vitamins: pyridoxine, pyridoxal, and pyridoxamine. After absorption, pyridoxine is converted to the active forms of pyridoxal and pyridoxamine phosphates. These vitamins are found in many foods, including meats, egg yolk, fish, fowl, whole grains (such as wheat germ), and vegetables. The B vitamins are important in heme synthesis and function as coenzymes in amino acid metabolism and glycogenolysis. As vitamin B_6 is partially destroyed by heat, overheating of infant formula makes infants particularly prone to vitamin B_6 deficiency.

Professional Considerations:
1. Consent form NOT required.
2. Preparation:
   A. Obtain a lavender-top tube and a paper bag.
3. Procedure:
   A. Draw a 7-ml blood sample. Place the sample immediately in a paper bag to protect it from light.
   B. Write the collection time on the laboratory requisition.
4. Postprocedure care:
   A. Send the specimen to the laboratory within 30 minutes.
   B. The plasma must be quickly separated and frozen.
5. Client and family teaching:
   A. Symptoms of B_6 deficiency may include colic, enhanced startle reflex, convulsions, and irritability.
6. Factors that affect results:
   A. Prolonged exposure of the specimen to light invalidates the results.
   B. Reject specimens received more than 30 minutes after collection.
7. Other data:
   A. Concurrent testing recommended for evaluation of vitamin B_6 status includes plasma 58-phosphate, plasma pyridoxal, and urinary 4-pyridoxic acid.
   B. Vitamin B_6 may be measured indirectly via tryptophan loading and measurement of subsequent xanthurenic acid in the urine.

Bibliography:

Inbal A, Avissar N, Shaklai M, et al.: Myopathy, lactic acidosis, and sideroblastic anemia: a new syndrome. Am J Med Genet 55(3):372–378, 1995.

Raiten DJ, Reynolds RD, Andon MB, et al.: Vitamin B metabolism in premature infants. Am J Clin Nutr 53(1):78–83, 1991.

VITAMIN B₁₂ (CYANOCOBALAMIN, EXTRINSIC FACTOR), SERUM

Norm:

		SI Units
Low	<100 pg/ml	<74 pmol/L
Indeterminate	100–200 pg/ml	74–147 pmol/L
Normal	200–1100 pg/ml	147–810 pmol/L
High	>1100 pg/ml	>810 pmol/L

Increased: Chronic obstructive pulmonary disease, congestive heart failure, diabetes, hepatic cellular damage, leukemia (chronic granulocytic), obesity, polycythemia vera, and renal failure (chronic).

Decreased: Atrophic gastritis, Crohn's disease, gastrectomy (with removal of parietal cells), hepatitis (alcoholic), inflammatory bowel disease, intestinal tapeworm, intrinsic factor deficiency (pernicious anemia), malabsorption, malnutrition, sickle cell anemia, and veganism. Drugs include antibacterials, anticonvulsants, antigout agents, antimalarials, antituberculosis agents, chemotherapeutics, diuretics, oral contraceptives, oral hypoglycemics, protozoacides, and sedatives.

Description: Vitamin B_{12} (cyanocobalamin) is a water-soluble vitamin obtained from dietary animal sources that is necessary for proper deoxyribonucleic acid (DNA) synthesis. It can be absorbed from the gastrointestinal tract only when intrinsic factor glycoprotein secreted from the stomach parietal cells is present. Although the body stores up to 12 months' worth of this vitamin in the liver, kidneys, and heart, rapid growth states or conditions causing rapid turnover of cells increase the body's need for it. Symptoms of vitamin B_{12} deficiency include anemia and neurologic abnormalities of extremity paresthesias.

Professional Considerations:

1. Consent form NOT required.
2. Preparation:
   A. This test should be performed prior to the Schilling test.
   B. Hold blood transfusion or B_{12} administration until blood is drawn, when possible.
   C. Ascertain baseline hematocrit.
   D. Tube: Red-top, red/gray-top, or gold-top, and a paper bag.
   E. *See Client and family teaching.*
3. Procedure:
   A. Draw a 1-ml blood sample. Place the tube immediately in a paper bag to protect it from light.
4. Postprocedure care:
   A. Send the specimen to the laboratory immediately. Samples must be quickly spun, with serum separated, frozen, and protected from light.
5. Client and family teaching:
   A. Fast overnight prior to the test.
6. Factors that affect results:
   A. Hemolysis or prolonged exposure of the specimen to light invalidates the results.
   B. Administration of radiographic dyes within 7 days prior to the test invalidates the results.
7. Other data:
   A. *See also Schilling Test, Diagnostic; and Vitamin B₁₂, Unsaturated Binding Capacity, Serum.*

Bibliography:

al-Momen AK: Diminished vitamin B12 levels in patients with severe sickle cell disease. J Intern Med *237*(6):551–555, 1995.

Carretti N, Eremita GA, Pizzichini M, et al.: Relation between erythropoietin and vitamin B12 in normal and anemic pregnant women. Gynecol Obstet Invest *39*(2):83–87, 1995.

Gimsing P: Cobalamin forms and analogues in plasma and myeloid cells during chronic myelogenous leukaemia related to clinical condition. Br J Haematol *89*(4):812–819, 1995.

Norman EJ: Screening for cobalamin deficiency (letter). Arch Fam Med *4*(4):304–305, 1995.

VITAMIN B₁₂, UNSATURATED BINDING CAPACITY (UBC), SERUM

Norm: 870–2000 pg/ml (640–1473 pmol/L, SI Units).

Increased: Hepatoma, leukemia (chronic myelogenous), myeloprolif-

erative state, polycythemia vera, pregnancy, and reactive leukocytosis. Drugs include oral contraceptives.

Decreased: Hypoproteinemia.

Description: Vitamin B_{12} (cyanocobalamin) is a water-soluble vitamin obtained from dietary animal sources that is necessary for proper deoxyribonucleic acid (DNA) synthesis. It is absorbed from the gastrointestinal tract only when bound by intrinsic factor glycoprotein secreted from the stomach parietal cells. After absorption, it is transported in the bloodstream by transcobalamin-binding proteins, primarily transcobalamin I. In this test, intrinsic factor is added to a mixture of the client's serum and radio labeled vitamin B_{12}. The mixture is incubated, and then the fraction of bound radio labeled vitamin B_{12} is measured by a scintillation counter after removal of the unbound vitamin. The results are an indication of the level of transcobalamin-binding proteins, which are known to be elevated in certain conditions (listed above).

Professional Considerations:

1. Consent form NOT required.
2. Preparation:
   A. Preschedule this test with the laboratory.
   B. Tube: Red-top, red/gray-top, gold-top, or lavender-top (depending on laboratory requirements).
3. Procedure:
   A. Draw a 7-ml blood sample.
4. Postprocedure care:
   A. Send the specimen to the laboratory immediately or else refrigerate it.
5. Client and family teaching:
   A. Results are normally available within 48 hours.
6. Factors that affect results:
   A. Clotting of the specimen may cause elevated results.
   B. Falsely elevated results may occur if intrinsic factor that is not highly purified is used.
7. Other data:
   A. *See also Vitamin B₁₂, Serum; and Schilling Test, Diagnostic.*

Bibliography:

Lucas MH, Elgazzar AH: Detection of protein bound vitamin B12 malabsorption. A case report and review of the literature. Clin Nucl Med *19*(11): 1001–1003, 1994.

Shor-Posner G, Morgan R, Wilkie F, et al.: Plasma cobalamin levels affect information processing speed in a longitudinal study of HIV-1 disease. Arch Neurol *52*(2):195–198, 1995.

VITAMIN C (ASCORBIC ACID), PLASMA OR SERUM

Norm:

		SI Units
Normal level	0.6–2 mg/dl	34–114 µmol/L
Possible deficiency	<0.3 mg/dl	<17 µmol/L
Deficiency	<0.2 mg/dl	<11 µmol/L

Increased: Drugs that include ascorbic acid.

Decreased: Alcoholism, hyperthyroidism, malabsorption, pregnancy, renal failure, and scurvy.

Description: Vitamin C is a water-soluble vitamin found in citrus fruits and leafy (raw) vegetables and tomatoes. It is absorbed from the diet through the small intestine and stored in the adrenal glands, kidney, spleen, liver, and leukocytes. Excess amounts of the vitamin are excreted in the urine. Vitamin C is important in cellular structure, collagen synthesis, capillary integrity, wound healing, intestinal iron absorption, and resistance to infection.

Professional Considerations:

1. Consent form NOT required.
2. Preparation:
   A. Clarify the type of tube needed with the testing laboratory, as requirements vary.
   B. Tube: CHILLED green-top, red-top, red/gray-top, gold-top, lavender-top, or black-top.
   C. Obtain a container of ice.
   D. *See Client and family teaching.*
3. Procedure:
   A. Draw a 10-ml blood sample according to specific laboratory requirements. Use a chilled tube.
   B. Place the specimen immediately on ice.
4. Postprocedure care:
   A. Send the specimen to the laboratory immediately. Serum or plasma must be promptly separated and frozen.
5. Client and family teaching:
   A. Fast overnight prior to the test.
   B. Results are normally available within 24 hours.
6. Factors that affect results:
   A. Chronic tobacco smoking decreases levels.
7. Other data:
   A. For clients ingesting inadequate vitamin C, scurvy can develop in about 90 days.

Bibliography:

Bates CJ: Plasma vitamin C assay: a European experience. EC FLAIR Concerted Action No. 10: Micronutrient Measurement, Absorption and Status. Int J Vitam Nutr Res *64*(4):283–287, 1994.

Essien, EU: Plasma levels of retinol, ascorbic acid and alpha-tocopherol in sickle cell anaemia. Cent Afr J Med *41*(2):48–50, 1995.

VITAMIN D (CHOLECALCIFEROL), PLASMA OR SERUM

Norm: Norms vary according to the test method used.

		SI Units
Serum vitamin D$_3$ 1,25-dihydroxy	25–45 pg/ml	60–108 nmol/L
Plasma vitamin D$_3$ 25-hydroxy		
Summer	15–80 ng/ml	37–200 nmol/L
Winter	14–42 ng/ml	35–105 nmol/L

Increased: Hyperparathyroidism, hypervitaminosis D, and sarcoidosis.

Decreased: Hepatic failure, hypoparathyroidism, malabsorption, osteomalacia, pseudohypoparathyroidism, renal failure, renal osteodystrophy, and rickets. Drugs include anticonvulsants and isoniazid.

Description: Vitamin D is a fat-soluble vitamin found as a dietary supplement in milk, and synthesized by the body from cholesterol in conjunction with exposure to sunlight. Vitamin D becomes biologically active through hepatic hydroxylation to 25-hydroxy vitamin D and then to 1,25-dihydroxy vitamin D through renal hydroxylation. It works in conjunction with calcitonin and parathyroid hormone and is necessary for proper dietary calcium absorption from the intestinal tract, for regulation of skeletal calcium resorption, and for release of parathyroid hormone.

Professional Considerations:

1. Consent form NOT required.
2. Preparation:
   A. Tube: Red-top, red/gray-top, or gold-top (for serum); or green-top (for plasma).
   B. *See Client and family teaching.*
3. Procedure:
   A. Draw a 3-ml blood sample.
4. Postprocedure care:
   A. None.
5. Client and family teaching:
   A. Fast overnight prior to the test.
   B. Results are normally available within 24 hours.
6. Factors that affect results:
   A. Insufficient dietary phosphorus intake causes decreased 1,25-dihydroxy vitamin D.
   B. Clients who have no exposure to sunlight may have decreased levels.
7. Other data:
   A. Concurrent measurement of parathyroid hormone is recommended.
   B. Hypervitaminosis D may be nephrotoxic.

Bibliography:

Beckman MJ, Johnson JA, Goff JP et al.: The role of dietary calcium in the physiology of vitamin D toxicity: excess dietary Vitamin D3 blunts parathyroid hormone induction of kidney 1-hydroxylase. Arch Biochem Biophy *319*(2):535–539, 1995.

Ito M, Koyama H, Ohshige A, et al.: Prevention of preeclampsia with calcium supplementation and vitamin D3 in an antenatal protocol. Int J Gynaecol Obstet *47*(2):115–120, 1994.

VITAMIN E (ALPHA-TOCOPHEROL), SERUM

Norm: 0.8–1.5 mg/dl (19–35 µmol/L, SI Units).

		SI Units
Adults	5–20 µg/ml	11.6–46.4 µmol/L
Children	3–15 µg/ml	7.0–34.8 µmol/L

Increased: Excessive intake of supplemental vitamin E.

Decreased: Chronic alcoholism, brown-bowel syndrome, certain neurologic degenerative diseases, and malabsorption due to intestinal bile deficiency (biliary atresia, cystic fibrosis).

Description: Vitamin E is a fat-soluble vitamin found widely in foods such as green vegetables, grains, eggs, oils, liver, chicken, and fish. This vitamin prevents oxidation of vitamin A, deoxyribonucleic acid (DNA), and cell membrane phospholipids by free radicals. It is necessary for proper reproductive function, muscle growth and development, and hemolytic resistance of red blood cell membranes. Deficiency of vitamin E causes hemolytic anemia and neurologic abnormalities.

Professional Considerations:

1. Consent form NOT required.
2. Preparation:
   A. Tube: Red-top, red/gray-top, or gold-top, and a paper bag.
3. Procedure:
   A. Draw a 10-ml blood sample. Label the tube, and place it promptly in a paper bag to protect it from light.
4. Postprocedure care:
   A. Send the specimen to the laboratory. Serum must be separated within 2 hours of collection.
5. Client and family teaching:
   A. Results are normally available within 72 hours.
6. Factors that affect results:
   A. Prolonged exposure of the specimen to light invalidates the results.
7. Other data:
   A. The specimen is stable at room temperature or refrigerated for 14 days, or frozen for up to a year.

Bibliography:

Choudhury N, Tan L, Truswell AS: Comparison of palmolein and olive oil: effects on plasma lipids and vitamin E in young adults. Am J Clin Nutr *61*(5):1043–1051, 1995.

Gross MD, Proudy CB, Jacobs DR Jr: Stability of carotenoids and alpha-tocopherol during blood collection and processing procedures. Clin Chem *41*(6, Pt 1):493–494, 1995.

VOLATILE SCREEN, BLOOD OR URINE

(see Toxicology, Volatiles Group by GLC, Blood or Urine)

VON WILLEBRAND FACTOR ANTIGEN (VWF AG, FACTOR VIII R:AG, FACTOR VIII RELATED ANTIGEN), BLOOD

Norm: 45–185% of control sample activity.

Usage: Differentiation between hemophilia A (classical hemophilia) and von Willebrand's disease when bleeding time tests are inconclusive.

Description: Von Willebrand's disease is an autosomal dominantly transmitted Factor VIII defect. It is a coagulation disorder that results in varying degrees of bleeding abnormalities. Coagulation Factor VIII has three properties, namely, procoagulant activity, antigenic activity, and von Willebrand factor activity. In this test, Factor VIII antigenic activity is determined by measurement of von Willebrand factor antigen (vWF Ag). In hemophilia A, vWF Ag activity is normal, but in von Willebrand's disease, vWF Ag is characteristically low (i.e., <40% of control sample activity).

Professional Considerations:

1. Consent form NOT required.
2. Preparation:
   A. Preschedule this test with the laboratory.
   B. Tube: 2.7-ml or 4.5-ml blue-top and a control tube, and a waste tube or syringe.
3. Procedure:
   A. Withdraw 2 ml of blood into a syringe or vacuum tube. Remove the syringe or tube, leaving the needle in place. Attach a second syringe, and draw a blood sample of 2.4 ml for a 2.7-ml tube or 4.0 ml for a 4.5-ml tube.
   B. Gently roll the tube several times to mix the blood with the anticoagulant.
4. Postprocedure care:
   A. Send the specimen to the laboratory immediately and refrigerate it until it is tested.
5. Client and family teaching:
   A. Results are normally available within 72 hours.
6. Factors that affect results:
   A. Hemolysis invalidates the results.
   B. Contamination of the specimen with tissue thromboplastins invalidates the results. This is the reason for the double-draw technique.
   C. Results are invalidated if the specimen is received by the laboratory more than 2 hours after collection.
7. Other data:
   A. None.

Bibliography:

Sabharwal AK, Bajaj SP, Ameri A, et al.: Tissue factor pathway inhibitor and von Willebrand factor antigen levels in adult respiratory distress syndrome and in a primate model of sepsis. Am J Respir Crit Care Med 151(3, Pt 1):758–767, 1995.

Yurdakok M, Gurakan B, Ergin H, et al.: Increased von Willebrand factor antigen in early respiratory distress syndrome [letter]. Am J Hematol 49(1):95–96, 1995.

VON WILLEBRAND FACTOR ASSAY, BLOOD

Norm: Aggregation occurs after addition of ristocetin to the sample.

Usage: Helps differentiate between hemophilia A (classical hemophilia) and von Willebrand's disease.

Description: Von Willebrand's disease is an autosomal dominantly transmitted Factor VIII defect. It is a coagulation disorder that results in varying degrees of bleeding abnormalities. Coagulation Factor VIII has three properties—namely, procoagulant activity (low or absent in hemophilia A), antigenic activity, and von Willebrand factor activity. The von Willebrand factor activity of Factor VIII enhances the formation of platelet plugs. In this test, the von Willebrand factor activity of Factor VIII is measured by using a modified platelet aggregation test. In normal clients or those with hemophilia A, the antibiotic, ristocetin, induces platelet aggregation on a test sample. In clients with von Willebrand's disease, however, addition of ristocetin to the client's serum does not result in platelet aggregation.

Professional Considerations:

1. Consent form NOT required.
2. Preparation:
   A. Preschedule this test with the laboratory.
   B. Tube: 2.7-ml or 4.5-ml blue-top and a control tube, and a waste tube or syringe.
3. Procedure: *The blood draw is best performed by a laboratory technician.*
   A. Withdraw 2 ml of blood into a syringe or vacuum tube. Remove the syringe or tube, leaving the needle in place. Attach a second syringe, and draw a blood sample of 2.4 ml for a 2.7-ml tube or 4.0 ml for a 4.5-ml tube.
   B. Gently roll the tube several times to mix the blood with the anticoagulant.
   C. *Serum should be immediately separated into a plastic vial and frozen before sending it to the laboratory.*
4. Postprocedure care:
   A. Send the specimen to the laboratory

immediately and refrigerate it until it is tested.

5. Client and family teaching:
   A. Results are normally available within 72 hours.
6. Factors that affect results:
   A. Hemolysis or clotting of the specimen invalidates the results.
   B. Contamination of the specimen with tissue thromboplastins invalidates the results. This is the reason for the double-draw technique.
   C. Results are invalidated if the specimen is received by the laboratory more than 2 hours after collection.
7. Other data:
   A. None.

Bibliography:

Baillod P, Gaucher C, Affolter B, et al.: New variant of type II von Willebrand's disease with structural abnormality of plasma von Willebrand factor in a patient with very mild bleeding history. Am J Hematol 49(1):21–28, 1995.

Rick ME: Laboratory diagnosis of von Willebrand's disease. Clin Lab Med 14(4):781–794, 1994.

V/Q SCAN
(see Lung Scan, Perfusion and Ventilation, Diagnostic)

VULVA SMEAR, DIAGNOSTIC
(see Pap Smear, Diagnostic)

WASHING CYTOLOGY, SPECIMEN
(see Bronchial Washing, Specimen, Diagnostic)

WATER DEPRIVATION TEST FOR VASOPRESSIN DEFICIENCY, DIAGNOSTIC
(see Concentration Test, Urine)

WATER LOADING TEST, DIAGNOSTIC

Norm: ≥500-ml urine output over 4 hours after water ingestion.

Urine Osmolality: < serum osmolality or <180 mOsm/kg by 5 hours after water ingestion.

Usage: Diagnosis of syndrome of inappropriate antidiuretic hormone secretion (SIADHS).

Description: The water loading test involves administering a large quantity of water, and then comparing the osmolality of timed urine and serum collections. In a normal client, increased fluid intake increases urine output and decreases urine osmolality. In clients with SIADHS, however, excess secretion of antidiuretic hormone causes a lower than normal urine output in response to the water loading, and a urine osmolality that does not decrease below serum osmolality.

Professional Considerations:
1. Consent form NOT required.

Risks:
Fluid overload, congestive heart failure. Complications of nasogastric tube insertion include bleeding, dysrhythmias, esophageal perforation, laryngospasm, and decreased mean PO_2.

Contraindications/Precautions:
Performed with extreme caution in clients with a history of congestive heart failure.

2. Preparation:
   A. The baseline serum sodium level should be at least 125 mEq/L before starting this test.
   B. Withhold diuretics for 12 hours prior to the test.
   C. Tube: Six (6) red-top, red/gray-top, or gold-top.
   D. Also obtain six (6) clean plastic specimen containers.
   E. Insert a nasogastric tube if the client will be unable to drink 1 L of water over a short period of time.
3. Procedure:
   A. Draw a 1-ml blood sample for the baseline serum osmolality. Obtain a 20-ml random urine sample in a clean plastic container for baseline urine osmolality.
   B. Have the client drink 1 L of water or 20 mL/kg body weight over 15–20 minutes, or instill it through a nasogastric tube.
   C. Document the quantity of urine output, starting with the time of water ingestion and ending 5 hours later.
   D. Obtain samples for serum and urine osmolality as in step A every hour × 5 hours. Label each tube sequentially, and write the collection time on the label.

4. Postprocedure care:
   A. Refrigerate the serum samples if they are not tested within 4 hours.
   B. Refrigerate all urine samples until they are tested.
5. Client and family teaching:
   A. The client will be asked to drink, or have instilled, at least 1 liter of water within 20 minutes.
6. Factors that affect results:
   A. Diuretics administered within 12 hours prior to the test invalidate the results.
7. Other data:
   A. None.

Bibliography:

Howanitz JH, Howanitz PJ, Henry JB: Clinical Diagnosis & Management by Laboratory Methods, 18th ed, JB Henry (ed). Philadelphia, WB Saunders, 1991, p 313.

Miller M: Inappropriate antidiuretic hormone secretion. Curr Ther Endocrinol Metab 5:186–189, 1994.

WEBER TEST, DIAGNOSTIC
(see Tuning Fork Test of Weber, Rinne, and Schwabach Tests, Diagnostic)

WEIL-FELIX AGGLUTININS, BLOOD

Norm: A less than fourfold rise in titer between acute and convalescent samples; or titer <1:160.

Usage: Aids in the diagnosis of rickettsial infections.

Description: A test performed for the purpose of detecting and differentiating rickettsial antibodies in the serum. Rickettsial organisms cause Rocky Mountain spotted fever, Q fever, Brill-Zinsser disease, epidemic typhus, murine typhus, scrub typhus, and rickettsial pox. Three *Proteus* antigens are known to cross-react in specific relationships with rickettsial antibodies. The test is performed by mixing serial dilutions of test serum with suspensions of *Proteus* strains OX-2, OX-19, and OX-K and observing for agglutination. A single titer >1:320 or a fourfold rise in titer between acute and convalescent samples is considered diagnostic.

Professional Considerations:

1. Consent form NOT required.
2. Preparation:
   A. Tube: Red-top, red/gray-top, or gold-top.

B. Specimens MAY be drawn during hemodialysis.
3. Procedure:
   A. Draw a 10-ml blood sample and label it as the acute sample. Repeat the test every 3–5 days. Draw a final sample in 10–14 days and label it as the convalescent sample.
4. Postprocedure care:
   A. None.
5. Client and family teaching:
   A. Return for serial sampling as prescribed, then in 10–14 days for final follow-up testing.
6. Factors that affect results:
   A. Hemolysis invalidates the results.
   B. Immunosuppressed clients may be infected but have low or negative titers.
   C. Antibiotic therapy causes low initial titers.
7. Other data:
   A. Because the test is based on a known cross-reaction, caution must be used in interpreting the results. Although differentiation between Rocky Mountain spotted fever and typhus fever is not possible with this test, interpretation of results can rule out certain rickettsial infections.
   B. *See also Febrile Agglutinins, Serum.*

Bibliography:

Amano K, Kyohno K, Aoki S, et al.: Serological studies of the antigenic similarity between typhus group rickettsiae and Weil-Felix test antigens. Microbiol Immunol 39(1):63–65, 1995.

Gray GC, Rodier GR, Matras-Maslin VC, et al.: Serologic evidence of respiratory and rickettsial infections among Somali refugees. Am J Trop Med Hyg 52(4):349–353, 1995.

Hammerschlag MR: Atypical pneumonias in children. Adv Pediatr Infect Dis 10:1–39, 1995.

Raoult D, Marrie T: Q fever. Clin Infect Dis 20(3):489–495, 1995.

WESTERGREN SEDIMENTATION RATE
(see Sedimentation Rate, Erythrocyte, Blood)

WESTERN BLOT
(see Acquired Immune Deficiency Syndrome Evaluation Battery, Diagnostic)

WESTERN EQUINE ENCEPHALITIS VIRUS SEROLOGY, SERUM

Norm: Negative. A less than fourfold rise in titer between acute and convalescent samples; H1 titer <1:10; no IgM antibody detected.

Positive: Aseptic meningitis and meningoencephalitis.

Description: Western equine encephalitis is caused by a group A arbovirus (arthropod-borne virus), specifically, togavirus, which results in inflammation of parts of the brain, meninges, and spinal cord in horses and humans. Occurrence is primarily in the Western Hemisphere and in summer to early fall. Mode of transmission to humans is from small birds and mammals through the bite of an infected mosquito. Symptoms are short in duration and may range from mild to fatal (10%) encephalitis symptoms (stiff neck, lethargy, sore throat, vomiting, stupor, coma, paralysis in children). Identification of the virus is performed through viral neutralization, complement fixation, hemagglutin inhibition, fluorescent antibody, and agar gel precipitation.

Professional Considerations:

1. Consent form NOT required.
2. Preparation:
   A. Tube: Red-top, red/gray-top, or gold-top.
3. Procedure:
   A. Draw a 7-ml blood sample as soon as possible after symptoms appear and label it as the acute sample. Repeat the test in 14 days and label it as the convalescent sample.
4. Postprocedure care:
   A. None.
5. Client and family teaching:
   A. The mode of transmission is by a mosquito bite. Wear insect-repellant spray or lotion on skin when outdoors.
   B. Return in 2 weeks for follow-up testing.
6. Factors that affect results:
   A. Cross-reactions may occur with eastern equine encephalitis virus, another group A togavirus.
7. Other data:
   A. Testing may also be performed on cerebrospinal fluid.
   B. Western equine encephalitis is not transmitted client to client.

Bibliography:

Fulhorst CF, Hardy JL, Eldridge BF, et al.: Natural vertical transmission of western equine encephalomyelitis virus in mosquitoes. Science 263(5147): 676–678, 1994.

Sellers RF, Maarouf AR: Weather factors in the prediction of western equine encephalitis epidemics in Manitoba. Epidemiol Infect 111(2):373–390, 1993.

Weaver SC, Hagenbaugh A, Bellew LA, et al.: A comparison of the nucleotide sequences of eastern and western equine encephalomyelitis viruses with those of other alphaviruses and related RNA viruses. Virology 202(2):1083, 1994.

WHITE BLOOD CELL COUNT DIFFERENTIAL, BLOOD
(see Differential Leukocyte Count, Peripheral Blood)

WHITE BLOOD COUNT (WBC), BLOOD
(see Differential Leukocyte Count, Peripheral Blood)

WHOLE-BLOOD CLOTTING TIME
(see Lee White Clotting Time, Blood)

WHOLE-BODY SCAN, DIAGNOSTIC
(see Bone Scan, Diagnostic)

WINTROBE SEDIMENTATION RATE, BLOOD
(see Sedimentation Rate, Erythrocyte, Blood)

WOUND CULTURE
(see Culture, Routine, Specimen)

WOUND, FUNGUS, CULTURE
(see Biopsy, Fungus, Culture or Body Fluid, Fungus, Culture)

WOUND, MYCOBACTERIA, CULTURE
(see Biopsy, Mycobacteria, Culture or Body Fluid, Mycobacteria, Culture)

XANTHURIC ACID, 24-HOUR, URINE

Norm: 6 mg/24 hours of xanthine excreted.

Increased: Disseminated carcinoma, leukemia/lymphoma therapy with Allopurinol (up to 750 mg/day excreted), nephropathy.

Decreased: Vitamin B_6 deficiency, Xanthine stones (genetic disorder), xanthinuria (autosomal recessive disorder).

Description: Xanthine is normally converted to uric acid by the enzyme xanthine oxidase and uric acid is then secreted into the urine. Allopurinol inhibits xanthine oxidase, blocking the synthesis of uric acid. This can lead to an increase in xanthuric acid (xanthine in its uric acid form) in the urine. Also, tryptophan loading will assess the status of vitamin B_6 because xanthuric acid is a major metabolite of the amino acid tryptophan.

Professional Considerations:

1. Consent form NOT required.
2. Preparation:
   A. Obtain a 3-L container for urine.
   B. Write the beginning time of collection on the laboratory requisition.
3. Procedure:
   A. Discard the first morning void.
   B. Save all the urine for the next 24 hours. If obtaining specimens from catheter bags, empty the urine into the collection container every 2 hours.
4. Postprocedure care:
   A. Write the ending time of collection on the laboratory requisition.
5. Client and family teaching:
   A. Save all the urine for 24 hours AFTER discarding the first morning void. If any urine is accidentally discarded, discard the entire specimen and restart the collection the next day.
   B. Urinate before defecating to avoid contaminating the specimen with stool or toilet tissue.
6. Factors that affect results:
   A. Increasing urinary pH (alkalinization) will increase solubility of xanthuric acid and increase excretion.
7. Other data:
   A. Study results found xanthuric crystals in the urine of 8 of 19 allopurinol-treated children undergoing treatment for acute lymphocytic leukemia.

Bibliography:

Andreoli SP, Clark JH, McGuire WA, et al.: Purine excretion during tumor lysis in children with acute lymphocytic leukemia receiving allopurinol: relationship to acute renal failure. J Pediatr *109:* 292–298, 1986.

Rieselbach RE: Nephrotoxicity caused by cancer chemotherapy: Xanthine nephropathy, p 880. *In* Nephrology, Vol 1, RR Robinson (ed). New York, Springer-Verlag, 1984.

Smith LH: Urolithiasis, Ch 25, pp 793–794. *In* Diseases of the Kidney, Vol 1, RW Schrier, CW Gottschalk (eds). Boston, Little, Brown, 1988.

Ueda N, Walker PD, Shah SV: Oxident stress in acute renal failure. Contemporary Issues Nephrol *30:*45–74, 1995.

XEROMAMMOGRAM
(see Mammography, Diagnostic)

X-RAY DIAGNOSTIC
(see Bone X-Ray, Diagnostic; Chest X-Ray, Diagnostic; Cardiac Radiography, Diagnostic; Eye Radiography, Diagnostic; Flat Plate X-Ray of Abdomen, Diagnostic; Pelvic X-Ray for Flat Ileum, Diagnostic; Sinus X-Rays, Diagnostic; and X-Ray of Skull, Chest, and Cervical Spine, Diagnostic)

X-RAY OF SKULL, CHEST, AND CERVICAL SPINE, DIAGNOSTIC

Norm: Negative for fracture or dislocation.

Usage: Trauma and determination of location and extent of suspected skull fracture and/or cervical spine damage.

Description: This procedure involves radiographic examination of the skull, chest, and cervical spine to detect skull and spinal injuries resulting from trauma. Fractures of the skull are classified by location and type. Types of skull fractures may be penetrating, depressed, bending, linear, or diastatic (involving the skull suture area[s]). The orbits are examined for the presence of free air, which indicates a fractured sinus area. Radiography of the chest and cervical spine identifies the seven cervical spine segments as well as the C7–T1 area and relationship. Definite indications for cervical spine x-rays include neck pain or a tender cervical area. Other indications may include decreased level of consciousness, paresthesias, decreased sensation, weakness, muscle spasm near the cervical area, or decreased anal tone.

Professional Considerations:

1. Consent form NOT required.
2. Preparation:
   A. Move the client only the minimal amount necessary to obtain the different radiographic views.
   B. Maintain strict body alignment throughout transport and transfer of the client. If uncooperative or combative, the client may need to be intubated, paralyzed, and mechanically ventilated to maintain alignment.

3. Procedure:
   A. *Skull x-ray:* Conventional plain-film radiography of the skull is performed, including the following views: posteroanterior, anteroposterior in Townes' projection, two lateral views, posteroanterior Water's, and lateral views designed to highlight the facial area.
   B. *Chest and cervical spine x-ray:* Conventional plain-film radiography of the cervical spine is performed, including the following views: anteroposterior, lateral, both obliques, and one that shows the ondontoid process. Risks versus benefits must be considered before taking flexion and extension views.
4. Postprocedure care:
   A. Maintain strict body alignment until radiograph results are known.
   B. Perform postsedation or paralytic monitoring per institutional protocol, if either was used.
5. Client and family teaching:
   A. Results are normally available within 24 hours or immediately in case of emergency.
   B. Body alignment should be maintained until results are known.
6. Factors that affect results:
   A. Linear skull fractures may not be detected if their location is not on the side of the skull closest to the film. They must be distinguished from vascular grooves of the skull.
   B. Skull suture area (diastatic) fractures are difficult to detect without a great deal of experience in radiographic interpretation.
   C. Skull x-ray interpretation should take into consideration clinical findings from scalp and soft tissue examination.

7. Other data:
   A. Nuclear medicine studies can help pinpoint fractures near the base of the skull that are not demonstrable by conventional radiography.
   B. Computed tomography of the spine may be needed to detect spinal fractures not demonstrable by conventional radiography.
   C. Because as many as half of spinal injuries occur below the cervical area, radiographs of the lower spine should also be taken.

Bibliography:

Fecht-Gramley, ME: Emergency! Pediatric head trauma. Am J Nurs 95(5):54, 1995.

Jonsson B, Petren-Mallmin M, Jonsson H Jr, et al.: Pathoanatomical and radiographic findings in spinal breast cancer metastasis. J Spinal Disord 8(1):26–38, 1995.

Rosehorn J, Duus B, Nielsen K, et al.: Is a skull x-ray necessary after milder head trauma? Br J Neurosurg 5(2):135–139, 1991.

Saddison D, Vanek VW, Racanelli JL: Clinical indications for cervical spine radiographs in alert trauma patients. Am Surg 57(6):366–369, 1991.

XYLOSE, BLOOD
(see d-Xylose Absorption Test, Diagnostic)

XYLOSE, URINE
(see d-Xylose Absorption Test, Diagnostic)

XYLOSE TOLERANCE TEST, DIAGNOSTIC
(see d-Xylose Absorption Test, Diagnostic)

YERSINIA ENTEROCOLITICA ANTIBODY, BLOOD

Norm: <1:160. A fourfold increase between acute and convalescent specimens (e.g., convalescent titer 1:1280) is diagnostic for yersiniosis.

Increased: Gastroenterocolitis or endocarditis due to *Yersinia* (yersiniosis), and terminal ileitis.

Decreased: Titers decrease to normal levels 2–6 months after recovery from *Yersinia* infections.

Description: *Yersinia enterocolitica* is a fungus found in animal carriers and bodies of water that is transmitted to humans via the fecal-oral route or by ingestion of food or water contaminated with the organism. *Y. enterocol-*

itica causes gastroenterocolitis accompanied by diarrhea, anorexia, fever, vomiting, headache, arthritis, and abscesses and may progress to septicemia. Incidence is more common in children and teens than in adults. In this test, an indirect Coombs' test is performed to identify the presence of the antibody to *Y. enterocolitica*.

Professional Considerations:

1. Consent form NOT required.
2. Preparation:
   A. Tube: Red-top, red/gray-top, or gold-top.
3. Procedure:
   A. Draw a 7-ml blood sample as soon as possible after symptoms appear. Label the sample as the acute specimen.

B. Repeat the test in 2–3 weeks and label the sample as the convalescent specimen.
4. Postprocedure care:
   A. None.
5. Client and family teaching:
   A. Return in 2–3 weeks for a convalescent blood sample.
   B. Because *Yersinia* infection is transmitted from stool to other persons, avoid contaminating your hands with stool and wash your hands vigorously for 15 seconds with antibacterial soap after each defecation. Cleanse the toilet seat with disinfectant after each defecation until the physician confirms that you are no longer contagious.
   C. *Yersinia* infection may be treated with amphotericin B.
6. Factors that affect results:
   A. Results may not be elevated in clients who are infected with *Yersinia* but who are immunosuppressed or receiving antifungal therapy.

7. Other data:
   A. Diagnosis should be confirmed via blood culture.
   B. Universal precautions are adequate for preventing transmission of *Yersinia* infection to others. Use strict universal precautions when handling feces of infected clients, as fecal shedding of *Yersinia* occurs throughout the period of active symptoms.
   C. Reactive arthritis may be triggered by *Yersinia*.

Bibliography:

Giamarellou H, Antoniadou A, Kanavos K, et al.: *Yersinia enterocolitica* endocarditis: case report and literature review. Eur J Clin Microbiol Infect Dis *14*(2):126–130, 1995.

Taccetti G, Trapani S, Ermini M, et al.: Reactive arthritis triggered by *Yersinia enterocolitica*: a review of 18 pediatric cases. Clin Exp Rheumatol *12*(6): 681–684, 1994.

ZETA SEDIMENTATION RATE, BLOOD
(see Sedimentation Rate, Erythrocyte, Blood)

ZETA SEDIMENTATION RATIO (ZSR), BLOOD
(see Sedimentation Rate, Erythrocyte, Blood)

ZINC, BLOOD

Norm:

		SI Units
All ages	70–120 µg/dl	10.7–18.4 µmol/L
Zinc deficiency	<70 µg/dl	<10.7 µmol/L

Toxic Level Symptoms and Treatment:

Symptoms of Zinc Toxicity: Cough, chest discomfort, tachycardia, hypertension, gastrointestinal irritation, nausea, vomiting, diarrhea, and metallic taste in the mouth.

Treatment of Zinc Toxicity:
Eliminate dietary zinc or reduce zinc additives to hyperalimentation. Peritoneal dialysis WILL remove excess zinc.

Symptoms of Zinc Deficiency: May progress from decreased weight, low sperm count, and impaired wound healing to alopecia, hypogonadism, ataxia, tremors, and impaired resistance to infection.

Treatment of Zinc Deficiency: Zinc replacement through diet, medication, or hyperalimentation.

Increased: Anemia, arteriosclerosis, coronary heart disease, dietary intake of acidic food or beverages from galvanized containers, industrial exposure to zinc (welding), and primary osteosarcoma of bone. Drugs include cisplatin, corticosteroids, estrogens, interferon, oral contraceptives (containing estrogen), phenytoin, and thiazides.

Decreased: Acrodermatitis enteropathica, alopecia, alcoholism, anemia (hemolytic), celiac sprue, cirrhosis, diarrhea, gallbladder disease, hepatic metastasis, hypoalbuminemia, hypogonadal dwarfism, infection (acute), leukemia, lymphoma, malabsorption, myocardial infarction, poor dietary intake, pregnancy (third trimester), receiving parenteral nutrition, renal failure (chronic), stress (acute), thalassemia major, typhoid fever, and tuberculosis (pulmonary). Drugs include antimetabolites, chlorthalidone, cisplatin, diuretics, estrogens, histidine, and penicillamine.

Description: Zinc is a nutritional trace metal important for cellular growth and metabolism. Both zinc toxicity and serious zinc deficiency are possible (see symptoms listed above). Zinc levels are usually measured as part of a heavy-metal screen for suspected zinc toxicity. Routine levels are measured for clients receiving parenteral nutrition and to monitor progress during replacement for zinc deficiency.

Professional Considerations:
1. Consent form NOT required.
2. Preparation:
   A. Obtain a stainless steel needle and a metal-free, navy-blue-top BD Vacutainer tube from the laboratory.
   B. Do NOT draw specimens during hemodialysis.

3. Procedure:
   A. Draw a 1-ml blood sample without hemolysis directly into the tube through a stainless steel needle.
4. Postprocedure care:
   A. Send the specimen to the laboratory promptly for spinning and separation of the serum into a metal-free container.
5. Client and family teaching:
   A. Results are normally available within 72 hours.
6. Factors that affect results:
   A. Collecting the specimen in a regular, rubber-top tube other than that specified above invalidates the results.
   B. Hemolysis invalidates results.
7. Other data:
   A. None.

Bibliography:

Arnaud J, Faure H, Bourlard P, et al.: Longitudinal changes in serum zinc concentrations and distribution after acute myocardial infarction. Clin Chim Acta 230(2):147–156, 1994.

Dolev E, Burstein R, Lubin F, et al.: Interpretation of zinc status indicators in a strenuously exercising population. J Am Diet Assoc 95(4):482–484, 1995.

Mocchegiani E, Provinciali M, Stefano G, et al.: Role of the low zinc bioavailability on cellular immune effectiveness in cystic fibrosis. Clin Immunol Immunopathol 75(3):214–224, 1995.

Williams NR, Rajput-Williams J, West JA, et al.: Plasma, granulocyte and mononuclear cell copper and zinc in patients with diabetes mellitus. Analyst 120(3):889–890, 1995.

Reportable Diseases

Reportable Disease (in many areas)	Report Immediately?	Quarantine Required? 1-800-362-2736	Sexually Transmitted?
AIDS	No	No	**Yes**
Amebiasis	No	No	No
Anthrax	No	No	No
Botulism	**Yes**	No	No
Brucellosis	No	No	No
Campylobacteriosis	No	No	No
Chlamydia trachomatis	No	No	No
Cholera	**Yes**	**Yes**	No
Ciguatera	No	No	No
Cyclosporosis	No	No	No
Dengue	No	No	No
Diphtheria	**Yes**	No	No
Disease outbreaks of public concern	**Yes**	**Possibly**	**Not usually**
E. coli infection	No	No	No
Encephalitis	No	No	No
Giardiasis (acute)	No	No	No
Gonorrhea	No	No	**Yes**
Granuloma inguinale	No	No	**Yes**
Group A streptococcal infection (invasive)	No	No	No
Guillain-Barré Syndrome	No	No	No
Haemophilus influenzae (invasive)	No	No	No
Hemolytic-uremic syndrome	No	No	No
Hemorrhagic fever	No	No	No
Hepatitis (A; B; Non-A, Non-B, unspecified)	No	**Yes**	No
Histoplasmosis	No	No	No
Influenza (report by number of cases)	No	No	No
Kawasaki disease/syndrome	No	No	No
Lead poisoning (>10 µg/dl)	No	No	No
Legionnaires' disease	No	No	No
Leprosy	No	No	No
Leptospirosis	No	No	No
Listeriosis	No	No	No
Lyme disease	No	No	No
Lymphogranuloma venereum	No	No	**Yes**
Malaria	No	No	No
Measles (rubella)	No	No	No
Measles (rubeola)	**Yes**	No	No
Meningitis (aseptic and bacterial)	No	No	No
Meningococcal infections (other)	No	No	No
Mumps	No	No	No
Paralytic shellfish poisoning	No	No	No
Parovirus (B19)	No	No	No
Pertussis (whooping cough)	No	No	No

Reportable Disease (in many areas)	Report Immediately?	Quarantine Required? 1-800-362-2736	Sexually Transmitted?
Pesticide poisoning	No	No	No
Plague	**Yes**	**Yes**	No
Poliomyelitis	**Yes**	No	No
Psittacosis	No	No	No
Rabies (human) or bite from animal that may be rabid	**Yes**	No	No
Relapsing fever	No	No	No
Reye syndrome	No	No	No
Rheumatic fever	No	No	No
Rocky Mountain spotted fever	No	No	No
Salmonellosis	No	No	No
Shigellosis	No	No	No
Syphilis	No	No	**Yes**
Tetanus	No	No	No
Toxic shock syndrome	No	No	No
Trichinosis	No	No	No
Tuberculosis	No	No	No
Tularemia	No	No	No
Typhoid fever (*Salmonella typhi*)	No	No	No
Yellow fever	**Yes**	No	**Yes**

Index